Dynamics of Bone and Cartilage Metabolism

Dynamics of Bone and Cartilage Metabolism

Edited by

MARKUS J. SEIBEL

Department of Medicine
Division of Endocrinology and Metabolism
University of Heidelberg Medical School
Heidelberg, Germany

SIMON P. ROBINS

Skeletal Research Unit
Rowett Research Institute
Aberdeen, United Kingdom

JOHN P. BILEZIKIAN

Departments of Medicine and Pharmacology
Division of Endocrinology
College of Physicians and Surgeons
Columbia University
New York, New York

ACADEMIC PRESS

San Diego   New York   Boston   London   Sydney   Tokyo   Toronto

Academic Press
a division of Harcourt Brace & Company
525 B Street, Suite 1900, San Diego, California 92101-4495, USA
http://www.apnet.com

Academic Press
24-28 Oval Road, London NW1 7DX, UK
http://www.hbuk.co.uk/ap/

Library of Congress Catalog Card Number: 98-89456

International Standard Book Number: 0-12-634840-5

PRINTED IN THE UNITED STATES OF AMERICA
99 00 01 02 03 04 EB 9 8 7 6 5 4 3 2 1

Contents

PART I Components of the Organic Extracellular Matrix of Bone and Cartilage

CHAPTER 1 Structure and Biosynthesis of Collagens
KLAUS VON DER MARK

CHAPTER 2 Fibrillogenesis and Maturation of Collagens
SIMON P. ROBINS

CHAPTER 3 Vitamin K-Dependent Proteins of Bone and Cartilage
CAREN M. GUNDBERG AND SATORU K. NISHIMOTO

CHAPTER 4 Noncollageneous Proteins: Glycoproteins and Related Molecules
DICK HEINEGÅRD, TORE SAXNE, AND PILAR LORENZO

CHAPTER 5 Proteoglycans and Glycosaminoglycans
TIM E. HARDINGHAM

CHAPTER 6   Growth Factors

CHAPTER 7   Cytokines and Prostaglandins

CHAPTER 8   Integrins and Adhesion Molecules

CHAPTER 9   Acid and Alkaline Phosphatases

CHAPTER 10   Matrix Proteases

PART II   Structure and Metabolism of the Extracellular Matrix of Bone and Cartilage

CHAPTER 11   Mineralization, Structure, and Function of Bone

CHAPTER 12   The Cells of Bone

CHAPTER 13   Parathyroid Hormone: Structure, Function, and Dynamic Actions

CHAPTER 14   PTHrP: Of Molecules, Mice, and Men

ANDREW C. KARAPLIS AND DAVID GOLTZMAN

CHAPTER 15   The Vitamin D Hormone and Its Nuclear Receptor: Genomic Mechanisms Involved in Bone Biology

GEERT CARMELIET, ANNEMIEKE VERSTUYF, EVIS DACI, AND ROGER BOUILLON

CHAPTER 16   Sex Steroid Effects on Bone Metabolism

SUNDEEP KHOSLA, THOMAS C. SPELSBERG, AND B. LAWRENCE RIGGS

CHAPTER 17   Physiology of Calcium and Phosphate Homeostasis

RENÉ RIZZOLI AND JEAN-PHILIPPE BONJOUR

CHAPTER 18   New Concepts in Bone Remodeling

DAVID W. DEMPSTER

PART III   Markers of Bone and Cartilage Metabolism

A. Quantification: Technical Aspects

Contributors

*Numbers in parentheses indicate the pages on which the authors'
contributions begin.*

Kristina Åkesson (637)
Department of Orthopedics, Malmö University Hospital,
S-205 02 Malmö, Sweden

Roy D. Altman (339)
Division of Rheumatology and Immunology, University
of Miami School of Medicine, Miami, Florida 33101

John P. Bilezikian (187, 571)
Departments of Medicine and Pharmacology, Division of
Endocrinology, College of Physicians and Surgeons,
Columbia University, New York, New York 10032

Jean-Jacques Body (591)
Supportive Care Clinic and Bone Diseases Clinic,
Institut Jules Bordet, Université Libre de Bruxelles,
1000 Brussels, Belgium

Jean-Philippe Bonjour (247)
Department of Medicine, Division of Pathophysiology,
University Hospital Cantonal, 1211 Geneva 4,
Switzerland

Adele L. Boskey (153)
Hospital for Special Surgery, New York,
New York 10021

Roger Bouillon (217)
Laboratory for Experimental Medicine and
Endocrinology, Katholieke Universiteit Leuven,
3000 Leuven, Belgium

Kim Brixen (427)
University Department of Endocrinology, Aarhus
Amtssygehus, Aarhus DK-8000, Denmark

Peter Bruckner (289)
Department of Physiological Chemistry and
Pathobiochemistry, Westfälische Wilhelms-Universität,
48149 Münster, Germany

Geert Carmeliet (217)
Laboratory for Experimental Medicine and
Endocrinology, Katholieke Universiteit Leuven,
3000 Leuven, Belgium

Ian M. Clark (137)
School of Biological Sciences, University of East
Anglia, Norwich NR4 7TJ, United Kingdom

Peter I. Croucher (83)
Department of Human Metabolism and Clinical
Biochemistry, Division of Biochemical and
Musculoskeletal Medicine, University of Sheffield
Medical School, Sheffield S10 2RX,
United Kingdom

Evis Daci (217)
Laboratory for Experimental Medicine and
Endocrinology, Katholieke Universiteit Leuven,
3000 Leuven, Belgium

Pierre D. Delmas (465)
University Claude Bernard of Lyon, INSERM
Unit 403, Hopital Edouard Herriot, 69003 Lyon,
France

David W. Dempster (261)
Department of Clinical Pathology,
Columbia University, Regional Bone Center,
Helen Hayes Hospital, West Haverstraw,
New York 10993

Jean-Pierre Devogelaer (301)
Department of Rheumatology, Saint Luc University Hospital, University of Louvain in Brussels, 1200 Brussels, Belgium

Marc K. Drezner (547)
Department of Endocrinology, Metabolism, and Nutrition, Duke University Medical Center, Durham, North Carolina 27710

Richard Eastell (401)
Bone Metabolism Group, University of Sheffield, Clinical Sciences Center, Northern General Hospital, Sheffield S5 7AU, United Kingdom

Eric F. Eikenberry (289)
Department of Pathology, University of Medicine and Dentistry of New Jersey, Robert Wood Johnson Medical School, Piscataway, New Jersey 08854

Erik F. Eriksen (427)
University Department of Endocrinology, Aarhus Amtssygehus, 8000 Aarhus, Denmark

Lorraine A. Fitzpatrick (187)
Endocrine Research Unit, Mayo Clinic and Mayo Foundation, Rochester, Minnesota 55905

Patrick Garnero (465)
INSERM Unit 403, Hopital Edouard Herriot, 69003 Lyon, France

Renate E. Gay (437)
WHO Collaborating Center for Molecular Biology and Novel Therapeutic Strategies, Department of Rheumatology, University Hospital Zürich, 8091 Zürich, Switzerland

Steffen Gay (437)
WHO Collaborating Center for Molecular Biology and Novel Therapeutic Strategies, Department of Rheumatology, University Hospital Zürich, 8091 Zürich, Switzerland

Joseph M. Gertner (649)
Serono Laboratories, Norwell, Massachusetts 02061

Mary B. Goldring (623)
Arthritis Research, Massachusetts General Hospital, Charlestown, Massachusetts 02129

Steven R. Goldring (623)
Deaconess Hospital, Harvard Medical School, Boston, Massachusetts 02215

David Goltzman (203)
Department of Medicine, McGill University, Calcium Research Laboratory, Royal Victoria Hospital, Montreal, Quebec H3A 1A1, Canada

Esther A. González (561)
Division of Nephrology, St. Louis University School of Medicine, St. Louis, Missouri 63110

Andreas Grauer (581)
Institute for Endocrinology and Nuclear Medicine, 60329 Frankfurt, Germany

Caren M. Gundberg (43)
Department of Orthopaedics and Rehabilitation, Yale University School of Medicine, New Haven, Connecticut 06520

Hafida El Hajjaji (301)
Laboratoire de Chimie Physiologique (Metabolic Research Group), Christian de Duve Institute of Cellular Pathology, 1200 Brussels, Belgium

Timothy E. Hardingham (71)
Wellcome Trust Centre for Cell-Matrix Research, School of Biological Sciences, University of Manchester, Manchester M13 9PT, United Kingdom

Hans Jörg Häuselmann (325)
Department of Rheumatology, Center for Experimental Rheumatology, University Hospital Zürich, 8091 Zürich, Switzerland

Erik Hedbom (325)
Department of Rheumatology, Center for Experimental Rheumatology, University Hospital, CH-8091 Zürich, Switzerland

Dick Heinegård (59)
Department of Cell and Molecular Biology, Lund University, 221 00 Lund, Sweden

Miep H. Helfrich (111)
Department of Medicine and Therapeutics, University of Aberdeen, Foresterhill, Aberdeen AB9 2ZD, United Kingdom

Paula Henthorn (127)
Department of Clinical Studies, Section of Medical Genetics, University of Pennsylvania School of Veterinarian Medicine, Philadelphia, Pennsylvania 19104

Michael A. Horton (111)
Bone and Mineral Centre, Department of Medicine, The Rayne Institute, London WC1E 6JJ, United Kingdom

Andrew C. Karaplis (203)
Department of Medicine, McGill University, Lady Davis Institute for Medical Research, Montreal, Quebec H3T 1E2, Canada

Sundeep Khosla (233)
Mayo Medical School, Mayo Clinic, Rochester, Minnesota 55905

Marius E. Kraenzlin (411)
Endocrine Clinic, 4055 Basel, Switzerland

Pheobe Leboy (127)
Department of Biochemistry, University of Pennsylvania School of Dental Medicine, Philadelphia, Pennsylvania 19104

Mary Ellen Lenz (453)
Department of Biochemistry, Rush Medical College, Rush-Presbyterian/St. Luke's Medical Center, Chicago, Illinois 60612

Jane B. Lian (165)
Department of Cell Biology, University of Massachusetts
Medical Center, Worcester, Massachusetts 01655

Joseph A. Lorenzo (97)
Division of Endocrinology and Metabolism, University
of Connecticut Health Center, Farmington,
Connecticut 06030

Pilar Lorenzo (59)
Department of Cell and Molecular Biology, Lund
University, 221 00 Lund, Sweden

Carlos J. Lozada (339)
University of Miami School of Medicine, Miami,
Florida 33136

Daniel-Henri Manicourt (301, 453)
Laboratoire de Chimie Physiologique (Metabolic
Research Group), Christian de Duve Institute of Cellular
Pathology and Department of Rheumatology, Saint Luc
University Hospital, University of Louvain in Brussels,
1200 Brussels, Belgium

Kevin J. Martin (561)
Division of Nephrology, St. Louis University School of
Medicine, St. Louis, Missouri 63110

Koichi Masuda (453)
Departments of Biochemistry and Orthopedic Surgery,
Rush Medical College, Rush-Presbyterian/St. Luke's
Medical Center, Chicago, Illinois 60612

José Luis Millán (127)
The Burnham Institute, La Jolla Cancer Research Center,
La Jolla, California 92037

Carolina A. Moreira Kulak (515, 527)
Department of Endocrinology, Federal University of
Parana, Hospital de Clinicas, Curitiba, Brazil

Jean E. Mulder (527)
Department of Medicine, College of Physicians and
Surgeons, Columbia University, New York,
New York 10032

Gillian Murphy (137)
School of Biological Sciences, University of East
Anglia, Norwich NR4 7TJ, United Kingdom

Kim E. Naylor (401)
Bone Metabolism Group, University of Sheffield,
Clinical Sciences Center, Northern General Hospital,
Sheffield S5 7AU, United Kingdom

Michel Neidhart (437)
WHO Collaborating Center for Molecular Biology and
Novel Therapeutic Strategies, Department of
Rheumatology, University Hospital Zürich, 8091 Zürich,
Switzerland

Satoru K. Nishimoto (43)
Department of Biochemistry, The University of
Tennessee College of Medicine, Memphis,
Tennessee 38163

Eric S. Orwoll (493)
Bone and Mineral Research Unit, Department of
Medicine, Oregon Health Sciences University, Portland
VA Medical Center, Portland, Oregon 97201

Huibert A. P. Pols (355)
Department of Internal Medicine, Erasmus University
Medical School, 3000 DR Rotterdam,
The Netherlands

Lawrence G. Raisz (97)
Division of Endocrinology and Metabolism,
University of Connecticut Health Center, Farmington,
Connecticut 06030

Ian R. Reid (505)
Department of Medicine, University of Aukland,
Auckland, New Zealand

B. Lawrence Riggs (233)
Mayo Clinic and Mayo Foundation, Rochester,
Minnesota 55905

Juha Risteli (275)
Department of Clinical Chemistry, University of Oulu,
90220 Oulu, Finland

Leila Risteli (275)
Department of Clinical Chemistry, University of Oulu,
90220 Oulu, Finland

René Rizzoli (247)
Department of Internal Medicine, Division of Bone
Diseases, WHO Collaborating Center for Osteoporosis
and Bone Diseases, University Hospital,
1211 Geneva 14, Switzerland

Simon P. Robins (31)
Skeletal Research Unit, Rowett Research Institute,
Bucksburn, Aberdeen AB21 9SB, United Kingdom

Clifford J. Rosen (479)
Maine Center for Osteoporosis Research and
Education, St. Joseph Hospital, Bangor,
Maine 04401

R. Graham G. Russell (83)
Department of Human Metabolism and Clinical
Biochemistry, Division of Biochemical and
Musculoskeletal Medicine, University of Sheffield
Medical School, Sheffield S10 2RX,
United Kingdom

Tore Saxne (59)
Department of Cell and Molecular Biology, Lund
University, S-221 00 Lund, Sweden

Heinrich Schmidt-Gayk (375)
Endocrine Laboratory, Laboratory Group,
69126 Heidelberg, Germany

Markus J. Seibel (411)
Department of Medicine, Division of Endocrinology
and Metabolism, University of Heidelberg,
69115 Heidelberg, Germany

Elizabeth Shane (515, 527)
Department of Medicine, College of Physicians and Surgeons, Columbia University, New York, New York 10032

Shonni J. Silverberg (571)
Department of Medicine, College of Physicians and Surgeons, Columbia University, New York, New York 10032

Peter A. Simkin (319)
Department of Medicine, Division of Rheumatology, University of Washington School of Medicine, Seattle, Washington 98195

Ethel Siris (581)
Department of Medicine, College of Physicians and Surgeons, Columbia University, New York, New York 10032

Thomas C. Spelsberg (233)
Mayo Medical and Graduate School, Rochester, Minnesota 55905

Gary S. Stein (165)
Department of Cell Biology, University of Massachusetts Cancer Center, University of Massachusetts Medical Center, Worcester, Massachusetts 01655

Eugène Jean-Marie Antoine Thonar (301, 453)
Departments of Biochemistry, Internal Medicine, and Orthopedic Surgery, Rush Medical College, Rush-Presbyterian/St. Luke's Medical Center, Chicago, Illinois 60612

André G. Uitterlinden (355)
Department of Internal Medicine, Erasmus University Medical School, 3000 DR Rotterdam, The Netherlands

Johannes P. T. M. van Leeuwen (355)
Department of Internal Medicine, Erasmus University Medical School, 3000 DR Rotterdam, The Netherlands

Annemieke Verstuyf (217)
Laboratory for Experimental Medicine and Endocrinology, Katholieke Universiteit Leuven, 3000 Leuven, Belgium

Klaus von der Mark (3)
Institute of Experimental Medicine, Friedrich Alexander University, 91054 Erlangen, Germany

Michael P. Whyte (605)
Metabolic Research Unit, Shriners Hospital for Children; and Division of Bone and Mineral Diseases, Washington University School of Medicine, St. Louis, Missouri 63110

Foreword

For many years, bone and cartilage were considered the "Cinderellas" of biology and medicine. Basic research was neglected and the little progress made was centered on calcium metabolism. There were few conferences, with one of the first series in the field being the Macy Conferences in the fifties. One of the reasons for this situation was the fact that both bone and cartilage were very difficult to study, particularly because the cells were embedded in a large amount of matrix and were often difficult to isolate. Investigations of patients were even more difficult, and the techniques available were few and time consuming.

In the last decades the situation has changed drastically. Skeletal tissues are today as "in" as other tissues. The interest has developed in an incredible way, which is well demonstrated by the number of attendees at conferences in the field, both preclinical and clinical. Thus, meetings of the American Society for Bone and Mineral Research, which counted a few hundred participants in 1979, are now attended by over 5000. Similarly, meetings on osteoporosis have developed from a few hundred participants in 1979 to more than 5000 recently.

There are several reasons for this dramatic change in the level of interest. The development of new techniques in biology has given insights into molecular mechanisms that one could not even have dreamt of a few decades ago. Discoveries of a new local endocrinology at the cellular level modulated by cytokines, the role of intracellular factors such as transcription factors, the intracellular cascade of information, all of which can now be investigated in bone and cartilage, have opened entirely new vistas. In clinical investigation, the development of markers for bone and cartilage turnover and techniques for measuring with precision and accuracy the amounts of bone mineral have been major contributors to progress. Indeed, these methods have not only facilitated the investigation and diagnosis of skeletal diseases but also provided the means to follow the efficacy of their treatment. These advances in monitoring drug efficacy in humans and animals have provided an impetus for the pharmaceutical industry to develop a series of new therapeutic agents. This, in turn, has led to increased interest in skeletal tissues and an increase in both public and pharmaceutical financing of basic and clinical research.

The aim of this book is to convey to the reader knowledge and understanding of these developments. It has the great merit of being constructed along the pathophysiological sequence: structure—biology at the various levels—mechanisms of the diseased functions—assessment of these functions—clinical aspects of the diseases. This approach should give both the student and the physician an improved understanding of skeletal diseases and the ability to provide more rational and efficacious treatments. Another merit of the book is that it covers both bone and cartilage in an integrated way, an option that has until now been rarely adopted.

The book is divided into 46 chapters written by outstanding specialists in their respective fields. Part I describes the structure, biosynthesis, and molecular biology of the extracellular matrices, as well as the main regulators of the turnover and function of these tissues, such as cytokines and other factors. Part II deals with the interrelationships between structure and function in both health and disease. These are presented at the molecular, cellular, and tissue level. Bone turnover, calcium metabolism, and their hormonal regulation as well as cartilage and joint physiology and pathophysiology are then described. Part III is based on the concepts developed in previous sections and deals first with the measurement of structure and function of both bone and cartilage, with special emphasis on the new biochemical and genetic markers. This is followed by a discussion of the etiology, diagnosis, and clinical follow-up of various human diseases involving the two tissues, with special emphasis on osteoporosis, rheumatoid arthritis, and osteoarthritis.

This logical approach and the extensive cross-referencing between chapters make this book easy to read and effective in providing information. These factors, together with the excellent choice of subjects and the high quality of the content, combine to make this volume a great asset in the available literature and a must for anyone interested in the field.

H. FLEISCH
Professor Emeritus of Pathophysiology
University of Berne
Berne, Switzerland

Preface

Pathophysiology may be described as the art and science of understanding life, manifest as an extremely complex yet logical system of individual actions and interactions. The skeleton represents a perfect example of this notion, as it consists of many different yet closely interrelated components that function well only when they function together. The two largest entities of the skeleton are the tissues of bone and cartilage. At first glance, bone and cartilage may appear to be distinct because of their anatomical locations and their functional properties. To a certain extent, this is an accurate perception. On closer examination, however, it is evident that both tissues share a great number of structural principles and components. For example, both bone and cartilage display similar metabolic processes, as reflected by similar or even identical markers of cellular or matrix turnover. Moreover, in some cases, perturbations of normal function will eventually result in diseases involving both cartilage and bone. For example, rheumatoid arthritis, a disorder involving cartilage breakdown, is often associated with local and general osteoporosis. Paget's disease of bone is often associated, sooner or later, with osteoarthritis. These are just two examples of the interdependence of bone and cartilage in the context of disease.

With these notions in mind, the editors of this volume met in the late summer of 1997 at the Hopcrofts Holt Hotel, an olde English inn near Oxford, UK, to discuss the concept of a new and comprehensive textbook on skeletal pathophysiology. The outward setting for this task could have not been more ideal. The rural location of this 600-year-old one-time post depot at a crossroad north of Oxford allowed undisturbed work sessions and long walks across the beautiful English countryside. Surrounded by tranquil summer gardens, we attempted to design a book that would cover the two major tissues of the weight-bearing skeleton, namely, bone and cartilage. At the same time, it was our explicit objective to design a book that would be comprehensive, ranging from basic aspects of tissue biochemistry, genetics, and metabolic regulation to the clinical application of this knowledge to defined pathologies of bone and joint disease. In short, we envisaged a book that would take readers on a journey dealing with all aspects of skeletal metabolism, starting with the individual components of bone and cartilage, their biochemical structure, synthesis, and degradation; progressing to their function, interactions, and regulation; and arriving at their utility and value as markers of cellular and tissue function, thus providing a clear biochemical basis for their use as disease markers.

To this end, we asked more than 75 internationally known specialists—basic scientists as well as clinicians active in research—to contribute to this book. The challenging task for all authors was to write a relatively short, readable, yet comprehensive chapter on the current state of knowledge in the field of their expertise. The goal was to present individual chapters that would stand alone but also, taken together, would form a mosaic providing a complete picture of bone and cartilage physiology both in health and in disease. Our intention has been to make this book a valuable resource not only for those involved in skeletal research but also for internists, rheumatologists, endocrinologists, orthopedic surgeons, clinical biochemists, and others interested and participating in the management of patients with bone and cartilage diseases.

xix

The book's 46 chapters are divided into three major sections that lead from basic to clinically applied science. Part I, "Components of the Organic Extracellular Matrix of Bone and Cartilage," provides an up-to-date and comprehensive account of our knowledge of the structure, biosynthesis, and molecular biology of the major components of bone and cartilage. Chapters include "tissue building blocks" such as the collagens, the vitamin K-dependent proteins, the non-collageneous glycoproteins, and the proteoglycans and glycosaminoglycans. Additional chapters are devoted to the major regulators of bone and cartilage metabolism, such as the cytokines, growth factors, phosphatases, and matrix proteases.

Part II of the book covers the "Structure and Metabolism of the Extracellular Matrix of Bone and Cartilage." It describes the supramolecular organization of bone and cartilage and demonstrates how structure and function are interwined. Current concepts of the mechanisms of skeletal mineralization, remodeling, and hormonal regulation are discussed in conjunction with a thorough characterization of the products derived from the metabolic activity of bone and cartilage. This section of the book establishes the basis for a clear understanding of the mechanisms involved in normal and abnormal tissue function. Separate chapters are designed, moreover, to cover the important issues of fluid dynamics and protein trafficking in joints, as well as animal and *in vitro* models of cartilage metabolism, damage, and repair.

Alterations in tissue function will inevitably result in changes in tissue metabolism. Structural and functional components of these processes in bone and cartilage may be used as markers of these changes. Part III thus deals with the utility of components specific to bone and cartilage as biomarkers of tissue turnover in health and disease. This application-oriented section begins with a detailed account of the methodological and technical aspects of the various biochemical and genetic markers, as well as with their measurements. This helps to place into context the currently used biochemical markers of bone and cartilage metabolism and describes the use of these components in the screening, diagnosis, and follow-up of defined clinical disorders. Twenty-two separate chapters cover a wide range of diseases affecting bone and cartilage metabolism, including the different forms of osteoporosis, metastatic bone disease, and arthritic diseases, as well as some of the less common growth and degenerative abnormalities. Each chapter focuses on etiology, management, and the clinical use of biochemical markers.

Bringing together such a large number of experts from diverse fields of research and from all directions of the globe was a great task of daunting proportion. Eventually, with the help of many, we succeeded. First, we are grateful to our authors, who despite a rather short deadline managed to complete their chapters on time. Numerous e-mails, faxes, and telephone calls were made; holidays and birthdays were spoiled; prefinal versions of chapters were exchanged; authors even traveled across the oceans to sit together and write—it was a tremendous experience and a great pleasure to work with all of you.

Also, we are grateful to Dr. Jasna Markovac and to Jenny Wrenn of Academic Press, who supported us and our task from the first moments until the book was completed. We hope you will agree with us that the result speaks for itself.

MARKUS J. SEIBEL, Heidelberg

SIMON P. ROBINS, Aberdeen

JOHN P. BILEZIKIAN, New York

June 1999

PART I

Components of the Organic Extracellular Matrix of Bone and Cartilage

CHAPTER 1

Structure, Biosynthesis, and Gene Regulation of Collagens in Cartilage and Bone

KLAUS VON DER MARK   Institute of Experimental Medicine and Connective Tissue Research,
Friedrich-Alexander University of Erlangen-Nuremberg, 91054 Erlangen, Germany

I. INTRODUCTION

Collagens provide the structural framework of bones and cartilages and are responsible for shape and biomechanical properties such as resistance to pressure, torsion, or tension. In 1998, 20 genetically distinct collagen types in vertebrates have been described with rather diverse structural features and supramolecular organizations. Based on these features, collagens may be grouped into seven or eight different families, including the fibril-forming collagens, FACIT collagens, network-forming collagens and others (see Table I). Not all of them are found in cartilage and bone; in these tissues the fibril-forming collagens are dominant. Collagen heterofibrils consisting of types I and V constitute the fibrillar backbones in bone and types II and XI collagen in cartilage. In cartilage, the collagen fibrils are decorated with

the FACIT collagen type IX and are interwoven with a microfibrillar meshwork made of type VI collagen, which may provide additional elasticity. In hypertrophic cartilage of the growth plate, a network-foming collagen, type X collagen, supports endochondral ossification. Since collagens provide the major organic component with 90% of the dry mass in bone and 60% of the dry mass in cartilage, it is obvious that defects in structure, biosynthesis, assembly, or turnover of collagens generally lead to severe connective tissue diseases such as osteoporosis, osteoarthritis, chondrodysplasias, or osteogenesis imperfecta.

In order to understand the dynamics of collagen metabolism in bone and cartilage and to gain insight into the various levels of transcriptional and translational regulation of collagen biosynthesis and turnover, it is necessary to understand not only the basic features of the structure of the

3

TABLE I.   The Collagen Families

Type	Subunits	Molecular forms	Tissue distribution	Characteristic features
			Fibril-forming collagens	
I	$\alpha1(I)$ $\alpha2(I)$	$[\alpha1(I)]_2\alpha2$	bone, dermis, tendon, ligaments	Forms fibers of high tensile strength; most abundant collagen
		$[\alpha1(I)]_3$	cornea, most other tissues dermis, dentin	Rare form
II	$\alpha1(II)$	$[\alpha1(II)]_3$	cartilage, notochord, vitreous body embryonic epithelia	Major cartilage collagen; forms heterofibrils with Col IX and XI; can induce arthritis
III	$\alpha1(III)$	$[\alpha1(III)]_3$	reticular fibres of most tissues (lung, liver, dermis, spleen, vessel wall etc.)	Often in mixed fibrils with type I collagen; abundant in elastic tissues; cys-bridges in triple helix
V	$\alpha1(V)$ $\alpha2(V)$ $\alpha3(V)$	$[\alpha1(V)]_3$ $[\alpha1(V)]_2\,\alpha3(V)$	*in vitro:* hamster lung cell cultures lung, cornea, bone, fetal membranes; together with type I collagen	Propeptide partially retained in the fibrils; forms heterofibrils with type I collagen; controls fibril diameter
XI	$\alpha1(XI)$ $\alpha2(XI)$ $\alpha3(XI)$	$\alpha1(XI)\alpha2(XI)\alpha3(XI)$ $[\alpha1(XI)]_2\,\alpha2(V)$	cartilage, vitreous body bone	Highly homologous to Col V; nucleates and controls cartilage coll. fibril formation; $\alpha3(XI)$ same gene as for $\alpha1(II)$
			Basement membrane collagens	
IV	$\alpha1(IV)$ $\alpha2(IV)$ $\alpha3(IV)$ $\alpha4(IV)$ $\alpha5(IV)$ $\alpha6(IV)$	$[\alpha1(IV)]_2\,\alpha2(IV)$ $[\alpha3(IV)]_2\,\alpha4(IV)$? ? ?	basement membranes glomerular basement membranes, neuromuscular junctions, glomerular basement membrane; lung, kidney	Flexible triple helix with many interruptions; forms super coiled three-dimensional networks; NC1 $\alpha3(IV)$ = Goodpasture antigen; mutations in $\alpha5(IV)$ Alport syndrome
			Microfibrillar collagen	
VI	$\alpha1(VI)$ $\alpha2(VI)$ $\alpha3(VI)$	$\alpha1(VI)\alpha2(VI)$ $\alpha3(VI)$	widespread, in dermis, cartilage, placenta, lung vessel wall, intervertebral disc	Contains VWF and Kunitz-type protein inhibitor domains; forms beaded filaments; highly disulfide cross-linked
			Anchoring fibrils	
VII	$\alpha1(VII)$	$\alpha1(VII)_3$	skin, oral mucosa, cervix dermal–epidermal junctions	Forms bundles made of dimers (terminal NC1) anchored in anchoring plaques and basement membrane
			Hexagonal network-forming collagens	
VIII	$\alpha1(VIII)$ $\alpha2(VIII)$	$[\alpha1(VIII)]_2\,\alpha2(VIII)$	endothelial cells Descemet's membrane	Molecules assemble into hexagonal network in Descemet's membrane; strong inter- and intramolecular interactions between NC1 domains
X	$\alpha1(X)$	$[\alpha1(X)]_3$	hypertrophic cartilage	Mutations in Col X–NC1 SMCD
			FACIT collagens	
IX	$\alpha1(IX)$ $\alpha2(IX)$ $\alpha3(IX)$	$\alpha1(IX)\alpha2(IX)\alpha3(IX)$	cartilage, vitreous humor splice variant without NC4 domain in cornea	Covalently linked to type II collagen fibrils; NC4 domain projects into cartilage matrix; contains chondroitin sulfate
XII	$\alpha1(XII)$	$[\alpha1(XII)]_3$	perichondrium, ligaments, tendon	Large cruciform-shaped NC3 domain; associated with type I collagen fibrils splice variants
XIV	$\alpha1(XIV)$	$[\alpha1(XIV)]_3$	dermis, tendon, vessel wall, placenta, lung, liver	Associated with type I collagen; splice variant without collagenous domain = undulin
			Transmembrane collagens	
XIII	$\alpha1(XIII)$	$[\alpha1(XIII)]_3$	epidermis, hair follicle, endomysium, intestines, chondrocytes, lung, liver	Transmembrane domain in NC4; splice variant homology to Col XV
XVII	$\alpha1(XVII)$	$[\alpha1(XVII)]_3$	dermal-epidermal junctions	Same as Bullous Pemphigoid antigen BPAG-2; NH_2 end inside the cell
			Multiplexins	
XV	$\alpha1(XV)$		kidney, pancreas; adrenal gland	NC1 domain homologous to aggrecan; three collagenous domains
XVI	$\alpha1(XVI)$	?	amnion, fibroblasts, keratinocytes	10 collagenous domains; NC domains begin with Cys-X-Y-Cys
XVIII	$\alpha1(XVIII)$	?	lung, liver	Related to Col XV C-terminal NC1 domain = endostatin
XIX	$\alpha1(XIX)$	?	Human rhabdomyosarcoma	C-terminal Col 1 domain homologous to Col IX, XII, XIV, and XVI

collagen molecules and their higher aggregates but also the structure of the collagen genes and their *cis*-acting regulatory elements, the various posttranslational modifications, and the mechanisms of processing and extracellular assembly. An overwhelming amount of literature has been published on these topics, but the scope of this chapter does not permit a detailed and complete presentation of our current knowledge on the mechanisms of collagen metabolism and its regulation in bone and cartilage. Fortunately, a number of excellent, comprehensive review articles and book chapters are available dealing with the structure and function of collagen types [1–8], with collagen genes [9, 10], collagen biosynthesis and regulation [11–13], and collagen degradation [14]. For more detailed and comprehensive information on collagens, the reader may be also referred to books and volumes on collagens and their genes [2, 15, 16]. In this chapter, I only shortly summarize basic and recent information on the structure of collagens and their genes and focus on aspects of collagen biosynthesis, including recent findings on *cis*-acting promoter, enhancer, and silencer elements of the major collagen genes and mechanisms of posttranslational modifications. No further information will be given on collagens that do not play a major role in cartilage and bone, such as types IV, VII, VIII, and XIII to XX. Aspects of extracellular assembly to supramolecular structures, in particular fibril formation and cross-link formation, will be dealt with in Chapters 2, 11, and 20. Collagen degradation by proteases will be covered in Chapter 10 on matrix proteases.

II. THE COLLAGEN FAMILIES

A. Structural and Functional Diversity

In 1998, at least 20 genetically distinct collagen types have been described in mammals (Table I). As many of them are composed of several α-subunits, at least 35 mammalian collagen genes are known, and more are likely to be discovered [4, 6–8, 17]. There is considerable complexity and diversity in the structure of the different collagen types, their splice variants, their triple helical and non-triple helical domains, and their assembly into extracellular matrix structures: fibrils, flexible meshworks, hexagonal sheets, beaded filaments, anchoring fibrils, and perhaps other, yet unknown structures.

The fibril-forming collagens, with five members and about 90% of the total collagens, represent the most abundant and widespread family of collagens in vertebrates. Type IV collagens with a more flexible triple helix assemble into supercoiled chicken wire-like meshworks restricted to basement membranes, and types VIII and X form hexagonal sheets. Type VI collagen is highly disulfide cross-linked and forms a meshwork of beaded filaments interwoven with collagen fibrils. Collagens IX, XII, and XIV associate as single molecules with collagen fibrils (FACIT-collagens) [6], while others (Col

XIII and XVII) span cell membranes. In most of the recently discovered collagens, the triple helical part seems to play a minor role and is dominated by complex, globular, or cross-shaped nontriple helical domains, and the question arises whether all triple helix-containing proteins, in particular the membrane-spanning collagens XIII and XVII, should be classified as "collagens" [18]; other triple helix-containing proteins such as C1q, acetylcholinesterase, or a macrophage scavenger receptor [19] have escaped the collagen nomenclature.

Much has been speculated but little is firmly established on the specific functions of collagen, even the classical, long-known fibril-forming collagens. Initial ideas on functions of collagens were mostly derived from their distribution in tissues and from *in vitro* experiments, e.g., cell and organ culture studies. Owing to their torsional stability and tensile strength, the major function of fibril-forming collagen is to support the tissue architecture and stability. Despite their structural similarity, however, the fibrillar collagen types I, II, and III have different, specific functions in different tissues, different immunological properties, and show specific interactions with different cell types. More recently, natural and artificially introduced mutations in human and animal collagen genes and the inactivation of collagen genes by homologous recombination in mice ("knockout mice") [20, 21] have provided valuable information on the role of some collagens in cartilage and bone. Surprising results of gene knockout experiments in mice or from human mutations have often caused a revision of common opinions on the function of various collagens; thus, after inactivation of the type II collagen gene Col2a1 in mice, normal embryonic development of notochord and somites and the eye was observed, although early expression of Col2a1 in embryonic epithelia [22–24] and several *in vitro* studies had strongly suggested a critical role of this collagen in early epithelial–mesenchymal interactions [25, 26]. On the other hand, the analysis of collagen mutants confirmed the proposed role of type XI collagen as regulatory components in the cartilage collagen fibril [27, 28]. More and valid information on the function of individual collagens and their domains can be expected from targeted mutations in distinct domains and tissue specific inactivation (conditional knock out) of collagen genes.

B. The Collagen Triple Helix

The key feature of all collagens is a coiled-coil structure in form of a right-handed triple helix of 1.5 nm diameter, composed of three polypeptide chains [1, 29–32] (Fig. 1). A structural requirement for the assembly of polypeptide chains into a collagen triple helix is a glycine residue in every third position, resulting in the $(Gly-X-Y)_n$ repeat structure characterizing all collagens. The α-chains form a stretched, left-handed helix with a pitch of 18 amino acid residues per turn

N-Propeptide   **C-Propeptide**

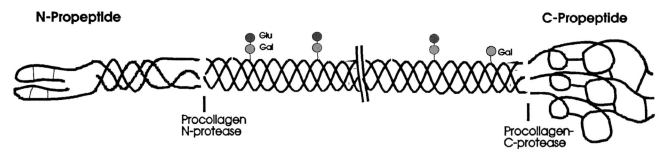

FIGURE 1   Procollagen type I. The N-propetide consists of a short triple helical part and a β-sheet at the N terminus.

[33] and assemble around a central axis in a way that all glycine residues are positioned in the center of the triple helix. The more bulky side chains of the other amino acids in the X and Y positions occupy the outer positions, where they are available for lateral interactions with neighboring collagen molecules to form fibrils. Another typical feature is the high content of proline and hydroxyproline (ca. 20%). The hydroxyl groups of 4-hydroxyproline are essential for the formation of intramolecular hydrogen bonds and thus critically determine the thermal stability of each collagen triple helix [34, 35]. The melting temperature of the type I collagen triple helix is 39°C at neutral pH [30], but can be considerably higher, e.g., 46°C in chicken type X collagen [36] or 65°C in the amino-terminal 7S domain of type IV collagen [37]. Triple helical domains vary considerably in their length: In fibril-forming collagens they span 300 nm corresponding to 1000 amino acid residues per processed α-chain. Interruptions of the $(Gly-X-Y-Gly-X-Y)_n$ structure by only one residue may cause a flexibility in the triple helix and render the helix susceptible to proteolytic attack, e.g., in collagen type IV. The native state of a triple helix may be measured by optical rotation, circular dichroism, or resistance to proteases such as pepsin, trypsin, or chymotrypsin [38]. This resistance of the native triple helix to proteases has been the basis for almost all biochemical isolation procedures of collagens in the past, using pepsin to destroy noncollagenous proteins while leaving the collagen triple helices intact.

Triple helical collagenous domains are also found in proteins such as C1q, acetycholine esterase, and MARCO, a macrophage scavenger receptor [18, 19].

covered "multiplexins" (collagens with *multiple* triple helix *in*terruptions [40], see Table I) the collagenous domains are short and separated by nine or ten noncollagenous domains. While the triple helix is a highly conserved structural protein element like the α-helix or the β-pleated sheet, there is considerably more structural and functional diversity among the noncollagenous domains of the different collagen families and types. For example, in the fibril-forming collagens, the largely globular C-propeptides are all homologous and serve as nucleation sites for chain assembly and triple helix formation, while the N-propeptides regulate the fibril size when retained in the molecule (see later). There is also sequence homology among the N-terminal NC domains of IX, XI, XII, and XVII collagens. Many noncollagenous domains, e.g., in collagen VI and XI, contain thrombospondin and von Willebrand factor-like domains or fibronectin type III repeats [41, 42]. The C-propeptide of type II collagen remains in cartilage after cleavage from the procollagen molecule as a stable molecule ("chondrocalcin") and may participate in cartilage calcification [43], while the C-propeptide of type XVIII collagen is retained after cleavage as a protein with anti-angiogenic properties (endostatin) [44]. Other collagens such as XII and XIV contain huge, cross-shaped domains at the amino end.

Thus, particularly in the non-fibril-forming collagens, the noncollagenous domains show more specific and important structural and functional features than the triple helical domains. The term "collagen" may even not be adequate for some triple helix-containing proteins, as it should be restricted to proteins with predominantly extracellular structural functions.

C. Noncollagenous Domains

In the fibril-forming collagens, the triple helix represents the majority of the collagen molecule but is always flanked by noncollagenous domains (NC domains) at both ends (Fig. 1). In some collagens such as the "FACIT" collagen (*fibril-associated collagens with interrupted triple helices* [39], see later) the collagenous domains are interrupted by two or three noncollagenous domains; in the more recently dis-

III. FIBRIL-FORMING COLLAGENS

Fibril-forming collagens, which include types I, II, III, V, and XI collagen, are defined by their ability to assemble in a quarter-staggered array to fibrils with diameters between 25 and 400 nm. Fibrils thicker than 50 nm show a characteristic banding pattern in the electron microscope with a periodicity of 65 to 67 nm (D-period) [30–32]. All fibril-forming collagens consist of a triple helical core 300 nm in length corresponding to α chains of about 1000 amino acid residues, flanked by short 15–30 amino acid-long telopeptides, and in the case of Col XI and V, by large parts of the amino-terminal propeptides. More information on the assembly to fibrils and their structure will be provided in Chapter 2; therefore, here I will focus on the structure, distribution, and biosynthesis of the constituent collagen molecules.

A. Type I Collagen

1. MOLECULAR STRUCTURE AND TISSUE DISTRIBUTION

Type I collagen is the most abundant, longest known, and best studied collagen in vertebrates. It forms 90% of the organic mass of bone and tendon and is the major collagen of skin, ligaments, cornea, and many interstitial connective tissues. The human type I procollagen is made of 2 proα1 chains of 1464 amino acid residues [45] and a somewhat shorter proα2 subunit (1366 amino acids) [46]. It is synthesized in large quantities by fibroblasts, osteoblasts [47], and odontoblasts [48], and to a lesser extent by nearly all other tissue cells [2, 5, 49]. It is present in reticular fibers of most parenchymal tissues such as lung, kidney, liver, muscle, or spleen, with the exception of hyaline cartilage, brain, and vitreous humor [49]. Much of our information on biochemical and biophysical properties, cross-linking, and biosynthesis of collagens is based on research on this collagen and may be applied to other collagens, although significant differences have been found in structural details, physiological properties, and regulatory principles. Although purified type I collagen can be reconstituted to cross-banded fibrils *in vitro*, *in vivo* it is mostly incorporated into heterofibrils containing either type III collagen (in skin and reticular fibers [50, 51]), or type V collagen (in bone, tendon, cornea, and other tissues [52–54]) or both. Adachi and Hayashi [55] have shown that inclusion of type V collagen reduces the fibril diameter of type I collagen fibrils; in embryonic chick cornea, for example, a content of 20% type V collagen limits the fibril diameter to 25 nm [56]. In contrast, in bone, collagen fibrils with a content of ~5% type V collagen reach diameters of 400 nm or more. Embedded in hydroxyapatite crystals and various bone-specific glycoproteins, type I/V heterofibrils reveal unmatched biomechanical properties concerning load bearing, tensile strength, and torsional resistance.

Besides its biomechanical properties, type I collagen is important as an adhesive substrate for many cells and plays a major role in tissue and organ development, in cell migration, proliferation, and differentiation, in wound healing, tissue remodeling, and hemostasis [56, 57]. For example, *in vitro* studies have shown that many epithelial and endothelial cells acquire a polar cell shape and develop a luminal structure when cultured in a three-dimensional hydrated collagen lattice [58, 59]. Cells recognize native type I collagen

via $\alpha 1\beta 1$ and $\alpha 2\beta 1$ integrins [60], which are transmembrane receptors and confer signals from the extracellular matrix to intracellular signal cascades and to the actin cytoskeleton [61–64]. Valuable and important information on the role of type I collagen has been gained from the Mov13 mouse strain in which the expression of $\alpha 1$(I) chains is blocked owing to an insertion of the Mulv13 moloney virus into the first intron [65, 66]. Homozygous embryos die at day 13.5 owing to vessel rupture, but early development of organs is normal in the absence of type I collagen. Organ culture of salivary glands or lung buds showed that branching morphogenesis is also normal in the absence of type I collagen [67], possibly owing to a supplementing effect by type III collagen. Interestingly, in organ culture of tooth and bone anlagen $\alpha 1$(I) collagen is expressed despite the insertion of the Moloney virus in the Col1a1 gene [48, 68]. This observation lead to the discovery of a bone-specific control of Col1a1 transcription which differs from the transcriptional control in fibroblasts (see later).

B. Type II Collagen

Type II collagen is found predominantly, but not exclusively, in hyaline cartilage [69, 70], where it accounts for approximately 90% of the total collagen. It is a homotrimeric molecule with the composition $[\alpha 1(\text{II})]_3$ with similar size and biochemical features as type I collagen [7, 71], but it contains considerably more hydroxylysine-linked galactosyl-glucosyl-disaccharides (10 residues per $\alpha 1$(II) versus 2 disaccharides per $\alpha 1$(I) chain). Type II collagen exists in two splice variants (Fig. 2); in IIB, the dominant form found in mature cartilage, exon 2 is spliced out, which codes for a 69 amino acid residue cysteine-rich domain in the N-terminal propeptide. It is retained in IIA, a transient embryonic form that was found in prechondrogenic mesenchyme, in perichondrium, and vertebrae [72–74]. Type II collagen is not only the major collagen of hyaline elastic [75] and fibrous cartilage [49] but also represents the major collagen of vitreous humor [76, 77] and the nucleus pulposus of intervertebral discs. Furthermore, type II collagen is synthesized transiently by many embryonic epithelia such as notochord [78], cornea epithelium [76, 79, 80], retina pigment epithelium, craniofacial mesenchyme, and endocardial and mesocardial tissues [24, 81, 82]. The transient expression of collagen type II in early embryonic epithelia has given rise to many speculations on its role in epithelial–mesenchymal interactions and development. Curiously, however, inactivation of the type II collagen gene in mice did not affect early embryonic development of the eye, the somites, or cranofacial tissues, but had severe, lethal consequences on cartilage formation and vertebral development [21]. Compared to other fibrillar collagens, type II collagen has unique antigenic properties: Antibodies raised against chicken type II collagen cross-react with type II collagens from all other species including human, mouse, rat,

Structural domains of fibril forming collagens

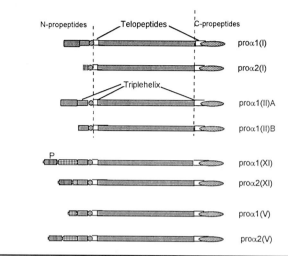

Microfibrillar collagen (type VI)

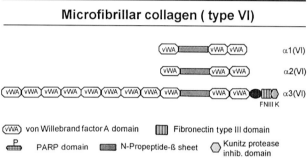

FIGURE 2   Structural domains of fibril forming collagen (procollagens) and the microfibrillar collagen type VI.

calf, dog, sheep, and shark [49, 71], indicating highly conserved antigenic epitopes in the type II collagen molecule. Another unique feature of type II collagen is its ability to induce arthritis in certain strains of mice and rats [83–86]. In accordance with this feature of type II collagen are numerous studies showing the development of autoantibodies against type II collagen in patients affected with rheumatoid arthritis [83, 87]. Although purified type II collagen is able to assemble into D-staggered, cross-banded collagen fibrils *in vitro* [88], native collagen fibrils in cartilage tissues are always heterofibrils containing ~5–10% type XI and type IX collagen [89, 90], which limit the fibril diameter to about 25 to 50 mm in embryonic cartilage [7, 27, 28, 56].

C. Type III Collagen

Collagen type III is a homotrimer with the composition $[\alpha 1(III)]_3$. It is characterized by interchain disulfide bridges of the triple helix close to the C terminus and is abundant in elastic tissue, predominantly in skin, reticular fibers of lung, liver, kidney parenchyme, and most other tissues [1, 2, 49].

Type III collagen was isolated first from pepsin-digested skin and separated forms type I collagen by fractional salt precipitation [91–93]. It colocalizes in all tissues and forms mixed fibrils with type I collagen [49] with few exceptions such as bone or chicken corneal stroma, which do not contain type III collagen [94]. Immuno-electronmicroscopical studies of the skin demonstrated that type III collagen can form both thin fibrils, separate from type I collagen fibrils [51], but thick type III collagen fibrils have also been observed [50]. In contrast to type I collagen, however, the N-propeptide of type III collagen is retained in the fibril, thus regulating the fibril diameter, similar to type V collagen [51]. Release of the highly immunogenic $\alpha 1(III)$ N-propeptide into tissue fluids or serum indicates fibrotic events and has been used as a marker for fibrosis and connective tissue turnover, e.g., in the liver [95–97].

D. Type V and XI Collagens

Type V and XI collagens and other α-chains may be considered a subfamily of structurally very closely related fibril-forming collagens with similar biochemical properties and similar functions in the organism. Type V collagen usually codistributes with type I collagen in bone, corneal stroma, interstitial matrix of smooth muscle, skeletal muscle, liver, lung, and placenta [98], while type XI collagen is attributed to cartilage collagen. Both collagens precipitate in their pepsin-treated form between 0.8 and 1.2 M NaCl at acidic pH, a feature that was decisive for their first discovery and separation from the dominant type I or type II collagens, respectively [99]. Five of the pro-α-chains of collagen V and XI are further characterized by large amino-terminal noncollagenous domains, which are partially retained in the fibrils [100, 101]. The sixth α-subunit $\alpha 3(XI)$, is nearly identical to $\alpha 1(II)$ and is translated from the same gene, but differs from $\alpha 1(II)$ by a higher degree of hydroxylation and glycosylation [99, 102–105]. The 400 amino acid residue globular domain of $\alpha 1$, $\alpha 2$, $\alpha 3(V)$ and $\alpha 1$ and $\alpha 2(XI)$ located between signal peptide and the short triple helix of the N-propeptide are about twice as large as the corresponding cysteine-rich region in $\alpha 1(I)$, $\alpha 1(II)$, or $\alpha 1(III)$ (Fig. 2). The domains are processed only partially after secretion, leaving stubs of 70–100 kDa in the fibril [101, 106, 107] that are critical for controlling fibril assembly and growth (see later). Complex alternative splicing occurs within the amino-terminal noncollagenous domains of $\alpha 1(XI)$ and $\alpha 2(XI)$ [108–110]. The high content of tyrosine sulfate in the N-propeptide of $\alpha 1$ and $\alpha 2(V)$ collagen chains is unusual [111]. With 40% of the tyrosine residues being O-sulfated, a strong regulating interaction with the more basic triple helical part is likely to stabilize the fibrillar complex. A proline- and arginine-rich subdomain (PARP domain) of the amino-propetides of $\alpha 1(XI)$ and $\alpha 2(XI)$ seems to be rather stable and persists in the cartilage matrix [112, 113]. In contrast to types I, II, and III collagen, the triple helical parts of types V and XI collagen are resistant to digestion with vertebrate collagenase (MMP1) but not to stromelysin [105, 114, 115].

Depending on the tissue, there is some heterogeneity in the composition of type V and XI molecules. Most tissues contain type V collagen molecules consisting of two $\alpha1(V)$ and one $\alpha2(V)$ chain, but $[\alpha1(V)]_3$ homotrimers have been isolated from tumor cells [116], and some tissues contain $\alpha1(V)$, $\alpha2(VI)$, $\alpha3(V)$ heterotrimers (see Table I). Also, type V/XI hybrid molecules containing $\alpha1(V)$ and $\alpha2(XI)$ collagen chains were described in articular cartilage [117], in bone [118] and in vitreous humor [119].

Immunohistochemical identification of type V collagen in tissue sections with antibodies requires demasking of the epitopes with acid or enzymes [52, 54], indicating a dense packing of type V collagen within the type I/V collagen heterofibrils [120]. Fibril reconstitution studies with mixtures of purified, native type V and type I collagen demonstrated that incorporation of 20% type V collagen into type I collagen reduces the fibril diameter to 25 nm [55], corresponding to the diameter of collagen fibrils in the chicken corneal stroma [121]. Similarly, antibody staining of type XI collagen in cartilage collagen fibrils by immunoelectronmicroscopy required mechanical or enzymatic loosening of fibrils [90]. The pivotal role of type XI collagen in the control of cartilage collagen fibril assembly became apparent from the analysis of the gene defect of the *cho* mouse mutant affected with an autosomal recessive chondrodysplasia: A point mutation in the

$\alpha1(XI)$ gene leading to chain determination caused absence of type VI collagen, resulting in a cartilage with irregular thick collagen fibrils, disorganized cartilage growth plate, and disturbed chondrocyte differentiation [27]. Similarly, an inframe deletion in the $\alpha2(XI)$ gene caused an autosomal recessive bone dysplasia or autosomal dominant Stickler syndrome [28].

IV. NONFIBRIL-FORMING COLLAGENS

A. Fibril-Associated Collagens with Interrupted Triple Helices (FACITs)

1. TYPE IX COLLAGEN

The first evidence for the presence of additional collagenous proteins in cartilage was seen in the form of various pepsin-resistant small collagenous fragments [103, 122, 123]. Combined protein-chemical and molecular biological efforts [124] led to the elucidation of the complex structure of type IX collagen. It is a heterotrimeric molecule consisting of $\alpha1(IX)$, $\alpha2(IX)$ and $\alpha3(IX)$ chains, with three triple helical segments that are interrupted and flanked by four globular domains, Col 1–Col 4 [71, 125, 126] (Fig. 3). Analysis of carefully dissected cartilage collagen fibrils by electron microscopy revealed that the highly cationic NC4 domain, the largest domain with 243 amino acid residues and pI of 9.7

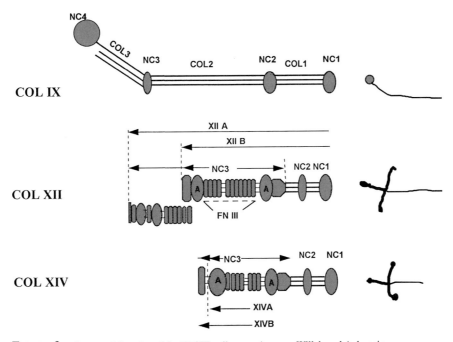

FIGURE 3   Structural domains of the FACIT collagens. A = von Willebrand A domain.

reaches out from the fibril where it presumably interacts with proteoglycans [127]. A "hinge region" in NC3 caused by additional amino acids in the NC3 domain of the $\alpha 2$(IX) chain allows flexibility in the molecule, which is covalently linked to the surface of cartilage collagen fibrils with the collagenous domains Col 1 and Col 2 [128]. The $\alpha 2$(IX) chain contains chondroitin sulfate side chain of varying size [89, 129], linked to a serine residue in the NC3 hinge region [130]. This CS chain is considerably longer in vitreous humor than in cartilage [131].

Owing to a second transcription start site between exon 6 and 7 in the $\alpha 1$(IX) collagen gene (see later), a shorter form of the $\alpha 1$(IX) collagen lacking the entire NC4 globular region is expressed in the cornea and vitreous humor [132, 133]. The importance of type IX collagen for the integrity of the cartilage matrix was underlined by the result of inactivation of the $\alpha 2$(IX) gene in mice. Animals homozygous for the deficiency in $\alpha 2$(XI) showed severe defects in cartilage development and revealed degenerative changes in adult articular cartilage similar to osteoarthritis [134].

2. TYPES XII AND XIV COLLAGEN

Type XII collagen is a homotrimeric molecule with sequence homologies to type IX collagen in the C-terminal NC1 and Col 1 domain but only two collagenous domains that associate with type I collagen fibrils. The large, cross-shaped NC3 domain at the amino end [135–138] reaches out into the perifibrillar space [139]; this domain contains VWFA domains, TSP, and FN type III domains (Fig. 3). Type XII collagen exists in two splice variants: The smaller IIB form with an $\alpha 1$(XII) chain of M_r 220 kDa is found in skin, periosteum, and perichondrium [138, 140]. The larger XIIA form with an α-chain of M_r 310 kDa was found in an epidermal cell line and contains a chondroitin sulfate chain. Collagen type XIV has a similar structure, although the cross-shaped NC3 domain is smaller than in Col XII [141–144]. A smaller form lacking the collagenous domains ("undulin") has also been isolated [145], but it is not clear whether this is a splice variant or a proteolytically processed form. Type XIV collagen colocalizes with type I collagen in skin, tendon, lung, liver, placenta, and vessel walls by immunofluorescence [145–148] and to some extent with type XII collagen in skin [149]. However, it does not bind to type I collagen directly, but via dermatan sulfate of decorin, which associates with type I collagen. While type XII collagen is located predominantly in the perichondrium and articular surface, type XIV collagen is more uniformly distributed throughout articular and tracheal cartilage [150].

B. Microfibrillar Collagens: Type VI Collagen

Type VI collagen is the major collagenous component of microfibrils in elastic fibers in a large variety of tissues including blood vessels (intima), skin, cornea, cartilage, placenta,

uterus, ciliary body, iris, etc. [151, 152]. The type VI collagen molecule is a highly glycosylated, cysteine-rich heterotrimer consisting of two α-chains of about 1000 amino acid residues [$\alpha 1$(VI) and $\alpha 2$(VI)], and a longer $\alpha 3$(VI) chain with about 3000 amino acid residues; the short triple helical core accounts only for about 20% of the molecule. It was discovered first in the form of pepsin-resistant "short chain" collagen with three α-subunits in smooth muscle and placenta [153, 154]. The three α-chains share three noncollagenous domains, which are homologous to the von Willebrand factor-A (VWF-A) domain [155–159]; the $\alpha 3$(VI) contains an additional eight VWF-A domains at the N terminus [160]. At least three of them are essential for collagen VI assembly and secretion [164]. The C-terminal domain of $\alpha 3$(VI) also contains a Kunitz-type inhibitor motif. Type VI collagen interacts with other matrix proteins and proteoglycans, e.g., hyaluronan, heparan sulfate, decorin, or NC2-proteoglycan [161–163].

Examination of type VI collagen in tissues or cell cultures by electron microscopy often reveals beaded filaments with 25 nm beads aligned in 100 nm intervals [165, 166]. Such structures can be assembled *in vitro* from type VI collagen tetramers, which connect and overlap at the globular ends when visualized by rotary shadowing [151, 152]. In tissues such as skin or cartilage, the type VI collagen forms a highly disulfide cross-linked, branched network, separate from interwoven fibrillar collagens [167]. In cartilage, type VI collagen is preferentially located in the pericellular space [151, 168]; it is enhanced in osteoarthritic cartilage [169], but has not been identified yet in calcified bone tissues. In some tissues such as nucleus pulposus and in some tumors type VI collagen filaments may assemble in a parallel fashion to give rise to sheets with the characteristic 100 nm periodicity [152].

The pericellular location of type VI collagen is consistent with its highly adhesive properties for many cell types. In contrast to other fibrillar collagens, several RGD sequences in the $\alpha 2$- and $\alpha 3$(VI) chain were found to be recognized by integrin receptors (see Chapter 8).

C. Network-Forming Collagens: Type X Collagen

Hypertrophic cartilage in the growth plate of fetal and juvenile long bones, ribs, and vertebrae contains a short-chain collagen, type X collagen [1, 170–176], which is unique to this tissue in the healthy organism and is only found elsewhere under pathological conditions, e.g., in osteoarthritic articular cartilage and in chondrosarcomas [177–180]. There is, however, recent evidence that type X collagen is also present in small amounts in the menisci and in the surface layer of articular cartilage of certain human, mouse, and dog joints.

Type X collagen is a homotrimeric collagen with a 130 nm triple helical core (460 amino acids per chain), a large C-terminal globular NC1 domain, and a short amino-terminal

NC2 globular region [175, 176]. It is homologous in both sequence and structure to type VIII collagen, which is produced by endothelial cells [181, 182]. Type VIII collagen assembles into sheets with a hexagonal arrangement in the Descemet's membrane [183], and *in vitro* reconstitution experiments with chicken type X collagen indicate that this collagen is able to form similar structures [184]. The three C-terminal NC1 domains of type X collagen molecule associate with unusually high affinity to dense globules. The NC1 domains are homologous to the complement factor C1q and TNFα [185]. Mutations in the NC1 domains lead to cartilage growth abnormalities and waddling gait in patients affected with Schmid type metaphyseal chondrodysplasia (SMCD) [186–189]. *In vitro* studies on the chain assembly of type X collagen demonstrated that the SMCD mutations severely affect triple helix assembly [190–192].

The function of type X collagen is not entirely clear. The severe cartilage and joint defects in SMCD patients clearly indicate a critical role for type X collagen in endochondral ossification; similar, transgenic expression of a truncated chicken type X collagen gene in mice cause growth plate abnormalities and a hunch back [193]; surprisingly, however, the phenotypic changes in the growth plate of two strains of type X collagen knockout mice were only moderate [194, 195]. There is also indirect evidence that type X collagen might be involved in matrix–vesicle-initiated calcification of hypertrophic cartilage [195].

D. Other Collagens

1. MULTIPLEXINS

Collagen types XV, XVI, XVII, XVIII, and XIX are composed of 8–12 collagenous domains interrupted by short noncollagenous domains, allowing a flexibility in the molecular shape that is not possible in fibril-forming collagens [4, 16, 196–199]. The cellular location and tissue distribution of most of these collagens has been described, but little is yet known of their possible functions. The C-terminal NC1 domain of Col XVIII, a basement membrane heparan sulfate proteoglycan, has received much attention recently as it persists as a separate entity in tissues and blood and was shown to inhibit angiogenesis by interfering with endothelial cell sprouting [44, 200].

The XIII collagen also exists as a transmembrane splice variant and can be localized on the surface of fibroblasts and other cells [201]. Similarly, type XVII is a transmembrane collagen with an amino-terminal noncollagenous part in the cytoplasm and multiple collagenous and noncollagenous domains in the extracellular space. Collagen XVII is located in hemidesmosomes at epithelial–mesenchymal interfaces and carries the Bullous pemphigoid autoantigen [202, 203]. Mutations in Col XVII may lead to mild forms of epidermolysis bullosa [204, 205].

V. COLLAGEN BIOSYNTHESIS

Most of our knowledge of the mechanisms of collagen biosynthesis is based on studies on fibril-forming collagens, in particular type I collagen. For this reason, this chapter focuses on biosynthesis events and mechanisms elucidated for the fibrillar collagens, but it is likely that most of it will apply also for other collagens.

A. Steps of Collagen Biosynthesis

1. TRANSCRIPTION AND ALTERNATIVE SPLICING

Although most collagen genes are transcribed only into one collagen gene product, e.g., types I, II, and IV collagen, some collagen genes may be transcribed into different mRNA species owing to several transcription start sites in some collagen genes, as in type IX collagen, and by alternative splicing. In the cornea and in the vitreous, a shorter form of type IX collagen is generated, owing to an alternative transcription start site between exons 6 and 7. Alternative splicing of collagen mRNAs was first described for type II collagen, which exists in an embryonic, longer form (IIB) and a shorter, adult form (IIA) from which exon 2 has been spliced out [72, 110, 206, 207]. More recently, alternative spliced forms have been reported for collagens VI, XI, XII, [208] and others, for example, type XIII with more than 12 splice variants [209]. Further heterogeneity among collagen mRNA species is introduced by heterogeneity in polyadenylation at the 3′ end. Thus, two α1(I) mRNA species of 4.8 and 5.8 kb in length can be observed in fibroblast cultures, and also for α2(I), α1(II), and α1(III) two different mRNA species are detected in cell cultures depending on the cell type [210].

2. TRANSLATION

Collagens are synthesized as procollagen molecules in the lumen of the rough endoplasmatic reticulum (RER), transported to the Golgi, and secreted (with the exception of membrane-spanning collagens) into the extracellular space via secretory vesicles (Fig. 4). The nascent pre-pro-α-chains protrude after translation from the ribosome-bound collagen mRNA into the lumen of the RER with the help of signal-recognition particles and receptors. Immediately after intrusion, the signal peptide is cleaved off, and the nascent procollagen chains are modified by hydroxylation and glycosylation before they align into triple helical procollagen molecules, which are secreted and processed before assembling into complex extracellular aggregates [211].

3. HYDROXYLATION AND GLYCOSYLATION

In the nascent procollagen chains about half of the proline residues in the Y position of the Gly-X-Y-triplets are

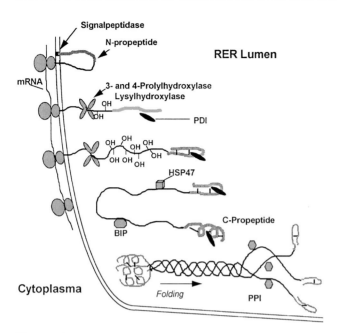

Figure 4 Biosynthesis of type I procollagen in the lumen of the rough endoplasmatic reticulum (RER). After completion of the triple helical procollagen molecule, the molecule is transported to the Golgi for processing of the N-linked oligosaccharides at the C-propetide (not shown), and then secreted in secretory vesicles. Cleavage of the N- and C-terminal propetides and crosslinking occurs outside the cell. PDI, protein disulphide isomerase; HSP47 and BIP, molecular chaperones; PPI, prolyl-peptidyl-cis-trans-isomerase.

converted to 4-hydroxyproline by the enzyme prolyl-4-hydroxylase [212–214]. Cofactors of hydroxylation are Fe^{2+}, α-ketoglutarate, oxygen and ascorbic acid. The extent of hydroxylation depends on the collagen type, species, and the cell and tissue type, and may change during development and aging or under pathological conditions. A few proline residues (all in the X position) may also be converted to 3-hydroxyproline by the enzyme prolyl-3-hydroxylase [212, 213]. The extent of lysine hydroxylation also varies considerably among collagen types. For example, two lysine residues in the $\alpha 1$(I) chain, both adjacent to the telopeptide region, and about 10 lysine residues in the $\alpha 1$(II) are hydroxylated to 5-hydroxylysine by the enzyme lysylhydroxylase [215]. Subsequently, glucosyl and galactosyl residues are transferred to the hydroxyl groups of hydroxylysine by glycosyl transferases to form glucosyl-galactosyl-disaccharides, and a mannose-rich oligosaccharide is coupled to a N-glycosylation receptor sequence in the C-propeptides of fibril-forming collagens.

4. Alignment of the Triple Helix

Assembly of the procollagen chains to triple helical molecules occurs after hydroxylation of the nascent chains and completion of the C-propeptides, which fold into the correct conformation stabilized by intrachain disulfide bonds

and assemble three α-chains to the procollagen trimer (Fig. 4) [216]. Chain assembly involves a two-stage recognition event in the fibril forming collagens. The first association and chain recognition is driven by the C-propeptides; essential for assembly are hydrophobic sequence patches with four hydrophobic amino acids that are conserved in their positions in all fibril-forming collagens. Assembly of the C-propeptides does not require the formation of interchain disulfide bonds [217], which form later after the assembly of the trimer. The formation of a native disulfide bond requires the catalysis by the enzyme protein disulfide isomerase (PDI) [218–220], which is identical to the β-subunit of prolyl-4-hydroxylase [213]. Rate limiting for the folding of the triple helix is the *cis-trans*-isomerization of prolyl peptide bonds in the α-chains [221], which is catalyzed by the enzyme peptidyl-prolyl *cis-trans*-isomerase (PPI) [222]. Critical support for a key role of PPI in collagen chain-folding was the observation that cyclosporin, an inhibitor of PPI and other cyclins, blocks folding of procollagen I and III in cell cultures [223]. After alignment of the C-propeptides, triple helix formation starts from the C terminus and progresses toward the N terminus; it is driven by a patch of three to four Gly-Pro-Hyp triplets located at the C terminus of the triple helix by providing a core stabilized by hydrogen bonds [35, 224]. Although the role of C-propeptides in chain assembly of fibril-forming collagens is firmly established, their role in chain selectivity in cells that produce several collagen types is not yet clear. Interestingly, only procollagen chains containing eight cysteines in the C-propeptide are able to form homotrimers [e.g., pro $\alpha 1$(I), $\alpha 1$(II), $\alpha 1$(III)], while procollagen chains lacking two or three of the eight cysteine residues such as pro-$\alpha 2$(I) can only form heterotrimers [225].

5. Chaperones Involved in Folding and Processing of Procollagen

Several chaperones such as BiP and HSP47 are involved in the posttranslational modification folding and processing of the procollagen molecule [226, 227]. The heat shock protein HSP47 binds cotranslationally to the nascent pro-α-chain in the RER and prevents unspecific chain folding and aggregation [226, 228]. Interestingly, it also binds to native, triple helical collagen molecules in the RER and controls bundle formation and transport to the Golgi apparatus and procollagen processing [229]. HSP47 is a heat shock protein and is expressed at 10-fold enhanced levels in chicken fibroblasts at 42–45°C [230]. Although it has a basic pI of 9.0, the glycoprotein binds to basic collagen chains and to native collagen with a K_d of 10^{-6} to 10^{-7} M, but with high on and off rates [231]. Originally it has been isolated by affinity chromatography on denatured collagen and was named colligin, a cellular protein binding to gelatin and type IV collagen [232].

A key enzyme required for the cross-linking of collagen α-chains and molecules is the enzyme lysyl oxidase [243], which catalyzes the oxidation of the ε-amino group of certain lysine and hydroxyline residues to aldehyde groups. More about this enzyme and its role in collagen cross-link formation will be provided in Chapter 2.

6. PROCOLLAGEN PROCESSING

Following secretion of procollagens in secretory vesicles, the C-propeptides of the fibril-forming collagen and the N-propeptides of type I, II, and partially also of type III collagen are cleaved by specific proteases. Both procollagen N-proteinase and procollagen-C-proteinases belong to a family of Zn^{2+}-dependent metalloproteinases M12 [13, 244]. The N-proteinase exists in two splice variants: a longer form of 140 kDa (pNP1) and a shorter form of 70 kDa (pNP-2) [245, 246]. Both cleave the N-propeptides of types I and II procollagen [247], but only in the native state, leaving the N-telopeptide in the hairpin loop configuration. The N-proteinase is structurally similar to atrolysin and adamalysin II and contains an RGD sequence and properdin-like repeats in the C-terminal part [13]. A N-proteinase that cleaves the N-propeptide of type III collagen has been described [248], but the final characterization of this enzyme has not been completed.

The procollagen-C-proteinase cleaves the C-propeptides of types I, II, and III collagen as well as laminin 5 and lysyl oxidase precursor [13]. Curiously, the enzyme is partially identical to bone morphogenetic protein 1 (BMP-1) or the mouse *tolloid* protease, and is related to *Drosophila tolloid*, Astacin, and BP10 [249, 250]. All these enzymes share the Zn^{2+}-binding proteinase domain, but the procollagen C-proteinases cCP-2 (mTld) ($M_r = 110$ kDa) or pCP-1 (BMP1) (70 kDa) differ in their C-terminal parts. The C-terminal procollagen propeptides that are cleaved off may remain in the tissue for some time. This has been shown in particular for type II collagen: The C-propeptide has been isolated from cartilage as an intact, disulfide-bounded entity that has been given the name chondrocalcin [43, 251, 252] as it is found in particular in calcified cartilage.

Besides the described C-proteinases of the BMP-1 type, other proteinases seem to be able to cleave procollagen-propeptides, e.g., cathepsin D [253]. This possibility must be taken in consideration in view of the recent finding that inactivation of both alleles of BMP-1 in mice did not dramatically alter procollagen processing but caused failure of body wall closure [250].

B. Translational and Posttranslational Regulation of Collagen Biosynthesis

1. EVIDENCE FOR TRANSLATIONAL REGULATION

Evidence for translational control of collagen mRNA was provided by the observation that chondrocytes contain un-translated $\alpha 1(I)$ mRNA [210, 254, 255]. The $\alpha 2(I)$ mRNA that was also present in chondrocytes was later found to be translated into a noncollagenous protein [256, 257] using a different reading frame. The mechanism and factors regulating this cartilage-specific translation is, however, still unknown. Another mechanism for regulation of collagen mRNA translation may be associated with the 3'-untranslated sequences. Polymorphic mRNA species exist for $\alpha 1(I)$, $\alpha 2(I)$, $\alpha 1(II)$, $\alpha 1(III)$, and $\alpha 1(IV)$; for example, Northern blotting of $\alpha 1(I)$ reveals two bands of 4.7 and 5.7 kb in the fibroblast monolayer [258, 259], which are expressed in different ratios depending on the cell type. This ratio increases significantly under the influence of TGF-β [260], which also increases the half life of the mRNA, which is normally 9–10 hrs. In collagen gels, however, only the smaller form of $\alpha 1(I)$ mRNA is expressed [261, 262]. The 3'-untranslated segment of collagen mRNA may be responsible for the stability and the translation rate of the mRNA [263].

2. REGULATION BY mRNA FOLDING

There is experimental evidence that translation initiation of $\alpha 1(I)$, $\alpha 2(I)$, $\alpha 1(II)$, and $\alpha 1(III)$ mRNA may be controlled by highly conserved nucleotide sequences close to the translation initiation codon. RNA patches of about 50 nucleotides contain inverted repeat sequences, which form stem loops or dimers and thus prevent translation initiation [264]. Deletion of these sequences in the $\alpha 2(I)$ mRNA *in vitro* did not, however, always affect mRNA translation [265].

3. FEEDBACK INHIBITION BY N- AND C-PROPEPTIDES

Studies on fibroblasts with Ehlers–Danlos syndrome VII as well as cell culture studies indicated that the N-propeptides of type I and III collagen induce feedback inhibition of type I collagen synthesis [266, 267]. The N-propeptide of $\alpha 1(I)$ specifically inhibited cell-free translation of $\alpha 1(I)$ mRNA [266], but curiously with fragmentation of the N-peptide into smaller fragments the inhibitory effect became nonspecific [268]. Providing strong support for a specific role of the N-propeptide was the observation that it binds specifically to fibroblast membranes and is taken up by endocytosis [268a]. Furthermore, expression of a metallothionein-inducible N-propeptide minigene in fibroblasts inhibited type I collagen synthesis [269].

The type I procollagen C-propeptide has also been implicated in the regulation of procollagen synthesis after internalization [270]. In contrast to the N-propeptide, however, it is transported to the nucleus and seems to control collagen gene expression at the transcriptional level, while smaller fragments of the C-propeptide may regulate collagen synthesis both negatively or positively at the postranscriptional level [271]. Similarly, the C-propeptide of type II collagen appears to inhibit translation of $\alpha 1(II)$ mRNA [272].

VI. COLLAGEN GENES AND TRANSCRIPTIONAL REGULATION

A. Genes Coding for Fibrillar Collagens

The genes coding for fibrillar collagens are highly conserved and are characterized by numerous short exons interrupted by fairly long introns. The triple helices of the genes of $\alpha1(I)$ (COL1A1 for the human gene, Col1a1 for the murine), of $\alpha2(I)$ (Col1a2), $\alpha1(II)$ (Col2a1), $\alpha1(III)$ (Col3a1), and all three chains of type V and XI collagen are encoded by 44 short exons. They are flanked by two longer exons at the $5'$ end coding for the N-propeptide and four exons at the $3'$ end coding for the conserved C-propeptide and $3'$ untranslated regions. The exons coding for triple helical sequences are all multiples of 9 bp corresponding to a Gly-Xaa-Yaa triplet; most common are 45, 54, and 109 bp [9, 10, 273, 274]. This highly conserved structure suggests that the fibrillar collagen genes have envolved from an ancestral multi-exon gene coding for collagen triplets. This feature is unique for fibril-forming collagens. Most of the non-fibril-forming collagens and invertebrate collagens are composed of fewer and larger exons. In contrast to the highly conserved size and number of exons in fibrillar collagen genes, there is considerable variation the intron length. For example, the gene COL1A1, coding for human proα1(I), has a total length of 18 kb, while the gene COL1A2 for α2(I) is 40 kb [275]. All genes coding for human fibrillar collagens are located on different chromosomes.

As in most regulated genes, transcription of collagen genes is regulated by multiple *cis*-acting elements including promoters, enhancers, and silencers. In all collagen genes investigated, the promoter region within 500 to 1000 bp $5'$ of the transcription start site that contains the binding site for the polymerase II and various transcription factors is critically important for expression. The activation of the promaximal promoter may be up- or down-regulated by additional enhancer or silencer elements further upstream of the promoter or located within the introns. Identification of these elements is currently a major task for elucidating the mechanisms of transcriptional regulation of collagen gene expression, including the identification of transcription factors and their role in growth factor or cytokine-induced receptor activation and signalling pathways [10, 276, 277].

1. Type I Collagen Genes

a. α1(I) Genes The regulatory elements in the type I collagen genes have been most extensively studied, but conflicting data have been published on the location and size of the minimal promoter and the role of an enhancer element in the first intron. The conflicts are primarily due to different methods and constructs used. Initial results were obtained from transient transfection studies of cell lines with reporter gene constructs containing fragments of the promoter and the first intron. The level of expression of the reporter genes, usually CAT, growth hormone, or luciferase, reflects the activity of the selected promoter, enhancer, and silencer elements, and the tissue specificity of the elements is assessed by transfecting different cell types that normally express type I collagen, e.g., fibroblasts or osteoblasts. More recently, the tissue-specific expression of *cis*-acting elements was analyzed in mice using LacZ as reporter genes, which allows the localization of reporter gene-expressing tissues through a color reaction. Studies by Sokolov *et al.* [278, 279], and Rossert *et al.* [280, 281] indicate that for human Col1A1 expression in skin a minimal promoter is required, which is located within -476 bp and -900 bp upstream of the transcription start site. In transgenic mice, the -476 bp promoter seems sufficient for tissue-specific expression even without intron sequences [278]. Interestingly, for expression of Col1A1 in bone, enhancer elements further $5'$ up to -2.3 kb are required [281]. This is in accordance with previous observations on differential regulation of Col1A1 in bone and teeth versus fibroblasts and other cells (see later).

Considerable efforts have been devoted in the past to identify positive and negative regulatory sequences in the first intron of $\alpha1(I)$ genes [276]. Several *cis*-acting intronic sequences with a highly conserved 29 bp domain involved in transcriptional regulation were located between $+292$ and $+670$ bp [282]. Between $+820$ and $+1093$ bp a silencer element is active when combined with a 332 bp promoter fragment. The effect of the intronic sequences varies with their size, location, and orientation within the reporter gene constructs and the cell type used for transfection. For example, while Slack *et al.* [283] reported that a reporter gene construct containing a 440 bp segment of the Col1A1 promoter lacked tissue specificity without the first intron, Sokolov *et al.* [278] found a 476 bp fragment of the Col1A1 promotor coupled to a human Col1A1 minigene allowed tissue-specific expression in transgenic mice without the first intron. Promoter elements shorter than 100 bp show tissue-specific expression of Col1A1 only when combined with sequences from the first intron.

The first evidence for a role of the first intron was obtained form the Mov13 mouse mutant, which was generated by infection with the Moloney virus [65, 66]. The insertion of the virus into the first intron of the Col1A1 gene caused complete block of Col1A1 transcription. Mice homozygous for the insertion of the virus did not contain any type I collagen (although the α2(I) gene was transcribed to mRNA) and died at day 13.5 due to vessel rupture [48, 65, 66]. Interestingly, however, the α1(I) gene was expressed in tooth and bone anlagen when cultured *in vitro*, indicating a different transcriptional regulation in osteoblasts and odontoblasts as compared to fibroblasts [67, 284]. In fact, Rossert *et al.* [280] and Pavlin *et al.* [285] located an enhancer element between -1656 and -1540 bp upstream of the transcription start site that promotes expression in osteoblasts. The transcription factor that binds to this element remains to be elucidated. Also, a TGF-β activating element (TAE) with nuclear factor-1 like sequences was located at -1600 bp upstream of the Col1A1 gene transcription start site; the TAE contained an activator protein-2 (AP-2) binding site [286]. Important for the regulation of Col1A1 expression in osteoblasts may be a vitamin D3-responsive element within the -3.6 kb promoter of rat Col1A1, which is down-regulated by vitamin D3 in ROS-osteoblasts but not in fibroblasts [285]. Similarly, glucocorticoids, which have been shown to down-regulate collagen synthesis, also decrease expression of Col1A1 promoter–reporter gene constructs [287, 288].

b. $\alpha 2(I)$ Genes

Similar to the Col1a1 gene, regulatory sequences have been described in the first intron of Col1α2 between $+418$ and $+524$ bp upstream of the transcription start site [289]. The intron of human COL1A2 suppressed reporter gene transcription in chicken fibroblasts, while the murine intron enhances transcription in mouse NIH 3T3 fibroblasts [289]; a -2000 bp promoter-lac Z-construct is active in osteoblasts. A NF-1 binding site mediates the inhibitory effect of TGF-β on the $\alpha 2(I)$ promoter [290]. TGF-β is one of the major factors stimulating type I collagen synthesis in fibroblasts (see later) [291, 292]. Some data suggest that an AP-1 site in the proximal promoter of COL1a2 is reponsible for the regulation of $\alpha 2(I)$ expression by TGF-β [293], while other data indicate that the transcription factor Sp1 but not Ap1 is required for early response of COL1A2 to TGF-β [294]. A proximal element within the human $\alpha 2(I)$ collagen promoter located between -161 to -125 bp relative to the transcription start site is responsible for down-regulation of Col1A2 promoter activity by interferon γ (IFNγ) [295]. This IFNγ response element (TaRE) is located between -265 and -241 bp. A potent far upstream enhancer element between 15 and 17 kb $5'$ of the Col1a2 gene strongly increased the expression of a reporter gene in transgenic mice in dermis, fascia, and other fibrous tissue [296]. The Col1a2 gene contains an alternative, cartilage-specific transcription start site with a 179 bp promoter in the third intron, which is transcribed in cartilage to a mRNA with an open reading frame but does not translate into a collagen [256, 297]. The role of this alternative transcript that is rapidly turned over in cartilage is yet unclear. Of particular interest is the mechanism controlling the shift from the use of the fibroblast-specific transcript pro-$\alpha 2(I)$ in chondroprogenitor cells to the use of the cartilage specific promoter in differentiated chondrocytes.

2. TYPE II COLLAGEN GENES

Unlike type I or III collagen, the expression of type II collagen is restricted to only few tissues, predominantly to cartilage and some embryonic epithelia; therefore the tissue-specific regulation of Col2a1 expression has received particular interest in the past. Horton *et al.* [298] observed that CAT reporter gene constructs containing only Col2a1 promoter fragments upstream of the transcription start site showed low expression levels, which was significantly increased when a 800 bp segment of the first intron was induced. The enhancer element consists of three high-mobility group (HMG)-binding sites located within a 48 bp sequence between $+1878$ and $+2345$ bp [299, 300]. Four tandem repeats or 12 tandem copies of an 18 bp subelement of this enhancer in combination with a 309 bp Col2a1 promoter allowed cell-specific expression of a β-galactosidase reporter gene in mouse chondrocyte [301]. The critical role of this enhancer is underlined by the finding that cartilage-specific expression in trasgene mice even occurs when the 309 bp Col2a1 promoter is replaced by a minimal β-globin promoter [299]. The localization of this enhancer element allowed the identification of SOX-9 as major transcription factor regulating type II collagen expression in chondrocyte [300–304]. SOX-9 is a member of DNA-binding proteins with high homology to SRY, the sex-determining gene C. The DNA-binding domain is encoded by a variant of the HMG box. In mouse chondrocytes, high levels of SOX-9 protein correlate with type II collagen-expressing cells, while dedifferentiated chondrocytes lack SOX-9 [303, 304]. Furthermore, a zinc-finger protein CII2FP was described, which binds to the enhancer within the first intron of Col2a1 and to Sp1, but the role of this protein in the control of COL2a1 expression remains to be elucidated. In the rat Col2a1 gene a strong enhancer activity was located within a 156 bp fragment between $+1288$ and $+2343$ bp in the first intron [305]. In the Col2a1 promoter a short sequence including two GC boxes between -68 to -145 bp was identified that binds an Sp 1-related factor and an enhancer-nuclear factor complex [306]. The complexity of the transcriptional regulation of the type II collagen gene is underlined by the finding of two silencer elements in the rat Col2a1 promoter that seem to inhibit Col2a1 expression in nonchondrocytic cells [307].

3. TYPE III COLLAGEN GENES

In the mouse Col3a1 gene two positive and one negative regulatory domains were located in the proximal promoter region. A 12 bp stretch at -122 to -106 bp recognized by an AP-1-like protein enhances transcription in DNA transfection assays [308], whereas the 22 bp segment B (-61 to -83 bp upstream of the transcription start site) binds a nuclear factor (BBF) extracted from Hela cells [309]. A negative regulatory element located between -350 and -300 bp repressed the activity of the promoter [310].

4. TYPE V AND XI COLLAGEN GENES

In contrast to the genes of type I, II, and III collagen, the human $\alpha 1(V)$ collagen gene Col5A1 [311] lacks obvious TATA and CAAT boxes and has a number of features characteristic of the promoters of housekeeping genes [312]. It has multiple transcription start sites, a high GC-content, and a number of consensus sites for the potential binding of the transcription factor SP1. The promoter seems to consist of an array of *cis*-acting elements, with a minimal promoter 212 bp upstream of the major transcription start site. The Col5a2 gene seems more closely related to the Col3a1 gene, but little is known of its regulating sequences [313]. Similar to the Col5a1 gene, the genes of the human type XI collagens COL11A1 and COL11A2 lack TATA boxes indicating that they are regulated through mechanisms similar to those for housekeeping genes [314, 315]. The human COL11A1 gene has several minor transcriptional start sites clustered around one major start site at 318 bp from the ATG codon [313].

A transcriptional complex containing potential binding sites for ubiquitous nuclear proteins such as AP2 and Sp 1 is closely related to a similar complex in the proximal promoter of the Col11a2 gene. The Col11a2 gene spans 30.5 kb with a minimum of 62 exons. Similar to Col5a2, its promotor is GC-rich with two potential Sp1-binding sites [109, 316]. A chondrocyte-specific enhancer element in the Col11a2 gene that resembles the Col2a1 enhancer confers tissue-specific expression [317].

B. Type VI Collagen Genes

The genes of the three type VI collagen subunits are similar to those of the fibril-forming collagens in that they are composed of numerous small exons that are multiples of 9 bp, in a range between 27 and 90 bp in the 19 exons coding for the triple helical part of chicken $\alpha 1(VI)$ and $\alpha 2(VI)$ [318, 319]. Multiple splice variants have been described for $\alpha 2(VI)$ and $\alpha 3(VI)$ in chicken and human: In the chicken $\alpha 2(VI)$ the major splice variant containing a VWFA domain at the carboxy-terminal globule is replaced by a FN-type III repeat in the minor splice variant, which is expressed only in aortic tissue [320]. For human $\alpha 2(VI)$ three protein variants have been described owing to alternative splicing at the C terminus [207]. The chicken $\alpha 3(VI)$ shows extensive size heterogeneity with five bands in SDS-PAGE due to alternative splicing of VWFA modules in the globular domain [321]. The $\alpha 3(VI)$ splice variants show different tissue distribution depending on age and developmental stage [322].

In the chicken $\alpha 1(VI)$ gene two major and several minor transcription start sites were found [323]. Within the basic, proximal promoter, which lacks TATA or CAAT boxes, three regulatory C-GGAGGG (GA box) boxes were identified that bind several transcription factors, including Sp1 and AP1 [324, 325] and AP2 [326]. These elements are responsible for up-regulation of $\alpha 1(VI)$ expression during C2C12 myoblast differentiation [325]. Expression of murine $\alpha 1(VI)$ promoter–reporter gene constructs in transgenic mice indicated that the -215 bp minimal promoter is not sufficient for expression in tissues [323, 327]. Additional *cis*-acting elements between -0.4 and 1.4 kb are required for tissue ex-

pression. The *cis*-acting elements at -46 to 5.4 kb are responsible for $\alpha 1(VI)$ expression in joints, while the region at -6.2 to 7.5 kb upstream of the transcription start site is required for expression in the muscle meninges [323] and other tissues except lung and uterus [327]. Two promoters control the transcription of the human $\alpha 2(VI)$ gene [326]. The chicken $\alpha 2(VI)$ collagen promoter encompasses four regulatory sites: S1, S2, and S3 are recognized by transcription factors of the Sp1-family, while site X binds a Mr 43 kDa transcription factor [328]. No data on the regulation of $\alpha 3(VI)$ expression are available so far. The type of *cis*-acting regulatory elements found in the type VI collagen genes differs completely from those found in the genes of fibril-forming collagen. This is consistent with the distinct regulation of type VI collagen expression in tissues and cell culture in comparison to collagens I, II, or III: All three type VI collagen genes are up-regulated in fibroblasts when grown at increasing densities in culture, while Col I and III levels do not change [329]. Conversely, the phorbolester cocarcinogen PMA reduces Col I and III levels but not Col VI expression. Similar to Col I and III, however, Col VI expression is increased in systemic sclerosis [330] and in keloids [331]. A strong up-regulation of collagen VI expression has been observed during chondrocyte differentiation [332]. In only one study has expression of $\alpha 1(VI)$ in osteoblast-like cells been documented; it is upregulated by interleukin-4. Interestingly, the $\alpha 3(VI)$ gene is not always coregulated with $\alpha 1(VI)$ and $\alpha 2(VI)$. $\alpha 3(VI)$ expression, not $\alpha 1(VI)$ nor $\alpha 2(VI)$, is up-regulated by TGF-β [333] or down-regulated by IFN-γ [334].

C. Type X Collagen Genes

Unlike genes coding for fibril-forming collagens or type VI collagen chains, the genes for type X collagen contain only 3 exons that are fairly conserved in all four species investigated: chicken [181], mouse [335–337], bovine [338], and human [339, 340]. Exon 1 contains 80–114 bp 5′ UTR sequences, exon 2 contains 159–169 bp, while exon 3 with 2136–2900 bp codes for the majority of the triple helical part, the entire C-terminal NC1-1 domain, and up to 939 (human) 3′ UTR sequences [341]. Nuclear run-on experiments as well as *in situ* hybridization studies indicate that collagen X expression is regulated strictly at the transcriptional level [342, 343].

As expected from the tight developmental control of collagen X expression in the fetal cartilage growth plate [171, 344], strong positive and negative regulatory *cis*-acting elements have been described in the promoter of collagen X genes, with major differences, however, between mammalian and chicken genes [341]. In chicken, multiple negative elements in the proximal promoter (-580 bp) restrict expression of the collagen X gene to hypertrophic chondrocytes [345–347]. A BMP-2, BMP-4, and BMP-7 responsive 529 bp element was located 2.4–2.9 kb upstream from the Col X transcription start site, which was necessary and sufficient for BMP-stimulated Col X expression in prehypertrophic chicken chondrocytes [348]. In the human promoter, however, a strong enhancer element located between −2200 and −2500 bp [349, 350] stimulates transcription of reporter gene constructs in hypertrophic chondrocytes, while a silencer element between −2500 and −3000 bp suppresses transcription in nonhypertrophic chondrocytes and fibroblasts [350]. In the mouse Col10a1 promoter an additional 2000 bp segment containing LINE elements, B1, B2, and LTR elements are inserted [341]; thus, the regulatory region corresponding to the known human promoter including the enhancer and silencer element are not yet known. In the proximal promoter a TATA box, one ETS binding site, and an AP-2 binding site are conserved between mouse, bovine, and human Col10a1 [340, 341]. Data by Harada et al. [350a] indicate that the murine Col10a1 promoter is up-regulated by osteogenic protein 1, which is mediated by a MEF2-like sequence. The murine Col10a1 has a second transcription start site and, correspondingly, another TATA box that is utilized only in the newborn mouse [336]. CCAAT boxes at −120 bp have been found so far only in the mammalian Col10a1 genes.

VII. FACTORS REGULATING COLLAGEN BIOSYNTHESIS

Numerous proteins factors, hormones and cytokines have been shown to inhibit collagen gene expression *in vivo* and *in vitro*, but only a few factors have been identified that unequivocally stimulate collagen synthesis [16, 276]. One of the longest known and best described factors stimulating type I and III collagen synthesis in fibroblasts, osteoblasts, hepatocytes, and many other cell types is TGF-β [291,351]. Separate chapters are devoted in this volume to the role of growth factors, hormones, and cytokines to cartilage and bone metabolism; therefore, only the key observations on the role of such factors in collagen metabolism are presented. Incubation of cells with TGF-β1 causes enhanced collagen type I mRNA levels not only by stimulating gene transcription but also by enhancing stability and translational activity of collagen mRNA [260]. TGF-β1 also enhances α1(I) mRNA levels in fibroblasts but, curiously, down-regulates mRNA levels in the presence of TGF-β3 [352] (see Table II). In contrast to collagens I and III, TGF-β inhibits expression of the type II collagen promoter–reporter genes [353–356]. Another growth factor that has been shown to enhance collagen V synthesis in gingival fibroblasts is PDGF [357–359], while EGF inhibits collagen type I synthesis in osteoblasts [360]. Further factors that inhibit collagen type I synthesis at both mRNA and protein levels in osteoblasts are vitamin D3 [285, 361–363] and PTH [364]. Also, overexpression of c-fos in

the MC3T3-E1 cell line inhibits α1(I) mRNA levels [363], while v-fos stimulates α1(III) gene expression in NIH3T3 cells [365]. Glucocorticoids generally suppress synthesis of collagens in fibroblasts [366–368], in hepatocytes [369, 370], and in cartilage [371]. In calvarial bone dexamethasone suppresses collagen production in long-term dexamethasone cultures, following an initial phase of stimulation [372, 373]. The effect of glucocorticoids can be complex in the presence of other factors; e.g., it potentiates the stimulatory effect of IGF-I on collagen synthesis [374].

Interleukin 1 (IL-1) increases type I and III collagen mRNA levels in cultures of human chondrocytes [375], probably owing to the presence of dedifferentiated chondrocytes, while it suppresses the α1 (II) mRNA levels [375, 376]. Interferon-γ (IFNγ) and TNFα both suppress type I collagen mRNA levels in fibroblasts [377–380]; IFNγ also reduces type II collagen mRNA levels in chondrocytes [376].

Ascorbic acid is an essential factor in collagen biosynthesis as it is involved in hydroxylation of proline and hydroxyproline [381]. But beyond this role, ascorbic acid has been shown to enhance collagen α2(I) mRNA levels 6-fold and to enhance mRNA stability in chicken tendon fibroblasts [382].

VIII. CONCLUSIONS

In active growth phases of embryonic development, during tissue repair and under certain pathological conditions such as fibrosis or keloid formation, the expression of most collagen genes is highly up-regulated and tissue specifically controlled at transcriptional level by growth factors and hormones, while under inflammatory and necrotic conditions collagen synthesis may be suppressed by cytokines [277]. To ensure tissue homeostasis with a constant collagen pool in the adult organism, a carefully controlled dynamic equilibrium between collagen biosynthesis and degradation is achieved by regulating both anabolic and catabolic pathways at various levels [16].

The collagen protein level in a tissue may be controlled by regulating gene transcription, mRNA translation, and posttranslational level, while collagen turnover can be regulated by controlling protease expression, activation, and inhibition by physiological protease inhibitors.

Despite almost two decades of research on collagen gene regulation, our knowledge of the tissue-specific regulation of collagen gene expression by growth factors, hormones, cytokines, and other physiological factors is still incomplete and relies largely on studies on the influence of various factors on collagen synthesis at mRNA or protein levels in cell or organ cultures. Since the regulation of individual collagen genes *in situ* is complex and multifactorial, conclusions drawn from cell culture studies are necessarily limited but have nevertheless provided valuable information on the potential regulatory mechanism of collagen metabolism.

TABLE II.   Cytokines, Growth Factors, and Oncogenes Modulating Collagen Biosynthesis

Factor	Collagens affected	Cellular targets	Type of response	Reference
TGF-β1	I, III	fibroblasts, hepatoblasts, dediff. chondrocytes, osteoblasts	increased mRNA level and stability enhanced translational activity of α2(I) mRNA (suppression of MMP activity	260; 291; 292; 351–353
	II	chondrocytes	suppression of Col2A1 gene transcription	354–357
	VI	fibroblasts	upregulates α3(VI), downregulates α1(VI) and α2(VI)	333, 334
TGF-β3	α1(I)	fibroblasts	stimulates α1(I) mRNA levels; downregulation in presence of TGF-β1	352
PDGF	collagen V	gingival fibroblasts	stimulation of collagen protein synthesis	358, 359
EGF	I	osteoblasts	inhibits collagen synthesis	360
IL-1	I, III	dediff chondrocytes, fibroblasts	enhanced mRNA levels	375
	II	chondrocytes	suppresses of CO2A1 transcription	376
IFNγ	I	fibroblasts	suppression of collagen synthesis and mRNA levels	377–380
	II	chondrocytes	suppression of α1(II) mRNA levels	377
Vitamin D3	I	osteoblasts	decreases α1(I) mRNA and protein levels	361–363
Glucocorticoids	α1(I)	fibroblasts and others	reduced transcription rate of α1(I), multifactorial complex effects	366–374
PTH	I	fetal rat calvaria	suppression of α1(I) mRNA levels	364
	II	proliferated chondrocytes	enhanced α1(II) mRNA levels	383
	II, X	hypertrophic chondrocytes	reduced mRNA levels	384
Retinoic acid	I, III	chondrocytes	enhanced mRNA level; enhanced transcription	385
	II	chondrocytes	suppression of COL2A1 transcription	386
	X	chondrocytes	transient stimulation of COL10A1 transcription	387
Ascorbate	all collagens	fibroblasts, chondrocytes, osteoblasts etc.	enhanced prolyl- and lysylhydroxylation stimulation of α2(I) mRNA transcription, enhanced mRNA stability	381, 283
v-fos	I, III	NIH3T3 fibroblasts	stimulates α1(III) gene expression	365
c-fos	I	osteoblasts	c-fos overexpression inhibits α1(I) mRNA levels in osteoblasts	363
TNFα	I	fibroblasts	suppression of α1(I) levels	377–379

References

1. Kühn, K. (1986). The collagen family-variations in the molecular and supramolecular structure. *Rheumatology* **10**, 29–69.
2. Mayne, R., and Burgeson, R. E. (1987). Structure and function of collagen types. *In* "Regulation of Matrix Accumulation" (R. P. Mecham, ed.). Academic Press, Orlando, FL.
3. Kielty, C. M., Hopkinson, I., and Grant, M. E. (1993). The collagen family: Structure, assembly and organization in the extracellular matrix. *In* "Connective Tissue and its Heritable Disorders" (P. M. Royce, and B. Steinmann, eds.), pp. 103–147. Wiley-Liss, New York.

4. Mayne, R., and Brewton, R. G. (1993). New members of the collagen superfamily. *Curr. Opin. Cell Biol.* **5**, 883–890.
5. van der Rest, M., Garrone, R., and Herbage, D. (1989). Collagen: A family of proteins with many facets. *In* "Advances in Molecular and Cell Biology" (E. Bittar, and H. Kleinman, eds.), pp. 1–67. JAI Press, Greenwich, CT.
6. van der Rest, M., and Garrone, R. (1991). Collagen family of proteins. *FASEB J.* **5**, 2814–2823.
7. Bruckner, P., and van der Rest, M. (1994). Structure and function of cartilage collagens. *Microsc. Res. Tech.* **28**, 378–384.
8. Hulmes, D. J. (1992). The collagen superfamily—diverse structures and assemblies. *Essays Biochem.* **27**, 49–67.

9. Sandell, L., and Boyd, C. D., eds. (1990). "Extracellular Matrix Genes." Academic Press, San Diego, CA.

10. Ramirez, F., and diLiberto, M. (1990). Complex and diversified regulatory programs control the expression of vertebrate collagen genes. *FASEB J.* **4**, 1616–1623.

11. Kivirikko, K. I. (1998). Collagen biosynthesis: A mini-review cluster. *Matrix Biol.* **16**, 355–356.

12. Nagata, K. (1998). Expression and function of heat shock protein 47: A collagen-specific molecular chaperone in the endoplasmic reticulum. *Matrix Biol.* **16**, 379–386.

13. Prockop, D. J., Sieron, A. L., and Li, S. W. (1998). Procollagen N-proteinase and procollagen C-proteinase. Two unusual metalloproteinases that are essential for procollagen processing probably have important roles in development and cell signaling. *Matrix Biol.* **16**, 399–408.

14. Johnson, L. L., Dyer, R., and Hupe, D. J. (1998). Matrix metalloproteinases. *Curr. Opin. Chem. Biol.* **2**, 466–471.

15. von der Mark, K., and Goodman, S. (1998). Adhesive glycoproteins. *In* "Connective Tissue and its Heritable Disorders" (B. Steinmann, and P. M. Royce, eds.), pp. 211–236. Wiley-Liss, New York.

16. Bateman, J. F., Lamandé, S. R., and Ramskans, J. A. M. (1996). Collagen superfamily. *In* "Extrazellular Matrix" (W. D. Comper, ed.), pp. 22–67. Harwood Academic Publishers, Chur, Switzerland.

17. Myers, J. C., Li, D., Bageris, A., Abraham, V., Dion, A. S., and Amenta, P. S. (1997). Biochemical and immunohistochemical characterization of human type XIX defines a novel class of basement membrane zone collagens. *Am. J. Pathol.* **151**, 1729–1740.

18. Kodama, T., Doi, T., Suzuki, H., Takahashi, K., Wada, Y., and Gordon, S. (1996). Collagenous macrophage scavenger receptors. *Curr. Opin. Lipidol.* **7**, 287–291.

19. Elomaa, O., Sankala, M., Pikkarainen, T., Bergmann, U., Tuuttila, A., Raatikainen-Ahokas, A., Sariola, H., and Tryggvason, K. (1998). Structure of the human macrophage MARCO receptor and characterization of its bacteria-binding region. *J. Biol. Chem.* **273**, 4530–4538.

20. Hagg, R., Hedbom, E., Mollers, U., Aszodi, A., Fassler, R., and Bruckner, P. (1997). Absence of the alpha1(IX) chain leads to a functional knock-out of the entire collagen IX protein in mice. *J. Biol. Chem.* **272**, 20650–20654.

21. Aszodi, A., Chan, D., Hunziker, E., Bateman, J. F., and Fassler, R. (1998). Collagen II is essential for the removal of the notochord and the formation of intervertebral discs. *J. Cell Biol.* **143**, 1399–1412.

22. von der Mark, K., and Glückert, K. (1990). Biochemische und molekularbiologische Aspekte zur Früherfassung humaner Arthrosen. *Orthopaedics*, **19**, 2–15.

23. Timpl, R., and Risteli, L. (1981). *In* "Immunochemistry of the Extracellular Matrix" (H. Furthmayr, ed.), Vol. 1, CRC Press, Boca Raton, FL.

24. Cheah, K. S., Lau, E. T., Au, P. K., and Tam, P. P. (1991). Expression of the mouse alpha 1(II) collagen gene is not restricted to cartilage during development. *Development* **111**, 945–953.

25. Gibson, G. J., and Kielty, C. M. G. S. L. G. E. (1983). Identification and partial characterization of three low-molecular-weight collegenous polypeptides synthesized by chondrocytes cultured within collagen gels in the absence and in the presence of fibronectin. *Biochem. J.* **211**, 417–426.

26. Greenburg, G., and Gospodarowicz, D. (1982). Inactivation of a basement-membrane component responsible for cell-proliferation but not for cell attachment. *Exp. Cell Res.* **140**, 1–14.

27. Li, Y., Lacerda, D. A., Warman, M. L., Beier, D. R., Yoshioka, H., Ninomiya, Y., Oxford, J. T., Morris, N. P., Andrikopoulos, K., and Ramirez, F. (1995). A fibrillar collagen gene, Col11a1, is essential for skeletal morphogenesis. *Cell* **80**, 423–430.

28. Vikkula, M., Mariman, E. C., Lui, V. C., Zhidkova, N. I., Tiller, G. E., Goldring, M. B., van Beersum, S. E., de Waal Malefijt, M. C., van

den Hoogen, F. H., and Ropers, H. H. (1995). Autosomal dominant and recessive osteochondrodysplasias associated with the COL11A2 locus. *Cell* **80**, 431–437.

29. Piez, K. A. (1998). Molecular and aggregate structure of the collagens. *In* "Extracellular Matrix Biochemistry" (K. A. Piez, and H. Reddi, eds). Elsevier, Amsterdam.

30. Traub, W., and Piez, K. A. (1971). The chemistry and structure of collagen. *Adv. Protein Chem.* **25**, 243–352.

31. Hulmes, D. J., and Miller, A. (1981). Molecular packing in collagen. *Nature* **293**, 239–234.

32. Hulmes, D. J., Miller, A., Parry, D. A., Piez, K. A., and Woodhead-Galloway, J. (1973). Analysis of the primary structure of collagen for the origins of molecular packing. *J. Mol. Biol.* **79**, 137–148.

33. Hofmann, H., Fietzek, P. P., and Kuhn, K. (1978). The role of polar and hydrophobic interactions for the molecular packing of type I collagen: A three-dimensional evaluation of the amino acid sequence. *J. Mol. Biol.* **125**, 137–165.

34. Berg, R. A., and Prockop, D. J. (1973). Purification of (14C) protocollagen and its hydroxylation by prolylhydroxylase. *Biochemistry* **12**, 3395–3401.

35. Berg, R. A., and Prockop, D. J. (1973). The thermal transition of a non-hydroxylated form of collagen. Evidence for a role for hydroxyproline in stabilizing the triple-helix of collagen. *Biochem. Biophys. Res. Commun.* **52**, 115–120.

36. Schmid, T. M., and Linsenmayer, T. F. (1984). Denaturation-renaturation properties of two molecular forms of short-chain cartilage collagen. *Biochemistry* **23**, 553–558.

37. Risteli, J., Baechinger, H. P., Engel, J., Furthmayr, H., and Timpl, R. (1980). 7S-collagen: Characterization of an unusual basement membrane structure. *Eur. J. Biochem.* **108**, 239–250.

38. Bruckner, P., and Prockop, D. J. (1981). Proteolytic enzymes as probes for the triple-helical conformation of procollagen. *Anal. Biochem.* **110**, 360–368.

39. Shaw, L. M., and Olsen, B. R. (1991). FACIT collagens: Diverse molecular bridges in extracellular matrices. *Trends Biochem. Sci.* **16**, 191–194.

40. Oh, S. P., Warman, M. L., Seldin, M. F., Cheng, S. D., Knoll, J. H., Timmons, S., and Olsen, B. R. (1994). Cloning of cDNA and genomic DNA encoding human type XVIII collagen and localization of the alpha 1(XVIII) collagen gene to mouse chromosome 10 and human chromosome 21. *Genomics* **19**, 494–499.

41. Yamagata, M., Yamada, K. M., Yamada, S. S., Shinomura, T., Tanaka, H., Nishida, Y., Obara, M., and Kimata, K. (1991). The complete primary structure of type XII collagen shows a chimeric molecule with reiterated fibronectin type III motifs, von Willebrand factor A motifs, a domain homologous to a noncollagenous region of type IX collagen, and short collagenous domains with an Arg-Gly-Asp site. *J. Cell Biol.* **115**, 209–221.

42. Bork, P. (1992). The modular architecture of vertebrate collagens. *FEBS Lett.* **307**, 49–54.

43. Poole, A. R., Pidox, J., Reiner, A., Choi, H., and Rosenberg, L. C. (1984). Association of an extracellular protein (chondrocalcin) with the calcification of cartilage in endochondral bone formation. *J. Cell Biol.* **98**, 54–65.

44. O'Reilly, M. S., Boehm, T., Shing, Y., Fukai, N., Vasios, G., Lane, W. S., Flynn, E., Birkhead, J. R., Olsen, B. R., and Folkman, J. (1997). Endostatin: An endogenous inhibitor of angiogenesis and tumor growth. *Cell* **88**, 277–285.

45. Tromp, G., Kuivaniemi, H., Stacey, A., Shikata, H., Baldwin, C. T., Jaenisch, R., and Prockop, D. J. (1988). Structure of a full-length cDNA clone for the prepro alpha 1(I) chain of human type I procollagen. *Biochem. J.* **253**, 633–640.

46. Kuivaniemi, H., Tromp, G., Chu, M. L., and Prockop, D. J. (1988). Structure of a full-length cDNA clone for the prepro alpha 2(I) chain of

human type I procollagen. Comparison with the chicken gene confirms unusual patterns of gene conservation. *Biochem. J.* **252**, 633–640.

47. Gerstenfeld, L. C., Chipman, S. D., Kelly, C. M., Hodgens, K. J., Lee, D. D., and Landis, W. J. (1988). Collagen expression, ultrastructural assembly, and mineralization in cultures of chicken embryo osteoblasts. *J. Cell Biol.* **106**, 979–989.

48. Kratochowil, K., von der Mark, K., Kollar, E. J., Jaenisch, R., Mooslehner, K., Schwarz, M., Haase, K., Gmacht, I., and Harbers, K. (1992). Retrovirus-induced insertional mutation in mov13 mice affects collagen-I expression in a tissue-specific manner. No Journal Found,

49. von der Mark, K. (1981). Localization of collagen types in tissues. *Int. Rev. Connect. Tissue Res.* **9**, 265–324.

50. Keene, D. R., Sakai, L. Y., Baechinger, H. P., and Burgeson, R. E. (1987). Type III collagen can be present on banded collagen fibrils regardless of fibril diameter. *J. Cell Biol.* **105**, 2393–2402.

51. Fleischmajer, R., MacDonald, E. D., Perlish, J. S., Burgeson, R. E., and Fisher, L. W. (1990). Dermal collagen fibrils are hybrids of type I and type III collagen molecules. *J. Struct. Biol.* **105**, 162–169.

52. von der Mark, K., and Oecalan, M. (1982). Immunofluorescent localization of type V collagen in the chick embryo with monoclonal antibodies. *Collagen Relat. Res.* **2**, 541–555.

53. Niyibizi, C., and Eyre, D. R. (1989). Bone type V collagen: Chain composition and location of a trypsin cleavage site. *Connect. Tissue Res.* **20**, 247–250.

54. Linsenmayer, T. F., Fitch, J. M., Schmid, T. M., Zak, N. B., Gibney, E., Sanderson, R. D., and Mayne, R. (1983). Monoclonal antibodies against chicken type V collagen: Production, specificity, and use for immunocytochemical localization in embryonic cornea and other organs. *J. Cell Biol.* **96**, 124–132.

55. Adachi, E., and Hayashi, T. (1985). In vitro formation of fine fibrils with a D-periodic banding pattern from type V collagen. *Collagen Relat. Res.* **5**, 225–232.

56. Hay, E. D. (1981). Collagen and embryonic development. *In* "Cell Biology of Extracellular Matrix" (E. D. Hay, ed.), pp. 379–409. Plenum, New York.

57. Kleinman, H. K., Rohrbach, D. H., Terranova, V. P., Varner, H. H., Hewitt, T. H., Grotendorst, G. R., Wilkes, C. M., Martin, G. R., Seppae, H., and Shiffmann, E. (1982). Collagenous matrices as determinants of cell function. *In* "Immunochemistry of the Extracellular Matrix" (H. Furthmayr, ed.), Vol. 2, pp. 151–174. CRC Press, Boca Raton, FL.

58. Lee, E. Y., Lee, H. P., Kaetzel, C. S., Parry, G., and Bissell, M. S. (1985). Interaction of mouse mammary epithelial cells with collagen substrata: Regulation of caseni gene expression and secretion. *Proc. Natl. Acad. Sci. U.S.A.* **82**, 1419–1423.

59. Montesano, R., Orci, L., and Vassalli, P. (1983). In vitro rapid organization of endothelial cells into capillary-like networks is promoted by collagen matrices. *J. Cell Biol.* **97**, 1648–1652.

60. Staatz, W. D., Rajpara, S. M., Wayner, E. A., Carter, W. G., and Santoro, S. A. (1989). The membrane glycoprotein Ia-IIa (VLA-2) complex mediates the Mg++-dependent adhesion of platelets to collagen. *J. Cell Biol.* **108**, 1917–1924.

61. Hemler, M. E. (1990). VIa proteins in the integrin family—structures, functions, and their role on leukocytes. *Annu. Rev. Immunol.* **8**, 365–400.

62. Ruoslahti, E. (1991). Integrins. *J. Clin. Invest.* **85**, 1–5.

63. Albelda, S. M., and Buck, C. A. (1990). Integrins and other cell adhesion molecules. *FASEB J.* **4**, 2868–2880.

64. Hynes, R. O. (1992). Integrins: Versatility, modulation, and signaling in cell adhesion. *Cell* **69**, 11–25.

65. Hartung, S., Jaenisch, R., and Breindl, M. (1986). Retrovirus insertion inactivates mouse alpha 1(I) collagen gene by blocking initiation of transcription. *Nature* **320**, 365–367.

66. Jaenisch, R., Harbers, K., Schnieke, A., Lohler, J., Chumakov, I., Jahner, D., Grotkopp, D., and Hoffmann, E. (1983). Germline integration of moloney murine leukemia virus at the Mov13 locus leads to recessive lethal mutation and early embryonic death. *Cell* **32**, 209–216.

67. Schwarz, M., Harbers, K., and Kratochwil, K. (1990). Transcription of a mutant collagen-i gene is a cell type and stage-specific marker for odontoblast and osteoblast differentiation. *Development* **108**, 717–726.

68. Kratochwil, K., Dziadek, M., Lohler, J., Harbers, K., and Jaenisch, R. (1986). Normal epithelial branching morphogenesis in the absence of collagen I. *Dev. Biol.* **117**, 596–606.

69. Miller, E. J. (1971). Isolation and characterization of a collagen from chick cartilage containing three identical alpha chains. *Biochemistry* **10**, 1652–1659.

70. Trelstad, R. L., Kang, A. H., Igarashi, S., and Gross, J. (1970). Isolation of two distinct collagens from chick cartilage. *Biochemistry* **9**, 4993–4998.

71. Mayne, R., and von der Mark, K. (1983). Collagens of cartilage. *In* "The Biochemistry of Cartilage," Vol. 1, pp. 181–214. Academic Press, New York.

72. Ryan, M. C., and Sandell, L. J. (1990). Differential expression of a cysteine-rich domain in the amino-terminal propeptide of type II procollagen by alternative splicing of messenger-RNA. *J. Biol. Chem.* **265**, 10334–10339.

73. Sandell, L. J., Nalin, A. M., and Reife, R. A. (1994). Alternative splice form of type II procollagen mRNA (IIA) is predominant in skeletal precursors and non-cartilaginous tissues during early mouse development. *Dev. Dyn.* **199**, 129–140.

74. Sandell, L. J., Morris, N., Robbins, J. R., and Goldring, M. B. (1991). Alternatively spliced type II procollagen mRNAs define distinct populations of cells during vertebral development: Differential expression of the amino-propeptide. *J. Cell Biol.* **114**, 1307–1319.

75. Madsen, K., von der Mark, K., van Menxel, M., and Friberg, U. (1984). Analysis of collagen types synthesized by rabbit ear cartilage chondrocytes in vivo and in vitro. *Biochem. J.* **221**, 189–196.

76. Trelstad, R. L., and Kang, A. H. (1974). Collagen heterogeneity in the avian eye: Lens, vitreous body, cornea and sclera. *Exp. Eye Res.* **18**, 395–406.

77. Newsome, D. A., Linsenmayer, T. F., and Trelstad, R. L. (1976). Vitreous body collagen. Evidence for a dual origin from the neural retina and hyalocytes. *J. Cell Biol.* **71**, 59–67.

78. Linsenmayer, T. F., Trelstad, R. L., and Gross, J. (1973). The collagen of chick embryonic notochord. *Biochem. Biophys. Res. Commun.* **53**, 39–45.

79. von der Mark, K., von der Mark, H., Timpl, R., and Trelstad, R. L. (1977). Immunofluorescent localization of collagen type-1, type-2 and type-3 in embryonic chick eye. *Dev. Biol.* **59**, 75–85.

80. Linsenmayer, T. F., Smith, G. N., and Hay, E. D. (1977). Synthesis of 2 collagen types by embryonic chick corneal epithelium in vitro. *Proc. Natl. Acad. Sci. U.S.A.* **74**, 39–43.

81. Thorogood, P., Bee, J., and von der Mark, K. (1986). Transient expression of collagen type II at epitheliomesenchymal interfaces during morphogenesis of the cartilaginous neurocranium. *Dev. Biol.* **116**, 497–509.

82. Wood, A., Ashhurst, D. E., Corbett, A., and Thorogood, P. (1991). The transient expression of type II collagen at tissue interfaces during mammalian craniofacial development. *Development* **111**, 955–968.

83. Stuart, J. M., Watson, W. C., and Kang, A. H. (1988). Collagen autoimmunity and arthritis. *FASEB J.* **2**, 2950–2956.

84. Holmdahl, R., Malmstrom, V., and Vuorio, E. (1993). Autoimmune recognition of cartilage collagens. *Ann. Med.* **25**, 251–264.

85. Holmdahl, R., Andersson, M., Goldschmidt, T. J., Gustafsson, K., Jansson, L., and Mo, J. A. (1990). Type II collagen autoimmunity

in animals and provocations leading to arthritis. *Immunol. Rev.* **118**, 193–232.

86. Andersson, M., Cremer, M. A., Terato, K., Burkhardt, H., and Holmdahl, R. (1991). Analysis of type II collagen reactive T cells in the mouse. II. Different localization of immunodominant T cell epitopes on heterologous and autologous type II collagen. *Scand. J. Immunol.* **33**, 505–510.

87. Watson, W. C., Cremer, M. A., Wooley, P. H., and Townes, A. S. (1986). Assessment of the potential pathogenicity of type II collagen autoantibodies in patients with rheumatoid arthritis. Evidence of restricted IgG3 subclass expression and activation of complement C5 to C5a. *Arthritis Rheum.* **29**, 1316–1321.

88. Fertala, A., Holmes, D. F., Kadler, K. E., Sieron, A. L., and Prockop, D. J. (1996). Assembly in vitro of thin and thick fibrils of collagen II from recombinant procollagen II. The monomers in the tips of thick fibrils have the opposite orientation from monomers in the growing tips of collagen I fibrils. *J. Biol. Chem.* **271**, 14864–14869.

89. Vaughan, L., Winterhalter, K. H., and Bruckner, P. (1985). Proteoglycan Lt from chicken embryo sternum identified as type IX collagen. *J. Biol. Chem.* **260**, 4758–4763.

90. Mendler, M., Eich-Bender, S. G., Vaughan, L., Winterhalter, K. H., and Bruckner, P. (1989). Cartilage contains mixed fibrils of collagen types II, IX and XI. *J. Cell Biol.* **108**, 191–197.

91. Chung, E., and Miller, E. J. (1974). Collagen polymorphism: Characterization of molecules with the chain composition (alpha 1 (3)03 in human tissues. *Science* **183**, 1200–1201.

92. Epstein, E. H., Jr. (1974). (Alpha 1(3))3 human skin collagen. Release by pepsin digestion and preponderance in fetal life. *J. Biol. Chem.* **249**, 3225–3231.

93. Miller, E. J., Epstein, E. H., Jr., and Piez, K. A. (1971). Identification of three genetically distinct collagens by cyanogen bromide cleavage of insoluble human skin and cartilage collagen. *Biochem. Biophys. Res. Commun.* **42**, 1024–1029.

94. Conrad, G. W., Dessau, W., and von der Mark, K. (1980). Synthesis of type-III collagen by fibroblasts from the embryonic chick cornea. *J. Cell Biol.* **84**, 501–512.

95. Nowack, H., Olsen, B. R., and Timpl, R. (1976). Characterization of the amino-terminal segment in type III procollagen. *Eur. J. Biochem.* **70**, 205–216.

96. Nowack, H., Rohde, H., and Timpl, R. (1976). Isolation of a procollagen peptide from amniotic fluid. *Hoppe-Seyler's Z. Physiol. Chem.* **357**, 601–604.

97. Paakko, P., Sormunen, R., Risteli, L., Risteli, J., Ala-Kokko, L., and Ryhanen, L. (1989). Malotilate prevents accumulation of type III pN-collagen, type IV collagen, and laminin in carbon tetrachloride-induced pulmonary fibrosis in rats. *Am. Rev. Respir. Dis.* **139**, 1105–1111.

98. Burgeson, R. E., El Adli, F. A., Kaitila, I. I., and Hollister, D. W. (1976). Fetal membrane collagens: Identification of two new collagen alpha chains. *Proc. Natl. Acad. Sci. U.S.A.* **73**, 2579–2583.

99. Burgeson, R. E., and Hollister, D. W. (1979). Collagen heterogeneity in human cartilage: Identification of several new collagen chains. *Biochem. Biophys. Res. Commun.* **87**, 1124–1131.

100. Fessler, L., Robinson, W. J., and Fessler, J. H. (1981). Biosynthesis of procollagen [pro α1(V)]$_2$ pro α2(V) by chick tendon fibroblasts and procollagen [pro α1(V)]$_3$ by hamster lung cell cultures. *J. Biol. Chem.* **256**, 9646–9651.

101. Fessler, J. H., Shigaki, N., and Fessler, L. I. (1985). Biosynthesis and properties of procollagens V. *Ann. N. Y. Acad. Sci.* **460**, 181–186.

102. Burgeson, R. E., Hebda, P. A., Morris, N. A., and Hollister, D. W. (1982). Human cartilage collagens. *J. Biol. Chem.* **257**, 7852–7856.

103. Reese, C. A., and Mayne, R. (1981). Minor collagens of chicken hyaline cartilage. *Biochemistry* **20**, 5443–5448.

104. von der Mark, K., van Menxel, M., and Wiedemann, H. (1982).

105. Eyre, D., and Wu, J.-J. (1987). Type XI or 1alpha, 2alpha, 3alpha collagen. *In* "Stucture and Function of Collagen Types" (R. Mayne and R. E. Burgeson, eds.), pp. 261–281. Academic Press, Orlando, FL.

106. Fessler, L. I., Kumamoto, C. A., Meis, M. E., and Fessler, J. H. (1981). Assembly and processing of procollagen V (AB) in chick blood vessels and other tissues. *J. Biol. Chem.* **256**, 9640–9645.

107. Fessler, L. I., Shigaki, N., and Fessler, J. H. (1985). Isolation of a new procollagen V chain from chick embryo tendon. *J. Biol. Chem.* **260**, 13286–13293.

108. Davies, G. B., Oxford, J. T., Hausafus, L. C., Smoody, B. F., and Morris, N. P. (1998). Temporal and spatial expression of alternative splice-forms of the alpha1 (XI) collagen gene in fetal rat cartilage. *Dev. Dyn.* **213**, 12–26.

109. Lui, V. C. H., Ng, L. J., Sat, E. W. Y., Nicholls, J., and Cheah, K. S. E. (1996). Extensive alternative splicing within the amino-propeptide coding domain of alpha2(XI) procollagen mRNAs. Expression of transcripts encoding truncated pro-alpha chains. *J. Biol. Chem.* **271**, 16945–16951.

110. Tsumaki, N., and Kimura, T. (1995). Differential expression of an acidic domain in the amino-terminal propeptide of mouse pro-alpha 2(XI) collagen by complex alternative splicing. *J. Biol. Chem.* **270**, 2372–2378.

111. Fessler, L. I., Brosh, S., Chapin, S., and Fessler, J. H. (1986). Tyrosine sulfation in precursors of collagen V. *J. Biol. Chem.* **261**, 5034–5040.

112. Neame, P.J., Young, C. N., and Treep, J. T. (1990). Isolation and primary structure of PARP, a 24-kDa proline- and arginine- rich protein from bovine cartilage closely related to the NH2-terminal domain in collagen alpha 1 (XI). *J. Biol. Chem.* **265**, 20401–20408.

113. Zhidkova, N. I., Brewton, R. G., and Mayne, R. (1993). Molecular cloning of PARP (proline/arginine-rich protein) from human cartilage and subsequent demonstration that PARP is a fragment of the NH2-terminal domain of the collagen alpha 2(XI) chain. *FEBS Lett.* **326**, 25–28.

114. Niyibizi, C., Chan, R., Wu, J. J., and Eyre, D. (1994). A 92 kDa gelatinase (MMP-9) cleavage site in native type V collagen. *Biochem. Biophys. Res. Commun.* **202**, 328–333.

115. Wu, J. J., Lark, M. W., Chun, L. E., and Eyre, D. R. (1991). Sites of stromelysin cleavage in collagen types II, IX, X, and XI of cartilage. *J. Biol. Chem.* **266**, 5625–5628.

116. Haralson, M. A., Mitchell, W. M., Rhodes, R. K., Kresina, T. F., Gay, R., and Miller, E. J. (1980). Chinese hamster lung cells synthesize and confine to the cellular domain a collagen composed solely of B chains. *Proc. Natl. Acad. Sci. U.S.A.* **77**, 5206–5210.

117. Eyre, D. R., Wu, J.-J., and Apon, S. (1987). A growing family of collagens in articular cartilage: Identification of 5 genetically distinct types. *J. Rheumatol.* **14**, 25–27.

118. Niyibizi, C., and Eyre, D. R. (1989). Identification of the cartilage alpha 1(XI) chain in type V collagen from bovine bone. *FEBS Lett.* **242**, 314–318.

119. Mayne, R., Brewton, R. G., Mayne, P. M., and Baker, J. R. (1993). Isolation and characterization of the chains of type V/type XI collagen present in bovine vitreous. *J. Biol. Chem.* **268**, 9381–9386.

120. Birk, D. E., Fitch, J. M., Babiarz, J. P., and Linsenmayer, T. F. (1988). Collagen type I and type V are present in the same fibril in the avian corneal stroma. *J. Cell Biol.* **106**, 999–1008.

121. Hay, E. D., and Revel, J. P. (1969). Fine structure of the developing avian cornea. *Monogr. Dev. Biol.* **1**, 1–144.

122. Shimokomaki, M., Duance, V. C., and Bailey, A. J. (1980). Identification of a new disulphide bonded collagen from cartilage. *FEBS Lett.* **121**, 51–54.

123. Ayad, S., Abedin, M. Z., and Grundy, S. M. (1981). Isolation and

Isolation and characterization of new collagens from chick cartilage. *Eur. J. Biochem.* **124**, 57–62.

characterization of an usual collagen from hyaline cartilage and intervertebral disc. *FEBS Lett.* **123**, 195–199.

124. Ninomiya, Y., and Olsen, B. R. (1984). Synthesis and characterization of cDNA encoding a cartilage-specific short collagen. *Proc. Natl. Acad. Sci. U.S.A.* **81**, 3014–3018.

125. van der Rest, M., Mayne, R., Ninomiya, Y., Seidah, N. G., Chrétien, M., and Olsen, B. R. (1985). The structure of type IX collagen. *J. Biol. Chem.* **260**, 220–225.

126. Mayne, R. (1989). Cartilage collagens—what is their function, and are they involved in articular disease. *Arthritis Rheum.* **32**, 241–246.

127. Vaughan, L., Mendler, M., Huber, S., Bruckner, P., Winterhalter, K. H., Irwin, M. I., and Mayne, R. (1988). D-periodic distribution of collagen type IX along cartilage fibrils. *J. Cell Biol.* **106**, 998–997.

128. van der Rest, M., and Mayne, R. (1988). Type IX collagen proteoglycan from cartilage is covalently cross-linked to type II collagen. *J. Biol. Chem.* **263**, 1615–1618.

129. Noro, A., Kimata, K., Oike, Y., Shinomura, T., Maeda, N., Yano, S., Takahashi, N., and Suzuki, S. (1983). Isolation and characterization of a third proteoglycan (PG-Lt) from chick embryo cartilage which contains disulfide-bonded collagenous polypeptide. *J. Biol. Chem.* **258**, 9323–9331.

130. Huber, S., Winterhalter, K. H., and Vaughan, L. (1988). Isolation and sequence-analysis of the glycosaminoglycan attachment site of type-IX collagen. *J. Biol. Chem.* **263**, 752–756.

131. Brewton, R. G., Wright, D. W., and Mayne, R. (1991). Structural and functional comparison of type IX collagen-proteoglycan from chicken cartilage and vitreous humor. *J. Biol. Chem.* **266**, 4752–4757.

132. Nishimura, I., and Muragaki, Y. (1989). Tissue-specific forms of type IX collagen-proteoglycan arise from the use of two widely separated promoters. *J. Biol. Chem.* **264**, 20033–20041.

133. Muragaki, Y., Nishimura, I., Henney, A., Ninomiya, Y., and Olsen, B. R. (1990). The alpha 1(IX) collagen gene gives rise to two different transcripts in both mouse embryonic and human fetal RNA. *Proc. Natl. Acad. Sci. U.S.A.* **87**, 2400–2404.

134. Fassler, R., Schnegelsberg, P. N., Dausman, J., Shinya, T., Muragaki, Y., McCarthy, M. T., Olsen, B. R., and Jaenisch, R. (1994). Mice lacking a1(IX) collagen develop non-inflammatory degenerative joint disease. *Proc. Natl. Acad. Sci. U.S.A.* **91**, 5070–5074.

135. Gordon, M. K., Gerecke, D. R., and Olsen, B. R. (1987). Type XII collagen: Distinct extracellular matrix component discovered by cRNA cloning. *Proc. Natl. Acad. Sci. U.S.A.* **84**, 6040–6044.

136. Dublet, B., Oh, S., Sugrue, S. P., Gordon, M. K., Gerecke, D. R., Olsen, D. R., and van der Rest, M. (1989). The structure of avian type-XII collagen—alpha-1 (XII) chains contain 190-kda non-triple helical amino-terminal domains and form homotrimeric molecules. *J. Biol. Chem.* **264**, 13150–13156.

137. Gordon, M. K., Castagnola, P., Dublet, B., Linsenmayer, T. F., van der Rest, M., Mayne, R., and Olsen, B. R. (1991). Cloning of a cDNA for a new member of the class of fibril-associated collagens with interrupted triple helices. *Eur. J. Biochem.* **201**, 333–338.

138. Lunstrum, G. P., Morris, N. P., McDonough, A. M., Keene, D. R., and Burgeson, R. E. (1991). Identification and partial characterization of two type XII-like collagen molecules. *J. Cell Biol.* **113**, 963–969.

139. Keene, D. R., Lunstrum, G. P., Morris, N. P., Stoddard, D. W., and Burgeson, R. E. (1991). Two type XII-like collagens localize to the surface of banded collagen fibrils. *J. Cell Biol.* **113**, 971–978.

140. Gerecke, D. R., Olson, P. F., Koch, M., Knoll, J. H., Taylor, R., Hudson, D. L., Champliaud, M. F., Olsen, B. R., and Burgeson, R. E. (1997). Complete primary structure of two splice variants of collagen XII, and assignment of alpha 1(XII) collagen (COL12A1), alpha 1(IX) collagen (COL9A1), and alpha 1(XIX) collagen (COL19A1) to human chromosome 6q12- q13. *Genomics* **41**, 236–242.

141. Dublet, B., and van der Rest, M. (1991). Type XIV collagen, a new homotrimeric molecule extracted from bovine skin and tendon, with a triple helical disulfide-bonded domain homologous to type IX and type XII collagens. *J. Biol. Chem.* **266**, 6853–6858.

142. Brown, J. C., Mann, K., Wiedemann, H., and Timpl, R. (1993). Structure and binding properties of collagen type XIV isolated from human placenta. *J. Cell Biol.* **120**, 557–567.

143. Aubert-Foucher, E., Font, B., Eichenberger, D., Goldschmidt, D., Lethias, C., and van der Rest, M. (1992). Purification and characterization of native type XIV collagen. *J. Biol. Chem.* **267**, 15759–15764.

144. Walchli, C., Trueb, J., Kessler, B., Winterhalter, K. H., and Trueb, B. (1993). Complete primary structure of chicken collagen XIV. *Eur. J. Biochem.* **212**, 483–490.

145. Schuppan, D., Cantaluppi, M. C., Becker, J., Veit, A., Bunte, T., Troyer, D., Schuppan, F., Schmid, M., Ackermann, R., and Hahn, E. G. (1990). Undulin, an extracellular matrix glycoprotein associated with collagen fibrils. *J. Biol. Chem.* **265**, 8823–8832.

146. Walchli, C., Koch, M., Chiquet, M., Odermatt, B. F., and Trueb, B. (1994). Tissue-specific expression of the fibril-associated collagens XII and XIV. *J. Cell Sci.* **107**, 669–681.

147. Ehnis, T., Dieterich, W., Bauer, M., Kresse, H., and Schuppan, D. (1997). Localization of a binding site for the proteoglycan decorin on collagen XIV (undulin). *J. Biol. Chem.* **272**, 20414–20419.

148. Font, B., Aubert-Foucher, E., Goldschmidt, D., Eichenberger, D., and van der Rest, M. (1993). Binding of collagen XIV with the dermatan sulfate side chain of decorin. *J. Biol. Chem.* **268**, 25015–25018.

149. Berthod, F., Germain, L., Guignard, R., Lethias, C., Garrone, R., Damour, O., van der Rest, M., and Auger, F. A. (1997). Differential expression of collagens XII and XIV in human skin and in reconstructed skin. *J. Invest. Dermatol.* **108**, 737–742.

150. Watt, S. L., Lunstrum, G. P., McDonough, A. M., Keene, D. R., Burgeson, R. E., and Morris, N. P. (1992). Characterization of collagen types XII and XIV from fetal bovine cartilage. *J. Biol. Chem.* **267**, 20093–20099.

151. von der Mark, H., Aumailley, M., Wick, G., Fleischmajer, R., and Timpl, R. (1984). Immunochemistry, genuine size and tissue localization of collagen VI. *Eur. J. Biochem.* **142**, 493–502.

152. Timpl, R., and Engel, J. (1987). Type VI collagen. *In* "Structure and Function of Collagen Types" (R. Mayne and R. E. Burgeson, eds.), pp. 105–143. Academic Press, Orlando, FL.

153. Chung, E., Rhodes, R. K., and Miller, E. J. (1976). Isolation of three collagenous components of probable basement membrane origin from several tissues. *Biochem. Biophys. Res. Commun.* **71**, 1167–1174.

154. Jander, R., Rauterberg, J., and Glanville, R. W. (1983). Further characterization of the three polypeptide chains of bovine and human short-chain collagen (intima collagen). *Eur. J. Biochem.* **133**, 39–46.

155. Chu, M.-L., Pan, T., Conway, D., Kuo, H.-J., Glanville, R. W., Timpl, R., Mann, K., and Deutzmann, R. (1989). Sequence analysis of alpha 1(VI) and alpha 2(VI) chains of human type VI collagen reveals internal triplication of globular domains similar to the A domains of von Willebrand factor and two alpha2(VI) chain variants that differ in the carboxy terminus. *EMBO J.* **8**, 1939–1946.

156. Chu, M. L., Pan, T. C., Conway, D., Kuo, H. J., Glanville, R. W., Timpl, R., Mann, K., and Deutzmann, R. (1989). Sequence analysis of alpha 1(VI) and alpha 2(VI) chains of human type VI collagen reveals internal triplication of globular domains similar to the A domains of von Willebrand factor and two alpha 2(VI) chain variants that differ in the carboxy terminus. *EMBO J.* **8**, 1939–1946.

157. Koller, E., Winterhalter, K. H., and Trueb, B. (1989). The globular domains of type VI collagen are related to the collagen-binding domains of cartilage matrix protein and von Willebrand factor. *EMBO J.* **8**, 1073–1077.

158. Bonaldo, P., Russo, V., Bucciotti, F., Bressan, G. M., and Colombatti, A. (1989). Alpha 1 chain of chick type VI collagen. The complete cDNA sequence reveals a hybrid molecule made of one short collagen

and three von Willebrand factor type A-like domains. *J. Biol. Chem.* **264**, 5575–5580.

159. Bonaldo, P., and Colombatti, A. (1989). The carboxyl terminus of the chicken alpha3 chain of collagen VI is a unique mosaic structure with glycoprotein lb-like, fibronectin type III, and Kunitz modules. *J. Biol. Chem.* **264**, 20235–20239.

160. Stokes, D. G., Saitta, B., Timpl, R., and Chu, M. L. (1991). Human alpha 3(VI) collagen gene. Characterization of exons coding for the amino-terminal globular domain and alternative splicing in normal and tumor cells. *J. Biol. Chem.* **266**, 8626–8633.

161. Burg, M. A., Tillet, E., Timpl, R., and Stallcup, W. B. (1996). Binding of the NG2 proteoglycan to type VI collagen and other extracellular matrix molecules. *J. Biol. Chem.* **271**, 26110–26116.

162. Bidanset, D. J., Guidry, C., Rosenberg, L. C., Choi, H. U., Timpl, R., and Hook, M. (1992). Binding of the proteoglycan decorin to collagen type VI. *J. Biol. Chem.* **267**, 5250–5256.

163. Specks, U., Mayer, U., Nischt, R., Spissinger, T., Mann, K., Timpl, R., Engel, J., and Chu, M. L. (1992). Structure of recombinant N-terminal globule of type VI collagen alpha 3 chain and its binding to heparin and hyaluronan. *EMBO J.* **11**, 4281–4290.

164. Lamande, S. R., Sigalas, E., Pan, T. C., Chu, M. L., Dziadek, M., Timpl, R., and Bateman, J. F. (1998). The role of the alpha3(VI) chain in collagen VI assembly. Expression of an alpha3(VI) chain lacking N-terminal modules N10-N7 restores collagen VI assembly, secretion, and matrix deposition in an alpha3(VI)-deficient cell line. *J. Biol. Chem.* **273**, 7423–7430.

165. Bruns, R. R., Press, W., Engvall, E. T., and Gross, J. (1986). Type VI collagen in extracellular, 100-nm periodic filaments and fibrils: Identification by immunoelectron microscopy. *J. Cell Biol.* **103**, 393–404.

166. Furthmayr, H., Wiedemann, H., Timpl, R., Odermatt, E., and Engel, J. (1983). Electron-microscopical approach to a structural model of intima collagen. *Biochem. J.* **211**, 303–311.

167. Keene, D. R., and Engvall, E. G. W. (1988). Ultrastructure of type VI collagen in human skin and cartilage suggests an anchoring function for this filamentous network. *J. Cell Biol.* **107**, 1995–2006.

168. Ayad, S., Evans, H., Weiss, J. B., and Holt, L. (1984). Type VI collagen but not type V collagen is present in cartilage. *Collagen Relat. Res.* **4**, 165–168.

169. Swoboda, B., Pullig, O., Kirsch, T., Kladny, B., Steinhauser, B., and Weseloh, G. (1998). Increased content of type-VI collagen epitopes in human osteoarthritic cartilage: Quantitation by inhibition ELISA. *J. Orthop. Res.* **16**, 96–99.

170. Schmid, T. M., and Conrad, H. E. (1982). A unique ow-molecular weight collagen secreted by cultured chick-embryo chondrocytes. *J. Biol. Chem.* **257**, 2444–2450.

171. Schmid, T. M., and Linsenmayer, T. F. (1985). Developmental acquisition of type X collagen in the embryonic chick tibiotarsus. *Dev. Biol.* **107**, 373–381.

172. Gibson, G. J., Schor, S. L., and Grant, M. E. (1982). The identification of a new cartilage collagen synthesized by chondrocytes cultured within collagen gels. *Connect. Tissue Res.* **9**, 207–208.

173. Capasso, O., Quarto, N., Descalci-Cancedda, F., and Cancedda, R. (1984). The low molecular weight collagen synthesized by chick tibial chondrocytes is deposited in the matrix both in culture and in vivo. *EMBO J.* **3**, 823–827.

174. Remington, M. C., Bashey, R. I., Brighton, C. T., and Jimenez, S. A. (1984). Biosynthesis of a disulphide bounded short-chain collagen by calf growth plate cartilage. *Biochem. J.* **224**, 227–233.

175. Schmid, T. M., and Linsenmayer, T. F. (1987). Type X collagen. *In* "Structure and Function of Collagen Types" (R. Mayne and R. E. Burgeson eds.), pp. 223–259. Academic Press, Orlando, FL.

176. Schmid, T. M., Cole, A. A., Chen, Q., Bonen, D. K., Luchene, L., and Linsenmayer, T. (1994). Assembly of type X collagen by hypertrophic chondrocytes. *In* "Extracellular Matrix Assembly and Structure" (P., Yurchenco, D. Birk, and R. Mecham, eds.), pp. 171–206. Academic Press, San Diego, CA.

177. von der Mark, K., Kirsch, T., Nerlich, A. G., Kub, A., Weseloh, G., Glückert, K., and Stöb, H. (1992). Type X collagen synthesis in human osteoarthritic cartilage: Indication of chondrocyte hypertrophy. *Arthritis Rheum.* **35**, 806–811.

178. Aigner, T., Reichenberger, E., Bertling, W., Kirsch, T., Stöb, H., and von der Mark, K. (1993). Type X collagen expression in osteoarthritic and rheumatoid articular cartilage. *Virchows Arch.* **63**, 205–211.

179. Girkontaite, J., Frischholz, S., Lammi, P., Wagner, K., Swoboda, B., Aigner, T., and von der Mark, K. (1996). Immunolocalization of type X collagen in normal fetal and adult osteoarthritic cartilage with monoclonal antibodies. *Matrix Biol.* **15**, 231–238.

180. Walker, G. D., Fischer, M., Gannon, J., Thompson, R. C., and Oegama, T. R. (1995). Expression of type X collagen in osteoarthritis. *J. Orthop. Res.* **13**, 4–12.

181. Luvalle, P., Ninomiya, Y., and Rosenblum, N. D. (1988). The type X collagen gene. *J. Biol. Chem.* **263**, 18378–18385.

182. Yamaguchi, N., Mayne, R., and Ninomiya, Y. (1991). The alpha 1 (VIII) collagen gene is homologous to the alpha 1 (X) collagen gene and contains a large exon encoding the entire triple helical and carboxyl-terminal non-triple helical domains of the alpha 1 (VIII) polypeptide. *J. Biol. Chem.* **266**, 4508–4513.

183. Sawada, H., Konomi, H., and Hirosawa, K. (1990). Characterization of the collagen in the hexagonal lattice of Descemet's membrane: Its relation to type VIII collagen. *J. Cell Biol.* **110**, 219–227.

184. Kwan, A. P. L., Cummings, C. E., Chapman, J. A., and Grant, M. E. (1991). Macromolecular organization of chicken type X collagen in vitro. *J. Cell Biol.* **114**, 597–605.

185. Brass, A., Kadler, K. E., Thomas, J. T., Grant, M. E., and Boot-Handford, R. P. (1992). The fibrillar collagens, collagen VIII, collagen X and the C1q complement proteins share a similar domain in their C-terminal non-collagenous regions. *FEBS Lett.* **303**, 126–128.

186. Warman, M. L., Abbott, M., Apte, S. S., Hefferon, T., McIntosh, I., Cohn, D. H., Hecht, J. T., Olsen, B. R., and Francomano, C. A. (1993). A type X collagen mutation causes Schmid metaphyseal chondrodysplasia. *Nat. Genet.* **5**, 79–82.

187. Wallis, G. A., Rash, B., Sweetman, W. A., Thomas, J. T., Super, M., Evans, G., Grant, M. E., and Boot-Handford, R. P. (1994). Amino acid substitutions of conserved residues in the carboxyl-terminal domain of a1(X) chain of type x collagen occur in two unrelated families with metaphyseal chondrodysplasia type Schmid. *Am. J. Hum. Genet.* **54**, 169–178.

188. Bonaventure, J., Chaminade, F., and Maroteaux, P. (1995). Mutations in three subdomains of the carboxy-terminal region of collagen type X account for most of the Schmid metaphyseal dysplasias. *Hum. Genet.* **96**, 58–64.

189. Chan, D., and Jacenko, O. (1998). Phenotypic and biochemical consequences of collagen X mutations in mice and humans. *Matrix Biol.* **17**, 169–184.

190. Chan, D., Weng, Y. M., Graham, H. K., Sillence, D. O., and Bateman, J. F. (1998). A nonsense mutation in the carboxyl-terminal domain of type X collagen causes haploinsufficiency in schmid metaphyseal chondrodysplasia. *J. Clin. Invest.* **101**, 1490–1499.

191. Chan, D., Weng, Y. M., Hocking, A. M., Golub, S., McQuillan, D. J., and Bateman, J. F. (1996). Site-directed mutagenesis of human type X collagen. Expression of alpha 1(X) NC1, NC2, and helical mutations in vitro and in transfected cells. *J. Biol. Chem.* **271**, 13566–13572.

192. Chan, D., Cole, W. G., Rogers, J. G., and Bateman, J. F. (1995). Type X collagen multimer assembly in vitro is prevented by a Gly618 to Val mutation in the alpha 1(X) NC1 domain resulting in Schmid metaphyseal chondrodysplasia. *J. Biol. Chem.* **270**, 4558–4562.

193. Jacenko, O., LuValle, P. A., and Olsen, B. R. (1993). Spondylometaphyseal dysplasia in mice carrying a dominant negative mutation in

a matrix protein specific for cartilage to bone transition. *Nature* **365**, 56–61.

194. Rosati, R., Horan, G. S., Pinero, G. J., Garofalo, S., Keene, D. R., Horton, W. A., Vuorio, E., deCrombrugghe, B., and Behringer, R.R. (1994). Normal long bone growth and development in type X collagen-null mice. *Nat. Genet.* **8**, 129–135.

195. Kwan, K. M., Pang, M. K., Zhou, S., Cowan, S. K., Kong, R. Y., Pfordte, T., Olsen, B. R., Sillence, D. O., Tam, P. P., and Cheah, K. S. (1997). Abnormal compartmentalization of cartilage matrix components in mice lacking collagen X: Implications for function. *J. Cell Biol.* **136**, 459–471.

196. Hagg, P. M., Horelli-Kuitunen, N., Eklund, L., Palotie, A., and Pihlajaniemi, T. (1997). Cloning of mouse type XV collagen sequences and mapping of the corresponding gene to 4B1-3. Comparison of mouse and human alpha 1 (XV) collagen sequences indicates divergence in the number of small collagenous domains. *Genomics* **45**, 31–41.

197. Rehn, M., and Pihlajaniemi, T. (1994). Alpha 1(XVIII), a collagen chain with frequent interruptions in the collagenous sequence, a distinct tissue distribution, and homology with type XV collagen. *Proc. Natl. Acad. Sci. U.S.A.* **91**, 4234–4238.

198. Oh, S. P., Kamagata, Y., Muragaki, Y., Timmons, S., Ooshima, A., and Olsen, B. R. (1994). Isolation and sequencing of cDNAs for proteins with multiple domains of Gly-Xaa-Yaa repeats identify a distinct family of collagenous proteins. *Proc. Natl. Acad. Sci. U.S.A.* **91**, 4229–4233.

199. Burgeson, R. E. (1988). New collagens, new concepts. *Annu. Rev. Cell Biol.* **4**, 551–577.

200. Sasaki, T., Fukai, N., Mann, K., Gohring, W., Olsen, B. R., and Timpl, R. (1998). Structure, function and tissue forms of the C-terminal globular domain of collagen XVIII containing the angiogenesis inhibitor endostatin. *EMBO J.* **17**, 4249–4256.

201. Hagg, P., Rehn, M., Huhtala, P., Vaisanen, T., Tamminen, M., and Pihlajaniemi, T. (1998). Type XIII collagen is identified as a plasma membrane protein. *J. Biol. Chem.* **273**, 15590–15597.

202. Swann, D. A., and Sotsman, S. (1980). Chemical composition of bovine vitreous humor collagen fibers. *Biochem. J.* **185**, 545–554.

203. Li, K., Tamai, K., Tan, E. M., and Uitto, J. (1993). Cloning of type XVII collagen. Complementary and genomic DNA sequences of mouse 180-kilodalton bullous pemphigoid antigen (BPAG2) predict an interrupted collagenous domain, a transmembrane segment, and unusual features in the 5′-end of the gene and the 3′-untranslated region of the mRNA. *J. Biol. Chem.* **268**, 8825–8834.

204. Gatalica, B., Pulkkinen, L., Li, K., Kuokkanen, K., Ryynanen, M., McGrath, J. A., and Uitto, J. (1997). Cloning of the human type XVII collagen gene (COL17A1), and detection of novel mutations in generalized atrophic benign epidermolysis bullosa. *Am. J. Hum. Genet.* **60**, 352–365.

205. Chavanas, S., Gache, Y., Tadini, G., Pulkkinen, L., Uitto, J., Ortonne, J. P., and Meneguzzi, G. (1997). A homozygous in-frame deletion in the collagenous domain of bullous pemphigoid antigen BP180 (type XVII collagen) causes generalized atrophic benign epidermolysis bullosa. *J. Invest. Dermatol.* **109**, 74–78; errata: *Ibid.*, No. 4, p. 613.

206. Ryan, M. C., Sieraski, M., and Sandell, L. J.(1990). The human type II procollagen gene: Identification of an additional protein-coding domain and location of potential regulatory sequences in the promoter and first intron. *Genomics* **8**, 41–48.

207. Saitta, B., Stokes, D. G., Vissing, H., Timpl, R., and Chu, M. L. (1990). Alternative splicing of the human alpha 2(VI) collagen gene generates multiple mRNA transcripts which predict three protein variants with distinct carboxyl termini. *J. Biol. Chem.* **265**, 6473–6480.

208. Lunstrum, G. P., McDonough, A. M., Marinkovich, M. P., Keene, D. R., Morris, N. P., and Burgeson, R. E. (1992). Identification and partial purification of a large, variant form of type XII collagen. *J. Biol. Chem.* **267**, 20087–20092.

209. Peltonen, S., Rehn, M., and Pihlajaniemi, T. (1997). Alternative splicing of mouse alpha1 (XIII) collagen RNAs results in at least 17 different transcripts, predicting alpha1 (XIII) collagen chains with length varying between 651 and 710 amino acid residues. *DNA Cell Biol.* **16**, 227–234.

210. Finer, M. H., Gerstenfeld, L. C., Young, D., Doty, P., and Boedtker, H. (1985). Collagen expression in embryonic chicken chondrocytes treated with phorbol myristate acetate. *Mol. Cell. Biol.* **5**, 1415–1424.

211. Fessler, J. H., Doege, K. J., Duncan, K. G., and Fessler, L. I. (1985). Biosynthesis of collagen. *J. Cell. Biochem.* **28**, 31–37.

212. Pihlajaniemi, T., Myllylä, R., and Kivirikko, K. I. (1991).Prolyl 4-hydroxylase and its role in collagen synthesis. *J. Hepatol.* **13** (Suppl. 3), S2–S7.

213. Kivirikko, K. I., and Pihlajaniemi, T. (1998).Collagen hydroxylases and the protein disulfide isomerase subunit of prolyl 4-hydroxylases. *Adv. Enzymol. Relat. Areas Mol. Biol.* **72**, 325–398.

214. Kivirikko, K. I., and Myllyharju, J. (1998). Prolyl 4-hydroxylases and their protein disulfide isomerase subunit. *Matrix Biol.* **16**, 357–368.

215. Myllylä, R., Pihlajaniemi, T., Pajunen, L., Turpeenniemi-Hujanen, T., and Kivirikko, K. I. (1991). Molecular cloning of chick lysyl hydroxylase. Little homology in primary structure to the two types of subunit of prolyl 4-hydroxylase. *J. Biol. Chem.* **266**, 2805–2810.

216. Doege, K. J., and Fessler, J. H. (1986). Folding of carboxyl domain and assembly of procollagen I. *J. Biol. Chem.* **261**, 8924–8935.

217. Bulleid, N. J., Wilson, R., and Lees, J. F. (1996). Type-III procollagen assembly in semi-intact cells: chain association, nucleation and triple-helix folding do not require formation of inter-chain disulphide bonds but triple-helix nucleation does require hydroxylation. *Biochem. J.* **317**, 195–202.

218. Bassuk, J. A., and Berg, R. A. (1989). Protein disulphide isomerase, a multifunctional endoplasmic reticulum protein. *Matrix* **9**, 244–258.

219. Freedman, R. B., Hirst, T. R., and Tuite, M. F. (1994). Protein disulphide isomerase: Building bridges in protein folding. *Trends Biochem. Sci.* **19**, 331–336.

220. Bulleid, N. J. (1993). Protein disulfide-isomerase: Role in biosynthesis of secretory proteins. *Adv. Protein Chem.* **44**, 125–150.

221. Bachinger, H. P., Bruckner, P., Timpl, R., Prockop, D. J., and Engel, J. (1980). Folding mechanism of the triple helix in type-III collagen and type-III pN-collagen. Role of disulfide bridges and peptide bond isomerization. *Eur. J. Biochem.* **106**, 619–632.

222. Lang, K., Schmid, F. X., and Fischer, G. (1987). Catalysis of protein folding by prolyl isomerase. *Nature* **329**, 268–270.

223. Steinmann, B., Bruckner, P., and Superti-Furga, A. (1991). Cyclosporin A slows collagen triple-helix formation in vivo: Indirect evidence for a physiologic role of peptidyl-prolyl cis-trans-isomerase. *J. Biol. Chem.* **266**, 1299–1303.

224. Inouye, K., Kobayashi, Y., Kyogoku, Y., Kishida, Y., Sakakibara, S., and Prockop, D. J. (1982). Synthesis and physical properties of (hydroxyproline-proline-glycine)10: hydroxyproline in the X-position decreases the melting temperature of the collagen triple helix. *Arch. Biochem. Biophys.* **219**, 198–203.

225. McLaughlin, S. H., and Bulleid, N. J. (1998). Molecular recognition in procollagen chain assembly. *Matrix Biol.* **16**, 369–377.

226. Nagata, K., and Hosokawa, N. (1996). Regulation and function of collagen-specific molecular chaperone, HSP47. *Cell Struct. Funct.* **21**, 425–430.

227. Prockop, D. J., and Tuderman, L. (1982). Posttranslational enzymes in the biosynthesis of collagen: Extracellular enzymes. *In* "Methods in Enzymology" (L. W. Cunningham and D. W. Frederiksen, eds.), Vol. 82, Part A, pp. 305–319. Academic Press, New York.

228. Nagata, K. (1996). Hsp47: A collagen-specific molecular chaperone. *Trends Biochem. Sci.* **21**, 22–26.

229. Nakai, A., Satoh, M., Hirayoshi, K., and Nagata, K. (1992).

Involvement of the stress protein HSP47 in procollagen processing in the endoplasmic reticulum. *J. Cell Biol.* **117**, 903–914.

230. Nagata, K., Saga, S., and Yamada, K. M. (1986). A major collagen-binding protein of chick embryo fibroblasts is a novel heat shock protein. *J. Cell Biol.* **103**, 223–229.

231. Natsume, T., Koide, T., Yokota, S., Hirayoshi, K., and Nagata, K. (1994). Interactions between collagen-binding stress protein HSP47 and collagen. Analysis of kinetic parameters by surface plasmon resonance biosensor. *J. Biol. Chem.* **269**, 31224–31228.

232. Ball, E. H., Jain, N., and Sanwal, B. D. (1997). Colligin, a collagen binding serpin. *Adv. Exp. Med. Biol.* **425**, 239–245.

233. Chessler, S. D., and Byers, P. H. (1993). BiP binds type I procollagen pro alpha chains with mutations in the carboxyl-terminal propeptide synthesized by cells from patients with osteogenesis imperfecta. *J. Biol. Chem.* **268**, 18226–18233.

234. Veijola, J., Annunen, P., Koivunen, P., Page, A. P., Pihlajaniemi, T., and Kivirikko, K. I. (1996). Baculovirus expression of two protein disulphide isomerase isoforms from *Caenorhabditis elegans* and characterization of prolyl 4-hydroxylases containing one of these polypeptides as their beta subunit. *Biochem. J.* **317**, 721–729.

235. Helaakoski, T., Veijola, J., Vuori, K., Rehn, M., Chow, L. T., Taillon-Miller, P., Kivirikko, K. I., and Pihlajaniemi, T. (1994). Structure and expression of the human gene for the alpha subunit of prolyl 4-hydroxylase. The two alternatively spliced types of mRNA correspond to two homologous exons the sequences of which are expressed in a variety of tissues. *J. Biol. Chem.* **269**, 27847–27854.

236. Annunen, P., Helaakoski, T., Myllyharju, J., Veijola, J., Pihlajaniemi, T., and Kivirikko, K. I. (1997). Cloning of the human prolyl 4-hydroxylase alpha subunit isoform alpha(II) and characterization of the type II enzyme tetramer. The alpha(I) and alpha(II) subunits do not form a mixed alpha(I)alpha(II)beta2 tetramer. *J. Biol. Chem.* **272**, 17342–17348.

237. Chvapil, M., and Ryan, J. N. (1972). Diverse effect of 1,10-phenanthroline and 2,2′-dipyridyl on the synthesis of collagen and noncollagenous proteins in in vivo and in vitro systems. *Biochim. Biophys. Acta* **273**, 208–211.

238. Bienkowski, R. S. (1989). Intracellular degradation of newly synthesized collagen. *Rev. Biol. Cell.* **21**, 423–443.

239. Tschank, G., Brocks, D. G., Engelbart, K., Mohr, J., Baader, E., Gunzler, V., and Hanauske-Abel, H. M. (1991). Inhibition of prolyl hydroxylation and procollagen processing in chick-embryo calvaria by a derivative of pyridine-2,4-dicarboxylate. Characterization of the diethyl ester as a proinhibitor. *Biochem. J.* **275**, 469–476.

240. Hanauske-Abel, H. M. (1991). Prolyl 4-hydroxylase, a target enzyme for drug development. Design of suppressive agents and the in vitro effects of inhibitors and proinhibitors. *J. Hepatol.* **13** (Suppl. 3), S8–S15.

241. Majamaa, K., Hanauske-Abel, H. M., Gunzler, V., and Kivirikko, K. I. (1984). The 2-oxoglutarate binding site of prolyl 4-hydroxylase. Identification of distinct subsites and evidence for 2-oxoglutarate decarboxylation in a ligand reaction at the enzyme-bound ferrous ion. *Eur. J. Biochem.* **138**, 239–245.

242. McCaffrey, T. A., Pomerantz, K. B., Sanborn, T. A., Spokojny, A. M., Du, B., Park, M. H., Folk, J. E., Lamberg, A., Kivirikko, K. I., and Falcone, D. J. (1995). Specific inhibition of elF-5A and collagen hydroxylation by a single agent. Antiproliferative and fibrosuppressive effects on smooth muscle cells from human coronary arteries. *J. Clin. Invest.* **95**, 446–455.

243. Hamalainen, E. R., Kemppainen, R., Pihlajaniemi, T., and Kivirikko, K. I. (1993). Structure of the human lysyl oxidase gene. *Genomics* **17**, 544–548.

244. Rawlings, N. D., and Barrett, A. J. (1995). Evolutionary families of metallopeptidases. *In* "Methods in Enzymology" (A. J. Barrett ed.), Vol. 248, 183–228. Academic Press, San Diego, CA.

245. Hojima, Y., McKenzie, J. A., van der Rest, M., and Prockop, D. J. (1989). Type I procollagen N-proteinase from chick embryo tendons. Purification of a new 500-kDa form of the enzyme and identification of the catalytically active polypeptides. *J. Biol. Chem.* **264**, 11336–11345.

246. Colige, A., Li, S. W., Sieron, A. L., Nusgens, B. V., Prockop, D. J., and Lapiere, C. M. (1997). cDNA cloning and expression of bovine procollagen I N-proteinase: A new member of the superfamily of zinc-metalloproteinases with binding sites for cells and other matrix components. *Proc. Natl. Acad. Sci. U.S.A.* **94**, 2374–2379.

247. Tuderman, L., and Prockop, D. J. (1982). Procollagen N-proteinase. Properties of the enzyme purified from chick embryo tendons. *Eur. J. Biochem.* **125**, 545–549.

248. Halila, R., and Peltonen, L. (1986). Purification of human procollagen type III N-proteinase from placenta and preparation of antiserum. *Biochem. J.* **239**, 47–52.

249. Li, S. W., Sieron, A. L., Fertala, A., Hojima, Y., Arnold, W. V., and Prockop, D. J. (1996). The C-proteinase that processes procollagens to fibrillar collagens is identical to the protein previously identified as bone morphogenic protein-1. *Proc. Natl. Acad. Sci. U.S.A.* **93**, 5127–5130.

250. Suzuki, N., Labosky, P. A., Furuta, Y., Hargett, L., Dunn, R., Fogo, A. B., Takahara, K., Peters, D. M., Greenspan, D. S., and Hogan, B. L. (1996). Failure of ventral body wall closure in mouse embryos lacking a procollagen C-proteinase encoded by Bmp1, a mammalian gene related to Drosophila tolloid. *Development* **122**, 3587–3595.

251. Choi, H. U., Tang, L. H., Johnson, T. L., Pal, S., Rosenberg, and Poole, A. R. (1983). Isolation and characterization of a 36.000 molecular weight subunit fetal cartilage matrix protein. *J. Biol. Chem.* **258**, 655–661.

252. Hinek, A., Reiner, A., and Poole, R. (1987). The calcification of cartilage matrix in chondrocyte culture: Studies of the C-propetide of type II collagen (chondrocalcin). *J. Cell Biol.* **104**, 1435–1441.

253. Helseth, D. L., Jr., and Veis, A. (1984). Cathepsin D-mediated processing of procollagen: Lysosomal enzyme involvement in secretory processing of procollagen. *Proc. Natl. Acad. Sci. U.S.A.* **81**, 3302–3306.

254. Focht, R. J., and Adams, S. L. (1984). Tissue specificity of type I collagen gene expression is determined at both transcriptional and post-transcriptional levels. *Mol. Cell. Biol.* **4**, 1843–1852.

255. Benya, P., and Padilla, P. D. (1986). Modulation of the rabbit chondrocyte phenotype by retinoic acid terminates type II collagen synthesis without inducing type I collagen: The modulated phenotype differs from that produced by subculture. *Dev. Biol.* **118**, 296–305.

256. Bennett, V. D., and Adams, S. L. (1990). Identification of a cartilage-specific promoter within intron-2 of the chick alpha-2(I) collagen gene. *J. Biol. Chem.* **265**, 2223–2230.

257. Bennett, V. D., and Adams, S. L. (1987). Characterization of the translational control mechanism preventing synthesis of alpha 2(I) collagen in chicken vertebral chondroblasts. *J. Biol. Chem.* **262**, 14806–14814.

258. Chu, M. L., de Wet, W., Bernard, M., and Ramirez, F. (1985). Fine structural analysis of the human pro-alpha 1 (I) collagen gene. Promoter structure, Alul repeats, and polymorphic transcripts. *J. Biol. Chem.* **260**, 2315–2320.

259. Saitta, B., Timpl, R., and Chu, M. L. (1992). Human alpha 2(VI) collagen gene. Heterogeneity at the 5′-untranslated region generated by an alternate exon. *J. Biol. Chem.* **267**, 6188–6196.

260. Penttinen, R. P., Kobayashi, S., and Bornstein, P. (1988). Transforming growth factor beta increases mRNA for matrix proteins both in the presence and in the absence of changes in mRNA stability. *Proc. Natl. Acad. Sci. U.S.A.* **85**, 1105–1108.

261. Eckes, B., Mauch, C., Huppe, G., and Krieg, T. (1993). Downregulation of collagen synthesis in fibroblasts within three-dimensional collagen lattices involves transcriptional and posttranscriptional mechanisms. *FEBS Lett.* **318**, 129–133.

262. Mauch, C., Hatamochi, A., Scharffetter, K., and Krieg, T. (1988). Regulation of collagen synthesis in fibroblasts within a three-dimensional collagen gel. *Exp. Cell Res.* **178**, 493–503.

263. Speth, C., and Oberbaumer, I. (1993). Expression of basement membrane proteins: Evidence for complex post-transcriptional control mechanisms. *Exp. Cell Res.* **204**, 302–310.

264. Rossi, P., and de Crombrugghe, B. (1987). Formation of a type I collagen RNA dimer by intermolecular base-pairing of a conserved sequence around the translation initiation site. *Nucleic Acids Res.* **15**, 8935–8956.

265. Bornstein, P., McKay, J., Devarayalu, S., and Cook, S. C. (1988). A highly conserved, 5′ untranslated, inverted repeat sequence is ineffective in translational control of the alpha 1(I) collagen gene. *Nucleic Acids Res.* **16**, 9721–9736; errata: *Ibid.*, No. 23, p. 11399.

266. Paglia, L. M., Wiestner, M., Duchene, M., Ouellette, L. A., Horlein, D., Martin, G. R., and Muller, P. K. (1981). Effects of procollagen peptides on the translation of type II collagen messenger ribonucleic acid and on collagen biosynthesis in chondrocytes. *Biochemistry* **20**, 3523–3527.

267. Paglia, L., Wilczek, J., de Leon, L. D., Martin, G. R., Horlein, D., and Muller, P. (1979). Inhibition of procollagen cell-free synthesis by amino-terminal extension peptides. *Biochemistry* **18**, 5030–5034.

268. Horlein, D., McPherson, J., Goh, S. H., and Bornstein, P. (1981). Regulation of protein synthesis: Translational control by procollagen-derived fragments. *Proc. Natl. Acad. Sci. U.S.A.* **78**, 6163–6167.

268a. Schlumberger, W., Thie, M., Volmer, H., Rauterberg, J., and Robenek, H. (1988). Binding and uptake of Col 1(I), a peptide capable of inhibiting collagen synthesis in fibroblasts. *Eur. J. Cell Biol.* **46**, 244–252.

269. Fouser, L., Sage, E. H., Clark, J., and Bornstein, P. (1991). Feedback regulation of collagen gene expression: A Trojan horse approach. *Proc. Natl. Acad. Sci. U.S.A.* **88**, 10158–10162.

270. Wu, C. H., Donovan, C. B., and Wu, G. Y. (1986). Evidence for pretranslational regulation of collagen synthesis by procollagen propeptides. *J. Biol. Chem.* **261**, 10482–10484.

271. Aycock, R. S., Raghow, R., Stricklin, G. P., Seyer, J. M., and Kang, A. H. (1986). Post-transcriptional inhibition of collagen and fibronectin synthesis by a synthetic homolog of a portion of the carboxyl-terminal propeptide of human type I collagen. *J. Biol. Chem.* **261**, 14355–14360.

272. Nakata, K., Miyamoto, S., Bernier, S., Tanaka, M., Utani, A., Krebsbach, P., Rhodes, C., and Yamada, Y. (1996). The c-propeptide of type II procollagen binds to the enhancer region of the type II procollagen gene and regulates its transcription. *Ann. N. Y. Acad. Sci.* **785**, 307–308.

273. Olson, B. R., and Nimni, M. E. (1981). Collagen. *In* "Molecular Biology." CRC Press, Boca Raton, FL.

274. Vuorio, E., and de Crombrugghe, B. (1990). The family of collagen genes. *Annu. Rev. Biochem.* **59**, 837–872.

275. Dewet, W., Bernard, M., Bensochanda, V., Chu, M. L., Dickson, L., Weil, D., and Ramirez, F. (1987). Organization of the human pro-alpha 2(I) collagen gene. *J. Biol. Chem.* **262**, 16032–16036.

276. Bornstein, P., and Sage, H. (1989). Regulation of collagen gene expression. *Prog. Nucleic. Acid. Res. Mol. Biol.* **37**, 67–106.

277. Slack, J. L., Liska, D. J., and Bornstein, P. (1993). Regulation of expression of the type I collagen genes. *Am. J. Med. Genet.* **45**, 140–151.

278. Sokolov, B. P., Ala-Kokko, L., Dhulipala, R., Arita, M., Khillan, J. S., and Prockop, D. J. (1995). Tissue-specific expression of the gene for type I procollagen (COL1A1) in transgenic mice. Only 476 base pairs of the promoter are required if collagen genes are used as reporters. *J. Biol. Chem.* **270**, 9622–9629.

279. Sokolov, B. P., Mays, P. K., Khillan, J. S., and Prockop, D. J. (1993). Tissue- and development-specific expression in transgenic mice of a type I procollagen (COL1A1) minigene construct with 2.3 kb of the promoter region and 2 kb of the 3′-flanking region. Specificity is independent of the putative regulatory sequences in the first intron. *Biochemistry* **32**, 9242–9249.

280. Rossert, J. A., Chen, S. S., Eberspaecher, H., Smith, C. N., and de Crombrugghe, B. (1996). Identification of a minimal sequence of the mouse pro-alpha 1(I) collagen promoter that confers high-level osteoblast expression in transgenic mice and that binds a protein selectively present in osteoblasts. *Proc. Natl. Acad. Sci. U.S.A.* **93**, 1027–1031.

281. Rossert, J., Eberspaecher, H., and de Crombrugghe, B. (1995). Separate cis-acting DNA elements of the mouse pro-alpha 1(I) collagen promoter direct expression of reporter genes to different type I collagen-producing cells in transgenic mice. *J. Cell Biol.* **129**, 1421–1432.

282. Liska, D. J., Robinson, V. R., and Bornstein, P. (1992). Elements in the first intron of the alpha 1(I) collagen gene interact with Sp1 to regulate gene expression. *Gene Expression* **2**, 379–389.

283. Slack, J. L., Liska, D. J., and Bornstein, P. (1991). An upstream regulatory region mediates high-level, tissue-specific expression of the human alpha 1(I) collagen gene in transgenic mice. *Mol. Cell. Biol.* **11**, 2066–2074.

284. Kratochwil, K., Ghaffari-Tabrizi, N., Holzinger, I., and Harbers, K. (1993). Restricted expression of Mov13 mutant alpha 1(I) collagen gene in osteoblasts and its consequences for bone development. *Dev. Dyn.* **198**, 273–283.

285. Pavlin, D., Bedalov, A., Kronenberg, M. S., Kream, B. E., Rowe, D. W., Smith, C. L., Pike, J. W., and Lichtler, A. C. (1994). Analysis of regulatory regions in the COL1A1 gene responsible for 1,25-dihydroxyvitamin D3-mediated transcriptional repression in osteoblastic cells. *J. Cell. Biochem.* **56**, 490–501.

286. Ritzenthaler, J. D., Goldstein, R. H., Fine, A., and Smith, B. D. (1993). Regulation of the alpha 1(I) collagen promoter via a transforming growth factor-beta activation element. *J. Biol. Chem.* **268**, 13625–13631.

287. Meisler, N., Keefer, K. A., Ehrlich, H. P., Yager, D. R., Myers-Parrelli, J., and Cutroneo, K. R. (1997). Dexamethasone abrogates the fibrogenic effect of transforming growth factor-beta in rat granuloma and granulation tissue fibroblasts. *J. Invest. Dermatol.* **108**, 285–289.

288. Meisler, N., Shull, S., Xie, R., Long, G. L., Absher, M., Connolly, J. P., and Cutroneo, K. R. (1995). Glucocorticoids coordinately regulate type I collagen pro alpha 1 promoter activity through both the glucocorticoid and transforming growth factor beta response elements: a novel mechanism of glucocorticoid regulation of eukaryotic genes. *J. Cell. Biochem.* **59**, 376–388.

289. Rossi, P., and deCrombrugghe, B. (1987). Identification of a cell-specific transcriptional enhancer in the first intron of the mouse alpha 2 (type I) collagen gene. *Proc. Natl. Acad. Sci. U.S.A.* **84**, 5590–5594.

290. D'Souza, R. N., Niederreither, K., and de Crombrugghe, B. (1993). Osteoblast-specific expression of the alpha 2(I) collagen promoter in transgenic mice: Correlation with the distribution of TGF-beta 1. *J. Bone Miner. Res.* **8**, 1127–1136.

291. Ignotz, R. A., Endo, T., and Massague, J. (1987). Regulation of fibronectin and type I collagen mRNA levels by transforming growth factor-beta. *J. Biol. Chem.* **262**, 6443–6446.

292. Ignotz, R. A., and Massague, J. (1986). Transforming growth factor-beta stimulates the expression of fibronectin and collagen and their incorporation into the extracellular matrix. *J. Biol. Chem.* **261**, 4337–4345.

293. Chung, K. Y., Agarwal, A., Uitto, J., and Mauviel, A. (1996). An AP-1 binding sequence is essential for regulation of the human alpha 2(I) collagen (COL1A2) promoter activity by transforming growth factor-beta. *J. Biol. Chem.* **271**, 3272–3278.

294. Greenwel, P., Inagaki, Y., Hu, W., Walsh, M., and Ramirez, F. (1997). Sp1 is required for the early response of alpha2(I) collagen to transforming growth factor-beta1. *J. Biol. Chem.* **272**, 19738–19745.

295. Higashi, K., Kouba, D. J., Song, Y. J., Uitto, J., and Mauviel, A. (1998). A proximal element within the human alpha 2(I) collagen (COL1A2) promoter, distinct from the tumor necrosis factor-alpha response element, mediates transcriptional repression by interferon-gamma. *Matrix Biol.* **16**, 447–456.

296. Bou-Gharios, G., Garrett, L. A., Rossert, J., Niederreither, K., Eberspaecher, H., Smith, C., Black, C., and Crombrugghe, B. (1996). A potent far-upstream enhancer in the mouse pro alpha 2(I) collagen gene regulates expression of reporter genes transgenic mice. *J. Cell Biol.* **134**, 1333–1344.

297. Pallante, K. M., Niu, Z., Zhao, Y., Cohen, A. J., Nah, H. D., and Adams, S. L. (1996). The chick alpha 2(I) collagen gene contains two functional promoters, and its expression in chondrocytes is regulated at both transcriptional and post-transcriptional levels. *J. Biol. Chem.* **271**, 25233–25239.

298. Horton, W., Miyashita, T., Kohno, K., Hassell, J. R., and Yamada, Y. (1987). Identification of a phenotype-specific enhancer in the first intron of the rat collagen II gene. *Proc. Natl. Acad. Sci. U.S.A.* **84**, 8864–8868.

299. Zhou, G., Garofalo, S., Mukhopadhyay, K., Lefebvre, V., Smith, C. N., Eberspaecher, H., and de Crombrugghe, B. (1995). A 182 bp fragment of the mouse pro alpha 1(II) collagen gene is sufficient to direct chondrocyte expression in transgenic mice. *J. Cell Sci.* **108**, 3677–3684.

300. Zhou, G., Lefebvre, V., Zhang, Z., Eberspaecher, H., and de Crombrugghe, B. (1998). Three high mobility group-like sequences within a 48-base pair enhancer of the Col2a1 gene are required for cartilage-specific expression in vivo. *J. Biol. Chem.* **273**, 14989–14997.

301. Lefebvre, V., Zhou, G., Mukhopadhyay, K., Smith, C. N., Zhang, Z., Eberspaecher, H., Zhou, X., Sinha, S., Maity, S. N., and de Crombrugghe, B. (1996). An 18-base-pair sequence in the mouse proalpha1(II) collagen gene is sufficient for expression in cartilage and binds nuclear proteins that are selectively expressed in chondrocytes. *Mol. Cell. Biol.* **16**, 4512–4523.

302. Lefebvre, V., and de Crombrugghe, B. (1998). Toward understanding SOX9 function in chondrocyte differentiation. *Matrix Biol.* **16**, 529–540.

303. Zhao, Q., Eberspaecher, H., Lefebvre, V., and de Crombrugghe, B. (1997). Parallel expression of Sox9 and Col2a1 in cells undergoing chondrogenesis. *Dev. Dyn.* **209**, 377–386.

304. Lefebvre, V., Huang, W., Harley, V. R., Goodfellow, P. N., and de Crombrugghe, B. (1997). SOX9 is a potent activator of the chondrocyte-specific enhancer of the pro alpha1(II) collagen gene. *Mol. Cell. Biol.* **17**, 2336–2346.

305. Mukhopadhyay, K., Lefebvre, V., Zhou, G., Garofalo, S., Kimura, J. H., and de Crombrugghe, B. (1995). Use of a new rat chondrosarcoma cell line to delineate a 119-base pair chondrocyte-specific enhancer element and to define active promoter segments in the mouse pro-alpha 1(II) collagen gene. *J. Biol. Chem.* **270**, 27711–27719.

306. Savagner, P., Krebsbach, P. H., Hatano, O., Miyashita, T., Liebman, J., and Yamada, Y. (1995). Collagen II promoter and enhancer interact synergistically through Sp1 and distinct nuclear factors. *DNA Cell Biol.* **14**, 501–510.

307. Savagner, P., Miyashita, T., and Yamada, Y. (1990). Two silencers regulate the tissue-specific expression of the collagen II gene. *J. Biol. Chem.* **265**, 6669–6674.

308. Ruteshouser, E. C., and de Crombrugghe, B. (1989). Characterization of two distinct positive cis-acting elements in the mouse alpha 1(II) collagen promoter. *J. Biol. Chem.* **264**, 13740–13744.

309. Ruteshouser, E. C., and de Crombrugghe, B. (1992). Purification of BBF, a DNA-binding protein recognizing a positive cis-acting element in the mouse alpha 1(III) collagen promoter. *J. Biol. Chem.* **267**, 14398–14404.

310. Mudryj, M., and de Crombrugghe, B. (1988). Deletion analysis of the mouse alpha 1(III) collagen promoter. *Nucleic Acids Res.* **16**, 7513–7526.

311. Takahara, K., Hoffman, G. G., and Greenspan, D. S. (1995). Complete structural organization of the human alpha 1 (V) collagen gene (COL5A1): Divergence from the conserved organization of other characterized fibrillar collagen genes. *Genomics* **29**, 588–597.

312. Lee, S., and Greenspan, D. S. (1995). Transcriptional promoter of the human alpha 1(V) collagen gene (COL5A1). *Biochem. J.* **310**, 15–22.

313. Truter, S., Di Liberto, M., Inagaki, Y., and Ramirez, F. (1992). Identification of an upstream regulatory region essential for cell type-specific transcription of the pro-alpha 2(V) collagen gene (COL5A2). *J. Biol. Chem.* **267**, 25389–25395.

314. Yoshioka, H., Inoguchi, K., Khaleduzzaman, M., Ninomiya, Y., Andrikopoulos, K., and Ramirez, F. (1995). Coding sequence and alternative splicing of the mouse alpha 1(XI) collagen gene (Col11a1). *Genomics* **28**, 337–340.

315. Yoshioka, H., Greenwel, P., Inoguchi, K., Truter, S., Inagaki, Y., Ninomiya, Y., and Ramirez, F. (1995). Structural and functional analysis of the promoter of the human alpha 1(XI) collagen gene. *J. Biol. Chem.* **270**, 418–424.

316. Lui, V. C., Ng, L. J., Sat, E. W., and Cheah, K. S. (1996). The human alpha 2(XI) collagen gene (COL11A2): completion of coding information, identification of the promoter sequence, and precise localization within the major histocompatibility complex reveal overlap with the KE5 gene. *Genomics* **32**, 401–412.

317. Bridgewater, L. C., Lefebvre, V., and de Crombrugghe, B. (1998). Chondrocyte-specific enhancer elements in the Col11a2 gene resemble the Col2a1 tissue-specific enhancer. *J. Biol. Chem.* **273**, 14998–15006.

318. Hayman, A. R., Koppel, J., and Trueb, B. (1991). Complete structure of the chicken alpha 2(VI) collagen gene. *Eur. J. Biochem.* **197**, 177–184.

319. Hayman, A. R., Koppel, J., Winterhalter, K. H., and Trueb, B. (1990). The triple-helical domain of alpha 2(VI) collagen is encoded by 19 short exons that are multiples of 9 base pairs. *J. Biol. Chem.* **265**, 9864–9868.

320. Walchli, C., Marcionelli, R., Odermatt, B. F., Peltonen, J., Vuorio, E., and Trueb, B. (1996). Expression and distribution of two alternatively spliced transcripts from the chicken alpha 2 (VI) collagen gene. *J. Cell. Biochem.* **63**, 207–220.

321. Doliana, R., Bonaldo, P., and Colombatti, A. (1990). Multiple forms of chicken alpha 3(VI) collagen chain generated by alternative splicing in type A repeated domains. *J. Cell Biol.* **111**, 2197–2205.

322. Doliana, R., Mucignat, M. T., Segat, D., Zanussi, S., Fabbro, C., Lakshmi, T. R., and Colombatti, A. (1998). Alternative splicing of VWFA modules generates variants of type VI collagen alpha 3 chain with a distinctive expression pattern in embryonic chicken tissues and potentially different adhesive function. *Matrix Biol.* **16**, 427–442.

323. Braghetta, P., Fabbro, C., Piccolo, S., Marvulli, D., Bonaldo, P., Volpin, D., and Bressan, G. M. (1996). Distinct regions control transcriptional activation of the alpha1(VI) collagen promoter in different tissues of transgenic mice. *J. Cell Biol.* **135**, 1163–1177.

324. Fabbro, C., Braghetta, P., Girotto, D., Piccolo, S., Volpin, D., and Bressan, G. M. (1999). Cell type-specific transcription of the alpha1(VI) collagen gene. Role of the ap1 binding site and of the core promoter. *J. Biol. Chem.* **274**, 1759–1766.

325. Piccolo, S., Bonaldo, P., Vitale, P., Volpin, D., and Bressan, G. M. (1995). Transcriptional activation of the alpha 1(VI) collagen gene during myoblast differentiation is mediated by multiple GA boxes. *J. Biol. Chem.* **270**, 19583–19590.

326. Saitta, B., and Chu, M. L. (1995). Characterization of the human alpha 1(VI) collagen promoter and its comparison with human alpha 2(VI) promoters. *Eur. J. Biochem.* **234**, 542–549.

327. Braghetta, P., Vitale, P., Piccolo, S., Bonaldo, P., Fabbro, C., Girotto, D., Volpin, D., and Bressan, G. M. (1997). Tissue-specific expression of promoter regions of the alpha1(VI) collagen gene in cell cultures and transgenic mice. *Eur. J. Biochem.* **247**, 200–208.

328. Willimann, T. E., Maier, R., and Trueb, B. (1995). A novel transcription factor and two members of the Sp 1 multigene family regulate

the activity of the alpha 2(VI) collagen promoter. *Matrix Biol.* **14**, 653–663.

329. Hatamochi, A., Aumailley, M., Mauch, C., Chu, M.-L., Timpl, R., and Krieg, T. (1989). Regulation of collagen VI expression in fibroblasts. Effects of cell density, cell-matrix interactions, and chemical transformation. *J. Biol. Chem.* **264**, 3494–3499.

330. Peltonen, J., Kahari, L., Jaakkola, S., Kahari, V. M., Varga, J., Uitto, J., and Jimenez, S. A. (1990). Evaluation of transforming growth factor beta and type I procollagen gene expression in fibrotic skin diseases by in situ hybridization. *J. Invest. Dermatol.* **94**, 365–371.

331. Peltonen, J., Hsiao, L. L., Jaakkola, S., Sollberg, S., Aumailley, M., Timpl, R., Chu, M. L., and Uitto, J. (1991). Activation of collagen gene expression in keloids: co-localization of type I and VI collagen and transforming growth factor-beta 1 mRNA. *J. Invest. Dermatol.* **97**, 240–248.

332. Quarto, R., Dozin, B., Bonaldo, P., Cancedda, R., and Colombatti, A. (1993). Type VI collagen expression is upregulated in the early events of chondrocyte differentiation. *Development* **117**, 245–251.

333. Heckmann, M., Aumailley, M., Chu, M. L., Timpl, R., and Krieg, T. (1992). Effect of transforming growth factor-beta on collagen type VI expression in human dermal fibroblasts. *FEBS Lett.* **310**, 79–82.

334. Heckmann, M., Aumailley, M., Hatamochi, A., Chu, M. -L., Timpl, R., and Krieg, T. (1989). Down-regulation of alpha3(VI) chain expression by gamma-interferon dereases synthesis and deposition of collagen type VI. *Eur. J. Biochem.* **182**, 719–726.

335. Elima, K., Eerola, I., Rosati, R., Metsäranta, M., Garofalo, S., Perälä, M., deCrombrugghe, B., and Vuorio, E. (1993). The mouse collagen X gene: Complete nucleotide sequence, exon structure and expression pattern. *Biochem. J.* **289**, 247–253.

336. Kong, R. Y., Kwan, K. M., Lau, E. T., Thomas, J. T., Boot-Handford, R. P., Grant, M. E., and Cheah, K. S. (1993). Intron-exon structure, alternative use of promoter and expression of the mouse collagen X gene, COL10A-1. *Eur. J. Biochem.* **213**, 99–111.

337. Apte, S. S., and Oslen, B. R. (1993). Characterization of the mouse type X collagen gene. *Matrix* **13**, 165–179.

338. Thomas, J. T., Kwan, A. P. L., Grant, M. E., and Boot-Handford, R. P. (1991). Isolation of cDNAs encoding the complete sequence of bovine type X collagen. *Biochem. J.* **273**, 141–148.

339. Thomas, J. T., Cresswell, C. J., Rash, B., Nicolai, H., Jones, T., Solomon, E., Grant, M. E., and Boot-Handford, R. P. (1991). The human collagen X gene. *Biochem. J.* **280**, 617–623.

340. Reichenberger, E., Beier, F., Luvalle, P., Olsen, B. R., von der Mark, K., and Bertling, W. (1992). Genomic organisation and full length cDNA sequence of human collagen X. *FEBS Lett.* **311**, 305–310.

341. Beier, F., Eerola, I., Vuorio, E., Luvalle, P., Reichenberger, E., Bertling, W., von der Mark, K., and Lammi, M.J. (1996). Variability in the upstream promoter and intron sequences of the human, mouse and chick type X collagen genes. *Matrix Biol.* **15**, 415–422.

342. Luvalle, P., Hayashi, M., and Olsen, B. B. (1989). Transcriptional regulation of type X collagen during chondrocyte maturation. *Dev. Biol.* **133**, 613–616.

343. Luvalle, P., Daniels, K., Hay, E. D., and Olsen, B. (1992). Type X collagen is transcriptionally activated and specifically localized during sternal cartilage maturation. *Matrix* **12**, 404–413.

344. Capasso, O., Tajana, G., and Cancedda, R. (1984). Location of 64K collagen producing chondrocytes in developing chick embryo tibiae. *Mol. Cell. Biol.* **4**, 1163–1168.

345. Luvalle, P., Iwamoto, M., Fanning, P., Pacifici, M., and Olsen, B. R. (1993). Multiple negative elements in a gene that codes for an extracellular matrix protein, collagen X, restrict expression to hypertrophic chondrocytes. *J. Cell Biol.* **121**, 1173–1179.

346. Dourado, G., and Luvalle, P. (1998). Proximal DNA elements mediate repressor activity conferred by the distal portion of the chicken collagen X promoter. *J. Cell. Biochem.* **70**, 507–516.

347. Long, F., Sonenshein, G. E., and Linsenmayer, T. F. (1998). Multiple transcriptional elements in the avian type X collagen gene. Identification of Sp1 family proteins as regulators for high level expression in hypertrophic chondrocytes. *J. Biol. Chem.* **273**, 6542–6549.

348. Volk, S. W., Luvalle, P., Leask, T., and Leboy, P. S. (1998). A BMP responsive transcriptional region in the chicken type X collagen gene. *J. Bone Miner. Res.* **13**, 1521–1529.

349. Chambers, D., Thomas, J. T., Boam, D., Wallis, G. A., Grant, M. E., and Boot-Handford, R. P. (1996). Sequence elements within intron 1 of the human collagen X gene do not contribute to the regulation of gene expression. *Ann. N. Y. Acad. Sci.* **785**, 227–230.

350. Beier, F., Vornehm, S., Pöschl, E., von der Mark, K., and Lammi, M. J. (1997). Localization of silencer and enhancer elements in the human type X collagen gene. *J. Cell Biochem.* **66**, 210–218.

350a. Harada, S., Sampath, T. K., Aubin, J. E., and Rodan, G. A. (1997). Osteogenic protein-1 up-regulation of the collagen X promoter activity is mediated by a MEF-2-like sequence and requires an adjacent AP-I sequence. *Mol. Endocrinol.* **11**, 1832–1845.

351. Roberts, A. B., and Sporn, M. B. (1993). Physiological actions and clinical applications of transforming growth factor-beta (TGF-beta). *Growth Factors* **8**, 1–9.

352. Murata, H., Zhou, L., Ochoa, S., Hasan, A., Badiavas, E., and Falanga, V. (1997). TGF-beta3 stimulates and regulates collagen synthesis through TGF-beta1-dependent and independent mechanisms. *J. Invest. Dermatol.* **108**, 258–262.

353. Slavin, J., Unemori, E., Hunt, T. K., and Amento, E. (1994). Transforming growth factor beta (TGF-beta) and dexamethasone have direct opposing effects on collagen metabolism in low passage human dermal fibroblasts in vitro. *Growth Factors* **11**, 205–213.

354. Bradham, D. M., in der Wiesche, B., Precht, P., Balakir, R., and Horton, W. (1994). Transrepression of type II collagen by TGF-beta and FGF is protein kinase C dependent and is mediated through regulatory sequences in the promoter and first intron. *J. Cell. Physiol.* **158**, 61–68.

355. Galera, P., Vivien, D., Pronost, S., Bonaventure, J., Redini, F., Loyau, G., and Pujol, J. P. (1992). Transforming growth factor-beta 1 (TGF-beta 1) up-regulation of collagen type II in primary cultures of rabbit articular chondrocytes (RAC) involves increased mRNA levels without affecting mRNA stability and procollagen processing. *J. Cell. Physiol.* **153**, 596–606.

356. Pujol, J. P., Galera, P., Pronost, S., Boumediene, K., Vivien, D., Macro, M., Min, W., Redini, F., Penfornis, H., and Daireaux, M. (1994). Transforming growth factor-beta (TGF-beta) and articular chondrocytes. *Ann. Endocrinol.* **55**, 109–120.

357. Throckmorton, D. C., Brogden, A. P., Min, B., Rasmussen, H., and Kashgarian, M. (1995). PDGF and TGF-beta mediate collagen production by mesangial cells exposed to advanced glycosylation end products. *Kidney Int.* **48**, 111–117.

358. Lepisto, J., Peltonen, J., Vaha-Kreula, M., Soderstrom, K., Niinikoski, J., and Laato, M. (1996). Selective modulation of collagen gene expression by different isoforms of platelet-derived growth factor in experimental wound healing. *Cell Tissue Res.* **286**, 449–455.

359. Lepisto, J., Peltonen, J., Vaha-Kreula, M., Niinikoski, J., and Laato, M. (1995). Platelet-derived growth factor isoforms PDGF-AA, -AB and -BB exert specific effects on collagen gene expression and mitotic activity of cultured human wound fibroblasts. *Biochem. Biophys. Res. Commun.* **209**, 393–399.

360. Hata, R., Sunada, H., Arai, K., Sato, T., Ninomiya, Y., Nagai, Y., and Senoo, H. (1988). Regulation of collagen metabolism and cell growth by epidermal growth factor and ascorbate in cultured human skin fibroblasts. *Eur. J. Biochem.* **173**, 261–267; errata: *Ibid.*, **175**(3), 679.

361. Genovese, C., Rowe, D., and Kream, B. (1984). Construction of DNA sequences complementary to rate alpha 1 and alpha 2 collagen

mRNA and their use in studying the regulation of type I collagen synthesis by 1,25-dihydroxyvitamin D. *Biochemistry* **23**, 6210–6216.

362. Rowe, D. W., and Kream, B. E. (1982). Regulation of collagen synthesis in fetal rat calvaria by 1,25-dihydroxyvitamin D3. *J. Biol. Chem.* **257**, 8009–8015.

363. Kuroki, Y., Shiozawa, S., Kano, J., and Chihara, K. (1995). Competition between c-fos and 1,25(OH)$_2$ vitamin D3 in the transcriptional control of type I collagen synthesis in MC3T3-E1 osteoblastic cells. *J. Cell. Physiol.* **164**, 459–464.

364. Kream, B. E., Lafrancis, D., Petersen, D. N., Woody, C., Clark, S., Rowe, D. W., and Lichtler, A. (1993). Parathyroid hormone represses alpha 1(I) collagen promoter activity in cultured calvariae from neonatal transgenic mice. *Mol. Endocrinol.* **7**, 399–408.

365. Setoyama, C., Hatamochi, A., Peterkofsky, B., Prather, W., and de Crombrugghe, B. (1986). V-fos stimulates expression of the alpha 1(III) collagen gene in NIH 3T3 cells. *Biochem. Biophys. Res. Commun.* **136**, 1042–1048.

366. Oikarinen, A. I., Vuorio, E. I., Zaragoza, E. J., Palotie, A., Chu, M. L., and Uitto, J. (1988). Modulation of collagen metabolism by glucocorticoids. Receptor-mediated effects of dexamethasone on collagen biosynthesis in chick embryo fibroblasts and chondrocytes. *Biochem. Pharmacol.* **37**, 1451–1462.

367. Oikarinen, A., Autio, P., Kiistala, U., Risteli, L., and Risteli, J. (1992). A new method to measure type I and III collagen synthesis in human skin in vivo: Demonstration of decreased collagen synthesis after topical glucocorticoid treatment. *J. Invest. Dermatol.* **98**, 220–225.

368. Russell, S. B., Trupin, J. S., Myers, J. C., Broquist, A. H., Smith, J. C., Myles, M. E., and Russell, J. D. (1989). Differential glucocorticoid regulation of collagen mRNAs in human dermal fibroblasts. Keloid-derived and fetal fibroblasts are refractory to down-regulation. *J. Biol. Chem.* **264**, 13730–13735.

369. Weiner, F. R., Czaja, M. J., Jefferson, D. M., Giambrone, M. A., Tur-Kaspa, R., Reid, L. M., and Zern, M. A. (1987). The effects of dexamethasone on in vitro collagen gene expression. *J. Biol. Chem.* **262**, 6955–6958.

370. Hansen, M., Stoltenberg, M., Host, N. B., Boesby, S., Lorenzen, I., and Bentsen, K. D. (1995). Glucocorticoids inhibit the synthesis rate of type III collagen, but do not affect the hepatic clearance of its aminoterminal propeptide (PIIINP). *Scand. J. Clin. Lab. Invest.* **55**, 543–548.

371. Silbermann, M. M. M. (1987). Dexamethasone impairs growth and collagen synthesis in condylar cartilage in vitro. *Bone Miner.* **2**, 87–106.

372. Advani, S., Lafrancis, D., Bogdanovic, E., Taxel, P., Raisz, L. G., and Kream, B. E. (1997). Dexamethasone suppresses in vivo levels of bone collagen synthesis in neonatal mice. *Bone* **20**, 41–46.

373. Kream, B. E., Tetradis, S., Lafrancis, D., Fall, P. M., Feyen, J. H., and Raisz, L. G. (1997). Modulation of the effects of glucocorticoids on collagen synthesis in fetal rat calvariae by insulin-like growth factor binding protein-2. *J. Bone Miner. Res.* **12**, 889–895.

374. Bird, J. L., and Tyler, J. A. (1994). Dexamethasone potentiates the stimulatory effect of insulin-like growth factor-I on collagen

production in cultured human fibroblasts. *J. Endocrinol.* **142**, 571–579.

375. Goldring, M., Birkhead, J., Sandell, L., Kimura, T., and Krane, S. (1988). Interleukin 1 supresses expression of cartilage-specific types II and IX collagens and increases types I and III collagens in human chondrocytes. *J. Clin. Invest.* **82**, 2026–2037.

376. Goldring, M. B., Fukuo, K., Birkhead, J. R., Dudek, E., and Sandell, L. J. (1994). Transcriptional suppression by interleukin-1 and interferon-gamma of type II collagen gene expression in human chondrocytes. *J. Cell. Biochem.* **54**, 85–99.

377. Scharffetter, K., Heckmann, M., Hatamochi, A., Mauch, C., Stein, B., Riethmuller, G., Ziegler-Heitbrock, H. W., and Krieg, T. (1989). Synergistic effect of tumor necrosis factor-alpha and interferon-gamma on collagen synthesis of human skin fibroblasts in vitro. *Exp. Cell Res.* **181**, 409–419.

378. Kahari, V. M., Chen, Y. Q., Su, M. W., Ramirez, F., and Uitto, J. (1990). Tumor necrosis factor-alpha and interferon-gamma suppress the activation of human type I collagen gene expression by transforming growth factor-beta 1. Evidence for two distinct mechanisms of inhibition at the transcriptional and posttranscriptional levels. *J. Clin. Invest.* **86**, 1489–1495.

379. Bird, J. L., and Tyler, J. A. (1995). Tumour necrosis factor alpha, interferon gamma and dexamethasone regulate IGF-I-maintained collagen production in cultured human fibroblasts. *J. Endocrinol.* **147**, 167–176.

380. Rosenbloom, J., Feldman, G., Freundlich, B., and Jimenez, S. A. (1986). Inhibition of excessive scleroderma fibroblast collagen production by recombinant gamma-interferon. Association with a coordinate decrease in types I and III procollagen messenger RNA levels. *Arthritis Rheum.* **29**, 851–856.

381. Pinnell, S. R. (1985). Regulation of collagen biosynthesis by ascorbic acid: A review. *Yale J. Biol. Med.* **58**, 553–559.

382. Schwarz, R. I. (1985). Procollagen secretion meets the minimum requirements for the rate-controlling step in the ascorbate induction of procollagen synthesis. *J. Biol. Chem.* **260**, 3045–3049.

383. Erdmann, S., Müller, W., Bahrami, S., Vornehm, S., Mayer, H., Bruckner, P., von der Mark, K., and Burkhardt, H. (1995), Differential effects of parathyroid hormone fragments on collagen gene expression in chondrocytes. *J. Cell Biol.* **135**, 1179–1191.

384. Crabb, I. D., O'Keefe, R. J., Puzas, J. E., and Rosier, R. N. (1992). Differential effects of parathyroid hormone on chick growth plate and articular chondrocytes. *Calcif. Tissue Int.* **50**, 61–66.

385. Benya, P., and Padilla, P. D. (1986). Modulation of the rabbit chondrocyte phenotype by retinoic acid terminates type II collagen synthesis without inducing type I collagen: The modulated phenotype differs from that produced by subculture. *Dev. Biol.* **118**, 296–305.

386. Pacifici, M., Golden, E. B., Iwamoto, M., and Adams, S. L. (1991). Retinoic acid treatment induces type X collagen gene expression in cultured chick chondrocytes. *Exp. Cell Res.* **195**, 38–46.

387. Dietz, U., Aigner, T., Bertling, W., and von der Mark, K. (1993). Alterations of collagen mRNA expression during retinoic acid induced chondrocyte modulation: Absence of untranslated alpha 1(I) mRNA in hyaline chondrocytes. *J. Cell. Biochem.* **52**, 57–68.

CHAPTER 2

Fibrillogenesis and Maturation of Collagens

SIMON P. ROBINS   Skeletal Research Unit, Rowett Research Institute, Bucksburn, Aberdeen AB21 9SB

I. INTRODUCTION

The biophysical characteristics of bone and cartilage are governed to a large degree by the properties of their
respective collagens, which constitute the majority of the protein content of these tissues. The properties of the collagens
are, in turn, a consequence primarily of their fibrillar structure, and the characteristics of collagen fibrils dictate not only
the biomechanical properties but also many other metabolic
processes, including susceptibility to degradation. The factors that control collagen fibrillogenesis and the subsequent
stabilization of the fibrils are therefore crucial to an understanding of the dynamics of bone and cartilage metabolism.

There are over 20 genetically distinct forms of collagen,
but for the present discussion we will be particularly concerned with those types that spontaneously self-assemble to
form fibrils: collagens I, II, III, V, and XI. Of these fibrillar
collagens, type I is the major component of bone and collagen II is the main collagenous component of cartilage. It
has become increasingly clear however, that collagen fibrils
rarely comprise a single collagen type and, in addition to
containing mixtures of fibrillar collagens, fibrils often incorporate a number of FACIT (fibril associated with interrupted
triple-helix) collagens, particularly types IX, XII, XIV, and
XIX. Such heterotypic fibrils are prevalent in cartilage but

their structure and assembly will not be discussed here in
detail (see Chapter 20).

Proteoglycans, such as decorin, fibromodulin, and biglycan, together with other matrix constituents, have important influences on collagen fibril formation and, although
the structure and biosynthesis of these components is discussed elsewhere in this volume (Chapters 4 and 5), their
influence on fibrillogenesis will be reviewed briefly. A major factor in the functional capacity of collagen fibrils is the
cross-linking process that imparts the tensile properties and
resistance to enzymatic degradation. The initial cross-linking
reactions and the spontaneous processes that lead to mature
collagen fibrils will be discussed in detail, but changes associated with true aging and senescence that might be defined
as being deleterious to function are beyond the scope of this
review. Several reviews have been published on collagen fibrillogenesis [1] and on cross-linking [2, 3].

II. FIBRILLOGENESIS

Most studies of fibril formation have been performed using collagen I and discussion here will be limited to this type
of collagen. The main steps involved in fibrillogenesis are
illustrated in Figure 1. As the collagen is synthesized and

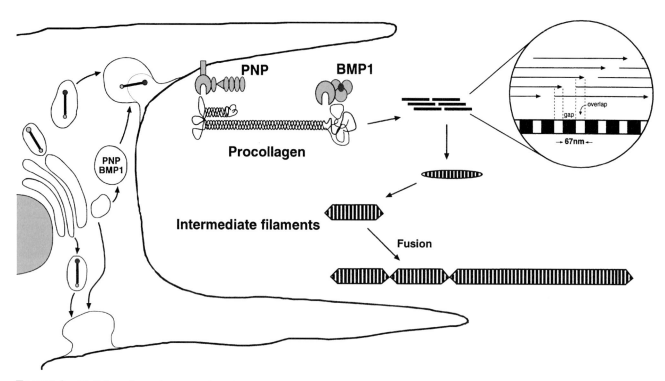

FIGURE 1   Fibril formation and structure: following secretion of procollagen, the propeptides are cleaved by an N-proteinase (PNP) and C-proteinase (BMP1); intermediate fibrils assemble with collagen monomers in a regular, quarter-staggered array (see inset) that gives rise to 67 nm banding; longer fibrils are formed by fusion of intermediates which may also occur laterally. The assembly process is influenced by interactions of both procollagen and the fibrils with proteoglycans and other matrix molecules (not shown).

secreted as a precursor procollagen molecule with globular extensions at both the N- and C-terminal ends (see Chapter 1), the initial events are removal of the extension propeptides, which occurs through the action of discrete proteinases at or close to the cell surface. One function of the propeptides is to prevent intracellular fibril formation, since the released triple-helical collagen monomers have an intrinsic property to self assemble into fibrils arranged in a quarter-staggered array. This organization is mainly an entropy-driven process occurring through disruption of ordered solvent molecules at the monomer surface and is enhanced by specific ionic interactions between neighboring molecules to give a 4D overlap (in Fig. 1). This gap and overlap structure gives rise to the 67 nm banding pattern revealed in the electron microscope after negative staining with phosphotungstic acid where the excess stain enters the gap regions of the fibril.

Procollagen N-proteinase acts at specific bonds in each chain resulting in the release of the intact propeptide. The same enzyme appears to process both procollagens I and II. The C-proteinase, which is identical to the protein initially identified as bone morphogenetic protein-1 (BMP-1), specifically cleaves procollagens I, II, and III at a single locus, releasing the propeptide intact. A procollagen C-proteinase enhancer (PCPE) has been isolated; this 55 kDa glycoprotein appears to exert some control on fibrillogenesis through interaction with the C-proteinase rather than with its substrate [4]. Both proteinases are members of a large family

of zinc-binding metalloproteinases [5]. Evidence shows that the N-proteinase binds to one of the FACIT collagens, type XIV [6], and the C-proteinase has been shown to bind the $\alpha_1\beta_1$ and $\alpha_2\beta_1$ integrins [7]. These proteinases may, therefore, have important biological functions in addition to their role in processing procollagens.

Much of the information currently available on the mechanisms of fibril assembly has come from cell-free systems using purified proteinases to generate collagen monomers *de novo* [8]. Under these conditions, after a relatively short "nucleation" period, intermediate filaments with a blunt (β) end and a pointed (α) end are formed, with growth occurring at the pointed end. Subsequently, growth of the fibril from the blunt end is initiated, giving rise to a parabola-shaped intermediate fibril. Initial studies showed that the intermediate filaments were bipolar with the N-terminals oriented towards both of the pointed ends, thus necessitating a change in orientation at some point along the filament. This type of intermediate filament was subsequently shown to occur *in vivo* [9] although the consequences of the polarity changes have not been established. Fibrils produced from acid-extracted collagen monomers are unipolar and the initial presence of the C-propeptide during fibril formation appears to have a major effect [1]. Both longitudinal and lateral growth of the collagen fibril is believed to occur through fusion of these intermediates. Some studies have shown that only unipolar intermediates undergo fusion; indeed, regulation of the formation of these two types of intermediates may have important influences on fibril growth. Other studies of developing chick tendon support the concept of fibril growth by fusion of fibril segments [10], but they also found a more rapid growth in length with development so that, in an 18-day tendon, no small, intermediate fibril segments were observed [11]. At this stage, analyses of serial sections by transmission electron microscopy showed that fibril ends were detected randomly along the fibril. This observation indicated that single fibrils did not span the full length of tendon and, in contrast to earlier stages of development, no fibrils shorter than 60 μm were detected [11]. As will be discussed later, these results also emphasize the importance of inter- as well as intrafibril cross-linking, since the former are essential in stabilizing the fibrils within the tendon fiber.

A. Factors Affecting Fibril Formation

The kinetics of removal of the propeptides clearly influences fibril formation [12], and transient retention of the N-propeptides has been suggested as a model to account for preferred fibril diameters at intervals of about 11 nm corresponding to cleavage of the propeptides at the surface [13, 14]. Once the propeptides have been removed, however, there are several other factors which affect the nature and rate of fibril formation.

1. TELOPEPTIDES

The short, nonhelical domains at each end of the molecule, the telopeptides, that contain the cross-linking sites (see Section III), are only 15 to 20 amino acids in length but their removal through enzyme treatment essentially abolishes the ability of the remaining triplehelical monomers to form banded fibrils [15]. Experiments in which either N-terminal or C-terminal telopeptides have been specifically removed indicate that the C-telopeptide is important for shortening the "nucleation" time and accelerating lateral accretion, whereas the N-telopeptide is associated with the attainment of the correct banding pattern [16].

2. OTHER FIBRILLAR COLLAGENS

In soft tissues, collagen I forms hybrid fibrils with other fibrillar collagens, particularly collagens III and V. Thus, cofibril formation with collagen III in skin is believed to regulate the diameter of fibrils and probably is associated with the longer retention of the propeptide for collagen type III [17]. Studies of the tissues from mice containing a mutant collagen III gene have demonstrated the crucial role of this molecule for adequate collagen type I fibrillogenesis [18]. In bone, however, collagen III is virtually absent, although about 5% of the collagen is type V. The latter collagen has been shown to form hybrid or heterotypic fibrils in cornea which again act to limit fibril size because of the partial processing of the

N-terminal propeptide of collagen V [19]. Loss of corneal morphology has been demonstrated in corneal fibroblasts where the levels of collagen V had been decreased by introducing a nonfunctional $\alpha 1$(V) gene [20]. The importance of heterotypic fibrils in cartilage collagen assembly is discussed in Chapter 20.

3. FACIT COLLAGENS

The fibril associated collagens with interrupted triple-helix (FACIT) are particularly important in cartilage, but this topic will be dealt with in Chapter 20. For collagen type I, interactions with the FACIT types XII and XIV have major effects in modulating the properties of soft tissues, but these collagens are essentially absent in bone. Collagen types XII and XIV are relatively large molecules with extended globular domains; rather than affecting fibrillogenesis directly in soft tissues, these molecules appear to mediate interactions between fibrils, thereby modulating the biomechanical properties of the tissue [21].

4. OTHER MATRIX CONSTITUENTS

Of the many influences from other matrix constituents on collagen fibrillogenesis, that exerted by the small, leucine-rich proteoglycans, decorin, fibromodulin, and biglycan (see Chapter 5), has probably received the most attention. That decorin plays a major role in collagen fibrillogenesis was demonstrated by the dramatic effects of a decorin gene "knockout" in mice where the phenotype exhibited skin fragility with abnormal morphology characterized by uncontrolled lateral fusion of collagen fibrils [22]. Following suggestions by Scott [23] that these proteoglycans limited the lateral extent of the fibril, models have been proposed in which arch-shaped decorin molecules bind to the collagen helix at the gap region, thereby promoting the correct alignment of the fibril and potentially limiting lateral accretion [24]. Other studies of collagen fibrillogenesis *in vitro* suggest, however, that the presence of decorin increases fibril diameter [25].

A matrix constituent that copurified with lysyl oxidase [26] was found to have marked effects on fibril formation; this 22 kDa protein, termed TRAMP (tyrosine-rich acidic matrix protein), accelerated the rate of fibrillogenesis *in vitro*, resulting in normally-banded fibrils as judged by electron microscopy [27]. It is conceivable that such matrix constituents have important functions in mineralized tissues, as TRAMP was found to be one of the major proteins in extracts of porcine dentine [28].

III. CROSS-LINKING

The formation of intermolecular cross-links within newly formed collagen fibrils conveys the structural stability necessary for tissue function. The main processes involved in the initial formation of intermediate, chemically reducible cross-links followed by maturation to more stable, nonreducible bonds have been established over several years. A number of questions remain, however, concerning the nature of the mature forms of bonds and the mechanisms of tissue-specific cross-link formation. It is clear that lysine-derived cross-links account for almost all cross-linking in young tissue and that their formation is driven by a single enzymatic process—the action of lysyl oxidase.

A. Lysyl Oxidase

Lysyl oxidase is one of a family of copper-dependent amine oxidase enzymes. For collagen, the enzyme catalyzes the conversion of lysine or hydroxylysine residues in the N- and C-telopeptides to aldehyde residues (Fig. 2). For many years, there was some debate concerning the cofactors necessary for activity, but evidence has demonstrated that the active center contains lysine tyrosyl quinone formed by the cross-linking of two amino acid side chains within the enzyme [29]. Early studies showed that lysyl oxidase acts extracellularly and requires as a substrate native collagen fibrils in a quarter-staggered array [30]. This observation led to suggestions that amino acid residues at the overlap sites in the helix of adjacent molecules in the fibril participate in the reaction; these sites are known to have highly conserved amino acid sequences [31]. Studies using synthetic peptide substrates have been interpreted in terms of charge neutralization at the site of oxidation [32].

Lysyl oxidase is synthesized as a precursor which undergoes posttranslational glycosylation [33]. The propeptide portion appears to be cleaved by the same metalloproteinase that cleaves the procollagen type I C-propeptide, BMP-1/C-proteinase, although the presence of the precursor peptide is not necessary for the folding and secretion of lysyl oxidase [34]. Despite its copper dependence, lysyl oxidase appears to be rather insensitive to nutritional copper deficiency, as judged by animal experiments [35]. Expression of the enzyme is, however, regulated by several cytokines including transforming growth factor-β [36]. The finding that the *ras* recision gene, *rrg*, encodes a form of lysyl oxidase and that interferon-induced reversion of transformed cells is accompanied by restoration of *rrg* expression [37] suggests that lysyl oxidase may also have important functions in tumor suppression.

B. Tissue Specificity of Cross-Linking

As shown in Figure 3, the two major pathways of cross-linking depend on whether the residue in the telopeptide is lysine or hydroxylysine. As will become evident later in this section, the presence of hydroxylysine in the telopeptide has a profound effect on the stability of the cross-links initially formed as well as on the final products. The types of cross-link formed are related to the tissue rather than to the collagen type, and the tissue specificity is governed primarily by enzymatic hydroxylation reactions in the telopeptides. Thus, in skin collagen, virtually no hydroxylysine is present in the telopeptides so that cross-linking proceeds through the aldimine route (Fig. 3) and ultimately to histidine-containing compounds. In cartilage and bone, a large proportion of the

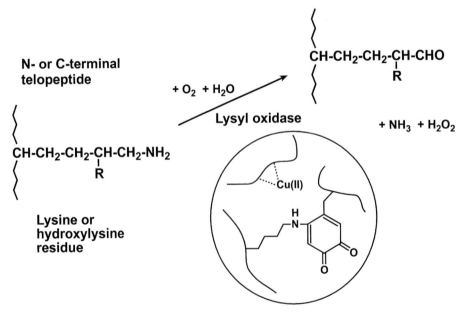

FIGURE 2   Lysyl oxidase action causes conversion of telopeptide lysine or hydroxylysine residues (R = H or OH, respectively) to aldehydes. The inset shows the lysyl tyrosyl quinone and Cu(II) at the active center of the enzyme.

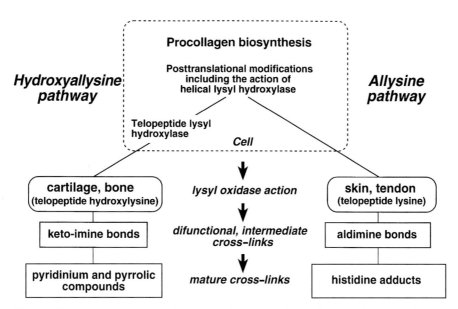

FIGURE 3   Collagen cross-linking is tissue specific. Hydroxylation of lysine in the telopeptide intracellularly gives rise to two pathways of extracellular cross-linking, the lysine aldehyde (allysine) pathway
and the hydroxyallysine pathway; the latter results in mainly pyridinium and pyrrolic cross-links in bone
and cartilage.

telopeptide lysines are hydroxylated, giving rise mainly to
keto-imine forms of cross-link which can lead to the formation of pyridinium cross-links on maturation.

Hydroxylation of lysine residues in the telopeptides clearly
has crucial effects on cross-linking. Indirect evidence from
a number of sources has suggested that the enzyme that hy-
droxylates lysine residues in the telopeptides is distinct from
that which acts on lysine residues destined to be in the helix.
Highly purified lysyl hydroxylase was found to be inactive
on isolated telopeptide [38] and, in various diseases or animal models, a disparity between changes in hydroxylation of
telopeptide and helical lysine residues was observed [39–41].
Further evidence for a telopeptide lysyl hydroxylase enzyme
was obtained by analysis of tissues from patients with a rare
form of osteogenesis imperfecta [42]. Bone from affected individuals contained normal amounts of hydroxylysine in the
helix but no pyridinium cross-links were detected, indicating a defect in the gene for telopeptide lysyl hydroxylase.
Although the gene for this novel enzyme has not yet been
identified, it has been located on chromosome 17 [42]. Interestingly, there appear to be tissue-specific forms of this
enzyme, as pyridinium cross-link formation in cartilage and
ligaments of the affected individuals was normal. Helical lysyl hydroxylase also has tissue-specific isotypes, of which
three have now been described [43]. Tissue differences in
the patterns of collagen cross-linking are therefore due to
variations in the expression and activities of telopeptide and
helical lysyl hydroxylases.

Some hydroxylysine residues in central parts of fibrillar
collagens destined to become the helix are further modified
enzymatically during synthesis by addition of galactosyl or

both galactosyl and glucosyl residues to the hydroxyl group
(see Chapter 1). These hydroxylysine glycosides may participate in cross-linking, giving rise to glycosylated forms of both
the difunctional cross-links and their maturation products.

C. Mechanisms of Cross-Linking

1. INTERMEDIATE DIFUNCTIONAL CROSS-LINKS

Following the action of lysyl oxidase, the lysine aldehyde (allysine) or hydroxylysine aldehyde (hydroxyallysine)
residues undergo spontaneous reactions according to the separate pathways indicated in Figure 4. For allysine, reaction
with a hydroxylysine or lysine residue in the helix results
in the formation of the aldimines, dehydro-hydroxylysinon-
orleucine (Δ-HLNL) or dehydro-lysinonorleucine (Δ-LNL),
respectively. These aldimine bonds provide the main structural stability in newly-formed dermal tissue but are readily
cleaved by heat or dilute acids, rendering such tissue completely soluble in dilute acetic acid. Another consequence of
the chemical lability of the aldimine bonds is that reduction
with borohydride is essential to stabilize the compounds to
the hydrolytic processes necessary for their isolation. The use
of radiolabelled borohydride was helpful initially in identifying the reduced compounds as HLNL and LNL [44].

The corresponding difunctional cross-links formed
through reactions of hydroxyallsine with helical hydroxylysine or lysine residues are stabilized by a spontaneous Amadori
rearrangement to produce hydroxylysino-5-keto-norleucine
(HLKNL) or lysino-5-keto-norleucine (LKNL), respectively

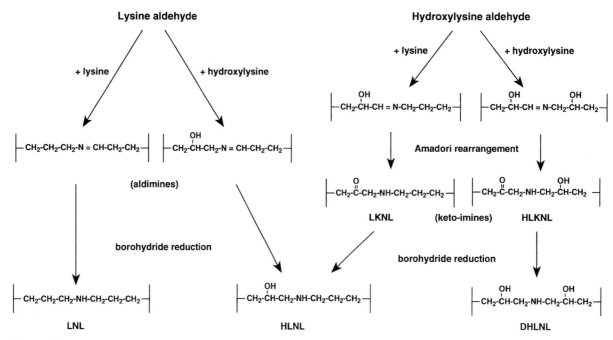

FIGURE 4   Difunctional cross-link formation occurs in different ways depending on the aldehyde. Telopeptide lysine aldehyde reacts with lysine or hydroxylysine residues in the helix to form aldimine (Schiff base) cross-links that give rise to LNL and HLNL on reduction with borohydride. When hydroxylysine aldehyde is present in the telopeptide, the products initially formed undergo an Amadori rearrangement to the more stable keto-imines, which on reduction give HLNL and DHLNL.

(Fig. 4). This rearrangement renders these compounds stable to the effects of mild acid treatment and peptides containing these cross-links have been isolated without borohydride reduction. After reduction, HLKNL and LKNL are converted to dihydroxy-lysinonorleucine (DHLNL) and hydroxylysinonorleucine (HLNL). The latter compound can therefore be derived from both the allysine and hydroxyallysine pathways (Fig. 4), but the products of the two pathways can be distinguished by identifying the products of a Smith degradation (periodate cleavage followed by borohydride reduction): in bone about 75% of HLNL is derived from hydroxyallysine [45].

Another difference between the lysine aldehyde and hydroxylysine aldehyde pathways of cross-linking is that the former compound can participate in an "aldol" condensation reaction to give an intramolecular cross-link between the α-chains of a single molecule. The structure of the aldol condensation product (ACP) undergoes further reactions yielding products that have been detected in tissues after reduction with borohydride. Hydroxyallysine does not form intramolecular aldols and no corresponding products from this pathway have been detected. The main product derived from the aldol that was identified in borohydride-reduced tissue was the compound histidino-hydroxymerodesmosine (HHMD); its creation involved the addition of hydroxylysine and histidine residues to the ACP [46]. Although evidence was presented that this compound was an artifact of the borohydride reduction process and that the nonreduced form did

not constitute a cross-link *in vivo* [47], contradictory results were reported subsequently [48]. This question still has not been fully resolved.

2. MATURATION OF INTERMEDIATE CROSS-LINKS

The reducible intermediate cross-links decrease in concentration during maturation and aging of the tissues [44]. Considerable effort over several years has been expended in attempting to define the way in which these bonds are modified during maturation and thereby establish the forms of cross-link present in older tissues. Initial studies indicating that reduction *in vivo* yields the same cross-links as those produced by borohydride reduction have been discounted. A proposed oxidative pathway of modification also has not been substantiated. As discussed in the following sections, the best characterized products of maturation are the pyridinium cross-links in bone and cartilage and a histidine adduct in soft tissues. There is also evidence for pyrrolic forms of cross-links (Fig. 5). It is important to bear in mind, however, that these processes have not been fully characterized and several questions remain, particularly with respect to kinetics and stoichiometry.

a. Pyridinium Cross-links   A fluorescent, 3-hydroxypyridinium compound in hydrolysates of bovine tendon was identified by Fujimoto and colleagues [49] as a trifunctional cross-link, termed pyridinoline. Although the function of pyridinoline as a cross-link initially was disputed [50], further

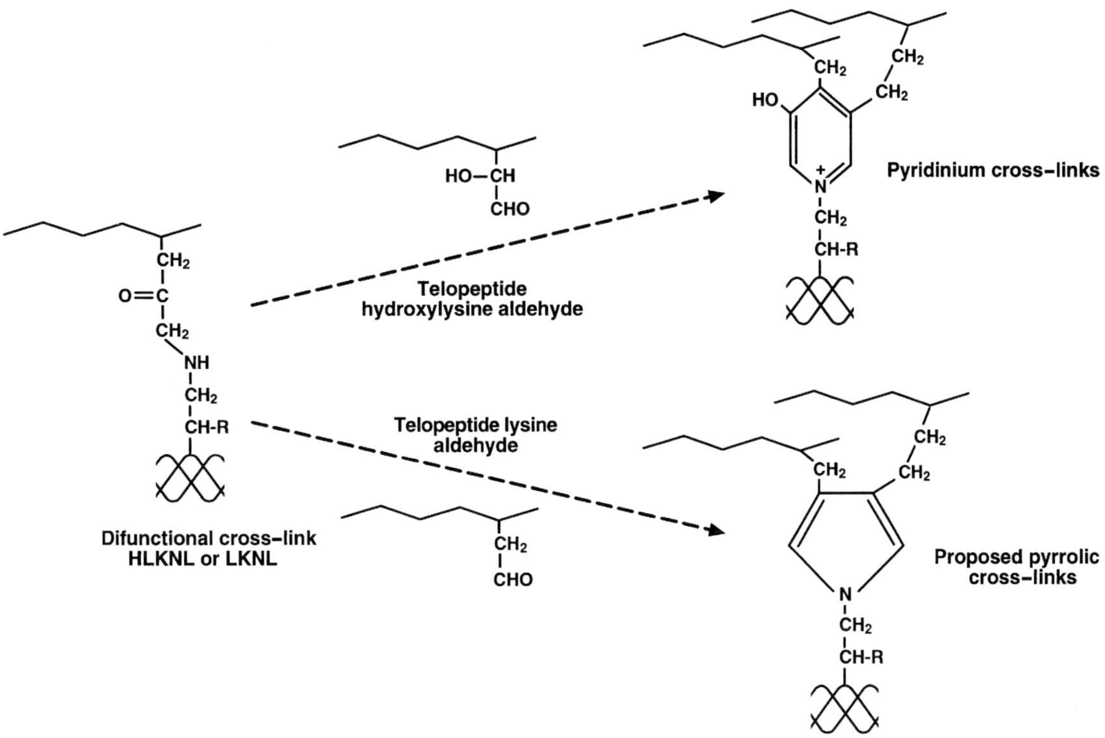

FIGURE 5 Pyridinium and pyrrolic cross-links are the best characterized products of maturation. The difunctional cross-links hydroxylysino-5-ketonorleucine (HLKNL) or lysino-5-ketonorleucine (LKNL), where R = −OH or −H, respectively, are converted to the different trifunctional cross-links depending on whether the telopeptide aldehydes are hydroxylated.

structural studies [51] and characterization of pyridinoline-containing peptides [52, 53] confirmed its existence as a cross-link in cartilage. An analog, named deoxypyridinoline, was discovered in bone [54]. Because the latter cross-link involved reaction of a lysine residue from the helix, it has been termed lysyl-pyridinoline, or LP, to distinguish this compound from pyridinoline derived from helical hydroxylysine, which is referred to as hydroxylysyl-pyridinoline or HP [55]. Two mechanisms for formation of the pyridinium cross-links have been proposed: one involving interaction between two intermediate keto-imine cross-links [56] and the other a reaction between the keto-imine and hydroxylysine aldehyde [51]. The chemistry of these two mechanisms is in fact very similar but there are important functional implications as will be discussed in Section III.E.

b. Pyrrolic Cross-links   The initial suggestion for the presence in collagen of pyrrolic cross-links came from work by Scott and colleagues [57] and was based on the formation of colored reaction products of collagen hydrolysates with Ehrlich's reagent (p-dimethylaminobenzaldehyde in acid solution). The initial work was difficult to interpret because the apparent concentrations of pyrrole cross-links in different tissues were not consistent with the known differences in cross-link pathways. Later studies of pyrrole-containing peptides [58] provided a firmer basis for the presence of these

cross-links, and identification of cross-linked peptides in tendon led to a proposed mechanism of formation [59]. This proposal suggests that in tissues where not all of the telopeptide lysine residues are hydroxylated, lysine aldehyde may interact with the intermediate keto-imine to form a pyrrolic trifunctional cross-link (Fig. 5). According to this mechanism, therefore, pyrrole cross-links should be absent from dermal tissue because of the lack of keto-imines and also from cartilage because the telopeptides are fully hydroxylated; this tissue distribution has been verified experimentally [3]. Bone has been shown to contain relatively large amounts of the pyrrolic cross-links [41], and preliminary evidence suggests that these are present in higher amounts within the N-terminal telopeptides in collagen type I [60]. All of the quantitative assessments are, however, based on color yields of standard compounds and, until the pyrrolic cross-links are fully characterized, some doubts about these figures remain. The main reason for the lack of characterization of the pyrrole compounds is their instability during the hydrolytic and chromatographic procedures necessary to isolate them. In particular, the pyrroles are susceptible to oxidation and polymerization reactions which result in diminishing yields during purification of these compounds. Some data from mass spectrometry of peptides from human bone collagen were interpreted as representing a hydrated, ring-cleaved product of a pyrrole-cross-linked peptide [60].

c. Kinetics of Cross-link Maturation There have been relatively few studies of the kinetics of cross-link maturation and most of these have involved administration of radioactively labelled lysine to rats. From these types of study, the half-life of the reducible, difunctional cross-links has been estimated as a few weeks [61]. Several groups have shown that the concentrations of reducible, intermediate cross-links remain much higher in bone than in other tissues, including skin and cartilage. The continual turnover of bone matrix, in contrast to the other tissues, undoubtedly contributes to this observation and results in the higher proportion of recently-synthesized collagen found in bone.

D. Effects of Mineralization on Cross-Linking

The structural features of collagen type I fibrils in bone that allow mineralization to occur have not been fully elucidated, and conflicting reports have been published. It is generally agreed, however, that the types and location of cross-linking are different in bone compared with soft tissues containing collagen type I, such as skin or tendon. Analyses of the C-telopeptide cross-linking during maturation of bovine bone indicated that some reducible, difunctional cross-links were converted to pyridinium bonds, but a proportion also was cleaved to free lysine and hydroxylysine aldehydes leading to the suggestion that mineralization itself induces structural alterations in the fibril and a decreased connectivity in C-terminal cross-linking [62]. Studies of mineralized tissues and model compounds indicated, however, that the apparent formation of aldehydes may, in fact, have been due to the method used to demineralize the bone prior to reduction with borohydride; extended treatment with alkaline EDTA altered the cross-link profile whereas demineralization in acid did not [41].

Because the concentrations of pyridinium cross-links in mammalian bone are relatively low throughout life in comparison with other tissues, such as cartilage [63], it has been suggested that the presence of mineral arrests maturation of difunctional cross-links into pyridinoline and deoxypyridinoline. Arguing against this contention is the fact that "aging" *in vitro* of mineralized bone (incubation in physiological saline at 37°C) converts precursor cross-links to their mature forms [64]; however, earlier studies indicated that there might be differences in the rate of reaction between mineralized and nonmineralized bone [65]. The formation of pyrrole cross-links provides a more complete network of mature cross-links and, although it has been suggested that the pyrroles are functionally the more important mature cross-link in avian bone [3], so far there is little evidence that this is the case for mammalian bone.

The natural mineralization of turkey leg tendon at around 12–14 weeks of age has been widely used as a model system for the study of structural changes in collagen type I during the addition of mineral [66]. Yamauchi and Katz [67]

made the intriguing discovery that there was a change in the pattern of pyridinium cross-links such that the nonmineralized portion contained primarily pyridinoline whereas the mineralized portion also contained a high proportion of deoxypyridinoline. Because this altered cross-linking pattern appears to involve changes in the intracellular hydroxylation of lysine residues, these results inferred that mineralization is accompanied by the production of a new matrix with modified postribosomal modifications. Similar changes in lysine hydroxylation and cross-link patterns were found to be associated with changes in thermal characteristics of the collagenous matrix [41]. These experiments serve to emphasize the fact that collagen type I capable of mineralization exhibits specific patterns of posttranslational hydroxylation which in turn are associated with particular cross-linking patterns, of which the presence of deoxypyridinoline is one characteristic.

E. Cross-Linking in Relation to Molecular Packing

Although there is still some debate as to the most appropriate molecular packing model for fibrillar collagen, the limitations imposed by the chemistry and location of the intermolecular cross-links has to be accommodated [68]. An arrangement of compressed pentafibrils in a pseudohexagonal lattice satisfies both the biochemical and X-ray diffraction data [69] and one form of this molecular arrangement is shown in Figure 6. For mineralized tissues, three-dimensional image reconstruction methods and electron microscopy combined with computed tomography have provided evidence that some mineral crystals span the hole regions of adjacent microfibrils [70], a configuration that requires all microfibrils to be in register with their hole regions aligned. The difunctional intermediate cross-links are known to stabilize the quarter-staggered overlap (between segments 1 and 5 in Fig. 6). During their maturation to trifunctional pyridinium or pyrrole cross-links, reactions can occur either with an aldehyde from another chain of the same molecule, giving an intrafibril cross-link or with a reactive group from an adjacent microfibril, giving an interfibrillar bond linking three molecules. Distinguishing between these possibilities is difficult biochemically, but these arrangements will have major effects on the functional properties of the tissue. It should be noted that the mechanism of formation of mature cross-links proposed by Eyre and colleagues [56, 60] with the reaction of two difunctional cross-links can only occur between microfibrils in register.

F. Biological Consequences of Intermolecular Collagen Cross-Linking

Inhibition of collagen cross-linking via the dietary lathyrogen, β-amino-proprionitrile (βAPN), provides graphic

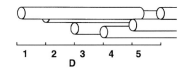

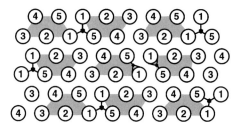

FIGURE 6   Inter- and intrafibrillar cross-links are shown by this schematic representation of quarter-staggered collagen molecules, 4.4D periods in length, where each segment is numbered (upper). One possible arrangement of compressed microfibrils (pentafilaments denoted by the shaded areas) is shown (lower) with interfibrillar cross-links between segments 1 and 5 at the periphery and intrafibrillar crosslinks toward the center.

evidence of the importance of the intermolecular bonds for proper tissue function. The lathyrogen, originally discovered as the toxic agent released *in vivo* after chronic ingestion of the sweet pea *Lathyrus oderatus*, is now known to be an irreversible inhibitor of the cross-link initiating enzyme, lysyl oxidase, and leads to severe malformations in the skeleton as well as to many other abnormalities. Following the discovery of this agent in 1959 [34], βAPN has been used extensively for both *in vivo* and *in vitro* experiments to provide noncrosslinked matrix proteins for research purposes. In addition to the developmental problems associated with a severe lack crosslinking, the quantity and nature of cross-links have profound effects on the susceptibility to proteolysis and the mechanical characteristics of collagen fibrils.

1. Susceptibility to Proteolysis

The triple helical structure of individual monomers within the collagen fibril is resistant to most proteolytic enzymes except specific collagenases or matrix metalloproteinases (see Chapter 10) which cleave through all three chains simultaneously at a point three quarters distance from the N-terminal end. Other enzymes, such as cathepsins and elastase, cleave the telopeptide portions of the molecule between the cross-linking site and the helix, thus depolymerizing the fibril. Evidence has been presented that cathepsin K, a product of osteoclasts, may also cleave collagen I within the helical region [71]. The presence of the lysine-derived crosslinks has, however, been shown to affect dramatically the susceptibility of the fibrils to proteolysis. Thus, for fibrils that were formed *in vitro* from soluble chick bone collagen, the susceptibility to proteolysis was related directly to the concentrations of difunctional cross-links in the fibrils introduced by the actions of purified lysyl oxidase [72].

Although these studies appeared to show that as little as one cross-link per ten collagen molecules was sufficient to impart a two- to three-fold resistance to collagenase digestion, this may be an underestimate because the cross-link values represent a figure for the whole fibril but the methods used will have introduced higher concentrations of cross-links at the surface. Maturation of fibrils leads to a lower susceptibility to enzyme degradation, and the formation of multifunctional cross-links that link more than two molecules (see Section III.E) may be important in giving rise to these properties. Distinct from maturational changes, the introduction of crosslinks between the helices of adjacent molecules through ageing processes, including advanced glycation end-product (AGE) reactions, leads to major changes in the properties of the fibrils [2].

The presence of a fibrillar network cross-linked at the telopeptides means that once cleavage of a peripheral molecule by collagenase has occurred the cleaved chains will remain attached for a period of time to the fibril through the crosslinks. At body temperature, the cleaved fragments denature and can be detected by specific antibodies that react only with sequence-dependent epitopes, thus providing a means to assess immunocytochemically patterns of degradation in tissues [73]. Similar techniques have been used to detect degradation patterns in cartilage [74].

2. Mechanical Properties

There is no doubt that cross-linking in collagen is primarily responsible for the strength of the fibrils, but the relative contributions of the different types of cross-links is less clear. Studies of the effects of partial lathyrism on the mechanical strength of embryonic avian bone indicated that a 10% decrease in the concentration of the difunctional ketoimine cross-link resulted in a 15% decrease in bone strength [64]. Similar studies have shown that the concentrations of pyridinoline are also related to the strength of adult bone in the rabbit [75] and rat [76]. It has been suggested that the pyrrole cross-links are more important than the pyridinium cross-links in determining the mechanical properties of bone [64], but this conclusion is based on experiments in avian bone which contains much smaller proportions of the pyridinium cross-links than that found in mammalian bone. In bovine tendon, the concentrations of the pyrrolic and pyridinium cross-links were found to have similar positive correlations with thermal stability [77], suggesting that both types of cross-link was performing a similar function. There appear to be differences in the relative proportions of crosslinks involving the N- and C-terminal telopeptides, with about 85% of the pyrroles being present at the N-terminus whereas the pyridinium cross-links were equally distributed [60]; it is unclear whether these differences affect the biomechanical properties. Whether the multifunctional cross-links are within or between fibrils is an important question in this respect (see Section III.E).

IV. CONCLUDING REMARKS

Much progress has been made in understanding the complex processes of collagen fibril formation and stabilization. The intracellular postribosomal modifications of collagen are key to many of the properties of the fibrillar collagens and these control many of the biophysical properties, including the propensity to mineralize and tissue strength. Although age-related changes have not been dealt with in this chapter, such changes may have important implications for diseases such as osteoporosis. Indeed, increased hydroxylation of lysines with age has been reported and this may contribute both to changes in crosslinking patterns and to altered levels of hydroxylysine glycosides [78]. The latter may give rise to the production of smaller collagen fibrils that have modified, less robust mechanical properties consistent with the changes seen in osteoporosis. Further studies are necessary, however, to confirm the functional effects of such changes in collagen processing and to consider these in relation to many other changes that occur. One age-related change in collagen structure is an aspartyl to isoaspartyl transformation within the C-terminal telopeptide of the collagen $\alpha 1(\text{I})$ chain [79]. This β-aspartyl peptide has proved useful as a biochemical marker (see Chapter 29). Similar transformations have been shown to occur within the N-telopeptide of the $\alpha 2(\text{I})$ chain [80], although the structural consequences, if any, of these changes are nuclear. More detailed studies of the functional consequences of structural changes in collagen and their changes with age provide many challenges for future research aimed at understanding skeletal diseases.

Acknowledgments

I am grateful to Dr. Karl Kadler for helpful discussions and for providing illustrations (http://www.empgu.man.ac.uk/emunit) which form the basis of Figure 1, and to the Scottish Office Agriculture, Environment, and Fisheries Department for support.

References

1. Kadler, K. E., Holmes, D. F., Trotter, J. A., and Chapman, J. A. (1996). Collagen fibril formation. *Biochem. J.* **316**, 1–11.

2. Reiser, K., McCormick, R. J., and Rucker, R. B. (1992). Enzymatic and nonenzymatic cross-linking of collagen and elastin. *FASEB J.* **6**, 2439–2449.

3. Knott, L., and Bailey, A. J. (1998). Collagen cross-links in mineralizing tissues: A review of their chemistry, function, and clinical relevance. *Bone* **22**, 181–187.

4. Hulmes, D. J., Mould, A. P., and Kessler, E. (1997). The CUB domains of procollagen C-proteinase enhancer control collagen assembly solely by their effect on procollagen C-proteinase/bone morphogenetic protein-1. *Matrix Biol.* **16**, 41–45.

5. Prockop, D. J., Sieron, A. L., and Li, S. W. (1998). Procollagen N-proteinase and procollagen C-proteinase. Two unusual metalloproteinases that are essential for procollagen processing probably have important roles in development and cell signaling. *Matrix Biol.* **16**, 399–408.

6. Colige, A., Beschin, A., Samyn, B., Goebels, Y., Vanbeeumen, J., Nusgens, B., and Lapiere, C. (1995). Characterization and partial amino acid sequencing of a 107-kDa procollagen I N-proteinase purified by affinity chromatography on immobilized type XIV collagen. *J. Biol. Chem.* **270**, 16724–16730.

7. Davies, D., Tuckwell, D. S., Calderwood, D. A., Weston, S. A., Takigawa, M., and Humphries, M. J. (1997). Molecular characterisation of integrin-procollagen C-propeptide interactions. *Eur. J. Biochem.* **246**, 274–282.

8. Kadler, K. E., Hojima, Y., and Prockop, D. J. (1987). Assembly of collagen fibrils de novo by cleavage of the type I pC-collagen with procollagen C-proteinase. Assay of critical concentration demonstrates that collagen self-assembly is a classical example of an entropy-driven process. *J. Biol. Chem.* **262**, 15696–15701.

9. Holmes, D. F., Lowe, M. P., and Chapman, J. A. (1994). Vertebrate (chick) collagen fibrils formed in vivo can exhibit a reversal in molecular polarity. *J. Mol. Biol.* **235**, 80–83.

10. Birk, D. E., Nurminskaya, M. V., and Zycband, E. I. (1995). Collagen fibrillogenesis in situ: fibril segments undergo post-depositional modifications resulting in linear and lateral growth during matrix development. *Dev. Dyn.* **202**, 229–243.

11. Birk, D. E., Zycband, E. I., Woodruff, S., Winkelmann, D. A., and Trelstad, R. L. (1997). Collagen fibrillogenesis in situ: Fibril segments become long fibrils as the developing tendon matures. *Dev. Dyn.* **208**, 291–298.

12. Mellor, S. J., Atkins, G. L., and Hulmes, D. J. S. (1991). Developmental changes in the type I procollagen processing pathway in chick-embryo cornea. *Biochem. J.* **276**, 777–784.

13. Hulmes, D. J. (1983). A possible mechanism for the regulation of collagen fibril diameter in vivo. *Collagen Relat. Res.* **3**, 317–321.

14. Chapman, J. A. (1989). The regulation of size and form in the assembly of collagen fibrils in vivo. *Biopolymers* **28**, 1367–1382.

15. Helseth, D. L., Jr., and Veis, A. (1981). Collagen self-assembly in vitro. Differentiating specific telopeptide-dependent interactions using selective enzyme modification and the addition of free amino telopeptide. *J. Biol. Chem.* **256**, 7118–7128.

16. Capaldi, M. J., and Chapman, J. A. (1982). The C-terminal extrahelical peptide of type I collagen and its role in fibrillogenesis in vitro. *Biopolymers* **21**, 2291–2313.

17. Fleischmajer, R., MacDonald, E. D., Perlish, J. S., Burgeson, R. E., and Fisher, L. W. (1990). Dermal collagen fibrils are hybrids of type I and type III collagen molecules. *J. Struct. Biol.* **105**, 162–169.

18. Liu, X., Wu, H., Byrne, M., Krane, S., and Jaenisch, R. (1997). Type III collagen is crucial for collagen I fibrillogenesis and for normal cardiovascular development. *Proc. Natl. Acad. Sci. U.S.A.* **94**, 1852–1856.

19. Linsenmayer, T., Gibney, E., Igoe, F., Gordon, M., Fitch, J., Fessler, L., and Birk, D. (1993). Type V collagen: Molecular structure and fibrillar organization of the chicken alpha 1(V) NH2-terminal domain, a putative regulator of corneal fibrillogenesis. *J. Cell. Biol.* **121**, 1181–1189.

20. Marchant, J. K., Hahn, R. A., Linsenmayer, T. F., and Birk, D. E. (1996). Reduction of type V collagen using a dominant-negative strategy alters the regulation of fibrillogenesis and results in the loss of corneal-specific fibril morphology. *J. Cell. Biol.* **135**, 1415–1426.

21. Nishiyama, T., McDonough, A. M., Bruns, R. R., and Burgeson, R. E. (1994). Type XII and XIV collagens mediate interactions between banded collagen fibers in vitro and may modulate extracellular matrix deformability. *J. Biol. Chem.* **269**, 28193–28199.

22. Danielson, K. G., Baribault, H., Holmes, D. F., Graham, H., Kadler, K. E., and Iozzo, R. V. (1997). Targeted disruption of decorin leads to abnormal collagen fibril morphology and skin fragility. *J. Cell Biol.* **136**, 729–743.

23. Scott, J. (1991). Proteoglycan—collagen interactions in connective tissues—ultrastructural, biochemical, functional and evolutionary aspects. *Int. J. Biol. Macromol.* **13**, 157–161.

24. Weber, I. T., Harrison, R. W., and Iozzo, R. V. (1996). Model structure of decorin and implications for collagen fibrillogenesis. *J. Biol. Chem.* **271**, 31767–31770.

25. Kuc, I. M., and Scott, P. G. (1997). Increased diameters of collagen fibrils precipitated in vitro in the presence of decorin from various connective tissues. *Connect. Tissue Res.* **36**, 287–296.

26. Cronshaw, A., MacBeath, J., Shackleton, D., Collins, J., Fothergill, G. L., and Hulmes, D. (1993). TRAMP (tyrosine rich acidic matrix protein), a protein that co-purifies with lysyl oxidase from porcine skin. Identification of TRAMP as the dermatan sulphate proteoglycan-associated 22K extracellular matrix protein. *Matrix* **13**, 255–266.

27. MacBeath, J., Shackleton, D., and Hulmes, D. (1993). Tyrosine-rich acidic matrix protein (TRAMP) accelerates collagen fibril formation in vitro. *J. Biol. Chem.* **268**, 19826–19832.

28. Domenicucci, C., Goldberg, H. A., and Sodek, J. (1997). Identification of lysyl oxidase and TRAMP as the major proteins in dissociative extracts of the demineralized collagen matrix of porcine dentine. *Connect. Tissue Res.* **36**, 151–163.

29. Wang, S. X., Mure, M., Medzihradszky, K. F., Burlingame, A. L., Brown, D. E., Dooley, D. M., Smith, A. J., Kagan, H. M., and Klinman, J. P. (1996). A crosslinked cofactor in lysyl oxidase: Redox function for amino acid side chains. *Science* **273**, 1078–1084.

30. Siegel, R. C. (1979). Lysyl oxidase. *Int. Rev. Connect. Tissue Res.* **8**, 73–118.

31. Fietzek, P. P., Allmann, H., Rauterberg, J., and Wachter, E. (1977). Ordering of cyanogen bromide peptides of type III collagen based on their homology to type I collagen: Preservation of sites for crosslink formation during evolution. *Proc. Natl. Acad. Sci. U.S.A.* **74**, 84–86.

32. Frischholz, S., Beier, F., Girkontaite, I., Wagner, K., Poschl, E., Turnay, J., Mayer, U., and von der Mark, K. (1998). Characterization of human type X procollagen and its NC-1 domain expressed as recombinant proteins in HEK293 cells. *J. Biol. Chem.* **273**, 4547–4555.

33. Trackman, P., Bedell, H. D., Tang, J., and Kagan, H. (1992). Post-translational glycosylation and proteolytic processing of a lysyl oxidase precursor. *J. Biol. Chem.* **267**, 8666–8671.

34. Levene, C. I., and Gross, J. (1959). Alterations in the state of molecular aggregation of collagen induced in chick embryos by beta-aminopropionitrile (lathyrus factor). *J. Exp. Med.* **110**, 771–790.

35. Rucker, R. B., Romero Chapman, N., Wong, T., Lee, J., Steinberg, F. M., McGee, C., Clegg, M. S., Reiser, K., Kosonen, T., Uriu Hare, J. Y., Murphy, J., and Keen, C. L. (1996). Modulation of lysyl oxidase by dietary copper in rats. *J. Nutr.* **126**, 51–60.

36. Boak, A. M., Roy, R., Berk, J., Taylor, L., Polgar, P., Goldstein, R. H., and Kagan, H. M. (1994). Regulation of lysyl oxidase expression in lung fibroblasts by transforming growth factor-beta 1 and prostaglandin E2. *Am. J. Respir. Cell Mol. Biol.* **11**, 751–755.

37. Kenyon, K., Contente, S., Trackman, P., Tang, J., Kagan, H., and Friedman, R. (1991). Lysyl oxidase and rrg messenger RNA. *Science* **253**, 802.

38. Royce, P. M., and Barnes, M. J. (1985). Failure of highly purified lysyl hydroxylase to hydroxylatelysyl residues in the non-helical regions of collagen. *Biochem. J.* **230**, 475–480.

39. Gerriets, J. E., Curwin, S. L., and Last, J. A. (1993). Tendon hypertrophy is associated with increased hydroxylation of nonhelical lysine residues at two specific cross-linking sites in type-I collagen. *J. Biol. Chem.* **268**, 25553–25560.

40. Steinmann, B., Eyre, D. R., and Shao, P. (1995). Urinary pyridinoline cross-links in Ehlers-Danlos syndrome type VI (letter). *Am. J. Hum. Genet.* **57**, 1505–1508.

41. Knott, L., Tarlton, J. F., and Bailey, A. J. (1997). Chemistry of collagen cross-linking: Biochemical changes in collagen during the partial mineralization of turkey leg tendon. *Biochem. J.* **322**, 535–542.

42. Bank, R. A., Robins, S. P., Breslau-Siderius, L. J., Bardoel, A. F. J., van der Sluijs, H. A., Pruijs, H. E. H., and TeKoppele, J. M. (1999). Defective collagen crosslinking in bone but not in ligament or cartilage in Bruck syndrome: Evidence for a bone-specific telopeptide lysyl hydroxylase on chromosome 17. *Proc. Natl. Acad. Sci. U.S.A.* **96**, 1054–1058.

43. Valtavaara, M., Szpirer, C., Szpirer, J., and Myllyla, R. (1998). Primary structure, tissue distribution, and chromosomal localization of a novel isoform of lysyl hydroxylase (lysyl hydroxylase 3). *J. Biol. Chem.* **273**, 12881–12886.

44. Bailey, A. J., Robins, S. P., and Balian, G. (1974). Biological significance of the intermolecular crosslinks of collagen. *Nature* **251**, 105–109.

45. Robins, S., and Bailey, A. (1975). The mechanism of stabilization of the reducible intermediate crosslinks. *Biochem. J.* **149**, 381–385.

46. Tanzer, M. L., Housley, T., Berube, L., Fairweather, R., Franzblau, C., and Gallop, P. M. (1973). Structure of two histidine-containing crosslinks from collagen. *J. Biol. Chem.* **248**, 393–402.

47. Robins, S., and Bailey, A. (1973). The characterisation of Fraction C, a possible artifact produced during the reduction of collagen fibres with borohydride. *Biochem. J.* **135**, 657–665.

48. Bernstein, P. H., and Mechanic, G. L. (1980). A natural histidine-based imminium crosslink in collagen and its location. *J. Biol. Chem.* **255**, 10414–10422.

49. Fujimoto, D., Moriguchi, T., Ishida, T., and Hayashi, H. (1978). The structure of pyridinoline, a collagen crosslink. *Biochem. Biophys. Res. Commun.* **84**, 52–57.

50. Elsden, D. F., Light, N. D., and Bailey, A. J. (1980). An investigation of pyridinoline, a putative collagen cross-link. *Biochem. J.* **185**, 531–534.

51. Robins, S. P. (1983). Crosslinking of collagen: Isolation, structural characterization and glycosylation of pyridinoline. *Biochem. J.* **215**, 167–173.

52. Robins, S. P., and Duncan, A. (1983). Crosslinking of collagen. Location of pyridinoline in bovine articular cartilage at two sites of the molecule. *Biochem. J.* **215**, 175–182.

53. Wu, J. J., and Eyre, D. R. (1984). Identification of hydroxypyridinium cross-linking sites in type II collagen of bovine articular cartilage. *Biochemistry* **23**, 1850–1857.

54. Ogawa, T., Ono, T., Tsuda, M., and Kawanashi, Y. (1982). A novel fluor in insoluble collagen: A crosslinking molecule in collagen molecule. *Biochem. Biophys. Res. Commun.* **107**, 1252–1257.

55. Eyre, D. R. (1984). Cross-Linking in collagen and elastin. *Annu. Rev. Biochem.* **53**, 717–748.

56. Eyre, D. R., and Oguchi, H. (1980). Hydroxypyridinium crosslinks of skeletal collagens: Their measurement, properties and a proposed pathway of formation. *Biochem. Biophys. Res. Commun.* **92**, 403–410.

57. Scott, J. E., Hughes, E. W., and Shuttleworth, A. (1981). A collagen-associated Ehrlich chromogen: A pyrrolic cross-link? *Biosci. Rep.* **1**, 611–618.

58. Scott, J. E., Qian, R., Henkel, W., and Glanville, R. W. (1983). An Ehrlich chromogen in collagen cross-links. *Biochem. J.* **209**, 263–264.

59. Kuypers, R., Tyler, M., Kurth, L. B., Jenkins, I. D., and Horgan, D. J. (1992). Identification of the loci of the collagen-associated Ehrlich chromogen in type I collagen confirms its role as a trivalent cross-link. *Biochem. J.* **283**, 129–136.

60. Hanson, D., and Eyre, D. (1996). Molecular site specificity of pyridinoline and pyrrole cross-links in type I collagen of human bone. *J. Biol. Chem.* **271**, 26508–26516.

61. Reiser, K. M., and Last, J. A. (1986). Biosynthesis of collagen crosslinks: *In vivo* labelling of neonatal skin, tendon, and bone in rats. *Connect. Tissue Res.* **14**, 293–306.

62. Otsubo, K., Katz, E. P., Mechanic, G. L., and Yamauchi, M. (1992). Cross-Linking connectivity in bone collagen fibrils: The COOH-terminal locus of free aldehyde. *Biochemistry* **31**, 396–402.

63. Eyre, D. R., Dickson, I. R., and VanNess, K. P. (1988). Collagen cross-linking in human bone and cartilage: Age-related changes in the content of mature hydroxypyridinium residues. *Biochem. J.* **252**, 495–500.

64. Knott, L., Whitehead, C. C., Fleming, R. H., and Bailey, A. J. (1995). Biochemical changes in the collagenous matrix of osteoporotic avian bone. *Biochem. J.* **310**, 1045–1051.

65. Eyre, D. R. (1981). Crosslink maturation in bone collagen. *Dev. Biochem.* **22**, 51–55.

66. Traub, W., Arad, T., and Weiner, S. (1989). Three-dimensional ordered distribution of crystals in turkey tendon collagen fibers. *Proc. Natl. Acad. Sci. U.S.A.* **86**, 9822–9826.

67. Yamauchi, M., and Katz, E. (1993). The post-translational chemistry and molecular packing of mineralizing tendon collagens. *Connect. Tissue Res.* **29**, 81–98.

68. Bailey, A. J., Light, N. D., and Atkins, E. D. T. (1980). Chemical cross-linking restrictions on models for the molecular organization of the collagen fibre. *Nature* **288**, 408–410.

69. Trus, B. L., and Piez, K. A. (1980). Compressed microfibril models of the native collagen fibril. *Nature* **286**, 300–301.

70. Landis, W., Hodgens, K., Song, M., Arena, J., Kiyonaga, S., Marko, M., Owen, C., and McEwen, B. (1996). Mineralization of collagen may occur on fibril surfaces: Evidence from conventional and high-voltage electron microscopy and three-dimensional imaging. *J. Struct. Biol.* **117**, 24–35.

71. Garnero, P., Borel, O., Byrjalsen, I., Ferreras, M., Drake, F. H., Mc-Queney, M. S., Foged, N. T., Delmas, P. D., and Delaisse, J. M. (1998). The collagenolytic activity of cathepsin K is unique amongst mammalian proteinases. *J. Biol. Chem.* **273**, 32347–32352.

72. Vater, C. A., Harris, E. D. J., and Siegel, R. C. (1979). Native cross-links in collagen fibrils induce resistance to human synovial collagenase. *Biochem. J.* **181**, 639–645.

73. Rucklidge, G. J., Riddoch, G. I., and Robins, S. P. (1986). Immunocytochemical staining of rat tissues with antibodies to denatured type I collagen: A technique for localizing areas of collagen degradation. *Collagen Relat. Res.* **6**, 185–193.

74. Dodge, G. R., and Poole, A. R. (1989). Immunohistochemical detection and immunochemical analysis of type II collagen degradation in human normal, rheumatoid, and osteoarthritic articular cartilages and in explants of bovine articular cartilage cultured with interleukin 1. *J. Clin. Invest.* **83**, 647–661.

75. Lees, S., Eyre, D. R., and Barnard, S. M. (1990). BAPN dose dependence of mature crosslinking in bone matrix collagen of rabbit compact bone: Corresponding sonic velocity and equatorial diffraction spacing. *Connect. Tissue Res.* **24**, 95–105.

76. Oxlund, H., Barckman, M., Ortoft, G., and Andreassen, T. T. (1995). Reduced concentrations of collagen cross-links are associated with reduced strength of bone. *Bone* **17**, 365S–371S.

77. Horgan, D. J., King, N. L., Kurth, L. B., and Kuypers, R. (1990). Collagen crosslinks and their relationship to the thermal properties of calf tendons. *Arch. Biochem. Biophys.* **281**, 21–26.

78. Bätge, B., Winter, C., Notbohm, H., Acil, Y., Brinckmann, J., and Müller, P. K. (1997). Glycosylation of human bone collagen in relation to lysylhydroxylation and fibril diameter. *J. Biochem.* **122**, 109–115.

79. Fledelius, C., Johnsen, A. H., Cloos, P. A. C., Bonde, M., and Qvist, P. (1997). Characterization of urinary degradation products derived from type I collagen. Identification of a beta-isomerized Asp-Gly sequence within the C-terminal telopeptide (alpha1) region. *J. Biol. Chem.* **272**, 9755–9763.

80. Brady, J. B., Ju, J., and Robins, S. P. (1998). Isoaspartyl bond formation within N-terminal sequences of collagen type I: Implications for their use as markers of collagen degradation. *Clin. Sci.* **96**, 209–215.

CHAPTER 3

Vitamin K-Dependent Proteins of Bone and Cartilage

CAREN M. GUNDBERG Department of Orthopaedics and Rehabilitation, Yale University School of Medicine, New Haven, Connecticut 06510

SATORU K. NISHIMOTO Department of Biochemistry, The University of Tennessee College of Medicine, Memphis, Tennessee 38163

I. ABSTRACT

The importance of vitamin K for the normal functioning of blood coagulation factors is well known. However, this vitamin is also involved in the physiological activation of various proteins that are not involved in hemostasis. Here we focus on the biochemistry and physiology of osteocalcin and matrix Gla protein (MGP), which are abundant in bone and cartilage, respectively. While osteocalcin biosynthesis is restricted to bone and dentin, MGP is synthesized in a variety of tissues and cell types. Two other vitamin K-dependent proteins, Gas6, which is involved in the regulation of cell proliferation, and protein S, an inhibitor of coagulation, have been shown to have a potential role in bone metabolism.

II. INTRODUCTION

The family of vitamin K-dependent gamma-carboxylated proteins is important in a variety of tissue and cellular functions. The formation of gamma-carboxyglutamic acid (Gla) occurs via a unique post-translational modification of specific peptide-bound glutamate residues in selective proteins. This reaction, which is required for the biological activities of all the vitamin K dependent proteins, is inhibited by warfarin (Fig. 1). Beside the vitamin K-dependent coagulation factors (prothrombin, and factors VII, IX, X), Gla-containing proteins include the anticoagulation factors, protein C and S, as well as protein Z, a plasma glycoprotein of unknown function. In addition, either carboxylase activity or vitamin K-dependent formation of Gla residues have been observed

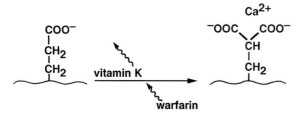

FIGURE 1 Gamma-carboxyglutamic acid (Gla). Vitamin K and CO_2 are required for the carboxylation of specific glutamic acid residues in osteocalcin. This reaction is inhibited by warfarin. The adjacent carboxyl groups of Gla are binding sites for Ca^{2+}.

in a wide variety of other tissues, including bone, kidney, intestine, placenta, pancreas, skin, spleen, lung, heart, blood vessels, spinal cord, and testis [1]. Accumulation of Gla-containing proteins in sites of pathological ectopic calcification has been observed [2–4]. It also has been shown that the carboxylating enzyme itself is vitamin K dependent and contains Gla residues [5].

Bone and cartilage were the first tissues after the liver where the Gla proteins were identified and characterized. Osteocalcin, the Gla protein exclusive to bone and dentin, is a small Ca^{2+}-binding protein that contains three Gla residues. Another Gla-containing species, matrix Gla protein (MGP) [6, 7], contains five Gla residues and exhibits some peptide sequence similarity to osteocalcin. MGP expression occurs in a broad variety of tissues, but only bone, cartilage, and calcified cartilage normally accumulate MGP. In addition, two other vitamin K-dependent proteins, Gas6 and protein S, have been identified in bone and cartilage [8, 9].

III. OSTEOCALCIN

A. Structure and Biosynthesis

Osteocalcin is a small protein (49 amino acids) synthesized by mature osteoblasts, odontoblasts, and hypertrophic chondrocytes. Osteocalcin is characterized by the presence of three residues of Gla. In human bone, however, the first potential Gla residue at position 17 is only partially carboxy-

lated (55–89%) whereas residues 21 and 24 are greater than 90% gamma-carboxylated. This is due to partial carboxylation of the protein during synthesis [10].

Combined chemical, immunochemical, and spectral investigations have provided a 3-dimensional model of osteocalcin structure. The model consists of two antiparallel alpha-helical domains, the "Gla helix" (residues 16–25) and the "Asp–Glu helix" (residues 30–41), connected by a peptide segment containing a beta-turn (residues 26–29) and stabilized by a disulfide bond. The adjacent carboxyl groups in the Gla residues are aligned such that they project from the helix in a plane, potentially facilitating the protein's adsorption to hydroxyapatite [11]. Millimolar levels of Ca^{2+} cause normal osteocalcin to change from a random-coil to an alpha-helical conformation. Not only must Gla residues be present, they must also be in helical register to fully achieve the adsorption specificity for hydroxyapatite. Thermally decarboxylated osteocalcin containing less than 0.5 residues Gla/molecule fails to demonstrate this conformational transition in the presence of calcium, and the protein's affinity for hydroxyapatite is reduced [12].

In all species, the protein is synthesized as an 11 kDa molecule consisting of a 23-residue hydrophobic signal peptide, a 26-residue propeptide, and the 49-residue mature protein. After the hydrophobic region is cleaved by a signal peptidase, proosteocalcin is gamma-carboxylated. The proregion contains a gamma-carboxylation recognition site homologous to corresponding regions in the vitamin K-dependent clotting factors (Fig. 2). Arg at position -1 and Phe at -16 are strictly conserved and appear to be critical for the binding of the vitamin K-dependent carboxylase enzyme to its substrates [13–15]. The importance of the propeptide region for functional carboxylation is illustrated by the finding of one individual with increased warfarin sensitivity who had an alanine to threonine mutation at residue -10 in the propeptide region of factor IX [16].

After carboxylation, the propeptide is removed and the mature protein is secreted [17]. The newly synthesized protein is primarily deposited in the extracellular matrix of bone but a small amount enters the blood. The circulating levels of osteocalcin are taken as a specific marker of osteoblastic activity (for reviews, see references [18–22]).

1	11	21	31	41	51	61	71	78
YE'SHESMESY	ELNPFINRRN	ANTFISPQQR	WRAKVQE'RIR	E'RSKPVHE'LN	RE'ACDDYRLC	E'RYAMVYGYN	AAYNRYF	(RKR RGTK)

QAGAKPSGAE	SSFAFVSKQE	GSEVVKRPRR -	YLYQWLGAP	VPYPDPLE'PR	RE'VCE'LNPDC	DELADHIGFQ	EAYRRFYGPV
-21	-11	-1 1	10	20	30	40	

FIGURE 2 Comparison of the primary sequences of human osteocalcin (bottom) and human MGP (top). Bold symbols indicate conserved regions, E' indicate gamma-carboxyglutamic acid, and italics indicate phosphoserines. Processing of the 84-amino-acid protein yields the 1–77 form isolated from human bone. A gamma-carboxylation recognition site is similar to corresponding regions in the vitamin K-dependent clotting factors. Arg (at position -1 in OC and $+30$ in MGP) and Phe (at -16 in OC and $+15$ in MGP) are strictly conserved and appear to be critical for the binding of the vitamin K-dependent carboxylase enzyme to its substrates. The Ala–Gly substitution at -10 in osteocalcin results in reduced affinity for the vitamin K–carboxylase enzyme.

B. Function

Although osteocalcin is one of the most abundant noncollagenous proteins in bone, the biological function of osteocalcin has not been precisely defined. Because of its specific interaction with hydroxyapatite, osteocalcin was thought to affect the growth or maturation of Ca^{2+}-phosphate mineral phases. Osteocalcin first appears coincident with the onset of mineralization and an increase in synthesis of the protein occurs in concert with hydroxyapatite deposition during skeletal growth [23, 24]. Immunolocalization studies show that the protein is distributed throughout the mineralized regions of bone matrix, dentin, and calcified cartilage [25–27]. However, an accumulation of evidence indicates that osteocalcin is not related to events that allow mineral deposition to occur, but rather that it participates in regulation of mineralization or bone turnover. Early studies showed that the protein could regulate the growth of the hydroxyapatite crystal in solution [28].

In vitro studies demonstrate that osteocalcin is a marker of late osteoblast differentiation [29–31]. When osteoblasts are grown in culture they produce a dense collagenous extracellular matrix [32, 33]. Alkaline phosphatase activity and MGP expression increase postproliferatively coincident with the onset of mineralization. As the extracellular matrix accumulates and mineralizes, synthesis of osteocalcin and other calcium binding proteins (e.g., osteopontin and bone sialoprotein) is initiated. Alkaline phosphatase activity subsequently decreases, but osteocalcin synthesis remains high throughout the life of the culture [34, 35]. In cultures in which mineralization is delayed, expression of osteocalcin is also delayed [29].

Recently, gene targeting has produced a mouse that has had the osteocalcin gene "knocked out." These mice are characterized by a progressive *increase* in bone mass, leading to bone of better biomechanical quality by 6–9 months. These mice exhibit an accelerated rate of bone formation without changes in osteoclast or osteoblast number [36]. The gradual appearance of this phenotype is consistent with the fact that osteocalcin content of bone is low in newborn rats (less than 4% of the adult level) and increases gradually with age [37]. No changes in mineral content of the bones of osteocalcin-depleted mice were detectable by von Kossa staining or histomorphometry. However, a more sensitive assay of mineralization, Fourier transform infrared microspectroscopy, revealed differences in the size and perfection of the crystallite [38]. In wild-type animals the crystals were larger and more "perfect" in the cortical bone than in trabecular bone. In contrast, in the osteocalcin knockout animals, the crystal size and perfection were the same in both the trabecular and cortical bone and resembled that of the wild-type trabecular bone. These findings are consistent with impaired mineral maturation in the osteocalcin deficient bone and imply the presence of newer (less remodeled) mineral. Similar findings were observed when ovariectomized wild-type and knockout mice were compared. Based on these findings, it appears that osteocalcin plays some as yet undefined role in regulating bone mineral turnover.

Other *in vivo* and *in vitro* studies support a role for osteocalcin in bone remodeling. First, disrupted collagen fibrillogenesis in the cloned mouse calvarial cell line MCT3T3-E1 results in increased turnover of the collagenous matrix, a decrease in alkaline phosphatase, but a five-fold increase in osteocalcin biosynthesis [39]. Second, the pattern of osteocalcin distribution in human osteons changes with gender and age, and localized reductions of osteocalcin in the extracellular matrix are associated with reduced cortical remodeling [40]. Several earlier studies have suggested that osteocalcin is involved in recruitment and activation of bone resorbing cells. The protein is a chemoattractant for peripheral mononuclear cells and osteoclast-like cells of giant cell tumors [41–43]. Incorporation of osteocalcin into synthetic hydroxyapatite particles placed onto the chick chorioallantoic membrane enhanced osteoclast formation [44]. Subcutaneously implanted bone particles that were osteocalcin deficient show a decrease in both progenitor cell recruitment and resorption of the bone particles [45]. Other researchers were unable to reproduce these findings, but large inflammatory responses that can obscure the more specific osteoclastic response were observed in their studies [46]. Furthermore, coating apatite with osteocalcin increases its resorption [47].

It is possible that osteocalcin may act in combination with other hydroxyapatite binding proteins as a signal for bone remodeling. Osteopontin, which potentiates osteoclast adhesion to mineral surfaces, forms a complex with osteocalcin *in vitro* [48, 49]. Altered expression of both osteocalcin and osteopontin have been reported in rat models of osteopetrosis in which osteoclastic resorption is impaired. Further studies in animals depleted of combinations of matrix proteins should provide clues to the function of osteocalcin and other bone specific proteins.

C. Gene Structure

The human osteocalcin gene is a single copy gene located at the distal long arm of chromosome 1 [50]. The structure and sequence of the gene in various species are similar [51], but multiple copies of the gene occur in the rat and mouse [52, 53]. In the rat, one or more copies of the gene have been found, depending upon the strain. The mouse osteocalcin cluster contains three genes, two of which encode osteocalcin and are expressed only in bone (OG1 and OG2), whereas a third gene, the osteocalcin related gene (ORG), is found in low levels in brain, lung, and kidney, but not in bone. ORG is expressed at day 10 in embryonic development, earlier than OG1 and OG2, which are expressed at day 17, the beginning of osteogenesis. The coding sequence of

ORG carries five amino acid substitutions, one at the propeptide cleavage site. ORG also contains an additional exon that is not translated, and a 3 kb insertion separates the ORG coding sequence from a bone-specific promoter. The insertion sequence has the structure of a typical retro virus, an attribute which leads to the downregulation of transcription, possibly explaining the low levels of expression of ORG in non-osseous tissues [53].

It has been suggested that the ORG gene product is nephrocalcin, a Gla-containing calcium oxalate crystal growth inhibitor found in kidney [4, 54, 55]. However, the primary sequence of this protein remains unknown, and human specific osteocalcin antibodies do not cross-react with partially purified human nephrocalcin [F. L. Coe, Y. Nakagawa, and C. Gundberg, unpublished observations]. Osteocalcin has also been detected in renal calculi in rats, but osteocalcin could not be found in the corresponding kidney tissue [56]. It is possible that the osteocalcin found in the renal calculi originated from circulating osteocalcin, which became entrapped as a consequence of the protein's high affinity for mineral.

Nevertheless, early studies demonstrated the presence of an 8–10 kDa Gla-containing protein in rat and bovine kidney [57, 58] that also did not cross-react with rat-and bovine-specific antibodies to osteocalcin [P. V. Hauschka, P. A. Friedman, and C. Gundberg, unpublished observations]. In the rat, the synthesis of the protein was responsive to $1,25(OH)_2D$ [59]. Deyl *et al.* [60] partially sequenced the Gla-containing protein in rat kidney, but it was not homologous to rat osteocalcin, although it showed some similarity to the bovine protein.

D. Regulation

Osteocalcin gene expression or protein synthesis is regulated by various hormones and growth factors [extensively reviewed in reference 61]. A specific vitamin D regulatory element has been identified in the osteocalcin promoter [62–65]. In most species, $1,25(OH)_2D$ upregulates osteocalcin biosynthesis. However, in the mouse, osteocalcin synthesis is suppressed by $1,25(OH)_2D$ [66–68]. Stimulation of osteocalcin by $1,25(OH)_2D$ in chicks is increased when cultures are derived from 12-day embryos, but decreased in 17-day embryos [69]. There is a significant nucleotide difference in the VDRE of the mouse gene and the lack of inducibility of mouse osteocalcin is likely attributable to the interaction of VDR receptor complex with corepressors. This vitamin D response element is also the mediator of positive regulation in response to retinoic acid [70]. Separate promoter regions are responsible for repression by glucocorticoid and TGFβ. On the other hand, cAMP influences osteocalcin gene expression by modulating mRNA stability [61, 71]. Some effectors (e.g., γ-interferon, IGF I or II, TNFα, and some metal ions) indirectly regulate osteocalcin through vitamin D

responsiveness [72]. Osteocalcin mRNA levels are also altered by estrogen, thyroxine, calcitonin, prostaglandin E2, or BMPs, but the specific mechanisms have not been defined and may be indirect [61].

Osteocalcin mRNA has also been detected in bone marrow megakaryocytes and peripheral blood platelets, liver, lung, and brain by reverse transcription-polymerase chain reaction, but translation into protein has not been verified [73, 74]. Like the mouse ORG gene, the mRNA levels observed in these tissues are three orders of magnitude lower than those found in bone. Furthermore, they are not vitamin D responsive, suggesting that control of expression is under a nonskeletal promoter. To date, bone and dentin are the only known sites of production of osteocalcin.

Osteoblast differentiation is marked by the sequential activation of many genes encoding the extracellular matrix proteins. Osteocalcin gene expression is tightly regulated at multiple levels, accounting for both tissue specificity and variations in expression during the osteoblast developmental sequence. Although there are species-specific differences in the regulation of osteocalcin, common patterns are present. Studies demonstrated that a series of elements contribute to basal expression of osteocalcin. The promoter of all osteocalcin genes has a TATA sequence. An intragenic silencer may be involved in regulating the basal levels during developmental stage-specific expression of the protein [75–77].

Because of the specificity of the osteocalcin gene for differentiated osteoblasts, several laboratories have used the osteocalcin promoter as a tool to identify osteoblast-specific *cis*-acting elements and transcription factors in human, rat, and mouse osteocalcin genes. A CBF (core-binding factor) consensus binding site was shown to be a regulatory element for osteoblast-specific transcriptional activation [78, 79]. CBF transcription factors comprise a family of heterodimeric proteins; the CBFα subunit binds DNA and is encoded by three distinct genes whereas the beta subunit is common. CBFα proteins are mammalian homologs of the *Drosophila* segmentation gene, *runt*. Recently, Cbfa1 was shown to be present only in osteoblast nuclear extracts and could regulate expression of multiple genes expressed in osteoblasts [80]. The importance of Cbfa1 in osteogenesis is shown by targeted disruption of Cbfa1 in mice, which resulted in a complete lack of ossification. Osteoblasts of the mutant mice expressed low levels of alkaline phosphatase but barely detectable levels of osteopontin and osteocalcin [81, 82]. The other factors involved in the regulation of temporal expression of osteoblastic genes are yet to be determined.

E. Catabolism

The catabolic fate of osteocalcin is of interest because of the use of circulating osteocalcin as a marker of bone formation in metabolic bone disease. Various fragments of osteocalcin are known to circulate, and these have been detected by antibodies originally made against the intact molecule (19). It is thought that the majority of circulating osteocalcin is composed of the intact molecule and a large N-terminal mid-molecule fragment [83, 84]. Although the large N-terminal mid-molecule fragment has not been directly sequenced, it is thought to encompass residues 1–43. This is based on the fact that osteocalcin contains a trypsin cleavage site at residue 43, and the two antibodies used to characterize this fragment are specific for residues 5–13 and for the 25–37 region. Recent data indicate that there are in fact other smaller (<30 residues) N-terminal immunoreactive species of osteocalcin in the serum in addition to the larger mid-molecule fragment [85, 86].

It has been suggested that the large N-terminal mid-molecule fragment is generated by proteolysis during circulation in the blood or during sample processing and storage. This is primarily based on the findings that (1) the fragment is detected immediately after blood sampling, and (2) osteocalcin levels decrease with incubation at room temperature when measured by conventional RIA or by intact assays, but values are stable with an assay that recognizes both the intact and large N-terminal mid-molecule fragment [83, 87]. However, the large N-terminal mid-molecule fragment was also detected in conditioned media from human osteoblast-like cells [83]. Whether this fragment was derived from proteolysis in the media or by intracellular processing has not been established. Studies by Taylor *et al.* [88] suggest that a unique fragment found in sera from patients with Paget's disease may have been derived from altered osteoblastic synthesis. It is possible that osteoblastic degradation of osteocalcin may serve as a mechanism to regulate osteocalcin concentration.

The breakdown of osteocalcin may also occur during osteoclastic dissolution of bone. Salo *et al.* [89] showed that osteocalcin-related immunoreactive material was liberated from resorption lacunae when osteoclasts were cultured on bovine bone. Whether this material was intact osteocalcin or comprised an immunoreactive fragment is not known, but in other studies osteocalcin has been shown to be a substrate for osteoclastic enzymes [90]. Cathepsins D, L, and H will degrade human osteocalcin to the 1–41, 4–43, 8–43, 4–49, and 8–49 fragments, and these can be recognized by many polyclonal antibodies [91]. In addition, plasmin cleaves osteocalcin to the 1–43 and 44–49 peptides both when the protein is in solution and when it is bound to hydroxyapatite, resulting in the detachment of the peptides from the crystal surface [92]. This protease, plasmin, which is associated with membranes of osteoblast-like cells, has a potential role in bone resorption by activating collagenase activity. Whether the generation of osteocalcin fragments during bone resorption is related to osteocalcin's potential biological function in regulating bone turnover is unknown.

IV. MATRIX GLA PROTEIN

A. Structure and Biosynthesis

MGP was the second vitamin K-dependent protein to be discovered in bone. MGP is likely to be the ancestral template for osteocalcin, as sharks contain MGP but not osteocalcin. Osteocalcin makes its first appearance with the bony fishes [93]. There are several similarities between osteocalcin and MGP. There is 20% identity between osteocalcin and the carboxy-terminal region of MGP (Fig. 2). Although MGP is γ-carboxylated at five sites, two of the Gla residues are adjacent to a disulfide bond as in osteocalcin, potentially facilitating interaction of MGP with hydroxyapatite. Finally, like osteocalcin, MGP contains a 19-amino-acid N-terminal hydrophobic transmembrane secretion signal that is cleaved during translocation into the rough endoplasmic reticulum [94].

A major difference between MGP and osteocalcin (and the other vitamin K-dependent proteins) is that MGP does not undergo amino-terminal proteolytic processing of a propeptide. Instead, the consensus sequence for γ-carboxylation resides in the N terminus of the mature protein. Because MGP retains the recognition sequence, decarboxylated MGP is an excellent substrate for *in vitro* assays of γ-carboxylase and is approximately 50 times better as a substrate than decarboxylated osteocalcin [95].

MGP also differs from osteocalcin in that all species examined from shark to human are phosphorylated on serines in the N terminus. These serines are in a consensus sequence of Ser-X-Glu/Ser(P), also found in milk caseins, salivary proteins, and some regulatory peptides (IL-6, proenkephalin A, growth factor binding protein 1) [96]. It is not known if MGP is a substrate for acid and alkaline phosphatases or whether the properties and function of MGP may be altered by dephosphorylation, similar to that observed in osteopontin when its degree of phosphorylation is altered [97]. For example, the degree of phosphorylation of MGP could provide flexible regulation of calcification inhibitory activity (see below).

Proteolytic processing of MGP occurs at the C terminus. Cleavage of the signal peptide leaves an 84-amino-acid long protein [94]. However, MGP is isolated from human bone only as the 77-amino-acid protein with a carboxy-terminal phenylalanine, whereas 1–79 and 1–83 forms are isolated from bovine bone. No MGP protein corresponding to the 1–84 sequence has ever been detected [98]. Intracellular processing of an 84-amino-acid MGP by the action of a carboxypeptidase would yield the 1–83 protein whereas the 1–77 and 1–79 forms could be derived from sequential proteolysis via a trypsin-like activity followed by removal of an arginine. As described for osteocalcin, it is possible that plasmin could remove the C-terminal cluster of positively charged amino acids, converting the MGP 84 to the truncated species found in tissues [92].

B. Tissue Localization

MGP is secreted in culture by osteoblasts, chondrocytes, cardiac myocytes, vascular endothelial cells, breast cells, fibroblasts, pneumocytes, and kidney cells. A number of tumor types express MGP (e.g., renal cell carcinoma, prostatic carcinoma, and testicular germ-cell tumors) [99]. *In vivo*, MGP mRNA has been found in most tissues examined, with the highest levels in kidney, heart, lung, and cartilage [100–104]. Once secreted, MGP can anchor to the extracellular mineralized matrix of cartilage, and bone. Accumulation of the protein occurs normally only in bone, cartilage, and calcified cartilage (Table I) [105, 106]. MGP is particularly abundant in calcified costal cartilage, in which it accounts for 35–40% of the total protein [93].

MGP content in calcified cartilage and bone matrix remains constant throughout adult life [105]. The final concentration of MGP attained in mature rat bone (0.4 mg/g) is about 10% of the osteocalcin level on a molar basis [37]. Measurable amounts of MGP in soft tissues are found only *in utero*, in the neonatal period, and in juvenile animals [105]. It is not known if the MGP in organs in which it is transiently found is γ-carboxylated, phosphorylated, and C-terminally proteolytically processed as is the MGP in mature bone or cartilage [96, 98]. MGP is measured in serum and appears similar to MGP isolated from bone and cartilage [98]. Nevertheless, because these studies relied upon immunological techniques, an antigenically masked or modified form of MGP could have been overlooked.

In situ hybridization analysis shows that MGP mRNA is present during embryonic development as early as day 10.5, prior to the onset of skeletal mineralization. Its expression is restricted to the epithelial mesenchymal interface, principally in lung and limb buds. By day 12.5, MGP is predominantly expressed in cartilage and blood vessels. In cells of the chondrocytic lineage, expression occurs in areas that will become ossified and in areas that will remain cartilaginous, such as the trachea and bronchi. Later, MGP is restricted to cartilaginous regions such as bronchi and trachea; alveolar cells do not express the protein. MGP mRNA is found in the media of arteries and in the aortic valve but not in heart. Low levels are also found in the kidney medulla [103, 107].

Skeletal expression of MGP occurs in resting, proliferative, and late hypertrophic chondrocytes but not in early hypertrophic chondrocytes. Although MGP expression is not observed in osteoblasts during embryonic development, primary cultures of rat and human osteoblasts have been shown to synthesize and secrete MGP. During osteoblast differentiation *in vitro*, MGP expression is maximal during maturation of the extracellular collagenous matrix which follows the downregulation of cellular proliferation [108]. Similarly, in osteosarcoma cell lines, MGP synthesis is often lower if differentiated osteoblast markers such as osteocalcin are high. A clonal line of rat osteosarcoma cells, ROS 25/1, which is

TABLE I.   Summary of MGP Protein Levels in Rat and Bovine Tissues of Varying Age

	mg/100 g tissue
Rat cartilages	
Costal	9.9[a]
Tracheal	8.0[a]
Vertebral disc	3.3[a]
Nasal septum	1.9[a]
Growth plate	3.2[b]
Rat tracheal cartilage	
Age: 6 months	1.5[e]
Age: 18 months	1.5[e]
Age: 30 months	1.5[e]
Bovine calcified cartilage	14.0[c]
Rat tibial bone	
Diaphysis + metaphysis	4.1[a]
Epiphysis	5.7[a]
Rat Long bones	
Age: birth (0 days)	5.0[d]
Age: 10 days	4.5[d]
Age: 20 days	4.5[d]
Adult	4.6[d]
Bovine bone	6.0[c]
Rat soft tissue	
Lung	0.109[b]
Heart	0.059[b]
Kidney (2 weeks)	0.014[b]
Kidney (>3 weeks)	<0.010[f]
Tendons, skin, liver, muscle	<0.010[a]

[a] MGP levels determined by radioimmunoassay on cleaned and dissected tissues from 1- to 2-month-old rats [105].

[b] MGP levels determined by radioimmunoassay on cleaned and dissected tissues from 2-week-old rats [106].

[c] MGP levels determined from protein recovery from 2-year-old steers [93].

[d] MGP levels determined by radioimmunoassay on pooled femur, tibia, radius, and ulna from 0- through 20-day-old rats [37].

[e] MGP levels determined by radioimmunoassay on intact trachea of 6- through 30-month-old normal and diet-restricted rats [105].

[f] MGP levels determined by radioimmunoassay on intact kidney from 0- to 90-day-old rats [102].

a poor osteocalcin producer, has been found to synthesize MGP subject to control by 1,25-dihydroxyvitamin D_3. Another cell line, ROS 17/2.8, which is distinguished by its synthesis of abundant osteocalcin, produces low levels of MGP normally [109, 110]. However, these cells shift their biosynthetic production away from osteocalcin toward exclusive production of MGP during 1 week of continuous exposure to 1,25-dihydroxyvitamin D_3 [111]. In other studies, MGP was detected by *in situ* hybridization in trabecular lining osteoblasts of the fracture callus [112, 113].

MGP is synthesized by arterial smooth muscle cells in adult human, adult cynomolgus monkey, and in developing mice [107, 114, 115]. In humans, the protein is deposited by smooth muscle cells near calcified areas of atherosclerotic plaque in association with lipid-rich matrices and in the media of arteries and atheromatous intima [115]. MGP synthesis increases with progression of atherosclerosis in a rabbit model [116].

C. Regulation

MGP synthesis is stimulated by many developmental, pathological, and morphological events. Many hormones and growth factors are able to regulate synthesis of MGP. Control of the gene is influenced by multiple overlapping, synergistic, and contradictory signals received by cells *in vivo*. These signals include nutritional stimuli such as vitamin K availability, and hormone and morphogenic factors such as retinoic acid (RA), 1,25-dihydroxyvitamin D_3, EGF, bFGF, and TGF-β. Few factors have been found to have a universal effect on MGP synthesis in all cells. The complexity of MGP gene expression is underscored by the many normal and pathological situations in which MGP is synthesized. Response to any particular regulatory event depends on the specific cell type, the presence of other regulatory molecules, and animal species.

The human MGP gene is present as a single copy on the short arm of chromosome 12 (12p). The gene is 3937 bp long from the transcriptional start site (major 5′ cap site) to the AATAAA polyadenylation signal. Four exons contribute the 615 nucleotides of the MGP mRNA, and 103 amino acids comprise the initial translation product [94]. Between mouse and man the intron–exon structure is highly conserved, as is the 5′ flanking nucleotide sequence. However, while the human gene contains a putative upstream regulatory element for vitamin D (VDRE), retinoic acid (RARE), and CAT box binding proteins (CCAAT), these are not present in the mouse gene [103].

The MGP-stimulatory response of skeletal cells to 1,25-dihydroxyvitamin D_3 is species and tissue dependent. 1,25-dihydroxyvitamin D_3 stimulates MGP synthesis in normal rat osteoblasts and chondrocytes [108] and in human and rat osteosarcoma cells [109, 111, 117, 118]. It does not stimulate MGP synthesis in normal human adult or fetal osteoblasts, fetal chondrocytes, or newborn fibroblasts [118]. The response in the mouse has not been tested.

Retinoic acid is a major regulator of MGP synthesis. It stimulates synthesis in skeletal cells [117–119] but inhibits synthesis in kidney epithelial cells [120]. The presence of the estrogen receptor can alter the response of breast cancer cells to retinoic acid. In MCF-7 human breast cancer cells with estrogen receptors, RA inhibits synthesis [120, 121], whereas RA-treatment of breast cancer cells either lacking or with low levels of the estrogen receptor results in an increase in MGP gene expression [121]. The different effects of RA on MGP synthesis in different cell types is not totally

understood. However, Kirfel *et al.* have demonstrated that the negative effects of RA on the synthesis of MGP in MCF-7 and NRK kidney cells may arise by binding of RAR/RXR to a novel negative responsive element (NRE) which functions to displace proximal promoter CCAAT binding proteins in these tissues [120].

Epithelial growth factor (EGF) and basic fibroblast growth factor inhibit MGP gene expression, whereas platelet-derived growth factor has no effect. TGF-β1 and OP-1 stimulate MGP synthesis [122–124]. In preosteoblasts the effect is specific for TGF-β1, as the closely related BMP-4 does not stimulate MGP synthesis [122].

D. Function of MGP

By analogy to osteocalcin, MGP has been considered to be a calcium and hydroxyapatite binding protein. This assumption derives from the presence of Gla and phosphoserine in MGP, its localization in mineralized matrices, and its synthesis by cells in regions near calcifying matrix. However, MGP function may be modulated through interaction with other extracellular proteins. Unlike osteocalcin, which is solubilized by dissolving the mineral, complete extraction of MGP from bone or cartilage requires chaotropic agents, suggesting strong interaction with organic components of the matrix [105, 106, 125]. MGP has oppositely charged amino and carboxyl termini that might interact to form macromolecular arrays such as that depicted in Figure 3. The biological function of MGP may involve ion-pair interaction with charged regions of proteins such as osteopontin, osteonectin, or collagen. However, quantitative mineral binding studies of MGP to mineral ions and hydroxyapatite or to other organic components of the matrix have not yet been published.

Studies have suggested that MGP functions as a regulator/inhibitor of mineralization. In mice with a nonfunctional MGP gene (MGP-null), excessive mineralization of arteries

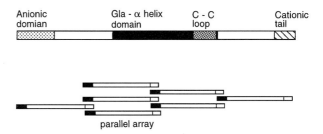

FIGURE 3   Diagram of potential interaction between MGP molecules. The N terminus is shown as an anionic domain due to the high density of negative charges from phosphoserines and Gla. The Gla-alpha helix domain contains the highest probability for alpha helix. Interactions of the anionic N-terminal domain and the cationic C terminus could initiate MGP aggregation and precipitation. This feature may be a key to its function on a molecular level.

and cartilage occurs, suggesting MGP normally functions to inhibit mineralization in these tissues [107]. Several phenotypic abnormalities were observed, which are consistent with the pattern of expression of MGP. First, growth plate cartilage from MGP-null mice exhibited disorganized columns of chondrocytes with calcification extending into the zone of proliferating chondrocytes. This resulted in the inability to appropriately replace the cartilage with normal bone matrix, and short stature, osteopenia, and fractures ensued in these animals. Nevertheless, because of its normal abundance in calcified cartilage and bone, it appears that the presence of MGP is not sufficient to inhibit mineralization in these tissues. Rather, MGP may serve to control the degree of mineral deposition in normally calcified tissue. Alternatively, MGP may only be passively adsorbed to mineralized tissue via its Gla residues, as has been shown for several of the vitamin K-dependent clotting factors [126]. It is also possible that MGP is modulated or activated by interaction with other components or by proteolytic processing or phosphorylation. Therefore, a direct role of MGP in bone remodeling or bone cell function needs to be explored.

The second phenotypic change in the MGP-null mice was the calcification of all elastic and muscular arteries. By 2–3 weeks after birth, the aortic media was calcified, resulting in disruption of normal artery wall tissue structure. Within 2 months of birth death resulted from rupture of the aorta, which contained apatite similar to that found in atherosclerotic lesions. However, no atherosclerotic plaques were observed in these animals. The calcified areas contained hypertrophic chondrocytes with typical cartilage matrix containing matrix vesicles, type II collagen, and proteoglycan, recapitulating the initial stages of skeletal calcification. The presence of chondrocytes may represent an attempt to repair structural failures in the calcified artery wall in response to compressive forces, similar to those that are known to encourage chondrocyte-like cells in healing tendon and bone.

Arterial calcification is a common complication associated with atherosclerosis. Several studies have demonstrated that cell cultures of calcifying vascular smooth muscle cells undergo osteoblast-like differentiation [127–129]. cAMP provokes the *in vitro* calcification of these cells and increases MGP synthesis as well as synthesis of other early markers of osteoblast differentiation [130]. It appears that the increase in MGP in human vascular calcification may be an invoked response to limit further deposition of mineral. It is interesting to note that mineralization of porcine heart valves compromises its usefulness as a substitute for damaged human valves [131, 132]. If MGP can act as a direct inhibitor of mineralization, it may be clinically useful as a component of prosthetic heart valve implants to inhibit mineralization.

No abnormalities were observed in embryonic and newborn MGP-null mice, despite the fact that the protein is expressed in affected tissues early during development. The necessity for alternative inhibitors of mineralization during development may derive from the fact that there is little placental transfer of vitamin K to the embryo. In the fetus and newborn, vitamin K is maintained at levels less than necessary to achieve full γ-carboxylation of vitamin K-dependent proteins. This begs the question, however, of the significance of early expression of the protein and suggests that MGP may have an alternative function, perhaps in influencing processes in cell differentiation. This suggestion comes from several observations. Large increases in MGP synthesis are found in post confluent cell culture [108, 111]. MGP levels decline 50–100 fold when rat kidney cells are subcultured 1:30 [133]. This induction may be due to interaction of the cells with the extracellular matrix. Rat preosteoblasts, differentiating skeletal cells, and kidney epithelial cells increase MGP synthesis in the presence of ascorbic acid after the deposition of a competent collagenous matrix [100, 108, 117]. Conversely, EGF downregulates the expression of MGP in post confluent cells at a time when collagen message is reduced [133]. It has been suggested that MGP may play some role in cell–cell interactions. However, early studies suggesting interaction with integrins have not been substantiated [134, 135].

It is tempting to speculate that MGP expression is linked to apoptosis of certain cell lineages. MGP is differentially expressed after 1,25-dihydroxyvitamin D_3 treatment in C6.9 rat glioma cells that undergo a cell death program when exposed to the hormone [136]. MGP synthesis is increased during apoptosis of prostate cells after androgen withdrawal [137]. It is also increased in several human cancers (Table II) [138, 139], and it is possible that MGP reflects apoptosis in these tumor cells [138, 139]. It is not clear what role, if any, MGP has in the conversion of normal cells to cancers, but the tumors found to express MGP may reflect upon the lineage of cells that transformed into tumor cells. Indeed, a potential role in apoptosis might explain the differential MGP expression in late hypertrophic chondrocytes in the growth plate, but not in early hypertrophic chondrocytes. Perhaps the inability to synthesize MGP in growth plates of MGP-null mice leads to disruption of apoptosis and contributes to the disorganization of the normal columnar orientation of the cells.

V. GAS6

A recently described growth factor, Gas6, is the latest member of the family of vitamin K-dependent proteins to have a potential role in bone. Gas6 (the product of *growth arrest specific gene 6*) is a polypeptide growth factor that is upregulated in response to serum starvation and down regulated during growth induction in cultured cells [140]. Gas6 displays significant sequence similarity to protein S (43% amino acid identity), a vitamin K-dependent protein and negative coregulator of the blood coagulation cascade.

TABLE II. *In Vivo* MGP Content, Localization, and mRNA Expression in Development, Pathological Calcification, or Cancer

Process	Observation	References
Development		
Chondrogenesis	mRNA in mouse resting, proliferative, late hypertrophic chondrocytes of growth plate, limb bud prechondrocytes	103
	newborn monkey protein more widely distributed than adult	15
	no change in rat protein levels from 6 to 30 months age	
Circulatory system	Protein in monkey vascular smooth muscle	113
	mRNA and protein in human artery vascular smooth muscle;	
	mRNA in mouse aortic valves and media of arteries	108
Kidney development	mRNA and protein in weanling rat kidney,	102–104
	mRNA in mouse kidney medulla;	
	mRNA and protein in rat kidney tubules peak after birth, then mRNA levels decrease after 1 month	
Lung morphogenesis	mRNA and protein in weanling rat lung	102–104
	mRNA in developing trachea, differentiating tubules, later in cartilaginous components of bronchi	
	mRNA levels in rat lung decrease rapidly after 1 month	
Pathologic calcifications		
Growth plate	MGP-null mice exhibit disorganized chondrocyte columns, abnormal calcification, short staure, and osteopenia	108
Arterial wall	MGP-null mice had chondrocyte-like cells in arteries, matrix vesicles, and calcification of all elastic and muscular arteries	108
Atherosclerosis	mRNA in human lesion, highest in macrophages and smooth muscle cells, and lumen lining endothelial cells. protein in the matrix around lipid-rich, calcified areas	114
	mRNA increases with progression of rabbit lesion	115
Fracture callus	mRNA in fibroblast-like and chondrocytes of early rat callus proliferating and hypertrophic chondrocytes and trabecular surface osteoblasts of 9-day rat callus	112
	protein seen in monkey osteoclasts	113
Calcifying pilomatricoma	mRNA enhanced in pilomatricoma tissues	138
Cancer and apoptosis		
Cancer	mRNA in malignant human breast cells	99, 138, 139
	mRNA in human breast cancers	
	mRNA in urogenital malignancies	
Apoptosis	mRNA induced by rat prostate apoptosis	137

Both proteins contain a Gla domain, a thrombin sensitive segment, an EGF-like domain. The C terminus is homologous to the steroid hormone-binding globulin protein. Protein S is expressed primarily in the liver, whereas Gas6 is widely expressed, with the highest levels in lung, intestine, heart, kidney, neural, and hematopoietic tissue [140]. A Gas6 splice variant has been identified and has a similar distribution pattern to that of Gas6 [141].

Gas6 and protein S act as ligands for the AUS class of tyrosine kinase receptors (RTK). The members of this receptor subfamily include Axl (also called Ufo and Ark), Tyro3 (also known as Rse, Brt, Tif, and Sky), and Mer (also called cEyk). These RTKs share about 35% similarity in amino acid sequence and a conserved general domain structure, suggesting that they are recognized by related ligands. These three related RTKs display differential patterns of expression. Tyro3 is most prominently expressed in the adult nervous system, although it is also expressed in kidney, ovary, testis, differentiating embryonic stem cells, and a number of hematopoietic cell lines. Axl and Mer are also expressed in the nervous system but are more widely expressed in peripheral tissues [142, 143].

The SHG domain of Gas6 is responsible for the binding of Gas6 to tyrosine kinase receptors. The Gla domain is important for receptor activation by the calcium-dependent binding of Gla residues to the phosphatidyl serines of the membrane [144, 145]. Although the exact physiological function for Gas6 and its receptors remains to be discovered, several studies show that they may be important for growth regulation. Gas6 has mitogenic activity for Schwann cells and NIH3T3 cells [146, 147]. Bellosta *et al.* found that Gas6 increased cell survival by protecting NIH3T3 cells from apoptosis induced by serum starvation [148]. Interestingly, there are several reports that Gas6 is important in vascular smooth muscle cells. Gas6 has Gla-dependent growth potentiating activity in vascular smooth muscle cells which may work in conjunction with G protein receptor mediated signaling pathways [149–151]. Gas6 also induces receptor-mediated chemotactic activity of smooth muscle cells [152]. Whether Gas6 and MGP are part of a vitamin K-dependent cascade involved in modifying the progression of atherosclerosis and arterial calcification remains to be determined.

Relevant to bone, a study by Nakamura *et al.* [8] showed that protein S and Gas6 were direct regulators of osteoclasts. Gas6 induced the rapid phosphorylation of endogenous Tyro3 receptors on osteoclasts derived from 10-day-old rabbits. Osteoclast activity, as assessed by pit area, was increased in a dose-dependent manner by both proteins, but differentiation of osteoclast precursors was not affected. In addition, the authors reported that bone marrow stromal cells express Gas6 and, furthermore, that its expression is regulated by parathyroid hormone and 1,25-dihydroxyvitamin D_3. These reports are interesting in light of the previous observation that protein S is secreted and synthesized by osteoblasts, suggesting that protein S (and perhaps Gas6) provides a link between the osteoblast and the osteoclast [9].

Gas6 has also been detected in human cartilage and chondrocytes. Furthermore, both Gas6 and conditioned medium from chondrocyte cultures stimulated Axl tyrosine phosphorylation in chondrocytes [153].

VI. VITAMIN K/WARFARIN

The presence of Gla-containing proteins in bone suggests that vitamin K may play a role in skeletal health. Several studies have directly assessed vitamin K status in healthy individuals and in those with osteoporosis. In one study, circulating vitamin K levels were significantly lower in elderly osteoporotic patients with fractures of the femoral neck than in those without fractures [154]. However, the results of studies assessing the direct effect of warfarin therapy on bone density in humans have been conflicting. Two studies showed no effect of warfarin at the spine and hip [155, 156] while another two studies showed modest reduction at these sites [157, 158]. In a recent large multi-center study there was no difference in spine or total hip BMD or fracture rate in 150 Caucasian women 65 years or older using warfarin compared to nonusers [159].

The current RDA for vitamin K_1 (80 μg/day) is based on maintenance of normal coagulation status as assessed by simple clotting times [160]. However, this test does not detect subclinical deficiency and does not consider nonliver vitamin K requirements. Several studies have shown that the degree of undercarboxylated osteocalcin in serum is the most sensitive measure of vitamin K nutritional status [161]. Using such methods, an association was observed between undercarboxylated osteocalcin and risk of hip fracture. However, vitamin D status in these subjects was not documented. It is not known if undercarboxylated osteocalcin or low vitamin K levels are an indicator of generalized poor total nutritional status in these studies.

The phenotype of the osteocalcin knockout precludes a direct role for osteocalcin *per se* in any potential negative effects of vitamin K deficiency on bone. Unlike the liver-derived clotting factors, osteocalcin is not maximally carboxylated even when subjects receive vitamin K at the RDA. Supplementation with 420 μg/d of phylloquinone results in a 41% increase in carboxylation of osteocalcin [162]. It has been shown that a patient with warfarin sensitivity had an alanine to threonine mutation at residue -10 in the propeptide region of factor IX. This alanine residue is invariantly found in all vitamin K-dependent proteins *except* osteocalcin, which has a glycine in the corresponding position. Both amino acid substitutions (Ala–Thr and Ala–Gly) resulted in reduced affinity for the vitamin K–carboxylase enzyme *in vitro* [5]. It is interesting to speculate that the osteoblast may have relatively greater vitamin K requirements than the liver to *impede* deposition of osteocalcin. Thus, naturally occurring undercarboxylation of osteocalcin may represent a selective advantage for the protection of bone. Nothing is known about the normal carboxylation status of the other vitamin K-dependent proteins involved with bone and cartilage. It is not known if MGP is maximally carboxylated in all tissues in which it is expressed and at all developmental stages.

Any effects of vitamin K deficiency or warfarin administration may be regulated in a cell-specific way, and the mechanism for control may depend on the function of the gene product. Warfarin increased levels of MGP mRNA in cultured ROS 25/1 osteosarcoma cells and in cultured rat pneumocytes but had no effect in pre-chondrocytes, and fetal calvarial bone organ culture MGP mRNA levels were unchanged [163, 164]. Furthermore, warfarin had opposing effects on osteocalcin and MGP mRNA levels in the same cells [163]. Rats chronically treated with warfarin show premature closure of the epiphyseal growth plate and a denser cortical bone shaft [165], likely reflecting the effect of the drug on expression of both MGP and osteocalcin. Furthermore, carboxylation may play differing roles in the intracellular fate of the various vitamin K-dependent proteins. Acarboxyprothrombin is retained by rat hepatocytes, but secreted to variable degrees by human and bovine cells [166]. On the other hand, the presence of Gla residues is not absolutely required for production of the mature circulating osteocalcin species [17, 109, 167].

Several studies suggest that extra-hepatic vitamin K-dependent proteins respond to vitamin K depletion or repletion differently than the liver derived vitamin K-dependent proteins, and this difference probably reflects the diverse biological functions of these proteins [168]. The differing requirements for vitamin K in different tissues is illustrated by studies indicating that placental transfer of vitamin K may be tightly regulated to allow for appropriate signaling pathways in embryogenesis [169]. Modern tools in molecular biology are leading to the discovery of additional vitamin K-dependent proteins. Two novel proline-rich Gla proteins (PRGP1 and PRGP2) have been identified; they are single-pass transmembrane proteins abundantly expressed in the spinal cord and thyroid [170]. It is highly likely that there are other vitamin K-dependent proteins that are as yet unknown. Potential involvement of Gla-containing proteins with signal transduction pathways and/or calcium homeostasis may be responsible for any underlying bone pathology resulting from vitamin K deficiency.

References

1. Suttie, J. W., ed. (1987). "Current Advances in Vitamin K Research." Elsevier, New York.
2. Levy, R. J., Gundberg, C. M., and Scheinman, R. (1983). The presence of the bone specific vitamin K dependent protein, osteocalcin, in calcified atheroscleratic plaque and mineralized heart valves. *Atherosclerosis* **46**, 49–56.
3. Lian, J. B., Skinner, M., Glimcher, M. J., and Gallop, P. M. (1976). The presence of gamma-carboxyglutamic acid in the proteins associated with ectopic calcification. *Biochem. Biophys. Res. Commun.* **73**, 349–355.
4. Nakagawa, Y., Abram, V., Kezdy, F. J., Kaiser, E. T., and Coe, F. L. (1983). Purification and characterization of the principal inhibitor of calcium oxalate monohydrate crystal growth in human urine. *J. Biol. Chem.* **258**, 12594–12600.
5. Berkner, L., and Pudota, B. N. (1998). Vitamin K-dependent carboxylation of the carboxylase. *Proc. Natl. Acad. Sci. U.S.A.* **95**, 466–471.
6. Price, P. A., Urist, M. R., and Otawara, Y. (1983). Matrix Gla protein, a new gamma-carboxyglutamic acid-containing protein which is associated with the organic matrix of bone. *Biochem. Biophys. Res. Commun.* **117**, 765–771.
7. Price, P. A., and Williamson, M. K. (1985). Primary structure of bovine matrix Gla protein, a new vitamin K dependent bone protein. *J. Biol. Chem.* **260**, 14971–14975.
8. Nakamura, Y. S., Hakeda, Y., Takakura, N., Kameda, T., Hamaguchi, I., Miyamoto, T., Kakudo, S., Nakano, T., Kumegawa, M., and Suda, T. (1998). Tyro 3 receptor tyrosine kinase and its ligand, gas6, stimulate the function of osteoclasts. *Stem Cells* **16**, 229–238.
9. Maillard, C., Berruyer, M., Serre, C. M., Dechavanne, M., and Delmas, P. D. (1992). Protein-S, a vitamin K-dependent protein, is a bone matrix component synthesized and secreted by osteoblasts. *Endocrinology* **130**, 1599–1604.
10. Cairns, J. R., and Price, P. A. (1994). Direct demonstration that the vitamin K-dependent bone Gla protein is incompletely gamma-carboxylated in humans. *J. Bone Miner. Res.* **9**, 1989–1997.
11. Hauschka, P. V., and Carr, S. A. (1982). Calcium-dependent alpha-helical structure in osteocalcin. *Biochemistry* **21**, 2538–2547.
12. Poser, J. W., and Price, P. A. (1979). A method for decarboxylation of gamma-carboxyglutamic acid in proteins: Properties of the decarboxylated gamma-carboxyglutamic acid protein from calf bone. *J. Biol. Chem.* **254**, 431–436.
13. Pan, L. C., and Price, P. A. (1985). The propeptide of rat bone gamma-carboxyglutamic acid protein shares homology with other vitamin K-dependent protein precursors. *Proc. Natl. Acad. Sci. U.S.A.* **82**, 6109.
14. Price, P. A., Fraser, J. D., and Metz-Virca, G. (1987). Molecular cloning of matrix Gla protein: Implications for substrate recognition by the vitamin K-dependent gamma-carboxylase. *Proc. Natl. Acad. Sci. U.S.A.* **84**, 8335–8339.
15. Jorgensen, M. J., Cantor, A. B., Furie, B. C., Brown, C. L., Shoemaker, C. B., and Furie, B. (1987). Recognition site directing vitamin K-dependent gamma-carboxylation resides on the propeptide of factor IX. *Cell* **48**, 185–191.
16. Chu, K., Wu, S. M., Stanley, T., Stafford, D. W., and High, K. A. (1996). A mutation in the propeptide of factor IX leads to a warfarin sensitivity by a novel mechanism *J. Clin Invest.* **98**, 1619–1625.
17. Gundberg, C. M., and Clough, M. E. (1992). The osteocalcin propeptide is not secreted *in vivo* or *in vitro*. *J. Bone Miner. Res.* **7**, 73–80.
18. Gundberg, C. M. (1993). Methods for the measurement of urinary gamma-carboxyglutamic acid and serum osteocalcin and their use in the clinical situation as markers of bone disease. *In* "Vitamin K and Vitamin K-Dependent Proteins" (M. J. Shearer and M. J. Seghatchian, eds.), pp. 297–328. CRC Press, Boca Raton, FL.
19. Calvo, M. S., Eyre, D., and Gundberg, C. M. (1996). Molecular basis and clinical application of biological markers of bone turnover. *Endocr. Revi.* **17**, 333–368.
20. Eriksen, E. F., Brixen, K., and Charles, P. (1995). New markers of bone metabolism: Clinical use in metabolic bone disease. *Eur. J. Endocrinol.* **132**, 251–263.
21. Delmas, P. D. (1990). Biochemical markers of bone turnover for the clinical assessment of metabolic bone disease. *Endocrinol. Metab. Clin. North Am.* **19**, 1–18.
22. Lian, J. B., and Gundberg, C. M. (1988). Osteocalcin: Biochemical considerations and clinical applications. *Clin. Orthop. Relat. Res.* **226**, 267–291.
23. Hauschka, P. V., and Reid, M. L. (1978). Timed appearance of a calcium-binding protein containing gamma-carboxyglutamic acid in developing chick bone. *Dev. Biol.* **65**, 426.
24. Lian, J. B., Roufosse, A. H., and Reit, B. (1982). Concentrations of osteocalcin and phosphoprotein as a function of mineral content and age in cortical bone. *Calcif. Tissue Int.* **34**, S82–S87.
25. Mark, M. P., Prince, C. W., Gay, S., Austin, R. L., Bhown, M., Finkelman, R. D., and Butler, W. T. (1987). A comparative immunocytochemical study on the subcellular distributions of 44 kDa bone phosphoprotein and bone gammacarboxyglumatic acid (Gla)-containing protein in osteoblasts. *J. Bone Miner. Res.* **2**, 337–346.
26. Boivin, G., Morel, G., Lian, J. B., Anthoinc-Terrier, C., Dubois, P. M., and Meunier, P. J. (1990). Localization of endogenous osteocalcin in neonatal rat bone and its absence in articular cartilage: Effect influence of warfarin treatment. *Virchows Arch. A: Pathol. Anat. Histopathol.* **417**, 505–512.
27. McKee, M. D., and Nanci, A. (1993). Ultrastructural, cytochemical and immunocytochemical studies of bone and its interfaces. *Cells Mater.* **3**, 219–243.
28. Hauschka P. V., and Gallop P. M. (1977). Purification and calcium-binding properties of osteocalcin, the gamma-carboxyglutamate-containing protein of bone. *In* "Calcium Binding Proteins and Calcium Function" (R. Wasserman *et al.*, eds.) p. 338. Elsevier/North-Holland, Amsterdam.
29. Owen, T. A., Aronow, M., Shalhoub, V., Barone, L. M., Wilming, L., Tassinari, M. S., Kennedy, M. B., Pockwinse, S., Lian, J. B., and Stein, G. S. (1990). Progressive development of the rat osteoblast phenotype in vitro: Reciprocal relationships in expression of genes associated

with osteoblast proliferation and differentiation during formation of the bone extracellular matrix. *J. Cell. Physiol.* **143**, 420.

30. Harris, S., Enger, R., Riggs, B., and Spelsberg, T. (1995). Development and characterization of a conditionally immortalized human fetal osteoblastic cell line. *J. Bone Miner. Res.* **10**, 178–184.

31. Pockwinse, S. M., Lawrence, J. B., Singer, R. H., Stein, J. L., Lian, J. B., and Stein, G. S. (1993). Gene expression at single cell resolution associated with development of the bone cell phenotype: Ultrastructural and in situ hybridization analysis. *Bone* **14**, 347–352.

32. Gerstenfeld, L. C., Chipman, S. D., Glowacki, J., and Lian, J. B. (1987). Expression of differentiated function by mineralizing cultures of chicken osteoblasts. *Dev. Biol.* **122**, 49–60.

33. Gerstenfeld, L., Lian, J., Gotoh, Y., Lee, D., Landis, W., McKee, M., Nanci, A., and Glimcher, M. (1989). Use of cultured embryonic chicken osteoblasts as a model of cellular differentiation and bone mineralization. *Connect. Tissue Res.* **21**, 215–222.

34. Zhou, H., Choong, P., McCarthy, R., Chou, S., Martin, T., and Ng, K. (1994). *In situ* hybridization to show sequential expression of osteoblast gene markers during bone formation in vivo. *J. Bone Miner. Res.* **9**, 1489–1499.

35. Stein, G. S., Lian, J. B., and Owen, T. A. (1990). Relationship of cell growth to the regulation of tissue-specific gene expression during osteoblast differentiation. *FASEB J.* **4**, 3111–3123.

36. Ducy, P., Desbois, C., Boyce, B., Pinero, G., Story, B., Dunstan, C., Smith, E., Bonadio, J., Goldstein, S., Gundberg, C., Bradley, A., and Karsenty, G. (1996). Increased bone formation in osteocalcin-deficient mice. *Nature* **382**, 448–452.

37. Otawara, Y., and Price, P. A. (1986). Developmental appearance of matrix GLA protein during calcification in the rat. *J. Biol. Chem.* **261**, 10828–10832.

38. Boskey, A. L., Gadaleta, S., Gundberg, C., Doty, S. B., Ducy, P., and Karsenty, G. (1998). FT-IR microspectroscopic analysis of bones osteocalcin-deficient mice provides insight into the function of osteocalcin. *Bone* **23**, 187–196.

39. Wenstrup, R. J., Fowlkes, J. L., Witte, D. P., and Florer, J. B. (1996). Discordant expression of osteoblast markers in MC3T3-E1 cells that synthesize a high turnover matrix. *J. Biol. Chem.* **271**, 10271–10276.

40. Ingram, R. T., Park, Y.-K., Clarke, B. L., and Fitzpatrick, L. A. (1994). Age- and gender-related changes in the distribution of osteocalcin in the extracellular matrix of normal male and female bone. *J. Clin. Invest.* **93**, 989–997.

41. Malone, J. D., Teitelbaum, S. L., Griffin, G. L., Senior, R. M., and Kahn, A. J. (1982). Recruitment of osteoblast precursors by purified bone matrix constituents. *J. Cell Biol.* **92**, 227–230.

42. Lian, J. B., Dunn, K., and Key, L. L. (1986). *In vitro* degradation of bone particles by human monocytes is decreased with the depletion of the vitamin K-dependent bone protein from the matrix. *Endocrinology* **118**, 1636–1642.

43. Chenu, C., Colucci, S., Grano, M., Zigrino, P., Barattolo, R., Zambonin, G., Baldini, N., Vergnaud, P., Delmas, P. D., and Zallone, A. Z. (1994). Osteocalcin induces chemotaxis, secretion of matrix proteins, and calcium-mediated intracellular signaling in human osteoclast-like cells. *J. Cell Biol.* **127**, 1149–1158.

44. Webber, D., Osdoby, P., Hauschka, P., and Krukowski, M. (1990). Correlation of an osteoclast antigen and ruffled border on giant cells formed in response to resorbable substrates. *J. Bone Miner. Res.* **5**, 401–410.

45. Lian, J. B., Tassinari, M., and Glowacki, J. (1984). Resorption of implanted bone prepared from normal and warfarin-treated rats. *J. Clin. Invest.* **73**, 1223–1226.

46. Serre, C. M., Price, P., and Delmas, P. D. (1995). Degradation of subcutaneous implants of bone particles from normal and warfarin-treated rats. *J. Bone Miner. Res.* **10**, 1158–1167.

47. Glowacki, J., Rey, C., Glimcher, M. J., Cox, K. A., and Lian, J. B.

(1991). A role for osteocalcin in osteoclast differentiation. *J. Cell. Biochem.* **45**, 292–302.

48. Reinholt, F. P., Hultenby, K., Oldberg, A., and Heinegard, D. (1990). Osteopontin—a possible anchor of osteoclasts to bone. *Proc. Natl. Acad. Sci. U.S.A.* **87**, 4473–4475.

49. Ritter, N. M., Farach-Carson, M. C., and Butler, W. T. (1992). Evidence for the formation of a complex between osteopontin and osteocalcin. *J. Bone Miner. Res.* **7**, 877–885.

50. Puchacz, E., Lian, J. B., and Stein, G. S. (1989). Chromosomal localization of the human osteocalcin gene. *Endocrinology* **124**, 2648–2650.

51. Yoon, K., Rutledge, S. J. C., Buenage, R. F., and Rodan, G. A. (1988). Characterization of the rat osteocalcin gene: Stimulation of promoter activity by 1,25-Dihydroxyvitamin D$_3$. *Biochemistry* **27**, 8521–8526.

52. Rahman, S., Oberdorf, A., Montecino, M., Tanhauser, S. M., Lian, J. B., Stein, G. S., Laipis, P. J., and Stein, J. L. (1993). Multiple copies of the bone-specific osteocalcin gene in mouse and rat. *Endocrinology* **133**, 3050–3053.

53. Bedbois, C., Hogue, D. A., and Karsenty, G. (1994). The mouse osteocalcin gene cluster contains three genes with two separate spatial and temporal patterns of expression. *J. Biol. Chem.* **269**, 1183–1190.

54. Nakagawa, Y., Abram, V., and Coe, F. L. (1984). Isolation of a calcium oxalate monohydrate crystal growth inhibitor from rat kidney and urine. *Am. J. Physiol.* **247**, F765–F772.

55. Nakagawa, Y., Ahmed, M., Hall, S. L., Deganello, S., and Coe, F. L. (1987). Isolation from human calcium oxalate renal stones of nephrocalcin, a glycoprotein inhibitor of calcium oxalate crystal growth. *J. Clin. Invest.* **79**, 1782–1787.

56. McKee, M. D., Nanci, A., and Khan, S. R. (1995). Ultrastructural immunodetection of osteopontin and osteocalcin as major matrix components of renal calculi. *J. Bone Miner. Res.* **10**, 1913–1929.

57. Hauschka, P. V., Friedman, P. A., Travarso, H. P., and Gallop, P. M. (1976). Vitamin K dependent gamma carboxyglutamic acid formatiom by kidney microsomes in vitro. *Biochem. Biophys. Res. Commun.* **71**, 1207–1213.

58. Friedman, P. A., Mitch, W. E., and Silva, P. (1982). Localization of renal vitamin K-dependent gamma-glutamyl carboxylase to tubule cells. *J. Biol. Chem.* **257**, 11037–11040.

59. Karl, P. I., and Friedman, P. A. (1983). Effects of parathyroid hormone and vitamin D on the renal vitamin K-dependent carboxylating system. *J. Biol. Chem.* **258**, 12783–12786.

60. Deyl, Z., Vancikova, O., and Macek, K. (1980). Gamma-carboxyglutamic acid-containing protein of rat kidney cortex changes with high fat diet, and molecular parameters. *Hoppe-Seyler's Z. Physiol. Chem.* **361**, 1767–1772.

61. Stein, G. S., Lian, J. B., van Wijnen, A. J., and Stein, J. L. (1997). The osteocalcin gene: A model for multiple parameters of skeletal-specific transcriptional control. *Mol. Biol. Rep.* **24**, 185–196.

62. Morrison, N. A., Shine, J., Fragonas, J. C., Verkest, V., McMenemy, L., and Eisman, J. A. (1989). 1,25-dihydroxyvitamin D-responsive element and glucocorticoid repression in the osteocalcin gene. *Science* **246**, 1158–1161.

63. Demay, M. B., Gerardi, J. M., DeLuca, H. F., and Kronenberg, H. M. (1990). DNA sequences in the rat osteocalcin gene that bind the 1,25-dihydroxyvitamin D$_3$ receptor and confer responsive to 1,25-dihydroxyvitamin D$_3$. *Proc. Natl. Acad. Sci. U.S.A.* **87**, 369–373.

64. Markose, E. R., Stein, J. L., Stein, G. S., and Lian, J. B. (1990). Vitamin D-mediated modifications in protein-DNA interactions at two promoter elements of the osteocalcin gene. *Proc. Natl. Acad. Sci. U.S.A.* **87**, 1701–1705.

65. Kerner, S. A., Scott, R. A., and Pike, J. W. (1989). Sequence elements in the human osteocalcin gene confer basal activation and inducible response to hormonal vitamin D$_3$. *Proc. Natl. Acad. Sci. U.S.A.* **86**, 4455–4459.

66. Lian, J. B., Shalhoub, V., Aslam, F., Frenkel, B., Green, J., Hamrah, M., Stein, G. S., and Stein, J. L. (1997). Species-specific glucocorticoid and 1,25 dihydroxyvitamin D responsiveness in mouse MC3T3-E1 osteoblasts: Dexamethasone inhibits osteoblast differentiation and vitamin D down-regulates osteocalcin gene expression. *Endocrinology* **138**, 2117–2127.

67. Carpenter, T. O., Moltz, K. C., Ellis, B., Andreoli, M., McCarthy, T. L., Centrella, M., Bryan, D., and Gundberg, C. (1998). Osteocalcin production in primary osteoblast cultures derived from normal and Hyp mice. *Endocrinology* **139**, 35–43.

68. Zhang, R., Ducy, P., and Karsenty, G. (1997). 1,25-Dihydroxyvitamin D$_3$ inhibits osteocalcin expression in mouse through an indirect mechanism. *J. Biol. Chem.* **272**, 110–116.

69. Gerstenfeld, L. C., Zurakowski, D., Schaffer, J. L., Nichols, D. P., Toma, C. D., Broess, M., Bruder, S. P., and Caplan, A. L. (1996). Variable hormone responsiveness of osteoblast populations isolated at different stages of embryogenesis and its relationship to the osteogenic lineage. *Endocrinology* **137**, 3957–3968.

70. Nishimoto, S. K., Salka, C., and Nimni, M. E. (1987). Retinoic acid and glucocorticoids enhance the effect of 1,25-dihydroxyvitamin D$_3$ on bone gamma-carboxyglutamic acid protein synthesis by rat osteosarcoma cells. *J. Bone Miner. Res.* **2**, 571–577.

71. Noda, M., Yoon, K., and Rodan, G. A. (1988). Cyclic AMP-mediated stabilization of osteocalcin mRNAa in rat osteoblast-like cell treated with parathyroid hormone. *J. Biol. Chem.* **263**, 18574–18577.

72. Egrise, D. Martin, D., Neve, P., Verhas, M., and Schoutens, A. (1990). Effects and interactions of 17B-estradiol, T$_3$ and 1,25 (OH)$_2$D$_3$ on cultured osteoblasts from mature rats. *Bone Miner.* **11**, 273–283.

73. Thiede, M. A., Smock, S. L., Petersen, D. N., Grasser, W. A., Thompson, D. D., and Nishimoto, S. K. (1994). Presence of messenger ribonucleic acid encoding osteocalcin, a marker of bone turnover, in bone marrow megakaryocytes and peripheral blood platelets. *Endocrinology* **135**, 929–937.

74. Fleet, J. C., and Hock, J. M. (1994). Identification of osteocalcin mRNA in non-osteoid tissue of rats and humans by reverse transcription-polymerase chain reaction. *J. Bone Miner. Res.* **9**, 1565–1573.

75. Li, Y. P., Chen, W., and Stashenko, P. (1995). Characterization of a silencer element in the first exon of the human osteocalcin gene. *Nucleic Acid Res.* **23**, 5064–5072.

76. Goto, K., Heymont, J. L., Klein-Nulend, J., Kronenberg, H. M., and Demay, M. B. (1996). Identification of an osteoblastic silencer element in the first intron of the rat osteocalcin gene. *Biochemistry.* **35**, 11005–11011.

77. Frenkel, B., Montecino, M., Stein, J. L., Lian, J. B., and Stein, G. S. (1994). A composite intragenic silencer domain exhibits negative and positive transcriptional control of the bone-specific osteocalcin gene: promoter and cell type requirements. *Proc. Natl. Acad. Sci. U.S.A.* **91**, 10923–10927.

78. Merriman, H. L., van Wijnen, A. J., Hiebert, S., Bidwell, J. P., Fey, E., Lian, J. B., Stein, J., and Stein, G. S. (1995). The tissue-specific nuclear matrix protein, NMP-2, is a member of the AML/CBF/PEBP2/Runt domain transcription factor family: Interactions with the osteocalcin gene promoter. *Biochemistry* **34**, 13125–13132.

79. Geoffroy, V., Ducy, P., and Karsenty, G. (1995). A PEBP2a/AML-1-related factor increases osteocalcin promoter activity through its binding to an osteoblast-specific cis-acting element. *J. Biol. Chem.* **270**, 30973–30979.

80. Ducy, P., Zhang, R., Geoffroy, V., Ridall, A. L., and Karsenty, G. (1997). Osf2/Cbfa1: A transcriptional activator of osteoblast differentiation. *Cell* **89**, 747–754.

81. Otto, F., Thornell, A. P., Crompton, T., Denzel, A., Gilmour, K. C., Rosewell, I. R., Stamp, G. W. H., Beddington, R. S. P., Mundlos, S., Olsen, B. R., Selby, P. B., and Owen, M. J. (1997). Cbfa1, a candidate gene for cleidocranial dysplasia syndrome, is essential for osteoblast differentiation and bone development. *Cell* **89**, 765–771.

82. Komori, T., Yagi, H., Nomura, S., Yamaguchi, A., Sasaki, K., Deguchi, K., Shimizu, Y., Bronson, R. T., Gao, Y. H., Inada, M., Sato, M., Okamoto, R., Kitamura, Y., Yoshiki, S., and Kishimoto, T. (1997). Targeted disruption of Cbfa1 results in a complete lack of bone formation owing to maturational arrest of osteoblasts. *Cell* **89**, 755–764.

83. Garnero, P., Grimaux, M., Seguin, P., and Delmas, P. D. (1994). Characterization of immunoreactive forms of human osteocalcin generated in vivo and in vitro. *J. Bone Miner. Res.* **9**, 255–264.

84. Rosenquist, C., Quist, P., Bjarnason, N., and Christiansen, C. (1995). Measurement of a more stable region of osteocalcin in serum by ELISA with two monoclonal antibodies. *Clin. Chem.* **41**, 1439–1445.

85. Chen, J. T., Hosoda, K., Hasumi, K., Ogata, E., and Shiraki, M. (1996). Serum N-terminal osteocalcin is a good indicator for estimating responders to hormone replacement therapy in postmenopausal women. *J. Bone Miner. Res.* **11**, 1784–1792.

86. Gorai, L., Hosoda, K., Taguchi, Y., Chacki, O., Nakavama, M., Yoh, K., Yamaii, T., and Minaguchi, H. (1997). A heterogeneity in serum osteocalcin N-terminal fragments in Paget's disease: A comparison with other biochemical indices in pre- and post-menopause. *J. Bone. Miner. Res.* **12**, T678.

87. Blumsohn, A., Hannon, R. A., and Eastell, R. (1995). Apparent instability of osteocalcin in serum as measured with different commercially available immunoassays. *Clin. Chem.* **41**, 318–320.

88. Taylor, A. K., Linkhart, S., Mohan, S., Christenson, R. A., Singer, F. R., and Baylink, D. J. (1990). Multiple osteocalcin fragments in human urine and serum as detected by a midmolecule osteocalcin radioimmunoassay. *J. Clin. Endocrinol. Metab.* **70**, 467–472.

89. Salo, J., Lehenkari, P., Mulari, M., Metsikkö, K., and Väänänen, H. K. (1997). Removal of osteoclast bone resorption products by transcytosis. *Science* **276**, 270–273.

90. Page, A. E., Hayman, A. R., Andersson, L. M. B., Chambers, T. J., and Warburton, M. J. (1993). Degradation of bone matrix proteins by osteoclast cathepsins. *Int. J. Biochem.* **25**, 545–550.

91. Baumgrass, R., Williamson, M. K., and Price, P. A. (1997). Identification of peptide fragments generated by digestion of bovine and human osteocalcin with the lysosomal proteinases cathepsin B, D, L, H, and S. *J. Bone. Miner. Res.* **12**, 447–455.

92. Novak, J. F., Hayes, J. D., and Nishimoto, S. K. (1997). Plasmin-mediated proteolysis of osteocalcin. *J. Bone. Miner. Res.* **12**, 1035–1042.

93. Rice, J. S., Williamson, M. K., and Price, P. A. (1994). Isolation and sequence of the vitamin K-dependent Matrix Gla Protein from the calcified cartilage of the soupfin shark. *J. Bone Miner. Res.* **9**, 567–576.

94. Cancela, M. L., Hsieh, C., Francke, U., and Price, P. A. (1990). Molecular structure, chromosome assignment, and promoter organization of the human matrix Gla protein gene. *J. Biol. Chem.* **265**, 15040–15048.

95. Engelke, J. E., Hale, J. E., Suttie, J. W., and Price, P. A. (1991). Vitamin K-dependent carboxylase: Utilization of decarboxylated bone Gla protein and matrix Gla protein as substrates. *Biochim. Biophys. Acta* **1078**, 31–34.

96. Price, P. A., Rice, J. S., and Williamson, M. K. (1994). Conserved phosphorylation of serines in the Ser-X-Glu/Ser(P) sequences of the vitamin K-dependent matrix Gla protein from shark, lamb, rat, cow and human. *Protein Sci.* **3**, 822–830.

97. Nemir, M., DeVouge, M. W., and Mukherjee, B. B. (1989). Normal rat kidney cells secrete both phosphorylated and nonphosphorylated forms of osteopontin showing different physiological properties. *J. Biol. Chem.* **264**, 18202–18208.

98. Hale, J. E., Williamson, M. K., and Price, P. A. (1991). Carboxyl-terminal proteolytic processing of matrix Gla protein. *J. Biol. Chem.* **266**, 21145–21149.

99. Levedakou, E. N., Strohmeyer, T. G., Effert, P. J., and Liu, E. T. (1992). Expression of the matrix Gla protein in urogenital malignancies. *Int. J. Cancer* **52**, 534–537.

100. Zhao, J., Araki, N., and Nishimoto, S. K. (1995). Quantification of matrix Gla protein by competitive polymerase chain reaction using glyceraldehyde-3-phosphate dehydrogenase as an internal control. *Gene* **155**, 159–165.

101. Zhao, J., and Nishimoto, S. K. (1995). An RNA-competitive polymerase chain reaction method for human matrix Gla protein mRNA measurement. *Anal. Biochem.* **228**, 162–164.

102. Zhao, J., and Nishimoto, S. K. (1996). Matrix Gla protein gene expression is elevated during postnatal development. *Matrix Biol.* **15**, 131–140.

103. Luo, G., D'Souza, R., Hogue, D., and Karsenty, G. (1995). The Matrix Gla protein gene is a marker of the chondrogenesis lineage during mouse development. *J. Bone Miner. Res.* **10**, 325–334.

104. Fraser, J. D., and Price, P. A. (1988). Lung, heart, and kidney express high levels of mRNA for the vitamin K-dependent protein matrix Gla protein. *J. Biol. Chem.* **263**, 11033–11036.

105. Nishimoto, S. K., Robinson, F. D., and Snyder, D. L. (1993). Effect of aging and dietary restriction on matrix Gla protein and other components of rat tracheal cartilage. *Matrix* **13**, 373–380.

106. Zhao, J., Araki, N., and Nishimoto, S. K. (1995). Quantification of matrix Gla protein by competitive polymerase chain reaction using glyceraldehyde-3-phosphate dehydrogenase as an internal control. *Gene* **155**, 159–165.

107. Luo, G., Ducy, P., McKee, M. D., Pinero, J. P., Loyer, E., Behringer, R. R., and Karsenty, G. (1997). Spontaneous calcification of arteries and cartilage in mice lacking Matrix Gla protein. *Nature* **386**, 78–81.

108. Barone, L. M., Owen, T. A., Tassinari, M. S., Bortell, R., Stein, G. S., and Lian, J. B. (1991). Developmental expression and hormonal regulation of the rat matrix Gla protein (MGP) gene in chondrogenesis and osteogenesis. *J. Cell. Biochem.* **46**, 351–365.

109. Fraser, J. D., Otawara, Y., and Price, P. A. (1988). 1,25-Dihydroxyvitamin D_3 stimulates the synthesis of matrix Gla protein by osteosarcoma cells. *J. Biol. Chem.* **263**, 911–916.

110. Nishimoto, S. K., and Price, P. A. (1980). Secretion of the vitamin K-dependent protein of bone by rat osteosarcoma cells. Evidence for an intracellular precursor. *J. Biol. Chem.* **255**, 6579–6583.

111. Fraser, J. D., and Price, P. A. (1990). Induction of matrix Gla protein synthesis by prolonged 1,25 dihyroxyvatamin D_3 treatment of osteosarcoma cells. *Calcif. Tissue Int.* **46**, 270–279.

112. Hirakawa, K., Hirota, S., Ikeda, T., Yamguchi, A., Takemura, T., Nagoshi, J., Yoshiki, S., Suda, T., Kitamura, Y., and Nomura, S. (1994). Localization of the mRNA for bone matrix proteins during fracture healing as determined by in situ hybridization. *J. Bone Miner. Res.* **9**, 1551–1559.

113. Sugimoto, M., Hirota, S., Sato, M., Kawahata, H., Tsukamoto, I., Yasui, N., Kitamura, Y., Ochi, T., and Nomura, S. (1998). Impaired expression of noncollagenous bone matrix protein mRNAs during fracture healing in ascorbic acid-deficient rats. *J. Bone Miner. Res.* **13**, 271–278.

114. Carlson, C. S., Tulli, H. M., Jayo, M. J., Loeser, R. F., Tracy, R. P., Mann, K. G., and Adams, M. R. (1993). Immunolocalization of noncollagenous bone matrix proteins in lumbar vertebrae from intact and surgically menopausal cynomolgus monkeys. *J. Bone Miner. Res.* **8**, 71–81.

115. Shanahan, C. M., Cary, N. R. B., Metcalf, J. C., and Weissberg, P. L. (1994). High expression of genes for calcification-regulating proteins in human atherosclerotic plaques. *J. Clin. Invest.* **93**, 2393–2402.

116. Sohma, Y., Suzuki, T., Sasano, H., Nagura, H., Nose, M., and Yamamoto, T. (1994). Expression of mRNA for matrix Gla protein during progression of atherosclerosis in aortae of watanabe heritable Hyperlipidemic rabbits. *J. Biochem.* **116**, 747–751.

117. Choong, P. F. M., Martin T. J., and Ng, K. W. (1993). Effects of ascorbic acid, calcitriol, and retinoic acid on the differentiation of preosteoblasts. *J. Orthop. Res.* **11**, 638–647.

118. Cancela, M. L., and Price, P. A. (1992). Retinoic acid induces matrix Gla protein gene expression in human cells. *Endocrinology* **130**, 102–108.

119. Cancela, M. L., Williamson, M. K., and Price, P. A. (1993). Retinoic acid increases MGP in rat plasma. *Nutr. Res.* **13**, 87–91.

120. Kirfel, J., Kelter, M., Cancela, M. L., Price, P. A., and Schule, R. (1997). Identification of a novel negative retinoic acid responsive element in the promoter of the human matrix Gla protein gene. *Proc. Natl. Acad. Sci. U.S.A.* **94**, 2227–2232.

121. Sheikh, M. S., Shao, Z.-M., Chen, J.-C., and Fontana, J. A. (1993). Differential regulation of matrix Gla protein (MGP) gene expression by retinoic acid and estrogen in human breast carcinoma cells. *Mol. Cell. Endocrinol.* **92**, 153–160.

122. Zhou, H., Hammonds, R. G., Findlay, D. M., Martin, T. J., and Ng, K. W. (1993). Differential effects of transforming growth factor-1 and bone morphogenetic protein 4 on gene expression and differentiated function of preosteoblasts. *J. Cell. Physiol.* **155**, 112–119.

123. Haaijman, A., D'Souza, R. N., Bronckers, A. L., Goei, S. W., and Burger, E. H. (1997). OP-1 (BMP-7) affects mRNA expression of type 1,11, X collagen, and matrix Gla protein in ossifying long bones in vitro. *J. Bone Mineral Res.* **12**, 1815–1823.

124. Zhao, J., and Warburton, D. (1997). Matrix Gla protein gene expression is induced by transforming growth factor-b in embryonic lung culture. *Am. J. Physiol.* **273**, L282–L287.

125. Price, P. A., Urist, M. R., and Otawara, Y. (1983). Matrix Gla protein, a new Gla-containing protein which is associated with the organic matrix of bone. *Biochem. Biophys. Res. Commun.* **117**, 765–771.

126. Thomsen, M. K., Wildgoose, P., Nilsson, P., and Hedner, U. (1993). Accumulation of the recombinant factor VIIa in rat bone: Importance of the Gla-domain and relevance to factor IX, another vitamin K-dependent clotting factor. *Pharmacol. Toxicol.* **73**, 127–132.

127. Tintut, Y., Parhami, F., Bostrom, K., Jackson, S. M., and Demer, L. L. (1998). cAMP stimulates osteoblast-like differentiation of calcifying vascular cells, potential signaling pathway for vascular calcification. *J. Biol Chem.* **273**, 7547–7553.

128. Proudfoot, D., Skepper, J. N., Shanahan, C. M., and Weissberg, P. L. (1998). Calcification of human vascular cells in vitro is correlated with high levels of matrix Gla protein and low levels of osteopontin expression. *Arterioscler. Thromb. Vasc. Biol.* **18**, 379–388.

129. Bostrom, K., Watson, K. E., Stanford, W. P., and Demer, L. L. (1995) Atherosclerotic calcification: Relation to developmental osteogenesis. *Am. J. Cardiol.* **75**, 88–91.

130. Giachelli, C. M., Bae, N., Almeida, M. Denhardt, D. T., Alpers, C. E., and Schwartz, S. M. (1993). Osteopontin is elevated during neointimal formation in rat arteries and is a novel component of human atherosclerotic plaques. *J. Clin. Invest.* **92**, 1686–1696.

131. Levy, R. J., Schoen, F. J., Levy, J. T., Nelson, A. C., Howard, S. L., and Oshry, L. J. (1983). Biologic determinants of dystrophic calcification and osteocalcin deposition in glutaraldehyde-preserved porcine heart valve leaflets implanted subcutaneously in rats. *Am. J. Pathol.* **113**, 143–155.

132. Levy, R. J., Qu, X., Underwood, T., Trachy, J., and Schoen, F. J. (1995). Calcification of valved aortic allografts in rats: Effects of age, crosslinking, and inhibitors. *J. Biomed. Mater. Res.* **29**, 217–226.

133. Cancela, M. L., Hu, B., and Price, P. A. (1997). Effect of cell density and growth factors on matrix Gla protein expression by normal rat kidney cells. *J. Cell. Physiol.* **171**, 125–134.

134. Loeser, R. F., and Wallin, R. (1992). Cell adhesion to matrix Gla protein and its inhibition by an Arg-Gly-Asp-containing peptide. *J. Biol. Chem.* **267**, 9459–9462.

135. Cancela, M. L., Williamson, M. K., and Price, P. A. (1994). The putative RGD-dependent cell adhesion activity of matrix Gla protein is due to higher molecular weight contaminants. *J. Biol. Chem.* **269**, 12185–12189.

136. Baudet, C., Perret, E., Delpech, B., Kaghad, M., Brachet, P., Wion, D.,

and Caput, D. (1998). Differentially expressed genes in C6.9 glioma cells during vitamin D-induced cell death program. *Cell Death Differ.* **5**, 116–125

137. Briehl, M. M., and Miesfeld, R. L. (1991). Isolation and characterization of transcripts induced by androgen withdrawal and apoptotic cell death in the rat ventral prostate. *Mol. Endocrinol.* **5**, 1381–1388.

138. Hirota, S., Ito, A., Nagoshi, J., Takeda, M., Kurata, A., Takatsuka, Y., Kohri, K., Nomura, S., and Kitamura, Y. (1995). Expression of bone matrix protein messenger ribonucleic acids in human breast cancers. *Lab. Invest.* **72**, 64–69.

139. Chen, L., O'Bryan, J. P., Smith, H. S., and Liu, E. (1990). Overexpression of matrix Gla protein mRNA in malignant human breast cells: Isolation by differential cDNA hybridization. *Oncogene* **5**, 1391–1395.

140. Manfioletti, G., Brancolini, C., Avanzi, G., and Schneider, C. (1993). The protein encoded by a growth arrest arrest-specific gene (gas6) is a new member of the vitamin K-dependent proteins related to protein S, a negative coregulator in the blood coagulation cascade. *Mol. Cell. Biol.* **13**, 4976–4985.

141. Marcandalli, P., Gostissa, M., Varnum, B., Goruppi, S., and Schneider, C. (1997). Identification and tissue expression of a splice variant for the growth arrest-specific gene gas6. *FEBS Lett.* **415**, 56–58.

142. Stitt, T. N., Conn, G., Gore, M., Lai, C., Bruno, J., Radziejewski, C., Mattsson, K., Fisher, J., Gles, D. R., Jones, P. F., Masiakowski, P., Ryan, T. E., Tobkes, N. J., Chen, D. H., DiStefano, P. S., Long, G. L., Basilico, C., Goldfarb, M. P., Lemke, G., Glass, D. J., and Yancopoulos, G. D. (1995). The anticoagulation factor protein S and its relative, gas6, are ligands for the tyro 3/axl family of receptor tyrosine kinases. *Cell* **80**, 661–670.

143. Crosier, P. S., Lewis, P. M., and Hall, L. R. (1994). Isolation of a receptor tyrosine kinase (DTK) from embryonic stem cells: Structure, genetic mapping and analysis of expression. *Growth Factors* **11**, 125–136.

144. Mark, M. R., Chen, J., Hammonds, R. G., Sadick, M., and Godowsk, P. J. (1996). Characterization of gas6, a member of the superfamily of G domain-containing proteins, as a ligand for Rse and Axl. *J. Biol. Chem.* **271**, 9785–8789.

145. Joseph, D. R. (1997). Sequence and functional relationships between androgen-binding protein/sex hormone-binding globulin and its homologs protein S, gas6, laminin, and agrin. *Steroids* **62**, 578–588.

146. Li, R., Chen, J., Hammonds, G., Phillips, H., Armanini, M., Wood, P., Bunge, R., Godowski, P. J., Sliwkowski, M. X., and Mather, J. P. (1996). Identification of gas6 as a growth factor for human Schwann cells. *J. Neurosci.* **16**, 2012–2019.

147. Goruppi, S., Ruaro, E., Varnum, B., and Schneider, C. (1997). Requirement of phosphatidylinositol 3-kinase-dependent pathway and Src for gas6-Axl mitogenic and survival activities in HIH 3T3 fibroblasts. *Mol. Cell Biol.* **17**, 4442–4453.

148. Bellosta, P., Zhang, Q., Goff, S. P., and Basilico, C. (1997). Signaling through the ARK tyrosine kinase receptor protects from apoptosis in the absence of growth stimulation. *Oncogene* **15**, 2387–2397.

149. Nakano, T., Higashino, K., Kikuchi, N., Kishino, J., Nomura, K., Fujita, H., Ohara, O., and Arita, H. (1995). Vascular smooth muscle cell-derived, Gla-containing growth-potentiating factor for Ca^{2+}-mobilizing growth factors. *J. Biol. Chem.* **270**, 5702–5705.

150. Nakano, T., Ishimoto, Y., Kishino, J., Umeda, M., Inoue, K., Nagata, K., Ohashi, K., Mizuno, K., and Arita, H. (1997). Cell adhesion to phosphatidylserine mediated by a product of growth arrest-specific gene 6. *J. Biol. Chem.* **272**, 29411–29414.

151. Nakano, T., Kawamoto, K., Kishino, J., Nomura, K., Higashino, K., and Arita, H. (1997). Requirement of gamma-carboxyglutamice acid residue for the biological activity of gas6: Contribution of endogenous gas6 to the proliferation of vascular smooth muscle cells. *Biochem. J.* **323**, 387–392.

152. Fridell, Y. W. C., Villa, J., Attar, E., and Liu, E. T. (1998). Gas6 induces axl-mediated chemotaxis of vascular smooth muscle cells. *J. Biol. Chem.* **273**, 7123–7126.

153. Loesser, R. F., Varnum, B. C., Carlson, C. S., Goldring, M. B., Liu, E. T., Sadiev, S., Kute, T. E., and Wallin, R. (1997). Human chondrocytes expression of growth-arrest-specific gene and the tyrosine kinase receptor axl: Potential role in autocrine signaling in cartilage. *Arthritis Rheum.* **40**, 1455–1465.

154. Hodges, S. J., Akesson, K., Vergnaud, P., Obrant, K., and Delmas, P. D. (1993). Circulating levels of vitamin K1 and K2 decreased in elderly women with hip fracture. *J. Bone Miner. Res.* **8**, 1241–1245.

155. Rosen, H. N., Maitland, L. A., Suttie, J. W., Manning, W. J., Glynn, R. J., and Greenspan, S. L. (1993). Vitamin K and maintenance of skeletal integrity in adults. *Am. J. Med.* **94**, 62–68.

156. Lafforque, P., Daver, L., Monites, J. R., Chagnaud, C., deBoissezon, M. C., and Aquaviva, P. C. (1997). Bone mineral density in patients given oral vitamin K antagonists. *Rev. Rhum. Mal. Osteo-Articulaires* **64**, 249–254.

157. Philip, W. J. U., Martin, J. C., Richardson, J. M., Reid, D. M., Webster, J., and Douglas, A. S. (1995). Decreased axial and peripheral bone density in patients taking long-term warfarin. *Q. J. Med.* **88**, 635–840.

158. Monreal, M., Olive, A., and Lafozz, E. (1991). Heparins, coumarin, and bone density. *Lancet* **338**, 706.

159. Jamal, S., Milani, G., Lipschutz, R., Stone, R., Browner, W. S., and Cummings, S. R. (1997). The therapeutic use of Warfarin does not influence post-menopausal osteoporosis. *J. Bone Miner. Res.* **12**, T512.

160. Food and Nutrition Board. (1989). "Recommended Dietary Allowances." 10th ed. National Academic Press, Washington, DC.

161. Sokoll, L. J., and Sadowski, J. A. (1996). Comparison of biochemical indexes for assessing vitamin K nutritional status in a healthy adult population. *Am. J. Clin. Nutr.* **63**, 566–573.

162. Sokoll, L. J., Booth, S. L., O'Brien, M. E., Davidson, K. W., Tsaioun, K. I., and Sadowski, J. A. Changes in serum osteocalcin, plasma phylloquinone, and urinary gamma-carboxyglutamic acid in response to altered intakes of dietary phylloquinone in human subjects. *Am. J. Clin. Nutr.* **65**, 779–784.

163. Barone, L. M., Aronow, M. A., Tassinari, M., Conlon, D., Canalis, E., Stein, G. S., and Lian, J. B. (1994). Differential effects of warfarin on mRNA levels of developmentally regulated vitamin K dependent proteins, osteocalcin, and matrix Gla protein in vitro. *J. Cell. Physiol.* **160**, 255–264.

164. Rannels, S. R., Cancela, M. L., Wolpert, E. B., and Price, P. A. (1993). Matrix Gla protein mRNA expression in cultured type II pneumocytes. *Am. J. Physiol.* **265**, L270–L278.

165. Price, P. A., and Williamson, M. K. (1981). Effects of warfarin on bone: Studies on the vitamin K-dependent protein of rat bone. *J. Biol. Chem.* **256**, 12754–12759.

166. Wu, W., Bancroft, J. D., and Suttie, J. W. (1996). Differential effects of warfarin on the intracellular processing of vitamin K-dependent proteins. *Thromb. Haemostasis* **76**, 46–52.

167. Nishimoto, S. K., and Price, P. A. (1985). The vitamin K-dependent bone protein is accumulated within cultured osteosarcoma cells in the presence of the vitamin K antagonist warfarin. *J. Biol. Chem.* **260**, 2832–2836.

168. Booth, S. L., and Suttie, J. W. (1998). Dietary intake and adequacy of vitamin K. *J. Nutr.* **128**, 785–788.

169. Saxena, S. P., Fan, T., Li, M., Israels, E. D., and Israels, L. G. (1997). A novel role for Vitamin K1 in a tyrosine phosphorylation cascade during chick embryogenesis. *J. Clin. Invest.* **99**, 602–607.

170. Kulman, J. D., Harris, J. E., Haldeman, B. A., and Davie, E. W. (1997). Primary structure and tissue distribution of two novel proline-rich gamma-carboxyglutamic acid proteins. *Proc. Natl. Acad. Sci. U.S.A.*, **94**, 9058–9062.

CHAPTER 4

Noncollagenous Proteins; Glycoproteins and Related Proteins

DICK HEINEGÅRD, PILAR LORENZO   Section for Connective Tissue Biology, Department of Cell and Molecular Biology, Lund University, S-221 00 Lund, Sweden

TORE SAXNE   Department of Rheumatology, Lund University, S-221 00 Lund, Sweden

I. INTRODUCTION

Over recent years, development in areas of cartilage and bone biology has provided expanding knowledge on a number of molecular constituents and in some cases also an understanding of functional properties, both with regard to bone and cartilage. Thus, we can view both tissues as composite materials with an organic major extracellular matrix, which provides the tissue properties. In bone, this organic matrix actually guides the deposits of minerals, essential for the tissue properties. The processes in the tissue are, however, governed by the cells that have to recognize events such as fatigue with resulting material insufficiency and also have to respond to altered requirements such as modified tissue load. Thus, the cells appear to sense alterations in the tissue via a variety of receptors, often integrins or special cell surface proteoglycans. To understand degradation of the tissue and consequences of extracellular matrix breakdown, it is important to know the organization of the molecules with regard to key elements in interactions. Also, in repair it is important that synthesis is coordinated such that a balance between newly produced molecules is optimal for their assembly into matrix structures.

As a background to the understanding of normal matrix biology and pathology in cartilage and bone, this chapter will describe key macromolecules and what is known about their functional roles. It should be kept in mind that the properties of cartilage and bone are quite different, both with regard to mechanics and with regard to composition. However, at the interface between the cartilage and the bone, it is imperative that molecules can interact between the two tissue structures to provide a tightly interwoven zone that is not sheared off, even by the high stress forces generated in the use of the joints.

59

II. CARTILAGE EXTRACELLULAR MATRIX

Cartilage matrix, schematically illustrated in Figure 1, consists of fibrillar networks, primarily of collagen II [1–3] and highly negatively charged molecules of aggrecan [4, 5] providing fixed charged density and therefore an osmotic environment that creates a swelling pressure [6, 7]. There are also a number of noncollagenous glycoproteins that apparently contribute to the regulation of tissue assembly and properties. In some cases these constitute small proteoglycans.

A. Aggrecan

As discussed in Chapter 5, aggrecan has a major role in providing fixed charge groups creating an osmotic environment in the cartilage, thus immobilizing water and restricting water flow. This is essential for the function of aggrecan in taking up and distributing load over the cartilage tissue and further onto the underlying bone. In fact, the charge density of aggrecan is so extreme that there is a very high swelling

pressure in the tissue [6, 7], which is resisted by the collagen network discussed below.

The tissue can thus be viewed as a composite of aggrecan within a fibrillar network. Aggrecan has more than a hundred negatively charged chondroitin sulfate side chains, each with some fifty carboxyl and fifty sulfate groups. The fibrillar network consists of collagen and attached, crossbridging and linking noncollagenous as well as collagenous matrix proteins.

B. The Collagen Network

The major functional property of the collagen network in cartilage is to provide tensional stability. To achieve this, the tissue contains collagen fibers apparently linked together by glycoproteins/proteoglycans. Such linking molecules may function to extend the collagen fibrillar network throughout the tissue. They may also serve to regulate fibrillogenesis by preventing accretion of new collagen molecules to a pre-existing or forming fibril. Indeed, inactivation of the genes for two of these collagen binding proteins (decorin and lumican) in mice leads to thicker and irregular collagen fibers in

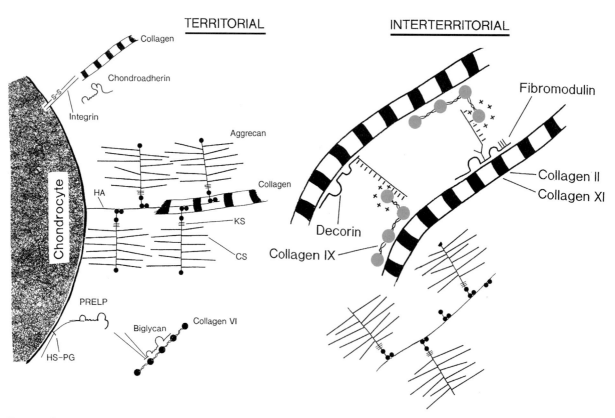

FIGURE 1   Illustration of cartilage matrix composition. The different molecular organization of territorial (close to cells) and interterritorial (distant from cells) matrices is depicted. Major constituents are proteoglycans and the collagen-based network, where collagen fibers contain numerous bound molecules that have roles in regulating assembly and maintaining function of the network. Interactions at the surface of the chondrocyte are likely to have roles in providing cells with information on matrix properties.

several tissues [8, 9]. However, the collagen fibers themselves contain two types of molecules, i.e., collagen II and a few percent of collagen XI that are closely related and that form the actual fibers [10]. Along the surface of these fibrils bound collagen IX is present [10, 11], a more complex collagen consisting of classical triple-helical domains interrupted by globular domains. This collagen may actually become covalently cross-linked to the collagen II fibers [12]. Of particular interest is that collagen IX may contain a glycosaminoglycan side chain bound to one of the non-triple-helical domains. Also, the N-terminal part of the α_1 chain [13] contains a large, globular, rather cationic domain. It has been shown that this extends out from the collagen fibril and provides a site for interactions with other anionic molecules in the matrix.

It is becoming clear that the molecules bound at the surface of the collagen fibers vary. Indeed, recent data indicate that there are fibers that lack collagen IX and others that lack decorin [14], the latter discussed later. There is a distinct and apparently separate collagen fibrillar system in cartilage made up of collagen VI molecules. The character of these molecules is quite distinct, with globular domains interrupting the triple helical structures [15, 16]. They form thinner fibrils that occur predominantly closer to the cells [17]. The function of this network is not clear.

C. Collagen-Associated Molecules

There are a number of noncollagenous molecules bound to the collagen fibrils in the tissue. These include decorin, fibromodulin, and lumican, all binding to fibers of collagen [18, 19], but in general not showing a great deal of specificity for a particular type of collagen. These molecules, as is discussed later, have structures of the protein core, suitable for binding to other matrix components. A related molecule, biglycan, appears not to primarily bind collagen II but binds tightly to collagen VI [C. Wiberg, E. Hedbom, and D. Heinegård, unpublished data].

Decorin, fibromodulin, and lumican are all members of a larger family of leucine-rich proteins with homologous structures (Fig. 2) [20]. These proteins have a central region of leucine-rich repeats (LRR), each of some 25 amino acid residues but somewhat variable in length. There are 10 or 11 such repeats in the proteins present in the extracellular matrix, although there are two exceptions (osteoglycin and epiphycan/PG-Lb) with shorter repeat regions. Structural details of this repeat region have been studied by X-ray crystallography of the ribonuclease inhibitor, an intracellular protein that shows homology but contains a larger number of repeats. For reference the reader is referred to the review by Deisenhofer [21, 22]. The repeat region is surrounded by two disulphide loop structures. In the N-terminal end there is usually an extension carrying either the glycosaminoglycan side chains in the case of decorin and biglycan [20] or tyrosine

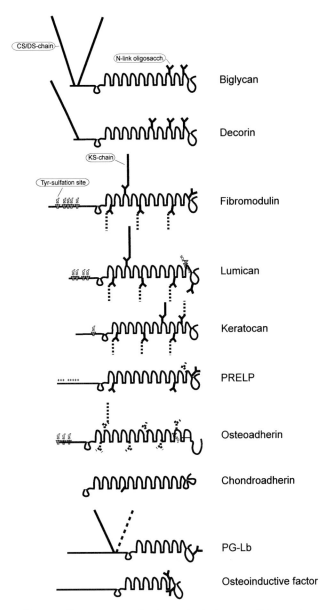

FIGURE 2   Illustration of LRR proteins in the extracellular matrix.

sulfate domains in the case of fibromodulin [23], lumican [24], osteoadherin [25], and probably also keratocan [26].

In PRELP the N-terminal peptide is rich in proline and arginine [27]. Preliminary data indicate that PRELP can actually bind heparin and heparan sulfate via this N-terminal extension (E. Bengtsson, A. Aspberg and D. Heinegård, unpublished data). The natural ligand in the tissue for this interaction remains to be identified. Furthermore, no ligand for binding to its leucine-rich repeat region has been identified. PRELP may, however, have a role at the cell surface interacting with heparan sulfate in syndecan, for example. This interaction may function in regulating cell signals. Indeed, it has been reported that PRELP can mediate cell binding, possibly involving heparan sulfate [28].

The one known exception containing no extension is chondroadherin [29]. In the C-terminal end, osteoadherin contains a long extension with a high abundance of acidic amino acids [25]. Thus, the members of this family of extracellular matrix leucine-rich repeat proteins include decorin, biglycan, fibromodulin, lumican, keratocan, PRELP, chondroadherin, and osteoadherin as well as two members with fewer repeats, i.e., osteoglycin and epiphycan [20], as is illustrated in Figure 2.

In addition to the protein domain binding to collagen, the molecules within the family, i.e., decorin, biglycan, fibromodulin, and lumican, all contain negatively charged domains, both in the forms of glycosaminoglycan side chains of dermatan sulfate/chondroitin sulfate (decorin, biglycan) and keratan sulfate (fibromodulin, lumican) as well as in the form of highly anionic tyrosine sulfate-rich structures (fibromodulin, lumican, and probably keratocan). These highly anionic structures indeed appear to form a second functional domain. Thus, as is illustrated in Figure 1, the protein core of these molecules appears to be bound to one collagen fiber such that the negatively charged side chain may participate in interactions with the neighboring fibril, either directly or via positively charged domains, e.g., in the form of the cationic NC4 domain of the α_1 chains of collagen IX bound to these fibers. Consequently, it is likely that these interactions will provide a tight, multiple-site linkage between adjacent collagen fibers stabilizing the network and the tissue. Thereby a highly tensile resistant structure is created that is likely to be of fundamental importance for the cartilage, since the highly negatively charged domain of the aggrecan molecules creates a swelling pressure that needs to be counteracted, in this case by a stable, stiff fibrillar network. It is conceivable that at some stage in processes of joint disease the stability of this network is impaired by proteolytic cleavage of the participating noncollagenous proteins. This may lead to the swelling of the tissue, as is often seen in osteoarthritis.

Another functional property has been ascribed to some members of the LRR family of proteins/proteoglycans. Biglycan, decorin, and fibromodulin have been shown to be able to bind TGF-β *in vitro* via their core proteins [30]. The physiological relevance of this interesting interaction is presently not known, although one can speculate on a role in growth, remodeling, and repair by releasing TGF-β.

Among the LRR matrix proteins, chondroadherin and osteoadherin have been shown to bind cells. This occurs via integrin $\alpha_2\beta_1$ for chondroadherin [31] and $\alpha_v\beta_3$ for osteoadherin [32]. Interestingly, cells binding to chondroadherin do not show spreading and cell division [28, 31], an effect commonly observed when cells bind via this integrin to collagen, for example. Thus, the molecule may have a role in regulating cell growth in the cartilage matrix. In support, its localization is predominantly close to cells in the pericellular environment [33].

D. Other Cartilage Extracellular Matrix Constituents

1. COMP

A prominent component in cartilage is COMP (cartilage oligomeric matrix protein). This protein is a homopentamer of five subunits, each with a protein molecular mass of just above 100,000 daltons [34–37]. These are joined via a coiled-coil domain near the N terminus [38] and the interaction is further stabilized by disulphide bonds. The protein has extensive homology to the thrombospondins but shows a more restricted tissue distribution to cartilage [34] and tendon [39, 40]. Recently, it has been shown that COMP interacts with triple helical collagen with a K_D of 10^{-9} in a Zn^{2+}-dependent manner [41]. Each of the five subunits contains one binding site in the C-terminal globular domain, thus potentially providing the protein with five interaction sites. Therefore, COMP may have a role in stabilizing the collagen network and/or in promoting the collagen fibril assembly. It has furthermore been proposed that COMP may bind chondrocytes [42]. However, the protein is predominantly present in the interterritorial compartment in adult articular cartilage at distance from the cells [43] and thus a primary role in this tissue does not appear to be cell binding. In contrast, the protein is found to be more abundant close to the cells in the proliferative region of the growth plate, where it thus may have a role in cell interactions [43].

Interestingly, there are calcium-binding repeats in COMP [41]. These appear to have a role in interactions, since the protein can be extracted from tissues using EDTA [35]. Furthermore, mutations in this domain cause growth abnormalities in pseudo-achondroplasia and multiple epiphyseal dysplasia [44–46]. These patients have a phenotype that becomes apparent only after birth, showing severe dysplasia and later osteoarthritis. One characteristic of these patients is lax joints, perhaps an effect of a function of COMP in the tendons and ligaments. The consequences of this defective Ca^{2+} binding are not apparent, although it appears that the collagen binding does not depend on Ca^{2+}. On the other hand, the chondrocytes show major lamellar deposits containing COMP and collagen IX [47]. It may be that one consequence of the COMP retention in the cells is that other key matrix proteins are also retained, creating a major molecular defect in the matrix.

2. MATRILINS

Cartilage matrix protein (CMP, matrilin-1) [48] is the first member of a new family with three known members, the matrilins [49]. These proteins contain von Willebrand factor A domains (vWFA). In the case of matrilin-1 [50], there are two such domains in each of the three identical subunits with a molecular weight of around 50,000. The three subunits are held together via a coiled-coil domain. The matrilins also contain one (matrilin-1) or several (four in matrilin-3) EGF repeat domains [49, 50].

Matrilins-1 and 3 are quite restricted to cartilage [49, 51] while matrilin-2 has a more general distribution. Interestingly, matrilin-1 has an even further restricted distribution in that it is not found in mechanically loaded tissues such as articular cartilage and the intervertebral disc, while it is particularly prominent in tracheal cartilage of older individuals [51]. The protein is present in the more immature cartilage of the femoral head during earlier phases of development and can be seen in the early bone anlagen [52]. However, at the time of the formation of articular cartilage, the protein is no longer found in this part of the tissue [51]. Its role in the cartilage is not clear, but its two vWFA homology domains (only one in matrilin-3) may mediate the indicated collagen binding capacity [53]. Furthermore, matrilin-1 was initially isolated because of its apparent ability to bind to aggrecan [54]. In subsequent studies it has been shown that the protein appears very tightly bound to distinct regions of aggrecan, possibly via a covalent bond [55]. In more recent work, it has been shown that matrilin-1 can be isolated from cartilage as a mixed polymer that contains subunits of matrilin-1 as well as matrilin-3 [56]. The functional significance of this heterocomplex is not understood.

3. CILP (CARTILAGE INTERMEDIATE LAYER PROTEIN)

This cartilage protein [57] is coded by a gene that is transcribed into a large message that includes two proteins. The major N-terminal portion is the ~92 kDa protein CILP, and the C-terminal portion represents a nucleotide pyrophosphohydrolase [58]. It appears that the precursor protein is cleaved in conjunction with its secretion from the cells to form the two proteins [58]. At this time there is no defined function of CILP, a protein that shares little homology with previously described proteins. Its distribution within the articular cartilage, however, suggests specific functions. Indeed CILP is not found equally throughout the cartilage and shows a restricted distribution to the middle-deep portion of the cartilage [57]. This indicates that this part of the tissue has some distinct functional requirements, where the presence of CILP contributes to the unique matrix properties important for meeting this challenge. Furthermore, CILP is markedly increased in both early and late osteoarthritis, perhaps an indication of an important role of the protein in repair/remodeling [P. Lorenzo, M. Bayliss, and D. Heinegård, unpublished work].

E. Other Proteins in Cartilage

There are a number of other proteins in cartilage that have been studied. These include a 39 kDa protein found predominantly in the more superficial parts of articular cartilage [59]. This protein is also found in other tissues.

A novel proteoglycan containing both keratan sulfate and chondroitin sulfate chains is primarily present in the superficial part of the articular cartilage and is also produced in the synovial capsule [60]. Little is known of its functional properties.

Fibronectin is present in cartilage and is interestingly upregulated in osteoarthritis [61]. The form present in cartilage is distinguished from that present in serum by being differently spliced [61, 62].

Fibulin-2 has been shown to be present, particularly in cartilage from growing individuals, although its function is not clear [63].

F. Concluding Remarks

The identification of an increasing number of matrix constituents and their characterization has resulted in new tools that can be used in the study of the normal biology of articular cartilage and that provide means for studies of pathobiology. An important future development should be to increase our understanding of the function of the individual proteins in order to correlate alterations in abundance with losses of components of functions in the cartilage. Furthermore, this could potentially also provide a means for developing procedures to stimulate their synthesis and thus help any repair process.

III. BONE EXTRACELLULAR MATRIX

A major feature of bone is its continuous remodeling. Therefore, the molecular constitutents of bone will be described in relation to this process. Load causes fatigue and often altered requirements on the tissue architecture. Thus, there is a characteristic bone remodeling cycle, schematically depicted in Figure 3, with the purpose of removing old, less functional bone and replacing this with fresh bone. Overall, this remodeling cycle has two phases. In the initial stage, bone breakdown is executed by the osteoclasts that adhere to the bone surface and create a secondary lysosome with an acid pH to dissolve the hydroxyapatite mineral. These cells contain a variety of lysosomal enzymes with the capacity to attack, degrade, and dissolve the organic matrix. The second, rebuilding phase depends on the recruitment of osteoblasts that lay down an osteoid, which becomes mineralized in a tightly regulated fashion.

Critical issues for understanding the normal regulation and dysregulation in disease of this cycle are how osteoclasts are recruited and become attached to the bone and how their activity is regulated; how osteoblasts or precursors are selectively recruited to the location where bone was previously removed, how they lay down a matrix, and particularly what initiates calcification. Current data on osteoclastic bone breakdown clearly indicate a role for the osteoblast in this phase. Thus,

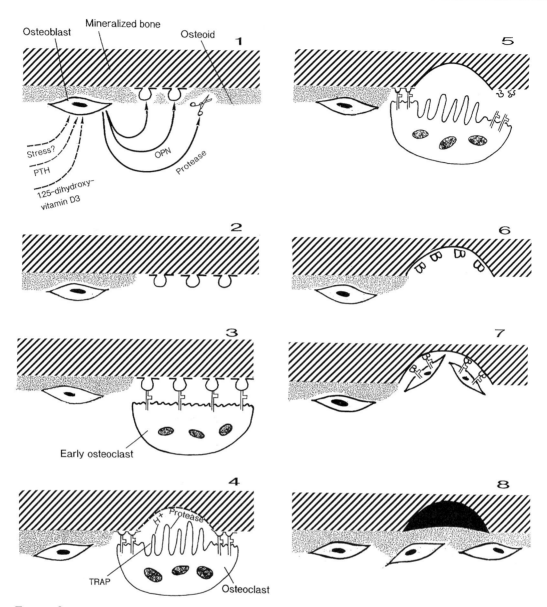

FIGURE 3 Schematic illustrations of the bone remodeling cycle. Matrix constituents having apparent roles in the various events are indicated. TRAP is tartrate-resistant phosphatase.

it appears that the osteoblast or lining cell is stimulated, most likely by local factors, possibly including stress, to secrete proteases to remove this osteoid and expose the mineralized bone surface. It is likely that in this process either cell-binding macromolecules are secreted and bound to the bone mineral surface or previously deposited such molecules become exposed.

Thus, from studies of osteoclast attachment, it has become clear that these cells can bind to osteopontin *in vitro* via their $\alpha_v\beta_3$ integrin [64]. In support of this, studies of osteoclasts by immunoelectron microscopy of bone tissue have shown that the $\alpha_v\beta_3$ integrin is localized in the clear zone [65], i.e., the site where the cells are attached to the underlying mineralized surface, and that osteopontin is selectively found op-

posing this part of the osteoclast [65]. In other studies, others, e.g., Teti, Zambonin-Zallone and collaborators [66, 67], have similarly shown the location of the $\alpha_v\beta_3$ integrin also to be in the clear zone area.

It thus appears from these studies that both the ligand and the receptor are found at corresponding locations. However, in one study, Lakkakorpi *et al.* [68] suggested that the $\alpha_v\beta_3$ integrin is actually predominantly localized to the ruffled border region. It is not clear what causes the difference, but this work contained no studies of ligands for the receptor. Neither was the force driving its location to this compartment discussed. In more recent studies, it has been shown that osteoclasts in bone of a mutant osteopetrotic rat (ia/ia) do not develop any significant ruffled border resorption region, and the surface facing the bone remains as a large clear zone area, especially without development of a resorptive ruffled border region. The $\alpha_v\beta_3$ integrin is localized to this entire area and osteopontin is found much enriched in the corresponding part of the opposing mineralized bone [68a]. The defect appears to block the secretory vesicles from emptying their contents into the extracellular matrix such that they become enriched on the cytosolic side of the plasma membrane

In summary, then, overwhelming data demonstrate that the only ligand that is localized at the attachment site, osteopontin, will bind to the $\alpha_v\beta_3$ integrin concentrated in the clear zone attachment area of the plasma membrane. Further information on the key role of the $\alpha_v\beta_3$ receptor and ligand is the fact that bone turnover can be interfered with by adding RGD-integrin-binding peptides [69, 70]. Also, it has been shown that osteopontin can be dephosphorylated by the tartrate-resistant acid phosphatase [71] secreted into the underlying extracellular area by osteoclasts [72]. Such dephosphorylated osteopontin has also been shown *in vitro* not to promote binding of osteoclasts [71], potentially a release mechanism for these cells. The role of osteoblasts is indicated by the fact that osteoblasts surrounding active osteoclasts have been shown to contain mRNA for osteopontin [73, 74]. It can thus be hypothesized that the cells actually lay down the osteopontin on the mineralized matrix and when the protein becomes exposed it promotes recruitment of the osteoclasts.

Interestingly, gene inactivation in mice of osteopontin produced no particular bone phenotype and apparently not osteopetrosis [75; A. Franzén and D. Heinegård, unpublished work]. It appears then that in this case another ligand has substituted for osteopontin, and one question is whether the $\alpha_v\beta_3$ receptor is still involved. Once the osteoclast has left the site of resorption, the next step is the recruitment of osteoblasts/osteoblast precursors. These cells must find an adhesion molecule at the surface of the "eroded" bone. However, an alternative may be that they secrete their own adhesion molecule, which in turn binds to some structure at the surface to which they are targeted. It is interesting that the bone surface that previously supported the osteoclast now instead will support an osteoblast. There are a number of candidate adhesion molecules. Collagen is abundantly present in the bone and can certainly bind cells via the $\alpha_1\beta_1$, $\alpha_2\beta_1$, and $\alpha_3\beta_1$ integrins [31, 76]. Fibronectin, although not particularly abundant at this site [74], would also have a potential for supporting cell binding via a number of integrins [77]. Other molecules that occur at this site in the bone and that are known to bind the integrins are of course osteopontin and BSP [64, 71] as well as osteoadherin [32]. All these proteins primarily bind cells via $\alpha_v\beta_3$ integrin, although osteopontin has been shown to bind to other integrins. The osteoblast certainly has the capacity to secrete these proteins [25, 78, 79]. Another alternative is that they remain present at the eroded bone surface. BSP is a potentially interesting candidate, since it has been shown to be particularly enriched in areas of bone

formation [73]. This includes seams and the bone–cartilage interface in the growth plate [73].

Osteoadherin, a bone-specific protein, appears to have the capacity to bind cells [32] via their $\alpha_v\beta_3$ integrin. Studies of the distribution of this bone protein in the tissue show its presence throughout the bone, albeit more enriched at the osteochondral junction [79a]. *In situ* hybridization shows that the protein is expressed by osteoblasts at the surface of trabecular bone [79a]. It should be emphasized that unfortunately there are no data to date to indicate whether one of these proteins actually has a primary role in the recruitment of osteoblasts or whether there are yet other proteins that have this primary role.

One protein with potential roles in regulating cellular activities, albeit not in binding the cells, is osteonectin (or SPARC) [80]. This protein is present in many connective tissues and has several names, e.g., osteonectin, its original name [81], BM-40 [82], and SPARC [83]. It is particularly abundant in bone. Studies *in vitro* have shown roles in modulating cell division and cell migration [80]. Another protein, the multimeric thrombospondin-1 also present in bone [84], has similar activities and may also actually bind cells [85–87]. The more detailed role of thrombospondin-1 in bone has to be further elucidated. In recent work, another member of this protein family, thrombospondin-2, was shown to have a role in bone homeostasis [88]. Thus, mice where the thrombospondin-2 gene was inactivated showed alterations in the bone mineral density [88].

The next event in the new bone formation is that the osteoblasts lay down an osteoid, nonmineralized matrix where the major constituent is collagen I, which forms fibers. These fibers contain molecules bound at their surface, i.e., fibromodulin, biglycan, and decorin as outlined above. It is particularly interesting that both decorin and fibromodulin bind to the gap region [89, 90], in view of the role that this part of the fiber has been postulated to have in mineral deposition. Indeed, it is known from work by several groups [91, 92] that collagen itself can actually support the mineralization. Although it is not clear what elicits this mineralization process one may hypothesize that removal of molecules occupying the gap zone may expose previously protected sites on the collagen. Thus, it is possible that an important event preceding mineralization is removal of decorin and fibromodulin. Indeed, in some very preliminary experiments we have found [K. Hultenby, F. P. Reinholt, and D. Heinegård, unpublished data], using immunolocalization at the ultrastructural level, that fibromodulin, while present in the osteoid on the collagen fibers, is not found in the mineralized bone. This loss of the protein from the tissue may represent an event preceding the mineralization but may alternatively represent a secondary phenomenon of changes in the conformation of the collagen network by the formation of mineral deposits.

A molecule that is unique to bone is osteocalcin [93, 94]. This is one of the few proteins that has posttranslational modifications in the form of gamma-carboxyglutamic acid residues (see Chapter 3). These residues provide the protein with particularly negatively charged clusters, which may promote binding to mineral deposits. Indeed, mice where the gene for osteocalcin has been inactivated show increased bone formation [95]. More exact details of interactions and functions of osteocalcin are not known despite much effort. Bone also contains numerous other molecules without defined functional properties. Many of these, including α_2HS [96, 97], are not synthetic products of the bone cells and are not further discussed here.

IV. CONCLUDING REMARKS

The increased knowledge of matrix constituents of bone and cartilage has provided an opportunity to develop assays for an increasing number of these molecules. Their continued study is likely to provide important insight into the understanding of the biology of the tissues and also to provide means for the study of events in tissues in normal remodeling as well as in pathological events in disease. This technology also offers opportunities for repeated analyses in the monitoring of evolving disease processes and in this defining characters of fragments produced. Thus, over recent years the so-called marker technology has developed. This aims at the measurement of, for example, fragments of matrix constituents released from their confinement in tissues as a result of a catabolic process. Quantitative assessment of such fragments has been shown to provide important information on early events leading to cartilage destruction in osteoarthritis [98] as well as rheumatoid arthritis [99, 100]. Future work can be anticipated to provide important tools for the diagnosis of disease in the musculoskeletal system, for monitoring the progress of disease, and for discerning mechanistic aspects.

References

1. Eyre, D. R. (1991). The collagens of articular cartilage. *Semin. Arthritis Rheum.* **21** (Suppl. 2), 2–11.
2. Mayne, R., van der Rest, M., Bruckner, P., *et al.* (1996). The collagens of cartilage (types II, IX, X and XI) and the type IX-related collagens of other tissues (types XII and XIV). *In* "Extracellular Matrix: A Practical Approach" (M. A. Haralson and J. R. Hassell, eds.), pp. 73–97. IRL Press at Oxford University Press, Oxford.
3. van der Rest, M., and Garrone, R. (1991). Collagen family of proteins. *FASEB J.* **5**, 2814–2823.
4. Hardingham, T. E., and Fosang, A. J. (1992). Proteoglycans: Many forms and many functions. *FASEB J.* **6**, 861–870.
5. Heinegård, D., Oldberg, Å.,Royce, P. M., and Steinmann, B, eds. (1998). Glycosylated matrix proteins. *In* "Connective Tissue and Its Heritable Disorders" (D. Heinegård *et al.*, eds.), pp. 189–209. Wiley-Liss, New York.
6. Mow, V., Setton, L., Brandt, K. D., Doherty, M., and Lohmander, L. S., eds. (1998). 7.2.4. Mechanical properties of normal and osteoarthritic articular cartilage. *In* "Osteoarthritis" (V. Mow *et al.*, eds.), pp. 108–122. Oxford University Press, New York.
7. Maroudas, A., and Freeman, M. A. R., eds. (1979). Physicochemical properties of articular cartilage. *In* "Adult Articular Cartilage" (A. Maroudas and M. A. R. Freeman, eds.) pp. 215–290. Pitman Medical Turnbridge Wells.
8. Danielson, K. G., Baribault, H., Holmes, D. F., Graham, H., Kadler, K. E., and Iozzo, R. V. (1997). Targeted disruption of decorin leads to abnormal collagen fibril morphology and skin fragility. *J. Cell Biol.* **136**, 729–743.
9. Chakravarti, S., Magnuson, T., Lass, J. H., Jepsen, K. J., LaMantia, C., and Carroll, H. (1998). Lumican regulates collagen fibril assembly: Skin fragility and corneal opacity in the absence of lumican. *J. Cell Biol.* **141**, 1277–1286.
10. Mendler, M., Eich-Bender, S. G., Vaughan, L., Winterhalter, K. H., and Bruckner, P. (1989). Cartilage contains mixed fibrils of collagen types II, IX, and XI. *J. Cell Biol.* **108**, 191–197.
11. Eyre, D., Wu, J.-J., Woods, P., Kuettner, K. E., Schleyerbach, R., Peyron, J. G., and Hascall, V. C., eds. (1992). Cartilage specific collagens. Structural studies. *In* "Articular Cartilage and Osteoarthritis" (D. Eyre *et al.*, eds.) pp. 118–131. Raven Press, New York.
12. Wu, J. J., Woods, P. E., and Eyre, D. R. (1992). Identification of cross-linking sites in bovine cartilage type IX collagen reveals an antiparallel type II-type IX molecular relationship and type IX to type IX bonding. *J. Biol. Chem.* **267**, 23007–23014.
13. Muragaki, Y., Nishimura, I., Henney, A., Ninomiya, Y., and Olsen, B. R. (1990). The $\alpha 1$(IX) collagen gene gives rise to two different transcripts in both mouse embryonic and human fetal RNA. *Proc. Natl. Acad. Sci. U.S.A.* **87**, 2400–2404.
14. Hagg, R., Bruckner, P., and Hedbom, E. (1998). Cartilage fibrils of mammals are biochemically heterogeneous: Differential distribution of decorin and collagen IX. *J. Cell Biol.* **142**, 285–294.
15. Ayad, S., Marriott, A., Morgan, K., and Grant, M. E. (1989). Bovine cartilage types VI and IX collagens. Characterization of their forms *in vivo. Biochem. J.* **262**, 753–761.
16. Chu, M.-L., Zhang, R.-Z., Pan, T.-C., Stokes, D., Conway, D., Kuo, H.-J., Glanville, R., Mayer, U., Mann, K., Deutzmann, R., and Timpl, R. (1990). Mosaic structure of globular domains in the human type VI collagen $\alpha 3$ chain: Similarity to von Willebrand factor, fibronectin, actin, salivary proteins and aprotinin type protease inhibitors. *EMBO J.* **9**, 385–393.
17. Kielty, C. M., Whittaker, S. P., Grant, M. E., and Shuttleworth, C. A. (1992). Type VI collagen microfibrils: Evidence for a structural association with hyaluronan. *J. Cell Biol.* **118**, 979–990.
18. Hedbom, E., and Heinegård, D. (1993). Binding of fibromodulin and decorin to separate sites on fibrillar collagens. *J. Biol. Chem.* **268**, 27307–27312.
19. Rada, J. A., Cornuet, P. K., and Hassell, J. R. (1993). Regulation of corneal collagen fibrillogenesis in vitro by corneal proteoglycan (Lumican and Decorin) core proteins. *Exp. Eye Res.* **56**, 635–648.
20. Hocking, A. M., Shinomura, T., and McQuillan, D. J. (1998). Leucine-rich repeat glycoproteins of the extracellular matrix. *Matrix Biol.* **17**, 1–19.
21. Kobe, B., and Deisenhofer, J. (1994). The leucine-rich repeat: A versatile binding motif. *Trends Biochem. Sci.* **19**, 415–421.
22. Kobe, B., and Deisenhofer, J. (1993). Crystal structure of porcine ribonuclease inhibitor, a protein with leucine-rich repeats. *Nature* **366**, 751–756.
23. Antonsson, P., Heinegård, D., and Oldberg, Å. (1991). Posttranslational modifications of fibromodulin. *J. Biol. Chem.* **266**, 16859–16861.
24. Blochberger, T. C., Vergnes, J.-P., Hempel, J., and Hassell, J. R. (1992). cDNA to chick lumican (corneal keratan sulfate proteoglycan) reveals homology to the small interstitial proteoglycan gene family and expression in muscle and intestine. *J. Biol. Chem.* **267**, 347–352.

25. Sommarin, Y., Wendel, M., and Heinegård, D. (1998). Osteoadherin, a cell-binding keratan sulfate proteoglycan in bone, belongs to the family of leucine rich repeat proteins of the extracellular matrix. *J. Biol. Chem.* **273**, 16723–16729.

26. Corpuz, L. M., Funderburgh, J. L., Funderburgh, M. L., Bottomley, G. S., Prakash, S., and Conrad, G. W. (1996). Molecular cloning and tissue distribution of keratocan. *J. Biol. Chem.* **271**, 9759–9763.

27. Bengtsson, E., Neame, P., Heinegård, D., and Sommarin, Y. (1995). The primary structure of a basic leucine rich repeat protein, PRELP, found in connective tissues. *J. Biol. Chem.* **270**, 25639–25644.

28. Sommarin, Y., Larsson, T., and Heinegård, D. (1989). Chondrocyte-matrix interactions. Attachment to proteins isolated from cartilage. *Exp. Cell Res.* **184**, 181–192.

29. Neame, P., Sommarin, Y., Boynton, R., and Heinegård, D. (1994). The structure of a 38 kDa leucine rich repeat protein (Chondroadherin) isolated from bovine cartilage. *J. Biol. Chem.* **269**, 21547–21554.

30. Hildebrand, A., Romaris, M., Rasmussen, L. M., Heinegård, D., Twardzik, D. R., Border, W. A., and Ruoslahti, E. (1994). Interaction of the small interstitial proteoglycans biglycan, decorin and fibromodulin with transforming growth factor β. *Biochem. J.* **302**, 527–534.

31. Camper, L., Heinegård, D., and Lundgren-Åkerlund, E. (1997). Integrin α2β1 is a receptor for the cartilage matrix protein chondroadherin. *J. Cell Biol.* **138**, 1159–1167.

32. Wendel, M., Sommarin, Y., and Heinegård, D. (1998). Bone matrix proteins. Isolation and characterization of a novel cell-binding keratan sulfate proteoglycan (Osteoadherin) from bovine bone. *J. Cell Biol.* **141**, 839–847.

33. Shen, Z., Heinegård, D., and Sommarin, Y. (1998). Chondroadherin expression changes in skeletal development. *Biochem. J.* **330**, 549–557.

34. Hedbom, E., Antonsson, P., Hjerpe, A., Aeschlimann, D., Paulsson, M., Rosa-Pimentel, E., Sommarin, Y., Wendel, M., Oldberg, Å., Heinegård, D. (1992). Cartilage matrix proteins. An acidic oligomeric protein (COMP) detected only in cartilage. *J. Biol. Chem.* **267**, 6132–6136.

35. Mörgelin, M., Heinegård, D., Engel, J., and Paulsson, M. (1992). Electron microscopy of native cartilage oligomeric matrix protein purified from the swarm rat chondrosarcoma reveals a five-armed structure. *J. Biol. Chem.* **267**, 6137–6141.

36. Zaia, J., Boynton, R. E., McIntosh, A., Marshak, D. R., Olsson, H., Heinegård, D., and Barry, F. (1997). Post-translational modifications in cartilage oligomeric matrix protein. Characterization of the N-linked oligosaccharides by matrix-assisted laser desorption ionization time-of-flight mass spectrometry. *J. Biol. Chem.* **272**, 14120–14126.

37. Oldberg, Å., Antonsson, P., Lindblom, K., and Heinegård, D. (1992). COMP (Cartilage Oligomeric Matrix Protein) is structurally related to the thrombospondins. *J. Biol. Chem.* **267**, 22346–22350.

38. Malashkevich, V. N., Kammerer, R. A., Efimov, V. P., Schulthess, T., and Engel, J. (1996). The crystal structure of a five-stranded coiled coil in COMP: A prototype ion channel? *Science* **274**, 761–765.

39. DiCesare, P., Hauser, N., Lehman, D., Pasumarti, S., and Paulsson, M. (1994). Cartilage oligomeric matrix protein (COMP) is an abundant component of tendon. *FEBS Lett.* **354**, 237–240.

40. Smith, R., Zunino, L., Webbon, P., and Heinegård, D. (1997). The distribution of cartilage oligomeric matrix protein (COMP) in tendon and its variation with tendon site, age and load. *Matrix Biol.* **16**, 255–271.

41. Rosenberg, K., Olsson, H., Mörgelin, M., and Heinegård, D. (1998). COMP shows high affinity, Zn-dependent interaction with triple helical collagen. *J. Biol. Chem.* **273**, 20397–20403.

42. DiCesare, P., Mörgelin, M., Mann, K., and Paulsson, M. (1994). Cartilage oligomeric matrix protein and thrombospondin I. Purification from articular cartilage, electron microscopic structure and chondrocyte binding. *Eur. J. Biochem.* **223**, 927–937.

43. Shen, Z., Heinegård, D., and Sommarin, Y. (1994). Distribution and expression of a cartilage matrix protein—COMP and a bone matrix protein—BSP show marked changes during rat femoral head development. *Matrix Biol.* **14**, 773–781.

44. Hecht, J. T., Nelson, L. D., Crowder, E., Wang, Y., Elder, F. F. B., Harrison, W. R., Francomano, C. A., Prange, C. K., Lennon, G. G., Deere, M., and Lawler, J. (1995). Mutations in exon 17B of cartilage oligomeric matrix protein (COMP) cause pseudoachondroplasia. *Nat. Genet.* **10**, 325–329.

45. Briggs, M. D., Hoffman, S. M. G., King, L. M., Olsen, A. S., Mohrenweiser, H., Leroy, J. G., Mortier, G. R., Rimoin, D. L., Lachman, R. S., Gaines, E. S., Cekleniak, J. A., Knowlton, R. G., and Cohn, D. H. (1995). Pseudoachondroplasia and multiple epiphyseal dysplasia due to mutations in the cartilage oligomeric matrix protein gene. *Nat. Genet.* **10**, 330–336.

46. Deere, M., Sanford, T., Ferguson, H. L., Daniels, K., and Hecht, J. T., (1998). Identification of twelve mutations in cartilage oligomeric matrix protein (COMP) in patients with pseudoachondroplasia. *Am. J. Med. Genet.* **80**, 510–513.

47. Maddox, B. K., Keene, D. R., Sakai, L. Y., Charbonneau, N. L., Morris, N. P., Ridgway, C. C., Boswell, B. A., Sussman, M. D., Horton, W. A., Bächinger, H. P., and Hecht, J. T. (1997). The fate of cartilage oligomeric matrix protein is determined by the cell type in the case of a novel mutation in pseudoachondroplasia. Cell type in the case of a novel mutation in pseudoachondroplasia. *J. Biol. Chem.* **272**, 30993–30997.

48. Paulsson, M., and Heinegård, D. (1981). Purification and structural characterization of a cartilage matrix protein. *Biochem. J.* **197**, 367–375.

49. Belluoccio, D., Schenker, T., Baici, A., and Paulsson, M. (1998). Characterization of human Matrilin-3 (MATN3). *Genomics* **53**, 391–394.

50. Argraves, W. S., Deák, F., Sparks, K. J., Kiss, I., and Goetinck, P. F. (1987). Structural features of cartilage matrix protein deduced from cDNA. *Proc. Natl. Acad. Sci. U.S.A.* **84**, 464–468.

51. Paulsson, M., and Heinegård, D. (1982). Radioimmunoassay of the 148-kilodalton cartilage protein. *Biochem. J.* **207**, 207–213.

52. Franzén, A., Heinegård, D., and Solursh, M. (1987). Evidence for sequential appearance of cartilage matrix proteins in developing mouse limbs and in cultures of mouse mesenchymal cells. *Differentiation* **36**, 199–210.

53. Winterbottom, N., Tondravi, M. M., Harrington, T. L., Klier, F. G., Vertel, B. M., and Goetinck, P. F. (1992). Cartilage matrix protein is a component of the collagen fibril of cartilage. *Dev. Dyn.* **193**, 266–276.

54. Paulsson, M., and Heinegård, D. (1979). Matrix proteins bound to associatively prepared proteoglycans from bovine cartilage. *Biochem. J.* **183**, 539–545.

55. Hauser, N., Paulsson, M., Heinegård, D., and Mörgelin, M. (1996). Interaction of cartilage matrix protein with aggrecan. Increased covalent crosslinking with tissue maturation. *J. Biol. Chem.* **271**, 32247–32252.

56. Wu, J. J., and Eyre, D. R. (1998). Matrilin-3 forms disulfide-linked oligomers with matrilin-1 in bovine epiphyseal cartilage. *J. Biol. Chem.* **273**, 17433–17438.

57. Lorenzo, P., Bayliss, M. T., and Heinegård, D. (1998). A novel cartilage protein (CILP), present in the mid-zone of human articular cartilage increases with age. *J. Biol. Chem.* **273**, 23463–23475.

58. Lorenzo, P., Neame, P., Sommarin, Y., and Heinegård, D. (1998). Cloning and deduced amino acid sequence of a novel cartilage protein, CILP, identifies a proform including a pyrophosphohydrolase (NTPPHase). *J. Biol. Chem.* **273**, 23469–23475.

59. Hakala, B. E., White, C., and Recklies, A. D. (1993). Human cartilage gp-39, a major secretory product of articular chondrocytes and synovial cells, is a mammalian member of a chitinase protein family. *J. Biol. Chem.* **268**, 25803–25810.

60. Schumacher, B. L., Block, J. A., Schmid, T. M., Aydelotte, M. B., and Kuettner, K. E. (1994). A novel proteoglycan synthesized and secreted

by chondrocytes of the superficial zone of articular cartilage. *Arch. Biochem. Biophys.* **311**, 144–152.

61. Zang, D.-W., Burton-Wurster, N., and Lust, G. (1994). Antibody specific for extra domain B of fibronectin demonstrates elevated levels of both extra domain B(+) and B(−) fibronectin in osteoarthritic canine cartilage. *Matrix Biol.* **14**, 623–633.

62. Burton-Wurster, N., and Lust, G. (1989). Molecular and immunologic differences in canine fibronectins from articular cartilage and plasma. *Arch. Biochem. Biophys.* **269**, 32–45.

63. Pan, T.-C., Sasaki, T., Zhang, R.-Z., Fässler, R., Timpl, R., and Chu, M.-L. (1993). Structure and expression of Fibulin-2, a novel extracellular matrix protein with multiple EGF-like repeats and consensus motifs for calcium binding. *J. Cell Biol.* **123**, 1269–1277.

64. Flores, M., Norgård, M., Heinegård, D., Reinholt, F., and Andersson, G. (1992). RGD-directed attachment of isolated rat osteoclasts to osteopontin, bone sialoprotein and fibronectin. *Exp. Cell Res.* **201**, 526–530.

65. Reinholt, F. P., Hultenby, K., Oldberg, Å., and Heinegård, D. (1990). Osteopontin—a possible anchor of osteoclasts to bone. *Proc. Natl. Acad. Sci. U.S.A.* **87**, 4473–4475.

66. Zambonin-Zallone, A., Teti, A., Gaboli, M., and Marchisio, P. C. (1989). Beta 3 subunit of vitronectin receptor is present in osteoclast adhesion structures and not in other monocyte-macrophage derived cells. *Connect. Tissue Res.* **20**, 143–149.

67. Miyauchi, A., Alvarez, J., Greenfield, E. M., Teti, A., Grano, M., Colucci, S., Zambonin-Zallone, A., Ross, F. P., Teitelbaum, S. L., and Cheresh, D. A. (1991). Recognition of osteopontin and related peptides by an alpha v beta 3 integrin stimulates immediate cell signals in osteoclasts. *J. Biol. Chem.* **266**, 20369–20374.

68. Lakkakorpi, P. T., Horton, M. A., Helfrich, M. H., Karhukorpi, E.-K., and Väänänen, H. K. (1991). Vitronectin receptor has a role in bone resorption but does not mediate tight sealing zone attachment of osteoclasts to the bone surface. *J. Cell Biol.* **115**, 1179–1186.

68a. Reinholt, F. P., Hultenby, K., Heinegård, D., Marks, Jr., and Andersson, G. (1999). *Exp. Cell Res.* (submitted for publication).

69. Horton, M. A., Taylor, M. L., Arnett, T. R., and Helfrich, M. H. (1991). Arg-Gly-Asp (RGD) peptides and the anti-vitronectin receptor antibody 23C6 inhibit dentine resorption and cell spreading by osteoclasts. *Exp. Cell Res.* **195**, 368–375.

70. Sato, M., Sardana, M. K., Grasser, W. A., Garsky, V. M., Murray, J. M., and Gould, R. J. (1990). Echistatin is a potent inhibitor of bone resorption in culture. *J. Cell Biol.* **111**, 1713–1723.

71. Ek-Rylander, B., Flores, M., Wendel, M., Heinegård, D., and Andersson, G. (1994). Dephosphorylation of osteopontin and bone sialoprotein by osteoclastic tartrate-resistant acid phosphatase. *J. Biol. Chem.* **269**, 14853–14856.

72. Reinholt, F. P., Mengarelli Widholm, S., Ek-Rylander, B., and Andersson, G. (1990). Ultrastructural localization of a tartrate-resistant acid ATPase in bone. *J. Bone Miner. Res.* **5**, 1055–1061.

73. Hultenby, K., Reinholt, F. P., Norgård, M., Oldberg, Å., Wendel, M., and Heinegård, D. (1994). Distribution and synthesis of bone sialoprotein in metaphyseal bone of young rats show a distinctly different pattern from that of osteopontin. *Eur. J. Cell Biol.* **63**, 230–239.

74. Hultenby, K., Reinholt, F. P., Oldberg, Å., and Heinegård, D. (1991). Ultrastructural immunolocalization of osteopontin in metaphyseal and cortical bone. *Matrix* **11**, 206–213.

75. Rittling, S. R., Matsumoto, H. N., McKee, M. D., Nanci, A., An, X. R., Novick, K. E., Kowalski, A. J., Noda, M., and Denhardt, D. T. (1998). Mice lacking osteopontin show normal development and bone structure but display altered osteoclast formation in vitro. *J. Bone Miner. Res.* **13**, 1101–1111.

76. Gullberg, D., Gehlsen, K. R., Turner, D. C., Åhlén, K., Zijenah, L. S., Barnes, M. J., and Rubin, K. (1992). Analysis of $\alpha_1\beta_1$, $\alpha_2\beta_1$ and $\alpha_3\beta_1$ integrins in cell-collagen interactions: Identification of conformation

dependent $\alpha_1\beta_1$ binding sites in collagen type I. *EMBO J.* **11**, 3865–3873.

77. Charo, I. F., Nannizzi, L., Smith, J. W., and Cheresh, D. A. (1990). The vitronectin receptor $\alpha v \beta 3$ binds fibronectin and acts in concert with $\alpha 5 \beta 1$ in promoting cellular attachment and spreading on fibronectin. *J. Cell Biol.* **111**, 2795–2800.

78. Oldberg, Å., Franzén, A., and Heinegård, D. (1986). Cloning and sequence analysis of rat bone sialoprotein (osteopontin) cDNA reveals an Arg-Gly-Asp cell-binding sequence. *Proc. Natl. Acad. Sci. U.S.A.* **83**, 8819–8823.

79. Oldberg, Å., Franzén, A., and Heinegård, D. (1988). The primary structure of a cell-binding bone sialoprotein. *J. Biol. Chem.* **263**, 19430–19432.

79a. Shen, Z., Gantcheva, Sommarin, Y., and Heinegård, D. (1999). Tissue distribution of a novel cell binding protein, osteoadherin, in the rat. Submitted for publication.

80. Lane, T. F., and Sage, E. H. (1994). The biology of SPARC, a protein that modulates cell-matrix interactions. *FASEB J.* **7**, 163–173.

81. Termine, J. D., Kleinman, H. K., Whitson, S. W., Conn, K. M., McGarvey, M. L., and Martin, G. R. (1981). Osteonectin, a bone-specific protein linking mineral to collagen. *Cell* **26**, 99–105.

82. Lankat-Buttgereit, B., Mann, K., Deutzmann, R., and Timpl, R. (1988). Cloning and complete amino acid sequences of human and murine basement membrane protein BM-40 (SPARC, osteonectin). *FEBS Lett.* **236**, 352–356.

83. Mason, I. J., Taylor, A., Williams, J. G., Sage, H., and Hogan, B. L. M. (1986). Evidence from molecular cloning that SPARC, a major product of mouse embryo parietal endoderm, is related to an endothelial cell 'culture shock' glycoprotein of M_r 43000. *EMBO J.* **5**, 1465–1472.

84. Robey, P. G., Young, M. F., Fisher, L. W., and McClain, T. D. (1989). Thrombospondin is an osteoblast-derived component of mineralized extracellular matrix. *J. Cell Biol.* **108**, 719–727.

85. Lawler, J., Weinstein, R., and Hynes, R. O. (1988). Cell attachment to thrombospondin: The role of ARG-GLY-ASP, calcium, and integrin receptors. *J. Cell Biol.* **107**, 2351–2361.

86. Bornstein, P. (1992). Thrombospondins: Structure and regulation of expression. *FASEB J.* **6**, 3290–3299.

87. Lawler, J., Duquette, M., Urry, L., McHenry, K., and Smith, T. F. (1993). The evolution of the thrombospondin gene family. *J. Mol. Evol.* **36**, 509–516.

88. Kyriakides, T. R., Zhu, Y. H., Smith, L. T., Bain, S. D., Yang, Z., Lin, M. T., Danielson, K. G., Iozzo, R. V., LaMarca, M., McKinney, C. E., Ginns, E. I., and Bornstein, P. (1998). Mice that lack thrombospondin 2 display connective tissue abnormalities that are associated with disordered collagen fibrillogenesis, an increased vascular density, and a bleeding diathesis. *J. Cell Biol.* **140**, 419–430.

89. Pringle, G. A., and Dodd, C. M. (1990). Immunoelectron microscopic localization of the core protein of decorin near the d and e bands of tendon collagen fibrils by use of monoclonal antibodies. *J. Histochem. Cytochem.* **38**, 1405–1411.

90. Hedlund, H., Mengarelli-Widholm, S., Heinegård, D., Reinholt, F. P., and Svensson, O. (1994). Fibromodulin—distribution and association with collagen. *Matrix* **14**, 227–232.

91. Glimcher, M. J., Lindh, E., and Thorell, J. (1989). Mechanisms of calcification in bone: Role of collagen fibrils and collagen-phosphoprotein complexes *in vitro* and *in vivo*. *In* "Clinical Impact of Bone and Connective Tissue Markers" (M. J. Glimcher *et al.*, eds.), pp. 137–170. Academic Press, London.

92. Traub, W., Arad, T., and Weiner, S. (1989). Three-dimensional ordered distribution of crystals in turkey tendon collagen fibers. *Proc. Natl. Acad. Sci. U.S.A.* **86**, 9822–9826.

93. Price, P. A., Otsuka, A. S., Poser, J. W., Kristaponis, J., and Raman, N. (1976). Characterization of a gamma-carboxyglutamic acid-containing protein from bone. *Proc. Natl. Acad. Sci. U.S.A.* **73**, 1447–1451.

94. Price, P. A., Lothringer, J. W., Baukol, S. A., and Reddi, A. H. (1981). Developmental appearance of the vitamin K-dependent protein of bone during calcification. *J. Biol. Chem.* **256**, 3781–3784.

95. Ducy, P., Desbois, C., Boyce, B., Pinero, G., Story, B., Dunstan, C., Smith, E., Bonadio, J., Goldstein, S., Gundberg, C., Bradley, A., and Karsenty, G. (1996). Increased bone formation in osteocalcin-deficient mice. *Nature* **382**, 448–452.

96. Dickson, I. R., Poole, A. R., and Veis, A. (1975). Localisation of plasma α_2HS glycoprotein in mineralising human bone. *Nature* **256**, 430–432.

97. McKee, M. D., Farach-Carson, M. C., Butler, W. T., Hauschka, P. V., and Nanci, A. (1993). Ultrastructural immunolocalization of noncollagenous (Osteopontin and Osteocalcin) and plasma (albumin and α_2HS-glycoprotein) proteins in rat bone. *J. Bone Miner. Res.* **8**, 485–496.

98. Petersson, I., Boegård, J., Dahlström, B., Svensson, B., Heinegård, D., and Saxne, T. (1998). Changes in cartilage and bone metabolism identified by serum markers in early osteoarthritis of the knee join. *Br. J. Rheumatol.* **37**, 46–50.

99. Saxne, T., Wollheim, F., Pettersson, H., and Heinegård, D. (1987). Proteoglycan concentration in synovial fluid: Prediction of future cartilage destruction in rheumatoid arthritis. *Br. Med. J.* **295**, 1447–1448.

100. Månsson, B., Ionescu, M., Poole, A. R., Heinegård, D., and Saxne, T. (1995). Cartilage and bone metabolism in rheumatoid arthritis: Differences between rapid and slow progression of disease identified by serum markers of cartilage metabolism. *J. Clin. Invest.* **95**, 1071–1077.

CHAPTER 5

Proteoglycans and Glycosaminoglycans

TIM HARDINGHAM   Wellcome Trust Centre for Cell-Matrix Research, School of Biological Sciences, University of Manchester, Manchester M13 9PT, United Kingdom

I. INTRODUCTION

Proteoglycans form a special class of glycoproteins with attached long unbranched and highly charged glycosaminoglycan chains [1, 2]. These chains are strongly hydrophilic and they dominate the physical properties of proteoglycans. Cartilage and bone are tissues that contain large expanded extracellular matrices, although they are of quite different structure and have different biological functions. The composition of the two tissues is strikingly different and this is particularly apparent amongst the proteoglycan components. Cartilage contains 70–75% water and it has a high proteoglycan content (5–7%), predominantly containing chondroitin sulfate, but also containing considerable amounts of keratan sulfate. In contrast, bone matrix is predominantly mineral; it contains only 10% water and it has a correspondingly low proteoglycan content (~0.1%) which again is predominantly chondroitin sulfate. This contrast in composition is also reflected in the proteoglycans present. In cartilage, the major proteoglycan is aggrecan, which is important in expanding and hydrating the matrix. There are also lesser amounts of the lower molecular weight leucine-rich proteoglycans, including decorin and fibromodulin, which are collagen fibril associated, and also biglycan. In bone, there is no aggrecan and the collagen fibril-associated proteoglycans and biglycan are the predominant forms. Aggrecan and the leucine-rich proteoglycans are secreted extracellular matrix proteoglycans that contribute to matrix organization and stability. The cells of bone and cartilage also contain some cell-surface integral membrane proteoglycans; however, as the cell-density is low, the tissue content of these proteoglycans is low and they will not be discussed further here.

II. GLYCOSAMINOGLYCANS

A. Chondroitin Sulfate/Dermatan Sulfate

The glycosaminoglycans are long chain unbranched polysaccharides consisting of repeating disaccharide units [2]. In chondroitin sulfate, the disaccharide contains D-N-acetylgalactosamine $\beta1$–4 D-glucuronate, in $\beta1$–3 linked units. There is usually one sulfate group per disaccharide on the 4 or 6 position of the galactosamine. There is also a low frequency of nonsulfated disaccharides and, even more rarely, disulfated disaccharides. The chains are synthesized attached via a characteristic xylose–galactose–galactose linkage region to serine residues on proteoglycans (Fig. 1) by the stepwise addition

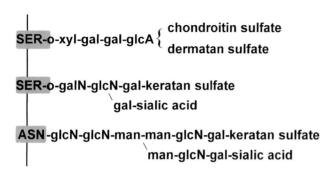

FIGURE 1   Glycosaminoglycan linkages to protein. Glycosaminoglycans are synthesized attached to proteoglycans during biosynthesis in the Golgi region of cells. Chondroitin sulfate/dermatan sulfate chains are attached to serine residue and have a similar linkage to heparan sulfate/heparin chains. Keratan sulfate occurs O-linked to serine (or threonine) and N-linked to asparagine.

of single sugar residues from nucleotide sugar intermediates to the non-reducing end of the growing chain, followed by sulfation as the chain grows. This takes place at a late stage of biosynthesis in the Golgi region of the cell immediately prior to secretion. Dermatan sulfate is synthesized as a chondroitin sulfate chain, in which some of the glucuronate residues in the chain are epimerized to iduronate intracellularly by inversion of the configuration of the carboxyl group at carbon 5 of the sugar ring. This moves the carboxyl group from an equitorial to an axial position and it may also be accompanied by 2-sulfation of the iduronate. The proportion of glucuronate residues that are changed to iduronate is quite variable, ranging from a few percent up to 90% of the total. The presence of iduronate residues has been shown to alter the chain conformation. Different properties have been identified in chains with block structures of glucuronate and iduronate sequences compared with those with more mixed alternating sequences, but how this influences the biological functions of the chains is unclear. The mechanisms controlling the biosynthesis and composition of chondroitin sulfate/dermatan sulfate chains are not well characterized, but because proteoglycans containing chondroitin sulfate and dermatan sulfate can be expressed by the same cells, there are clearly mechanisms for targeting the nascent proteins to receive different GAG chain structures.

B. Keratan Sulfate

Keratan sulfate contains a different disaccharide unit than that of chondroitin sulfate. It consists of D-galactose, $\beta 1$–3 D-N-acetylglucosamine, in $\beta 1$–4 linked units. This is also known as a lactosamine repeat and is found in a broad class of glycoproteins including ovarian mucins. However, in keratan sulfate the chain is sulfated during synthesis primarily at the 6 position of the galactose, and some N-acetylglucosamine residues are also 6-sulfated. The lactosamine chains that form

keratan sulfate are synthesized on two types of protein linkage (Fig. 1). The lactosamine chain can be formed as an extension of an oligosaccharide O-linked to threonine, but it can also be synthesized as an extension of an N-linked oligosaccharide of the complex type, attached to asparagine. Both types of keratan sulfate are found in the proteoglycans of cartilage and bone (see below).

C. Disaccharide Sequences in Glycosaminoglycan Chains

There is increasing evidence that glycosaminoglycan chains are not randomly sulfated or epimerized polymers and that they contain distinct patterns that may include some unique sequences. Monoclonal antibodies have been produced that recognize unusual sequences in chondroitin sulfate (CS) chains, and these reveal distinctive tissue distributions of the epitopes [3]. The abundance of some CS epitopes has also been shown to change during tissue development and in disease, such as in the cartilage in experimental joint disease [3]. A study of CS epitopes in synovial fluid from joints with trauma-induced ligament damage also showed increased expression of these epitopes [4]. So, although the structures of GAGs are based on repeating disaccharides, the selective sulfation of chondroitin sulfate and keratan sulfate chains and the epimerization of glucuronate to iduronate in dermatan sulfate chains produces chains with wide variations in structure and properties. These results also suggest that the cellular synthesis of glycosaminoglycans is much more closely controlled than has been previously suspected and that much has yet to be understood about the significance of the many well-documented changes in GAG composition that occur during tissue development, during aging, and that accompany pathology. Further progress in this area depends on the development of improved methods for determining sequences in GAG chains.

III. PROTEOGLYCANS IN CARTILAGE

Proteoglycans make a major contribution to the biomechanical properties of cartilage and this is particularly important at the articular surface, where the tissue has a load bearing function. It is the structure and organization of the macromolecules in the extracellular matrix that provide these properties [5] and they result from the composite structure of cartilage and the contribution made by fibrillar and nonfibrillar components. The collagen fibrillar network is made of fine fibers which have no preferred orientation in the mid zone of the cartilage. At the articular surface, the fibers are parallel to the surface and with one preferred orientation, and they are more perpendicular to the surface in deeper zones. The collagen provides a framework for the tissue that gives

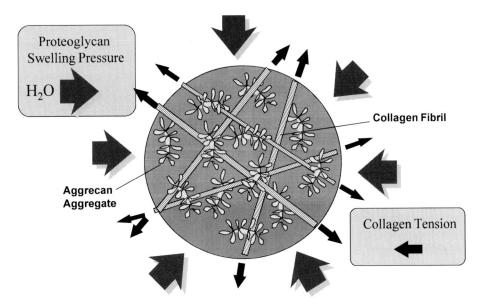

FIGURE 2   The combined properties of collagens and proteoglycans in articular cartilage.

it shape and form. The triple helical collagen molecules are organized into fibrils with overlapping and cross linking of adjacent molecules, and the fibrils laterally associate into longer fibers. The structure of collagen gives it impressive tensile properties and this is utilized in cartilage in a special way to produce a tissue that is not only strong in tension but also resistant to compression. This is achieved by filling the interfibrillar matrix with a very high content of proteoglycan, primarily aggrecan.

The aggrecan at high concentration draws water into the tissue as it creates a large osmotic swelling pressure (Fig. 2). This occurs because all of the negatively charged anionic groups on aggrecan carry with them mobile counter ions such as Na^+. This creates a large difference in concentration of ions inside cartilage compared with outside and an imbalance amongst the freely diffusible anions and cations. Water is drawn into the tissue because of this osmotic imbalance and because aggrecan is too large and immobile to redistribute itself. The water thus swells and expands the aggrecan-rich matrix. This places the collagen network under tension and an equilibrium is achieved when tension in the collagen network balances the swelling pressure (i.e., when no more water enters the tissue because the force is insufficient to stretch the collagen network any further). At this equilibrium, with the tissue swollen with water, it has good compressive resilience, as any new load on the tissue now places the collagen network under further tension. Another feature of the composite collagen/aggrecan organization is also important; not only is aggrecan greatly restricted in its ability to move within the matrix and the collagen/aggrecan network is stiff and resists deformation, but aggrecan also offers great resistance to any fluid flow and redistribution of water. The tissue thus behaves largely as a stiff elastic polymer resistant to sudden impact loading, but it also shows some slow inelastic deformation with sustained loads [6]. However, removal of all loads leads to a redistribution of water and a return to the preloading equilibrium position. The articular cartilage thus forms a tough but compliant load-bearing surface, and these characteristics depend on the integrity of the collagen network and the retention within it of a high concentration of aggrecan (Fig. 2).

IV. AGGRECAN

A. Aggrecan Structure

Aggrecan is a proteoglycan with a core protein of high molecular weight ($\sim$250,000) encoded by a single gene that is expressed predominantly in cartilaginous tissues [1, 2]. It has three globular and two extended domains (Fig. 3). It is highly glycosylated with $\sim$90% carbohydrate, mainly in two types of glycosaminoglycan chains, chondroitin sulfate and keratan sulfate (Table I). Each aggrecan contains $\sim$100 chondroitin sulfate chains, which are typically $\sim$20 kDa each, and the chains are either 4-sulfated, 6-sulfated, or usually both. There are fewer keratan sulfate chains (up to 60) and they are usually of shorter length (5–15 kDa). The chondroitin sulfate chains are all attached to the long extended domain between globular domains 2 and 3, but the keratan sulfate is more widely distributed. It is most abundant in a keratan sulfate-rich region just C-terminal to the G2 domain. Keratan sulfate is attached elsewhere on both extended domains and on the globular domains G1 and G2. Aggrecan also contains a variable number of O-linked oligosaccharides and N-linked oligosaccharides. The O-linked oligosaccharides have a linkage to protein similar to keratan sulfate and it appears that

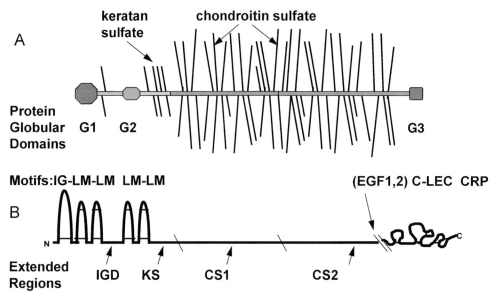

FIGURE 3   Aggrecan structure. (A) Globular protein and attached glycosaminoglycan chain structure. (B) Protein domain structure. Folded modules: IG, immunoglobulin fold; LM, link module; EGF1,2, epidermal growth factor modules; C-LEC, C-type lectin module; CRP, complement regulatory protein module. Extended domains: IGD, interglobular domain; KS, keratan sulfate-rich region; CS1,2, chondroitin sulfate attachment regions.

during biosynthesis, some O-linked oligosaccharides are extended and sulfated to form keratan sulfate chains. Variation in the proportion extended to form keratan sulfate and the length of the chains synthesized is thus likely to account for the large differences in the content of keratan sulfate in aggrecan from different cartilaginous tissues.

The primary gene product of aggrecan, the protein core, is variably glycosylated by the chondrocytes in which it is expressed to yield secreted macromolecules that show a broad range of composition. They always contain a high glycosaminoglycan content but contain variable numbers of chains of variable lengths and different patterns of sulfation. Although it is clear that many factors affect the synthesis of glycosaminoglycan chains and oligosaccharides, it is not yet fully understood how the composition of aggrecan relates to

the age and site of the tissue, or to the range of growth factors and cytokines acting on the chondrocytes in which it is expressed.

All three of the globular domains of the aggrecan protein contain sequences that are highly conserved amongst aggrecans from different vertebrate species, but the extended domains are less well conserved [2]. There is, for example, considerable variation in the length of the keratan sulfate-rich region amongst different species, and even this region has considerable polymorphisms in the human population [7]. This suggests that small variations in the large amount of glycosaminoglycan present on aggrecan are of little consequence to its major function, but that the functions of the globular structures are more sensitive to changes in sequence. While the G1 and G2 domains have related structures (see below), the G3 domain is distinctly different and contains four quite different protein modules. The likely function of this domain in matrix organization has yet to be determined (see below).

TABLE I.   Aggrecan Composition

	Molecular weight	Number of chains	% of total
Aggrecan	1–4 million	1	100
Protein	245,000	1	5–10
Chondroitin sulfate	10,000–30,000	100	70–90
Keratan sulfate	5,000–20,000	20–50	5–20

Polyanion Properties: Sulfate groups ~4500 mole per mole
Carboxyl groups ~4200 mole per mole
Total charged groups ~8700 mole per mole

B. Molecular Interactions Involved in Aggregation

The globular N-terminal protein domain (G1) of aggrecan contains a lectin-like binding site with high affinity for hyaluronan and is responsible for the formation of aggregates [8]. As hyaluronan is a long unbranched polysaccharide chain, with an average molecular weight of up to several million, each chain can bind a large number of aggrecans to form aggregates up to several hundred million in molecular weight [9]. The binding of each aggrecan to hyaluronan is further stabilized by a small glycoprotein (45 kDa), referred to as link protein [10, 11].

The G1 domain of aggrecan contains three protein motifs, an immunoglobulin fold (Ig-fold), and two copies of a hyaluronan-binding motif, or link module, also referred to as the proteoglycan tandem repeat (PTR) (Fig. 3). This module is present in tandem in all members of the hyaluronan-binding family of proteoglycans and in link protein, but it is also present as a single copy in the cell surface hyaluronan-binding receptor, CD-44, and in TSG-6, a secreted matrix protein, whose synthesis is induced by inflammatory cytokines. The structure of the recombinant link module from TSG-6 has now been determined by NMR to be related to the mammalian type-C lectin family of carbohydrate binding motifs [12]. Link protein has a structure very similar to the aggrecan G1 domain, as it contains an Ig-fold and two link modules, which suggests that they share a common gene ancestor. The structure of the G2 domain of aggrecan poses interesting, unresolved questions as it too is structurally related to G1 and link protein. Although lacking an Ig-fold, it contains two copies of the link module. However, no hyaluronan-binding properties of the G2 domain have been detected [13] and there is no clear role for a second hyaluronan-binding site on aggrecan in the formation of aggregates.

The binding of aggrecan to hyaluronan exhibits a high affinity, with a $K_d = 2 \times 10^{-8}$ M. The affinity remains high throughout the pH range 6–9, but it is dissociated at pH 3. At neutral pH, the binding is reversibly dissociated at temperatures up to 65°C, but at higher temperatures it slowly denatures irreversibly. The G1 domain renatures after exposure to many denaturing agents, including guanidine hydrochloride, urea, and potassium thiocyanate. It also survives treatment with solvents, such as ethanol, acetone, or ether without loss of activity, and it is also resistant to proteinase attack. Reduction of the disulphide bonds in the G1 domain efficiently abolishes binding to hyaluronan, but after reduction, their reoxidation under nondenaturing conditions can lead to a significant recovery of binding activity. These properties all suggest that the native structure of the G1 domain is resistant to denaturation and is strongly thermodynamically preferred, such that it reforms from denatured conditions with high efficiency [14]. The G1 domain of aggrecan thus appears to be a tough, stable structure suited to its long lifetime in the extracellular matrix.

C. The Function of Link Protein

Link protein in the aggregate structure strengthens the aggrecan–hyaluronan bond by forming a ternary complex involving both an interaction with hyaluronan mediated by the PTR and an interaction with the G1 domain through their

Ig-folds. Thus, aggregates formed in the presence of link protein do not dissociate significantly at physiological ionic strength and pH. Thermal stability is also enhanced as no dissociation of link protein-stabilized aggregates is detected up to 55–60°C, while at higher temperatures the link protein appears to denature irreversibly. The interaction between the Ig-folds of link protein and G1 in the aggregate structure appears to "lock" aggrecan onto the hyaluronan chain to form the compact ternary unit of the native aggregate structure. It is interesting that polyclonal antibodies to link protein do not detect it well in the intact aggregates, suggesting that the major epitopes on link protein are concealed in the native structure [15]. In contrast, polyclonal antibodies to the G1 domain are generally able to interact with G1 epitopes in aggregates without hindrance, showing that the epitopes in this case are more available.

D. The Role of Aggregation in Cartilage Structure and Function

Aggrecan is synthesized and secreted continuously by chondrocytes (Fig. 4). It follows the same intracellular pathways of synthesis as other secretory proteins [1, 2]. The mRNA is translated on membrane-bound ribosomes into the RER, followed by translocation to the Golgi for the main steps of O-glycosylation and glycosaminoglycan chain synthesis. The glycosaminoglycans appear to be synthesized rapidly on aggrecan as part of a highly concerted process that occurs just before secretion. There is no intracellular storage of the finished molecule prior to its release. Link protein, although it is less glycosylated and has no glycosaminoglycan chains, is also synthesized along the same intracellular pathway. However, hyaluronan is not synthesized within these same compartments in the cell, but is formed by synthase enzymes that are located in the plasma membrane, such that it is synthesized and secreted directly into the extracellular matrix [16]. Aggrecan (and link protein) thus encounter hyaluronan only after their secretion by the chondrocyte into the extracellular matrix. Aggregation is thus an extracellular mechanism for the assembly of aggrecan into higher order structures (Fig. 4). As this favours its retention within the cartilage extracellular matrix, it plays a major role in maintaining the large difference in concentration of aggrecan between cartilage matrix and the surrounding tissue, thereby supporting the tissue's biomechanical properties.

E. Molecular Organization in Aggregates

Determination of the stoichiometry of aggregation showed that when hyaluronan was saturated with bound aggrecan, the weight ratio was about 1 to 140. This suggests that for each mole of aggrecan (M_r 2 million) bound to hyaluronan

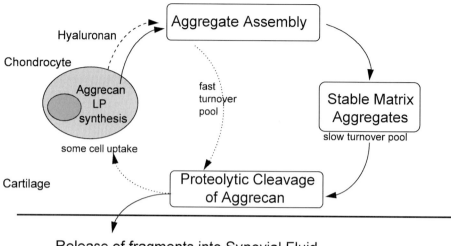

FIGURE 4   Aggrecan turnover in articular cartilage. Aggrecan is continuously synthesized by chondrocytes and secreted and assembled into aggregates in the cartilage matrix. There is also slow continuous turnover by extracellular proteinase action. Some aggrecan fragments accumulate in cartilage matrix, but most are released from the tissue into the synovial fluid.

there was a minimum hyaluronan mass of ∼7000. This corresponds to each aggrecan occupying a section of hyaluronan of 32–36 sugars. Electron microscopy of aggregates [9] prepared in monolayer films to contrast the glycosaminoglycan chains (Kleinschmidt technique) shows their structure has a large number of aggrecan monomers attached to a central filament of hyaluronan. In preparations visualized by rotary shadowing [17] to reveal the globular protein domains, the isolated G1 domain bound to hyaluronan with no evidence of cooperativity. In rotary shadowed images of the isolated aggrecan G1-G2 fragment bound to hyaluronan, the G2 domain always remained separate from the G1 domain and away from the hyaluronan. In the presence of link protein, the packing density of G1-G2 did not change, but the shadowed protein now appeared as a continuous coating on the central hyaluronan chain and not as discrete globular complexes. This appearance, of a continuous protein coat on the hyaluronan, is also seen in rotary shadowed preparations of intact aggregates, which may imply some cooperative association between adjacent G1-link protein complexes along the hyaluronan chain [18].

F. Functions of the G1-G2 Region in Aggrecan Turnover

The extended segment between G1 and G2 appears rather stiffened, as its length in rotary shadowed images is remarkably constant (21 ± 3 nm) [17]. This segment contains some keratan sulphate, which may contribute to its extended structure. This region also contains the major sites for proteinase attack on aggrecan, which is important in both normal and cytokine-stimulated catabolism by extracellular proteinases [2] (Fig. 4). Proteolytic cleavage in this region releases the G2 domain along with the attached large glycosaminoglycan-bearing region from the aggregate. Tight packing of the G1 domain and link protein on hyaluronan in the aggregate structure and their resistance to proteinases leads to a progressive increase with age of hyaluronan coated with G1 and link protein in the tissue. This is readily evident in extracts of old human cartilage, where it has been estimated that only half the G1 domain in the tissue is still part of large aggrecan molecules [19]. It is interesting to note that in young developing cartilage, the amount of hyaluronan is about 1% of the aggrecan, an optimum content to bind all the aggrecan at maximum density into large aggregates. It may also imply that the synthesis and turnover of hyaluronan and aggrecan in cartilage are closely coordinated. There is a progressive increase in hyaluronan in cartilage with age to almost 10% of the aggrecan. This increase occurs, at least in part, because a large proportion of the hyaluronan is occupied with the accumulated G1 domain fragments of aggrecan and link protein.

G. G3 Domain

The C-terminal G3 domain of aggrecan contains a composite structure of three protein motifs (Fig. 3). The motifs include a complement regulatory protein domain at the C-terminus, an adjacent mammalian type C-lectin domain, and two alternatively spliced epidermal growth factor-like domains. In a nanomelic chick with severe skeletal malformation, a primary defect in aggrecan was identified that resulted in a stop codon in the translated region towards G3 and resulted in the expression of a truncated aggrecan that was not glycosylated or secreted [20]. This led to the proposal that the G3 domain was required for the intracellular translocation of aggrecan from the RER to the Golgi, as this was necessary for the synthesis of glycosaminoglycan chains and their secretion. Aggrecan gene constructs lacking the G3 region, but containing the CS region and the aggrecan G1 domain, have been shown to be secreted less well [21]. However, the high conservation of all the motifs in the G3 region amongst aggrecan from different species and amongst all known members of the aggrecan family suggests that more specific interactive properties are likely to be present and that these may play an additional role in extracellular matrix organization.

The EGF domains in aggrecan are alternatively spliced, but the function of this is unclear. The EGF-1 domain that was first reported for human aggrecan is expressed in about 25% of human transcripts but is expressed infrequently in other species, whereas a second EGF-2 only occurs in about 5% of human transcripts but is present in most species [22]. Other members of the aggrecan family, versican, neurocan, and brevican, all contain EGF domains, but there is no evidence of alternative splicing. EGF domains in some modular matrix proteins have been shown to have growth factor activity and they may provide protein ligand binding sites. The three domains present in G3 are similar to those present in the selectins, where there are specific carbohydrate binding properties in which the EGF domain appears important for the lectin binding specificity. In the investigations of aggrecan mRNA, few transcripts containing any EGF motifs have been detected. This raises the question of whether there are conditions under which the alternatively spliced EGF forms that confer specific interactive properties are expressed. Although weak carbohydrate binding of recombinant G3 was detected [23], other results have shown that the C-lectin domains of all the aggrecan family members interact with tenascin-R [24]. This was shown to be a protein-protein interaction with no carbohydrate involvement and binding was with the fibronectin type-III repeats in tenascin. The natural ligands for aggrecan G3 domain in cartilage may thus be proteins rather than carbohydrates. Preparations of aggrecan from cartilage have been shown by rotary electron microscopy to contain less than half of the molecules with an intact G3 domain, and the G3 content of articular cartilage falls with age [25]. It is thus clear that in mature tissue, much of the function of aggrecan in the matrix does not rely on an intact G3 domain, but the G3 domain could be important during cartilage development or in responses to tissue damage, when an additional ligand interaction site on aggrecan may help to confer additional stability on the matrix.

The glycosaminoglycan attachment region of aggrecan between the G2 and G3 domains is the least well-conserved part of the protein. There are significant differences in the amino acid sequence amongst different species. For example, adjacent to the G2 domain is a keratan sulfate-rich region that contains characteristic hexapeptide repeats; there are 23 in bovine aggrecan, 12 in human aggrecan, and only some poorly conserved repeats in rodent and chicken aggrecans [26]. This results in a large variation in the maximum keratan sulfate content found in aggrecan from these different species. There is also evidence of significant polymorphism in the KS-repeats investigated in the human population [7]. Keratan sulfate is also found attached to the protein outside this KS-rich region, but chondroitin sulfate is found exclusively within the CS1/CS2 region between G2 and G3. The CS1 region contains 20 amino acid repeats, of which there are 15 in the rat and 29 in human aggrecan [27]. The CS-2 region has repeats of about 100 amino acids that are more highly variable. These sequence changes result in variations in aggrecan protein molecular mass; for example, the protein of human aggrecan is considerably larger than that of the rat (255 kDa compared with 225 kDa).

V. LEUCINE-RICH PROTEOGLYCANS IN CARTILAGE AND BONE

A. The Leucine-Rich Family

Members of the leucine-rich family of proteoglycans are found in most tissues of the body. They are characterized by containing repeating leucine-rich motifs within the protein sequence structure that are similar to a consensus sequence identified in a broad family of proteins ranging from mammalian RNAse inhibitor and FSH receptor, through *Drosophila* Toll and chaopterin proteins, to yeast adenylate cyclase [28]. All these family members contain multiple leucine-rich repeats that vary in number from three to thirty. The structure of the first member to be crystallized [29], RNAse inhibitor, showed the leucine-rich motif to form a β sheet/α helix structure, which packs with the β sheets parallel when several are present to give a curved structure resembling a doughnut with a bite taken out. Decorin and biglycan were the first leucine-rich proteoglycans to be cloned, but other members now include fibromodulin, lumican, and epiphycan (proteoglycan Lb) (Table II). They fall into a subfamily that shows some general sequence similarities. The exception is epiphycan, which contains fewer leucine-rich repeats, has different cysteine positions, and is more closely related to osteoglycin (osteoinductive factor). Decorin and biglycan are present in the matrices of most tissues, although as noted below they have different distributions within tissues. Fibromodulin has a more restricted distribution in cartilage, tendon, and sclera, but it is less abundant in bone and skin. Lumican, as its name implies, is found in the cornea, but it is also expressed in muscle and intestine and is poorly expressed in cartilage and bone.

TABLE II.   Small Leucine-Rich Proteoglycans

	Protein, kDa	LRR	GAG	N-Glyc	S-Tyr	Binding TGFb	Binding Collagen
Decorin	40	10	CS/DS	No	3	yes	yes
Biglycan	40	10	CS/DS	No	2	yes	no
Fibromodulin	42	10	KS	Yes	3–5	yes	yes
Lumican	38	10	KS	Yes	3–5	?	yes
Keratocan	38	10	KS	Yes	3–5	?	?
PRELP	44	10	KS	No	3–4	?	?
Osteoadherin	42	10	KS	Yes	3–5	?	?
Epiphycan	35	6	CS/DS	Yes	3–4	?	no
Osteoglycin	35	6	KS	Yes	2–3	?	?

LRR, number of leucine-rich repeats; GAG, number and type of glycosaminoglycans; N-Glyc, number of N-glycosylation sites; S-Tyr, number of potential tyrosine sulfation sites; Binding, known binding to TGFβ and to fibrillar collagens. Reproduced with permission from Iozzo [28], Crit, Rev. Biochem. Mol. Biol. **32**, 141–174, 1997. Copyright CRC Press, Boca Raton, Florida.

Other nonproteoglycan members of the leucine-rich family of proteins have been detected in cartilage. These include osteoadherin, a 42 kDa protein with 10 leucine-rich repeats, which has been shown to mediate cell attachment but does not facilitate cell spreading. PRELP is a proline/arginine-rich and leucine-rich protein which has also been cloned and shown to be most closely related to fibromodulin.

B. Decorin and Biglycan

Decorin contains a single site for GAG attachment at a serine four residues from the N terminus. Biglycan has two sites for GAG attachment; both are close to the N terminus and outside the region of leucine-rich repeats [30]. The glycosaminoglycan chains attached during biosynthesis are the chondroitin sulfate/dermatan sulfate type, and the GAG structure varies with the tissue and cell type in which the molecule is synthesized. For example, in bone the chains are chondroitin sulfate and free of iduronate, whereas in skin the chains invariably are dermatan sulfate and contain iduronate. Articular cartilage also contains dermatan sulfate, but in laryngeal cartilage the decorin contains only chondroitin sulfate. The functional significance of this variation in GAG chain structure is not yet explained. In spite of the close structural relationship between decorin and biglycan there is much to suggest that they have quite different functions [28]. Immunolocalization of decorin and biglycan during embryonic development shows that despite being frequently expressed in the same tissue at the same time, they have contrasting distributions [31]. Decorin is most abundant in matrix, whereas biglycan is mainly pericellular. Where cells mainly express decorin, they poorly express biglycan and *vice versa*. This suggests that decorin and biglycan differ in the interactions that determine their matrix distribution and that their expression is controlled independently.

The properties of decorin have been investigated more thoroughly than those of biglycan or of the other leucine-rich repeat proteoglycans. Decorin was shown to delay collagen fibril formation *in vitro* and was shown to bind to collagen fibrils at the d and e region of the gap zone [32]. This was a property of the protein, as removal of the GAG chain had no effect on collagen binding. Fibromodulin was subsequently shown also to bind to fibrillar collagen, also in the gap zone, but at an independent site [33]. In contrast, biglycan appears not to affect collagen fibril formation *in vitro* and to lack strong affinity for collagen in its protein. The crystal structure of ribonuclease inhibitor permitted a model of decorin to be proposed, which formed an open ring structure to which a collagen triple helix would bind by occupying the central hole [34] (Fig. 5). The effects of decorin on collagen fibril

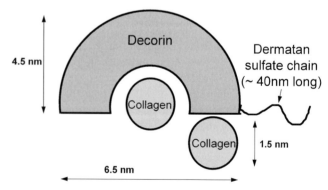

FIGURE 5   Model of decorin interaction with fibrillar collagens. Decorin has been modelled by Weber *et al.* [34] based on the leucine-rich repeat structure of ribonuclease inhibitor. This reveals an open ring structure that may interact with a collagen triple helix as shown. This may provide a basis for the binding of the leucine-rich repeat proteoglycans to collagens.

formation is evident in a mouse model in which decorin expression was transgenically disrupted [35]. The major phenotype was fragile skin with collagen fibers of irregular and abnormal diameter. It is, however, interesting to note that the cartilage and bone in these animals showed no gross defects. Any consequences of the lack of decorin were either more subtle or its role in fibril development is compensated by other mechanisms in these tissues.

Decorin has also been shown to interact with type VI collagen, which is a short chain collagen that forms beaded filaments [36]. Under the conditions tested with collagens coated on plastic, decorin showed little binding to fibrillar collagens I, II, and III, although binding to type VI was high affinity and highly specific. Decorin was also able to compete with binding between type VI collagen and type II collagen. The complement protein, C1q, was also shown to be bound by decorin and this was suggested to be close to, but not within, the collagenous sequences that form the stalk-like segments of this hexameric protein. It was also shown to inhibit complement activation through C1, and this required the GAG chain in addition to the protein core [37].

Decorin also has been reported to bind to fibronectin, which is inhibited by a decorin derived peptide NKISK [38]. Decorin binds to the cell-binding domain of fibronectin and it can inhibit fibronectin-mediated cell adhesion. Decorin is also taken up avidly by cells via receptor-mediated endocytosis. Heparan sulfate may facilitate this process, which is inhibited by heparin, and biglycan appears to be taken up by the same mechanism [39].

Decorin, biglycan, and fibromodulin have been shown to bind TGFβ with both high affinity (K_d 1–20 nM) and lower affinity sites [40]. The interaction was with the protein and removal of the GAG chain increased binding. The interaction was strongest with the active TGFβ dimer and was weak with the inactive latent precursor molecule. Both bone and cartilage are known to contain TGFβ bound in their matrices and the leucine-rich proteoglycans may provide sites for their localization. As TGFβ stimulates matrix protein production by chondrocytes and osteoblasts, a matrix store of this factor that might be released at times of matrix damage could be part of a mechanism for an early response to stimulate cells for tissue repair. Bone matrix decorin has been reported to bind TGFβ and enhance its inhibitory effect on the proliferation of osteoblastic cells [41] and on monocytes [42], but in other systems TGFβ induction of biglycan synthesis was inhibited by decorin [42].

The range of properties identified for decorin suggests a whole range of ways in which it may contribute to matrix organization. It may also help to regulate factors that control cell function. Some of these properties are shared with biglycan, but the weight of evidence shows decorin and biglycan to behave quite differently. Even in their isolation from tissue, biglycan was distinguished from decorin because it self-associated into oligomeric species in solution and bound more

strongly on hydrophobic octyl-Sepharose chromatography [43]. Investigation of the expression of decorin and biglycan in different tissues during embryogenesis by *in situ* hybridization reveals an interesting pattern where frequently both are expressed in the same cells, but the strong expression of one is accompanied by weak expression of the other [31]. In the developing limb cartilage, biglycan was found in the outer rim of cartilage, which lacked decorin, whereas the central region of cartilage was more rich in matrix and contained decorin and lacked biglycan. The surrounding noncartilaginous tissue contained biglycan, but lacked decorin. As development proceeded, biglycan was enriched in the territorial capsule of chondrocytes, whereas decorin was predominantly found in the interterritorial matrix. In mature cartilage, the content of biglycan decreased with age, whereas that of decorin increased. Biglycan expression was stimulated by TGFβ, but decorin was inhibited [44]. There is much evidence to show that these structurally related proteoglycans have quite different tissue functions in the extracellular matrix, but there is not yet a complete picture of what the different functions are.

C. Fibromodulin

Fibromodulin contains leucine-rich repeat sequences similar to those of decorin and biglycan, but it contains no Ser-Gly GAG attachment sequence. However, it does contain four N-linked oligosaccharide acceptor sequences and it has been shown that these can be substituted with N-linked keratan sulfate chains [45]. These site are within the leucine-rich repeat region, but there is also a tyrosine-rich sequence close to the N terminus which can be sulfated. Fibromodulin can thus be highly anionically charged even though it carries no CS/DS GAG chain. As it binds to fibrillar collagen at an independent site to decorin [33], it may have a role complementary to decorin in matrix organization.

D. Other Leucine-Rich Family Members and Nonglycanated Forms

Lumican is a leucine-rich repeat proteoglycan that is present in the cornea but is largely absent from cartilage and bone. It is most similar in sequence to fibromodulin, it contains N-linked keratan sulfate, but it lacks the tyrosine-rich sequence. It is also a fibrillar collagen-binding proteoglycan.

Investigation of tissue extracts from cartilage [46] and intervertebral disc [47] have revealed leucine-rich repeat proteoglycans lacking the glycosaminoglycan chains. This may arise because in decorin and biglycan, the N-terminal peptide, which includes the site of GAG attachment, has been shown to be sensitive to mild proteolytic cleavage. The removal of the peptide with the attached GAG chain could thus occur as a result of proteolytic action in the extracellular matrix. However, molecules may also be synthesized and secreted lacking GAG chains and this may be controlled during cell expression. More detailed analysis of structure and biosynthesis is required to show which of these alternative explanations is the major cause of the nonglycanated forms and also if they have any functional significance.

References

1. Hardingham, T. E., and Fosang, A. J. (1992). Proteoglycans: Many forms, many functions. *FASEB J.* **6**, 861–870.
2. Fosang, A. J., and Hardingham, T. E. (1996). Matrix proteoglycans. *In* "Extracellular Matrix" (W. D. Comper, ed.), Vol. 2, pp. 200–229. Harwood Academic Publishers, The Netherlands.
3. Caterson, B., Mahmoodian, F., Sorrell, J. M., Hardingham, T. E., Bayliss, M. T., Carney, S. L., Ratcliffe, A., and Muir, H. (1990). Modulation of native chondroitin sulphate structure in tissue development and in disease. *J. Cell Sci.* **97**, 411–417.
4. Hazell, P. K., Dent, C., Fairclough, J. A., Bayliss, M. T., and Hardingham, T. E. (1995). Changes in glycosaminoglycan epitope levels in knee joint fluid following injury. *Arthritis Rheum.* **38**, 953–959.
5. Hardingham, T. E. (1998). Articular cartilage. *In* "Oxford Textbook of Rheumatology" (P. J. Maddison, D. A. Isenberg, P. Woo, and D. N. Glass, eds.), pp. 405–420. Oxford Medical Publications, Oxford, UK.
6. Mow, V. C., Hou, J. S., Owens, J. M., and Ratcliffe, A. (1990). Biphasic and quasilinear viscoelastic theories for hydrated soft tissues. *In* "Biomechanics of Diarthrodial Joints" (V. C. Mow, A. Ratcliffe, and S. L.-Y. Woo, eds.), pp. 215–260. Springer-Verlag, New York.
7. Doege, K. J., Coulter, S. N., Meek, L. M., Maslen, K., and Wood, J. G. (1997). A human-specific polymorphism in the coding region of the aggrecan gene. Variable number of tandem repeats produce a range of core protein sizes in the general population. *J. Biol. Chem.* **272**, 13974–13979.
8. Hardingham, T. E., and Muir, H. (1972). The specific interaction of hyaluronic acid with cartilage proteoglycans. *Biochim. Biophys. Acta* **279**, 401–405.
9. Buckwalter, J. A., and Rosenberg, L. A. (1982). Direct evidence for the variable length of the chondroitin sulfate-rich region of the proteoglycan subunit core protein. *J. Biol. Chem.* **257**, 9830–9839.
10. Hascall, V. C., and Sajdera, S. W. (1969). Proteinpolysaccharide complexes from bovine nasal cartilage. *J. Biol. Chem.* **244**, 2384–2396.
11. Hardingham, T. E. (1979). The role of link-protein in the structure of cartilage proteoglycan aggregates. *Biochem. J.* **177**, 237–247.
12. Kohda, D., Morton, C. J., Parkar, A. A., Hatanaka, H., Inagaki, F. M., Campbell, I. D., and Day, A. J. (1996). Solution structure of the link module: A hyaluronan-binding domain involved in extracellular matrix stability and cell migration. *Cell* **86**, 767–775.
13. Fosang, A. J., and Hardingham, T. E. (1989). Isolation of the N-terminal globular domains from cartilage proteoglycan: Identification of G2 domain and its lack of interaction with hyaluronate and link protein. *Biochem. J.* **261**, 801–809.
14. Hardingham, T. E. (1981). Proteoglycans: Their structure, interactions and molecular organization in cartilage. *Biochem. Soc. Trans.* **9**, 489–497.
15. Ratcliffe, A., and Hardingham, T. E. (1983). Cartilage proteoglycan binding and link protein: Radioimmunoassays and the detection of masked determinants in aggregates. *Biochem. J.* **213**, 371–378.
16. Spicer, A. P., and McDonald, J. A. (1998). Characterization and molecular evolution of a vertebrate hyaluronan synthase gene family. *J. Biol. Chem.* **272**, 1923–1932.
17. Morgelin, M., Paulsson, M., Hardingham, T. E., Heinegard, D., and

Engel, J. (1988). Cartilage proteoglycans: Assembly with hyaluronate and link protein as studied by electron microscopy. *Biochem. J.* **253**, 175–185.
18. Morgelin, M., Paulsson, M., Heinegard, D., Aebi, U., and Engel, J. (1995). Evidence of a defined spatial arrangement of hyaluronan in the central filament of cartilage proteoglycan aggregates. *Biochem. J.* **307**, 595–601.
19. Hardingham, T. E., and Bayliss, M. T. (1990). Proteoglycans of articular cartilage: Changes in aging and joint disease. *Semin. Arthritis Rheum.* **20**, 12–33.
20. Vertel, B. M., Walters, L. M., Grier, B., Maine, N., and Goetinck, P. F. (1993). Nanomelic chondrocytes synthesise, but fail to translocate, a truncated aggrecan precursor. *J. Cell Sci.* **104**, 939–948.
21. Luo, W., Kuwada, T. S., Chandrasekaran, L., Zheng, J., and Tanzer, M. L. (1996). Divergent secretory behaviour of the opposite ends of aggrecan. *J. Biol. Chem.* **271**, 16447–16450.
22. Fulop, C., Walcz, E., Valyon, M., and Glant, T. T. (1993). Expression of alternatively spliced epidermal growth factor-like domains in aggrecan of different species. *J. Biol. Chem.* **268**, 17377–17383.
23. Saleque, S., Ruiz, N., and Drickamer, K. (1993). Expression and characterization of a carbohydrate-binding fragment of rat aggrecan. *Glycobiology* **3**, 185–190.
24. Asberg, A., Miura, R., Bourdoulous, S., Shimonaka, M., Heinegard, D., Schachner, M., Ruoslahti, E., and Yamaguchi, Y. (1997). The C-type lectin domains, a family of aggregating chondroitin sulfate proteoglycans, bind tenascin-R by protein-protein interactions independant of carbohydrate moiety. *Proc. Natl. Acad. Sci. U.S.A.* **94**, 10116–10121.
25. Dudhia, J., Davidson, C. M., Wells, T. M., Vynios, D. H., Hardingham, T. E., and Bayliss, M. T. (1996). Age related changes in the content of the carboxy-terminal region of aggrecan in human articular cartilage. *Biochem. J.* **313**, 933–940.
26. Antonsson, P., Heinegard, D., and Oldberg, A. (1989). The keratan sulfate-enriched region of bovine cartilage proteoglycan consists of a consequetively repeated hexapeptide motif. *J. Biol. Chem.* **264**, 16170–16173.
27. Doege, K. J., Sasaki, M., Horigan, E., Hassell, J. R., and Yamada, Y. (1991). Complete coding sequence and deduced primary structure of the human large aggregating proteoglycan, aggrecan. Human specific repeats and alternatively spliced forms. *J. Biol. Chem.* **266**, 894–902.
28. Iozzo, R. V. (1997). The family of the small leucine-rich proteoglycans: Key regulators of matrix assembly and cell growth. *Crit. Rev. Biochem. Mol. Biol.* **32**, 141–174.
29. Kobe, B., and Deisenhofer, J. (1995). A structural basis for the interactions between leucine-rich repeats and protein ligands. *Nature* **374**, 183–186.
30. Fisher, L. W., Termine, J. D., and Young, M. F. (1989). Deduced protein sequence of bone small proteoglycan I (biglycan) shows homology with proteoglycan II (decorin) and several non-connective tissue proteins in a variety of species. *J. Biol. Chem.* **264**, 4571–4576.
31. Bianco, P., Riminucci, M., Young, M. F., Termine, J. D., and Robey, P. G. (1990). Expression and localisation of the two small proteoglycans biglycan and decorin in developing human skeletal and non-skeletal tissues. *J. Histochem. Cytochem.* **38**, 1549–1563.
32. Pringle, G. A., and Dodd, C. M. (1990). Immunoelectron microscopic localization of the core protein of decorin near the d and e bands of tendon collagen fibrils by the use of monoclonal antibodies. *J. Histochem. Cytochem.* **38**, 1405–1411.
33. Hedbom, H., and Heinegard, D. (1993). Binding of fibromodulin and decorin to separate sites on fibrillar collagens. *J. Biol. Chem.* **268**, 27307–27312.
34. Weber, I. T., Harrison, R. W., and Iozzo, R. V. (1997). Model structure of decorin and implications for collagen fibrillogenesis. *J. Biol. Chem.* **271**, 31767–31770.

35. Danielson, K. G., Baribault, H., Holmes, D. F., Graham, H., Kadler, K. E., and Iozzo, R. V. (1997). Targetted disruption of decorin leads to abnormal collagen morphology and skin fragility. *J. Cell Biol.* **136**, 729–743.

36. Bidanset, D. J., Guidry, C., Rosenberg, L. C., Choi, H. U., Timpl, R., and Hook, M. (1992). Binding of the proteoglycan decorin to collagen type VI. *J. Biol. Chem.* **267**, 5250–5256.

37. Krumdieck, R., Hook, M., Rosenberg, L. C., and Volanakis, J. E. (1992). The proteoglycan decorin binds C1q and inhibits the activity of the C1 complex. *J. Immunol.* **149**, 3695–3701.

38. Schmidt, G., Hausser, G., and Kresse, H. (1991). Interaction of the small proteoglycan decorin with fibronectin. Involvement of the sequence NKISK of the core protein. *Biochem. J.* **280**, 411–414.

39. Hausser, H., Ober, B., Quentin-Hoffmann, E., Schmidt, B., and Kresse, H. (1992). Endocytosis of different members of the small chondroitin/dermatan sulfate proteoglycan family. *J. Biol. Chem.* **267**, 11559–11564.

40. Hildebrand, A., Romaris, M., Rasmussen, L. M., Heinegard, D., Twardzik, D. R., Border, W. A., and Ruoslahti, E. (1994). Interaction of the small interstitial proteoglycans biglycan, decorin and fibromodulin with transforming growth factor β. *Biochem. J.* **302**, 527–534.

41. Takeuchi, Y., Kodama, Y., and Matsumoto, T. (1994). Bone matrix decorin binds transforming growth factor-β and enhances its bioactivity. *J. Biol. Chem.* **269**, 32634–32638.

42. Hausser, H., Groning, A., Haslik, A., Schonherr, E., and Kresse, H. (1994). Selective inactivity of TGF-β/decorin complexes. *FEBS Lett.* **353**, 243–245.

43. Choi, H. U., Johnson, T. L., Pal, S., Tang, L. H., Rosenberg, L. C., and Neame, P. J. (1989). Characterization of dermatan sulfate proteoglycans, DS-PGI and DS-PGII, from bovine articular cartilage and skin isolated by octyl-sepharose chromatography. *J. Biol. Chem.* **264**, 2876–2884.

44. Roughly, P. J., Melching, L. I., and Recklies, A. D. (1994). Changes in the expression of decorin and biglycan in human articular cartilage with age and regulation by TGF-β. *Matrix Biol.* **14**, 51–59.

45. Plaas, A. H. K., Neame, P. J., Nivens, C. M., and Reiss, L. (1990). Identification of the keratan sulfate attachment sites on bovine fibromodulin. *J. Biol. Chem.* **265**, 20634–20640.

46. Sampaio, L. de O., Bayliss, M. T., Hardingham, T. E., and Muir, H. (1988). Dermatan sulphate proteoglycan from human articular cartilage. *Biochem. J.* **254**, 757–764.

47. Johnstone, B., Markopoulos, M., Neame, P., and Caterson, B. (1993). Identification and characterization of glycanated and non-glycanated forms of biglycan and decorin in the human intervertebral disc. *Biochem. J.* **292**, 661–666.

CHAPTER 6

Growth Factors

PETER I. CROUCHER AND R. GRAHAM G. RUSSELL

Department of Human Metabolism and Clinical Biochemistry, Division of Biochemical and Musculoskeletal Medicine, University of Sheffield Medical School, Sheffield, S10 2RX, United Kingdom

I. INTRODUCTION

The factors that regulate the behavior of the cells responsible for the development and normal maintenance of bone and cartilage are diverse. They include soluble factors, such as hormones and cytokines, proteinases, and adhesion molecules, each of which are discussed in more detail in other chapters. One major group of molecules that are of fundamental importance in the regulation of these tissues are the growth factors (Table I). The growth factors comprise a number of families including the insulin-like growth factors (IGF), members of the transforming growth factor-beta (TGF-β) superfamily, the fibroblast growth factors (FGF), the platelet-derived growth factors (PDGF), and members of the epidermal growth factor family (EGF). Members of these families are generally produced locally where they can act as autocrine or paracrine regulators of growth and/or differentiation. In addition, these molecules may play an important role in mediating the effects of circulating factors, particularly hormones, on target tissues. The identification of growth factors in bone matrix and the demonstration that many of these factors can be produced by osteoblasts has led to an increase in the number of studies dedicated to determining the role of these factors in bone. However, it should be remembered that many of these observations are based upon cell culture studies that may not be relevant *in vivo*. Moreover, there may be important differences between species and responses may differ depending upon the system used. Furthermore, observed responses, even though mediated via binding of the growth factor to its specific receptor, may be indirect in that they depend upon the secondary induction of other factors, including other growth factors or prostaglandins. The role of growth factors in the regulation of bone development and remodeling is the subject of this chapter.

II. INSULIN-LIKE GROWTH FACTORS

The insulin-like growth factors-I and -II (IGF-I and IGF-II) are polypeptide hormones structurally related to insulin. They form three members of the insulin-like growth factor family which share approximately 50% amino acid sequence identity. IGF-I is synthesized primarily in the liver under the influence of growth hormone and accounts for most of the chondrocyte stimulating activity found in serum. IGF-I was formerly known as somatomedin C. The IGFs are nonglycosylated single chain polypeptides with a molecular mass of 7600 that exist in serum primarily associated with IGF binding proteins (IGFBPs), and with an acid labile protein, as complexes of approximately 150 kDa. Since the original discovery of IGFBPs [1], a total of six binding proteins have been identified and named IGFBP-1 to -6 [2–6]. The

83

TABLE I.   Growth Factors That May Affect Bone
and Cartilage

Insulin-like growth factor I and II (IGF-I and -II)

Transforming growth factor-β1-3 (TGF-β1-3)

Bone morphogenetic proteins (BMPs)

Cartilage-derived morphogenetic proteins (CDMPs)

Fibroblast growth factor acidic / basic (FGF-1 and -2)

Heparin-binding secretory transforming protein-1 (hst-1, FGF-4)

Platelet-derived growth factor AA, AB, and BB
    (PDGF-AA, -AB, and -BB)

Epidermal growth factor (EGF)

Transforming growth factor-α (TGF-α)

Vascular endothelial growth factor (VEGF)

most abundant form is IGFBP-3, which is the main binding protein in serum. Although the precise function of each of the IGFBPs has not been fully established, they are themselves under endocrine regulation and play important roles in regulating the distribution of IGFs in tissues and can have both stimulatory and inhibitory effects on IGF function [6]. Since IGFs will bind with greater affinity to the IGFBPs than to the IGF receptor, the binding proteins serve as a potential reservoir for IGF. The affinity of the binding proteins for IGF can be modulated by proteolytic activity, thereby releasing IGF for interaction with its receptor. The IGF-I receptor is structurally related to the insulin receptor and comprises two extracellular alpha subunits and two transmembrane beta subunits which have tyrosine kinase activity. The IGF-II receptor is identical to the mannose-6-phosphate receptr. IGF-I binds with highest affinity to the IGF-I receptor, although it can also bind to the insulin and IGF-II receptors. IGF-II can associate with both IGF-I and IGF-II receptors although it has a higher affinity for the IGF-II receptor.

IGF-I and -II have been shown to be synthesised by osteoblasts [7–9] and to be present in the bone matrix [10]. The production of IGFs by osteoblasts can be regulated by a number of factors [11]. Parathyroid hormone can stimulate the production of IGF-I and 17β-estradiol has been shown to promote expression of the IGF-I mRNA [12–14], whereas 1,25-dihydroxyvitamin D_3, cortisol, and a number of local growth factors, including FGF-2, TGF-β1, and PDGF, inhibit IGF-I production by rodent osteoblasts [11, 15–17]. In contrast, parathyroid hormone, 17β-estradiol, and 1,25-dihydroxyvitamin D_3 along with other hormones, have no effect on IGF-II secretion [18] although, FGF-2, TGF-β1, and PDGF can decrease IGF-II production [19]. Interestingly, BMP-7 has been shown to stimulate production of IGF-II by human osteosarcoma cells [20]. IGFs produced by osteoblasts can be deposited in the bone matrix and this is thought to be mediated by the IGFBPs which are also produced by

osteoblast-like cells [21, 22] and regulted by hormones and local growth factors [22–24]. During bone resorption, IGFs may be released from bone and made available to modulate the behaviour of the cells involved in bone remodeling.

IGFs have been shown to promote bone resorption in neonatal murine calvariae [25] and fetal long bones [26]. IGF-1 and IGF-II can also promote the formation of osteoclasts in bone marrow cultures [25, 27] but have no effect on the activity of isolated osteoclasts [25]. These observations have led to the suggestion that the IGFs can promote bone resorption, albeit indirectly, via an effect on osteoblasts. These effects are likely to be mediated via IGF-I and -II receptors which have been shown to be expressed by osteoblast-like cells [28–31]. IGFs have been shown to promote the proliferation of isolated osteoblast-like cells and osteoblasts in organ culture [32, 33]. Furthermore, both IGF-I and -II promote the synthesis of bone matrix in organ culture and up-regulate type I collagen expression in isolated osteoblast-like cells [33–36].

The effect of IGF has been examined *in vivo* in a number of rodent models. Tobias *et al.* [37] demonstrated that daily subcutaneous injections of IGF-I promoted longitudinal bone growth and an increase in periosteal bone formation; however, this was associated with a decrease in trabecular bone formation. In contrast, Bagi *et al.* [38, 39] reported that IGF-I, when administered as a complex with IGFBP-3, could promote both trabecular and periosteal bone formation. Interestingly, Machwate *et al.* [40] were able to show that IGF-I could partially prevent the trabecular bone loss associated with disuse; however, IGF-I had no effect on control animals.

III. THE TRANSFORMING GROWTH FACTOR-BETA SUPERFAMILY

Transforming growth factor-beta (TGF-β) was originally identified as a factor that transformed the phenotype of fibroblasts *in vitro* [41]. It has become apparent that members of the TGF-β superfamily have a number of diverse and complex activities in a wide range of tissues. These include effects on cell growth and proliferation, on apoptosis, and on differentiation and the induction of new gene expression. The transforming growth factor-beta superfamily comprises a large number of structurally related gene products divided into a number of closely related groups. These include the TGF-β family, activins and inhibins, mullerian inhibiting substance, the bone morphogenetic proteins (BMPs), the cartilage-derived morphogenetic proteins, the *Drosophila* decapentaplegic gene product (*dpp*), the Vgr gene products, and glial cell line-derived neurotrophic factor. Given the size of this gene family, our comments will be confined to those members of the family that have been shown to be important in regulating bone or cartilage biology.

A. Transforming Growth Factor-Beta

The TGF-β family consists of three mammalian gene products (TGF-β1–3), a gene identified in chicken as TGF-β4, and an additional member of the family identified in *Xenopus laevis* (TGF-β5). Although mammalian cells can express each of the three isoforms, the majority of information has been generated with TGF-β1. Each of the isoforms exist as 25 kDa dimers which share more than 70% amino acid identity. TGF-β is produced as a latent complex of approximately 100 kDa which comprises two molecules, each containing mature TGF-β associated with a precursor which is also known as latency associated peptide (LAP). In addition, this latent TGF-β complex has also been shown to be associated with a binding protein with a molecular mass of 190 kDa in fibroblasts and 130 kDa in platelets. The mechanism of activation of latent TGF-β to active TGF-β has not been clearly established. However, studies have shown that parathyroid hormone, glucocorticoids, and local growth factors can promote cells to activate latent TGF-β. In some studies activation has been shown to be mediated by the production of plasmin which cleaves the precursor from the mature molecule [42, 43].

Members of the TGF-β family elicit their biological effect via interactions with specific TGF-β receptors. Two TGF-β receptors (TβRI and TβRII) with masses of 53 and 70 kDa, respectively, have been described [44]. Further analysis has demonstrated both receptors to be functional serine/threonine kinases that are thought to operate as a heterodimer [45, 46], with the TβRII required for ligand binding and both TβRI and TβRII needed for signaling. Studies have suggested that the functional signaling complex is likely to be a tetramer consisting of two TβRI and two TβRII molecules [47]. Interestingly, the type II receptor can bind both TGF-β1 and TGF-β3 but it has less affinity for TGF-β2. An additional receptor, the type III reeptor (betaglycan), appears to be required to present TGF-β2 to the type I/type II signaling complex [48]. The TGF-β receptor complex is known to interact with specific signaling mediators. Studies in *Drosophila* of the decapentaplegic gene identified a gene named *Mothers against dpp* (*Mad*) which is thought to mediate this signaling [49]. *Mad* has been shown to be a homologue of the *small body size* (*sma*) genes of *C. elegans* [50]. At least eight mammalian members of this gene family have also been identified [51] and these are now known as the Smad family of mediators of TGF-β signaling [52]. These molecules translocate to the nucleus where they can activate gene transcription. Although the functions of individual members of this family have not been fully established, it is likely that they mediate specific signals from individual members of the TGF-β superfamily. Indeed, Smad2 and Smad3 are thought to mediate TGF-β signaling. Furthermore, two other described members of this family, Smad6 and Smad7, inhibit TGF-β signaling [53, 54].

The role of TGF-β in bone has been the subject of considerable research interest. Early studies demonstrated the presence of two cartilage inducing factors (CIP-A and -B) in demineralized bone matrix [55], which were subsequently shown to be identical to TGF-β1 and TGF-β2, respectively [56, 57]. Bone has been shown to be a major source of TGF-β1, with reports estimating there to be as much as 200 μg of TGF-β1 per kg of tissue. Osteoblasts produce both the 100 kDa TGF-β precursor [58] and a complex containing the 190 kDa TGF-β binding protein [59]. The latter complex has been suggested to be deposited in bone during synthesis [60]. Factors that promote bone resorption, including 1,25-dihydroxyvitamin D$_3$, parathyroid hormone, and interleukin-1, have been shown to promote the release of TGF-β from fetal rat or neonatal calvarie [61]. In addition, inhibition of bone resorption also prevents release of TGF-β [61]. These data suggest that TGF-β is liberated as bone is resorbed; however, osteoclasts themselves have been shown to produce TGF-β. Northern blot analysis demonstrated the presence of the mRNA for each of the TGF-β2, TGF-β3, and TGF-β4 isoforms in avian osteoclasts, although TGF-β2 was reported to be the principal secreted form [62]. Zheng *et al.* [63] have also shown that osteoclast-like cells derived from giant cell tumors of bone express the mRNA for TGF-β1. Osteoclasts can activate latent TGF-β *in vitro* [62, 64]; however, the identity of the proteinase responsible for this remains unclear [62]. Although active TGF-β can be released during bone resorption, the effect of this factor has not been fully established because responses appear dependent upon the dose of TGF-β studied and the experimental system used. Chenu *et al.* [65] demonstrated that TGF-β could inhibit the formation of osteoclast-like cells *in vitro*, a response that was suggested to be mediated by preferentially stimulating the differentiation of cells towards a granulocytic phenotype rather than cells with characteristics of osteoclasts. Shinar and Rodan [66] also reported a decrease in osteoclast-like cell formation in murine bone marrow cultures; however, at low concentrations, TGF-β was reported to increase osteoclast-like cell formation. The effects of TGF-β on bone resorption in organ culture have also been conflicting. TGF-β has been reported to stimulate an increase in bone resorption in a murine neonatal calvaria system [67, 68]. In contrast, high doses of TGF-β cause an inhibition of bone resorption in fetal rat long bones [68, 69]. However, in an ovariectomized rat model, direct injection of TGF-β into the bone marrow space caused a significant decrease in both the osteoclast surface and numbers of osteoclasts, suggesting that *in vivo*, TGF-β may inhibit bone resorption [70].

Although TGF-β appears to have variable effects on bone resorption, a significant body of data has demonstrated that this molecule may be important in promoting bone formation. Multiple daily injections of TGF-β1 onto the parietal bones of neonatal rats or into the subcutaneous tissue overlying the calvaria of mice have been show to result in an increase in bone formation at the site of injection [71–73]. Beck *et al.* [74] demonstrated that a single application of TGF-β could induce healing of skull defect in rabbits. Rosen *et al.* [75] have demonstrated that systemic administration of TGF-β2 to both juvenile and adult rats could also stimulate bone formation. Although the mechanism of increased bone formation is unclear, it has been suggested that TGF-β promotes the proliferation and recruitment of new osteoblasts. In support of this, several studies have shown that TGF-β is chemotactic for bone cells such as rat osteosarcoma and osteoblast-like cells derived from fetal rat calvaria [76, 77]. However, the effect of TGF-β1 on the proliferation of osteoblast-like cells is somewhat unclear, with reports demonstrating either increases [78–80] or decreases in the proliferation of osteoblast-like cells [81, 82], and biphasic effects dependent upon cell density [83]. However, these data are confounded by the fact that many of the cells examined in these studies were osteosarcoma cells or more differentiated osteoblasts rather than osteoblast precursors. Studies have also shown that TGF-β can modulate the differentiated function of these cells. These include studies that demonstrate that TGF-β can both stimulate and inhibit the production or expression of alkaline phosphatase, type I collagen, and osteonectin [82, 84, 85]. However, the effects of TGF-β1 on expression of osteocalcin production and mineralization appear more consistent. A number of reports have demonstrated that TGF-β inhibits the expression [85, 86] and synthesis of osteocalcin in osteoblast-like cells [86]. Furthermore, studies have also shown a decrease in the formation of bone nodules *in vitro* [85, 87, 88].

B. Bone Morphogenetic Proteins

The bone morphogenetic proteins are a large family of prteins that share common structural features with TGF-β1 and other members of the TGF-β superfamily. Members of the BMP family can be further divided into a number of related subgroups based upon sequence identity (Table II) [89–96]. BMP family members are synthesized as precursors which are proteolytically processed to yield a mature protein containing seven conserved cysteine residues. Functionally, BMPs exist as homodimers that are linked by disulfide bonds, although a functional heterodimer has been reported [97]. In a similar manner to the TGF-β isoforms, members of the BMP family bind to type I and type II receptors, both of which are required for signal transduction. Two different type I BMP receptors have been identified: BMP receptor-IA (BMPR-IA, also known as ALK-3 (activin receptor-like kinase-3)) and BMP receptor-IB (BMPR-IB or ALK-6) [98, 99]. Although these two receptors are specific for BMP family members, several members can also bind to the activin type I receptor (ActR-I or ALK-2) [98]. A BMP type II receptor (BMPR-II) has also been identified which is specific

TABLE II.   Members of the Bone Morphogenetic Protein Family.

Prototype members / Subfamily	Members	References
BMP2 / BMP4	BMP-2	[90]
	BMP-4	[90]
	Dpp (*Drosophilia*)	[91]
BMP-3 / osteogenin	BMP-3 / osteogenin	[90]
	BMP3a / GDF-10	[92]
BMP7 / Osteogenic protein-1 (OP-1)	BMP-5	[93]
	BMP-6 / Vgr-1	[93]
	BMP-7 / OP-1	[93, 94]
	BMP-8 / OP-2	[95]
Cartilage-derived morphogenetic protein-1 and -2 (CDMP)	BMP-12 /GDF 7	
	BMP-13 / CDMP-2 /GDF 6	[96]
	BMP-14 / CDMP-1 /GDF 5	[96]
Unclassified members	BMP-9 /	
	BMP-10	
	BMP-15	

Note. This is a limited list and could include a separate, but related, subgroup, the growth/differentiation factors (GDFs). A more definitive list can be found in Reddi [89].

for BMPs [100, 101]; however, some BMPs can also bind to the activin type II receptors, albeit with reduced affinity [102]. Like TGF-β, signal transduction is mediated by members of the Smad family, with Smad1 and Smad5 being specifically implicated in BMP signaling.

Urist [103] made the important discovery that demineralized bone induced new bone formation when implanted into ectopic sites in rodents. Subsequent studies demonstrated that members of the BMP family contributed to this activity and that this family of molecules may play an important role in bone development [104]. BMPs -2, -4, -5, and -7 can all induce new bone formation *in vivo* [105–107] and heterodimers of the different members, including BMP4/7, increase this activity [108]. BMPs appear to initiate a complex cascade of events leading to new bone formation, which includes the migration of mesenchymal cells to these sites, their differentiation to chondroblasts and chondrocytes, mineralization of cartilage, angiogenesis, osteoblast differentiation, bone formation, and subsequently, remodeling of this bone [89]. BMPs may be required to initiate these events, which are subsequently supported by other factors; alternatively, they may modulate the behavior of cells at more than one stage. Several members of the BMP family have been shown to exhibit a chemotactic activity. For example, Cunningham *et al.* [109] demonstrated that BMP-3 and BMP-4 can promote migration of human monocytes. Furthermore, BMP-2, but not BMP-4 and BMP-6, are chemotactic for human osteoblasts [110]. BMPs have been shown to determine the differentiation pathways of uncommitted mesenchymal cells. Wang *et al.* [111] demonstrated that BMP-2 could promote he differentiation of C3H10T1/2 cells, which is a murine mesenchymal cell line, into cells with characteristics of osteoblasts or adipocytes. High concentrations of BMP-2 promoted differentiation into osteoblasts whereas low concentrations favored differentiation into adipocytic cells [111]. Furthermore, Katagiri *et al.* [112] reported that BMP-2 treatment of C2C12 myoblastic cells resulted in an increase in the expression of alkaline phosphatase, osteocalcin, and PTH dependent cAMP production and a concomitant reduction in myotube formation. In addition, BMP-6 was shown to promote the differentiation of a rat mesenchymal cell line into cells with characteristics of osteoblasts [113]. BMPs also have effects on committed osteoblast precursors with a number of reports demonstrating that BMPs-2, -3, -4, -6, and -7 can promote differentiation to an osteoblast phenotype, including the upregulation of alkaline phosphatase activity, type I collagen synthesis, and the expression of osteocalcin [107, 114–118]. Studies have shown that BMPs can regulate the production of IGFs by bone cells. BMP-2 upregulates the expression of IGF-I and -II and downregulates the expression of IGFBP-5 in rat calvarial osteoblasts [119, 120]. BMP-7 promotes expression of IGF-II but not IGF-I in human osteosarcoma cells [20]. Furthermore, BMP-7 stimulates production of IGFBP-3 and -5 but inhibits IGFGP-4 production in these cells, suggesting that BMP-7 can regulate the IGF system in a number of different ways [20].

The importance of BMPs in skeletal development have been exemplified by the demonstration that mutations in the BMP-5 gene in mice lead to the short ear phenotype [121], whereas mutations in GDF-5 (BMP-14) lead to the development of brachypodism [122]. Thomas *et al.* [123] have reported that a mutation in CDMP-1, the human homolog of GDF-5, is associated with a chondrodysplasia characterized by shortening of the bones of the appendicular skeleton and abnormalities of the bones in the hands and feet (Hunter–Thomson type). Furthermore, it has been suggested that abnormalities in the BMP-2 and -4 genes may be associated with fibrodysplasia ossificans progressiva because mutations in the *Drosophila* homolog, *dpp*, result in similar abnormalities [124].

IV. FIBROBLAST GROWTH FACTORS

The fibroblast growth factors are a family of heparin binding growth factors that are potent regulators of proliferation and differentiation. The family is thought to consist of at least nine members which share 30–50% amino acid sequence identity and contain two conserved cysteine residues. The prototypes of this family are acidic and basic FGF (FGF-1 and FGF-2, respectively) which were originally identified as factors in extracts of pituitary that stimulated the growth of 3T3 cells [125, 126]. The two proteins that comprised this

activity (FGF-1 and FGF-2) have different isoelectric points and share approximately 55% amino acid sequence identity. FGF-1 is approximately 16–18 kDa in size, whereas FGF-2 is slightly larger, approximately 18 kDa, although larger forms have been identified. Neither FGF-1 or -2 possesses a signal sequence suggesting that these two members of the family are not released via the classical pathway. However, studies have confirmed that they are released from cells by mechanisms that do not involve cell death and that inhibitors of exocytosis can prevent this release [127]. Extracellular FGF can bind to heparin or to heparan sulfate and can therefore be sequestered into the extracellular matrix which acts as a reservoir of this growth factor; alternatively, it can be found bound to the cell surface. FGFs elicit a biological response by interacting with members of the FGF receptor (FGFR) family of transmembrane tyrosine kinases. There are four members of the FGFR family, all of which have a similar general structure; however, alternate mRNA splicing can lead to a large number of isoforms of these receptors [128]. The mechanism by which FGF binds to its receptor and signals to the cell has not been fully determined. Studies have shown that FGF can bind to FGFRs in the absence of heparan sulfate [129]. However, binding of FGF to heparan sulfate appears to increase the affinity of FGF for its receptor [130] and is important for subsequent receptor dimerization and activation [128]. This has led to the suggestion that heparan sulfate acts as a low affinity receptor for FGF by binding FGF and allowing its presentation to the high affinity FGFR for signaling. Thus, the receptor complex consists of two FGFR molecules, one heparan sulfate molecule and either one or two FGF molecules [128].

The FGF/FGFR system is thought to play an important role in skeletal biology. Indeed, FGF-2 is synthesized by osteoblasts [131, 132], is stored in the bone matrix, and can be released during bone resorption [131, 133]. FGF-1 and -2 have been reported to stimulate bone resorption in organ culture [134, 135]. Furthermore, FGF-2 has been shown to stimulate the formation of osteoclasts in murine bone marrow cultures [136]. FGF-2 also stimulates the proliferation of osteoblasts and bone marrow stromal cells *in vitro* [137–141]. However, the effect of these molecules on characteristics of the osteoblast phenotype appears to depend on the system examined. FGF-2 inhibits alkaline phosphatase, osteocalcin, and type I collagen expression in osteoblast-like cells *in vitro* [139, 142–144], although the effects may depend on the concentrations studied because high doses of FGF appear to decrease collagen synthesis and low doses promote synthesis [139]. In contrast, in bone marrow stromal cell cultures, FGF appears to promote alkaline phosphatase expression and the formation of mineralized deposits within these cultures [140, 141, 145]. These observations are consistent with recent studies *in vivo* which suggest that systemic administration of FGF-2 results in an increase in the number of osteoblasts and new bone formation [146–148].

Interestingly, these effects were predominantly in endosteal bone and not on the periosteal surface. FGF-1 and FGF-4 (hst-1) have also been shown to promote an increase in bone formation [146]. Other studies have shown that FGFs can also regulate the production of other growth factors by osteoblast-like cells. FGF-2 has been shown to decrease IGF-I and -II and IGFBP production by MC3T3-E1 cells [149, 150]. In contrast, studies have shown that FGF-2 can promote the production of TGF-β1 by osteoblasts [151].

As with the BMPs, the importance of the FGF/FGFR system in bone development has been demonstrated by the identification of genetic mutations that lead to skeletal abnormalities. These mutations are often found in the receptors for FGF and are typified by the creation of an unpaired cysteine residue which can lead to ligand-independent dimerization and constitutive activation [152]. Mutations in FGFR-1 and -2 are found in the craniosynostosis syndromes [152, 153], including Aperts [154], Pfeiffer [155, 156], Jackson-Weiss [157], and Crouzons syndromes [158]. Mutations in FGFR-3 have also been shown to lead to skeletal abnormalities. These include a point mutation (Gly380Arg) in the transmembrane region of FGFR-3 that leads to the development of achondroplasia [159] and mutations in the tyrosine kinase domain, Asn540Lys and Lys650Glu, that lead to hypochondroplasia and thanatophoric dysplasia, respectively [160, 161].

V. PLATELET-DERIVED GROWTH FACTORS

Platelet derived growth factors are dimeric polypeptide growth factors with a molecular mass of approximately 30 kDa [162]. PDGF is encoded by two separate genes, PDGF-A and PDGF-B, that reside on separate chromosomes but can form three disulfide-linked dimers, PDGF-AA, -BB and -AB [163]. Alternate spliced forms of the PDGF-A chain have been identified and shown to give rise to products of different size that may also differ in function [164, 165]. PDGF elicits its biological response by interacting with specific cell surface receptors. These comprise two distinct subunits, α and β, that from either homo- or hetero-dimers, giving rise to three distinct forms of the PDGF receptor, termed the $\alpha\alpha$ receptor, the $\beta\beta$ receptor, and the $\alpha\beta$ receptor. PDGF-AA binds to the $\alpha\alpha$ receptor, PDGF-AB can bind to both $\alpha\alpha$ and $\alpha\beta$ receptors, whereas PDGF-BB can bind to each of the three forms of the receptor [166].

Early studies demonstrated that human osteosarcoma cells expressed both PDGF-A and -B chains [162, 163, 167]. Other studies have revealed that normal osteoblasts also express the mRNA and protein for the PDGF-A chain [168–170] and the mRNA for the PDGF-B chain [171]. The expression of the mRNA for the PDGF-B can be upregulated by treatment with TGF-β1 but not by PDGF-BB itself, or by IGF-I or FGF-2 [171]. PDGF can be deposited in bone

matrix (133) and be released during bone resorption or it can be released by osteoblasts to act in either a paracrine or autocrine manner. Indeed, both PDGF-AA and -BB can bind to osteoblasts [172–175], and studies have shown that both osteoblasts and bone-lining cells express the PDGF-α receptor *in situ* [170]. Reports suggest that expression of these receptors can be regulated by pro-inflammatory cytokines because interleukin-1β and tumor necrosis factor-α can downregulate PDGF-AA binding by reducing expression of PDGF α receptor on normal human osteoblasts [174, 176]. Each of the three isoforms of PDGF can promote the proliferation of osteoblasts [172, 174, 175]. Although PDGF-BB appears more potent than PDGF-AA in rodent osteoblasts [175], this does not appear to be the case in human osteoblasts [174]. PDGF has also been shown to promote collagen synthesis [172], but these effects are likely to be secondary to their effect on cell proliferation [173]. In long-term culture, continuous exposure to PDGF decreases alkaline phosphatase expression, type I collagen, and the appearance of mineralized nodules, which is consistent with an inhibitory effect on the differentiated function of the osteoblast [177]. However, short-term exposure to PDGF has the opposite effect and simulates mineralized nodule formation [178], which is consistent with the effects observed *in vivo*. The local administration of PDGF following osteotomy has been shown to accelerate healing and promote bone formation [179]. Furthermore, systemic administration of PDGF has been shown to prevent bone loss in ovariectomized rats, an effect that is accompanied by an increase in osteoblast number [180].

PDGF has also been shown to have effects on bone resorption. Tashjian *et al.* [181] demonstrated that partially purified PDGF promoted resorption of neonatal mouse calvariae, an effect that was thought to be mediated by an increase in the local production of PGE$_2$. Subsequent studies demonstrated that PDGF-AB and PDGF-BB, but not PDGF-AA, have the ability to promote bone resorption [182]. PDGF can also promote the production on interleukin-6, a factor that has been implicated in promoting bone resorption by rodent osteoblasts [183]. Furthermore, studies have shown that PDGF-BB, but not PDGF-AA, can upregulate osteoblast expression of collagenase-1 which may contribute to the degradation of type I collagen and the activation of bone resorption [184].

VI. ADDITIONAL GROWTH FACTORS

The growth factors described in the previous sections represent those factors that have been most widely studied in bone. However, a number of other growth factors have also been shown to have effects on the cells of bone. These include members of the epidermal growth factor family, such as epidermal growth factor (EGF), transforming growth factor-α (TGF-α), and vascular endothelial growth factor (VEGF, also known as vascular permeability factor).

EGF and TGF-α are structurally related glycoproteins that have been reported to have similar effects on bone. EGF receptors have been shown to be expressed by osteoblast-like cells [185, 186] and treatment of such cells with EGF results in an increase in cell proliferation [187] and the production of PGE$_2$ [188]. Similarly, TGF-α can also promote PGE$_2$ production in osteoblastic cells [189]. EGF and TGF-α have also been shown to promote bone resorption *in vitro* [67, 190–192]. Studies have also demonstrated that TGF-α can stimulate bone resorption *in vivo* and that this may contribute to the development of hypercalcemia of malignancy [193].

VEGF is a polypeptide growth factor that specifically promotes the proliferation of vascular endothelial cells, an effect that is mediated via specific VEGF receptors known as flt-1 and KDR. Studies have shown that both rodent and human osteoblast-like cells express the mRNA for VEGF and also produce the VEGF protein [194–196]. Futhermore, the expression of VEGF is promoted by prostaglandins, 1,25-dihydroxyvitamin D$_3$, and IGF-I [194–196]. Because blood vessels and endothelial cells are found closely associated with osteoblasts, the VEGF produced by these cells may promote both endothelial cell proliferation and the paracrine production of other growth factors [197].

VII. SUMMARY

The 1990s have seen significant advances in our understanding of the role of growth factors in skeletal development and the normal regulation of bone remodeling. It is clear that these factors play a very important role, although in many cases the precise functions of individual growth factors remain unclear. However, we now know that many of these factors are produced by osteoblasts and deposited in bone matrix. The release of these factors during bone resorption makes them available to regulate the cells involved in bone remodeling and they may therefore act as important coupling factors (Fig. 1). Clearly, one of the predominant effects of growth factors is to promote the proliferation and recruitment of osteoblast precursors, yet they also have other important effects. These include being able to promote the chemotaxis of osteoblasts, thereby recruiting these cells to sites of bone remodeling, and to regulate the differentiated function of osteoblasts, although the particular response appears to depend on the systems examined and the growth factors studied. Although our understanding of the role of growth factors in promoting bone formation has improved, we understand less about their effects on bone resorption. A number of growth factors are able to modulate bone resorption, but their precise role has not been determined. It is likely that in the next few years our understanding of the role of specific growth factors and their relative contributions to the physiological and pathological regulation of bone development and remodeling

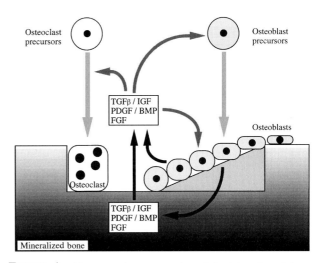

FIGURE 1 Diagrammatic representation of the interactions between growth factors and the cells of bone. Growth factors can be produced by osteoblasts, where they can either interact with cells directly or be deposited in bone matrix for later release following osteoclastic bone resorption. Growth factors released into the local environment can modulate the proliferation and differentiation of osteoblast precursors and also have direct effects on osteoblasts. Equally, these factors can influence the recruitment of osteoclasts and affect bone resorption.

will continue to improve. However, these molecules clearly play a fundamental role in these processes.

References

1. Hintz, R. L., and Liu, F. (1977). Demonstration of specific plasma protein binding sites for somatomedin. *J. Clin. Endocrinol. Metab.* **45**, 988–955.

2. Drop, S. L. S., Kortleve, D. J., and Guyda, H. J. (1984). Isolation of a somatomedin-binding protein from pre-term amniotic fluid. Development of a radioimmunoassay. *J. Clin. Endocrinol. Metab.* **59**, 899–907.

3. Martin, J. L., and Baxter, R. C. (1986). Insulin like growth factor binding protein from human plasma, purification and characterization. *J. Biol. Chem.* **261**, 8754–8760.

4. Brown, A. L., Chiariotti, L., Orlowski, C. C., Mehlman, T., Burgess, W. H., Ackerman, E. J., Bruni, C. B., and Rechler, M. M. (1989). Nucleotide sequence and expression of a cDNA encoding a fetal rat binding protein for insulin-like growth factors. *J. Biol. Chem.* **264**, 5148–5154.

5. Shimasaki, S., Shimonaka, M., Zhang, H. P., and Ling, N. (1991). Identification of five different insulin-like growth factor binding proteins (IGFBPs) from adult rat serum and molecular cloning of a novel IGFBP in rat and human. *J. Biol. Chem.* **266**, 10646–10653.

6. Clemmons, D. R. (1997). Insulin-like growth factor binding proteins and their role in controlling IGF action. *Cytokine Growth Factor Rev.* **8**, 45–62.

7. McCarthy, T. L., Centrella, M., and Canalis, E. (1990). Cyclic AMP induces insulin-like growth factor I synthesis in osteoblast-enriched cultures. *J. Biol. Chem.* **265**, 15353–15356.

8. Mohan, S., Bautista, C. M., Herring, S. J., Linkart, T. A., and Baylink, D. J. (1990). Development of valid methods to measure insulin-like growth factors-I and -II in bone cell-conditioned medium. *Endocrinology* **126**, 2534–2542.

9. Okazaki, R., Canover, C. A., Harris, S. A., Spelsberg, T. C., and Riggs, B. L. (1995). Normal human osteoblast-like cells consistently express genes for insulin-like growth factors I and II but transformed human osteoblast cell lines do not. *J. Bone Miner. Res.* **10**, 788–795.

10. Frolik, C. A., Ellis, L. F., and Williams, D. C. (1988). Isolation and characterization of insulin-like growth factor-II from human bone. *Biochem. Biophys. Res. Commun.* **151**, 1011–1018.

11. Canalis, E. (1993). Insulin like growth factors and the local regulation of bone formation. *Bone* **14**, 273–276.

12. McCarthy, T. L., Centrella, M., and Canalis, E. (1989). Parathyroid hormone enhances the transcipt and polypeptide levels of insulin-like growth factor I in osteoblast-enriched cultures from fetal rat bone. *Endocrinology* **124**, 1247–1253.

13. Linkhart, T. A., and Mohan, S. (1989). Parathyroid hormone stimulates release of insulin-like growth factor-I (IGF-I) and IGF-II from neonatal mouse calvaria in organ culture. *Endocrinology* **125**, 1484–1491.

14. Ernst, M., Heath, J. K., and Rodan, G. A. (1989). Estradiol effects on proliferation, messenger ribonucleic acid for collagen and insulin-like growth factor-I, and parathyroid hormone-stimulated adenylate cyclase activity in osteoblastic cells from calvariae and long bones. *Endocrinology* **125**, 825–833.

15. Scharla, S. H., Strong, D. D., Mohan, S., Baylink, D. J., and Linkhart, T. A. (1991). 1,25-dihydroxyvitamin D_3 differentially regulates the production of insulin-like growth factor I (IGF-I) and the IGF-binding protein-4 in mouse osteoblasts. *Endocrinology* **129**, 3139–3146.

16. McCarthy, T. L., Centrella, M., and Canalis, E. (1990). Cortisol inhibits the synthesis of insulin-like growth factor I in skeletal cells. *Endocrinology* **126**, 1569–1575.

17. Canalis, E., Pash, J., Gabbitas, B., Rydziel, S., and Varghese, S. (1993). Growth factors regulate the synthesis of insulin-like growth factor-I in bone cell cultures. *Endocrinology* **133**, 33–38.

18. Canalis, E., Centrella, M., and McCarthy, T. L. (1991). Regulation of insulin-like growth factor-II production by bone cultures. *Endocrinology* **129**, 2457–2462.

19. Gabbitas, B., Pash, J., and Canalis, E. (1994). Regulation of insulin-like growth factor-II synthesis in bone cell cultures by skeletal growth factors. *Endocrinology* **135**, 284–289.

20. Knutsen, R., Honda, Y., Strong, D. D., Sampath, T. K., Baylink, D. J., and Mohan, S. (1995). Regulation of insulin-like growth factor system components by osteogenic protein-1 in human bone cells. *Endocrinology* **136**, 857–865.

21. Mohan, S., Bautista, C. M., Wergedal, J., and Baylink, D. J. (1989). Isolation of an inhibitory insulin-like growth factor (IGF) binding protein from bone cell-conditioned medium: A potential local regulator of IGF action. *Proc. Natl. Acad. Sci. U.S.A.* **86**, 8338–8342.

22. Chen, T. L., Chang, L. Y., Bates, R. L., and Perlman, A. J. (1991). Dexamethasone and 1,25(OH)$_2$D$_3$ modulation of insulin-like growth factor binding proteins in rat osteoblast-like cell cultures. *Endocrinology* **128**, 73–80.

23. Chen, T. L., Liu, F., Bates, R. L., and Hintz, R. L. (1991). Further characterization of insulin-like growth factor binding proteins in rat osteoblast-like cell cultures. Modulation by 17β-estradiol and human growth hormone. *Endocrinology* **128**, 2489–2496.

24. Chen, T. L., Chang, L. Y., DiGregorio, D. A., Perlman, A. J., and Huang, Y. F. (1993). Growth factor modulation of insulin-like growth factor-binding proteins in rat osteoblast-like cells. *Endocrinology* **133**, 1382–1389.

25. Hill, P. A., Reynolds, J. J., and Meikle, M. C. (1995). Osteoblasts mediate insulin-like growth factor-I and -II stimulation of osteoclast formation and function. *Endocrinology* **136**, 124–131.

26. Slootweg, M. C., Most, W. M., van Beek, E., Schot, L. P. C., Papapoulous, S. E., and Lowik, C. W. G. M. (1992). Osteoclast formation together with interleukin-6 production in mouse long bones is increased by insulin-like growth factor-I. *J. Endocrinol.* **132**, 433–438.

27. Mochizuki, H., Hakeda, Y., Wahatsuki, N., Usui, N., Akashi, S., Sato, T., Tanaka, K., and Kumegawa, M. (1992). Insulin-like growth factor-I supports formation and activation of osteoclasts. *Endocrinology* **131**, 1075–1080.

28. Mohan, S., Linkhart, T., Rosenfield, R., and Baylink, D. (1989). Characterisation of the receptor for insulin-like growth factor II in bone cells. *J. Cell. Physiol.* **140**, 169–176.

29. Centrella, M., McCarthy, T. L., and Canalis, E. (1990). Receptors for insulin-like growth factors-I and -II in osteoblast-enriched cultures from fetal rat bone. *Endocrinology* **126**, 39–44.

30. Slootweg, M. C., Hoogerbrugge, C. M., de Poorter, T. L., Duursma, S. A., and van Buul-Offers, S. C. (1990). The presence of classical insulin-like growth factor (IGF) type-I and -II receptors on mouse osteoblasts: Autocrine/paracrine growth effect of IGFs? *J. Endocrinol.* **125**, 271–277.

31. Cantrell, P. R., Frolik, C. A., Ellis, L. F., and Williams, D. C. (1991). Binding of insulin-like growth factors to cultured rat calvarial cells with differing biologic responses. *J. Bone Miner. Res.* **6**, 851–857.

32. Fournier, B., Ferralli, J. M., Price, P. A., and Schlaeppi, J. M. (1993). Comparison of the effects of insulin-like growth factors-I and -II on the human osteosarcoma cell line OHS-4. *J. Endocrinol.* **136**, 173–180.

33. Hock, J. M., Centrella, M., and Canalis, E. (1988). Insulin-like growth factor I has independent effects on bone matrix formation and cell replication. *Endocrinology* **122**, 254–260.

34. Pfeilschifter, J., Oechsner, M., Naumann, A., Gronwald, R. G. K., Minne, H. W., and Ziegler, R. (1990). Stimulation of bone matrix apposition in vitro by local growth factors: A comparison between insulin-like growth factor I, platelet-derived growth factor, and transforming growth factor β. *Endocrinology* **127**, 69–75.

35. Schmid, C., Guler, H.-P., Rowe, D., and Froesch, E. D. (1989). Insulin-like growth factor I regulates type I procollagen messenger ribonucleic acid steady state levels in bone of rats. *Endocrinology* **125**, 1575–1580.

36. Strong, D. D., Beachler, A. L., Wergedal, J. E., and Linkhart, T. A. (1991). Insulin-like growth factor II and transforming growth factor β regulate collagen expression in human osteoblastlike cells in vitro. *J. Bone Miner. Res.* **6**, 15–23.

37. Tobias, J. H., Chow, J. W. M., and Chambers, T. J. (1992). Opposite effects of insulin-like growth factor-I on the formation of trabecular and cortical bone in adult female rats. *Endocrinology* **131**, 2387–2392.

38. Bagi, C. M., Brommage, R., Deleon, L., Adams, S., Rosen, D., and Sommer, A. (1994). Benefit of systemically administered rhIGF-I and rhIGF-I/IGFBP-3 on cancellous bone in ovariectomized rats. *J. Bone Miner. Res.* **9**, 1301–1312.

39. Bagi, C. M., Deleon, E., Brommage, R., Adams, S., Rosen, D., and Sommer, A. (1995). Systemic administration of rhIGF-I or rhIGF-I/-IGFBP-3 increases cortical bone and lean body mass in ovariectomized rats. *Bone* **16**, 263S–269S.

40. Machwate, M., Zerath, E., Holy, X., Pastoureau, P., and Marie, P. J. (1994). Insulin-like growth factor-I increases trabecular bone formation and osteoblastic cell proliferation in unloaded rats. *Endocrinology* **134**, 1031–1038.

41. Roberts, A. B., Anzano, M. A., Lamb, L. C., Smith, J. M., and Sporn, M. B. (1981). New class of transforming growth factors potentiated by epidermal growth factor. *Proc. Natl. Acad. Sci. U.S.A.* **78**, 5339–5343.

42. Sato, Y., and Rifkin, D. B. (1989). Inhibition of endothelial cell movement by pericytes and smooth muscle cells: Activation of a latent transforming growth factor-β1-like molecule by plasmin during coculture. *J. Cell Biol.* **109**, 309–315.

43. Lyons, R. M., Gentry, L. E., Purchio, A. F., and Moses, H. L. (1990). Mechanism of activation of latent recombinant transforming growth factor β1 by plasmin. *J. Cell Biol.* **110**, 1361–1397.

44. Cheifetz, S., Like, B., and Massagué, J. (1986). Cellular distribution of type I and type II receptors for transforming growth factor-β. *J. Biol. Chem.* **261**, 9972–9978.

45. Lin, H. Y., Wang, X.-F., Ng-Eaton, E., Weinberg, R. A., and Lodish, H. F. (1992). Expression cloning of the TGFβ type II receptor, a functional transmembrane serine/threonine kinase. *Cell* **68**, 775–785.

46. Bassing, C. H., Yingling, J. M., Howe, D. J., Wang, T., He, W. W., Gustafson, M. L., Shah, P., Donahoe, P. K., and Wang, X.-F. (1994). A transforming growth factor β type I receptor that signals to activate gene expression. *Science* **263**, 87–89.

47. Weiss-Garcia, F., and Massagué, J. (1996). Complementation between kinase-defective and activation defective TGF-β receptors reveals a novel form of receptor cooperativity essential for signaling. *EMBO J.* **15**, 276–289.

48. Alevizopoulos, A., and Mermod, N. (1997). Transforming growth factor-β: The breaking open of a black box. *BioEssays* **19**, 581–591.

49. Sekelsky, J. J. Newfeld, S. J., Raftery, L. A., Chartoff, E. H., and Gelbart, W. M. (1995). Genetic characterization and cloning of mothers against *dpp*, a gene required for decapentaplegic function in *Drosophila melanogaster. Genetics* **139**, 1347–1358.

50. Savage, C., Das, P., Finelli, A. L., Townsend, S. R., Sun, C.-Y., Baird, S. E., and Padgett, R. W. (1996). *Caenorhabditis elegans* genes *sma-2, sma-3* and *sma-4* define a conserved family of transforming growth factor β pathway components. *Proc. Natl. Acad. Sci. U.S.A.* **93**, 790–794.

51. Kawabata, M., Imamura, T., and Miyazono, K. (1998). Signal transduction by bone morphogenetic proteins. *Cytokine Growth Factor Rev.* **9**, 49–61.

52. Derynck, R., Gelbart, W. M., Harland, R. M., Heldin, C.-H., Kern, S. E., Massague, J., Melton, D. A., Mlodzik, M., Padgett, R. W., Roberts, A. B., Smith, J., Thomsen, G. H., Vogelstein, B., and Wang, X.-F. (1996) Nomenclature: Vertebrate mediators of TGFβ family signals. *Cell* **87**, 173.

53. Imamura, T., Takase, M., Nishihara, A., Hanai, J-I., Oeda, E., Kawabata, M., and Miyazono, K. (1997). Smad6 inhibits signaling by the TGF-β superfamily. *Nature* **389**, 622–626.

54. Nakao, A., Afrakhte, M., Moren, A., Nakyama, T., Christian, J. L., Heuchel, R., Itoh, S., Kawabata, M., Heldin, N.-E., Heldin, C.-H., and ten Dijke, P. (1997). Identification of Smad7, a TGF-β1 inducible antagonist of TGF-β signalling. *Nature* **389**, 631–635.

55. Seyedin, S. M., Thomas, T. C., Thompson, A. Y., Rosen, D. M., and Piez, K. A. (1985). Purification and characterization of two cartilage-inducing factors from bovine demineralised bone. *Proc. Natl. Acad. Sci. U.S.A.*, **82**, 2267–2271.

56. Seyedin, S. M., Thompson, A. Y., Bentz, H., Rosen, D. M., McPherson, J. M., Conti, A., Siegel, N. R., Galluppi, G. R., and Piez, K. A. (1986). Cartilage-inducing factor-A. Apparent identity to transforming growth factor-β. *J. Biol. Chem.* **261**, 5693–5695.

57. Centrella, M., McCarthy, T. L., and Canalis, E. (1991). Transforming growth factor-beta and remodeling of bone. *J. Bone J. Surg.* **73**, 1418–1428.

58. Bonewald, L. F., Wakefield, L., Oreffo, R. O. C., Escobedo, A., Twardzik, D. R., and Mundy, G. R. (1991). Latent forms of transforming growth factor-beta (TGF-β) derived from bone cultures. Identification of a naturally occuring 100-kDa complex with similarity to recombinant latent TGF-β. *Mol. Endocrinol.* **5**, 741–751.

59. Dallas, S. L., Park-Snyder, S., Miyazono, K., Twardzik, D., Mundy, G. R., and Bonewald, B. L. (1994). Characterization and autoregulation of latent transforming growth factor β (TGF-β) complexes in osteoblast-like cell lines: Production of a latent complex lacking the latent TGFβ-binding protein (LTBP). *J. Biol. Chem.* **269**, 6815–6822.

60. Bonewald, L. F., and Dallas, S. L. (1994). Role of active and latent transforming growth factor β in bone formation. *J. Cell. Biochem.* **55**, 350–357.

61. Pfeilschifter, J., and Mundy, G. R. (1987). Modulation of type β transforming growth factor activity in bone cultures by osteotropic hormones. *Proc. Natl. Acad. Sci. U.S.A.* **84**, 2024–2028.

62. Oursler, M. J. (1994). Osteoclast synthesis and secretion and activation of latent transforming growth factor β. *J. Bone Miner. Res.* **9**, 443–451.

63. Zheng, M. H., Fan, Y., Wysocki, S. J., Lau, A. T.-T., Robertson, T., Beilharz, M., Wood, D. J., and Papadimitriou, J. M. (1994). Gene expression of transforming growth factor-β1 and its type II receptor in giant cell tumors of bone. *Am. J. Pathol.* **145**, 1095–1104.

64. Oreffo, R. O. C., Mundy, G. R., Seyedin, S. M., and Bonewald, L. F. (1989). Activation of the bone derived latent TGF beta complex by isolated osteoclasts. *Biochem. Biophys. Res. Commun.* **158**, 817–823.

65. Chenu, C., Pfeilschifter, J., Mundy, G. R., and Roodman, G. D. (1988). Transforming growth factor β inhibits formation of osteoclast-like cells in long-term human marrow cultures. *Proc. Natl. Acad. Sci. U.S.A.* **85**, 5683–5687.

66. Shinar, D. M., and Rodan, G. A. (1990). Biphasic effects of transforming growth factor-β on the production of osteoclast-like cells in mouse bone marrow cultures: The role of prostaglandins in the generation of these cells. *Endocrinology* **126**, 3153–3158.

67. Tashjian, A. H., Voelkel, E. F., Lazzaro, M., Singer, F. R., Roberts, A. B., Derynck, R., Winkler, M. E., and Levine, L. (1985). α and β human transforming growth factors stimulate prostaglandin production and bone resorption in cultured mouse calvaria. *Proc. Natl. Acad. Sci. U.S.A.* **82**, 4535–4538.

68. Dieudonne, S. C., Foo, P., Van Zoelen, E. J. J., and Burger, E. H. (1991). Inhibiting and stimulating effects of TGF-β1 on osteoclastic bone resorption in fetal mouse bone organ cultures. *J. Bone Miner. Res.* **6**, 479–487.

69. Pfeilschifter, J. P., Seyedin, S., and Mundy, G. R. (1988). Transforming growth factor beta inhibits bone resorption in fetal rat long bone cultures. *J. Clin. Invest.* **82**, 680–690.

70. Beaudreuil, J., Mbalaviele, G., Cohen-Solal, M., Morieux, C., De Vernejoul, M. C., and Orcel, P. (1995). Short-term local injections of transforming growth factor-β1 decrease ovariectomy-stimulated osteoclastic resorption *in vivo* in rats. *J. Bone Miner. Res.* **10**, 971–977.

71. Noda, M., and Camilliere, J. J. (1989). *In vivo* stimulation of bone formation by transforming growth factor-β. *Endocrinology* **124**, 2991–2994.

72. Mackie, E. J., and Trechsel, U. (1990). Stimulation of bone formation *in vivo* by transforming growth factor-β: Remodeling of woven bone and lack of inhibition by indomethacin. *Bone* **11**, 295–300.

73. Marcelli, C., Yates, A. J., and Mundy, G. R. (1990). *In vivo* effects of human recombinant transforming growth factor β on bone turnover in normal mice. *J. Bone Miner. Res.* **10**, 1087–1096.

74. Beck, L. S., DeGuzman, L., Lee, W. P., Xu, Y., McFatridge, L. A., Gillett, N. A., and Amento, E. P. (1991). TGF-β1 induces bone closure of skull defects. *J. Bone Miner. Res.* **6**, 1257–1265.

75. Rosen, D., Miller, S. C., Deleon, E., Thompson, A. Y., Bentz, H., Mathews, M., and Adams, S. (1994). Systemic administration of recombinant transforming growth factor beta 2 (rTGF-β2) stimulates parameters of cancellous bone formation in juvenile and adult rats. *Bone* **15**, 355–359.

76. Lucas, P. A. (1989). Chemotactic response of osteoblast-like cells to transforming growth factor beta. *Bone* **10**, 459–463.

77. Pfeilschifter, J., Wolf, O., Naumann, A., Minne, H. W., Mundy, G. R., and Ziegler, R. (1990). Chemotactic response of osteoblastlike cells to transforming growth factor β. *J. Bone Miner. Res.* **5**, 825–830.

78. Robey, P. G., Young, M. F., Flanders, K. C., Roche, N. S., Kondaiah, P., Reddi, A. H., Termine, J. D., Sporn, M. B., and Roberts, A. (1987). Osteoblasts synthesize and respond to transforming growth factor type-β (TGF-β) *in vitro. J. Cell Biol.* **105**, 457–463.

79. Uneno, S., Yamamoto, I., Yamamuro, T., Okumura, H., Ohta, S., Lee, K., Kasai, R., and Konishi, J. (1989). Transforming growth factor β modulates proliferation of osteoblastic cells: Relation to its effect on receptor levels for epidermal growth factor. *J. Bone Miner. Res.* **4**, 165–171.

80. Chen, T. L., Bates, R. L., Dudley, A., Hammonds, R. G., and Amento, E. P. (1991). Bone morphogenetic protein-2b stimulation of growth and osteogenic phenotypes in rat osteoblast-like cells: Comparison with TGF-β1. *J. Bone Miner. Res.* **6**, 1387–1393.

81. Pfeilschifter, J., D'Souza, S. M., and Mundy, G. R. (1987). Effects of transforming growth factor beta on osteoblastic osteosarcoma cells. *Endocrinology* **121**, 212–218.

82. Noda, M., and Rodan, G. (1986). Typeβ transforming growth factor inhibits proliferation and expression of alkaline phosphatase in murine osteoblast-like cells. *Biochem. Biophys. Res. Commun.* **140**, 56–65.

83. Centrella, M., McCarthy, T. L., and Canalis, E. (1987). Transforming growth factor β is a bidirectional regulator of replication and collagen synthesis in osteoblast-enriched cell cultures from fetal rat bone. *J. Biol. Chem.* **262**, 2869–2874.

84. Noda, M., and Rodan, G. A. (1987). Type β transforming growth factor (TGF-β) regulation of alkaline phosphatase expression and other phenotype-related mRNAs in osteoblastic rat osteosarcoma cells. *J. Cell. Physiol.* **133**, 426–437.

85. Harris, S. E., Bonewald, L. F., Harris, M. A., Sabatini, M., Dallas, S., Feng, J. Q., Ghosh-Choudhury, N., Wozney, J., and Mundy, G. R. (1994). Effects of transforming growth factor β on bone nodule formation and expression of bone morphogenetic protein 2, osteocalcin, osteopontin, alkaline phosphatase, and type I collagen mRNA in long-term cultures of fetal calvarial osteoblasts. *J. Bone Miner. Res.* **9**, 855–863.

86. Pirskanen, A., Jaaskelainen, T., and Maenpaa, P. H. (1994). Effects of transforming growth factor β1 on the regulation of osteocalcin synthesis in human MG-63 osteosarcoma cells. *J. Bone Miner. Res.* **9**, 1635–1642.

87. Antosz, M. E., Bellows, C. G., and Aubin, J. E. (1989). Effects of transforming growth factor β and epidermal growth factor on cell proliferation and the formation of bone nodules in isolated fetal rat calvaria cells. *J. Cell. Physiol.* **140**, 386–395.

88. Chen, T. L., and Bates, R. L. (1993). Recombinant human transforming growth factor beta 1 modulates bone remodeling in a mineralizing bone organ culture. *J. Bone Miner. Res.* **8**, 423–434.

89. Reddi, A. H. (1997). Bone morphogenetic proteins: An unconventional approach to isolation of first mammalian morphogens. *Cytokine Growth Factor Rev.* **8**, 11–20.

90. Wozney, J. M., Rosen, V., Celeste, A. J., Mitsock, L. M., Whitters, M. J., Kriz, R. W., Hewick, R. M., and Wang, E. A. (1988). Novel regulators of bone formation: molecular clones and activities. *Science* **242**, 1528–1534.

91. Padgett, R. W., St. Johnston, R. D., and Gelbart, W. M. (1987). A transcript from a *Drophila* pattern gene predicts a protein homologous to the transforming growth factor-β family. *Nature,* **325** 81–84.

92. Cunningham, N. S., Jenkins, N. A., Gilbert, D. J., Copeland, N. G., Reddi, A. H., and Lee, S.-J. (1995). Growth/differentiation factor-10: A new member of the transforming growth factor-β superfamily related to bone morphogenetic protein-3. *Growth Factors* **12**, 99–109.

93. Celeste, A. J., Iannazzi, J. A., Taylor, R. C., Hewick, R. M., Rosen, V., Wang, E. A., and Wozney, J. M. (1990). Identification of transforming growth factor-β family members present in bone. *Proc. Natl. Acad. Sci. U.S.A.* **87**, 9843–9847.

94. Ozkaynak, E., Rueger, D. C., Drier, E. A., Corbett, C., Ridge, R. J., Sampath, T. K., and Oppermann, H. (1990). OP-1 cDNA encodes an osteogenic protein in the TGF-β family. *EMBO J.* **9**, 2085–2093.

95. Ozkaynak, E., Schnegelsberg, P. N. J., Jin, D. F., Clifford, G. M., Warren, F. D., Drier, E. A., and Oppermann, H. (1992). Osteogenic protein-2: A new member of the TGF-β superfamily expressed early in embryogenesis. *J. Biol. Chem.* **267**, 25220–25227.

96. Chang, S. C., Hoang, B., Thomas, J. T., Vukicevic, S., Luyten, F. P., Ryba, N. J. P., Kozak, C. A., Reddi, A. H., and Moos, M. (1994). Cartilage-derived morphogenetic proteins. New members of the trans-

forming growth factor-β superfamily predominantly expressed in long bones during embryonic development. *J. Biol. Chem.* **269**, 28227–28234.

97. Sampath, T. K., Coughlin, J. E., Whetstone, R. M., Banach, D., Corbett, C., Ridge, R. J., Ozkaynak, E., Oppermann, H., and Rueger, D. C. (1990). Bovine osteogenic protein is composed of dimers of OP-1 and BMP-2A, two members of the transforming growth factor-β superfamily. *J. Biol. Chem.* **265**, 13198–13250.

98. ten Dijke, P., Yamashita, H., Sampath, T. K., Reddi, A. H., Estevez, M., Riddle, D. L., Ichijo, H., Heldin, C.-H., and Mijazono, K. (1994). Identification of type I receptors for osteogenic protein-1 and bone morphogenetic protein-4. *J. Biol. Chem.* **269**, 16985–16988.

99. Koenig, B. B., Cook, J. S., Wolsing, D. H., Ting, J., Tiesman, J. P., Correa, P. E., Olson, C. A., Pecquet, A. L., Ventura, F., Grant, R. A., Chen, G.-X., Wrana, J. L., Massague, J., and Rosenbaum, J.S. (1994). Characterization and cloning of a receptor for BMP-2 and BMP-4 from NIH 3T3 cells. *Mol. Cell. Biol.* **14**, 5961–5974.

100. Rosenzweig, B. L., Imamura, T., Okadome, T., Cox, G. N., Yamashita, H., ten Dijke, P., Heldin, C.-H., and Miyazono, K. (1995). Cloning and characterization of a human type II receptor for bone morphogenetic proteins. *Proc. Natl. Acad, Sci. U.S.A.* **92**, 7632–7636.

101. Liu, F., Ventura, F., Doody, J., and Massague, J. (1995). Human type II receptor for bone morphogenetic proteins (BMPs): Extension of the two-kinase receptor model to the BMPs. *Mol. Cell. Biol.* **15**, 3479–3486.

102. Yamashita, H., ten Dijke, P., Huylebroeck, D., Sampath, T. K., Andries, M., Smith, J. C., Heldin, C.-H., and Miyazono, K. (1995). Osteogenic protein-1 binds to activin type II receptors and induces certain activin-like effects. *J. Cell Biol.* **130**, 217–226.

103. Urist, M. R. (1965). Bone: Formation by autoinduction. *Science* **150**, 893–899.

104. Sakou, T. (1998). Bone morphogenetic proteins: From basic studies to clinical approaches. *Bone* **22**, 591–603.

105. Wang, E. A., Rosen, V., D'Alessandro, J. S., Bauduy, M., Cordes, P., Harada, T., Israel, D. I., Hewick, R. M., Kerns, K. M., LaPan, P., Luxenberg, D. P., McQuaid, D., Moutsatsos, I. K., Nove, J., and Wozney, J. M. (1990). Recombinant human bone morphogenetic protein induces bone formation. *Proc. Natl. Acad. Sci. U.S.A.* **87**, 220–2224.

106. D'Alessandro, J. S., Cox, K. A., Israil, D. I., LaPan, P., Moutsatsos, I. K., Nove, J., Rosen, V., Ryan, M. C., Wozney, J. M., and Wang, E. A. (1991). Purification, characterization and activities of recombinant bone morphogenetic protein-5. *J. Bone Miner. Res.* **6**, S153.

107. Sampath, T. K., Maniacal, J. C., Hauschka, P. V., Jones, W. K., Sasak, H., Tucker, R. F., White, K. H., Coughlin, J. E., Tucker, M. M., Pang, R. H. L., Corbett, C., Ozkaynak, E., Oppermann, H., and Rueger, D. C. (1992). Recombinant human osteogenic protein-1 (hOP-1) induces new bone formation *in vivo* with a specific activity comparable with natural bovine osteogenic protein and stimulates osteoblast proliferation and differentiation in vitro. *J. Biol. Chem.* **267**, 20352–20362.

108. Aono, A., Hazama, M., Notoya, K., Taketomi, S., Yamasaki, H., Tsukuda, R., Sasaki, S., and Fujisawa, Y. (1995). Potent ectopic bone-inducing activity of bone morphogenetic protein -4/7 heterodimer. *Biochem. Biophys. Res. Commun.* **210**, 670–677.

109. Cunningham, N. S., Paralkar, V., and Reddi, A. H. (1992). Osteogenin and recombinant bone morphogenetic protein 2B are chemotactic for human monocytes and stimulated transforming growth factor β1 mRNA expression. *Proc. Natl. Acad. Sci. U.S.A.* **89**, 11740–11744.

110. Lind, M., Eriksen, E. F., and Bunger, C. (1996). Bone morphogenetic protein-2 but not bone morphogenetic protein-4 and -6 stimulates chemotactic migration of human osteoblasts, human marrow osteoblasts, and U2-OS cells. *Bone* **18**, 53–57.

111. Wang, E. A., Israel, D. I., Kelly, S., and Luxemberg, D. P. (1993). Bone morphogenetic protein-2 causes commitment and differentiation in C3H10T1/2 and 3T3 cells. *Growth Factors* **9**, 57–71.

112. Katagiri, T., Yamaguchi, A., Komaki, M., Abe, E., Takahashi, N., Ikeda, T., Rosen, V., Wozney, J. M., Fujisawa-Sehara, A., and Suda, T. (1994). Bone morphogenetic protein-2 converts the differentiation pathway of C2C12 myoblasts into the osteoblast lineage. *J. Cell Biol.* **127**, 1755–1766.

113. Gitelman, S. E., Kirk, M., Ye, J.-Q., Filvaroff, E. H., Kahn, A. J., and Derynck, R. (1995). Vgr-1/BMP-6 induces osteoblastic differentiation of pluripotential mesenchymal cells. *Cell Growth Differ.* **6**, 827–836.

114. Takuwa, Y., Ohse, C., Wang, E. A., Wozney, J. M., and Yamashita, K. (1991). Bone morphogenetic protein-2 stimulates alkaline phosphatase activity and collagen synthesis in cultured osteoblastic cells, MC3T3-E1. *Biochem. Biophys. Res. Commun.* **174**, 96–101.

115. Maliakal, J. C., Asahina, I., Hauschka, P. V., and Sampath, T. K. (1994). Osteogenic protein-1 (BMP-7) inhibits cell proliferation and stimulates the expression of markers characteristic of osteoblast phenotype in rat osteosarcoma (17/2.8) cells. *Growth Factors* **11**, 227–234.

116. Hughes, F. J., Collyer, J., Stanfield, M., and Goodman, S. (1995). The effect of bone morphogenetic protein-2, -4 and -6 on differentiation of rat osteoblast cells *in vitro*. *Endocrinology* **136**, 2671–2677.

117. Chen, T. L., Bates, R. L., Dudley, A., Hammonds, R., and Amento, E. P. (1991). Bone morphogenetic protein-2b stimulation of growth and osteogenic phenotypes in rat osteoblast-like cells: Comparison with TGF-β1. *J. Bone Miner. Res.* **6**, 1387–1393.

118. Zhou, H., Hammonds, R., Findlay, D. M., Martin, T. J., and Ng, K. W. (1993). Differential effects of transforming growth factor-beta 1 and bone morphogenetic protein 4 on gene expression and differentiated function of preosteoblasts. *J. Cell. Physiol.* **155**, 112–119.

119. Canalis, E., and Gabbitas, B. (1994). Bone morphogenetic protein 2 increases insulin-like growth factor I and II transcripts and polypeptide levels in bone cell cultures. *J. Bone Miner. Res.* **9**, 1999–2005.

120. Gabbitas, B., and Canalis, E. (1995). Bone morphogenetic protein-2 inhibits the synthesis of insulin-like growth factor-binding protein-5 in bone cell cultures. *Endocrinology* **136**, 2397–2403.

121. Kingsley, D. M., Bland, A. E., Grubber, J. M., Marker, P. C., Russell, L. B., Copeland, N. G., and Jenkins, N. A. (1992). The mouse short ear skeletal morphogenesis locus is associated with defects in a bone morphogenetic member of the TGF beta superfamily. *Cell* **71**, 339–410.

122. Storm, E. E., Huynh, T. V., Copeland, N. G., Jenkins, N. A., Kingsely, D. M., and Lee, S.-J. (1994). Limb alterations in *brachypodism* mice due to mutations in a new member of the TGFβ-superfamily. *Nature* **368**, 639–643.

123. Thomas, J. T., Lin, K., Nandedkar, M., Camargo, M., Cervenka, J., and Luyten, F. P. (1996). A human chondrodysplasia due to a mutation in a TGF-β superfamily member. *Nat. Genet.* **12**, 315–317.

124. Kaplan, F. S., Tabas, J. A., and Zasloff, M. A. (1990). Fibrodysplasia ossificans progressiva: A clue from the fly? *Calcif. Tissue Int.* **46**, 117–125.

125. Armelin, H. A. (1973). Pituitary extracts and steroid hormones in the control of 3T3 growth. *Proc. Natl. Acad. Sci. U.S.A.* **70**, 2702–2706.

126. Gospodarowicz, D. (1974). Localization of a fibroblast growth factor and its effect alone and with hydrocortisone on 3T3 cell growth. *Nature* **326**, 123–127.

127. Migantti, P., Morimoto, T., and Rifkin, D. G. (1992). Basic fibroblast growth factor, a protein devoid of secretory signal sequence, is released by cells via a pathway independent of the endoplasmic reticulum-golgi complex. *J. Cell. Physiol.* **151**, 81–93.

128. Green, P. J., Walsh, F. S., and Doherty, P. (1996). Promiscuity of fibroblast growth factor receptors. *BioEssays* **18**, 639–646.

129. Roghani, M., Mansukhani, A., Dell'Era, P., Bellosta, P., Basilico, C., Rifkin, D. B., and Moscatelli, D. (1994). Heparin increases the affinity of bFGF for its receptor, but is not required for binding. *J. Biol. Chem.* **269**, 3976–3984.

130. Ornitz, D. M., and Leder, P. (1992). Ligand specificity and heparin dependence of fibroblast growth factor receptors 1 and 3. *J. Biol. Chem.* **267**, 16305–16311.

131. Globus, R. K., Plouet, J., and Gospodarowicz, D. (1989). Cultured bovine bone cells synthesise basic fibroblast growth factor and store it in their extracellular matrix. *Endocrinology* **124**, 1539–1547.

132. Hurley, M. J., Abreu, C., Gronowicz, G., Kawaguchi, H., and Lorenzo, J. (1994). Expression and regulation of basic fibroblast growth factor mRNA levels in mouse osteoblastic MC3T3-E1 cells. *J. Biol. Chem.* **268**, 9392–9396.

133. Hauschka, P. V., Mavrakos, A. E., Iafrati, M. D., Doleman, S. E., and Klagsbrun, M. (1986). Growth factors in bone matrix. Isolation of multiple types by affinity chromatography on heparin-sepharose. *J. Biol. Chem.* **261**, 12665–12674.

134. Shen, V., Kohler, G., Huang, J., Huang, S. S., and Peck, W. A. (1989). An acidic fibroblast growth factor stimulates DNA synthesis, inhbits collagen and alkaline phosphatase synthesis and induces resorption in bone. *Bone Miner.* **7**, 407–408.

135. Simmons, H. A., and Raisz, L. G. (1991). Effects of acid and basic fibroblast growth factor and heparin on resorption of cultured fetal rat long bones. *J. Bone Miner. Res.* **6**, 1301–1305.

136. Hurley, M. M., Lee, S. K., Raisz, L. G., Bernecker, P., and Lorenzo, J. (1998). Basic fibroblast growth factor induces osteoclast formation in murine bone marrow cultures. *Bone* **22**, 309–316.

137. Globus, R. K., Patterson-Buckendahl, P., and Gospodarowicz, D. (1988). Regulation of bovine bone cell proliferation by fibroblast growth factor and transforming growth factor β. *Endocrinology* **123**, 98–105.

138. Rodan, S. B., Wesolowski, G., Thomas, K. A., Yoon, K., and Rodan, G. A. (1989). Effects of acidic and basic fibroblast growth factors on osteoblastic cells. *Connect. Tissue Res.* **20**, 283–288.

139. Canalis, E., Centrella, M., and McCarthy, T. (1988). Effects of basic fibroblast growth factor on bone formation *in vitro*. *J. Clin. Invest.* **81**, 1572–1577.

140. Pitaru, S., Kotev-Emeth, S., Noff, D., Kaffuler, S., and Savion, N. (1993). Effect of basic fibroblast growth factor on the growth and differentiation of adult bone marrow cells: Enhanced development of mineralized bone-like tissue in culture. *J. Bone Miner. Res.* **8**, 919–929.

141. Martin, I., Muraglia, A., Campanile, G., Cancedda, R., and Quarto, R. (1997). Fibroblast growth factor-2 supports *ex vivo* expansion and maintenance of osteogenic precursors from human bone marrow. *Endocrinology* **138**, 4456–4462.

142. Rodan, S. B., Wesolowski, G., Yoon, K., and Rodan, G. A. (1989). Opposing effects of fibroblast growth factor and pertussis toxin on alkaline phosphatase, osteopontin, osteocalcin, and type I collagen mRNA levels in ROS 17/2.8 cells. *J. Biol. Chem.* **264**, 19934–19941.

143. Hurley, M. M., Kessler, M., Gronowicz, G., and Raisz, L. G. (1992). The interaction of heparin and basic fibroblast growth factor on collagen synthesis in 21-day fetal rat calvariae. *Endocrinology* **130**, 2675–2682.

144. Hurley, M. M., Abreu, C., Harrison, J. R., Lichtler, A. C., Raisz, L. G., and Kream, B. E. (1993). Basic fibroblast growth factor inhibits type I collagen gene expression in osteoblastic MC3T3-E1 cells. *J. Biol. Chem.* **268**, 5588–5593.

145. Noff, D., Pitaru, S., and Savion, N. (1989). Basic fibroblast growth factor enhances the capacity of bone marrow cells to form bone-like nodules in vitro. *FEBS Lett.* **250**, 619–621.

146. Mayahara, H., Ito, T., Nagai, H., Miyajima, H., Tsukuda, R., Taketomi, S., Mizoguchi, J., and Kato, K. (1993). *In vivo* stimulation of endosteal bone formation by basic fibroblast growth factor in rats. *Growth Factors* **9**, 73–80.

147. Nakamura, T., Hanada, K., Tamura, M., Shibanushi, T., Nigi, H., Tagawa, M., Fukomoto, S., and Matsumoto, T. (1995). Stimulation of endosteal bone formation by systemic injections of recombinant basic fibroblast growth factor in rats. *Endocrinology* **136**, 1276–1284.

148. Nagai, H., Tsukuda, T., and Mayahara, H. (1995). Effect of basic fibroblast growth factor (bFGF) on bone formation in growing rats. *Bone* **16**, 367–373.

149. Canalis, E., Pash, J., Gabbitas, B., Rydziel., S., and Varghese, S. (1993). Growth factors regulate the synthesis of insulin-like growth factor-I in bone cell cultures. *Endocrinology* **133**, 33–88.

150. Hurley, M. J., Abreu, C., and Hakeda, Y. (1995). Basic fibroblast growth factor regulates IGF-I binding proteins in the clonal osteoblastic cell line MC3T3-E1. *J. Bone Miner. Res.* **10**, 222–230.

151. Noda, M., and Vogel, R. (1989). Fibroblast-growth factor enhances type β1 transforming growth factor gene expression in osteoblast-like cells. *J. Cell Biol.* **109**, 2529–2535.

152. Burke, D., Wilkes, D., Blundell, T. L., and Malcolm, S. (1998). *Fibroblast* growth factor receptors: lessons from the genes. *Trends Biochem. Sci.* **23**, 59–62.

153. Muenke, M., and Schell, U. (1995). Fibroblast-growth factor receptor mutations in human skeletal disorders. *Trends Genet.* **11**, 308–313.

154. Wilke, A. O. M. Slaney, S. F., Oldridge, M., Poole, M. D., Ashworth, G. J., Hockley, A. D., Hayward, R. D., David, D. J., Pulleyn, L. J., Rutland, P., Malcolm, S., Winter, R. M., and Reardon, W. (1995). Apert syndrome results from localized mutations of FGFR2 and is allelic with Crouzon syndrome. *Nat. Genet.* **9**,165–172.

155. Muenke, M., Schell, U., Hehr, A., Robin, N. H., Losken, H. W., Schinzel, A., Pulleyn, L. J., Rutland, P., Reardon, W., Malcolm, S., and Winter, R. M. (1994). A common mutation in the fibroblast growth factor receptor 1 gene in Pfeiffer syndrome. *Nat. Genet.* **8**, 269–274.

156. Rutland, P., Pulleyn, L. J., Reardon, W., Baraitser, M., Hayward, R., Jones, B., Malcolm, S., Winter, R. M., Oldridge, M., Slaney, S. F., Poole, M. D., and Wilkie, A. O. M. (1994). Identical mutations in the FGFR2 gene cause both Pfeiffer and Crouzon syndrome phenotypes. *Nat. Genet.* **9**, 173–176.

157. Jabs, E. W. Li, X., Scott, A. F., Meyers, G., Chen, W., Eccles, M., Mao, J.-I., Charnas, L. R., Jackson, C. E., and Jaye, M. (1994). Jackson-Weiss and Crouzon syndromes are allelic with mutations in fibroblast growth factor receptor 2. *Nat. Genet.* **8**, 275–279.

158. Readon, W., Winter, R. M., Rutland, P., Pulleyn, L. J., Jones, B. M., and Malcolm, S. (1994). Mutations in the fibroblast growth factor receptor 2 gene cause Crouzon syndrome. *Nat. Genet.* **8**, 98–103.

159. Rousseau, F., Bonaventure, J., Legeai-Mallet, L., Pelet, A., Rozet, J.-M., Maroteauz, P., Le Merrer, M., and Munnich, A. (1994). Mutations in the gene encoding fibroblast growth factor receptor-3 in achondroplasia. *Nature* **371**, 252–254.

160. Bellus, G. A., McIntosh, I., Smith, E. A., Aylsworth, A. S., Kaitila, I., Horton, W. A., Greenshaw, G. A., Hecht, J. T., and Francomano, C. A. (1995). A recurrent mutation in the tyrosine kinase domain of fibroblast growth factor receptor 3 causes hypochondroplasia. *Nat. Genet.* **10**, 357–359.

161. Tavormina, P. L., Shiang, R., Thompson, L. M., Zhu, Y.-Z., Wilkin, D. J., Lachman, R. S., Wilcox, W. R., Rimoin, D. L., Cohn, D. H., and Wasmuth, J. J. (1995). Thanatophoric dysplasia (types I and II) caused by distinct mutations in fibroblast growth factor receptor 3. *Nat. Genet.* **9**, 321–328.

162. Heldin, C-H., Johnsson, A., Wennergren, S., Wernstedt, C., Betsholtz, C., and Westermark, B. (1986). A human osteosarcoma cell line secretes a growth factor structurally related to a homodimer of PDGF A-chains. *Nature* **319**, 511–514.

163. Betsholz, C., Johnson, A., Heldin, C.-H., Westermark, B., Lind, P., Urdea, M. S., Eddy, R., Shows, T. B., Pholpott, K., Mellor, A. L., Knott, T. J., and Scott, J. (1986). cDNA sequence and chromosomal localization of human platelet-derived growth factor A-chain and its expression in tumour lines. *Nature* **320**, 695–699.

164. Tong, B. D., Auer, D. E., Jaye, M., Kaplow, J. M., Ricca, G., McConathy, E., Dronhan, W., and Deuel, T. F. (1987). cDNA clones reveal differences between human glial and endothelial cell platelet-derived growth factor A-chains. *Nature* **328**, 619–621.

165. Collins, T., Bonthron, D. T., and Orkin, S. H. (1987). Alternative RNA splicing affects function of encoded platelet-derived growth factor A chain. *Nature* **328**, 621–624.

166. Seifert, R. A., Hart, C. E., Phillips, P. E., Forstrom, J. W., Ross, R., Murray, M. J., and Bowen-Pope, D. F. (1989). Two distinct subunits associate to create isoform-specific platelet-derived growth factor receptors. *J. Biol. Chem.* **264**, 8771–8778.

167. Graves, D. T., Owen, A. J., Barth, R. K., Tempst, P., Winoto, A., Fors, L., Hood, L. E., and Antoniades, H. N. (1984). Detection of *c-sis* transcripts and synthesis of PDGF-like proteins by human osteosarcoma cells. *Science* **226**, 972–974.

168. Graves, D. T., Valentin-Opran, A., Delgado, R., Valente, A. J., Mundy, G., and Piche, J. (1989). The potential role of platelet-derived growth factor as an autocrine or paracrine factor for human bone cells. *Connect. Tissue Res.* **23**, 209–218.

169. Rydziel, S., Shaikh, S., and Canalis, E. (1994). Platelet-derived growth factor-AA and -BB (PDGF-AA and -BB) enhance the synthesis of PDGF-AA in bone cell cultures. *Endocrinology* **134**, 2541–2546

170. Horner, A., Bord, S., Kemp, P., Grainger, D., and Compston, J. E. (1996). Distribution of platelet-derived growth factor (PDGF) A chain mRNA, protein, and PDGF-a receptor in rapidly forming bone. *Bone* **19**, 353–362.

171. Rydziel, S., and Canalis, E. (1996). Expression and growth factor regulation of platelet-derived growth factor B transcripts in primary osteoblast cell cultures. *Endocrinology* **137**, 4115–4119.

172. Centrella, M., McCarthy, T. L., and Canalis, E. (1989). Platelet derived growth factor enhances deoxyribonucleic acid and collagen synthesis in osteoblast-enriched cultures from fetal rat parietal bone. *Endocrinology* **125**, 13–19.

173. Centrella, M., McCarthy, T. L., Kusmik, W. F., and Canalis, E. (1991). Relative binding and biochemical effects of heterodimeric and *homodimeric* isoforms of platelet-derived growth factor in osteoblast-enriched cultures from rat fetal bone. *J. Cell. Physiol.* **147**, 420–426.

174. Gilardetti, R. S., Chaibi, M. S., Stroumza, C. J., Williams S. R., Antoniades, H. N., Carnes, D. C., and Graves, D. T. (1991). High affinity binding of PDGF-AA and PDGF-BB to normal human osteoblastic cells and modulation by interleukin-1. *Am. J. Physiol.* **261**, C980–C985.

175. Pfeilschifter, J., Krempien, R., Naumann, A., Gronwald, R. G. K., Hoppe, J., and Ziegler, R. (1992). Differential effects of platelet-derived growth factor isoforms on plasminogen activator activity in fetal rat osteoblasts due to isoform-specific receptor functions. *Endocrinology* **130**, 2059–2066.

176. Kose, K. N., Xie, J. F., Carnes, D. L. and Graves, D. T. (1996). Proinflammatory cytokines down-regulate platelet-derived growth-factor-alpha receptor gene expresssion in human osteoblastic cells. *J. Cell. Physiol.* **166**, 188–197.

177. Yu, X. H., Hsieh, S. C., Bao, W., and Graves, D. T. (1997). Temporal expression of PDGF receptors and PDGF regulatory effects on osteoblastic mineralizing cultures. *Am. J. Physiol.* **41**, C1709–C1716.

178. Hsieh, S. C., and Graves, D. T. (1998). Pulse application of platelet-derived growth factor enhances formation of a mineralizing matrix while continuous application is inhibitory. *J. Cell. Biochem.* **69**, 169–180.

179. Nash, T. J., Howlett, C. R., Martin, C., Steele, J., Johnson, K. A., and Hicklin, D. J. (1994). Effect of platelet-derived growth factor in tibial osteotomies in rabbits. *Bone* **15**, 203–208.

180. Mitlak, B. H., Finkelman, R. D., Hill, E. L., Li, J., Martin, B., Smith, T., D'Andrea, M., Antoniades, H. N., and Lynch, S. E. (1996). The effect of systemically administered PDGF-BB on the rodent skeleton. *J. Bone Miner. Res.* **11**, 238–247.

181. Tashjian, A., Hohmann, E., Antoniades, H., and Levine, L. (1982). Platelet-derived growth factor stimulates bone resorption via a prostaglandin-mediated mechanism. *Endocrinology* **111**, 118–124.

182. Cochran, D. L., Rouse, C. A., Lynch, S. E., and Graves, D. T. (1993). Effects of platelet-derived growth factor isoforms on calcium release from neonatal mouse calvariae. *Bone* **14**, 53–58.

183. Franchimont, N., and Canalis, E. (1995). Platelet-derived growth factor stimulates the synthsis of interleukin-6 in cells of the osteoblast lineage. *Endocrinology* **136**, 5469–5474.

184. Varghese, S., Delany, A. M., Liang, L., Gabbitas, B., Jeffrey, J. J., and Canalis, E. (1996). Transcriptional and posttranslational regulation of interstitial collagenase by platelet-derived growth factor BB in bone cell cultures. *Endocrinology* **137**, 431–437.

185. Ng, K. W., Partridge, N. C., Niall, H., and Martin, T. J. (1983). Epidermal growth factor receptors in clonal lines of a rat osteogenic sarcoma and in osteoblast-rich rat bone cells. *Calcif. Tissue Int.* **35**, 298–303.

186. Shupnik, M. A., and Tashjian, A. H. (1982). Epidermal growth factor and phorbol ester actions on human osteosarcoma cells. *J. Biol. Chem.* **257**, 12161–12164.

187. Ng, K. W., Partridge, N. C., Niall, H., and Martin, T. J. (1983). Stimulation of DNA synthesis by epidermal growth factor in osteoblast-like cells. *Calcif. Tissue Int.* **35**, 624–628.

188. Yokota, K., Kusaka, M., Ohshima, T., Yamamoto, S., Kurihara, N., Yoshino, T., and Kumagawa, M. (1986). Stimulation of prostaglandin E_2 synthesis in cloned osteoblastic cells of mouse (MC3T3-E1) by epidermal growth factor. *J. Biol. Chem.* **261**, 15410–15415.

189. Harrison, J. R., Lorenzo, J. A., Kawaguchi, H., Raisz, L. G., and Pilbeam, C. (1994). Stimulation of prostaglandin E_2 production by interleukin-1α and transforming growth factor α in osteoblastic MC3T3-E1 cell. *J. Bone Miner. Res.* **9**, 817–823.

190. Raisz, L. G., Simmons, H. A., Sandberg, A. L., and Canalis, E. (1980). Direct stimulation of bone resorption by epidermal growth factor. *Endocrinology* **107**, 207–212.

191. Ibbotson, K. J., Harrod, J., Gowen, M., D'Souza, S., Smith, D. D., Winkler, M. E., Derynck, R., and Mundy, G. R. (1985). Stimulation of bone resorption *in vitro* by synthetic transforming growth factor α. *Science* **228**, 1007–1009.

192. Stern, P. H., Krieger, N. S., Nissenson, R. A., Williams R. D., Winkler, M. E., Derynck, R., and Strewler, G. J. (1985). Human transforming growth factor alpha stimulates bone resorption *in vitro*. *J. Clin. Invest.* **76**, 2016–2020.

193. Yates, A. J., Boyce, B. F., Favarato, G., Aufdemorte, T. B., Marcelli, C., Kester, M. B., Walker, R., Langton, B. C., Bonewald, L. F., and Mundy, G. R. (1992). Expression of human transforming growth factor α by chinese hamster ovarian tumors in nude mice causes hypercalcemia and increased osteoclastic bone resorption. *J. Bone Miner. Res.* **7**, 847–853.

194. Harada, S-I., Nagy, J. A., Sullivan, K. A., Thomas, K. A., Endo, N., Rodan, G. A., and Rodan, S. B. (1994). Induction of vascular endothelial growth factor by prostalandin E_2 and E_1 in osteoblasts. *J. Clin. Invest.* **93**, 2490–2496.

195. Wang, D. S., Yamazaki, K., Nohtomi, K., Shizume, K., Ohsumi, K., Shibuya, M., Demura, H., and Sato, K. (1996). Increase of vascular endothelial growth factor mRNA expression by 1,25-dihydroxyvitamin D_3 in human osteoblast-like cells. *J. Bone Miner. Res.* **11**, 472–479.

196. Goad, D. L., Rubin, J., Wang, H., Tashjian, A. H., and Patterson, C. (1996). Enhanced expression of vascular endothelial growth factor in human SaOS-2 osteoblast-like cells and murine osteoblasts induced by insulin-like growth factor I. *Endocrinology* **137**, 2262–2268.

197. Wang, D. S., Miura, M., Demura, H., and Sato, K. (1997). Anabolic effects of 1,25-dihyroxyvitamin D_3 on osteoblasts are enhanced by vascular endothelial growth factor produced by osteoblasts and by growth factors produced by endothelial cells. *Endocrinology* **138**, 2953–2962.

CHAPTER 7

Cytokines and Prostaglandins

JOSEPH A. LORENZO AND LAWRENCE G. RAISZ
The University of Connecticut Health Center, Farmington, Connecticut 06030

I. ABSTRACT

The role of prostaglandins and cytokines in bone and cartilage metabolism is evolving. This chapter summarizes recent discoveries in this field. Special emphasis is placed on the role of prostaglandins in cartilage metabolism and on the role of interleukin-1, tumor necrosis factor, and interleukin-6 in the development of osteoporosis. In addition, the role of leukotrienes in bone metabolism is discussed, as well as the potential role of other cytokines in bone and cartilage function.

II. THE ROLE OF PROSTAGLANDINS AND LEUKOTRIENES IN BONE AND CARTILAGE METABOLISM

A. Introduction

Prostaglandins act as local regulators of skeletal metabolism and have been shown to play key roles in both physiologic regulation and the pathologic response to inflammation. Studies of prostaglandins and bone have been the subject of several reviews which can provide additional references [1, 2]. Hence, this chapter will present only additional key references from recent studies. However, the role of prostaglandins in cartilage metabolism has not been reviewed recently and this chapter will provide a more extensive examination of this topic.

B. Regulation of Prostaglandin Synthesis

Cells of the osteoblastic lineage have been shown to produce abundant prostaglandins, and this production is highly regulated by cytokines, growth factors, and mechanical forces [1–6]. Chondrocytes can also produce prostaglandins, and regulation by hormones, growth factors, cytokines, and mechanical forces has been demonstrated [7–13]. Studies of endogenous prostaglandin production in intact animals or organ cultures are complicated by the fact that cells of hematopoietic lineage, particularly macrophages [14], as well as the adjacent muscle and vessels, are also abundant producers of prostanoids. In inflammation, marrow cells, as well as synovial cells, may contribute prostaglandins, which act on bone and cartilage. The major products of all of these cell types are prostaglandins of the E and F series (PGE_2 and $PGF_{2\alpha}$), and prostacyclin (PGI_2) may also be an important product, particularly of osteocytes. Production of

97

leukotrienes also occurs, but has been much less well studied [15].

Regulation of eicosanoid production is largely through changes in the inducible enzyme prostaglandin G/H synthase-2 or cyclooxygenase-2 (COX-2) [16–18]. Regulation at the level of arachidonate release by phospholipase may be important in inflammatory responses and also for initial responses in which release of arachidonate results in prostaglandin production from the constitutive prostaglandin G/H synthase-1 or cyclooxygenase-1 (COX-1).

C. Osteoblasts

Cells of the osteoblastic lineage are probably the major source of endogenous prostaglandins in the skeleton and certainly have been the most extensively studied. Systemic hormones, cytokines, and growth factors all regulate prostaglandin production. Moreover, prostaglandins themselves can increase their own production, thus providing an amplification system for small or transient stimuli [19]. While most of the stimulators of bone resorption increase prostaglandin production, this effect appears to have variable importance in the resorptive response. For example, 1,25-dihydroxyvitamin D has a relatively small effect on prostaglandin production in organ cultures, and its resorptive response appears to be quite independent of PGE_2. On the other hand, in mixed cell cultures, which produce osteoclasts, some inhibition of production can be observed with nonsteroidal anti-inflammatory drugs (NSAIDs) that block prostaglandin synthesis [20]. The importance of prostaglandins in osteoclastogenesis may not be restricted to the cells of the osteoblastic lineage since osteoclast precursors can also produce prostaglandin. It is likely that the level of endogenous prostaglandin production in bone from both cell lineages determines the early replication and differentiation of osteoclast precursors.

Stimulation of prostaglandin production by PTH, cytokines such as IL-1 and TNF, and growth factors such as FGF and TGFβ, as well as prostaglandins themselves, all appear to be associated with induction of COX-2, largely by direct transcriptional effects. There are fewer compounds which inhibit endogenous prostaglandin synthesis. Glucocorticoids, retinoic acid, and interleukins 4 and 13 have all been shown to have inhibitory effects on induction of COX-2 by various agonists [6].

The stimulation of bone formation by impact loading appears to be prostaglandin dependent. Impact loading has been shown to increase prostaglandin production in human bone *in vivo* [21]. This may be mediated by fluid shear stress, which can induce COX-2 in cell culture [3].

Reports of the effects of nitric oxide on prostaglandin production in bone are conflicting. Both stimulation and inhibition of the response to cytokines, lipopolysaccharide, and fluid shear stress have been reported, while in some studies no interaction was found [22–25]. In osteoarthritic cartilage a spontaneous increase in COX-2 expression was observed, which was inhibited by nitric oxide [26].

D. Chondrocytes

The fact that prostaglandins play an important role in inflammatory arthritis has led to cell culture studies that examine the production of prostaglandins by chondrocytes. Interpretation of *in vivo* studies, however, is complicated by the fact that in inflammation, the adjacent synovial cells are also likely to produce prostaglandins. Increased prostaglandin production in isolated chondrocyte cultures has been demonstrated with IL-1 and TNFα [7, 17]. Moreover, these two cytokines may by synergistic in their ability to stimulate prostaglandin production by increasing COX-2 levels. However, the effects of IL-1 on cartilage cells may be independent from, or even opposed by, prostaglandin production. For example, the stimulation of matrix metalloproteinase-9 production by IL-1 is blocked by prostaglandins [27]. Growth factors may also influence prostaglandin synthesis in cartilage cells. In contrast to its effects on osteoblasts, TGFβ inhibits the IL-1 effect on prostaglandin production in isolated chondrocytes [11]. On the other hand, FGF produces a synergistic increase in PG production with IL-1 [10]. Fluid shear stress has not been extensively studied but does appear to increase prostaglandin synthesis in cartilage cells and in osteoblasts [13]. 1,25-dihydroxyvitamin D stimulates prostaglandin production in growth cartilage with little effect in the resting zone, whereas 24,25-dihydroxyvitamin D was found to inhibit prostaglandin production in the resting zone with little effect on growth zone cells [12, 28].

E. Effects of Prostaglandin on Bone

Although the effects of PGs on bone are complex, the most important effects appear to be stimulation of bone resorption and formation. This is not simply due to an increase in coupled bone turnover. Rather, it involves stimulation at multiple sites. Thus, exogenous prostaglandins in animals cause an increase in periosteal as well as endosteal bone formation and a stimulation of endocortical and intracortical resorption [29]. These stimulatory processes appear to involve both the replication and the differentiation of precursor cells [30]. However, there may be different pathways involved. Studies in cell culture suggest that PGs have a mitogenic effect on osteoblast precursors as well as an effect to increase their differentiation [31]. In addition, in some systems PGE_2 inhibits replication. The anabolic effect can be observed in the presence of glucocorticoids and may even be enhanced by glucocorticoid treatment, which has been shown to increase the cyclic AMP response to PGs. The stimulation of bone formation and resorption can be mimicked by cyclic AMP analogs and appears to be largely mediated through protein kinase A [30]. There is an inhibitory effect of PGs on osteoblast collagen synthesis, which appears to be mediated by protein kinase C [32]. The receptors for these processes have not been fully identified. The EP_2 or EP_4 receptors have been implicated in the stimulatory effects, while an FP receptor has been implicated in the inhibition of collagen synthesis [33, 34]. Mitogenic effects may also be mediated through an FP receptor [35]. The anabolic effect of prostaglandins may depend, at least in part, on their ability to stimulate growth factor production in bone. Both IGF and IGF binding protein 5 (IGF-BP5) can be stimulated by prostaglandins [36, 37]. Prostaglandins can also increase FGF-2 mRNA levels, and this could be the basis for an additional amplification system since FGF can stimulate PG production [38].

F. Effects of Prostaglandin on Cartilage

Reports of PG effects on cartilage are inconsistent, possibly because different cell types or stages of differentiation, as well as different species and culture conditions, respond differently. Prostaglandins are essential mediators in the induction of cartilage cells during development [39]. This effect on cartilage differentiation and chondrogenesis is mediated by cyclic AMP. Prostaglandins have been shown to increase thymidine incorporation and the expression of alkaline phosphatase in cartilage cells, and both cyclic AMP and protein kinase C pathways have been implicated in this response [40, 41]. Biphasic effects on chondrocytes have been reported [42]. For example, studies have shown that $PGF_{2\alpha}$ is mitogenic, whereas in some bone cell lines PGE_1 inhibits mitogenesis. IGF-1 may be involved in the cartilage response and in the osteoblast response [40]. Prostaglandins have been shown to have a biphasic effect on collagen synthesis, with stimulation at low doses being associated with an increase in IGF-1 levels and with the production of IGF-BP3 and IGF-BP4 [41, 43]. Increased proteoglycan production has also been observed in cartilage cells treated with PGs [12]. However, the receptors that mediate this response have not been fully identified in cartilage [44]. Based on the role of cyclic AMP in other tissues, EP_2, EP_4, or prostacyclin (IP) receptors may be involved.

G. Leukotrienes in Bone Metabolism

Studies on the role of leukotrienes in skeletal metabolism are limited. There is evidence that leukotriene B4 (LTB4) can stimulate bone resorption, and other leukotrienes may have similar but less potent effects [45]. Inhibition of 5-lipoxygenase can impair bone resorption after tooth extraction, and this may be related to an effect on mast cells [15]. Osteogenic

sarcoma cells produce LTC4, and LTB4 levels, along with other cytokines, are increased in tissue samples from patients with osteomyelitis [46]. LTB-4 has also been shown to inhibit cell proliferation in rat osteoblastic cells, although its effects on human osteosarcoma cells are biphasic [47]. It will be important to elucidate further the role of LTB-4 in cartilage as well as in bone, since inhibition of PG synthesis, particularly selective inhibition of COX-2, may lead to a diversion of arachidonic acid into leukotriene pathways.

H. Conclusions

There is now ample evidence that prostaglandins play a central role as local regulators of physiologic responses and as mediators of pathologic responses in bone and cartilage. However, the relative importance of this role, compared to that of other local mediators, remains to be established. Moreover, the fact that prostaglandins are multifunctional regulators makes it difficult to determine what specific effects any given perturbation is likely to have. Some of the differences in prostaglandin response may be mediated by different receptors in skeletal cells, as well as by different signal transduction pathways. Further understanding of these receptors and pathways may lead to new insights into the role of eicosanoids and how these mechanisms can be manipulated to achieve therapeutic goals.

III. THE ROLE OF CYTOKINES IN BONE AND CARTILAGE METABOLISM

The cytokines that have been most extensively studied for their ability to regulate bone and cartilage function are interleukin-1 (IL-1), tumor necrosis factor (TNF), and interleukin-6 (IL-6). These agents have potent effects in a variety of *in vivo* and *in vitro* assays and this chapter will focus on their actions in bone and cartilage. In addition, the role of other cytokines will be briefly reviewed.

A. Effects of Interleukin-1 on Bone

Interleukin-1 (IL-1) is encoded by two separate gene products (α and β) that have identical activities [48]. This cytokine is the most potent peptide stimulator of *in vitro* bone resorption that has yet been identified [49] and it has potent *in vivo* effects [50]. It increases prostaglandin synthesis in bone [49, 51], which may augment its resorptive activity [52]. The *in vitro* effects of IL-1 on bone formation appear to be inhibitory [53–55], although it does stimulate DNA synthesis in both bone organ cultures and primary cultures of human bone cells [54, 56].

IL-1 is produced in bone [57] and IL-1 activity is present in bone marrow serum [58, 59]. Macrophages are a likely source of local bone IL-1 [60]. In addition, osteoblasts and osteoclasts may also produce IL-1 [61, 62].

A natural inhibitor of IL-1, IL-1 receptor antagonist (IL-1ra), is an analog of IL-1 that binds but does not activate the type 1 IL-1 receptor [63–65]. IL-1ra blocks the ability of IL-1 to stimulate resorption and PGE_2 production in bone organ cultures [66]. Increased release of IL-1ra has been demonstrated from peripheral blood monocytes (PBM) of both normal and osteoporotic postmenopausal women [67]. Decreased levels of IL-1ra are also reported in the bone marrow of some women with a rapid-loss form of osteoporosis [68].

There are two known receptors for IL-1, type I and type II [69]. All known biologic responses to IL-1 appear to be mediated exclusively through the type I receptor [70]. IL-1 receptor type I requires interaction with a second protein, interleukin-1 receptor accessory protein (IRAcP), to generate post-receptor signals [71–73]. However, binding of ligand to the IL-1 type I receptor occurs in the absence of IRAcP. IL-1 receptor type II appears to have no agonist activity. However, there is convincing evidence that it is a decoy receptor that prevents activation of IL-1 receptor type I [74]. IL-1 receptor type II can be released and circulate in serum as a soluble binding protein that inhibits interactions of IL-1 with the type I receptor [75, 76]. IL-1 receptor type II can also synergize with IL-1ra to inhibit activation of the IL-1 receptor type I [77].

IL-1 appears to be involved in the development of osteoporosis. Increased IL-1 bioactivity was found in the conditioned medium of PBM from some patients with a high-turnover form of this disease [78]. One group has found that *in vivo* estrogen treatment reduced the amount of IL-1 that was released from cultured PBM [79]. However, similar studies have failed to confirm this finding [80, 81]. Our group [58] and another laboratory [59] demonstrated that IL-1α bioactivity in the marrow serum of ovariectomized mice increased compared to sham controls or ovariectomized mice that were treated with estrogens. Importantly, this increase in activity resulted from factors in the marrow serum that modulated the response of bone cells to IL-1α and not to changes in IL-1α levels.

Studies of the regulation of IL-1 by estrogens in humans have been inconsistent. One group demonstrated that IL-1 levels in serum were increased 4 weeks after ovariectomy [82]. However, others failed to find a correlation between serum IL-1α, IL-1β, or IL-1ra levels and indices of bone turnover in either pre- or post-menopausal women [83] or between osteoporotic women and normal women [84].

In vivo administration of IL-1ra inhibited the bone loss that occurred in ovariectomized rats [85]. This effect was most pronounced 4 weeks after ovariectomy and was much less at earlier times. In addition, treatment of mice for 2 weeks

after ovariectomy with IL-1ra decreased the ability of marrow cell cultures to form osteoclast-like cells and inhibited the excretion of pyridinoline cross links (a marker of bone resorption) *in vivo* [86]. Confirmation of a role of IL-1 in estrogen-withdrawal bone loss came from studies of mice that do not respond to IL-1 because they lack the signal transmitting IL-1 receptor type I (IL-1 R1 KO mice). It was found that, in contrast to wild-type animals, IL-1 R1 KO mice did not lose bone mass after ovariectomy [87]. The finding that production of IL-1 receptor type II, the decoy IL-1 receptor, is upregulated by estrogen treatment [88, 89] is one potential mechanism by which estrogen might influence the IL-1 system. It is possible that estrogen regulates bone mass by increasing IL-1 receptor type II expression independent of any direct effects on IL-1 production. This response would decrease the ability of bone cells to respond to IL-1 and blunt the potent catabolic effects of IL-1 on bone mass.

B. Effects of Interleukin-1 on Cartilage

IL-1 is a potent regulator of cartilage cell function. It inhibits cartilage cell replication, colony formation in soft agar, and proteoglycan synthesis [90, 91], while it stimulates production of matrix metalloproteinases, which degrade cartilage collagen [92]. IL-1 also regulated expression of 1,25-dihydroxyvitamin D receptors and type X collagen production in growth plate chondrocytes but had little effect on type II collagen synthesis [93]. IL-1 may be involved in the regulation of growth plate cartilage since it is made by these cells [94]. Production of IL-1 in rat growth plate cartilage was altered by the vitamin D status of the animals [95]. This mechanism may be involved in growth. However, it is not critical since mice that cannot respond to IL-1 grow normally [96].

C. Effects of Tumor Necrosis Factor on Bone

Like IL-1, tumor necrosis factor (TNF) is a family of two related polypeptides (α and β) [97–101]. TNFα and β, have similar biologic activities and both are potent stimulators of bone resorption [102, 103] and inhibitors of bone collagen synthesis [53, 102, 104]. TNFα is produced by human osteoblast-like cell cultures [105] and IL-1, GM-CSF, and lipopolysaccharide stimulate its production.

Like IL-1, TNF binds to two cell surface receptors, the TNF receptor 1, or p55, and the TNF receptor 2, or p75 [106]. In contrast to IL-1, both receptors transmit biologic responses. Bones from mice that lack either IL-1 receptor type I or TNF receptor 1 are similar to those of wild-type mice except for a 36% increase in the total bone area of IL-1 receptor type I KO mice [96].

TNF also appears to mediate the effects of estrogen on bone. One group found that estrogen treatment modulated

TNF production *in vitro* in human osteoblast cultures [107]. However, another group failed to find an effect of estrogen on TNF protein production in human osteoblast-like cell cultures [108]. Spontaneous production of TNF in cultured peripheral monocytes from women who had recently undergone ovariectomy was increased compared to levels from cells that were assayed preovariectomy [109]. Bone resorbing activity in LPS-stimulated peripheral blood monocyte conditioned medium (CM) is increased in cultures from postmenopausal women and this effect relies, to some degree, on TNF in the CM [110]. Treatment of mice with soluble recombinant TNF receptor, an inhibitor of TNF action, reduced the ability of ovariectomy to decrease bone mass [111]. Likewise, mice that overexpressed a soluble form of TNF receptor 1 did not lose bone mass after ovariectomy [112].

D. Effects of Tumor Necrosis Factor on Cartilage

Like IL-1, TNFα stimulates production of degradative enzymes in cartilage and inhibits cartilage synthesis [113, 114]. Both TNF and IL-1 are implicated as mediators of inflammatory arthritis [115]. In costal chondrocytes, TNF decreased alkaline phosphatase and DNA synthesis [116]. *In vivo* fracture healing in rat ribs was inhibited by TNFα treatment [117]. This effect was due to a decrease in cartilaginous callus formation and possibly to a decrease in the differentiation of mesenchymal cells into chondroblasts [117].

E. Effects of Interleukin-6 on Bone

IL-6 has a wide variety of activities on immune cell function and on the replication and differentiation of a number of cell types [118, 119]. Osteoblastic cells produce IL-6 and IL-6 receptors [120–122]. In the majority of studies, production of IL-6 is minimal in the basal state but is stimulated by agents that also stimulate resorption [120–122].

Another source of IL-6 in the bone microenvironment is bone marrow stromal cells, which can produce IL-6 after they are stimulated with IL-1 and TNF [123]. The receptor for IL-6 is composed of two parts: a specific IL-6 binding protein (IL-6 receptor), which can be either membrane bound or soluble, and gp-130, an activator protein that is common to a number of cytokine receptors [124]. Production of the specific IL-6 receptor may be regulated since it does not appear to be expressed on bone cells at all times [125]. Soluble IL-6 receptor binds IL-6 and this complex can then activate cells that contain the gp-130 signal peptide [124, 125].

The ability of IL-6 to stimulate bone resorption *in vitro* is variable and depends on the assay system that is examined [121, 126]. The reasons for these discrepancies are unknown. It appears that a major effect of IL-6 is to regulate osteoclast

progenitor cell differentiation into mature osteoclasts [127, 128]. The ability of IL-1 and TNF, but not parathyroid hormone or 1,25-dihydroxyvitamin D, to stimulate osteoclast-like cell development in human marrow cultures appears dependent on endogenous IL-6 production [129]. Implanting Chinese hamster ovary (CHO) cells that had been genetically engineered to express murine IL-6 into nude mice produced a syndrome of hypercalcemia, cachexia, leukocytosis, and thrombocytosis [130]. The effects of IL-6 on resorption in this model were weak and were significantly potentiated when the animals were also implanted with PTH-rP secreting CHO cells [131]. A major effect of IL-6 in these *in vivo* models was to increase the number of early osteoclast precursors (CFU-GM) in the marrow. IL-6 appears to mediate some of the increased resorption and bone pathology that is seen in the clinical syndromes of Paget's disease [132], hypercalcemia of malignancy [133], fibrous dysplasia [134], giant cell tumors of bone [135], and Gorham-Stout disease [136].

IL-6 has only mild effects on bone growth parameters. It inhibited collagen and noncollagen protein synthesis and percent collagen synthesis in UMR-106 cells. However, the maximal inhibitory effect on collagen synthesis was small (27%). In contrast, IL-6 did not affect parameters of growth in another cell line (ROS 17/2.8) and in human osteoblast-like cells [137]. IL-6 together with its soluble receptor enhanced expression of insulin-like growth factor-I (IGF-1), collagenase 3, and IGF-1 binding protein-5 in osteoblasts [138–140]. IL-6 also inhibited bone nodule mineralization but not nodule formation in an assay that measured the differentiation of rat osteoprogenitor cells [141].

IL-6 has been linked to postmenopausal osteoporosis. However, as with IL-1 and TNF, results are conflicting. One group [123] demonstrated that TNF or IL-1 treatment increased IL-6 bioactivity in the conditioned medium of both stromal cells and a variety of osteoblast-like cell populations, and that pretreatment with 17β estradiol inhibited this response. However, others failed to find any modulation of osteoblast stimulated IL-6 production with estrogen treatment [107, 108]. Regulation of the transcriptional activity of the IL-6 promoter by estrogen and androgens has been demonstrated in a 225 bp 5$'$ proximal segment [142, 143].

The involvement of IL-6 in estrogen withdrawal bone loss has also been examined *in vivo*. One group [144] demonstrated that injection of a monoclonal antibody against IL-6 into ovariectomized mice for 4 weeks inhibited both the bone loss and increases in osteoclast formation. In addition, they found that IL-6 levels in bone marrow cultures from ovariectomized animals were increased compared to normal animals. However, another group could not demonstrate an increase in IL-6 in similar cultures with ovariectomized animals [86], nor could they find an effect of anti-IL-6 monoclonal antibody on estrogen withdrawal bone loss in mice 2 weeks post-ovariectomy [145]. IL-6 knockout mice, which make no IL-6, have increased basal bone turnover rates compared to normal animals and they fail to increase bone turnover or to lose bone mass after ovariectomy or orchiectomy [146, 147].

In two reports, ovariectomy had no detectable effect on IL-6 production in the mouse marrow [148, 149]. In contrast, one group did find ovariectomy to increase IL-6 protein levels in marrow serum [59]. It is also possible that the changes in bone that occur after ovariectomy are mediated through effects of estrogen on cellular responses to IL-6 [150].

F. Effects of Interleukin-6 on Cartilage

IL-6 is produced in cartilage in response to treatment with inflammatory cytokines such as IL-1 and TNF [115]. IL-6 production is increased by treatment with growth hormone or insulin-like growth factor-1 (IGF-1) in growth plate chondrocyte cultures [151]. However, in human articular cartilage cultures, IGF-1 had no effect on IL-6 production [152]. IL-6 is not critical for skeletal growth because IL-6 deficient mice grow normally [146]. IL-6 also enhances cartilage production of tissue inhibitor of metalloproteinase 1 (TIMP-1), a factor that blocks the activity of metalloproteinases, which degrade cartilage [153, 154] (see Chapter 10).

G. Effects of Other Interleukin-6 Family Members on Bone

IL-6 is a member of a group of cytokines that share the gp-130 activator protein in their receptor complex [155, 156]. In addition, each family member utilizes unique ligand receptors to generate specific binding. Besides IL-6, the cytokines in this family include interleukin 11 (IL-11), leukemia inhibitory factor (LIF), oncostatin M (OSM), ciliary neurotrophic factor (CNTF), and cardiotrophin-1 (CT-1). Except for CT-1, receptors for all other IL-6 family members have been detected in bone marrow stromal or osteoblastic cells [157]. IL-11-specific receptors are also present in osteoclast-like cells that are generated *in vitro* [156].

The effects of IL-6 family members vary with the cytokine and the system that is examined. The following is a summary of what is known about the actions of this group of factors on bone.

1. INTERLEUKIN-11

IL-11 is produced by bone cells in response to a variety of resorption stimuli [158]. It stimulates osteoclast formation in murine bone marrow cultures [159] and bone resorption in a variety of *in vitro* assays [160, 161]. Interestingly, it had no effect on isolated mature osteoclasts. IL-11-stimulated bone resorption in explant cultures was dependent on prostaglandin

and lipoxygenase synthesis as well as on synthesis of matrix metalloproteinases [160]. Studies of the effects of IL-11 on bone formation are limited. However, it inhibited osteoblast differentiation in a bone nodule formation assay [162].

2. LEUKEMIA INHIBITORY FACTOR

LIF is produced by bone cells in response to a number of resorption stimuli [163–165]. However, production can be variable and depends on the model system that is studied. The effects of LIF on bone resorption are also variable. In one *in vitro* model, LIF stimulated resorption by a mechanism that was prostaglandin dependent [166], whereas in other assays, it had inhibitory effects [167, 168]. LIF stimulated DNA synthesis in bone [169] and inhibited bone nodule formation and expression of osteoblastic markers in stromal cells [141]. Local injections of LIF *in vivo* increased both resorption and formation parameters and increased the thickness of treated bones [170]. In mice that lack the specific LIF receptor, and hence cannot respond to LIF, bone volume was reduced and osteoclast numbers were increased six-fold [171]. Thus, *in vivo* data seems to indicate that LIF is predominantly an anabolic factor in bone.

3. ONCOSTATIN M

Oncostatin M (OSM) stimulated multinuclear cell formation in murine and human bone marrow cultures [125, 172]. However, these cells appeared to be macrophage polykaryons and not osteoclasts [172]. In contrast, OSM inhibited osteoclast-like cell formation that was stimulated by 1,25-dihydroxyvitamin D in human marrow cultures [172] and it decreased bone resorption rates in fetal mouse long bone cultures [173]. *In vivo*, overexpression of oncostatin M in transgenic mice induced a phenotype of osteopetrosis [174]. Hence, it appears that OSM is an inhibitor of osteoclast formation and bone resorption [175].

OSM mRNA is made by bone cells [176]. In rodent osteoblastic cells, it stimulated DNA and IL-6 synthesis and inhibited collagen and alkaline phosphatase production [173]. It also blocked the induction of apoptosis in an osteoblastic cell line (MC3T3-E1) [177]. These results suggest that oncostatin M maintains osteoblastic cells in a proliferating and less differentiated state.

The role of IL-6 family members in osteoclast formation has been reexamined in light of data demonstrating that mice lacking the gp-130 activator protein have increased numbers of osteoclasts in their bones [178]. Since gp-130 is an activator of signal transduction for all members of the IL-6 family, this finding argues that at least some IL-6 family members have a predominantly inhibitory effect on osteoclast formation and bone resorption. Available data implicate oncostatin M [173] and possibly LIF [167, 168] as the major inhibitors of resorption in this family of cytokines.

H. Effects on Interleukin-6 Family Members on Cartilage

LIF is produced in human articular chondrocytes by treatment with IL-1, IL-6, and TNF [179]. In turn, treatment of these cells with LIF increased production of IL-6 [180]. Hence, a positive feedback loop may exist. IL-6, LIF, OSM, CNTF, and IL-11 suppressed proteoglycan synthesis in cultures of pig articular cartilage, and OSM and LIF also stimulated proteoglycan degradation [181]. These results demonstrate that members of this family can regulate cartilage turnover.

I. Effects of Interferon γ on Bone and Cartilage

Interferon γ (INFγ) has a wide variety of biologic activities. *In vitro*, INFγ inhibits bone resorption [182, 183]. This effect appears to be more specific for the response to IL-1 and TNF compared to PTH or 1,25-dihydroxyvitamin D [184]. INFγ can synergistically augment IL-1- or TNF-stimulated nitric oxide (NO) production by cultured osteoblasts [185]. NO appears to be a biphasic regulator of osteoclast-mediated bone resorption that stimulates at low concentrations and inhibits at high concentrations [185]. It is likely that part or all of the potent inhibitory effects of INFγ on IL-1- and TNF-mediated resorption results from effects on NO synthesis since INFγ together with IL-1 or TNF synergistically stimulates NO production to high levels in bone.

INFγ, IL-1, and TNFα inhibit type II collagen synthesis in human articular and costal chondrocytes [186, 187]. The effects of IL-1 and INFγ appear to be mainly transcriptional [188]. INFγ also inhibits production of metalloproteinases and cartilage degradation [189] in human chondrocytes and it decreases cell proliferation and proteoglycan synthesis [190, 191]. Hence, the net effect of INFγ on cartilage is an inhibition of both synthesis and turnover.

J. Additional Cytokines That Are Produced in Bone or That Have Effects on Bone or Cartilage Cell Function

A variety of additional cytokines have been shown to either be produced by bone cells or to have effects on bone cell function. Interleukin-8 (IL-8) and monocyte chemotactic peptide-1 (MCP-1) are members of the chemokine family of cytokines. Both are produced in bone cells in a regulated manner [192–194]. IL-8 is produced by human osteoblast-like cells, the human osteosarcoma cell line MG-63, and by human bone marrow stromal cells [108, 192]. Production of IL-8 in these cells was augmented by treatment with either IL-1 or TNF and was synergistically increased by their combination.

MCP-1 is produced by stimulated osteoblasts [193]. IL-1 and TNF strongly enhanced MCP-1 production in human and murine osteoblastic cells [194]. In contrast, TGF-β and IL-6 were weak stimuli in human osteoblastic cells [193].

Interleukins 4, 10, and 13 are members of a group of locally acting factors that have been termed inhibitory cytokines. Transgenic mice that overexpress IL-4 have a phenotype of osteoporosis [195]. This effect may result from both an inhibition of osteoclast formation and activity [196, 197] and an inhibition of bone formation [198]. In cartilage, IL-4 inhibited matrix degradation that was stimulated by IL-1 and it enhanced TIMP-1 expression [153].

Treatment of bone marrow cell cultures with IL-10 suppressed the production of osteoblastic proteins and prevented the onset of mineralization [199]. IL-10 also inhibits the formation of osteoclast-like cells in bone marrow cultures without affecting macrophage formation or the resorptive activity of mature osteoclasts [200]. IL-13 and IL-4 inhibit bone resorption stimulated by IL-1 by decreasing the production of prostaglandins and the activity of cyclooxygenase-2 [201]. IL-4 and IL-13 also induce chemotaxis in osteoblastic cells [202]. Interleukin-18 is expressed by osteoblastic cells and inhibits osteoclast formation through its ability to stimulate granulocyte macrophage colony stimulating factor (GM-CSF) [203], which is produced by T cells in response to IL-18 treatment [204].

References

1. Kawaguchi, H., Pilbeam, C. C., Harrison, J. R., and Raisz, L.G. (1995). The role of prostaglandins in the regulation of bone metabolism. *Clin. Orthop. Relat. Res.* **313**, 36–46.
2. Pilbeam, C. C., Harrison, J. R., and Raisz, L. G. (1996). Prostaglandins and bone metabolism. *In* "Principles of Bone Biology" (J. P. Bilezikian, L. G. Raisz, and G. A. Rodan, eds.), pp. 715–728. Academic Press, San Diego, CA.
3. Klein-Nulend, J., Burger, E. H., Semeins, C. M., Raisz, L. G., and Pilbeam, C. C. (1997). Pulsating fluid flow stimulates prostaglandin release and inducible prostaglandin G/H synthase mRNA expression in primary mouse bone cells. *J. Bone Miner. Res.* **12**(1), 45–51.
4. Tai, H., Miyura, C., Pilbeam, C. C., Tamura, T., Ohsugi, Y., Koishihara, Y., Kubodera, N., Kawagughi, H., Raisz, L. G., and Suda, T. (1997). Transcriptional induction of cyclooxygenase-2 in osteoblasts is involved in interleukin-6-induced osteoclast formation. *Endocrinology* **138**(6), 2372–2379.
5. Pilbeam, C., Rao, Y., Voznesensky, O., Kawaguchi, H., Alander, C., Raisz, L. G., and Herschman, H. (1997). Transforming growth factor-b1 regulation of prostaglandin G/H synthase-2 expression in osteoblastic MC3T3-E1 cells. *Endocrinology* **138**(11), 4672–4682.
6. Kawaguchi, H., Nemoto, K., Raisz, L. G., Harrison, J. R., Voznesensky, O., and Alander, C. B. (1996). Interleukin-4 inhibits prostaglandin G/H synthase-2 and cytosolic phospholipase A2 induction in neonatal mouse parietal bone cultures. *J. Bone Miner. Res.* **11**(3), 358–366.
7. Arner, E. C., and Pratta, M. A. (1989). Independent effects of interleukin-1 on proteoglycan breakdown, proteoglycan synthesis, and prostaglandin E2 release from cartilage in organ culture. *Arthritis Rheum.* **32**, 288–297.

8. Berenbaum, F., Jacques, C., Thomas, G., Corvol, M. T., Bereziat, G., and Masliah, J. (1996). Synergistic effect of interleukin-1 β and tumor necrosis factor α on PGE$_2$ production by articular chondrocytes does not involve PLA2 stimulation. *Exp. Cell. Res.* **222**, 379–384.

9. Chin, J. E., and Lin, J. A. (1988). Effects of recombinant human interleukin-1 b on rabbit articular chondrocytes. Stimulates of prostanoid release and inhibition of cell growth. *Arthritis Rheum.* **31**, 1290–1296.

10. Chin, J. E., Hatfield, C. A., Krzesicki, R. F., and Herblin, W. F. (1991). Interactions between interleukin-1 and basic fibroblast growth factor on articular chondrocytes. Effects on cell growth, prostanoid production, and receptor modulation. *Arthritis Rheum.* **34**, 314–324.

11. Fawthrop, F. W., Frazer, A., Russell, R. G., and Bunning, R. A. (1997). Effects of transforming growth factor b on the production of prostaglandin E and caseinase activity of unstimulated and interleukin-1-stimulated human articular chondrocytes in cultures. *Br. J. Rheum.* **36**, 729–734.

12. Schwartz, Z., Gilley, R. M., Sylvia, V. L., Dean, D. D., and Boyan, B. D. (1998). The effect of prostaglandin D$_2$ on costochondral chondrocyte differentiation is mediated by cyclic adenosine $3',5'$ monophosphate and protein kinase C. *Endocrinology* **139**, 1825–1834.

13. Smith, R. L., Donlon, B. S., Gupta, M. K., Mohtai, M., Das, P., Carter, D., Cooke, J., Gibbons, G., Hutchinson, N., and Schurman, D. J. (1995). Effects of fluid-induced shear on articular chondrocyte morphology and metabolism in vitro. *J. Orthop. Res.* **13**, 824–831.

14. Dayer, J. M., Ricard-Blum, S., Kaufmann, M. T., and Herbage, D. (1986). Type IX collagen is a potent inducer of PGE$_2$ and interleukin-1 production by human monocyte macrophages. *FEBS Lett.* **198**, 208–212.

15. Franchi-Miller, C., and Saffar, J. L. (1995). The 5-lipoxygenase inhibitor BWA4C impairs osteoclastic resorption in a synchronized model of bone remodeling. *Bone* **17**, 185–191.

16. Geng, Y., Blanco, F. J., Cornelisson, M., and Lotz, M. (1995). Regulation of cyclooxygenase-2 expression in normal human articular chondrocytes. *J. Immunol.* **155**, 796–801.

17. Lyons-Giordano, B., Pratta, M., Galbraith, W., Davis, G. L., and Arner, E. C. (1993). Interleukin-1 differentially modulates chondrocyte expression of cyclooxygenase-2 and phospholipase A2. *Exp. Cell Res.* **206**, 58–62.

18. Siegle, I., Klein, T., Backman, J. T., Saal, J. G., Nusing, R. M., and Fritz, P. (1998). Expression of cyclooxygenase 1 and cyclooxygenase 2 in human synovial tissue: Differential elevation of cyclooxygenase 2 in inflammatory joint diseases. *Arthritis Rheum.* **41**, 122–129.

19. Pilbeam, C. C., Raisz, L. G., Voznesensky, O., Alander, C. B., Delman, B. N., and Kawaguchi, H. (1995). Autoregulation of inducible prostaglandin G/H synthase in osteoblastic cells by prostaglandins. *J. Bone Miner. Res.* **10**(3), 406–414.

20. Hurley, M. M., Lee, S. K., Raisz, L. G., Bernecker, P., and Lorenzo, J. (1998). Basic fibroblast growth factor induces osteoclast formation in murine bone marrow cultures. *Bone* **22**(4), 309–316.

21. Thorsen, K., Kristoffersson, A. O., Lerner, U. H., and Lorentzon, R. P. (1996). In situ microdialysis in bone tissue. Stimulation of prostaglandin E$_2$ release by weight-bearing mechanical loading. *J. Clin. Invest.* **98**(11), 2446–2449.

22. Jarvinen, T. A, Moilanen, T., Jarvinen, T. L., and Moilanen, E. (1996). Endogenous nitric oxide and prostaglandin E$_2$ do not regulate the synthesis of each other in interleukin-1 b-stimulated rat articular cartilage. *Inflammation* **20**, 683–692.

23. Klein-Nulend, J., Semeins, C. M., Ajubi, N. E., Nijweide, P. J., and Burger, E. H. (1995). Pulsating fluid flow increases nitric oxide (NO) synthesis by osteocytes but not periosteal fibroblasts: Correlation with prostaglandin up-regulation. *Biochem. Biophys. Res. Commun.* **217**, 640–648.

24. Manfield, L., Jang, D., and Murrell, G. A. (1996). Nitric oxide enhances cyclooxygenase activity in articular cartilage. *Inflammation Res.* **45**, 254–258.

25. Smalt, R., Mitchell, F. T., Howard, R. L., and Chambers, T. J. (1997). Induction of NO and prostaglandin E$_2$ in osteoblasts by wall-shear stress but not mechanical strain. *Am. J. Physiol.* **36**, E751–E758.

26. Amin, A. R., Attur, M., Patel, R., Thakker, G. D., Marshall, P. J., Rediske, J., Stuchin, S. A., Patel, I. R., and Abramson, S. B. (1997). Superinduction of cyclooxygenase-2 activity in human osteoarthritis-affected cartilage. Influence of nitric oxide. *J. Clin. Invest.* **99**, 1231–1237.

27. Ito, A., Nose, T., Takahashi, S., and Mori, Y. (1995). Cyclooxygenase inhibitors augment the production of pro-matrix metalloproteinase 9 (progenatinase B) in rabbit articular chondrocytes. *FEBS Lett.* **360**, 75–79.

28. Schwartz, Z., Swain, L. D., Kelly, D. W., Brooks, B., and Boyan, B. D. (1992). Regulation of prostaglandin E$_2$ production by vitamin D metabolites in growth zone and resting zone chondrocyte cultures is dependent on cell matruation. *Bone* **13**, 395–401.

29. Ma, Y. F., Li, X. J., Jee, W. S., McOsker, J., Liang, X. G., Setterberg, R., and Chow, S. Y. (1995). Effects of prostaglandin E$_2$ and F$_{2a}$ on the skeleton of osteopenic ovariectomized rats. *Bone* **17**, 549–554.

30. Woodiel, F. N., Fall, P. M., and Raisz, L. G. Anabolic effects of prostaglandins in cultured fetal rat calvariae: Structure-activity relations and signal transduction pathway. *J. Bone Miner. Res.* **11**(9), 1249–1255.

31. Scutt, A., Bertram, P., and Brautigam, M. (1996). The role of glucocorticoids and prostaglandin E$_2$ in the recruitment of bone marrow mesenchymal cells to the osteoblastic lineage: Positive and negative. *Calcif. Tissue Int.* **59**, 154–162.

32. Fall, P. M., Breault, D. T., and Raisz, L. G. (1994). Inhibition of collagen synthesis by prostaglandins in the immortalized rat osteoblastic clonal cell cline, Pyla: Structure activity relations and signal transduction mechanisms. *J. Bone Miner. Res.* **9**, 1935–1943.

33. Nemoto, K., Bernecker, P. M., Pilbeam, C. C., and Raisz, L. G. (1995). Expression of regulation of prostaglandin F receptor mRNA in rodent osteoblastic cells. *Prostaglandins* **50**(5/6), 349–358.

34. Nemoto, K., Pilbeam, C. C., Bilak, S. R., and Raisz, L. G. (1997). Molecular cloning and expression of a rat prostaglandin E$_2$ subtype. *Prostaglandins* **54**, 713–725.

35. Hakeda, Y., Hotta, T., and Kurihara, N. (1987). Prostaglandin E$_2$ and F$_{2?}$ stimulate differentiation and proliferation, respectively, of clonal osteoblastic MC3T3-E1 cells by different second messengers in vitro. *Endocrinology* **121**, 1966–1974.

36. Raisz, L. G., Fall, P. M., Gabbitas, B. Y., McCarthy, T. L., Kream, B. E., and Canalis, E. (1993). Effects of prostaglandin E$_2$ on bone formation in cultured fetal rat calvariae: Role of insulin-like growth factor-1. *Endocrinology* **133**, 1504–1510.

37. Hakeda, Y., Kawaguchi, H., Hurley, M., Pilbeam, C. C., Abreu, C., Linkhart, T. A., Mohan, S., Kumegawa, M., and Raisz, L. G. (1996). Intact insulin-like growth factor binding protein-5 (IGFBP-5) associates with bone matrix and the soluble fragments of IGFBP-5 accumulated in culture medium of neonatal mouse calvariae by parathyroid hormone and prostaglandin E$_2$ treatment. *J. Cell. Physiol.* **166**, 370–379.

38. Kawaguchi, H., Pilbeam, C. C., Gronowicz, G., Abreu, C., Fletcher, B. S., Herschman, H. R., Raisz, L. G., and Hurley, M. M. (1995). Transcriptional induction of prostaglandin G/H synthase-2 by basic fibroblast growth factor. *J. Clin. Invest.* **96**(1), 923–930.

39. Kosher, R. A., and Gay, S. W. (1985). The effect of prostaglandins on the cyclic AMP content of limb mesenchymal cells. *Cell Differ.* **17**, 159–167.

40. DiBattista, J. A., Dore, S., Martel-Pelletier, J., and Pelletier, J. P. (1996). Prostaglandin E$_2$ stimulates incorporation of proline into collagenase

digestible proteins in human articular chondrocytes: Identification of an effector autocrine loop involving insulin-like growth factor I. *Mol. Cell. Endocrinol.* **123**, 27–35.

41. DiBattista, J. A., Dore, S., Morin, N., and Abribat, T. (1996). Prostaglandin E$_2$ up- regulates insulin-like growth factor binding protein-3 expression and synthesis in human articular chondrocytes by a cAMP-independent pathway: Role of calcium and protein kinase A and C. *J. Cell. Biochem.* **63**, 320–333.

42. Lowe, G. N., Fu, Y. H., McDougall, S., Polendo, R., Williams, A., Benya, P. D., and Hahn, T. J. Effects of prostaglandins on deoxyribonucleic acid and aggrecan synthesis in the RCJ 3.1C5.18 chondrocyte cell line: Role of second messengers. *Endocrinology* **137**, 2208–2216.

43. DiBattista, J. A., Dore, S., Morin, N., He, Y., Pelletier, J. P., and Martel-Pelletier, J. (1997). Prostaglandin E$_2$ stimulates insulin-like growth factor binding protein-4 expression and synthesis in cultured human articular and chondrocytes: Possible mediation by Ca(++)-calmodulin regulated processes. *J. Cell. Biochem.* **65**, 408–419.

44. deBrum-Fernandes, A. J., Morisset, S., Bkaily, G., and Patry, C. (1996). Characterization of the PGE$_2$ receptor subtype in bovine chondrocytes in culture. *Br. J. Pharmacol.* **118**, 1597–1604.

45. Garcia, C., Boyce, B. F., Gilles, J., Dallas, M., Qiao, M., Mundy, G. R., and Bonewald, L. F. (1996). Leukotriene B4 stimulates osteoclastic bone resorption both in vitro and in vivo. *J. Bone Miner. Res.* **11**, 1619–1627.

46. Klosterhlfen, B., Peters, K. M., Tons, C., Hauptmann, S., Klein, C. L., and Kirkpatrick, C. J. (1996). Local and systemic inflammatory mediator release in patients with acute and chronic post-traumatic osteomyelites. *J. Trauma* **40**, 372–378.

47. Ren, W., and Dziak, R. (1991). Effects of leukotrienes on osteoblastic cell proliferation. *Calcif. Tissue Int.* **49**, 197–201.

48. Dinarello, C. A. 1991. Interleukin-1 and interleukin-1 antagonism. *Blood* **77**, 1627–1652.

49. Lorenzo, J. A., Sousa, S., Alander, C., Raisz, L. G., and Dinarello, C. A. (1987). Comparison of the bone-resorbing activity in the supernatants from phytohemagglutinin-stimulated human peripheral blood mononuclear cells with that of cytokines through the use of an antiserum to interleukin 1. *Endocrinology* **121**, 1164–1170.

50. Sabatini, M., Boyce, B., Aufdemorte, T., Bonewald, L., and Mundy, G. R. (1988). Infusions of recombinant human interleukins 1 alpha and 1 beta cause hypercalcemia in normal mice. *Proc. Natl. Acad. Sci. U.S.A.* **85**, 5235–5239.

51. Sato, K., Fujii, Y., Kasono, K., Saji, M., Tsushima, T., and Shizume, K. (1986). Stimulation of prostaglandin E$_2$ and bone resorption by recombinant human interleukin 1 alpha in fetal mouse bones. *Biochem. Biophys. Res. Commun.* **138**, 618–624.

52. Klein, D. C., and Raisz, L. G. (1970). Prostaglandins: Stimulation of bone resorption in tissue culture. *Endocrinology* **86**, 1436–1440.

53. Smith, D. D., Gowen, M., and Mundy, G. R. (1987). Effects of interferon-gamma and other cytokines on collagen synthesis in fetal rat bone cultures. *Endocrinology* **120**, 2494–2499.

54. Canalis, E. (1986). Interleukin-1 has independent effects on deoxyribonucleic acid and collagen synthesis in cultures of rat calvariae. *Endocrinology* **118**, 74–81.

55. Stashenko, P., Dewhirst, F. E., Rooney, M. L., Desjardins, L. A., and Heeley, J. D. (1987). Interleukin-1 Beta is a potent inhibitor of bone formation in vitro. *J. Bone Miner. Res.* **2**, 559–565.

56. Gowen, M., Wood, D. D., and Russell, G. G. (1985). Stimulation of the proliferation of human bone cells in vitro by human monocyte products with interleukin-1 activity. *J. Clin. Invest.* **75**, 1223–1229.

57. Lorenzo, J. A., Sousa, S. L., Van Den Brink-Webb, S. E., and Korn, J. H. (1990). Production of both interleukin-1 α and β by newborn mouse calvaria cultures. *J. Bone Miner. Res.* **5**, 77–83.

58. Kawaguchi, H., Pilbeam, C. C., Vargas, S. J., Morse, E. E., Lorenzo, J. A., and Raisz, L. G. (1995). Ovariectomy enhances and estrogen replacement inhibits the activity of bone marrow factors that stimulate prostaglandin production in cultured mouse calvaria. *J. Clin. Invest.* **96**, 539–548.

59. Miyaura, C., Kusano, K., Masuzawa, T., Chaki, O., Onoe, Y., Aoyagi, M., Sasaki, T., Tamura, T., Koishihara Y., Ohsugi, Y., and Suda, T. (1995). Endogenous bone-resorbing factors in estrogen deficiency: Cooperative effects of IL-1 and IL-6. *J. Bone Miner. Res.* **10**, 1365–1373.

60. Horowitz, M. C., Philbrick, W. M., and Jilka, R. L. (1989). IL-1 release from cultured calvarial cells is due to macrophages. *J. Bone Miner. Res.* **4**(S1), 556 (abstr.).

61. Keeting, P. E., Rifas, L., Harris, S. A., Colvard, D. S., Spelsberg, T. C., Peck, W. A., and Riggs, B. L. (1991). Evidence for interleukin-1 beta production by cultured normal human osteoblast-like cells. *J. Bone Miner. Res.* **6**, 827–833.

62. O'Keefe, R. J., Teo, L. A., Singh, D., Puzas, J. E., Rosier, R. N., and Hicks, D. G. (1997). Osteoclasts constitutively express regulators of bone resorption: an immunohistochemical and in situ hybridization study. *Lab. Invest.* **76**, 457–465.

63. Eisenberg, S. P., Evans, R. J., Arend, W. P., Verderber, E., Brewer, M. T., Hannum, C. H., and Thompson, R. C. (1990). Primary structure and functional expression from complementary DNA of a human interleukin-1 receptor antagonist. *Nature* **343**, 341–346.

64. Hannum, C. H., Wilcox, C. J., Arend, W. P., Joslin, F. G., Dripps, D. J., Heimdal, P. L., Armes, L. G., Sommer, A., Eisenberg, S. P., and Thompson R. C. (1990). Interleukin-1 receptor antagonist activity of a human interleukin-1 inhibitor. *Nature* **343**, 336–340.

65. Arend, W. P., Welgus, H. G., Thompson, R. C., and Eisenberg, S. P. (1990). Biological properties of recombinant human monocyte-derived interleukin 1 receptor antagonist. *J. Clin. Invest.* **85**, 1694–1697.

66. Seckinger, P., Klein-Nulend, J., Alander, C., Thompson, R. C., Dayer, J. M., and Raisz, L. G. (1990). Natural and recombinant human IL-1 receptor antagonists block the effects of IL-1 on bone resorption and prostaglandin production. *J. Immunol.* **145**, 4181–4184.

67. Pacifici, R., Vannice, J. L., Rifa, L., and Kimble, R. B. (1993). Monocytic secretion of interleukin-1 receptor antagonist in normal and osteoporotic women: Effects of menopause and estrogen/progesterone therapy. *J. Clin. Endocrinol. Metab.* **77**, 1135–1141.

68. Abrahamsen, B., Shalhoub, V., Larson, E., Eriksen, E. F., Beck-Nielsen, H., and Marks, S. C., Jr. (1996). IL-1 beta and IL-1RA gene expression in transiliac bone biopsies: Correlation with bone loss and histomorphometry in healthy postmenopausal women. *J. Bone Miner. Res.* **11**, S105 (abstr.).

69. Dinarello, C. A. (1993). Blocking interleukin-1 in disease. *Blood Purif.* **11**, 118–127.

70. Sims, J. E., Gayle, M. A., Slack, J. L., Alderson, M. R., Bird, T. A., Giri, J. G., Colotta, F., Re, F., Mantovani, A., Shanebeck, K., Grabstein, K. H., and Dower S. K. (1993). Interleukin 1 signaling occurs exclusively via the type I receptor. *Proc. Natl. Acad. Sci. U.S.A.* **90**, 6155–6159.

71. Korherr, C., Hofmeister, R., Wesche, H., and Falk, W. (1997). A critical role for interleukin-1 receptor accessory protein in interleukin-1 signaling. *Eur. J. Immunol.* **27**, 262–267.

72. Wesche, H., Korherr, C., Kracht, M., Falk, W., Resch, K., and Martin, M. U. (1997). The interleukin-1 receptor accessory protein (IL-1RAcP) is essential for IL-1-induced activation of interleukin-1 receptor-associated kinase (IRAK) and stress-activated protein kinases (SAP kinases). *J. Biol. Chem.* **272**, 7727–7731.

73. Huang, J., Gao, X., Li, S., and Cao, Z. (1997). Recruitment of IRAK to the interleukin 1 receptor complex requires interleukin 1 receptor accessory protein. *Proc. Natl. Acad. Sci. U.S.A.* **94**, 12829–12832.

74. Colotta, F., Re, F., Muzio, M., Bertini, R., Polentarutti, N., Sironi, M., Giri, J. G., Dower, S. K., Sims, J. E., and Mantovani, A. (1993). Interleukin-1 type II receptor: A decoy target for IL-1 that is regulated by IL-4. *Science* **261**, 472–475.

75. Colotta, F., Dower, S. K., Sims, J. E., and Mantovani, A. (1994). The type II 'decoy' receptor: A novel regulatory pathway for interleukin 1. (Review). *Immunol. Today* **15**, 562–566.

76. Giri, J. G., Wells, J., Dower, S. K., McCall, C. E., Guzman, R. N., Slack, J., Bird, T. A., Shanebeck, K., Grabstein K. H., and Sims, J. E. (1994). Elevated levels of shed type II IL-1 receptor in sepsis. Potential role for type II receptor in regulation of IL-1 responses. *J. Immunol.* **153**, 5802–5809.

77. Burger, D., Chicheportiche, R., Giri, J. G., and Dayer, J. M. (1995). The inhibitory activity of human interleukin-1 receptor antagonist is enhanced by type II interleukin-1 soluble receptor and hindered by type 1 interleukin-1 soluble receptor. *J. Clin. Invest.* **96**, 38–41.

78. Pacifici, R., Rifas, L., Teitelbaum, S., Slatopolsky, E., McCracken, R., Bergfeld, M., Lee, W., Avioli, L. V., and Peck, W. A. 1987. Spontaneous release of interleukin 1 from human blood monocytes reflects bone formation in idiopathic osteoporosis. *Proc. Natl. Acad. Sci. U.S.A.* **84**, 4616–4620.

79. Pacifici, R., Rifas, L., McCracken, R., Vered, I., McMurtry, C., Avioli, L. V., and Peck, W. A. (1989). Ovarian steroid treatment blocks a postmenopausal increase in blood monocyte interleukin 1 release. *Proc. Natl. Acad. Sci. U.S.A.* **86**, 2398–2402.

80. Stock, J. L., Coderre, J. A., McDonald, B., and Rosenwasser, L. J. (1989). Effects of estrogen in vivo and in vitro on spontaneous interleukin-1 release by monocytes from postmenopausal women. *J. Clin. Endocrinol. Metab.* **68**, 364–368.

81. Hustmeyer, F. G., Walker, E., Xu, X. P., Girasole, G., Sakagami, Y., Peacock, M., and Manolagas, S. C. (1993). Cytokine production and surface antigen expression by peripheral blood mononuclear cells in postmenopausal osteoporosis. *J. Bone Miner. Res.* **8**, 1135–1141.

82. Fiore, C. E., Falcidia, E., Foti, R., Motta, M., and Tamburino, C. (1994). Differences in the time course of the effects of oophorectomy in women on parameters of bone metabolism and interleukin-1 levels in the circulation. *Bone Miner.* **20**, 79–85.

83. McKane, W. R., Khosla, S., Peterson, J. M., Egan, K., and Riggs, B. L. (1994). Circulating levels of cytokines that modulate bone resorption: Effects of age and menopause in women. *J. Bone Miner. Res.* **9**, 1313–1318.

84. Khosla, S., Peterson, J. M., Egan, K., Jones, J. D., and Riggs, B. L. (1994). Circulating cytokine levels in osteoporotic and normal women. *J. Clin. Endocrinol. Metab.* **79**, 707–711.

85. Kimble, R. B., Vannice, J. L., Bloedow, D. C., Thompson, R. C., Hopfer, W., Kung, V. T., Brownfield, C., and Pacifici, R. (1994). Interleukin-1 receptor antagonist decreases bone loss and bone resorption in ovariectomized rats. *J. Clin. Invest.* **93**, 1959–1967.

86. Kitazawa, R., Kimble, R. B., Vannice, J. L., Kung, V. T., and Pacifici, R. (1994). Interleukin-1 receptor antagonist and tumor necrosis factor binding protein decrease osteoclast formation and bone resorption in ovariectomized mice. *J. Clin. Invest.* **94**, 2397–2406.

87. Lorenzo, J. A., Naprta, A., Rao, Y., Alander, C., Glaccum, M., Widmer, M., Gronowicz, G., Kalinowski, J., and Pilbeam, C. C. (1998). Mice lacking the type I interleukin-1 receptor do not lose bone mass after ovariectomy. *Endocrinology* **139**, 3022–3025.

88. Pilbeam, C., Rao, Y., Alander, C., Voznesensky, O., Okada, Y., Sims, J. E., Raisz, L., and Lorenzo, J. (1997). Downregulation of mRNA expression for the "Decoy" interleukin-1 receptor 2 by ovariectomy in mice. *J. Bone Miner. Res.* **12** (Suppl. 1), S433 (abstr.).

89. Sunyer, T., Lewis, J., and Osdoby, P. (1997). Estrogen decreases the steady state levels of the IL-1 signaling receptor (Type I) while increasing those of the IL-1 decoy receptor (Type II) mRNAs in human osteoclast-like cells. *J. Bone Miner. Res.* **12** (Suppl. 1), S135 (abstr.).

90. Iwamoto, M., Koike, T., Nakashima, K., Sato, K., and Kato, Y. (1989). Interleukin 1: A regulator of chondrocyte proliferation. *Immunol. Lett.* **21**, 153–156.

91. Morales, T. I., and Hascall, V. C. (1989). Effects of interleukin-1 and lipopolysaccharides on protein and carbohydrate metabolism in bovine articular cartilage organ cultures. *Connect. Tissue Res.* **19**, 255–275.

92. Grumbles, R. M., Shao, L., Jeffrey, J. J., and Howell, D. S. (1996). Regulation of rat interstitial collagenase gene expression in growth cartilage and chondrocytes by vitamin D3, interleukin-1 beta, and okadaic acid. *J. Cell. Biochem.* **63**, 395–409.

93. Kato, Y., Nakashima, K., Iwamoto, M., Murakami, H., Hiranuma, H., Koike, T., Suzuki, F., Fuchihata, H., Ikehara, Y., and Noshiro, M. (1993). Effects of interleukin-1 on syntheses of alkaline phosphatase, type X collagen, and 1,25-dihydroxyvitamin D3 receptor, and matrix calcification in rabbit chondrocyte cultures. *J. Clin. Invest.* **92**, 2323–2330.

94. Horan, J., Dean, D. D., Kieswetter, K., Schwartz, Z., and Boyan, B. D. (1996). Evidence that interleukin-1, but not interleukin-6, affects costochondral chondrocyte proliferation, differentiation, and matrix synthesis through an autocrine pathway. *J. Bone Miner. Res.* **11**, 1119–1129.

95. Dean, D. D., Schwartz, Z., Muniz, O. E., Arsenis, C. H., Boyan, B. D., and Howell, D. S. (1997). Interleukin-1alpha and beta in growth plate cartilage are regulated by vitamin D metabolites in vivo. *J. Bone Miner. Res.* **12**, 1560–1569.

96. Vargas, S. J., Naprta, A., Glaccum, M., Lee, S. K., Kalinowski, J., and Lorenzo, J. A. (1996). Interleukin-6 expression and histomorphometry of bones from mice deficient for receptors for interleukin-1 or tumor necrosis factor. *J. Bone Miner. Res.* **11**, 1736–1744.

97. Beutler, B., and Cerami, A. (1986). Cachectin and tumour necrosis factor as two sides of the same biological coin. *Nature* **320**, 584–588.

98. Oliff, A. (1988). The role of tumor necrosis factor (cachectin) in cachexia. *Cell* **54**, 141–142.

99. Beutler, B., and Cerami, A. (1987). Cachectin: More than a tumor necrosis factor. *N. Engl. J. Med.* **316**, 379–385.

100. Old, L. J. (1985). Tumor necrosis factor (TNF). *Science* **230**, 630–632.

101. Paul, N. L., and Ruddle, N. H. (1988). Lymphotoxin. *Annu. Rev. Immunol.* **6**, 407–438.

102. Bertolini, D. R., Nedwin, G. E., Bringman, T. S., Smith, D. D., and Mundy, G. R. (1986). Stimulation of bone resorption and inhibition of bone formation in vitro by human tumour necrosis factors. *Nature* **319**, 516–518.

103. Tashjian, A. H., Jr., Voelkel, E. F., Lazzaro, M., Goad, D., Bosma, T., and Levine, L. (1987). Tumor necrosis factor-alpha (Cachectin) stimulates bone resorption in mouse calvaria via a prostaglandin-mediated mechanism. *Endocrinology* **120**, 2029–2036.

104. Canalis, E. (1987). Effects of tumor necrosis factor on bone formation in vitro. *Endocrinology* **121**, 1596–1604.

105. Gowen, M., Chapman, K., Littlewood, A., Hughes, D., Evans, D., and Russell, R. G. G. (1990). Production of tumor necrosis factor by human osteoblasts is modulated by other cytokines, but not by osteotropic hormones. *Endocrinology* **126**, 1250–1255.

106. Fiers, W. (1993). Tumor necrosis factor. *In* "The Natural Immune System: Humoral Factors" (E. Sim, ed.), pp. 65–119. IRL Press at Oxford University Press, Oxford.

107. Rickard, D., Russell, G., and Gowen, M. (1992). Oestradiol inhibits the release of tumour necrosis factor but not interleukin 6 from adult human osteoblasts in vitro. *Osteoporosis Int.* **2**, 94–102.

108. Chaudhary, L. R., Spelsberg, T. C., and Riggs, B. L. (1992). Production of various cytokines by normal human osteoblast-like cells in response to interleukin-1β and tumor necrosis factor-α: Lack of regulation by 17β-estradiol. *Endocrinology* **130**, 2528–2534.

109. Pacifici, R., Brown, C., Puscheck, E., Friedrich, E., Slatopolsky, E., Maggio, D., McCracken, R., and Avioli, L. V. (1991). Effect of surgical menopause and estrogen replacement on cytokine release from human blood mononuclear cells. *Proc. Natl. Acad. Sci. U.S.A.* **88**, 5134–5138.

110. Cohen-Solal, M. E., Graulet, A. M., Denne, M. A., Gueris, J., Baylink, D., and De Vernejoul, M.C. (1993). Peripheral monocyte culture supernatants of menopausal women can induce bone resorption: Involvement of cytokines. *J. Clin. Endocrinol. Metab.* **77**, 1648–1653.

111. Kimble, R. B., Bain, S. D., Kung, V., and Pacifici, R. (1995). Inhibition of IL-6 activity in genetically normal mice does not prevent ovariectomy-induced bone loss. *J. Bone Miner. Res.* **10**, S160 (abstr.).

112. Ammann, P., Rizzoli, R., Bonjour, J. P., Bourrin, S., Meyer, J. M., Vassalli, P., and Garcia I. (1997). Transgenic mice expressing soluble tumor necrosis factor-receptor are protected against bone loss caused by estrogen deficiency. *J. Clin. Invest.* **99**, 1699–1703.

113. Saklatvala, J. (1986). Tumour necrosis factor alpha stimulates resorption and inhibits synthesis of proteoglycan in cartilage. *Nature* **322**, 547–549.

114. Lefebvre, V., Peeters-Joris, C., and Vaes, G. (1991). Production of gelatin-degrading matrix metalloproteinases ('type IV collagenases') and inhibitors by articular chondrocytes during their dedifferentiation by serial subcultures and under stimulation by interleukin-1 and tumor necrosis factor α. *Biochim. Biophys. Acta Mol. Cell Res.* **1094**, 8–18.

115. Shinmei, M., Masuda, K., Kikuchi, T., and Shimomura, Y. (1989). Interleukin 1, tumor necrosis factor, and interleukin 6 as mediators of cartilage destruction. *Semin. Arthritis Rheum.* **18**, 27–32.

116. Enomoto, M., Pan, H. O, Kinoshita, A., Yutani, Y., Suzuki, F., and Takigawa, M. (1990). Effects of tumor necrosis factor alpha on proliferation and expression of differentiated phenotypes in rabbit costal chondrocytes in culture. *Calcif. Tissue Int.* **47**, 145–151.

117. Hashimoto, J., Yoshikawa, H., Takaoka, K., Shimizu, N., Masuhara, K., Tsuda, T., Miyamoto, S., and Ono, K. (1989). Inhibitory effects of tumor necrosis factor alpha on fracture healing in rats. *Bone* **10**, 453–457.

118. Akira, S., Hirano, T., Taga, T., and Kishimoto, T. (1990). Biology of multifunctional cytokines: IL-6 and related molecules (IL-1 and TNF). *FASEB J.* **4**, 2860–2867.

119. Hirano, T., Akira, S., Taga, T., and Kishimoto, T. (1990). Biological and clinical aspects of interleukin 6. *Immunol. Today* **11**, 443–449.

120. Feyen, J. H., Elford, P., Di Padova, F. E., and Trechsel, U. (1989). Interleukin-6 is produced by bone and modulated by parathyroid hormone. *J. Bone Miner. Res.* **4**, 633–638.

121. Lowik, C. W., Van der Pluijm, P. G., Bloys, H., Hoekman, K., Bijvoet, O. L., Aarden, L. A., and Papapoulos, S. E. (1989). Parathyroid hormone (PTH) and PTH-like protein (PLP) stimulate interleukin-6 production by osteogenic cells: A possible role of interleukin-6 in osteoclastogeneis. *Biochem. Biophys. Res. Commun.* **162**, 1546–1552.

122. Ishimi, Y., Miyaura, C., Jin, C. H., Akatsu, T., Abe, E., Nakamura, Y., Yamaguchi, A., Yoshiki, S., Matsuda, T., Hirano, T., Kishimoto, T., and Suda, T. (1990). IL-6 is produced by osteoblasts and induces bone resorption. *J. Immunol.* **145**, 3297–3303.

123. Girasole, G., Jilka, R. L., Passeri, G., Boswell, S., Boder, G., Williams, D. C., and Manolagas, S. C. (1992). 17β-Estradiol inhibits interleukin-6 production by bone marrow-derived stromal cells and osteoblasts in vitro: A potential mechanism for the antiosteoporotic effect of estrogens. *J. Clin. Invest.* **89**, 883–891.

124. Kishimoto, T., Taga, T., and Akira, S. (1994). Cytokine signal transduction. *Cell* **76**, 253–262.

125. Tamura, T., Udagawa, N., Takahashi, N., Miyaura, C., Tanaka, S., Yamada, Y., Koishihara, Y., Ohsugi, Y., Kumaki, K., Taga, T., Kishimoto, T., and Suda, T. (1993). Soluble interleukin-6 receptor triggers osteoclast formation by interleukin 6. *Proc. Natl. Acad. Sci. U.S.A.* **90**, 11924–11928.

126. Al-Humidan, A., Ralston,S. H., Hughes, D. E., Chapman, K., Aarden, L., Russell, R. G. G., and Gowen, M. (1991). Interleukin-6 does not stimulate bone resorption in neonatal mouse calvariae. *J. Bone Miner. Res.* **6**, 3–8.

127. Roodman, G. D. (1992). Interleukin-6: An osteotropic factor? *J. Bone Miner. Res.* **7**, 475–478.

128. Manolagas, S. C., and Jilka, R. L. (1995). Mechanisms of disease: Bone marrow, cytokines, and bone remodeling–Emerging insights into the pathophysiology of osteoporosis. *N. Engl. J. Med.* **332**, 305–311.

129. Devlin, R. D., Reddy, S. V., Savino, R., Ciliberto, G., and Roodman, G. D. (1998). IL-6 mediates the effects of IL-1 or TNF, but not PTHrP or 1,25(OH)$_2$D$_3$, on osteoclast-like cell formation in normal human bone marrow cultures. *J. Bone Miner. Res.* **13**, 393–399.

130. Black, K., Garrett, I. R., and Mundy, G. R. (1991). Chinese hamster ovary cells transfected with the murine interleukin-6 gene cause hypercalcemia as well as cachexia, leukocytosis and thrombocytosis in tumor bearing nude mice. *Endocrinology* **128**, 2657–2659.

131. De La Mata, J., Uy, H. L., Guise T. A., Story, B., Boyce, B. F., Mundy, G. R., and Roodman, G. D. (1995). Interleukin-6 enhances hypercalcemia and bone resorption mediated by parathyroid hormone-related protein in vivo. *J. Clin. Invest.* **95**, 2846–2852.

132. Roodman, G. D., Kurihara, N., Ohsaki, Y., Kukita, A., Hosking, D., Demulder, A., Smith, J. F., and Singer, F. R. (1992). Interleukin 6. A potential autocrine/paracrine factor in Paget's disease of bone. *J. Clin. Invest.* **89**, 46–52.

133. Guise, T. A., and Mundy, G. R. (1998). Cancer and bone. *Endocr. Rev.* **19**, 18–54.

134. Yamamoto, T., Ozono, K., Kasayama, S., Yoh, K., Hiroshima, K., Takagi, M., Matsumoto, S., Michigami, T., Yamaoka, K., Kishimoto, T., and Okada, S. (1996). Increased IL-6-production by cells isolated from the fibrous bone dysplasia tissues in patients with McCune-Albright syndrome. *J. Clin. Invest.* **98**, 30–35.

135. Reddy, S. V., Takahashi, S., Dallas, M., Williams, R. E., Neckers, L., and Roodman, G. D. (1994). Interleukin-6 antisense deoxyoligonucleotides inhibit bone resorption by giant cells from human giant cell tumors of bone. *J. Bone Miner. Res.* **9**, 753–757.

136. Devlin, R. D., Bone, H. G., III, and Roodman, G. D. (1996). Interleukin-6: A potential mediator of the massive osteolysis in patients with Gorham-Stout disease. *J. Clin. Endocrinol. Metab.* **81**, 1893–1897.

137. Littlewood, A. J., Aarden, L. A., Evans, D. B., Russell, R. G., and Gowen, M. (1991). Human osteoblastlike cells do not respond to interleukin-6. *J. Bone Miner. Res.* **6**, 141–148.

138. Franchimont, N., Gangji, V., Durant, D., and Canalis, E. (1997). Interleukin-6 with its soluble receptor enhances the expression of insulin-like growth factor-I in osteoblasts. *Endocrinology* **138**, 5248–5255.

139. Franchimont, N., Rydziel, S., Delany, A. M., and Canalis, E. (1997). Interleukin-6 and its soluble receptor cause a marked induction of collagenase 3 expression in rat osteoblast cultures. *J. Biol. Chem.* **272**, 12144–12150.

140. Franchimont, N., Durant, D., and Canalis, E. (1997). Interleukin-6 and its soluble receptor regulate the expression of insulin-like growth factor binding protein-5 in osteoblast cultures. *Endocrinology* **138**, 3380–3386.

141. Malaval, L., Gupta, A. K., Liu, F., Delmas, P. D., and Aubin, J. E. (1998). LIF, but not IL-6 regulates osteoprogenitor differentiation in rat calvaria cell cultures: Modulation by dexamethasone. *J. Bone Miner. Res.* **13**, 175–184.

142. Ray, A., Prefontaine, K. E., and Ray, P. (1994). Down-modulation of interleukin-6 gene expression by 17β- estradiol in the absence of high affinity DNA binding by the estrogen receptor. *J. Biol. Chem.* **269**, 12940–12946.

143. Pottratz, S. T., Bellido, T., Mocharla, H., Crabb, D., and Manolagas, S. C. (1994). 17β-estradiol inhibits expression of human interleukin-6 promoter-reporter constructs by a receptor-dependent mechanism. *J. Clin. Invest.* **93**, 944–950.

144. Jilka, R. L., Hangoc, G., Girasole, G., Passeri, G., Williams, D. C., Abrams, J. S., Boyce, B., Boxmeyer, H., and Manolagas, S. C. (1992). Increased osteoclast development after estrogen loss: Mediation by interleukin-6. *Science* **257**, 88–91.

145. Kimble, R. B., Bain, S., and Pacifici, R. (1997). The functional block of TNF but not of IL-6 prevents bone loss in ovariectomized mice. *J. Bone Miner. Res.* **12**, 935–941.

146. Poli, V., Balena, R., Fattori, E., Markatos, A., Yamamoto, M., Tanaka, H., Ciliberto, G., Rodan, G.A., and Costantini, F. (1994). Interleukin-6 deficient mice are protected from bone loss caused by estrogen depletion. *EMBO J.* **13**, 1189–1196.

147. Bellido, T., Jilka, R. L., Boyce, B. F., Girasole, G., Boxmeyer, H., Dalrymple, S. A., Murray, R., and Manalogas, S. C. (1995). Regulation of interleukin-6, osteoclastogenesis, and bone mass by androgens. The role of the androgen receptor. *J. Clin. Invest.* **95**, 2886–2895.

148. Vargas, S. J., Naprta, A., Lee, S. K., Kalinowski, J., Kawaguchi, H., Pilbeam, C. C., Raisz, L. G., and Lorenzo, J. A. (1996). Lack of evidence for an increase in interleukin-6 expression in adult murine bone, bone marrow, and marrow stromal cell cultures after ovariectomy. *J. Bone Miner. Res.* **11**, 1926–1934.

149. VanBezooijen, R. L., Farih-Sips, H. C., Papapoulos, S. E., and Lowik, C. W. (1998). IL-1alpha, IL-1beta, IL-6, and TNF-alpha steady-state mRNA levels analyzed by reverse transcription-competitive PCR in bone marrow of gonadectomized mice. *J. Bone Miner. Res.* **13**, 185–194.

150. Lin, S. C., Yamate, T., Taguchi, Y., Borba, V. C., Girasole, G., O'Brien, C. A., Bellido, T., Abe, E., and Manolagas, S. C. (1997). Regulation of the gp80 and gp130 subunits of the IL-6 receptor by sex steroids in the murine bone marrow. *J. Clin. Invest.* **100**, 1980–1990.

151. Saggese, G., Federico, G., and Cinquanta, L. (1993). In vitro effects of growth hormone and other hormones on chondrocytes and osteoblast-like cells. *Acta Paediatr.* **82** (Suppl. 391), 54–59; discussion: 60.

152. Guerne, P. A., Carson, D. A., and Lotz, M. (1990). IL-6 production by human articular chondrocytes. Modulation of its synthesis by cytokines, growth factors, and hormones in vitro. *J. Immunol.* **144**, 499–505.

153. Shingu, M., Miyauchi, S., Nagai, Y., Yasutake, C., and Horie, K. (1995). The role of IL-4 and IL-6 in IL-1-dependent cartilage matrix degradation. *Br. J. Rheumatol.* **34**, 101–106.

154. Lotz, M., and Guerne, P.-A. (1991). Interleukin-6 induces the synthesis of tissue inhibitor of metalloproteinases-1/erythroid potentiating activity (TIMP-1/EPA). *J. Biol. Chem.* **266**, 2017–2020.

155. Manolagas, S. C., Bellido, T., and Jilka, R. L. (1995). New insights into the cellular, biochemical, and molecular basis of postmenopausal and senile osteoporosis: Roles of IL-6 and gp130. *Int. J. Immunopharmacol.* **17**, 109–116.

156. Romas, E., Udagawa, N., Zhou, H., Tamura, T., Saito, M., Taga, T., Hilton, D. J., Suda, T., Ng, K. W., and Martin, T. J. (1996). The role of gp130-mediated signals in osteoclast development: Regulation of interleukin 11 production by osteoblasts and distribution of its receptor in bone marrow cultures. *J. Exp. Med.* **183**, 2581–2591.

157. Bellido, T., Stahl, N., Farruggella, T. J., Borba, V., Yancopoulos, G. D., and Manolagas, S. C. (1996). Detection of receptors for interleukin-6, interleukin-11, leukemia inhibitory factor, oncostatin M, and ciliary neurotrophic factor in bone marrow stromal osteoblastic cells. *J. Clin. Invest.* **97**, 431–437.

158. Elias, J. A., Tang, W., and Horowitz, M. C. (1995). Cytokine and hormonal stimulation of human osteosarcoma interleukin-11 production. *Endocrinology* **136**, 489–498.

159. Girasole, G., Passeri, G., Jilka, R. L., and Manolagas, S. C. (1994). Interleukin-11: A new cytokine critical for osteoclast development. *J. Clin. Invest.* **93**, 1516–1524.

160. Hill, P. A., Tumber, A., Papaioannou, S., and Meikle, M. C. (1998). The cellular actions of interleukin-11 on bone resorption *in vitro*. *Endocrinology* **139**, 1564–1572.

161. Morinaga, Y., Fujita, N., Ohishi, K., Zhang, Y., and Tsuruo, T. (1998). Suppression of interleukin-11-mediated bone resorption by cyclooxygenases inhibitors. *J. Cell. Physiol.* **175**, 247–254.

162. Hughes, F. J., and Howells, G. L. (1993). Interleukin-11 inhibits bone formation in vitro. *Calcif. Tissue Int.* **53**, 362–364.

163. Marusic, A., Kalinowski, J. F., Jastrzebski, S., and Lorenzo, J. A. (1993). Production of Leukemia inhibitory factor mRNA and protein by malignant and immortalized bone cells. *J. Bone Miner. Res.* **8**, 617–624.

164. Greenfield, E. M., Horowitz, M. C., and Lavish, S. A. (1996). Stimulation by parathyroid hormone of interleukin-6 and leukemia inhibitory factor expression in osteoblasts is an immediate-early gene response induced by cAMP signal transduction. *J. Biol. Chem.* **271**, 10984–10989.

165. Ishimi, Y., Abe, E., Jin, C. H., Miyaura, C., Hong, M. H., Oshida, M., Kurosawa, H., Yamaguchi, Y., Tomida, M., Hozumi, M., and Suda, T. (1992). Leukemia inhibitory factor/differentiation-stimulating factor (LIF/D-factor): Regulation of its production and possible roles in bone metabolism. *J. Cell. Physiol.* **152**, 71–78.

166. Reid, I. R., Lowe, C., Cornish, J., Skinner, S. J., Hilton, D. J., Willson, T. A., Gearing, D. P., and Martin, T. J. (1990). Leukemia inhibitory factor: A novel bone-active cytokine. *Endocinology* **126**, 1416–1420.

167. Lorenzo, J. A., Sousa, S. L., and Leahy, C. L. (1990). Leukemia inhibitory factor (LIF) inhibits basal bone resorption in fetal rat long bone cultures. *Cytokine* **2**, 266–271.

168. Van Beek, E., Van der Wee-Pals, L., van de Ruit, M., Nijweide, P., Papapoulos, S., and Lowik, C. (1993). Leukemia inhibitory factor inhibits osteoclastic resorption, growth, mineralization, and alkaline phosphatase activity in fetal mouse metacarpal bones in culture. *J. Bone Miner. Res.* **8**, 191–198.

169. Cornish, J., Callon, K. E., Edgar, S. G., and Reid, I. R. (1997). Leukemia inhibitory factor is mitogenic to osteoblasts. *Bone* **21**, 243–247.

170. Cornish, J., Callon, K., King, A., Edgar, S., and Reid, I. R. (1993). The effect of leukemia inhibitory factor on bone *in vivo*. *Endocrinology* **132**, 1359–1366.

171. Ware, C. B., Horowitz, M. C., Renshaw, B. R., Hunt, J. S., Liggitt, D., Koblar, S. A., Gliniak, B. C., McKenna, H. J., Papayannopoulou, T., Thoma, B., Cheng, L., Donovan, P. J., Peschon, J. J., Bartlett, P. F., Willis, C. R., Wright, B. D., Carpenter, M. K., Davison, B. L., and Gearing, D. P. (1995). Targeted disruption of the low-affinity leukemia inhibitory factor receptor gene causes placental, skeletal, neural and metabolic defects and results in perinatal death. *Development* **121**, 1283–1299.

172. Heymann, D., Guicheux, J., Gouin, F., Cottrel, M., and Daculsi, G. (1998). Oncostatin M stimulates macrophage-polykaryon formation in long-term human bone-marrow cultures. *Cytokine* **10**, 98–109.

173. Jay, P. R., Centrella, M., Lorenzo, J., Bruce, A. G., and Horowitz, M. C. (1996). Oncostatin-M: A new bone active cytokine that activates osteoblasts and inhibits bone resorption. *Endocrinology* **137**, 1151–1158.

174. Malik, N., Haugen, H. S., Modrell, B., Shoyab, M., and Clegg, C. H. (1995). Developmental abnormalities in mice transgenic for bovine oncostatin M. *Mol. Cell. Biol.* **15**, 2349–2358.

175. Mundy, G. R. (1996). An OAF by any other name. *Endocrinology* **137**, 1149–1150.

176. Bilbe, G., Roberts, E., Birch, M., and Evans, D. B. (1996). PCR phenotyping of cytokines, growth factors and their receptors and bone matrix proteins in human osteoblast-like cell lines. *Bone* **19**, 437–445.

177. Jilka, R. L., Weinstein, R. S., Bellido, T., Parfitt, A. M., and Manolagas, S. C. (1998). Osteoblast programmed cell death (apoptosis): Modulation by growth factors and cytokines. *J. Bone Miner. Res.* **13**, 793–802.

178. Kawasaki, K., Gao, Y. H., Yokose, S., Kaji, Y., Nakamura, T., Suda, T., Yoshida, K., Taga, T., Kishimoto, T., Kataoka, H., Yuasa, T., Norimatsu, H., and Yamaguchi, A. (1997). Osteoclasts are present in gp 130-deficient mice. *Endocrinology* **138**, 4959–4965.

179. Henrotin, Y. E., De, G. D., Labasse, A. H., Gaspar, S. E., Zheng, S. X., Geenen, V. G., and Reginster, J. Y. (1996). Effects of exogenous IL-1 beta, TNF alpha, IL-6, IL-8 and LIF on cytokine production by human articular chondrocytes. *Osteoarthritis Cartilage* **4**, 163–173.

180. Villiger, P. M., Geng, Y., and Lotz, M. (1993). Induction of cytokine expression by leukemia inhibitory factor. *J. Clin. Invest.* **91**, 1575–1581.

181. Hui, W., Bell, M., and Carroll, G. (1996). Oncostatin M (OSM) stimulates resorption and inhibits synthesis of proteoglycan in porcine articular cartilage explants. *Cytokine* **8**, 495–500.

182. Peterlik, M., Hoffmann, O., Swetly, P., Klaushofer, K., and Koller, K. (1985). Recombinant gamma-interferon inhibits prostaglandin-mediated and parathyroid hormone-induced bone resorption in cultured neonatal mouse calvaria. *FEBS Lett.* **185**, 287–290.

183. Gowen, M., and Mundy, G. R. (1986). Actions of recombinant interleukin 1, interleukin 2, and interferon-gamma on bone resorption in vitro. *J. Immunol.* **136**, 2478–2482.

184. Gowen, M., Nedwin, G. E., and Mundy, G. R. (1986). Preferential inhibition of cytokine-stimulated bone resorption by recombinant interferon gamma. *J. Bone Miner. Res.* **1**, 469–474.

185. Ralston, S. H., Ho, L.-P., Helfrich, M. H., Grabowski, P. S., Johnston, P. W., and Benjamin, N. (1995). Nitric oxide: A cytokine-induced regulator of bone resorption. *J. Bone Miner. Res.* **10**, 1040–1049.

186. Goldring, M. B., Sandell, L. J., Stephenson, M. L., and Krane, S. M. (1986). Immune interferon suppresses levels of procollagen mRNA and type II collagen synthesis in cultured human articular and costal chondrocytes. *J. Biol. Chem.* **261**, 9049–9056.

187. Reginato, A. M., Sanz-Rodriguez, C., Diaz, A., Dharmavaram, R. M., and Jimenez, S. A. (1993). Transcriptional modulation of cartilage-specific collagen gene expression by interferon gamma and tumour necrosis factor alpha in cultured human chondrocytes. *Biochem. J.* **294**, 761–769.

188. Goldring, M. B., Fukuo, K., Birkhead, J. R., Dudek, E., and Sandell, L. J. (1994). Transcriptional suppression by interleukin-1 and interferon-gamma of type II collagen gene expression in human chondrocytes. *J. Cell Biochem.* **54**, 85–99.

189. Andrews, H. J., Bunning, R. A. D., Plumpton, T. A., Clark, I. M., Russell, R. G. G., and Cawston, T. E. (1990). Inhibition of interleukin-1-induced collagenase production in human articular chondrocytes in vitro by recombinant human interferon-gamma. *Arthritis Rheum.* **33**, 1733–1738.

190. Verbruggen, G., Malfait, A. M., Veys, E. M., Gyselbrecht, L., Lambert, J., and Almqvist K. F. (1993). Influence of interferon-gamma on isolated chondrocytes from human articular cartilage. Dose dependent inhibition of cell proliferation and proteoglycan synthesis. *J. Rheumatol.* **20**, 1020–1026.

191. Dodge, G. R., Diaz, A., Sanz-Rodriguez, C., Reginato, A. M., and Jimenez, S. A. (1998). Effects of interferon-gamma and tumor necrosis factor alpha on the expression of the genes encoding aggrecan, biglycan, and decorin core proteins in cultured human chondrocytes. *Arthritis Rheum.* **41**, 274–283.

192. Chaudhary, L. R., and Avioli, L. V. (1995). Dexamethasone regulates IL-1-beta and TNF-alpha-induced interleukin-8 production in human bone marrow stromal and osteoblast-like cells. *Calcif. Tissue Int.* **55**, 16–20.

193. Zhu, J.-F., Valente, A. J., Lorenzo, J. A., Carnes, D., and Graves, D. T. (1994). Expression of monocyte chemoattractant protein 1 in human osteoblastic cells stimulated by proinflammatory mediators. *J. Bone Miner. Res.* **9**, 1123–1130.

194. Takeshita, A., Hanazawa, S., Amano, S., Matumoto, T., and Kitano, S. (1993). IL-1 induces expression of monocyte chemoattractant JE in clonal mouse osteoblastic cell line MC3T3-E1. *J. Immunol.* **150**, 1554–1562.

195. Lewis, D. B., Liggitt, H. D., Effmann, E. L., Motley, S. T., Teitelbaum, S. L., Jepsen, K. J., Goldstein, S. A., Bonadio, J., Carpenter, J., and Perlmutter, R. M. (1993). Osteoporosis induced in mice by overproduction of interleukin 4. *Proc. Natl. Acad. Sci. U.S.A.* **90**, 11618–11622.

196. Shioi, A., Teitelbaum, S. L., Ross, F. P., Welgus, H. G., Suzuki, H., Ohara, J., and Lacey, D. L. (1991). Interleukin 4 inhibits murine osteoclast formation in vitro. *J. Cell. Biochem.* **47**, 272–277.

197. Nakano, Y., Watanabe, K., Morimoto, I., Okada, Y., Ura, K., Sato, K., Kasono, K., Nakamura, T., and Eto, S. (1994). Interleukin-4 inhibits spontaneous and parathyroid hormone-related protein-stimulated osteoclast formation in mice. *J. Bone Miner. Res.*, **9**, 1533–1539.

198. Okada, Y., Morimoto, I., Ura, K., Nakano, Y., Tanaka, Y., Nishida, S., Nakamura, T., and Eto, S. (1998). Short-term treatment of recombinant murine interleukin-4 rapidly inhibits bone formation in normal and ovariectomized mice. *Bone* **22**, 361–365.

199. Van Vlasselaer, P., Borremans, B., Van Der Heuvel, R., Van Gorp, U., and De Waal Malefyt, R. (1993). Interleukin-10 inhibits the osteogenic activity of mouse bone marrow. *Blood* **82**, 2361–2370.

200. Owens, J., and Chambers, T. J. (1995). Differential regulation of osteoclast formation: interleukin 10 (cytokine synthesis inhibitory factor) suppresses formation of osteoclasts but not macrophages in murine bone marrow cultures. *J. Bone Miner. Res.* **10**, S220 (abstr.).

201. Onoe, Y., Miyaura, C., Kaminakayashiki, T., Nagai, Y., Noguchi, K., Chen, Q. R., Seo, H., Ohta, H., Nozawa, S., Kudo, I., and Suda, T. (1996). IL-13 and IL-4 inhibit bone resorption by suppressing cyclooxygenase-2-dependent prostaglandin synthesis in osteoblasts. *J. Immunol.* **156**, 758–764.

202. Lind, M., Deleuran, B., Yssel, H., Fink-Eriksen, E., and Thestrup-Pedersen, K. (1995). IL-4 and IL-13, but not IL-10, are chemotactic factors for human osteoblasts. *Cytokine* **7**, 78–82.

203. Udagawa, N., Horwood, N. J., Elliott, J., Mackay, A., Owens, J., Okamura, H., Kurimoto, M., Chambers, T. J., Martin, T. J., and Gillespie, M. T. (1997). Interleukin-18 (interferon-gamma-inducing factor) is produced by osteoblasts and acts via granulocyte/macrophage colony-stimulating factor and not via interferon-gamma to inhibit osteoclast formation. *J. Exp. Med.* **185**, 1005–1012.

204. Horwood, N. J., Udagawa, N., Elliott, J., Grail, D., Okamura, H., Kurimoto, M., Dunn, A. R., Martin, T., and Gillespie, M. T. (1998). Interleukin 18 inhibits osteoclast formation via T cell production of granulocyte macrophage colony-stimulating factor. *J. Clin. Invest.* **101**, 595–603.

CHAPTER 8

Integrins and Adhesion Molecules

M. H. HELFRICH   Department of Medicine and Therapeutics, University of Aberdeen, Foresterhill,
Aberdeen AB25 2ZD, United Kingdom

M. A. HORTON   Bone and Mineral Centre, Department of Medicine, The Rayne Institute,
London WC1E 6JJ, United Kingdom

I. ABSTRACT

Adhesion molecules play an important role in the development and function of all bone cell types. Here we discuss the repertoire of integrins, cadherins, Ig superfamily members, and cell surface proteoglycans expressed by osteoblasts, osteocytes, osteoclasts, and chondrocytes. Detailed information is available regarding integrin expression and, in particular, osteoclast integrin function has been well studied. Information about expression of other classes of adhesion molecules, however, is fragmented. The available data are summarized and possible functions for adhesion molecules in skeletal cells are discussed in this chapter.

II. INTRODUCTION

Connective tissue cells in general and bone and cartilage cells in particular are surrounded by an abundance of extracellular matrix. Chondroblasts, osteoblasts, and to a lesser extent osteocytes are responsible for the synthesis of the majority of the organic components of this matrix, whereas osteoclasts mainly degrade the matrix. The function of bone and cartilage cells reflects the matrix components which surround them and conversely, the composition of the matrix (i.e., the structure of cartilage and bone) is highly dependent upon the cellular function of chondroblasts, osteoblasts, and osteoclasts. Cell-matrix and cell-cell interactions are mediated by adhesion molecules and much information has become available regarding the expression and role of one class of adhesion molecules in bone, the integrins. Much less is known about possible roles for other classes of adhesion molecules, but it is clear that a number of nonintegrin adhesion molecules, including cadherins and members of the immunoglobulin family, are expressed in bone and cartilage cells. Adhesion molecules not only play a part in the function of fully differentiated cells in the skeleton, but are also increasingly implicated in their developmental pathways (for examples of possible roles for adhesion molecules in bone, see Fig. 1). In this chapter, we discuss the expression and function of the major adhesion molecules in bone and cartilage, focusing on data obtained with human tissue and discussing data from rodents and other species where little or no information in human tissue is available.

III. MOLECULAR STRUCTURE OF ADHESION MOLECULES

The main classes of adhesion molecules implicated in bone and cartilage turnover are given in Table I. Adhesion molecules are classified according to structural homologies [1, 2] and some basic features of the main groups are discussed below.

A. Integrins

The integrin family consists of receptors that share as basic structure two noncovalently linked transmembrane glycoproteins (α and β subunits). Both subunits have a single transmembrane domain and, with the exception of $\beta4$, have short cytoplasmic regions. Electron microscopic studies on the fibronectin receptor $\alpha5\beta1$ [3] showed that the large extracellular domain is organized as a globular head supported by a stalk, and both parts are composed of the α and β subunits. The ligand binding site is localized in the globular domain and requires determinants on the α and β subunit. The external dimensions of the receptor are $\sim 10 \times 20$ nm. This basic three-dimensional structure has now been confirmed in a number of integrins. Initial classification of integrins based on shared β subunits proved too rigid because both α and β subunits may be associated with more than one partner, thus forming receptors with distinct ligand binding capabilities. At present, 22 integrins are known, formed from 16 different α and eight different β subunits. The β subunits have higher cDNA sequence homology than the α subunits. They contain 56 cysteine residues (except $\beta4$ which has 48), which are organized into four 40-amino-acid long segments that are internally disulphide bonded. Their molecular masses range from 90–110 kDa, except for $\beta4$ which has a much longer cytoplasmic domain and hence a molecular mass of 210 kDa. The α subunits contain seven homologous repeating domains, with three or four of these containing divalent cation binding sites. These cation binding sites, together with one such site in the β subunit, are critically important for ligand binding and also play a role in receptor stability. Some subunits (CD11 a,b,c, $\alpha1$, and $\alpha2$) contain an extra 200 amino acids inserted between repeats 2 and 3, known as the I domain. Most other α subunits are posttranslationally cleaved into heavy and light fragments which are disulphide linked. Ligands for integrins include a wide range of extracellular matrix proteins and immunoglobulin family members such as VCAM and ICAM. Most integrins can bind more than one ligand and often this is through recognition of a common sequence. In many extra-

cellular matrix molecules this is an RGD peptide sequence, although in other proteins, sequences such as DGEA (in collagen) or LDV (in fibronectin) are the recognition sites for integrins. Integrins are linked to the cytoskeleton via interaction of the β subunit with actin-binding proteins α-actinin, vinculin, and talin. The cytoplasmic domain of the β subunit also associates with a signaling complex comprising kinases, phosphatases, and various adaptor proteins. Most information regarding signaling via integrins has come from studies in cells such as fibroblasts and osteosarcoma cell lines which produce focal contacts *in vitro*. Here, the most studied kinase present is focal adhesion kinase FAK which associates directly with the β subunit. Upon occupation of the integrin receptor, FAK is targeted to focal adhesions where it associates with the cytoskeleton and is activated by autophosphorylation. Downstream signaling pathways include association of Src family kinases with phosphorylated FAK and engagement of the Ras-MAP kinase pathway [4].

B. Cadherins

Cadherins are a rapidly growing family of calcium-dependent proteins that play prominent roles in morphogenesis. They are divided into at least three subsets of receptors: the classical cadherins, desmocollins, and desmogleins [5, 6]. In addition, protocadherins and a number of *Drosophila* gene products with cadherin-like sequences are part of this family. Cadherins are calcium-dependent single chain transmembrane glycoproteins that share several regions of high homology, with the greatest homology found in the short cytoplasmic domain. The extracellular domain contains 3-5 repeats of around 110 amino acids which contain negatively charged, calcium-binding motifs in the first three repeats and conserved cysteine residues in the fifth repeat. Cadherins are divided into subclasses (main members are E-, N-, M- and P-cadherin), all of which share this common structure and have molecular masses of around 100–130 kDa. The ligand binding site of cadherins is the conserved HAV motif located at the N-terminal region of the molecule in the first conserved extracellular repeat. Cadherins are mediators of cell–cell adhesion and bind ligand mainly in a homophilic manner, although heterophilic binding between different cadherin molecules is possible. As with integrins, cells often express a repertoire of different cadherins simultaneously. On the cell surface, cadherins tend to be concentrated at cell-cell junctions where they can associate with members of the Src kinase family leading to activation of signaling pathways [1]. The main function of cadherins is in the organization of solid tissues and during morphogenesis.

C. Ig Family Members

The immunoglobulin (Ig) family of receptors all share a basic motif consisting of an Ig fold of between 70 and 110 amino acids [7, 8] organized into two antiparallel β sheets which seem to serve as a scaffold on which unique determinants can be displayed. There is considerable variation in the primary structure of the members of this family and hence in their molecular masses, but their tertiary structure is well conserved. There are well over 70 members of this family known, all with different numbers of the basic Ig repeats. Their functions are wide ranging; some members function as true signal transducing receptors, whereas others have predominantly adhesive functions. Ligands for Ig family members include other Ig family members (identical, as well as nonidentical members), but also members of the integrin family and components of the extracellular matrix. Signaling pathways activated by Ig family members are not well established yet, but as discussed above, they appear to include Src kinases [1].

D. Syndecans

Syndecans are a family of cell surface proteoglycans. They are characterized by a shared heparan sulfate attachment sequence at the N terminus of their single polypeptide chain. There is little homology in the rest of their extracellular domain, but their single transmembrane domain and cytoplasmic domains are highly conserved. The cytoplasmic domain contains four conserved tyrosine residues, suggesting that phosphorylation of this domain could occur and could be involved in signal transduction events. However, syndecans are thought to function predominantly as coreceptors for other receptors such as integrins, members of the fibroblast growth factor family, and vascular endothelial cell growth factor, which all need heparan sulfate for signaling (see Chapter 6). In such situations, the signaling is thought to occur via the cytoplasmic domains of associated receptors rather than via the syndecan molecule [9]. There are four mammalian syndecans known, with syndecan-1 best studied so far. Syndecan-1 can function as a cell-matrix receptor binding various matrix proteins (type I collagen, fibronectin, tenascin), and in addition it can bind members of the FGF family. It appears that in different cell types, syndecan-1 can have different patterns of glycosaminoglycans attached to its core protein, which influences the ligand binding capabilities. Thus, where in one cell type syndecan-1 may contain heparan sulfate as well as chondroitin sulfate side chains and bind collagen, this may not be the case in another cell type in which it has heparan sulfate side chains only. The functions of syndecans are varied and include roles in cell-matrix interaction and cell proliferation [10].

E. CD44

CD44, also known as the hyaluronate receptor, is a family of transmembrane glycoproteins with molecular masses of 85–250 kDa. They share an N-terminal region which is related to the cartilage proteoglycan core and link proteins. Alternative splicing of ten exons and extensive posttranslational modification such as glycosylation and addition of chondroitin sulfate produces the wide variety of CD44 proteins. Chondroitin sulfate-containing variants can bind fibronectin, laminin, and collagen in addition to hyaluronate, and CD44 binding to osteopontin has also been reported [11]. Finally, CD44 may also bind homotypically. CD44 functions, therefore, in a variety of ways, including in cell–cell interactions (homing of lymphocytes or cell clustering), but also in cell–matrix adhesion. Malignant transformation of cells leads to upregulation of CD44 expression, and metastatic tumors often express an altered repertoire of CD44 variants.

F. Selectins

Selectins are a family of three closely related glycoproteins (P- and E-selectin are expressed in endothelial cells and L-selectin is expressed in leukocytes). Their common structure consists of an N-terminal Ca^{2+}-dependent lectin-type domain, an EGF domain and variable numbers of short repeats homologous to complement binding sequences, a single transmembrane region, and a short cytoplasmic domain. Their molecular masses range from 74–240 kDa, with differently glycosylated forms expressed in different cell types. In general, the function of selectins is in leukocyte trafficking. They are thought to be involved in the earliest stages of leukocyte extravasation, where binding of the selectin ligand on the leukocyte to selectins expressed on the endothelial surface results in "rolling" of leukocytes over the endothelial surface. These functions have now been confirmed in selectin knockout mice for L- and P-selectin. In a double knock-out for E- and P-selectin, it appeared that E-selectin also contributed to leukocyte homeostasis [12]. Other functions for selectins include roles in $\beta2$ integrin activation and O_2^- production by leukocytes [8]. Selectin ligands are specific oligosaccharide sequences in sialated and often sulfated glycans, such as sialyl-Lewis^x. There is, however, still considerable uncertainty about the natural ligands for selectins, since most ligands have been identified in *in vitro* assays, using recombinant selectins presented in multimeric form or in clustered arrays, which increases affinity for ligand but has no known *in vivo* equivalent. In addition, few of the ligands thus identified have been shown to mediate biological interactions [13]. Some molecules which seem to fulfill most of the criteria for true selectin ligands (i.e., with confirmation of a biological role) are P-selectin glycoprotein ligand-1 (PSGL-1), which, when expressed in the neutrophil surface in a properly glycosylated and tyrosine sulfated form, can bind to P-selectin in vasular endothelium and to L-selectin on other neutrophils and enable "rolling" over either surface. CD34, GlyCAM-1, and MAdCAM-1 are other candidate ligands (again, when correctly glycosylated and sulfated) for L-selectin. The signal transduction pathways linked to selectins are only partially elucidated and have been reviewed in Crockett-Torabi [14]. As with the other classes of adhesion molecules discussed above, they include tyrosine phosphorylation cascades and increases in intracellular calcium concentrations.

IV. ADHESION MOLECULES IN CELLS OF THE OSTEOBLAST LINEAGE

A. Integrins

In vivo, osteoblasts in normal human bone have been reported to express $\beta1$ and $\beta5$ integrins (e.g., [15–17]), but there are controversies regarding the α subunits associated with $\beta1$ and concerning expression of $\alpha v\beta3$ (Table I). $\beta2$, $\beta4$, and $\beta6$ integrins have not been reported in osteoblastic cells. There are also considerable differences between various reports on the integrin repertoire expressed by osteoblasts *in situ*, by human osteoblast cultures, or by osteoblastic cell lines, and these are most likely due to the heterogeneity of the cell population under study and the different culture conditions employed. Moreover, there is preliminary information regarding the impact of osteoblast activation status (e.g., synthetic osteoblast versus bone lining cell), anatomical site (e.g., endochondral versus intramembranous bone), or disease, but no definitive studies are published. For example, it has been

TABLE I. Expression of Adhesion Molecules in Osteoblasts and Osteocytes

Adhesion molecule expressed	Osteoblasts *in vivo*	Key references	Osteoblasts *in vitro*[a]	Key references	Osteocytes *in vivo*	Key references	Species[b]
Integrins							
$\alpha1$ (CD49a)	+ (−)	[17] ([16, 49])	+	[17, 133–135]	−	[16]	H, R, Ch
$\alpha2$ (CD49b)	− (+)	[16, 17] ([49, 136])	+	[18, 134, 135, 137]	−	[16, 136]	H, P
$\alpha3$ (CD49c)	− (+)	[15, 16] ([17])	+ (−)	[17, 18, 134, 135, 137] ([15])	−	[16]	H
$\alpha4$ (CD49d)	+ (−)	[15, 16] ([17, 49])	+ (−)	[15, 135, 138] ([17])	+/−	[15, 16]	H
$\alpha5$ (CD49e)	+ (−)	[15, 16, 49, 136] ([17])	+ (−)	[15, 18, 135, 138, 139] ([17])	+	[15, 16]	H
$\alpha6$ (CD49f)	−	[16, 17, 49]	− (+)	[17, 138] ([18, 134])	−	[16]	H
$\beta1$ (CD29)	+	[16, 17, 49]	+	[17, 18, 21, 139]	+	[16, 20, 21]	H, R, Ch
$\beta2$ (CD18)	−	[17, 49]	−	[17, 138]	−	[16]	H
$\beta3$ (CD61)	−	[16, 17, 49]	+ (−)	[15, 18] ([17, 138])	−	[16]	H
$\beta4$ (CD104)	−	[16, 49]	ND		−	[16]	H
$\beta5$	+	[59]	+ (−)	[15, 134, 135, 139] ([30])	+/−	[15, 30]	H, R
αv (CD51)	+ (−)	[15, 16] ([17])	+	[15, 17, 18, 138, 139]	+/−	[15, 16]	H
$\alpha v\beta3$ (CD51/CD61)	−	[16, 49]	+/−	[134, 135]	−	[16]	H
$\alpha v\beta1$ (CD51/CD29)	ND		+	[135]	ND		H
αL (CD11a)	−	[17, 138]	−	[17, 138]	ND		H
αM (CD11b)	−	[17, 138]	−	[17, 138]	ND		H
Cadherins							
E-Cadherin	ND		−	[31]	ND		H
Cadherin-4	ND		+	[31]	ND		H
Cadherin-11 or Ob-Cadherin	ND		+	[31, 33, 33a]	ND		H, R
N-Cadherin	ND		+	[31]	ND		H
Cell surface proteoglycans							
Syndecan-1	ND		+	[38–40]	+	Helfrich, unpublished	H
Syndecan-2	ND		+	[38–40]	ND		H
Syndecan-4	ND		+	[38–40]	ND		H
CD44	+	[42, 43, 81]	+	[42, 45]	+	[41–44, 81]	H, R
Immunoglobulin family members							
ICAM-1 (CD54)	ND		+	[35]	ND		H
VCAM-I (CD106)	ND		+	[35]	ND		H
LFA-3	ND		+	[35]	ND		H
NCAM (CD56)	+	[34]	ND		−	[34]	Ch

Note. +, receptor expressed (immunocytochemically or biochemically). −, receptor not found to be expressed; +/−, expression levels very low or result unclear; ND, not tested. Where conflicting data exist, the most frequently reported pattern is given, with differing data between brackets with associated references between brackets.

[a] Pooled data from primary osteoblast cultures and osteosarcoma cell lines; differences between primary cultures and transformed osteoblasts and between various osteosarcoma lines have been reported, in particular in expression of $\alpha1$, $\alpha2$, $\alpha4$, and $\alpha6$ integrin [137, 138, 140].

[b] H, human; P, primate; R, rodent; Ch, chick.

clearly demonstrated that *in vitro*, the substrate on which cells are cultured directly influences the pattern of integrin expression by osteoblasts [18, 19]. Generally, cultured osteoblasts express a wider integrin repertoire than osteoblasts *in situ* and in particular, increased expression of the collagen binding integrin $\alpha2\beta1$, the fibronectin receptor $\alpha5\beta1$, and the vitronectin receptor $\alpha v\beta3$ is seen in cultured osteoblasts [15, 17]. It is unclear whether increased expression of these integrins has an equivalent in bone pathology, since osteoblast integrin expression in bone disease is relatively unexplored. Integrin expression in osteocytes has not been studied extensively, but there are some data from immunocytochemical analyses of human bone sections and from functional studies in the chick (Table I). Difficulties in interpretating immunocytochemical staining in bone sections, in particular for cells embedded within matrix, have been reported by many authors and this may well have contributed to the current controversies in integrin phenotype of osteoblasts/osteocytes. Future comprehensive studies which combine immunocytochemical, biochemical, and molecular techniques could resolve this issue, although absence of isolation or culture procedures for human osteocytes so far prohibits their biochemical and functional analysis.

In the chick, where isolation procedures for osteocytes have been developed, the osteocytes and osteoblasts were shown to bind to a comprehensive range of extracellular matrix proteins *in vitro* in a $\beta1$- and partially RGD-dependent way [20]. The exact receptor involved could not be determined because of lack of α chain-specific antibodies for avian integrins. Expression of $\beta1$ integrin has been confirmed in mammalian osteocytes [16, 21].

Functional studies on osteoblast integrins have included adhesion assays to a variety of extracellular matrix molecules and inhibition by RGD-containing peptides. In keeping with their extensive repertoire of integrins, rodent and human osteoblasts were found to adhere to osteopontin, bone sialoprotein, vitronectin, and fibronectin in an RGD-dependent way (with fibronectin requiring much higher concentrations of peptide for inhibition), whereas binding to type I collagen and thrombospondin was less inhibited by RGD peptides [15, 22, 23]. In organ cultures of mineralizing fetal rat parietal bone, RGD peptides decreased bone formation, which was accompanied by a decrease in $\alpha2$ and $\beta1$ expression and disruption of the organization in the osteoblast layer [24]. Downregulation of $\alpha2$ and $\beta1$ integrin expression in osteoblasts by glucocorticoids has also been noted with similar disruption in osteoblast organization, whereas IGF-1 increased $\beta1$ expression in osteoblasts and calcified bone formation [21, 25]. Functional studies on osteoblast integrins have included reports on their role in osteoblast differentiation. Moursi *et al.* [26] demonstrated convincingly that osteoblast–fibronectin interaction was a critical event in the differentiation of fetal rat osteoblasts in an *in vitro* model, and although the receptor involved was not formally identified, the importance of

the central cell-binding domain of fibronectin in this effect suggested that the specific fibronectin receptor $\alpha5\beta1$ was involved. These results confirm earlier work suggesting a role for $\alpha5\beta1$ in differentiation of the human osteoblastic cell line MG63 [27–29]. In addition to fibronectin, collagen is also implicated in osteoblast differentiation. Ganta *et al.* [30] showed that ascorbic acid deficiency, which leads to underhydroxylation of type I collagen, resulted in downregulation of $\alpha2\beta1$ in osteoblasts and dysregulation of differentiation and mineralization in cultures of rat calvaria. Clearly, in addition to providing an anchor for osteoblasts to the bone matrix, integrin-ligand interactions play a role in the differentiation of osteoblasts and, via yet unknown signaling pathways, in the expression of differentiation-associated genes.

B. Cadherins

Cell–cell interactions between osteoblastic cells themselves and osteoblasts and haemopoietic cells within the bone marrow compartment are known to be important in bone metabolism. Such interactions are likely to be governed by adhesion molecules such as cadherins. The repertoire of cadherins expressed by bone cells has not been systematically investigated, but a number of cadherins have been reported to be expressed (e.g., cadherin-4, cadherin-11, and N-cadherin). HAV peptides inhibited osteoblast matrix formation *in vitro*, suggesting a role for cadherins in osteoblastic activity [31, 32]. Also, a novel cadherin cloned from osteoblasts, Ob-cadherin [33], is expressed in osteoblasts as well as some other tissues, but is now known to be identical to cadherin-11 [33a]. Functional studies on Ob-cadherin have so far not been reported.

C. Ig Family Members

There is very limited information about expression of Ig family members in bone cells. Expression of NCAM (in chick), ICAM-1, VCAM-1, and LFA-3 (in human) has been reported [34, 35]. There is circumstantial evidence for expression of NCAM in human osteoblasts from studies in multiple myeloma. It was shown that direct cell–cell contact between human osteoblasts and myeloma cells, which express high levels of NCAM, resulted in stimulation of IL-6 production by osteoblasts. This effect could be blocked in part with NCAM antibodies [36]. These experiments suggest that human osteoblasts express NCAM and that the receptor may be involved in activation of gene regulation in these cells, although it must be remembered that other ligands for NCAM, such as heparan sulfate-containing molecules, are also expressed in osteoblasts (see below) and could have mediated this effect. Similarly, however, crosslinking of ICAM-1 or VCAM-1 resulted in the production of bone resorbing cytokines by osteoblasts [35], suggesting that in general, expression of Ig family members by osteoblasts may lead to direct cellular interaction with immune cells, which express their ligands (Table IV), and subsequently to activation of production of bone resorbing cytokines. There is also some evidence (discussed below) that VCAM-1 is involved in the development of osteoclasts *in vitro*, an effect that could be direct, or indirect via osteoblastic cells. Clearly we need to know more about the expression and functional roles of this important class of adhesion molecules in bone.

D. Syndecans

The expression of syndecans in bone has only recently received attention. Syndecan-3 expression seems predominantly confined to cartilage (see below) and periosteum during endochondral bone formation, although low levels were seen in osteoblasts and osteocytes close to periosteal surfaces [37]. mRNA for the three cloned human forms of syndecan, syndecan-1, -2, and -4, was found in a primary human osteoblast culture and a number of osteoblast cell lines [38–40]. Culture of osteoblastic cells under conditions that induced differentiation resulted in a decrease of syndecan-1 levels [39]. Osteocytes, however, still had detectable levels of syndecan-1, as shown by immunostaining with antibody B-B4 (M. H. Helfrich, unpublished data). Syndecan-2 has been implicated in the mitogenic effect of GM–CSF on human osteoblastic cells [38]. A role of syndecans in presentation of growth factors to their receptors could prove to be their most prominent function in bone, but this falls outside the scope of this chapter; however, syndecan-1 could also be an additional adhesion receptor regulating interaction of osteoblastic cells with the extracellular matrix, in particular with type I collagen. Demonstration of such a role awaits further functional studies.

E. CD44

CD44 has been found in humans and rodents to be expressed in osteoblasts and osteocytes at all stages of maturation; however, there appears to be a clear increase in expression levels with increasing maturation in this cell lineage, with low levels expressed in preosteoblastic cells and very high levels expressed in osteocytes [41, 42]. Detailed localization studies have shown that CD44 expression in mature osteoblasts is confined to cytoplasmic processes only [43]. By a variety of immunological and molecular techniques, only the standard form of CD44, CD44H, was found to be expressed in osteoblasts and osteocytes in rat bone [42, 44]; however, several isoforms of CD44 were described in the human osteoblastic cell line MG63 [45]. Expression of CD44 in cells of the osteoblastic lineage correlates well with the presence of hyaluronate in surrounding tissues [44], suggesting that the receptor may function as a hyaluronate binding

protein. *In vitro*, osteoblastic cells have indeed been shown to be able to bind to and degrade hyaluronate in the transition zone from cartilage to bone in the growth plate by a CD44-dependent mechanism [45]. However, a variety of other known ligands for CD44 (e.g., type I collagen, fibronectin, laminin, and osteopontin) are also produced by osteoblasts (Chapters 1–4) and osteocytes [46] and colocalize with the receptor, indicating that a much wider range of functions for this molecule may exist.

F. Selectins

There are no published data on expression of selectins in osteoblasts or their precursors. As discussed for osteoclasts below, selectins may well play a role in extravasation of the mesenchymal precursors of osteoblasts. In the absence of definitive markers for osteoblast precursors, however, such information is unavailable.

V. ADHESION MOLECULES IN OSTEOCLASTS

A. Integrins

The integrin repertoire expressed in mature osteoclasts is well defined and has been the subject of several reviews [47, 48]. Immunocytochemical, biochemical, and functional assays have been used to confirm the expression of three major integrin receptors in human osteoclasts: $\alpha v\beta 3$, $\alpha 2\beta 1$, and $\alpha v\beta 1$ (e.g. [49–52]), whereas expression of other subunits has been largely excluded (Table II). A novel β subunit expressed in osteoclasts has been described [53], and there is also evidence for an alternatively spliced $\beta 1$ subunit in osteoclasts [54]. The exact receptors formed with these novel subunits and their ligand binding properties still need to be elucidated.

Detailed localization studies have tried to determine whether an integrin is present in and possibly responsible for maintenance of the tight sealing zone in resorbing osteoclasts, but the data so far are conflicting. Although some studies have excluded the presence of $\alpha v\beta 3$ [48, 55] and $\alpha 2\beta 1$ [56] in the sealing zone, others have reported the presence of αv and/or $\beta 3$ subunits at this site [57–59]. It is clear, however, that none of the integrin receptors is enriched in the clear zone of resorbing osteoclasts and that the receptors are in fact most abundant on the basolateral membrane, where they may act as true receptors coupled to signal transduction pathways [56, 60, 61]. There is also high expression of integrins on the ruffled border membrane in resorbing osteoclasts [56, 60], suggesting that cell–matrix interactions at that site may be involved in the progression, or cessation, of resorption.

The role of the vitronectin receptor $\alpha v\beta 3$ in osteoclast biology has been extensively studied. It has become clear that

TABLE II. Expression of Adhesion Molecules in Osteoclasts

Adhesion molecule expressed	Mature osteoclasts *in vivo*	Osteoclast progenitors *in vitro*[a]	Key references	Species[b]
Integrins				
α2β1 (CD49b/CD19)	+		[47, 50]	H, R
αvβ3 (CD51/CD61)	+		[47, 50, 77]	H, R, Ch
αvβ1 (CD51/CD19)	+		[47, 50]	H, R
α1, α4, α6-9	−		[47]	H, R
α3 (CD49c)	− (+)		[47] ([141])	H
α5 (CD49d)	− (+)		[47] ([16, 77, 136, 141])	H, R, P, Ch
β2 (CD18), β4 (CD104), β6-β8	−		[47]	H, R
αvβ5	−	+	[47, 48]	H, R, Ch
αMβ2	−	+	[47, 48]	H, R
αL(CD11a), αX(CD11c)	−		[47]	H
Cadherins				
E-cadherin	+	+	[78]	R
N-cadherin	−		[78]	R
P-cadherin	−		[78]	R
Cell surface proteoglycans				
CD44	+	+	[41, 51, 81, 82]	H, R
Immunoglobulin family members				
ICAM-1 (CD54)	+		[51]	H
VCAM-I (CD106)	−	+	[142]	R

Note. +, receptor expressed (immunocytochemically or biochemically); −, receptor not found to be expressed. Where conflicting data exist, the most frequently reported pattern is given, with differing data between brackets with associated references between brackets. References given are mainly review papers.

[a] Data on osteoclast precursors are indirect, derived mainly from functional studies in heterogeneous cell populations.

[b] H, human; P, primate; R, rodent; Ch, chick.

mammalian osteoclasts can adhere to a wide range of extracellular matrix proteins known to be expressed in bone and bone marrow using this receptor (Table IV) and that an RGD peptide sequence forms the recognition site for the receptor in all these ligands. Which protein constitutes the natural ligand of osteoclasts in bone remains to be determined. Colocalization studies have suggested that osteopontin is a candidate [62], because it was found to be enriched underneath the clear zones of resorbing osteoclasts. However, since osteoclasts actively synthesize osteopontin [63], this finding should be interpreted with some reservation. RGD-containing peptides and snake venoms (echistatin and kistrin) have been shown to inhibit osteoclast polarization, activity, and formation *in vitro* [64–67] and they, as with vitronectin receptor antibodies, also block bone resorption in various rodent models *in vivo* [68–71] (reviewed in Horton and Rodan) [47]. *In vitro*, occupation of the vitronectin receptor by antibodies or RGD peptides causes osteoclasts to retract and detach from the matrix, similar to the shape changes observed after administration of the potent antiresorptive peptide hormone calcitonin. In mammalian osteoclasts, this effect is preceded by a rise in intracellular calcium [72, 73], localized predominantly in the nucleus [72].

It remains to be elucidated exactly which downstream signaling pathways are associated with the osteoclast polarization that follows integrin-mediated adhesion to matrix and is essential for bone resorption. Several candidate molecules, such as c-src, integrin-linked kinase (ILK), phosphatidyl-inositol 3-kinase (PI-3 kinase), and FAK, are expressed at high levels in osteoclasts [74]. Mice with a c-src knockout have severe osteopetrosis due to a lack of ruffled border formation in osteoclasts, clearly implicating this molecule in the signaling cascade leading to polarization of osteoclasts. Both PI-3 kinase and ILK have been shown to be associated with the cytoskeleton in osteoclasts attached to bone matrix, and both coimmunoprecipitate with αvβ3 in bone-adherent osteoclasts [75, 76], suggesting that these molecules may also play a role. Whether FAK is important in osteoclast function is less clear since no osteoclast abnormalities are seen in the FAK knockout mouse.

α2β1 in mammalian osteoclasts functions predominantly as a receptor for type I collagen. In contrast to other cell types, adhesion of osteoclasts to collagen appears to be RGD-dependent [56, 64], although this could possibly be explained as a dominant-negative effect of RGD occupation of the abundant αvβ3 receptors on osteoclasts. Antibodies to α2 and β1 integrin inhibit resorption by human osteoclasts *in vitro*, but not to the same extent as antivitronectin receptor antibodies. Avian osteoclasts express abundant β1 integrin but do not adhere to collagen [77]. Avian osteoclasts probably use β1 integrin predominantly in association with α5 as a fibronectin-binding receptor.

The role of $\alpha v \beta 1$ on osteoclasts has not been explored in functional assays since no receptor complex-specific antibodies are available at present. This receptor is far less abundant than $\alpha v \beta 3$ and $\alpha 2 \beta 1$ in osteoclasts [50]. By analogy with other cell types, it is likely that $\alpha v \beta 1$ functions as a receptor for collagen or fibronectin in osteoclasts.

B. Cadherins

There is very limited information about cadherin expression in osteoclasts. Mbalaviele *et al.* [78] reported expression of E-cadherin, and absence of P- and N-cadherin, in mature human and mouse osteoclasts. This study also suggests that in the mouse in an *in vitro* system, osteoclast development, and in particular osteoclast fusion, requires expression of E-cadherin, although it remains to be firmly established whether this is at the level of the osteoclast precursor or whether E-cadherin expression is required in the accessory cells (osteoblasts and/or stromal cells, which are known to be crucially important in formation of multinucleated osteoclasts and are known to express cadherins). Although no comprehensive studies have been reported, it would not be surprising if cadherins did not play a prominent role in mature osteoclasts, since these are motile cells that do not form stable cell-cell interactions. During osteoclast formation, however, there may be roles for a wider range of cadherin family members.

C. Ig Family Members

Data on the expression of receptors of the Ig family in osteoclasts are limited. There is functional evidence implicating ICAM-1 and VCAM-1 in osteoclast development [79], but such effects may well be mediated indirectly via effects on osteoblastic cells or stromal cells (as discussed above for cadherins). Mature osteoclasts do not appear to express Ig family receptors and their presence on immature osteoclasts has not formally been established because accurate markers for preosteoclasts do not exist. Until such markers are available or systems for analyzing osteoclast development in isolation are established (rather than in cocultures of undifferentiated precursors with a stromal layer, or with bone rudiments [80]), it will be difficult to assess the precise role of any osteoclast-expressed adhesion molecule during development.

D. Syndecans

There is as yet no information about expression of syndecans in mature osteoclasts or for a role during osteoclast development.

E. CD44

CD44 is highly expressed in osteoclasts *in vivo* [41, 51, 81]. Detailed studies of sites of expression are so far confined to rodent osteoclasts, where expression is at the basolateral membrane rather than at the clear zone or ruffled border of resorbing osteoclasts [81]. One functional study addressing the role of CD44 in mature osteoclasts and during osteoclast development has been reported. Kania [82] described how mouse osteoclast formation *in vitro* was inhibited by CD44 antibodies, whereas the resorptive capacity of mature osteoclasts was not affected. Because CD44 has a widespread expression in marrow cells and in osteoblasts (discussed above), it remains to be established whether CD44 inhibition has a direct effect on osteoclast precursors, or is mediated via other haemopoietic cells or accessory cells in this *in vitro* system. A number of ligands for CD44 are expressed in the osteoclast environment (Table IV), including a range of extracellular matrix proteins. There is no definitive information about the isoforms of CD44 expressed in osteoclasts and this will require further molecular studies on highly purified cells, or by single cell PCR techniques. Such information would be necessary if CD44 was considered as a therapeutic target to inhibit osteoclast formation.

F. Selectins

There are no reports describing the expression of selectins on mature osteoclasts. Selectins are likely, however, to have a role during osteoclast development. Osteoclast precursors are known to be present in the circulation because mature, resorbing osteoclasts can be generated *in vitro* from mononuclear cells in blood. It remains unclear how osteoclast precursors *in vivo* reach the sites in bone where they differentiate into fully active osteoclasts, but this must at some point include extravasation, a process which, for all lymphoid cells at least, initially involves selectin-mediated interaction with endothelial cells, followed by integrin-mediated processes. Clearly this is an issue which needs to be investigated because it might offer therapeutic potential in diseases where osteoclast formation is uncontrolled.

VI. ADHESION MOLECULES IN CHONDROCYTES

A. Integrins

As for cells of the osteoblast lineage, the reported integrin phenotype of chondrocytes is complex, with additional inconsistency between publications [83–87] (Table III). A

TABLE III.   Expression of Adhesion Molecules in Cartilage

Adhesion molecule expressed	Chondrocyte *in vivo*	Chondrocyte *in vitro*	Species[a]	Key references
Integrins				
$\alpha1$ (CD49a)	+	+	H, P, R, C, Ot	[85, 86, 88, 91, 92, 106]
$\alpha2$ (CD49b)	+	+	H, R, C	[83–85, 106]
$\alpha3$ (CD49c)	+/−	ND	H, P, Ot	[85, 86, 88, 91, 92, 106]
$\alpha4$ (CD49d)	+	+	H	[88]
$\alpha5$ (CD49e)	+	+	H, P, R, Ch, Ot	[83–85, 88, 91, 92, 106]
$\alpha6$ (CD49f)	+	ND	H	[83, 85]
$\beta1$ (CD29)	+	+	H, P, R, Ch, Ot	[83–85, 88, 91, 92, 105, 106]
$\beta2$ (CD18)	+	ND	H	[85]
$(\alpha v)\beta3$ (CD61)	−(+/−)	+/−	H	[85, 86]
$\beta4$ (CD104)	−	ND	H	[91]
$(\alpha v)\beta5$	+	ND	H	[85, 86]
$\beta6$	−	ND	H	[85]
αv (CD51)	+	+	H, R	[83, 85, 86, 91, 92, 105]
Cadherins				
N-Cadherin	+	+	Ch	[109–111]
Cadherin-11	−	ND	R	[108]
Cell surface proteoglycans				
Syndecan-3	+	+	Ch	[118–120]
CD44	+	+	H, R	[121–125]
Immunoglobulin family members				
ICAM-1 (CD54)	+	ND	H	[114, 115]
NCAM (CD56)	+	+	R, Ch	

[a] H, human; P, primate; R, rodent; Ch, chick; Ot, other.

synthesis of the literature suggests that human chondrocytes express the $\beta1$ integrins $\alpha1$, $\alpha2$, $\alpha3$, $\alpha5$, and $\alpha6$, but not $\alpha4$. $\beta2$, $\beta4$, and $\beta6$ are absent; analysis of $\beta7$-9 and CD11 has not been reported. Some studies have shown high expression of αv integrin. As in osteoblasts (see above), this is mainly as $\alpha v\beta5$ and not the $\alpha v\beta3$ dimer; however, a subpopulation of superficial articular chondrocytes were found to be $\alpha v\beta3$ positive [86]. These complexities could well relate in part to variation in sampling site, use of fetal versus adult material, species differences, culture artifacts, or influences of disease on phenotypes; indeed, the first possibility is borne out by the study of Salter *et al.* [85] where the distribution of integrin clearly differs by site (human articular, epiphyseal, and growth plate chondrocytes were studied). Likewise, changes have been reported in *in vitro* cultured chondrocytes [88–90].

The role of cell adhesion molecules in cartilage is thus relatively unclear (though the current state of knowledge regarding the function of some cell adhesion molecules is summarized in Table IV). From first principles, these could include roles in cartilage differentiation during fetal development, response to mechanical forces (for example in articular cartilage, menisci), maintenance of tissue architecture and integrity including matrix synthesis and assembly and cell adhesion, and regulation of chondrocyte gene expression. Additionally, there is likely to be a role of cell adhesion

molecules in responses of cartilage to injury and disease [91, 92]. The changes in distribution of both integrin and matrix proteins [85] in different zones of cartilage suggest a role in chondrocyte differentiation from mesenchymal precursors [93, 94] and/or interaction with matrix, or a specialized function such as a response to mechanical stresses. There have been few studies to investigate these possibilities.

Extensive studies have been performed to address the role of $\alpha5\beta1$ in chondrocyte interaction with fibronectin [83, 84, 95–100]. Function-blocking antibodies and RGD peptides have been shown to inhibit cell adhesion to fibronectin and its fragments, thus modifying chondrocyte behavior and cartilage function. Likewise, chondrocyte recognition of collagen (including types I, II, and VI) has been studied *in vitro* [83, 84, 96, 99–102] and shown to be mediated via $\beta1$ integrins: $\alpha1\beta1$ for adhesion to type I [89, 103] and type VI [103] and $\alpha3\beta1$ [89, 90, 103] or $\alpha2\beta1$ [102] for adhesion to type II.

There is also increasing evidence for a connection between chondrocyte adhesion to extracellular matrix proteins, especially fibronectin, chondrocyte-synovial cell interaction [104], regulation of integrin expression and function by cytokines such as IL1, TGFβ, and IGF1, and the release of matrix metalloproteinases [105] and hence cartilage breakdown [95, 98, 103, 106, 107]. Such events are likely to be involved in the pathogenesis of the cartilage destruction seen in osteoarthritis and rheumatoid arthritis.

B. Cadherins

Cadherin-11 is expressed in mesenchymal cells migrating from the neuroectodermal ridge which form presumptive cartilage (and in other morphogenetic events) in the developing mouse [108]. Likewise, N-cadherin is expressed in prechondrocytic cells in avian limb buds, but not in mature cartilage [109–111]. *In vitro* culture of mesenchymal cells suggests a functional role for N-cadherin in early chondrogenesis [110, 111] and its function may be regulated by calciotropic factors such as vitamin D and TGFβ [112]. There is no published literature on cadherin in human cartilage development.

C. Ig Family Members

N-CAM distribution is similar to that of N-cadherin in early cartilage development [111, 113]. Again, there are no data for mature human cartilage. A further Ig-superfamily molecule, ICAM-1, is expressed by chondrocytes, particularly after activation by cytokines such as IL1 and interferon [114, 115]. These results support a role for ICAM in mediating T cell-chondrocyte interactions [116] at sites of inflammatory joint destruction [117]. There is no information on the expression of VCAM in cartilage, other than its expression in associated vascular tissue and pannus in arthritis.

D. Syndecans

Syndecan-3 expression has been analyzed in developing avian limb buds; there are few data in mammals or for other syndecan forms. Syndecan-3 is highly expressed in proliferating chondrocytes below the tenascin C-rich layer of articular chondrocytes; decreased levels are found in hypertrophic cartilage [118]. High levels are also found in forming perichondrium (and later in periosteum) in the developing avian limb [119] and it has been suggested that, with tenascin C, syndecan-3 is involved in establishing or maintaining boundaries during skeletogenesis [120].

E. CD44

CD44 is expressed by cartilage and has been studied for a variety of sites and species [41, 44, 121]. The predominant isoform detected is the standard CD44H variant; epithelial CD44E is not found [122]. There is some evidence from the use of function blocking antibodies that CD44 is involved in chondrocyte pericellular matrix assembly [123, 124]. The range of extracellular matrix molecules recognized by CD44 in cartilage is unclear, though interaction with hyaluronate is likely. CD44 is upregulated during cartilage catabolism (for example, on IL1α treatment of bovine articular cartilage) and chondrocytes have been shown to actively

take up hyaluronate via CD44-mediated endocytosis; thus, it is reasonable to speculate that this molecule plays a regulatory role in cartilage matrix turnover in health and in disease [125, 126].

F. Selectins

There is no information on selectin expression in chondrocytes.

VII. RECEPTOR–LIGAND INTERACTION OF BONE CELL ADHESION MOLECULES

There is no conclusive evidence for receptor-ligand interactions from *in vivo* studies or studies in knock-out mice, or from human genetic diseases; however, adhesion studies *in vitro* have pointed to large numbers of possible ligands for osteoblast, osteoclast, and chondrocyte adhesion molecules. In addition, colocalization of receptor and ligand by immunocytochemistry in bone sections has given further indications as to which interactions may indeed occur *in vivo*. The available data are summarized in Table IV.

VIII. A POSSIBLE ROLE FOR BONE CELL ADHESION MOLECULES IN SENSING MECHANICAL STRAIN

Osteocytes and osteoblasts are known to be highly responsive to mechanical effects on bone, and one of the mechanisms by which they may sense such effects is via the adhesion molecules that allow them to attach to extracellular matrix and to each other. In other cell systems it has been demonstrated that twisting or turning of integrin molecules directly affects gene transcription [127]. Stretching of cells (i.e., change of cell shape) has also been shown to affect gene transcription and cell survival [128], and it has been demonstrated that cell shape is largely controlled by extracellular matrix [129]. It is therefore tempting to speculate that positive mechanical effects on bone cells resulting in bone formation may be mediated indirectly via adhesion receptors and/or cellular shape changes resulting from the bone deformation. In contrast, the absence of mechanical stimuli may lead to a decrease in bone mass and this may be the result of a lack of "cellular stretch," particularly in osteocytes and bone lining cells, which may lead to apoptotic cell death [128, 130]. The capacity of bone to (re)model in response to mechanical strain is thought to depend on osteocyte viability. Bone tissue with a large number of apoptotic osteocytes is unlikely to respond adequately to mechanical strain and has been suggested to be

TABLE IV.   Possible Receptor–Ligand Interactions for Major Bone Cell Adhesion Molecules

Receptor	Cell type	Ligands bound[a]	Possible function	Key references
Integrins				
$\alpha v \beta 3$	Osteoclast	Osteopontin, bone sialoprotein, fibronectin, vitronectin, fibrinogen, denatured collagen, P1 fragment of laminin	Matrix adhesion Polarization Cessation of resorption	[56, 77, 143–145]
$\alpha 1 \beta 1$	Chondrocyte	Type I collagen, type VI collagen	Matrix adhesion	[89, 103]
$\alpha 2 \beta 1$	Osteoclast	Native collagens[b]	Matrix adhesion	[56]
	Osteoblast	Native collagen	Matrix adhesion Differentiation	[30, 137]
	Chondrocyte	Type II collagen	Matrix adhesion	[102]
$\alpha 3 \beta 1$	Chondrocyte	Type II collagen	Matrix adhesion	[89, 90, 103]
$\alpha 5 \beta 1$	Osteoblast	Fibronectin (RGD)	Osteoblast differentiation	[26]
	Chondrocyte	Fibronectin (RGD)	Cartilage breakdown	[83–86, 88, 91, 92, 106]
Cadherins				
N-cadherin	Osteoblast	N-cadherin	Osteoblast development, bone formation	[32]
	Chondrocyte	N-cadherin	Cartilage development	[109–111]
E-cadherin	Osteoclast	E-cadherin	Osteoclast formation	[78]
Cadherin-4	Osteoblast	Cadherin-4	Osteoblast development, bone formation	[32]
Ob-cadherin	Osteoblast	Ob-cadherin	Osteoblast development osteoblast function?	[33]
Immunoglobulin family members				
ICAM-1	Osteoblast	LFA-1 on leukocytes	Osteoblast differentiation, production of cytokines	[35]
VCAM-1	Osteoblast	$\alpha 4$ integrins on leukocytes	Osteoblast differentiation, production of cytokines	[35]
ICAM-1	Chondrocyte	LFA-1 on leukocytes?	Cartilage breakdown	[114, 115]
Cell surface proteoglycans				
Syndecan-1	Osteoblast/osteocyte	Type I collagen, tenascin-c?	Matrix adhesion? osteoblast differentiation? role in mechanosensing?	[39, 40, 146]
Syndecan-2	Osteoblast	GM-CSF	Osteoblast differentiation	[38]
Syndecan-3	Chondrocyte	Tenascin-c	Cartilage development	[108, 119, 120]
CD44	Osteoclast	Hyaluronate? osteopontin? type I collagen? fibronectin?	Osteoclast formation, osteoclast migration? osteoclast–osteoblast interaction?	[82]
	Osteoblast(progenitor)	Hyaluronate, osteopontin? type I collagen? fibronectin?	Hyaluronate degradation matrix adhesion	[45]
	Chondrocyte	Hyaluronate	Pericellular matrix assembly	[121, 122, 124]

[a] Shown is the range of ligands demonstrated to be bound in *in vitro* adhesion assays. There is no definitive information on the natural ligands in bone for these molecules. Where no data are available, molecules known to be able to bind the receptor in other cells and known to be expressed in the matrix surrounding the bone cells are given followed by a question mark.

[b] Not in avian osteoclasts.

preferentially resorbed [10]. Removal of apoptotic cells from bone is an unexplored area, but may, by analogy with removal of apoptotic neutrophils from inflamed sites, involve recognition by $\alpha v \beta 3$ on phagocytes. It has been suggested that osteoclasts may fulfill such a role in bone and that apoptotic osteocytes may give direction to the bone (re)modeling process [10]. Ultrastructural evidence has been presented for engulfment of osteocytes by osteoclasts [131], although at present it is unclear whether osteocyte death preceded uptake by osteoclasts. Currently largely speculative, the mechanisms whereby bone cells sense and respond to mechanical strain are the subject of intense investigation and these studies should reveal whether an adhesion-related mechanism, or any of the other proposed mechanisms [132] plays a role.

IX. CONCLUSION

Bone and cartilage cells express a wide variety of adhesion molecules. Integrin expression has been studied extensively, but there is a lack of information on the expression of other adhesion molecule family members. There is also little information on the expression and function of adhesion molecules of all classes during osteoblast and osteoclast development, largely because we currently lack adequate markers to identify immature bone cells. Adhesion molecules fulfill many functions in skeletal cells and are linked to a variety of intracellular signaling pathways. Although no unique osteoblast or osteoclast adhesion molecule has been identified to date, therapeutic strategies based on selectively inhibiting highly expressed receptors, such as $\alpha v \beta 3$ in osteoclasts, have proved to be successful in inhibition of excessive bone resorption. Better knowledge of the expression and roles of adhesion molecules in bone pathology is vital to designing similar therapeutic strategies for other bone cell types.

References

1. Ruoslahti, E., and Öbrink, B. (1996). Common principles in cell adhesion. *Exp. Cell Res.* **227**, 1–11.
2. Pigott, R., and Power, C. (1993). "The Adhesion Molecule Facts Book." Academic Press, London.
3. Nermut, M. V., Green, N. M., Eason, P., Yamada, S. S., and Yamada, K. M. (1988). Electron microscopy and structural model of human fibronectin receptor. *EMBO J.* **7**, 4093–4099.
4. Clark, E. A., and Brugge, J. S. (1995). Integrins and signal transduction pathways: The road taken. *Science* **268**, 233–239.
5. Takeichi, M. (1991). Cadherin cell adhesion receptors as a morphogenetic regulator. *Science* **251**, 1451–1455.
6. Cowin, P. (1994). Unraveling the cytoplasmic interactions of the cadherin superfamily. *Proc. Natl. Acad. Sci. U.S.A.* **91**, 10759–10761.
7. Hynes, R. O. (1992). Integrins: Versatility, modulation, and signaling in cell adhesion. *Cell* **69**, 11–25.
8. Barclay, A. N., Birkeland, M. L., Brown, M. H., Beyers, A. D., Davis, S. J., Somoza, C., and Williams, A. F. (1993). "The Leukocyte Antigen Facts book." Academic Press, San Diego, CA.
9. Elenius, K., and Jalkanen, M. (1994). Function of the syndecans—a family of cell surface proteoglycans. *J. Cell Sci.* **107**, 2975–2982.
10. Tomkinson, A., Reeve, J., Shaw, R. W., and Noble, B. S. (1997). The death of ostocytes via apoptosis accompanies estrogen withdrawal in human bone. *J. Clin. Endocrinol. Metab.* **82**, 3128–3135.
11. Weber, G. F., Ashkar, S., Glimcher, M. J., and Cantor, H. (1996). Receptor-ligand interaction between CD44 and osteopontin (Eta-1). *Science* **271**, 509–512.
12. Frenette, P. S., and Wagner, D. D. (1997). Insights into selectin function from knockout mice. *Thromb. Haemostasis* **78**, 60–64.
13. Varki, A. (1997). Selectin ligands: Will the real ones please stand up? *J. Clin. Invest.* **99**, 158–162.
14. Crockett-Torabi, E. (1998). Selectins and mechanisms of signal transduction. *J. Leukocyte Biol.* **63**, 1–14.
15. Grzesik, W. J., and Robey, P. G. (1994). Bone matrix RGD glycoproteins: Immunolocalization and interaction with human primary osteoblastic bone cells in vitro. *J. Bone Miner. Res.* **9**, 487–496.
16. Hughes, D. E., Salter, D. M., Dedhar, S., and Simpson, R. (1993). Integrin expression in human bone. *J. Bone Miner. Res.* **8**, 527–533.
17. Clover, J., Dodds, R. A., and Gowen, M. (1992). Integrin subunit expression by human osteoblasts and osteoclasts in situ and in culture. *J. Cell Sci.* **103**, 267–271.
18. Sinha, R. K., and Tuan, R. S. (1996). Regulation of human osteoblast integrin expression by orthopedic implant materials. *Bone* **18**, 451–457.
19. Gronowicz, G., and McCarthy, M. B. (1996). Response of human osteoblasts to implant materials: Integrin-mediated adhesion. *J. Orthop. Res.* **14**, 878–887.
20. Aarden, E. M., Nijweide, P. J., van der Plas, A., Alblas, M. J., Mackie, E. J., Horton, M.A., and Helfrich, M. H. (1996). Adhesive properties of isolated chick osteocytes in vitro. *Bone* **18**, 305–313.
21. Gohel, A. R., Hand, A. R., and Gronowicz, G. A. (1995). Immunogold localization of β1-integrin in bone: Effect of glucocorticoids and insulin-like growth factor I on integrins and osteocyte formation. *J. Histochem. Cytochem.* **43**, 1085–1096.
22. Puleo, D. A., and Bizios, R. (1991). RGDS tetrapeptide binds to osteoblasts and inhibits fibronectin-mediated adhesion. *Bone* **12**, 271–276.
23. Majeska, R. J., Port, M., and Einhorn, T. A. (1993). Attachment to extracellular matrix molecules by cells differing in the expression of osteoblastic traits. *J. Bone Miner. Res.* **8**, 277–289.
24. Gronowicz, G. A., and DeRome, M. E. (1994). Synthetic peptide containing Arg-Gly-Asp inhibits bone formation and resorption in a mineralizing organ culture system of fetal rat parietal bones. *J. Bone Miner. Res.* **9**, 193–201.
25. Doherty, W. J., DeRome, M. E., McCarthy, M. B., and Gronowicz, G. A. (1995). The effect of glucocorticoids on osteoblast function. The effect of corticosterone on osteoblast expression of β1 integrins. *J. Bone Jt. Surg., Am.* **77**, 396–404.
26. Moursi, A. M., Damsky, C. H., Lull, J., Zimmerman, D., Doty, S. B., Aota, S., Globus, and RK. (1996). Fibronectin regulates calvarial osteoblast differentiation. *J. Cell Sci.* **109**, 1369–1380.
27. Dedhar, S., Mitchell, M. D., and Pierschbacher, M. D. (1989). The osteoblast-like differentiated phenotype of a variant of MG-63 osteosarcoma cell line correlated with altered adhesive properties. *Connect. Tissue Res.* **20**, 49–61.
28. Dedhar, S. (1989). Signal transduction via the β1 integrins is a required intermediate in interleukin-1 beta induction of alkaline phosphatase activity in human osteosarcoma cells. *Exp. Cell Res.* **183**, 207–214.
29. Dedhar, S., Argraves, W. S., Suzuki, S., Ruoslahti, E., and Pierschbacher, M. D. (1987). Human osteosarcoma cells resistant to detachment by an Arg-Gly-Asp-containing peptide overproduce the fibronectin receptor. *J. Cell Biol.* **105**, 1175–1182.
30. Ganta, D. R., McCarthy, M. B., and Gronowicz, G. A. (1997). Ascorbic acid alters collagen integrins in bone culture. *Endocrinology* **138**, 3606–3612.
31. Cheng, S. L., Lecanda, F., Davidson, M. K., Warlow, P. M., Zhang, S. F., Zhang, L., Suzuki, S., St. John, T., and Civitelli, R. (1998). Human osteoblasts express a repertoire of cadherins, which are critical for BMP-2-induced osteogenic differentiation. *J. Bone Miner. Res.* **13**, 633–644.
32. Chen, S., Lecanda, F., Warlow, P. M., Avioli, L. V., and Civitelli, R. (1996). Cell-cell contact through cadherins is critical for human osteoblast differentiated function. *J. Bone Miner. Res.* **11**, S263.
33. Okazaki, M., Takeshita, S., Kawai, S., Kikuno, R., Tsujimura, A., Kudo, A., and Amann, E. (1994). Molecular cloning and characterization of OB-cadherin, a new member of cadherin family expressed in osteoblasts. *J. Biol. Chem.* **269**, 12092–12098.
33a. Takeichi, M. (1995). Morphogenetic roles of classic cadherins. *Curr. Opin. Cell. Biol.* **7**, 619–627.
34. Lee, Y. S., and Chuong, C. M. (1992). Adhesion molecules in skeletogenesis: I. Transient expression of neural cell adhesion molecules (NCAM) in osteoblasts during endochondral and intramembranous ossification. *J. Bone Miner. Res.* **7**, 1435–1446.
35. Tanaka, Y., Morimoto, I., Nakano, Y., Okada, Y., Hirota, S., Nomura, S., Nakamura, T., and Eto, S. (1995). Osteoblasts are regulated by the cellular adhesion through ICAM-1 and VCAM-1. *J. Bone Miner. Res.* **10**, 1462–1469.
36. Barillé, S., Collette, M., Bataille, R., and Amiot, M. (1995). Myeloma cells upregulate interleukin-6 secretion in osteoblastic cells through cell-to-cell contact but downregulate osteocalcin. *Blood* **86**, 3151–3159.

37. Koyama, E., Shimazu, A., Leatherman, J. L., Golden, E. B., Nah, H. D., and Pacifici, M. (1996). Expression of syndecan-3 and tenascin-C: Possible involvement in periosteum development. *J. Orthop. Res.* **14**, 403–412.

38. Modrowski, D., Lomri, A., Baslé, M. F., and Marie, J. P. (1997). Syndecan-2 binds GM-CSF and controls its mitogenic activity in human osteoblastic cells. *J. Bone Miner. Res.* **12**, S159.

39. Birch, M. A., and Skerry, T. M. (1997). Syndecan expression in human bone cells. *Bone* **20**, 68S.

40. Birch, M. A., and Skerry, T. M. (1997). Syndecan expression by osteosarcoma cell lines is regulated by cytokines but not osteotropic hormones. *J. Bone Miner. Res.* **12**, 1527.

41. Hughes, D. E., Salter, D. M., and Simpson, R. (1994). CD44 expression in human bone: A novel marker of osteocytic differentiation. *J. Bone Miner. Res.* **9**, 39–44.

42. Jamal, H. H., and Aubin, J. E. (1996). CD44 expression in fetal rat bone: In vivo and in vitro analysis. *Exp. Cell Res.* **223**, 467–477.

43. Nakamura, H., and Ozawa, H. (1996). Immunolocalization of CD44 and the ERM family in bone cells of mouse tibiae. *J. Bone Miner. Res.* **11**, 1715–1722.

44. Noonan, K. J., Stevens, J. W., Tammi, R., Tammi, M., Hernandez, J. A., and Midura, R. J. (1996). Spatial distribution of CD44 and hyaluronan in the proximal tibia of the growing rat. *J. Orthop. Res.* **14**, 573–581.

45. Pavasant, P., Shizari, T. M., and Underhill, C. B. (1994). Distribution of hyaluronan in the epiphysial growth plate: turnover by CD44-expressing osteoprogenitor cells. *J. Cell Sci.* **107**, 2669–2677.

46. Aarden, E. M., Wassenaar, A. M., Alblas, M. J., and Nijweide, P. J. (1996). Immunocytochemical demonstration of extracellular matrix proteins in isolated osteocytes. *Histochem. Cell Biol.* **106**, 495–501.

47. Horton, M. A., and Rodan, G. A. (1996). Integrins as therapeutic targets in bone disease. In "Adhesion Receptors as Therapeutic Targets" (M. A. Horton, ed.), pp. 223–245. CRC Press, Boca Raton, FL.

48. Rodan, S. B., and Rodan, G. A. (1997). Integrin function in osteoclasts. *J. Endocrinol.* **154**, S47–S56.

49. Horton, M. A., and Davies, J. (1989). Perspectives: Adhesion receptors in bone. *J. Bone Miner. Res.* **4**, 803–808.

50. Nesbitt, S., Nesbit, A., Helfrich, M., and Horton, M. (1993). Biochemical characterization of human osteoclast integrins. Osteoclasts express $\alpha v\beta 3$, $\alpha 2\beta 1$, and $\alpha v\beta 1$ integrins. *J. Biol. Chem.* **268**, 16737–16745.

51. Athanasou, N. A., and Quinn, J. (1990). Immunophenotypic differences between osteoclasts and macrophage polykaryons: Immunohistological distinction and implications for osteoclast ontogeny and function. *J. Clin. Pathol.* **43**, 997–1003.

52. Horton, M. A., and Helfrich, M. H. (1992). Antigenic markers of osteoclasts. In "Biology and Physiology of the Osteoclast" (B. R. Rifkin and C. V. Gay, eds.), pp. 33–54. CRC Press, Boca Raton, FL.

53. Kumar, C. S., James, I. E., Wong, A., Mwangi, V., Feild, J. A., Nuthulaganti, P., Connor, J. R., Eichman, C., Ali, F., Hwang, S. M., Rieman, D. J., Drake, F. H., and Gowen, M. (1997). Cloning and characterization of a novel integrin $\beta 3$ subunit. *J. Biol. Chem.* **272**, 16390–16397.

54. Townsend, P. A., and Horton, M. A. (1995). Identification of a potentially novel osteoclast integrin β chain. *Bone* **17**, S319–S320.

55. Väänänen, H. K., and Horton, M. (1995). The osteoclast clear zone is a specialized cell-extracellular matrix adhesion structure. *J. Cell Sci.* **108**, 2729–2732.

56. Helfrich, M. H., Nesbitt, S. A., Lakkakorpi, P. T., Barnes, M. J., Bodary, S. C., Shankar, G., Mason, W. T., Mendrick, D. L., Väänänen, H. K., and Horton, M. A. (1996). Beta 1 integrins and osteoclast function: Involvement in collagen recognition and bone resorption. *Bone* **19**, 317–328.

57. Neff, L., Amling, M., Tanaka, S., Gailit, J., and Baron, R. (1996). Both the αv and $\beta 3$ integrin subunits are present in the sealing zone of resorbing osteoclasts. *J. Bone Miner. Res.* **11**, S290.

58. Nakamura, I., Gailit, J., and Sasaki, T. (1996). Osteoclast integrin $\alpha v\beta 3$ is present in the clear zone and contributes to cellular polarization. *Cell Tissue Res.* **286**, 507–515.

59. Hultenby, K., Reinholt, F. P., and Heinegård, D. (1993). Distribution of integrin subunits on rat metaphyseal osteoclasts and osteoblasts. *Eur. J. Cell Biol.* **62**, 86–93.

60. Lakkakorpi, P. T., Helfrich, M. H., Horton, M. A., and Väänänen, H. K. (1993). Spatial organization of microfilaments and vitronectin receptor, $\alpha v\beta 3$, in osteoclasts. A study using confocal laser scanning microscopy. *J. Cell Sci.* **104**, 663–670.

61. Lakkakorpi, P. T., Horton, M. A., Helfrich, M. H., Karhukorpi, E. K., and Väänänen, H. K. (1991). Vitronectin receptor has a role in bone resorption but does not mediate tight sealing zone attachment of osteoclasts to the bone surface. *J. Cell Biol.* **115**, 1179–1186.

62. Reinholt, F. P., Hultenby, K., Oldberg, Å., and Heinegård, D. (1990). Osteopontin—a possible anchor of osteoclasts to bone. *Proc. Natl. Acad. Sci. U.S.A.* **87**, 4473–4475.

63. Dodds, R. A., Connor, J. R., James, I. E., Rykaczewski, E. L., Appelbaum, E., Dul, E., and Gowen, M. (1995). Human osteoclasts, not osteoblasts, deposit osteopontin onto resorption surfaces: An in vitro and ex vivo study of remodeling bone. *J. Bone Miner. Res.* **10**, 1666–1680.

64. Nakamura, I., Takahashi, N., Sasaki, T., Jimi, E., Kurokawa, T., and Suda, T. (1996). Chemical and physical properties of the extracellular matrix are required for the actin ring formation in osteoclasts. *J. Bone Miner. Res.* **11**, 1873–1879.

65. Horton, M. A., Taylor, M. L., Arnett, T. R., and Helfrich, M. H. (1991). Arg-Gly-Asp (RGD) peptides and the anti-vitronectin receptor antibody 23C6 inhibit dentine resorption and cell spreading by osteoclasts. *Exp. Cell Res.* **195**, 368–375.

66. van der Pluijm, G., Mouthaan, H., Baas, C., de Groot, H., Papapoulos, S., Löwik, C., and C. (1994). Integrins and osteoclastic resorption in three bone organ cultures: Differential sensitivity to synthetic Arg-Gly-Asp peptides during osteoclast formation. *J. Bone Miner. Res.* **9**, 1021–1028.

67. Sato, M., Sardana, M. K., Grasser, W. A., Garsky, V. M., Murray, J. M., and Gould, R. J. (1990). Echistatin is a potent inhibitor of bone resorption in culture. *J. Cell Biol.* **111**, 1713–1723.

68. Fisher, J. E., Caulfield, M. P., Sato, M., Quartuccio, H. A., Gould, R. J., Garsky, V. M., Rodan, G. A., and Rosenblatt, M. (1993). Inhibition of osteoclastic bone resorption in vivo by echistatin, an "arginyl-glycyl-aspartyl" (RGD)-containing protein. *Endocrinology* **132**, 1411–1413.

69. King, K. L., D'Anza, J. J., Bodary, S., Pitti, R., Siegel, M., Lazarus, R. A., Dennis, M. S., Hammonds, R. G., Jr., and Kukreja, S. C. (1994). Effects of kistrin on bone resorption in vitro and serum calcium in vivo. *J. Bone Miner. Res.* **9**, 381–387.

70. Crippes, B. A., Engleman, V. W., Settle, S. L., Delarco, J., Ornberg, R. L., Helfrich, M. H., Horton, M. A., and Nickols, G. A. (1996). Antibody to $\beta 3$ integrin inhibits osteoclast-mediated bone resorption in the thyroparathyroidectomized rat. *Endocrinology* **137**, 918–924.

71. Engleman, V. W., Nickols, G. A., Ross, F. P., Horton, M. A., Griggs, D. W., Settle, S. L., Ruminski, P. G., and Teitelbaum, S. L. (1997). A peptidomimetic antagonist of the $\alpha v\beta 3$ integrin inhibits bone resorption in vitro and prevents osteoporosis in vivo. *J. Clin. Invest.* **99**, 2284–2292.

72. Shankar, G., Davison, I., Helfrich, M. H., Mason, W. T., and Horton, M. A. (1993). Integrin receptor-mediated mobilisation of intranuclear calcium in rat osteoclasts. *J. Cell Sci.* **105**, 61–68.

73. Zimolo, Z., Wesolowski, G., Tanaka, H., Hyman, J. L., Hoyer, J. R., and Rodan, G. A. (1994). Soluble $\alpha v\beta 3$-integrin ligands raise $[Ca^{2+}]_i$ in rat osteoclasts and mouse-derived osteoclast-like cells. *Am. J. Physiol.* **266**, C376–C381.

74. Suda, T., Nakamura, I., Jimi, E., and Takahashi, N. (1997). Regulation of osteoclast function. *J. Bone Miner. Res.* **12**, 869–879.

75. Lakkakorpi, P. T., Wesolowski, G., Zimolo, Z., Rodan, G. A., and Rodan, S. B. (1997). Phosphatidylinositol 3-kinase association with the

osteoclast cytoskeleton, and its involvement in osteoclast attachment and spreading. *Ex. Cell Res.* **237**, 296–306.

76. Lakkakorpi, P. T., Dedhar, S., Mostachfi-Vasseghi, H., Rodan, G. A., and Rodan, S. B. (1996). Association of integrin-linked kinase (ILK) with β3-integrin and its activation and translocation to the cytoskeleton upon osteoclast attachment to bone. *J. Bone Miner. Res.* **11**, S287.

77. Ross, F. P., Chappel, J., Alvarez, J. I., Sander, D., Butler, W. T., Farach-Carson, M. C., Mintz, K. A., Robey, P. G., Teitelbaum, S. L., and Cheresh, D. A. (1993). Interactions between the bone matrix proteins osteopontin and bone sialoprotein and the osteoclast integrin αvβ3 potentiate bone resorption. *J. Biol. Chem.* **268**, 9901–9907.

78. Mbalaviele, G., Chen, H., Boyce, B. F., Mundy, G., and Yoneda, T. (1995). The role of cadherin in the generation of multinucleated osteoclast from mononuclear precursors in murine marrow. *J. Clin. Invest.* **95**, 2757–2765.

79. Horton, M. A., Townsend, P., and Nesbitt, S. (1996). Cell surface attachment molecules in bone. *In* "Principles of Bone Biology," pp. 217–230. Academic Press, San Diego, CA.

80. Nijweide, P. J., and De Grooth, R. (1992). Ontogeny of the osteoclast. *In* "Biology and Physiology of the Osteoclast" (B. R. Rifkin and C. V. Gay, eds.), pp. 81–104. CRC Press, Boca Raton, FL.

81. Nakamura, H., Kenmotsu, S., Sakai, H., and Ozawa, H. (1995). Localization of CD44, the hyaluronate receptor, on the plasma membrane of osteocytes and osteoclasts in rat tibiae. *Cell Tissue Res.* **280**, 225–233.

82. Kania, J. R., Kehat-Stadler, T., and Kupfer, S. R. (1997). CD44 antibodies inhibit osteoclast formation. *J. Bone Miner. Res.* **12**, 1155–1164.

83. Durr, J., Goodman, S., Potocnik, A., von der Mark, H., and von der Mark, K. (1993). Localization of β1-integrins in human cartilage and their role in chondrocyte adhesion to collagen and fibronectin. *Exp. Cell Res.* **207**, 235–244.

84. Enomoto, M., Leboy, P. S., Menko, A. S., and Boettiger, D. (1993). Beta 1 integrins mediate chondrocyte interaction with type I collagen, type II collagen, and fibronectin. *Exp. Cell Res.* **205**, 276–285.

85. Salter, D. M., Godolphin, J. L., and Gourlay, M. S. (1995). Chondrocyte heterogeneity: Immunohistologically defined variation of integrin expression at different sites in human fetal knees. *J. Histochem. Cytochem.* **43**, 447–457.

86. Woods, V. L., Jr., Schreck, P. J., Gesink, D. S., Pacheco, H. O., Amiel, D., Akeson, W. H., and Lotz, M. (1994). Integrin expression by human articular chondrocytes. *Arthritis Rheum.* **37**, 537–544.

87. Salter, D. M., Hughes, D. E., Simpson, R., and Gardner, D. L. (1992). Integrin expression by human articular chondrocytes. *Br. J. Rheumatol.* **31**, 231–234.

88. Loeser, R. F., Carlson, C. S., and McGee, M. P. (1995). Expression of beta 1 integrins by cultured articular chondrocytes and in osteoarthritic cartilage. *Exp. Cell Res.* **217**, 248–257.

89. Shakibaei, M. (1995). Integrin expression on epiphyseal mouse chondrocytes in monolayer culture. *Histol. Histopathol.* **10**, 339–349.

90. Shakibaei, M., Abou-Rebyeh, H., and Merker, H. J. (1993). Integrins in ageing cartilage tissue in vitro. *Histol. Histopathol.* **8**, 715–723.

91. Lapadula, G., Iannone, F., Zuccaro, C., Grattagliano, V., Covelli, M., Patella, V., Lo Bianco, G., and Pipitone, V. (1997). Integrin expression on chondrocytes: Correlations with the degree of cartilage damage in human osteoarthritis. *Clin. Exp. Rheumatol.* **15**, 247–254.

92. Forster, C., Kociok, K., Shakibaei, M., Merker, H. J., Vormann, J., Gunther, T., and Stahlmann, R. (1996). Integrins on joint cartilage chondrocytes and alterations by ofloxacin or magnesium deficiency in immature rats. *Arch. Toxicol.* **70**, 261–270.

93. Hirsch, M. S., and Svoboda, K. K. (1996). Beta 1 integrin antibodies inhibit chondrocyte terminal differentiation in whole sterna. *Ann. N.Y. Acad. Sci.* **785**, 267–270.

94. Tavella, S., Bellesse, G., Castagnola, P., Martin, I., Piccini, D., Doliana, R., Colombatti, A., Cancedda, R., and Tacchetti, C. (1997). Regulated

95. Clancy, R. M., Rediske, J., Tang, X., Nijher, N., Frenkel, S., Philips, M., and Abrahamson, S. B. (1997). Outside-in signaling in the chondrocyte. Nitric oxide disrupts fibronectin-induced assembly of a subplasmalemmal actin/rho A/focal adhesion kinase signaling complex. *J. Clin. Invest.* **100**, 1789–1796.

96. Shimizu, M., Minakuchi, K., Kaji, S., and Koga, J. (1997). Chondrocyte migration to fibronectin, type I collagen, and type II collagen. *Cell Struct. Funct.* **22**, 309–315.

97. Homandberg, G. A., and Hui, F. (1994). Arg-Gly-Asp-Ser peptide analogs suppress cartilage chondrolytic activities of integrin-binding and nonbinding fibronectin fragments. *Arch. Biochem. Biophys.* **310**, 40–48.

98. Xie, D., and Homandberg, G. A. (1993). Fibronectin fragments bind to and penetrate cartilage tissue resulting in proteinase expression and cartilage damage. *Biochim. Biophys. Acta* **1182**, 189–196.

99. Enomoto-Iwamoto, M., Iwamoto, M., Nakashima, K., Mukudai, Y., Boettinger, D., Pacifici, M., Kurisu, K., and Suzuki, F. (1997). Involvement of α5β1 integrin in matrix interactions and proliferation of chondrocytes. *J. Bone Miner. Res.* **12**, 1124–1132.

100. Loeser, R. F. (1993). Integrin-mediated attachment of articular chondrocytes to extracellular matrix proteins. *Arthritis Rheum.* **36**, 1103–1110.

101. Camper, L., Heinegård, D., and Lundgren-Akerlund, E. (1997). Integrin α2β1 is a receptor for the cartilage matrix protein chondroadherin. *J. Cell Biol.* **138**, 1159–1167.

102. Holmvall, K., Camper, L., Johansson, S., Kimura, J. H., and Lundgren-Akerlund, E. (1995). Chondrocyte and chondrosarcoma cell integrins with affinity for collagen type II and their response to mechanical stress. *Exp. Cell Res.* **221**, 496–503.

103. Loeser, R. F. (1997). Growth factor regulation of chondrocyte integrins. Differential effects of insulin-like growth factor 1 and transforming growth factor beta on α1β1 integrin expression and chondrocyte adhesion to type VI collagen. *Arthritis Rheum.* **40**, 270–276.

104. Ramachandrula, A., Tiku, K., and Tiku, M. L. (1992). Tripeptide RGD-dependent adhesion of articular chondrocytes to synovial fibroblasts. *J. Cell Sci.* **101**, 859–871.

105. Arner, E. C., and Tortorella, M. D. (1995). Signal transduction through chondrocyte integrin receptors induces matrix metalloproteinase synthesis and synergizes with interleukin-1. *Arthritis Rheum.* **38**, 1304–1314.

106. Yonezawa, I., Kato, K., Yagita, H., Yamauchi, Y., and Okumura, K. (1996). VLA-5-mediated interaction with fibronectin induces cytokine production by human chondrocytes. *Biochem. Biophys. Res. Commun.* **219**, 261–265.

107. Loeser, R. F. (1994). Modulation of integrin-mediated attachment of chondrocytes to extracellular matrix proteins by cations, retinoic acid, and transforming growth factor beta. *Exp. Cell Res.* **211**, 17–23.

108. Simonneau, L., Kitagawa, M., Suzuki, S., and Thiery, J. P. (1995). Cadherin 11 expression marks the mesenchymal phenotype: Towards new functions for cadherins? *Cell Adhes. Commun.* **3**, 115–130.

109. Oberlender, S. A., and Tuan, R. S. (1994). Spatiotemporal profile of N-cadherin expression in the developing limb mesenchyme. *Cell Adhes. Commun.* **2**, 521–537.

110. Oberlender, S. A., and Tuan, R. S. (1994). Expression and functional involvement of N-cadherin in embryonic limb chondrogenesis. *Development* **120**, 177–187.

111. Tavella, S., Raffo, P., Tacchetti, C., Cancedda, R., and Castagnola, P. (1994). N-CAM and N-cadherin expression during in vitro chondrogenesis. *Exp. Cell Res.* **215**, 354–362.

112. Tsonis, P. A., Del Rio-Tsonis, K., Millan, J. L., and Wheelock, M. J. (1994). Expression of N-cadherin and alkaline phosphatase in chick limb bud mesenchymal cells: Regulation by 1,25-dihydroxyvitamin D3 or TGF-beta 1. *Exp. Cell Res.* **213**, 433–437.

113. Hitselberger Kanitz, M. H., Ng, Y. K., and Iannaccone, P. M. (1993). Distribution of expression of cell adhesion molecules in the mid to late gestational mouse fetus. *Pathobiology* **61**, 13–18.

114. Bujia, J., Behrends, U., Rotter, N., Pitzke, P., Wilmes, E., and Hammer, C. (1996). Expression of ICAM-1 on intact cartilage and isolated chondrocytes. *In Vitro Cell. Dev. Biol. Anim.* **32**, 116–122.

115. Davies, M. E., Dingle, J. T., Pigott, R., Power, C., and Sharma, H. (1991). Expression of intercellular adhesion molecule 1 (ICAM-1) on human articular cartilage chondrocytes. *Connect. Tissue Res.* **26**, 207–216.

116. Horner, A., Davies, M. E., and Franz, B. (1995). Chondrocyte-peripheral blood mononuclear cell interactions: The role of ICAM-1. *Immunology* **86**, 584–590.

117. Seidel, M. F., Keck, R., and Vetter, H. (1997). ICAM-1/LFA-1 expression in acute osteodestructive joint lesions in collagen-induced arthritis in rats. *J. Histochem. Cytochem.* **45**, 1247–1253.

118. Shimazu, A., Nah, H. D., Kirsch, T., Koyama, E., Leatherman, J. L., Golden, E. B., Kosher, R. A., and Pacifici, M. (1996). Syndecan-3 and the control of chondrocyte proliferation during endochondral ossification. *Exp. Cell Res.* **229**, 126–136.

119. Seghatoleslami, M. R., and Kosher, R. A. (1996). Inhibition of in vitro limb cartilage differentiation by syndecan-3 antibodies. *Dev. Dyn.* **207**, 114–119.

120. Koyama, E., Leatherman, J. L., Shimazu, A., Nah, H. D., and Pacifici, M. (1995). Syndecan-3, tenascin-C, and the development of cartilaginous skeletal elements and joints in chick limbs. *Dev. Dyn.* **203**, 152–162.

121. Stevens, J. W., Noonan, K. J., Bosch, P. P., Rapp, T. B., Martin, J. A., Kurriger, G. L., Maynard, J. A., Daniels, K. J., Solursh, M., Tammi, R., Tammi, M., and Midura, R. J. (1996). CD44 in growing normal and neoplastic rat cartilage. *Ann. N. Y. Acad. Sci.* **785**, 333–336.

122. Salter, D. M., Godolphin, J. L., Gourlay, M. S., Lawson, M. F., Hughes, D. E., and Dunne, E. (1996). Analysis of human articular chondrocyte CD44 isoform expression and function in health and disease. *J. Pathol.* **179**, 396–402.

123. Knudson, C. B. (1993). Hyaluronan receptor-directed assembly of chondrocyte pericellular matrix. *J. Cell Biol.* **120**, 825–834.

124. Knudson, W., Aguiar, D. J., Hua, Q., and Knudson, C. B. (1996). CD44-anchored hyaluronan-rich pericellular matrices: An ultrastructural and biochemical analysis. *Exp. Cell Res.* **228**, 216–228.

125. Chow, G., Knudson, C. B., Homandberg, G., and Knudson, W. (1995). Increased expression of CD44 in bovine articular chondrocytes by catabolic cellular mediators. *J. Biol. Chem.* **270**, 27734–27741.

126. Hua, Q., Knudson, C. B., and Knudson, W. (1993). Internalization of hyaluronan by chondrocytes occurs via receptor-mediated endocytosis. *J. Cell Sci.* **106**, 365–375.

127. Wang, N., and Ingber, D. E. (1994). Control of cytoskeletal mechanics by extracellular matrix, cell shape and mechanical tension. *Biophys. J.* **66**, 2181–2189.

128. Ruoslahti, E. (1997). Stretching is good for a cell. *Science* **276**, 1345–1346.

129. Chen, C. S., Mrksich, M., Huang, S., Whitesides, G. M., and Ingber, D. E. (1997). Geometric control of cell life and death. *Science* **276**, 1425–1428.

130. Noble, B. S., Stevens, H., Mosley, J. R., Pitsillides, A. A., Reeve, J., and Lanyon, L. (1997). Bone loading changes the number and distribution of apoptotic osteocytes in cortical bone. *J. Bone Miner. Res.* **12**, S111.

131. Elmardi, A. S., Katchburian, M. V., and Katchburian, E. (1990). Electron microscopy of developing calvaria reveals images that suggest that osteoclasts engulf and destroy osteocytes during bone resorption. *Calcif. Tissue Int.* **46**, 239–245.

132. Aarden, E. M., Burger, E. H., and Nijweide, P. J. (1994). Function of osteocytes in bone. *J. Cell. Biochem.* **55**, 287–299.

133. Brighton, C. T., and Albelda, S. M. (1992). Identification of integrin cell-substratum adhesion receptors on cultured rat bone cells. *J. Orthop. Res.* **10**, 766–773.

134. Nissinen, L., Pirilä, L., and Heino, J. (1997). Bone morphogenetic protein-2 is a regulator of cell adhesion. *Exp. Cell Res.* **230**, 377–385.

135. Saito, T., Albelda, S. M., and Brighton, C. T. (1994). Identification of integrin receptors on cultured human bone cells. *J. Orthop. Res.* **12**, 384–394.

136. Steffensen, B., Duong, A. H., Milam, S. B., Potempa, C. L., Winborn, W. B., Magnuson, V. L., Chen, D., Zardeneta, G., and Klebe, R. J. (1992). Immunohistological localization of cell adhesion proteins and integrins in the periodontium. *J. Periodontol.* **63**, 584–592.

137. Riikonen, T., Koivisto, L., Vihinen, P., and Heino, J. (1995). Transforming growth factor-beta regulates collagen gel contraction by increasing $\alpha2\beta1$ integrin expression in osteogenic cells. *J. Biol. Chem.* **270**, 376–382.

138. Clover, J., and Gowen, M. (1994). Are MG-63 and HOS TE85 human osteosarcoma cell lines representative models of the osteoblastic phenotype? *Bone* **15**, 585–591.

139. Salter, D. M., Robb, J. E., and Wright, M. O. (1997). Electrophysiological responses of human bone cells to mechanical stimulation: Evidence for specific integrin function in mechanotransduction. *J. Bone Miner. Res.* **12**, 1133–1141.

140. Vihinen, P., Riikonen, T., Laine, A., and Heino, J. (1996). Integrin $\alpha2\beta1$ in tumorigenic human osteosarcoma cell lines regulates cell adhesion, migration, and invasion by interaction with type I collagen. *Cell Growth Differ.* **7**, 439–447.

141. Grano, M., Zigrino, P., Colucci, S., Zambonin, G., Trusolino, L., Serra, M., Baldini, N., Teti, A., Marchisio, P. C., and Zallone, A. Z. (1994). Adhesion properties and integrin expression of cultured human osteoclast-like cells. *Exp. Cell Res.* **212**, 209–218.

142. Duong, L. T., Tanaka, H., and Rodan, G. A. (1994). VCAM-1 involvement in osteoblast-osteoclast interaction during osteoclast differentiation. *J. Bone Miner. Res.* **9**, S131.

143. Helfrich, M. H., Nesbitt, S. A., Dorey, E. L., and Horton, M. A. (1992). Rat osteoclasts adhere to a wide range of RGD (Arg-Gly-Asp) peptide-containing proteins, including the bone sialoproteins and fibronectin, via a $\beta3$ integrin. *J. Bone Miner. Res.* **7**, 335–343.

144. Flores, M. E., Norgård, M., Heinegård, D., Reinholt, F. P., and Andersson, G. (1992). RGD-directed attachment of isolated rat osteoclasts to osteopontin, bone sialoprotein, and fibronectin. *Exp. Cell Res.* **201**, 526–530.

145. Horton, M. A., Spragg, J. H., Bodary, S. C., and Helfrich, M. H. (1994). Recognition of cryptic sites in human and mouse laminins by rat osteoclasts is mediated by $\beta3$ and $\beta1$ integrins. *Bone* **15**, 639–646.

146. Webb, C. M., Zaman, G., Mosley, J. R., Tucker, R. P., Lanyon, L. E., and Mackie, E. J. (1997). Expression of tenascin-C in bones responding to mechanical load. *J. Bone Miner. Res.* **12**, 52–58.

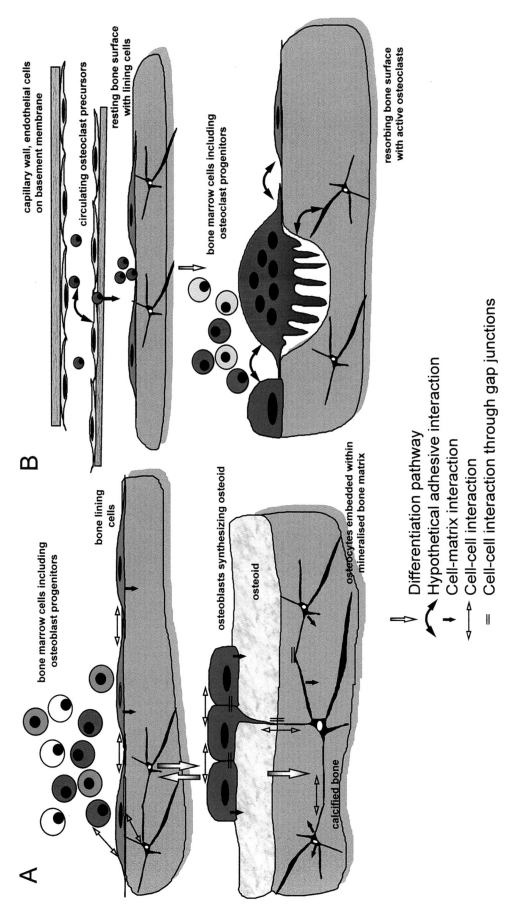

CHAPTER 8 FIGURE 1 Possible adhesive interactions between osteoblasts and other cell types and osteoblasts and matrix are shown in (A). These include cell–cell interactions with osteocytes which may be important in the anabolic response to mechanical loading and the transition from a resting surface with lining cells (top) to an active surface with osteoblasts synthesizing matrix. Cell–matrix interactions are known to influence osteoblast function, and such interactions may conceivably be with bone proteins incorporated within the osteoid or with soluble proteins. In (B), cell–cell and cell–matrix adhesive interactions of osteoclasts are shown. These include the as-yet-uninvestigated possible interactions of osteoclast progenitors with endothelial cells and the basement membrane of vessels (top). Resorbing osteoclasts have predominantly cell–matrix interactions, although it can not be excluded that they may establish transient cell–cell contacts with adjoining osteoblasts or lining cells. Uptake of apoptotic osteocytes has also been documented, and this may involve cell recognition mediated by adhesion receptors. Not shown in this figure are the cell–matrix interactions, which clearly are important for cell motility of nonresorbing osteoclasts. Also not shown are the largely hypothetical roles for adhesion molecules in cartilage cells, which are discussed in the text.

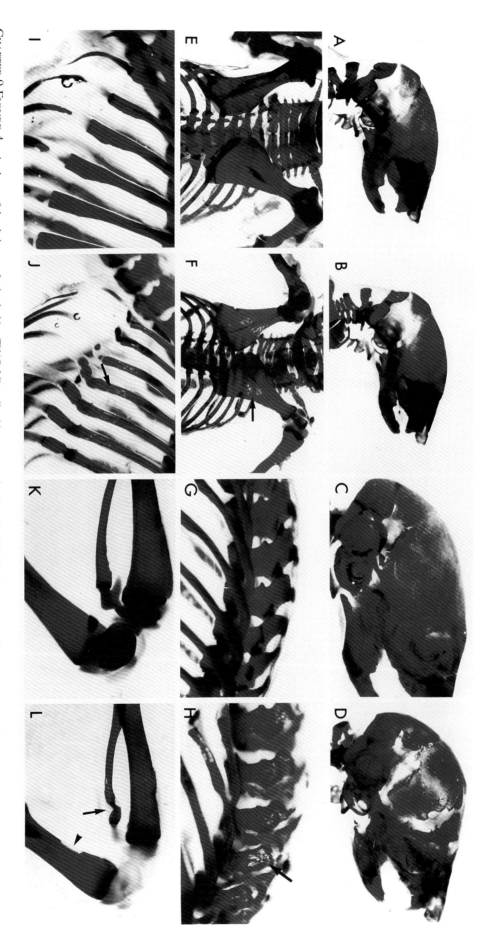

CHAPTER 9 FIGURE 4   Analyses of the skeletons of mice lacking TNAP. Mineralized bone was stained in red with alizarin red and cartilage was stained in blue with alcian blue. (A) Skull of 0-day-old TNAP+/+ newborn. (B) TNAP-/- littermate of A. (C) Skull of 8-day-old TNAP+/-. (D) TNAP-/- littermate of C. (E) Scapulas of 8-day-old TNAP+/-. (F) TNAP-/- littermate of E had unusual demineralization in the center of scapulas (arrow). (G) Vertebral bones of 8-day-old TNAP+/-. (H) TNAP-/- littermate of G. The arrow shows poor structure of the vertebral bone. (I) Rib bones of 8-day-old TNAP+/-. (J) TNAP-/- littermate of I; had deformity and poor mineralization (arrow). (K) Tibia, fibula, and femur of 8-day-old TNAP+/-. (L) TNAP-/- littermate of K. Arrow shows deformity in fibula, probably due to a fracture. Arrowhead shows demineralization.

CHAPTER 9

Acid and Alkaline Phosphatases

PAULA S. HENTHORN Section of Medical Genetics, Department of Clinical Studies-Philadelphia,
University of Pennsylvania School of Veterinary Medicine,
Philadelphia, Pennsylvania 19104

JOSÉ L. MILLÁN The Burnham Institute, La Jolla Cancer Research Center, La Jolla, California 92037

PHOEBE LEBOY Department of Biochemistry, University of Pennsylvania School of Dental Medicine,
Philadelphia, Pennsylvania 19104

I. INTRODUCTION

Acid and alkaline phosphatases are enzymes that are expressed in a variety of tissues, but each is a widely used marker for a particular bone cell type (osteoclast and osteoblast, respectively). Each is encoded by a single gene and, despite years of study, the functions of these enzymes are still speculative.

II. ACID PHOSPHATASES

The acid phosphatase expressed at high levels in osteoclasts is a form referred to as tartrate-resistant acid phosphatase (TRAP; EC 3.1.2.1), purple acid phosphatase, or type 5 acid phosphatase. This acid phosphatase is also expressed at high levels in monocyte-derived macrophages, hairy cell leukemia cells, cells from Gaucher patients, and placenta and at low levels in many tissues. A TRAP referred to as uteroferrin is expressed at high levels in pig uterine endometrium after progesterone induction [1]. TRAPs are iron-binding glycoproteins that appear to be secreted in placenta and bone, and they are lysosomal in location in other cell types.

A. cDNA and Gene Structure

1. cDNAs and Deduced Proteins

Full-length TRAP cDNAs have been isolated from human placenta, rat calvaria, and pig uterine endometrium, and a full-length mouse cDNA sequence has been deduced from the mouse TRAP gene sequence. Table I presents a list of TRAP cDNAs and genes which have been sequenced, along with their Genbank identification numbers. All TRAP cDNAs are approximately 1.4 kb in length and encode polypeptides ranging from 306 to 325 amino acids, of which the first 20 constitute a signal peptide. There are two potential N-linked glycosylation signals and a putative lysosomal targeting sequence that are conserved in all cDNAs. An alignment of the deduced TRAP polypeptide sequences of all four species can be found in Cassady [2].

127

TABLE I.   Vertebrate Tartrate-Resistant Acid Phosphatase cDNA and Gene Sequences

Name (GENBANK ID)	Species	Sequence	Tissue	Reference
PIGTRAP	Pig	cDNA	Spleen/endometrium	Ling and Roberts, 1993 [4]
PIGUFMR	Pig	cDNA	Uterus	Simmen *et al.*, 1989 [8]
PIGUFG	Pig	Promoter region	[Gene]	Simmen *et al.*, 1989 [8]
PIGUTBIND	Pig	Promoter region	[Gene]	Gonzalez *et al.*, 1994 [79]
RATTTRAP	Rat	cDNA	Calvarium	Ek-Rylander *et al.*, 1991 [80]
HUMACP5	Human	cDNA	Placenta	Ketcham *et al.*, 1989 [81]
HSMRACP5	Human	cDNA	Placenta	Lord *et al.*, 1990 [3]
HSTRAP	Human	Gene (exons 1–4)	[Gene]	Cassady *et al.*, 1993 [2]
HSTRAP5FR	Human	5′ flanking region	[Gene]	Fleckenstein *et al.*, 1996 [15]
HUMTRAPB	Human	5′ flanking region	[Gene]	Reddy *et al.*, 1995 [6]
MUSAP5A	Mouse	Gene (all exons)	[Gene]	Cassady *et al.*, 1993 [2]
MUSTRAP	Mouse	Promoter region	[Gene]	Reddy *et al.*, 1993 [2]

2. GENE AND PROMOTER STRUCTURE

The human TRAP gene has been localized to 19p13.2–13.3 [3]. Only a single TRAP gene is detected by blot hybridization analysis [3, 4], and the existence of only one gene that is expressed in multiple tissues is also supported by sequence analysis of partial and full length cDNA clones isolated from different tissues in the same species (see preceding section). The entire genes have been cloned from pig, human, and mouse, and are all relatively small genes (Fig. 1). The mouse and human TRAP genes have the same exon/intron structure, with the first exon containing only 5′ untranslated sequences, the second exon beginning with the ATG start codon, and the rest of the protein-coding region residing in three additional exons. The pig gene is composed of only three exons, with a noncoding first exon, a second exon that encodes the same amino acids as exons 2, 3, and 4 of the human and mouse genes, and a third exon that is analogous to exon 5 in human and mouse (Fig. 1).

The promoter regions in mouse, human, and pig have also been isolated. All have a major transcription start site upstream of the first (noncoding) exon. In mouse tissues and in an endometrial cell line, there is evidence of weak promoter activity from within intron 1 [5, 6]. Numerous consensus binding sites for various transcription factors have been identified in these upstream regions, including Sp1, Ap1, Pu.1, and GT1 (summarized by Reddy *et al.* [7]), while the pig TRAP promoter also contains progesterone and estrogen receptor complex binding sites [8]. However, since there is limited sequence homology between the TRAP promoter regions from different species, comparisons provide little insight into which of these binding sites may be important.

B. Control of Gene Expression

In bone, TRAP is selectively expressed at high levels by osteoclasts, and it is the most commonly used histochemical marker for assessing bone resorption [9]. However, it was first identified from patients with hairy cell leukemia and is used as a diagnostic marker for both this disease and osteoclastomas [10]. While clinically useful for these two malignancies, it is important to be aware that TRAP is also expressed by subsets of normal macrophages and granulocytes [10].

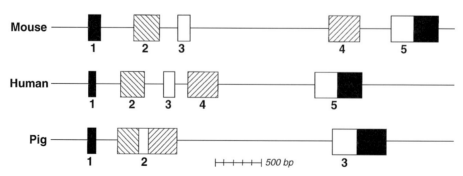

FIGURE 1   Comparison of the exon structure of the tartrate-resistant acid phosphatase genes from mouse, human, and pig. Exons are indicated by boxes, with noncoding regions filled in black. Analogous regions of coding sequence are indicated by identical hatching or white filling in the exon boxes.

Because measurement of serum TRAP levels might be used as a noninvasive method to monitor the degree of bone resorption, there has been considerable interest in improving techniques for TRAP quantitation. However, Ballanti *et al.* [11] have reported that spectrophotometic assays of TRAP activity in serum have low sensitivity compared with histomorphometric analysis of stained sections. Serum assays suffer from the additional disadvantage that it is not possible to distinguish osteoclast TRAP from that produced by other cell types. Several antibodies which react with human TRAP have been developed [12–14]. Such reagents may permit more sensitive methods for following bone resorption via immunoassay of serum TRAP.

As is true for other iron-transport and iron-binding proteins, TRAP levels are modulated by iron availability. In both human and mouse systems, iron-saturated transferrin increases TRAP expression at the level of transcription whereas hemin decreases levels of TRAP [7, 15, 16]. The mouse TRAP promoter has been examined for regulatory elements by Reddy and colleagues [7, 16]. Mouse TRAP promoter-luciferase constructs transfected into HRE H9 rabbit endometrial cells show transcriptional stimulation by iron with constructs containing a 600 bp region 1.2–1.8 kb upstream of the mouse TRAP gene [17]. Conversely, both hemin and its protoporphyrin moiety (protoporphyrin IX) inhibit transcription with these constructs [16]. Both of these modulators affect transcription from the upstream P1 promoter but not the downstream P2 promoter. Gel retardation and Southwestern blot studies suggest that the hemin/protoporphyrin inhibition involves repression via a hemin-responsive regulatory protein binding to a 27 bp segment of the mouse TRAP 5′-flanking region at bp −1815 to −1789 [16]. However, no iron response region which would account for the observed iron stimulation of TRAP transcription has been identified thus far. The human TRAP promoter, like the mouse promoter, contains a putative binding site for a hemin-responsive protein [15], but the mechanism for transcriptional regulation of the human TRAP gene by iron is unknown [10].

C. Function of Acid Phosphatase

1. Role in Bone Resorption

The concept that TRAP expression is important for bone resorption initially derived from Minkin's observation that it is expressed at high levels in mature, multinucleate osteoclasts active at resorbing bone surfaces [9]. When organ cultures of newborn mouse calvaria were stimulated by PTH or 1,25-dihydroxyvitamin D3, Minkin observed that bone resorption was accompanied by significant increases in TRAP activity released by osteoclasts. Subsequently, Zaidi and co-workers [18] showed that antibodies raised against placental TRAP (uteroferrin) markedly inhibited both TRAP activity of osteoclasts and bone resorption. Ultrastructural studies

demonstrated that TRAP is found at bone surfaces facing the ruffled border zone, and in osteoclasts it is localized in lysosome-like structures [19]. These observations are consistent with the concept that TRAP is exported from osteoclasts to areas of active bone resorption. However, the mechanism by which TRAP promotes bone resorption is currently unknown [10].

One theory is that TRAP released from osteoclasts dephosphorylates noncollagenous proteins in bone matrix and therefore alters proteins required for osteoclast attachment to bone surfaces. Ek-Rylander and co-workers have demonstrated that TRAP is capable of dephosphorylating osteopontin, osteonectin, and bone sialoprotein [20, 21], and that dephosphorylated osteopontin can no longer promote osteoclast attachment [20]. It is therefore plausible that TRAP might modulate osteoclast adhesion or migration. Another theory is that free radicals generated by TRAP activity may promote dissolution of bone mineral [22]. Since it can dephosphorylate proteins with phosphorylated tyrosine, serine, and threonine residues, intracellular TRAP might also be capable of modulating cell signal transduction systems [10]. TRAP is an iron-containing protein which requires reduced Fe^{2+} for activity; addition of the iron-chelator desferrioxamine inhibits the increase in TRAP observed when monocytes from human peripheral mononuclear cells are placed in culture [17]. In the placenta, TRAP (uteroferrin) is thought to function as an iron-transport protein [1], and it is possible that it might serve a similar function in osteoclasts.

2. Evidence from Knockout Mice

Because solid information on the molecular function of TRAP is limited, the availability of a model system lacking TRAP activity has been eagerly awaited. Hayman *et al.* [23] have reported initial studies of mice which contain a targeted disruption of the gene. Animals homozygous for the null allele showed shortened and deformed long bones and axial skeleton, but skull development and tooth eruption was normal. These are characteristics of a defect in endochondral bone formation. Consistent with this conclusion, histomorphometric analyses revealed widened and disorganized growth plates along with delayed cartilage mineralization. Intramembranous bone in the skull showed increased density, and long bones of older mice both homozygous and heterozygous for the mutation had increased mineral density, suggesting a defect in bone remodeling. Osteoclasts from the mutant mice had diminished resorptive activity as measured by *in vitro* pit assays. The conclusion from these studies is that TRAP is required both for cartilage mineralization preceding endochondral ossification during development and for bone turnover in adult animals [23]. It will be of great interest to see what these TRAP knock-out mice can tell us about the mechanism by which this enzyme promotes bone resorption.

III. ALKALINE PHOSPHATASES

A. Isoenzymes, cDNAs, and Gene Structure

The alkaline phosphatase (AP) expressed in bone is one of several isoenzymes of alkaline phosphatase found in mammalian tissues (Fig. 2). The genes encoding the various isoforms are the result of various gene duplication events during evolution, as outlined in Figure 2 for the mouse and human APs. In humans, the APs are encoded by four genes that are named after the tissues in which they are predominantly expressed. Tissue-nonspecific alkaline phosphatase (TNAP) is expressed at highest levels in liver, bone, and kidney (hence the alternative name L/B/K AP), in the placenta during the first trimester of pregnancy, and at lower levels in numerous other tissues [24]. Although products of the same gene, the AP isoforms from liver, bone, and kidney can be distinguished by tissue-specific variations in posttranslational modifications

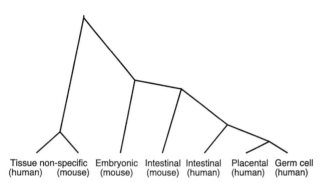

Tissue non-specific (human)   Embryonic (mouse)   Intestinal (mouse)   Intestinal (human)   Placental (human)   Germ cell (human)

FIGURE 2   A model of the evolutionary relationships between mouse and human tissue alkaline phosphatase genes.

[25]. The other three isoforms, placental (PLAP), placental-like or germ cell (GCAP), and intestinal (IAP) alkaline phosphatase, show much more restricted tissue expression; hence, the general term tissue-specific APs. These forms are encoded by three genes located together on the distal long arm of human chromosome 2 [26, 27] and are closely related, showing within 90% identical nucleotide and 87% identical amino acid sequences. The mRNA molecules are all about 2.5 kb in length and encode peptides ranging from 518 to 535 amino acids from which an amino-terminal signal peptide of approximately 20 amino acids is cleaved. No definitive functions have been assigned to any of the tissue specific AP isozymes, although several have been postulated [24, 28, 29]. A helpful alignment of the human AP protein sequences can be found in the review by Millan and Fishman [29].

The tissue-specific AP isoenzymes are much more thermostable than the TNAP enzyme, and they can also be specifically assayed using various uncompetitive low molecular weight inhibitors and immunologic reagents (reviewed by Harris [28] and by Millan and Fishman [29]; also see Section II.C.2.b.). Polyclonal antisera raised against the various tissue-specific forms cross-react with one another but not with TNAP, and monoclonal antibodies that differentially detect all four forms have been derived [28]. The biochemical and immunologic differences in the different AP isoforms make it possible to obtain clinically useful information on the probable source of TNAP in serum, and thus to distinguish bone disorders from liver malignancies and renal diseases.

cDNA clones for tissue-nonspecific alkaline phosphatase have been isolated from various tissues from different mammals, including human, cow, cat, mouse, and rat. Table II provides Genbank accession numbers and references for TNAP sequences. All encode a polypeptide of 524 amino acids,

TABLE II.   Vertebrate Tissue-Nonspecific Alkaline Phosphatase cDNA and Gene Sequences

Name (GENBANK ID)	Species	Sequence	Tissue	Reference
BOVAP	Bovine	cDNA	Kidney	Garattini *et al.*, 1987 [82]
FCU31569	Cat	cDNA	T-lymphocyte	Ghosh and Mullins, 1995 [83]
GGU19108	Chick	cDNA	Liver	Crawford *et al.*, 1995 [60]
HSAPHOL	Human	cDNA	Liver	Kishi *et al.*, 1989 [37]
HUMALPL	Human	Promoter region	(Gene)	Weiss *et al.*, 1988 [31]
HSALKPHOS	Human	Untranslated exon	Kidney [exon 1b]	Nosjean *et al.*, 1997 [84]
MMLBKTAP	Mouse	Promoter region	(Gene)	Terao *et al.*, 1990 [34]
MUSALPL1	Mouse	cDNA	L cells	Brown *et al.*, 1990 [85]
S57541	Mouse	Promoter region	[Gene]	Studer *et al.*, 1991 [35]
RATPHOA	Rat	cDNA	ROS17/2.8 osteosarcoma	Noda *et al.*, 1987 [86] Thiede *et al.*, 1988 [87]
RNALP	Rat	cDNA	Liver	Misumi *et al.*, 1988 [88]
RNALPHPR	Rat	Promoter region	[Gene]	Zernik *et al.*, 1990 [36]

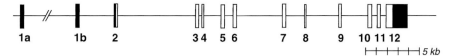

FIGURE 3 Organization of the human tissue nonspecific alkaline phosphatase gene. Exons are indicated by boxes, with noncoding regions filled in black. The unknown distance (greater than 25 kb) between exons 1a and 1b is indicated by parallel diagonal lines.

including the 17-amino-acid signal peptide. Aside from mouse and rat, which are 97% identical at the amino acid level and 93% identical over the nucleotides in the protein coding region, the other pairwise combinations of mammalian TNAP cDNAs display approximately 90% identical amino acid residues and 83 to 89% identical nucleotides. Like the tissue-specific isoforms, the TNAP mRNAs are approximately 2.5 kb in length. However, the tissue-nonspecific and tissue-specific mRNAs do not cross-hybridize. TNAP mRNAs isolated from different tissues have divergent sequences in the 5' untranslated region due to the alternate use of two different 5' noncoding exons.

The TNAP gene is located on the distal short arm of human chromosome 1, is composed of 13 exons, and occupies over 50 kbp of DNA (Fig. 3). The first two exons of the gene are noncoding and are separated from one another and from the exon that contains the ATG translation initiation site (exon 2) by relatively large introns, as first demonstrated in the rat [30]. The TNAP genes and promoter regions have been cloned and sequenced from human, rat, and mouse [31–35]. The 5'-most exon (referred to here as exon 1a) from human and rat have approximately 66% identical bases [33], while sequence homology cannot be detected between the 1b exons (3' noncoding exon) in these two species.

The major transcription start site and surrounding sequences of the 5'-most promoter 1a of the TNAP gene have been determined for human [31, 33, 36] and mouse [34]. There is some evolutionary sequence conservation of this promoter, with the rat versus human sequences showing 78% sequence identity over the first 200 bp and over 50% identity over the first 600 bp [34]. All three species have a TATA-like sequence located approximately 25 bases upstream of the major transcription start site, contain three or four consensus binding sites for the transcription factor Sp1, and are very GC-rich [30, 31, 33, 34]. Multiple copies of a purine-rich repeat were noticed in both human and mouse promoters [31, 34] and are also present in the rat promoter [33]. While numerous transcription factor binding sequences can be found, there is little mutagenesis or DNA binding data that support the use of any of these sequences.

The 1b exon and its promoter were first recognized in rat [30, 33] and have also been identified and sequenced in human and mouse [32, 34, 37–39]. The sequences upstream of exon 1b are not conserved between humans and rodents. The upstream promoter regions, however, do have some common features. For instance, none of the 1b promoters have a TATA sequence or CAAT box sequences. Elements that have been identified include two variant Sp1 sites in the rat 1b promoter [33] and a glucocorticoid response element (GRE) 2 kb upstream of the transcription start site in the human 1b promoter [32].

B. Control of Gene Expression

Exons 1a and 1b are incorporated into the mRNA in a mutually exclusive fashion that results from the fact that each exon has its own promoter sequence. This results in two types of mRNA, each encoding an identical polypeptide, that have different 5' untranslated sequences. The promoter usage has primarily been inferred by examination of the structure of TNAP cDNAs isolated from various tissues. In human and rat TNAP, the upstream promoter (1a) is preferentially utilized in osteoblasts and the downstream promoter (1b) is preferred in kidney and liver [30, 35, 37, 40]. However, in mice, the upstream promoter is used in all tissues expressing significant amounts of TNAP [35]. Although the 5' flanking regions of human, rat, and mouse TNAP have been analyzed in transient transfection assays, these studies have provided little insight into the mechanism for tissue-specific regulation.

The proximal 610 bp fragment of the human 1a promoter has been examined in detail both in a human osteosarcoma cell line expressing high levels and in HeLa cells expressing low levels of both TNAP mRNA and enzyme activity [41]. The 610 bp fragment had approximately the same promoter activity in transient transfections as a 4500 bp promoter fragment and showed similar activity in both cell types. Subsequent transfection experiments comparing SAOS osteosarcoma cells with HepG2 liver cells indicated that, although the endogenous TNAP mRNA levels differ by 1000-fold between the two cell lines, the transcription rate with promoter-reporter constructs was approximately equal in both cell types [42]. One possible explanation is that cultured liver cells can initiate transcription from the bone-type 1a promoter introduced by plasmid transfection, whereas the endogenous TNAP gene is transcribed using the downstream 1b promoter utilized in normal liver. This would argue that promoter-reporter transfection studies of the AP gene may not accurately reflect *in vivo* transcriptional control mechanisms. Alternatively, the authors suggest that the differential TNAP gene expression in these two cell types was due to differences in posttranscriptional control mechanisms [42].

Studies using agents which increase TNAP activity have provided evidence for both transcriptional and posttranscriptional regulation of the enzyme. Among these agents are retinoic acid, dexamethasone, and granulocyte colony-stimulating factor [43, 44]. All of these inducers promote transcription of TNAP from the upstream 1a promoter. In the case of retinoic acid, this transcriptional regulation presumably works via a retinoic acid-responsive element [45, 46]. There is also evidence that TNAP transcription in nonexpressing tissues of mice is repressed *in vivo* by methylation at the 1a promoter [46]. Because sequence analysis of the rat and human 1a promoters indicates a high level of methylatable CpG sites [36, 47], it is likely that negative regulation by methylation is a general mechanism for suppressing TNAP transcription in many tissues. Consistent with the hypothesis that suppression is responsible for the absence of TNAP in nonexpressing cells, intertypic cell hybrids between human TE-85 osteosarcoma and mouse fibrosarcoma show the low AP levels characteristic of the fibrosarcoma [48]. These results suggest that negative regulators from the fibroblasts are capable of extinguishing the high TNAP produced by the osteosarcoma cells.

Evidence for posttranscription regulation of TNAP is more indirect. Heath and colleagues [45] showed that while the preosteoblastic rat cell line RCT-1 will transcribe the TNAP gene in the absence of retinoic acid, enzyme activity requires the presence of retinoic acid. Subsequent studies showed that retinoic acid induced a modest increase in transcription rate along with a markedly greater increase in spliced, mature TNAP mRNA. These results argue that retinoic acid increases enzyme activity both by increasing the transcription rate and by stabilizing newly synthesized TNAP mRNA [49].

There is also evidence for regulation of TNAP at translational or posttranslational stages. Comparison of rat marrow stromal cell osteogenesis induced by dexamethasone and retinoic acid indicated that while dexamethasone causes parallel increases in TNAP mRNA and activity, retinoic acid induction of AP activity was considerably greater than the increases in mRNA levels [50]. Phosphate levels which increase the TNAP activity in SAOS osteosarcoma cells are found to decrease TNAP mRNA [51]. Conversely, although high levels of AP mRNA are found in mouse heart and diaphragm, these tissues show low levels of enzyme activity [35]. Neutrophils have high levels of TNAP mRNA and protein [44]; however, the protein is sequestered in an intracellular compartment until the cell is stimulated [52, 53]. As these reports make clear, it is unwise to draw conclusions about transcriptional regulation of alkaline phosphatase genes based solely on assays of enzyme activity.

Because the expression of TNAP in osteoblasts is linked to differentiation, some agents which cause elevated enzyme levels in these cells may do so by increasing expression of osteoblast-specific transcription factors or by relieving osteogenic suppression rather than by acting directly on the TNAP gene. Osteosarcoma/fibroblast cell hybrids regain elevated TNAP when treated with a combination of 1,25-dihydroxyvitamin D3 and TGFβ, suggesting that this combination diminishes repression of the TNAP gene [54]. Other reagents, such as ascorbic acid (vitamin C) and the bone morphogenetic proteins, may also act indirectly by stimulating osteogenic pathways. For example, ascorbic acid has been shown to increase TNAP mRNA in MC3T3-E1 cells by a slow mechanism requiring increased extracellular collagen synthesis which, in turn, promotes increased osteoblast differentiation [55]. Studies have suggested that this mechanism involves activation of a promoter element by the osteogenic transcription factor OSF-2/CBFA-1 [56]. It is clear that detailed analyses of TNAP promoter function using cell transfection and trangenic animal techniques will be necessary to define the regulatory sequences controlling TNAP expression in bone and other tissues. One factor impeding such studies is the presence of a very large (25–50 kb) intron separating exon 1a and 1b. This intron, which has not been analyzed or sequenced in any species, may contain regulatory elements controlling 1a and 1b promoter function.

C. Function of Alkaline Phosphatase

1. GENETIC AND GENE KNOCK-OUT EVIDENCE

The genetic disease hypophosphatasia demonstrates that diminished levels of TNAP are associated with defective bone mineralization (see Chapter 43 for a complete discussion and references). More detailed analyses of TNAP function have been possible using mice in which both copies of the TNAP gene have been inactivated [57, 58]. Mice deficient in the TNAP gene mimic the most severe forms of hypophosphatasia (i.e., perinatal and infantile hypophosphatasia) [58]. These TNAP−/− mice are growth impaired, develop epileptic seizures and apnea, and die before weaning with evidence of cranial and pulmonary hemorrhages. Examination of the tissues indicates abnormal bone mineralization, morphological changes in the osteoblasts, aberrant development of the lumbar nerve roots, disturbances in intestinal physiology, increased apoptosis in the thymus, and an abnormal spleen. Skeletal preparations of embryos and newborns revealed no bone abnormalities at birth. However, the staining of 8-day-old TNAP−/− bones clearly showed poor mineralization in the parietal bones, scapulae, vertebral bones, and ribs (Fig. 4, see color insert). Evidence of spontaneous fractures was evident in the fibulae. Fractures in the rib bones and broken incisors were also observed. The bone abnormalities worsen progressively with age.

The epileptic seizures in these TNAP knock-out mice can be corrected by administration of lipophylic forms of vitamin B_6, providing experimental evidence that alkaline phosphatase is involved in vitamin B_6 metabolism [57] and that pyridoxal-5′-phosphate is a natural substrate of TNAP. Accumulation of pyridoxal-5′-phosphate results in altered neurotransmitter levels and abnormalities in neuron function [57]. These observations, combined with the pleiotropic phenotypic abnormalities displayed by the mouse models, suggest that TNAP also plays a critical role in nonskeletal development.

Hui *et al.* [59] have suggested that high expression of TNAP may induce cellular changes associated with induction of terminal differentiation. This is consistent with long-standing observations that many tissues go through an AP-positive stage during embryonic development and then lose AP activity after differentiation [24]. Direct evidence that TNAP is required for embryonic differentiation is provided by studies demonstrating that inhibition of TNAP blocks early development of avian feather germs [60]. It is possible that TNAP functions as a protein phosphatase during development, and it therefore may alter intracellular signal transduction systems involved in cell differentiation [59, 61].

2. AP FUNCTION INFERRED FROM PROTEIN STRUCTURE

As mentioned in Section III.A, the tissue-specific and tissue-nonspecific alkaline phosphatases are encoded by a multigene family with a common ancestor. The coding regions of the TSAP genes display 90–98% identity at the protein level, while there exists only 50% sequence similarity between TNAP and the TSAP isozymes. The enzymes are synthesized as propeptides varying in length from 524 (TNAP) to 535 (PLAP/GCAP) amino acids. A hydrophobic signal peptide (17 to 22 amino acids in length) precedes the amino terminal sequence of the mature protein. Two putative glycosylation sites (Asn122 and Asn249) exist in the PLAP and GCAP molecules, three sites (Asn122, Asn249, and Asn410) in IAP, and five putative sites (Asn123, Asn213, Asn254, Asn286, and Asn413) in TNAP. GCAP has been shown, by site-directed mutagenesis experiments, to undergo glycosylation at both putative sites [62], but the structure and number of carbohydrate chains in the other APs remain to be determined.

The AP active site residues have been identified based on homology of the human AP sequences with that of the *E. coli* AP molecule for which a detailed structure has been established by X-ray crystallography [63]. Residues involved in the active site of the enzyme (i.e., Ser92, Asp91, Arg166) and the ligands coordinating to Zn^{2+} metal ions 1 and 2 and the Mg^{2+} ion are conserved. These homologies suggest that the catalytic mechanism of eukaryotic APs is similar to that of the *E. coli* enzyme. However, bacterial AP structure cannot be used to provide information on several aspects of eukaryotic AP properties: membrane insertion, inhibition, or interaction with extracellular proteins.

a. Membrane Insertion Eukaryotic APs are membrane-bound enzymes anchored to the exterior of the cytoplasmic membrane via a glycosyl phosphatidylinositol (GPI) anchor [64]. Asp484 was identified as the point of attachment of this anchor in PLAP [65]. Since Asp484 is perfectly conserved in GCAP and IAP, we can predict the same attachment site for these isozymes. However, the situation will, most likely, be different for TNAP as well as for the TSAPs of other species. Evidence indicates that the bovine IAPs may be attached via residue 480 [66].

b. Uncompetitive Inhibition Mammalian APs are inhibited stereo-specifically by L-amino acids and peptides through an uncompetitive mechanism [67]. TSAPs are generally inhibited by L-Phe, some even by L-Leu, whereas TNAPs are inhibited by L-homoarginine and levamisole but not by L-Phe. By far the best characterized of the TSAP isozymes are human PLAP and GCAP, which differ by only 12 of their 513 amino acids [68]. PLAP and GCAP are inhibited uncompetitively by L-Phe with equal efficiency, whereas GCAP displays much higher affinity for L-Leu [69]. The molecular mechanism for this isozyme-specific property has been attributed to a single E429G substitution in the GCAP molecule [70, 71]. The transition of Glu429 (in PLAP) to Gly429 (in GCAP), which generates the increase in L-Leu sensitivity, is accompanied by a major change in conformation of a loop region containing residue 429 as measured by a battery of conformation-specific monoclonal antibodies. These mutagenesesis studies have determined that the uncompetitive inhibition mechanism of PLAP and GCAP by L-Phe and L-Leu occurs through three interaction points of the inhibitor: the carboxylic group attacks the active site Arg166 during catalysis, the amino group of the inhibitor interacts with zinc 1 in the active site, while the side chain of the inhibitor is stabilized by the loop containing residue 429 [71].

c. Interaction with Extracellular Proteins Evidence has accumulated which suggests that APs may have a protein–protein interaction domain. Chicken TNAP [72, 73] has been reported to bind to collagen type I, II, and X, while human PLAP binds to IgG [74]. Based on sequence comparisons, a surface loop region harboring residue 429 was identified as a region of homology [75] between APs and Mac1, p150, Von Willebrand factor, complement factor B, and cartilage matrix protein, which are proteins known to interact with collagen. Site-directed mutagenesis and domain exchange experiments provided evidence that this loop domain, besides modulating the uncompetitive inhibition properties of APs, is primarily responsible for the heat-stability properties of TNAP and TSAPs and also accounts for at least half the binding affinity of mouse TNAP to collagen [76]. It appears that APs may have biological roles different or in addition to their catalytic functions. How this protein interaction domain may contribute to the *in vivo* roles of these isozymes is, however, not known at present.

Mammalian APs, like the *E. coli* molecule, are dimeric metaloenzymes composed of two identical subunits each containing two Zn^{2+} and one Mg^{2+} ions in the active site. The existence of cooperativity between AP subunits has been investigated intensively in the *E. coli* enzyme and evidence for the existence of positive cooperativity has been presented [77]. Studies using site-directed mutants and heterodimeric PLAP/GCAP isozymes have indicated that mammalian AP dimers display negative cooperativity when partially demetalated, whereas both AP monomers can function independently when both subunits are properly metalated. Fully metalated mammalian APs behave like noncooperative allosteric enzymes where the stability and catalytic properties of each monomer are controlled by the conformation of the second subunit [78].

An important property of mammalian APs that remains to be explained in terms of structure is what amino acid residues specify their high catalytic rate constants? There is one log difference in K_{cat} between the *E. coli* AP ($\sim$30 U/mg) and human PLAP or GCAP ($\sim$300 U/mg) and an additional log difference between the human isozymes and the bovine intestinal AP (bIAP I) ($\sim$3400 U/mg). Studies comparing the structure of two bovine intestinal APs of high and low catalytic turnover have conclusively demonstrated that substitutions at position 322 in these isozymes can have pronounced effects on the K_{cat} [72]. These data represent a significant first step toward characterizing this important difference between bacterial and mammalian APs.

References

1. Janickila, A. J., Yaziji, H., Lear, S. C., Martin, A. W., and Yam, L. T. (1996). Localization of tartrate-resistant acid phosphatase in human placenta. *Histochem. J.* **28**, 195–200.
2. Cassady, A. I., King, A. G., Cross, N. C., and Hume, D. A. (1993). Isolation and characterization of the genes encoding mouse and human type-5 acid phosphatase. *Gene* **130**, 201–207.
3. Lord, D. K., Cross, N. C., Bevilacqua, M. A., Rider, S. H., Gorman, P. A., Groves, A. V., Moss, D. W., Sheer, D., and Cox, T. M. (1990). Type 5 acid phosphatase. Sequence, expression and chromosomal localization of a differentiation-associated protein of the human macrophage. *Eur. J. Biochem.* **189**, 287–293.
4. Ling, P., and Roberts, R. M. (1993). Uteroferrin and intracellular tartrate-resistant acid phosphatase are the products of the same gene. *J. Biol. Chem.* **268**, 6896–6902.
5. Reddy, S. V., Scarcez, T., Windle, J. J., Leach, R. J., Hundley, J. E., Chirgwin, J. M., Chou, J. Y., and Roodman, G. D. (1993). Cloning and characterization of the 5′-flanking region of the mouse tartrate-resistant acid phosphatase gene. *J. Bone Miner. Res.* **8**, 1263–1270.
6. Reddy, S. V., Kuzhandaivelu, N., Acosta, L. G., and Roodman, G. D. (1995). Characterization of the 5′-flanking region of the human tartrate-resistant acid phosphatase (TRAP) gene. *Bone* **16**, 587–593.
7. Reddy, S. V., Hundley, J. E., Windle, J. J., Alcantara, O., Linn, R., Leach, R. J., Boldt, D. H., and Roodman, G. D. (1995). Characterization of the mouse tartrate-resistant acid phosphatase (TRAP) gene promoter. *J. Bone Miner. Res.* **10**, 601–606.
8. Simmen, R. C., Srinivas, V., and Roberts, R. M. (1989). cDNA sequence, gene organization, and progesterone induction of mRNA for uteroferrin, a porcine uterine iron transport protein. *DNA* **8**, 543–554.
9. Minkin, C. (1982). Bone acid phosphatase: Tartrate-resistant acid phosphatase as a marker of osteoclast function. *Calcif. Tissue Int.* **34**, 285–290.
10. Fleckenstein, E., and Drexler, H. G. (1997). Tartrate-resistant acid phosphatase: Gene structure and function. *Leukemia* **11**, 10–13.
11. Ballanti, P., Minisola, S., Pacetti, M. T., Scarnecchia, L., Rosso, R., Mazzuoli, G. F., and Bonucci, E. (1997). Tartrate-resistant acid phosphatase activity as osteoclastic marker: Sensitivity of cytochemical assessment and serum assay in comparison with standardized osteoclast histomorphometry. *Osteoporosis Int.* **7**, 39–43.
12. Chamberlain, P., Compston, J. E., Cox, T. M., Hayman, A. R., Imrie, R. C., Reynolds, K. J., and Holmes, S. D. (1995). Generation and characterization of monoclonal antibodies to human type-5 tartrate-resistant acid phosphatase: Development of a specific immunoassay of the isozyme in serum. *Clin. Chem.* **41**, 1495–1499.
13. Halleen, J., Hentunen, T. A., Hellman, J., and Vaananen, H. K. (1996). Tartrate-resistant acid phosphatase from human bone: Purification and development of an immunoassay. *J. Bone Miner. Res.* **11**, 1444–1452.
14. Janickila, A. J., Cardwell, E. M., and Yam, L. T. (1997). Characterization of monoclonal antibodies specific to human tartrate-resistant acid phosphatase. *Hybridoma* **162**, 175–182.
15. Fleckenstein, E., Dirks, W., Dehmel, U., and Drexler, H. G. (1996). Cloning and characterization of the human tartrate-resistant acid phosphatase (TRAP) gene. *Leukemia* **10**, 637–643.
16. Reddy, S. V., Alcantara, O., Roodman, G. D., and Boldt, D. H. (1996). Inhibition of tartrate-resistant acid phosphatase gene expression by hemin and protoporphyrin IX. Identification of a hemin-responsive inhibitor of transcription. *Blood* **88**, 2288–2297.
17. Alcantara, O., Reddy, S. V., Roodman, G. D., and Boldt, D. H. (1998). Transcriptional regulation of the tartrate-resistant acid phosphatase (TRAP) gene by iron. *Biochem. J.* **298**, 421–425.
18. Zaidi, M., Moonga, B., Moss, D. W., and MacIntyre, I. (1989). Inhibition of osteoclastic acid phosphatase abolishes bone resorption. *Biochem. Biophys. Res. Commun.* **159**, 68–71.
19. Reinholt, F. P., Widholm, S. M., Ek-Rylander, B., and Andersson, G. (1990). Ultrastructural localization of a tartrate-resistant acid ATPase in bone. *J. Bone Miner. Res.* **5**, 1055–1061.
20. Ek-Rylander, B., Flores, M., Wendel, M., Heinegård, D., and Andersson, G. (1994). Dephosphorylation of osteopontin and bone sialoprotein by osteoclastic tartrate-resistant acid phosphatase. Modulation of osteoclast adhesion *in vitro*. *J. Biol. Chem.* **269**, 14853–14856.
21. Andersson, G., and Ek-Rylander, B. (1995). The tartrate-resistant purple acid phosphatase of bone osteoclasts—a protein phosphatase with multivalent substrate specificity and regulation. *Acta Orthop. Scand.* **66**, 189–194.
22. Hayman, A. R., Warburton, M. J., Pringle, J. A., Coles, B., and Chambers, T. J. (1989). Purification and characterization of a tartrate-resistant acid phosphatase from human osteoclastomas. *Biochem. J.* **261**, 601–609.
23. Hayman, A. R., Jones, S. J., Boyde, A., Foster, D., Colledge, W. H., Carlton, M. B., Evans, M. J., and Cox, T. M. (1996). Mice lacking tartrate-resistant acid phosphatase (Acp 5) have disrupted endochondral ossification and mild osteopetrosis. *Development* **122**, 3151–3162.
24. McComb, R. B., and Bowers, G. N. (1979). "Alkaline Phosphatase." Plenum, New York.
25. Van Hoof, V. O., and De Broe, M. E. (1994). Interpretation and clinical significance of alkaline phosphatase isozyme patterns. *Crit. Rev. Clin. Lab. Sci.* **31**, 197–293.
26. Smith, M., Weiss, M. J., Griffin, C. A., Murray, J. C., Buetow, K. H., Emanuel, B. S., Henthorn, P. S., and Harris, H. (1988). Regional assignment of the gene for human liver/bone/kidney alkaline phosphatase to chromosome 1p36.1-p34. *Genomics* **2**, 139–143.
27. Martin, D., Tucker, D. F., Gorman, P. A., Sheer, D., Spurr, N. K., and

Trowsdale, J. (1987). The human placental alkaline phosphatase gene and related sequences map to chromosome 2 band q37. *Ann. Hum. Genet.* **51**, 145–152.

28. Harris, H. (1990). The human alkaline phosphatases: What we know and what we don't know. *Clin. Chim. Acta* **186**, 133–150.

29. Millan, J. L., and Fishman, W. H. (1995). Biology of human alkaline phosphatases with special reference to cancer. *Crit. Rev. Clin. Lab. Sci.* **32**, 1–39.

30. Toh, Y., Yamamoto, M., Endo, H., Fujiyata, A., Misumi, Y., and Ikehara, Y. (1989). Sequence divergence of 5′ extremities in rat liver alkaline phosphatase mRNAs. *J. Biochem.* **105**, 61–65.

31. Weiss, M. J., Ray, K., Henthorn, P. S., Lamb, B., Kadesch, T., and Harris, H. (1988). Structure of the human liver/bone/kidney alkaline phosphatase gene. *J. Biol Chem.* **263**, 12002–12010.

32. Matsuura, S., Kishi, F., and Kajii, T. (1990). Characterization of a 5′-flanking region of the human liver/bone/kidney alkaline phosphatase gene: Two kinds of mRNA from a single gene. *Biochem. Biophys. Res. Commun.* **168**, 993–1000.

33. Toh, Y., Yamamoto, M., Endo, H., Misumi, Y., and Ikehara, Y. (1989). Isolation and characterization of a rat liver alkaline phosphatase gene: A single gene with two promoters. *Eur. J. Biochem.* **182**, 231–237.

34. Terao, M., Studer, M., Giannì, M., and Garattini, E. (1990). Isolation and characterization of the mouse liver/bone/kidney-type alkaline phosphatase gene. *Biochem. J.* **268**, 641–648.

35. Studer, M., Terao, M., Giannì, M., and Garattini, E. (1991). Characterization of a second promoter for the mouse liver/bone/kidney-type alkaline phosphatase gene: Cell and tissue specific expression. *Biochem. Biophys. Res. Commun.* **179**, 1352–1360.

36. Zernik, J., Thiede, M. A., Twarog, K., Stover, M. L., Rodan, G. A., Upholt, W. B., and Rowe, D. W. (1990). Cloning and analysis of the 5′ region of the rat bone/liver/kidney/placenta alkaline phosphatase gene—a dual function promoter. *Matrix* **10**, 38–47.

37. Kishi, F., Matsuura, S., and Kajii, T. (1989). Nucleotide sequence of the human liver-type alkaline phosphatase cDNA. *Nucleic Acids Res.* **17**, 2129.

38. Uhler, M. D., and Stofko, R. E. (1990). Induction of alkaline phosphatase in mouse L cells by overexpression of the catalytic subunit of cAMP-dependent protein kinase. *J. Biol. Chem.* **265**, 13181–13189.

39. Terao, M., and Mintz, B. (1987). Cloning and characterization of a cDNA coding for mouse placental alkaline phosphatase. *Proc. Natl. Acad. Sci. U.S.A.* **84**, 7051–7055.

40. Zernik, J., Kream, B., and Twarog, K. (1991). Tissue-specific and dexamethasone-inducible expression of alkaline phosphatase from alternative promoters of the rat bone/liver/kidney/placenta gene. *Biochem. Biophys. Res. Commun.* **176**, 1149–1156.

41. Kiledjian, M., and Kadesch, T. (1990). Analysis of the human liver/bone/kidney alkaline phosphatase promoter in vivo and in vitro. *Nucleic Acids Res.* **18**, 957–961.

42. Kiledjian, M., and Kadesch, T. (1991). Post-transcriptional regulation of the human liver/bone/kidney alkaline phosphatase gene. *J. Biol. Chem.* **266**, 4207–4213.

43. Rodan, G. A., and Rodan, S. B. (1983). Expression of the osteoblastic phenotype. *Bone Miner. Res.* **2**, 244–285.

44. Sato, N., Takahashi, Y., and Asano, S. (1994). Preferential usage of the bone-type leader sequence for the transcripts of liver/bone/kidney-type alkaline phosphatase gene in neutrophilic granulocytes. *Blood* **83**, 1093–1101.

45. Heath, J. K., Suva, L. J., Yoon, K., Kiledjian, M., Martin, T. J., and Rodan, G. A. (1992). Retinoic acid stimulates transcriptional activity from the alkaline phosphatase promoter in the immortalized rat calvarial cell line, RCT-1. *Mol. Endocrinol.* **6**, 636–646.

46. Escalante-Alcalde, D., Recillas-Targa, F., Hernández-García, D., Castro-Obregón, S., Terao, M., Garattini, E., and Covarrubias, L. (1996). Retinoic acid and methylation cis-regulatory elements control the mouse tissue non-specific alkaline phosphatase gene expression. *Mech. Dev.* **57**, 21–32.

47. Weiss, M. J., Ray, K., Fallon, M. D., Whyte, M. P., Fedde, K. N., Lafferty, M. A., Mulivor, R., and Harris, H. (1989). Analysis of liver/bone/kidney alkaline phosphatase mRNA, DNA, and enzymatic activity in cultured skin fibroblasts from 14 unrelated patients with severe hypophosphatasia. *Am. J. Hum. Genet.* **44**, 686–694.

48. Johnson-Pais, T. L., and Leach, R. J. (1992). Extinction of liver/bone/kidney alkaline phosphatase in osteosarcoma hybrid cells. *Somatic Cell Mol.Genet.* **18**, 423–430.

49. Zhou, H., Manji, S. S., Findlay, D. M., Martin, T. J., Heath, J. K., and Ng, K. W. (1994). Novel action of retinoic acid. Stabilization of newly synthesized alkaline phosphatase transcripts. *J. Biol. Chem.* **269**, 22433–22439.

50. Leboy, P. S., Beresford, J. N., Devlin, C., and Owen, M. E. (1991). Dexamethasone induction of osteoblast mRNAs in rat marrow stromal cell cultures. *J. Cell. Physiol.* **146**, 370–378.

51. Kyeyune-Nyombi, E., Nicolas, V., Strong, D. D., and Farley, J. (1995). Paradoxical effects of phosphate to directly regulate the level of skeletal alkaline phosphatase activity in human osteosarcoma (SaOS-2) cells and inversely regulate the level of skeletal alkaline phosphatase mRNA. *Calcif. Tissue Int.* **56**, 154–159.

52. Kobayashi, T., and Robinson, J. M. (1991). A novel intracellular compartment with unusual secretory properties in human neutrophils. *J. Cell Biol.* **113**, 743–756.

53. Cain, T. J., Liu, Y., Takizawa, T., and Robinson, J. M. (1995). Solubilization of glycosyl-phosphatidylinositol-anchored proteins in quiescent and stimulated neutrophils. *Biochim. Biophys. Acta* **1235**, 69–78.

54. Johnson-Pais, T. L., and Leach, R. J. (1996). 1,25-dihydroxyvitamin D_3 and transforming growth factor-β act synergistically to override extinction of liver/bone/kidney alkaline phosphatase in osteosarcoma hybrid cells. *Exp. Cell Res.* **226**, 67–74.

55. Franceschi, R. T., Iyer, B. S., and Cui, Y. (1994). Effects of ascorbic acid on collagen matrix formation and osteoblast differentiation in murine MC3T3-E1 cells. *J. Bone Miner. Res.* **9**, 843–854.

56. Xiao, G., Cui, Y., Ducy, P., Karsenty, G., and Franceschi, R. T. (1997). Ascorbic-acid-dependent activation of the osteocalcin promoter in MC3T3-E1 preosteoblasts: Requirement for collagen matrix synthesis and the presence of an intact OSE2 sequence. *Mol. Endocrinol.* **11**, 1103–1113.

57. Waymire, K. G., Mahuren, J. D., Jaje, J. M., Guilarte, T. R., Coburn, S. P., and MacGregor, G. R. (1995). Mice lacking tissue non-specific alkaline phosphatase die from seizures due to defective metabolism of vitamin B-6. *Nat. Genet.* **11**, 45–51.

58. Narisawa, S., Fröhlander, N., and Millán, J. L. (1997). Inactivation of two mouse alkaline phosphatase genes and establishment of a model of infantile hypophosphatasia. *Dev. Dyn.* **208**, 432–446.

59. Hui, M. Z., Sukhu, B., and Tenenbaum, H. C. (1996). Expression of tissue non-specific alkaline phosphatase stimulates differentiated behaviour in specific transformed cell populations. *Anat. Rec.* **244**, 423–436.

60. Crawford, K., Weissig, H., Binette, F., Millán, J. L., and Goetinck, P. F. (1995). Tissue-nonspecific alkaline phosphatase participates in the establishment and growth of feather germs in embryonic chick skin cultures. *Dev. Dyn.* **204**, 48–56.

61. Shinozaki, T., Watanabe, H., Arita, S., and Chigira, M. (1995). Amino acid phosphatase activity of alkaline phosphatase—A possible role of protein phosphatase. *Eur. J. Biochem.* **227**, 367–371.

62. Watanabe, T., Wada, N., and Chou, J. Y. (1992). Structural and functional analysis of human germ cell alkaline phosphatase by site-specific mutagenesis. *Biochemistry* **31**, 3051–3058.

63. Sowadski, J. M., Handschumacher, M. D., Murthy, H. M. K., Foster, B. A., and Wyckoff, H. W. (1985). Refined structure of alkaline phosphatase from *E. coli* at 2.8Å resolution. *J. Mol. Biol.* **186**, 417–433.

64. Low, M. G., and Saltiel, A. R. (1988). Structural and functional roles of glycosylphosphatidylinositol in membranes. *Science* **239**, 268–275.

65. Micanovic, R., Bailey, C. A., Brink, L., Gerber, L., Pan, Y. C. E., Hulmes, J. D., and Udenfriend, S. (1988). Aspartic acid-484 of nascent placental

alkaline phosphatase condenses with a phosphatidylinositol glycan to become the carboxyl terminus of the mature enzyme. *Proc. Natl. Acad. Sci. U.S.A.* **85**, 1398–1402.

66. Manes, T., Hoylaerts, M. F., Muller, R., Lottspeich, F., Holke, W., and Millan, J. L. (1998). Genetic complexity, structure, and characterization of highly active bovine intestinal alkaline phosphatases. *J. Biol Chem.* **273**, 23353–23360.

67. Fishman, W. H., and Sie, H.-G. (1971). Organ-specific inhibition of human alkaline phosphatase isozymes of liver, bone, intestine, and placenta: L-phenylalanine, L-tryptophan and L-homoarginine. *Enzymologia* **41**, 140–167.

68. Millan, J. L., and Manes, T. (1988). Seminoma-derived Nagao isozyme is encoded by a germ cell alkaline phosphatase gene. *Proc. Natl. Acad. Sci. U.S.A.* **85**, 3024–3028.

69. Doellgast, G. J., and Fishman, W. H. (1976). L-Leucine, a specific inhibitor of a rare human placental alkaline phosphatase phenotype. *Nature* **259**, 49–51.

70. Watanabe, T., Wada, N., Kim, E. E., Wyckoff, H. W., and Chou, J. Y. (1991). Mutation of a single amino acid converts germ cell alkaline phosphatase to placental alkaline phosphatase. *J. Biol. Chem.* **266**, 21174–21178.

71. Hoylaerts, M. F., Manes, T., and Millan, J. L. (1992). Molecular mechanism of uncompetitive inhibition of human placental and germ cell alkaline phosphatase. *Biochem. J.* **286**, 23–30.

72. Vittur, F., Stagni, N., Moro, L., and De Bernard, B. (1984). Alkaline phosphatase binds to collagen: A hypothesis on the mechanism of extravesicular mineralization in epiphyseal cartilage. *Experientia* **40**, 836–837.

73. Wu, L. N. Y., Genge, B. R., Lloyd, G. C., and Wuthier, R. E. (1991). Collagen binding proteins in collagenase-released matrix vesicles from cartilage. *J. Biol. Chem.* **266**, 1195–1203.

74. Makiya, R., and Stigbrand, T. (1992). Placental alkaline phosphatase has a binding site for the human immunoglobulin-G Fc portion. *Eur. J. Biochem.* **205**, 341–345.

75. Tsonis, P. A., Argraves, W. S., and Millan, J. L. (1998). A putative functional domain of human placental alkaline phosphatase predicted from sequence comparison. *Biochem. J.* **254**, 623–624.

76. Bossi, M., Hoylaerts, M. F., and Millán, J. L. (1993). Modifications in a flexible surface loop modulate the isozyme-specific properties of mammalian alkaline phosphatases. *J. Biol. Chem.* **268**, 25409–25416.

77. Olafsdottir, S., and Chlebowski, J. F. (1989). A hybrid *E. coli* alkaline phosphatase formed on proteolysis. *J. Biol. Chem.* **264**, 4529–4535.

78. Hoylaerts, M. F., Manes, T., and Millan, J. L. (1997). Mammalian alkaline phosphatases are allosteric enzymes. *J. Biol. Chem.* **272**, 22781–22787.

79. Gonzalez, B. Y., Michel, F. J., and Simmen, R. C. (1994). A regulatory element within the uteroferrin gene 5′-flanking region binds a pregnancy-associated uterine endometrial protein. *DNA Cell Biol.* **13**, 365–376.

80. Ek-Rylander, B., Bill, P., Norgard, M., Nilsson, S., and Andersson, G. (1991). Cloning, sequence, and developmental expression of a type 5, tartrate-resistant, acid phosphatase of rat bone. *J. Biol. Chem.* **266**, 24684–24689.

81. Ketcham, C. M., Roberts, R. M., Simmen, R. C., and Nick, H. S. (1989). Molecular cloning of the type 5, iron-containing tartrate-resistant acid phosphatase from human placenta. *J. Biol. Chem.* **264**, 557–563.

82. Garattini, E., Hua, J. C., and Udenfriend, S. (1987). Cloning and sequencing of bovine kidney alkaline phosphatase cDNA. *Gene* **59**, 41–46.

83. Ghosh, A. K., and Mullins, J. I. (1995). cDNA encoding a functional feline liver/bone/kidney-type alkaline phosphatase. *Arch. Biochem. Biophys.* **322**, 240–249.

84. Nosjean, O., Koyama, I., Goseki, M., Roux, B., and Komoda, T. (1997). Human tissue non-specific alkaline phosphatases: Sugar-moiety-induced enzymatic and antigenic modulations and genetic aspects. *Biochem. J.* **321**, 297–303.

85. Brown, N. A., Stofko, R. E., and Uhler, M. D. (1990). Induction of alkaline phosphatase in mouse L cells by overexpression of the catalytic subunit of cAMP-dependent protein kinase. *J. Biol. Chem.* **265**, 13181–13189.

86. Noda, M., Thiede, M., Buenaga, R. F., Yoon, K., Weiss, M., Henthorn, P., Harris, H., and Rodan, G. A. (1987). cDNA cloning of alkaline phosphatase from a rat osteosarcoma (ROS 17/2.8) cells. *J. Bone Miner. Res.* **2**, 161–164.

87. Thiede, M. A., Yoon, K., Golub, E. E., Noda, M., and Rodan, G. A. (1988). Structure and expression of rat osteosarcoma (ROS 17/2.8) alkaline phosphatase: Product of a single copy gene. *Proc. Natl. Acad. Sci. U.S.A.* **85**, 319–323.

88. Misumi, Y., Tashiro, K., Hattori, M., Sakaki, Y., and Ikehara, Y. (1988). Primary structure of rat liver alkaline phosphatase deduced from its cDNA. *Biochem. J.* **249**, 661–668.

CHAPTER 10

Matrix Proteinases

IAN M. CLARK AND GILLIAN MURPHY

School of Biological Sciences, University of East Anglia, Norwich NR4 7TJ, United Kingdom

I. INTRODUCTION

Proteolysis of the extracellular matrix (ECM) of tissues is a feature of the normal remodeling associated with physiological processes such as morphogenesis, growth, and wound healing. Degradation of the ECM is also associated with many pathologies including arthritic diseases, osteoporosis, and periodontal disease. More recently, the concept of the role of proteinases in the modulation of cell–cell and cell–ECM interactions as a means of signalling to the cell and the determination of cell phenotype has emerged. This more subtle activity is clearly of importance not only in developmental processes, but also in diseases such as atherosclerosis and tumor invasion and metastasis.

Endopeptidases are thought to be the key enzymes in ECM degradation, and in vitro evidence suggests that members of all four major classes (metallo-, serine, cysteine, and aspartate at the active site) can cleave individual components of the ECM (Table IA, IB). Although the emphasis on different proteinase activities varies according to the situation, the metalloproteinases appear to have the most ubiquitous role in matrix turnover. In this review, we will summarize the role of other proteinase types and describe the metalloproteinases in more detail.

II. ASPARTIC PROTEINASES

Cathepsin D, a lysosomal enzyme [1], is the major aspartic proteinase involved in matrix degradation. It has optimal proteolytic activity at acid pH between 3 and 5, showing little activity at neutral pH. It can degrade proteoglycan core protein, gelatin, and collagen telopeptides, but not native triple helical collagen. Although early reports indicated that cathepsin D might be involved in the extracellular degradation of matrix molecules, later studies have demonstrated that its role is confined to the intracellular breakdown of phagocytosed matrix molecules. For example, pepstatin, an inhibitor of cathepsin D, and anticathepsin D antiserum do not inhibit vitamin A-induced cartilage breakdown in vitro [2]; in rat osteoclasts, cathepsin D was immunolocalized in granules or vacuoles, but negligible staining was seen along resorption lacunae and in eroded bone matrix, in contrast to the staining pattern seen for other cathepsins [3].

III. CYSTEINE PROTEINASES

The cysteine proteinases which degrade extracellular matrix components include cathepsins B, L, S, K, and calpains

137

TABLE IA.   Proteolysis of the Extracellular Matrix

Proteinase class	Matrix substrates	Inhibitors	pH range
Serine			
Plasmin	Fibrin, fibronectin, aggrecan, pro MMPs	α_2 antiplasmin	Neutral
Tissue plasminogen activator	Plasminogen	PAI-1, PAI-2	"
Urokinase-type plasminogen activator	Plasminogen	PAI-1, PAI-2, PN-1	"
Neutrophil elastase	Most ECM components, proMMPs	α_1-PI	"
Proteinase 3	Similar to elastase	α_1-PI, elafin	"
Cathepsin G	Aggrecan, elastin collagen II, proMMPs	α_1-PI	"
Plasma kallikrein	proUPA, proMMP1, MMP3	Aprotinin	"
Tissue kallikrein	proMMP8	Kallistatin	"
Tryptase	Collagen VI, fibronectin, proMMP3	Trypstatin	"
Chymase	Many ECM components, proMMP1, MMP3	α_1-PI	"
Granzymes	Aggrecan		
Cysteine			
Cathepsin B	Collagen telopeptides, collagen IX, XI, aggrecan	Cystatins	5.0–6.5
Cathepsin L	As cathepsin B, elastin	Cystatin	4.0–6.5
Cathepsin S	As cathepsin B, elastin	Cystatin	6.0–6.5
Cathepsin K	Collagen telopeptides, elastin	Cystatin	Neutral
Calpains	Proteoglycan, fibronectin, vitronectin	Calpastatin	Neutral
Aspartate			
Cathepsin D	Many phagocytosed ECM components	Pepstatin	3.0–6.0

I and II. Cathepsins B, L, and S are lysosomal enzymes with acid pH optima; ultrastructural studies using the electron microscope have demonstrated their involvement in intracellular degradation of phagocytosed matrix molecules. However, they may also function as extracellular proteinases at pH closer to neutral.

The lysosomal active form of cathepsin B is unstable at neutral pH, but both procathepsin B and a higher M_r, active form (which may be a noncovalent complex between cleaved propeptide and active enzyme) are secreted extracellularly from stimulated connective tissue cells and activated macrophages; these are more stable and possibly active at near neutral pH. A study of cathepsin B activity in synovial fluid demonstrated a higher level of activity in rheumatoid arthritis (RA) fluid than in osteoarthritis (OA) fluid, with 42 kDa proenzyme and 29 kDa active enzyme being present [4]. Human osteoblasts are reported to secrete a form of cathepsin B

that is stable at neutral pH and can be induced with IL-1 and PTH [5].

At acid pH *in vitro*, cathepsins B, L, and S cleave the telopeptides of type I and II collagen, causing depolymerization; they also cleave proteoglycan core protein, gelatin, and nonhelical regions of types IX and XI collagen [6, 7]. Cathepsins L and S are both potently elastolytic, and at neutral pH, cathepsin S has elastolytic activity comparable with that of neutrophil elastase [7]. Cathepsin S is stable over a broader pH range than cathepsin B or L. If cathepsins B and L are added to cartilaginous matrix at near neutral pH, then proteoglycan and collagen are released [8]. Indeed, cathepsin B has been shown to be increased in lysosomes of OA chondrocytes compared to normal, and also extracellularly at sites of cartilage degradation in OA [9]. A lipophilic cathepsin B inhibitor can block proteoglycan release induced by interleukin 1 in an explant model and this can also be blocked by

TABLE IB. Proteolysis of the Extracellular Matrix

MMP number	Enzyme	M_r, latent	M_r, active	Known substrates
MMP-1	Interstitial collagenase-1	55,000	45,000	Collagens I, II, III, VII, VIII, X; gelatin; aggrecan; versican; proteoglycan link protein; casein; α_1-proteinase inhibitor; α_2-macroglobulin (α_2M); pregnancy zone protein; ovostatin; nidogen; myelin basic protein (MBP); proTNF; L-Selectin; MMP-2; MMP-9
MMP-8	Neutrophil collagenase	75,000	58,000	Collagens I, II, III, V, VII, VIII, X; gelatin; aggrecan; α_1-proteinase inhibitor; α_2-antiplasmin; fibronectin
MMP-13	Collagenase-3	60,000	48,000	Collagens I, II, III, IV gelatin; plasminogen activator inhibitor 2; aggrecan; perlecan; tenascin
MMP-18	*Xenopus* collagenase	55,000	?	
MMP-3	Stromelysin-1	57,000	45,000	Collagens III, IV, IX, X; gelatin; aggrecan; versican, perlecan; nidogen; proteoglycan link protein; fibronectin; laminin; elastin; casein; fibrinogen; antithrombin-III; α_2M; ovostatin; α_1-proteinase inhibitor; MBP; proTNF; MMP-1; MMP-7; MMP-8; MMP-9; MMP-13
MMP-10	Stromelysin-2	57,000	44,000	Collagens III, IV, V; gelatin; casein; aggrecan; elastin; proteoglycan link protein; fibronectin; MMP-1; MMP-8
MMP-11	Stromelysin-3	51,000	44,000	α_1-proteinase inhibitor
MMP-19		?	?	Aggrecan
MMP-20	Enamelysin			Amelogenin
MMP-2	72 kDa gelatinase	72,000	66,000	Collagens I, IV, V, VII, X, XI, XIV; gelatin; elastin; fibronectin; aggrecan; versican; proteoglycan link protein; MBP; proTNF; α_1-proteinase inhibitor; MMP-9; MMP-13
MMP-9	92 kDa gelatinase	92,000	86,000	Collagens IV, V, VII, X, XIV; gelatin; elastin; aggrecan; versican; proteoglycan link protein; fibronectin; nidogen; α_1-proteinase inhibitor; MBP; pro TNF
MMP-7	Matrilysin (PUMP-1)	28,000	19,000	Collagens IV, X; gelatin; aggrecan; proteoglycan link protein; fibronectin; laminin; entactin; elastin; casein; transferrin; MBP; α_1-proteinase inhibitor; proTNF; MMP-1; MMP-2; MMP-9
MMP-12	Macrophage metalloelastase	5,400	45,000/ 22,000	Collagen IV; gelatin; elastin α_1-proteinase inhibitor; fibronectin; vitronectin; laminin; proTNF; MBP
MMP-14	MT-MMP-1	66,000	56,000	Collagens I, II, III; gelatin; casein; elastin; fibronectin; laminin B chain; vitronectin; aggrecan; dermatan sulfate proteoglycan; MMP-2; MMP-13; proTNF
MMP-15	MT-MMP-2	72,000	?	MMP-2; gelatin; fibronectin; tenascin; nidogen; laminin
MMP-16	MT-MMP-3	64,000	52,000	MMP-2
MMP-17	MT-MMP-4	?	?	

MMP inhibitors, perhaps revealing a role for the cathepsin in the activation of proMMP [10].

In endochondral bone formation, it has been proposed that the complete degradation of type X collagen requires both the action of MMP-13 from the chondrocyte and then cathepsin B from the osteoclast [11].

In bone resorption by osteoclasts, studies with specific inhibitors in a murine calvarial assay suggest that cathepsins L and S might act both intracellularly and extracellularly, but that cathepsin B only acts in the intracellular compartment, possibly via activation of other proteinases [12].

In rat osteoclasts, cathepsin B and L immunostained along lacunae with strong extracellular staining of both on collagen fibrils and the bone matrix under the ruffled border, with a stronger signal for cathepsin L than for cathepsin B [3]. A further ultrastructural study using specific inhibitors also suggested that cathepsin L played a key role in bone resorption by cultured osteoclasts [13].

A new cysteine proteinase, cathepsin K (previously called cathepsin O or O2), has been discovered in osteoclasts. Cathepsin K has 56% sequence homology with cathepsin S; it has a pH optimum of 6–6.5, similar to that of cathepsin S, but has activity over a broader range, remaining largely active at neutral pH. It degrades elastin, collagen telopeptides, and gelatin better than the other cysteine proteinase cathepsins [7, 14]. Inhibitors of cathepsin K have been shown to reduce bone resorption *in vivo* or *in vitro* [15] and an antisense approach blocks osteoclastic bone resorption *in vitro* [16]. It has been suggested that only cathepsin K, and not cathepsins B, L, or S, is abundantly expressed in human osteoclasts and that this enzyme is responsible for osteoclastic bone resorption [17]. Interestingly, pycnodyostosis, an osteochondrodysplasia, is caused by mutation in the cathepsin K gene [18].

A family of cysteine proteinase inhibitors, the cystatins, have also been described [19]. Their role in controlling the turnover of cartilage and bone is largely unknown; however, cystatin C is reported to inhibit bone resorption in different *in vitro* systems due to inhibition of osteoclastic proteolytic enzymes and to be produced by bone cells [20].

Calpains are cytosolic, Ca^{2+}-dependent, cysteine proteinases with neutral pH optima. Calpain I and II require micromolar and millimolar Ca^{2+} respectively for activation. These enzymes can degrade proteoglycan, fibronectin, and vitronectin [21]. Calpains have been shown to be raised in RA and OA synovial fluid and tissues [22] and in some animal models of arthritis [23]. Calpastatin, a specific cellular inhibitor of calpains, has been identified as an autoantigen in some RA patients [24].

IV. SERINE PROTEINASES

A. Leukocyte Enzymes

Neutrophil elastase, cathepsin G, and proteinase 3 are found in the azurophil granules of polymorphonuclear leukocytes. They are synthesized as precursors in promyelocytes of bone marrow during development [25]. Granule contents may be discharged into the extracellular space during inflammation where they have the opportunity to degrade matrix. These enzymes have pH optima between 7 and 9 and can degrade many components of the matrix. Neutrophil elastase and proteinase 3 are both potently elastolytic; neutrophil elastase and cathepsin G degrade the telopeptides of fibrillar collagens and type IV collagen. All three enzymes can degrade other matrix glycoproteins, gelatin, and proteoglycan core protein [26–28]. Proteinase 3 is an autoantigen in Wegener's granulomatosis [29].

The role of these enzymes in cartilage degradation may only be in specialized situations where they can escape inhibition by synovial fluid inhibitors, for example during joint sepsis. Beige mice lack both PMN elastase and cathepsin G, but still undergo severe cartilage loss during antigen-induced arthritis [30]. Rabbits depleted of neutrophils by nitrogen mustard show the same rate of cartilage degradation in arthritis models as the nontreated animals [31].

A number of inhibitors of these enzymes exist, including the general proteinase inhibitor α_2-macroglobulin. The major specific serum inhibitor of PMN elastase is α_1 proteinase inhibitor which also inhibits proteinase 3 [32]. α_1 antichymotrypsin and secreted leukocyte proteinase inhibitor (SLPI) inhibit both PMN elastase and cathepsin G; SLPI has been isolated from cartilage [33]. Thrombospondin 1, a matrix protein, is also a potent inhibitor of PMN elastase and cathepsin

G; this molecule is found to be induced in RA synovium proportionally to the numbers of surrounding leukocytes [34].

Cross talk may exist between proteinase families via action on proteinase inhibitors (e.g., serpins may be inactivated by MMPs and neutrophil elastase may inactivate TIMPs) [35, 36] (see Section V.C).

B. Plasminogen Activators and Plasmin

The conversion of plasminogen (Pg, 90 kDa) to plasmin by plasminogen activators (PA) is a key step in connective tissue remodeling because plasmin can degrade a number of matrix macromolecules (aside from fibrin, plasmin can degrade the core protein of proteoglycan, fibronectin, laminin, and type IV collagen) [37] and can also take part in the activation of proMMPs (e.g., proMMP-1 and -3). There are two types of PA, tissue-type (tPA) and urokinase-type (uPA). tPA (70 kDa) is mainly associated with endothelial cells but is also produced by fibroblasts and chondrocytes; it also binds to extracellular matrix components such as laminin, fibronectin, and thrombospondin [38]. tPA is the major activator of Pg in fibrinolysis. uPA (54 kDa, two subunits of 30 kDa and 24 kDa which are disulphide bonded) is produced by many connective tissue cells. It binds a specific cell surface receptor (uPAR) via a growth factor domain in uPA, and this enhances activation of cell-associated Pg and protects the uPA from inhibition. uPA may also have mitogenic effects via this receptor [39].

Inhibitors of plasmin and PA come from the serpin superfamily [32]. α_2-Antiplasmin is the major plasmin inhibitor in plasma. α_1-Proteinase inhibitor and α_2-antichymotrypsin are also active against plasmin [40].

PA inhibitors (PAIs) control the rate of plasmin production in the local extracellular environment. PAI-1, originally isolated from endothelial cells, is produced by a number of cell types and is present in platelets; it inhibits both tPA and uPA, but forms more stable complexes with the former [41]. PAI-1 binds to the pericellular matrix which enhances its extracellular stability and therefore may inhibit proteolysis in this environment. PAI-2 is a better inhibitor of uPA than tPA; it is present in plasma and is expressed by a number of cell types including macrophages [42]. PAI-3 is also an inhibitor of activated protein C and is less well characterized [43]. Finally, protease nexin 1 (PN-1) inhibits uPA and tPA with the PN-1:proteinase complex binding a specific cell surface receptor via the inhibitor, followed by internalization and degradation [44].

In synovial fluid, uPA, PAI-1, and uPAR levels are all elevated in RA compared to OA, and in OA compared to normal, though there was no direct association with clinical parameters [45]. There is also evidence for local production of uPA and PAI-1, with synovial fluid levels elevated compared to levels in plasma. At the invasive pannus front in the

RA synovium, uPA, uPAR, PAI-1, and PAI-2 are all induced compared to normal tissue [46, 47].

Plasminogen added to chondrocyte cultures causes an increase in interleukin-1-induced matrix degradation, implicating PA in this process; indeed, IL-1 induces uPA and PAI-1 in these cells. Similarly, plasminogen added to IL-1-stimulated cartilage explants potentiates increased collagen and proteoglycan loss, and this can be blocked with PA inhibitors or MMP inhibitors. Hence, there may be a cascade of enzyme activation with PA activating plasminogen and plasmin activating MMPs [48, 49]. Furthermore, intra-articular injection of protease nexin-1 blocks IL-1 or FGF-induced proteoglycan loss from rabbit knee. Tranexamic acid (TEA), another antiplasmin agent, used orally, has the same effect [50]. TEA treatment of RA patients also decreased urinary collagen cross links [51].

Osteoblasts also produce uPA, tPA, PAI-1, and uPAR, and their synthesis is regulated by osteotropic hormones [52, 53]. It has been postulated that they function as activators of proMMPs or latent growth factors in bone remodeling, or that uPA may be acting as a mitogen via its growth factor domain. Similarly, the direct resorptive activity of osteoclasts does not require tPA or uPA, but the latter may be involved in migration of the preosteoclasts to the mineral surface [54].

C. Mast Cell Proteinases

Mast cell granules contain tryptase, chymase, and cathepsin G. Tryptase has a trypsin-like specificity and degrades collagen type VI and fibronectin. Chymase has a chymotrypsin-like specificity and degrades a number of matrix substrates. Both enzymes have been implicated in the activation of pro-MMPs [55]. Activated, degranulated mast cells have been localized to regions of cartilage erosion in RA [56].

D. Granzymes

Granzyme A and B are serine proteinases that are stored in the granules of activated cytotoxic T-cells and NK cells. Granzyme B has been reported to degrade aggrecan in the extracellular matrix synthesized by chondrocytes [57]. Granzyme A-and B-expressing lymphocytes have been localized in the synovium of patients with RA and OA, and may be increased in RA tissue [58].

V. METALLOPROTEINASES

A. Non-MMP Metalloproteinases

At least three classes of zinc-dependent endopeptidase activity have been implicated in the degradation of cell surface molecules and the ECM [59]: the matrix metalloproteinase (MMP) family, the reprolysin-related proteinases (a disintegrin and metalloprotease [ADAM] or metalloprotease-like, disintegrin-like, cysteine-rich protein [MDC]) that contain both a metalloproteinase and a disintegrin domain, and the astacin-related proteinases. Membrane bound and secreted forms of these enzymes have been described. Little is known about the latter two families in cartilage and bone, although McKie et al. [60] have reported mRNA for some of the ADAMs in cartilage and bone cells. Inoue et al. [61] have shown that ADAM 11, 12, 15, and 19 are expressed by osteoblasts and ADAMs 11 and 15 by osteoclasts. These proteins have proposed functions in the proteolytic processing of cell surface ectodomains, in membrane fusion events, and in cell–cell, cell–matrix interactions [62]. Proteolysis of the aggrecan core protein occurs within the interglobular domain; amino-terminal sequencing of cleavage products has identified two main sites of proteolysis [63, 64]. Cleavage at the Asn341–Phe342 bond has been attributed to the action of the matrix metalloproteinases [65]; however, cleavage at the Glu373–Ala374 bond appears to be predominant in RA and also in stimulated cartilage explants in vitro. The enzyme catalysing this cleavage has been named "aggrecanase" but its identity remains unclear. Recently it has been reported that aggrecanase activity can be found in the culture medium of stimulated cartilage explants, but similar activity has also been identified on chondrocyte membranes [66]. The inhibition profile of the reported activities suggests that aggrecanase may be a metalloproteinase, but not a matrix metalloproteinase, and therefore may possibly belong to the reprolysin family. Indeed, a meeting report [67] suggests that an ADAM termed ADMP-1 (aggrecan-degrading metalloprotease-1) or ADAM-TS4 can perform the Glu373–Ala374 cleavage specific to "aggrecanase." This is member of a subfamily of ADAMs that are not membrane associated and contain thrombospondin-like repeats. It seems likely that a number of members of the subgroup will have the ability to cleave aggrecan in this way. The astacins discovered to date include the enzyme that cleaves the carboxy-terminal propeptides of the fibrillar collagens during collagen assembly (bone morphogenetic protein-1; [68]) and others involved in cell differentiation and pattern formation during development. Studies have provided direct morphological and functional links between the proteolytic activity of bone morphogenetic protein-1 and the ECM [69].

B. Matrix Metalloproteinases

The MMPs are key ECM-degrading proteinases and have been divided into subgroups according to their structure and function. Sixteen individual enzymes have been described (Table IB). The MMPs have a common domain structure with a signal peptide, a propeptide, a catalytic domain, a hinge region, and a haemopexin-like C-terminal domain. Individual

MMPs have variations on this general structure: the MT-MMPs (MMPs 14–17) have a transmembrane domain and cytoplasmic tail at the C-terminal end and, in common with MMP11, have a sequence containing a potential furin-cleavage site at the N-terminal end of the catalytic domain. Matrilysin lacks the C-terminal domain and hinge region, the gelatinases have an insert of three fibronectin type II repeats in the catalytic domain, and MMP9 has a collagen-like sequence at one end of the catalytic domain.

The collagenases-1, -2, and -3, MMP1, MMP8, and MMP-13 have the specific ability to degrade fibrillar collagens within the native triple helix. They also have limited ability to cleave other proteins, with MMP13 being the most active with significant activity against type IV collagen and denatured collagens (gelatins). The catalytic domains of collagenases alone retain proteolytic activity but they do not digest native triple-helical collagen. The gelatinases MMP2 and MMP9 actively degrade denatured collagens, and MMP2 has low but significant activity on soluble native fibrillar collagens. MMP2 and MMP9 also degrade soluble type IV collagen, but activity on more native preparations is extremely weak [70]. Both enzymes degrade type V collagen, elastin, aggrecan, and other matrix proteins to a limited extent.

The stromelysin subgroup, MMP3 and MMP10, cleave a number of matrix components, notably aggrecan, fibronectin, laminin, and type IV collagen. MMP3 has limited activity against collagens III, IX, and X and the telopeptides of collagens I, II, and XI [71]. Stromelysin 3, MMP11, has some of the substrate specificity of the other stromelysins, but its activity is so weak that its role as a proteinase may be against a specific, as yet unidentified, substrate. Matrilysin, MMP7, and metalloelastase MMP12 are also somewhat similar to the stromelysins, but are more active. MT-MMPs 1–3 (MMP14–16) are also known to cleave a number of ECM proteins, as do the other newer MMPs (Table IB).

Crystal structures have been obtained for the catalytic domains of human MMP1 [72–74], human MMP3 [75], and human MMP8 [76–78] complexed with synthetic inhibitors, and for the catalytic domain of human MMP1 in the absence of inhibitors [79]. The structures of these enzymes suggest that the type II fibronectin-like repeats that form the gelatin-binding domain of the gelatinases occur on a highly exposed loop far away from the active site cleft, and they are unlikely to disrupt the structure of the gelatinase catalytic domain [79]. The catalytic domains are spherical or ellipsoidal and have an active site cleft containing a catalytic zinc ion at the bottom. The structure is stabilized by a second zinc ion and a calcium ion. The three-dimensional structure of the catalytic domain of human MMP3 has also been determined by NMR [80–82]. Some of the differences in substrate specificity can be accounted for by variations in the six specificity subsites in the active site cleft and in sequences around the entrance to the cleft. The S1' pocket (the first specificity subsite on the carboxy-terminal side of the substrate scissile bond) is

deeper in MMP3 [75, 81] and larger in MMP8 [76, 78] than in MMP1.

The hinge region varies in length between the different MMPs. The crystal structure of porcine MMP1 showed the hinge to be highly exposed and to have no secondary structure [83]. In the collagenases, this region is proline-rich and may mimic the triple helix of collagen and contribute to the binding of MMP8 to type I collagen [84]. It has been suggested that collagenases trap triple helical collagen by folding the catalytic and C-terminal domains around the collagen; the length of the hinge region is vital in order to position the active site cleft correctly for cleavage [85, 86].

The crystal structures of full-length porcine MMP1 [83], C-terminal domain human MMP3 [86], and C-terminal domain human MMP2 [87] showed their haemopexin-like domains to comprise four similar units that form a four-bladed β-propeller structure. This propeller is stabilized by a disulphide bridge between the first and fourth units and has cations, postulated to be calcium, and chloride ions at the core. The whole structure has a disc-like shape with a funnel-like tunnel running through the short axis [86, 87]. On gelatinase A there is a surface patch of positive residues extending from the exit side of the tunnel across propeller blade III that has been proposed as an anchoring point for TIMP-2 [87]. The haemopexin-like domain contributes towards the specificity of the collagenases. Studies on the isolated N-terminal domain of MMP1 [88] and on truncated mutants of human collagenases and on collagenase/stromelysin-1 chimeric enzymes have shown that the ability of collagenase-1 [89] and MMP8 [90] to cleave native type I collagen is influenced by the C-terminal domain. This domain is also involved in the binding of active MMPs to TIMPs [88, 89, 91, 92] and in the binding of latent and active MMP3 [89] and MMP8 [93] to extracellular matrix molecules. The C-terminal domains of MMPs 2 and 9 allow them to form complexes with certain of the TIMPs when latent. Unlike the full-length molecule, MMP2 lacking the C-terminal domain cannot complex TIMP-2 and can not be activated by preparations of cell membranes [91].

The genes encoding MMP1, MMP3, MMP7, MMP9, and MMP10 have a TATA box and a TPA-responsive element (TRE), a sequence that binds to Fos and Jun (AP1), which is thought to mediate the induction of these MMPs by inflammatory cytokines such as IL-1 and TNF-α. MMP2 appears to be constitutively produced by cells in culture and is not generally significantly modulated by cytokines. The 5'-flanking region of MMP2 has no TATA box or identifiable TRE sequence, but it does contain a p53 sensitive sequence and an adenovirus E1A-responsive element resembling the AP2 binding site and two "silencer" regions [94]. Glucocorticoids, retinoids, and TGFβ repress the expression of at least MMP1 and MMP3 in connective tissue fibroblasts [95, 96]. Agents may induce the expression of one MMP while repressing expression of another. Furthermore, the effect of any one agent may differ

TABLE II. Factors That Modulate Expression of MMP and TIMP Genes

Gene	Inducing agent	Repressing agent
MMP-1	interleukin-1	transforming growth factor β
	tumour necrosis factor α	retinoic acid
	epidermal growth factor	oestrogen
	basic fibroblast growth factor	progesterone
	platelet-derived growth factor	interferon γ
	lipopolysaccharide	dexamethasone
	phorbol ester	
	colchicine	
	cytochalasin B	
	concanavalin A	
	calcium pyrophosphate	
	calcium ionophore A23187	
	UV irradiation	
TIMP-1	transforming growth factor β	dexamethasone
	interleukin-6	concanavalin A
	interleukin-11	
	oncostatin M	
	leukemia inhibitory factor	
	basic fibroblast growth factor	
	epidermal growth factor	
	interleukin-1	
	progesterone	
	oestrogen	
	retinoic acid	
	phorbol ester	
	lipopolysaccharide	
TIMP-2	progesterone	transforming growth factor β
		lipopolysaccharide
TIMP-3	transforming growth factor β	oncostatin M
	epidermal growth factor	
	platelet-derived growth factor	
	phorbol ester	
	dexamethasone	

with cell type; this makes it difficult to predict the effects of blocking cytokine/growth factor action. Table II shows some of the factors which modulate expression of the MMP-1 gene.

The extracellular regulation of MMP activity is a key feature of their function. The regulation of zymogen activation is possibly the most critical level of control of enzyme activity. The MMPs have latency conferred on them by their propeptide domain, which effectively blocks the active site in the catalytic domain. In the latent enzyme, a cysteine residue in the N-terminal propeptide PRCGVPDV sequence coordinates with the catalytic zinc ion, preventing water from occupying this site. In the active enzyme, water coordinated with this zinc ion is important in the mechanism of peptide bond hydrolysis. Upon enzymic cleavage in the prodomain, the Zn^{2+}-cysteine complex becomes destabilized, and a conformational change results in autoproteolysis of the entire propeptide [97]. Most of the MMPs are secreted in their latent forms and activation takes place outside the cell. MMP11

is an exception to this; it is activated intracellularly by furin prior to secretion [98]. The MT-MMPs have a furin-cleavage site (RXKR) similar to that of MMP11 and may also be activated before leaving the cell.

In vitro, the MMPs can be activated by chemical agents that modify cysteine residues, such as the organomercurial 4-aminophenylmercuric acetate (APMA). Activation may also occur when the conformation of the proenzyme is perturbed, as is evident from the SDS-activation of proMMP2 and pro-MMP9 during zymography. *In vivo*, however, activation probably takes place upon the enzymic cleavage of the propeptide. This cleavage may be an autolytic step, as occurs with proMMP2 at high concentrations *in vitro* [99], but more usually requires a second proteolytic activity. As can be seen from Table III, many of the MMPs share common activators and many are activated by other MMPs. This has given rise to speculation that the MMPs are involved in activation cascades [100]. An important cascade is initiated by the action of plasminogen activator (tPA or uPA) on plasminogen, which results in the active enzyme plasmin. This enzyme can activate several MMPs, as depicted in Figure 1. MMP2 is not involved in the plasmin cascade and appears to be regulated differently than the plasmin-activated MMPs. It is not cleaved by trypsin, chymotrypsin, plasmin, thrombin, elastase, cathepsin G, plasma kallikrein, or MMP3 [101, 102]. The mechanism involving MT-MMPs described earlier appears to be the most likely pathway for MMP2 activation and may lead to the activation of MMP13 and MMP9 [103].

C. Tissue Inhibitors of Metalloproteinases

There is a group of specific inhibitors of the MMPs called the TIMPs (tissue inhibitors of metalloproteinases). Four TIMPs have been described to date: TIMP-1 [104], a 28 kDa glycosylated protein; TIMP-2 [105], a 22 kDa nonglycosylated protein; TIMP-3 [106–112], a 21–27 kDa protein that binds to the extracellular matrix [96, 100]; and TIMP-4 [113, 114], the human form of which was cloned from a cDNA library and expressed as a 22 kDa recombinant protein [113]. TIMP-4 is more closely related to TIMP-2 and -3 than to TIMP-1 [114].

The TIMPs have 12 conserved cysteines, giving a protein structure of six loops that can be divided into two subdomains [115]. TIMP-1 has the shape of an elongated wedge in which the long edge, consisting of five different chains, occupies the active site cleft of MMP3 in the complex and is responsible for around 75% of the interactions between TIMP and MMP3. The central disulphide-linked segments, Cys1–Val4 and Ser68–Val69, bind either side of the MMP catalytic zinc, with Cys1 side-chain-ligation of the zinc [115].

In addition to their ability to bind to active MMPs, the TIMPs can bind to certain latent MMPs. TIMP-1 binds to MMP9 [116, 117] and TIMP-2 and -3 bind to MMP2 [91,

TABLE III.   Activation of MMPs

Human MMP	MMP number	Exogenous activators	Activating
Collagenase-1	1	Plasmin, kallikrein, chymase, MMP-3	MMP-2
Collagenase-2	8	Plasmin, MMP-3, MMP-10	Not known
Collagenase-3	13	Plasmin, MMP-2, MMP-3, MMP-14	MMP-2, MMP-9
Stromelysins-1, -2	3, 10	Plasmin, kallikrein, chymase, tryptase, elastase, cathepsin G	MMP-1, MMP-9, MMP-8, MMP-13
Stromelysin-3	11	Furin	Not known
Matrilysin	7	Plasmin, MMP-3	MMP-3
Metalloelastase	12	Plasmin	Not known
Gelatinase A	2	MMP-1, MMP-7, MMP-14, MMP-15, MMP-16	MMP-9, MMP-13
Gelatinase B	9	Plasmin, neutrophil elastase, MMP-3, MMP-2, MMP-13	Not known
MT1-MMP	14	Furin	MMP-2, MMP-13
MT2-MMP	15	Probably a proprotein convertase	MMP-2
MT3-MMP	16	Probably a proprotein convertase	MMP-2
MT4-MMP	17	Probably a proprotein convertase	Not known
MMP-19	19	Not known	Not known

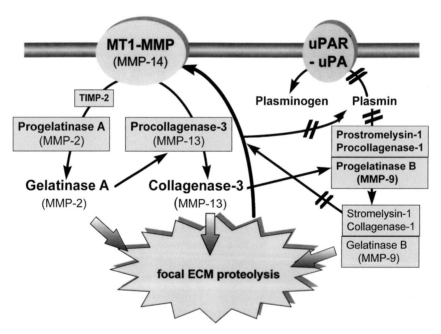

FIGURE 1   This scheme shows the cellular matrix metalloproteinase activation cascades that occur pericellularly. The activation of proMMPs is largely limited to the pericellular environment where cell-associated proteinases can function in a privileged environment away from an excess of proteinase inhibitors. Key initiators of the MMP activation cascades are thought to be MT-MMPs and plasmin-mediated proteolysis. The generation of partially active or active MMPs allows a cascade of cleavages to generate fully active enzymes. The efficiency of these interactions is dependent upon mechanisms for the concentration of MMPs at the cell surface or on the extracellular matrix. Figure courtesy of Dr. V. Knäuper, School of Biological Sciences, University of East Anglia, UK.

118–123]. The C-terminal loops of TIMP-1 are involved in the binding of this inhibitor to MMP9 [121]. Similarly, the C-terminal domain of TIMP-2 is essential for binding to MMP2, which may occur through interactions between a negatively charged "tail" on TIMP-2 [123] and a positively charged area on the haemopexin domain of MMP2 [87]. Since proMMP2 complexed to TIMP-2 is less prone to autoactivation, it was suggested that TIMP-2 acts to stabilize the proenzyme [124–126]; however, research has implicated TIMP-2 in the activation of proMMP2 by cells [127, 128]. ProMMP9 complexed to TIMP-1 resists activation by MMP3 [117] but can be activated by organomercurial compounds, albeit more slowly than noncomplexed proMMP9 [116, 129, 130].

TIMP-1 is produced by many cell types and can also be upregulated by a variety of factors such as serum, bFGF, EGF, TGFβ, IL-6 family members, retinoids, progesterone, and phorbol ester; expression is repressed by dexamethasone. In murine embryonic development, TIMP-1 is expressed at sites of osteogenesis in the limbs, ribs, digits, skull, and vertebrae [131]. TIMP-2 is often constitutively produced by cells and does not generally show a response to actions of cytokines. However, where expression is regulated, it is often in the opposite direction to TIMP-1 and -3; e.g., expression of TIMP-2 is repressed by TGFβ in various cell types. TIMP3 has been shown to be induced by factors such as EGF, PDGF, TGFβ, phorbol ester, and dexamethasone [131]. Table II shows some of the factors that regulate TIMP gene expression.

The TIMP-1, -2, and -3 promoters have potential Sp1-binding sites and share other features that are suggestive of housekeeping genes; however, TIMP-1 and -3 are known to be highly stimulus responsive. The TIMP-1 promoter has an AP-1 and PEA3 motif in close proximity, reminiscent of the inducible MMP genes described earlier; this gene also appears to have important regulatory sequences downstream of the transcription start sites. The murine TIMP-3 gene has six upstream AP-1 sites which may be involved in basal expression of the gene, although there appears to be conflicting data from the murine and human genes. The murine gene also has a putative p53 binding site but this appears to be nonfunctional. The TIMP-2 gene has a promoter proximal AP-1 motif, but this appears not to have a major role in basal expression of the gene [131].

D. α_2-Macroglobulin

α_2-Macroglobulin (α_2M) is a plasma proteinase inhibitor that is able to inhibit almost all proteinases including MMPs. Human α_2M is a 720 kDa tetrameric protein consisting of four 180 kDa subunits. Each subunit contains an exposed "bait" region, a sequence that can be cleaved by virtually all proteinases. Human MMP1 cleaves human α_2M at the Gly–Leu bond in the bait region sequence –Gly–Pro–Glu–Gly^{679}–Leu–Arg–Val–Gly–, which strongly resembles the collagenase-1 cleavage site in calf skin collagen α1(I) and α2(I) chains [132]. This cleavage leads to a conformational change in the α_2M, which traps the proteinase to the exclusion of large substrates; small (peptide) substrates may still be cleaved. Inhibition by α_2M is irreversible. α_2M-proteinase complexes are cleared from the circulation by a specific receptor that is a low-density lipoprotein receptor-related protein. Aside from its function as a proteinase inhibitor, α_2M has been shown to bind a variety of cytokines such as PDGF, TGFβ, bFGF, and IL-1β, whence it may act as a carrier protein [133, 134]. Interestingly, α_2M can inhibit urokinase-type plasminogen activator (uPA) when it is in solution but not when it is bound to uPA receptors at the cell surface, probably due to steric hindrance preventing the engulfing of the uPA by the α_2M [135]. The presence of this inhibitor thus localizes uPA activity to the cell surface.

E. MMPs and TIMPs in Cartilage and Bone

Extracts of cartilage from osteoarthritic patients show markedly increased expression of MMPs, with smaller increases in TIMPs; both are elevated compared to normal cartilage [136]. An imbalance of MMP and TIMP activity is implicated in cartilage loss. Similarly, MMP levels are elevated in the synovium and cartilage of RA patients [137]. In the septic joint, high levels of MMP–TIMP complexes have been found in the synovial fluid, with active MMPs present but free TIMPs absent; rapid cartilage destruction is seen in these patients [138].

Growth factors such as IL-1, TNFα, bFGF, PDGF, OSM, and ATRA stimulate MMP expression in cartilage and also induce cartilage resorption; factors such as TGFβ, IGF-I, IL-4, IL-10, and IL-13 may oppose these effects.

In cartilage breakdown, proteoglycan loss is rapid and reversible. In contrast, collagen loss is essentially irreversible [139] and therefore its prevention may represent a major therapeutic goal. The enzyme responsible for proteoglycan release from cartilage was thought to be stromelysin-1 (MMP-3), but analysis of proteoglycan fragments released from resorbing cartilage implicate another enzyme, "aggrecanase," whose identity is not fully established.

TIMP-1 and -2 have been shown to prevent collagen release in an *ex vivo* cartilage resorption model, suggesting the involvement of collagenase MMPs in this event; the same inhibitors were unable to prevent proteoglycan loss, perhaps indicative of the nonMMP nature of aggrecanase. Synthetic MMP inhibitors can prevent both proteoglycan and collagen loss, but they achieve the former only at high concentrations where their specificity may be doubtful [140].

In a further study, a strong correlation between inhibition of proteoglycan loss and inhibition of stromelysin-1 (MMP-3) has been reported, although again high concentrations of stromelysin inhibitors were needed (approximately

1000 times greater concentration was required to inhibit proteoglycan loss compared to inhibition of MMP-3). A strong correlation has been reported between inhibition of collagenase activity and inhibition of collagen release from cartilage explants; no correlation was observed with inhibition of stromelysin or gelatinase [141].

The identity of the collagenase MMP responsible for cartilage collagen loss is unknown. Collagenase-1 (MMP-1) and collagenase-3 (MMP-13) can be synthesized by chondrocytes, and collagenase-2 (MMP-8) may also be expressed by these cells. There is some evidence that specific MMP-13 inhibitors can block interleukin-1-induced collagen loss.

MMPs have been implicated in bone turnover, either via removal of osteoid to allow osteoclastic bone resorption or more directly as osteoclast enzymes.

In fetal rat calvarial osteoblasts, a variety of growth factors have been shown to alter expression of collagenase (MMP-13) and also to modulate bone resorption in calvarial explant assays; inducing agents include PTH, bFGF, ATRA, PDGF, and IL-6 and suppressing factors include IGF-I and -II, TGFβ, and BMP-2. Some of these factors (bFGF, TGFβ, and BMP-2) also induce expression of TIMP-1 and -3 [142]. Human osteoblasts have been reported to express at least MMP-1, -2, -3, -9, -10, -13, and -14 [143]. Synthetic MMP-inhibitors have been demonstrated to suppress bone resorption [144].

In human development, MMP-13 is expressed in mineralizing skeletal tissue, in hypertrophic chondrocytes, and in osteoblasts involved in ossification. In osteoblasts, MMP-14 and MMP-2 were colocalized with MMP-13. In postnatal tissues, MMP-13 is expressed at sites of remodeling such as bone cysts and ectopic bone and cartilage formation, while in RA patients strong expression is seen in cartilage. MMP-13 was therefore proposed to function in the degradation of type II collagen in primary ossification, skeletal remodeling, and joint disease [145]. Similar patterns of expression are seen in developing rat and mouse bone; rat osteoblasts possess a scavenger receptor which removes MMP-13 from the extracellular space [142].

Expression of MMPs particularly MMP-9, but also MMP-1, -2, -3, -13 and -14 [146] has also been noted in osteoclasts. Indeed, some inhibition of bone resorption by MMP inhibitors has been shown even on osteoid-free bone [144].

References

1. Dunn, B. M. (1990). Structure and function of the aspartic proteinases. Genetics, structures and mechanisms. *Adv. Exp. Med. Biol.* **306**, 1–585.
2. Hembry, R. M., Knight, C. G., Dingle, J. T., and Barrett, A. J. (1982). Evidence that extracellular cathepsin D is not responsible for the resorption of cartilage matrix in culture. *Biochim. Biophys. Acta* **714**, 307–312.
3. Goto, T., Kiyoshima, T., Moroi, R., Tsukuba, T., Nishimura, Y., Himeno, M., Yamamoto, K., and Tnaka, T. (1994). Localisation of cathepsin B, cathepsin D and cathepsin L in rat osteoclast by immuno-light and immunoelectron microscopy. *Histochemistry* **101**, 33–40.
4. Duffy, J. M., Walker, B., Guthrie, D., Grimshaw, J., McNally, G., Grimshaw, J. T., Spedding, P. L., and Mollan, R. A. B. (1994). The detection, quantification and partial characterisation of cathepsin B-like activity in human pathological synovial fluids. *Biochemistry* **32**, 429–434.
5. Aisa, M. C., Rahman, S., Senin, U., Maggio, D., and Russell, R. G. G. (1996). Cathepsin B activity in normal human osteoblast-like cells and human osteoblastic osteosarcoma cells (MG-63)—regulation by interluekin-1-beta and parathyroid hormone. *Biochim. Biophys. Acta* **1290**, 29–36.
6. Maciewicz, R. A., Wotton, S. F., Etherington, D. J., and Duance, V. C. (1990). Susceptibility of the cartilage collagens type II, type IX and type XI to degradation by the cysteine proteinases, cathepsin B and cathepsin L. *FEBS Lett.* **269**, 189–193.
7. Brömme, D., Okamoto, K., Wang, B. B., and Biroc, S. (1996). Human cathepsin O2, a matrix protein-degrading cysteine protease expressed in osteoclasts. *J. Biol. Chem.* **271**, 2126–2132.
8. Maciewicz, R. A., and Wotton, S. F. (1991). Degradation of cartilage matrix components by the cysteine proteinases, cathepsin B and cathepsin L. *Biomed. Biochim. Acta* **50**, 561–564.
9. Baici, A., Lang, A., Horler, D., Kissling, R., and Merlin, C. (1995). Cathepsin B in osteoarthritis—cytochemical and histochemical analysis of human femoral head cartilage. *Ann. Rheum. Dis.* **54**, 289–297.
10. Buttle, D. J., Handley, C. J., Ilic, M. Z., Saklatvala, J., Murata, M., and Barrett, A. J. (1993). Inhibition of cartilage proteoglycan release by a specific inactivator of cathepsin B and an inhibitor of matrix metalloproteinases—evidence for 2 converging pathways of chondrocyte-mediated proteoglycan degradation. *Arthritis Rheum.* **36**, 1709–1717.
11. Sires, U. I., Schmid, T. M., Fliszar, C. J., Wang, Z. Q., Gluck, S. L., and Welgus, H. G. (1995). Complete degradation of type X collagen requires the combined action of interstitial collagenase and osteoclast-derived cathepsin B. *J. Clin. Invest.* **95**, 2089–2095.
12. Hill, P. A., Buttle, D. J., Jones, S. J., Boyde, A., Murata, M., Reynolds, J. J., and Meikle, M. C. (1994). Inhibition of bone resorption by selective inactivators of cysteine proteinases. *J. Cell. Biochem.* **56**, 118–130.
13. Debari, K., Sasaki, T., Udagawa, N., and Rifkin, B. R. (1995). An ultrastructural evaluation of the effects of cysteine proteinase inhibitors on osteoclastic resorptive functions. *Calcif. Tissue Int.* **56**, 566–570.
14. Bossard, M. J., Thaddeus, T. A., Thompson, S. K., Amegadzie, B. Y., Hannings, C. R., Jones, C., Kurdyla, J. T., McNulty, D. E., Drake, F. H., Gowen, M., and Levy, M. A. (1996). Proteolytic activity of human osteoclast cathepsin K. *J. Biol. Chem.* **271**, 12517–12524.
15. Votta, B. J., Levy, M. A., Badger, A., Bradbeer, J., Dodds, R. A., James, I. E., Thompson, S., Bossard, M. J., Carr, T., Connor, J. R., Tomaszek, T. A., Szewczuk, L., Drake, F. H., Veber, D. F., and Gowen, M. (1997). Peptide aldehyde inhibitors of cathepsin K inhibit bone resorption both in vitro and in vivo. *J. Bone Miner. Res.* **12**, 1396–1406.
16. Inui, T., Ishibashi, O., Inaoka, T., Origane, Y., Kumegawa, M., Kokubo, T., and Yamamura, T. (1997). Cathepsin K antisense oligodeoxynucleotide inhibits osteoclastic bone resorption. *J. Biol. Chem.* **272**, 8109–8112.
17. Drake, F. H., Dodds, R. A., James, I. E., Connor, J. R., Debouck, C., Richardson, S., Leerykaczewski, E., Coleman, L., Rieman, D., Barthlow, R., Hastings, G., and Gowen, M. (1996). Cathepsin K, but not cathepsin B, cathepsin L or cathepsin S, is abundantly expressed in human osteoclasts. *J. Biol. Chem.* **271**, 12511–12516.
18. Gelb, B. D., Shi, G. P., Chapman, H. A., and Desnick, R. J. (1996). Pycnodyostosis, a lysosomal disease caused by cathepsin K deficiency. *Science* **273**, 1236–1238.
19. Barrett, A. J. (1987). The cystatins: A new class of peptidase inhibitors. *Trends Biochem. Sci.* **12**, 193–196.

20. Lerner, U. H., Johansson, L., Ransjo, M., Rosenquist, J. B., Reinholt, F. P., and Grubb, A. (1997). Cystatin C, an inhibitor of bone resorption produced by osteoblasts. *Acta Physiol. Scand.* **161**, 81–92.

21. Ménard, H. A., and El-Amine, M. (1996). The calpain-calpastatin system in rheumatoid arthritis. *Immunol. Today* **17**, 545–547.

22. Yamamoto, S., Shimizu, K., Niibayashi, H., Yasuda, T., and Yamamuro, T. (1994). Immunocytochemical demonstration of calpain in synovial cells in human arthritic synovial joints. *Biomed. Res.* **15**, 77–88.

23. Szomor, Z., Shimizu, K., Fujimori, Y., Yamamoto, S., and Yamamuro, T. (1995). Appearance of calpain correlates with arthritis and cartilage destruction in collagen-induced arthritic knee joints of mice. *Ann. Rheum. Dis.* **54**, 477–483.

24. Despres, N., Talbot, G., Plouffe, B., Boire, G., and Ménard, H. A. (1995). Detection and expression of a cDNA clone that encodes a polypeptide containing 2 inhibitory domains of human calpastatin and its recognition by rheumatoid arthritis sera. *J. Clin. Invest.* **95**, 1891–1896.

25. Salvesen, G., and Enghild, J. J. (1991). Zymogen activation, specificity and genomic structures of human neutrophil elastase and cathepsin G reveal a new branch of the chymotrypsinogen superfamily of serine proteinases. *Biomed. Biochim. Acta* **50**, 665–671.

26. Starkey, P. M., Barrett, A. J., and Burleigh, M. C. (1977). The degradation of articular collagen by neutrophil proteinases. *Biochim. Biophys. Acta* **483**, 386–397.

27. Rao, N. V., Wehner, N. G., Marshall, B. C., Gray, W. R., Gray, B. H., and Hoidal, J. R. (1991). Characterisation of proteinase-3 (PR-3), a neutrophil serine proteinase. *J. Biol. Chem.* **266**, 9540–9548.

28. McDonnell, J., Lobner, J. M., Knight, W. B., Lark, M. W., Green, B., Poe, M., and Moore, V. L. (1993). Comparison of the proteoglycanolytic activities of human leukocyte elastase and human cathepsin G in vitro and in vivo. *Connect. Tissue Res.* **30**, 1–9.

29. Campanelli, D., Melchior, M., Fu, Y. P., Nakata, M., Shuman, H., Nathan, C., and Gabay, J. E. (1990). Cloning of a cDNA for proteinase 3: A serine protease, antibiotic, and autoantigen from human neutrophils. *J. Exp. Med.* **172**, 1709–1715.

30. Schalkwijk, J., Joosten, L. A. B., Van den Berg, W. B., and Van de Putte, L. B. A. (1990). Antigen-induced arthritis in beige (Chediak-Higashi) mice. *Ann. Rheum. Dis.* **49**, 607–610.

31. Pettipher, E. R., Henderson, B., Hardingham, T. E., and Ratcliffe, A. (1989). Cartilage proteoglycan depletion in acute and chronic antigen-induced arthritis. *Arthritis Rheum.* **32**, 601–607.

32. Potempa, J., Korzus, E., and Travis, J. (1994). The serpin superfamily of proteinase inhibitors: structure, function and regulation. *J. Biol. Chem.* **269**, 15957–15960.

33. Thompson, R. C., and Ohlsson, K. (1986). Isolation, properties and complete amino acid sequence of human secretory leukocyte protease inhibitor, a potent inhibitor of leukocyte elastase. *Proc. Natl. Acad. Sci. U.S.A.* **83**, 6692–6696.

34. Gotis-Graham, I., Hogg, P. J., and McNeil, H. P. (1997). Significant correlation between thrombospondin 1 and serine proteinase expression in rheumatoid synovium. *Arthritis Rheum.* **40**, 1780–1787.

35. Mast, A. E., Enghild, J. J., Nagase, H., Suzuki, K., Pizzo, S. V., and Salvesen, G. (1991). Kinetics and physiological relevance of the inactivation of α_1-proteinase inhibitor, α_1-antichymotrypsin and antithrombin III by matrix metalloproteinases-1 (tissue collagenase), -2 (72-kDa gelatinase/type IV collagenase), and -3 (stromelysin). *J. Biol. Chem.* **266**, 15810–15816.

36. Okada, Y., Watanabe, S., Nakanishi, I., Kishi, J., Hayakawa, T., Watorek, W., Travis, J., and Nagase, H. (1988). Inactivation of tissue inhibitor of metalloproteinases by neutrophil elastase and other serine proteinases. *FEBS Lett.* **229**, 157–160.

37. Dano, K., Andreasen, P. A., Grondahl-Hansen, J., Kristensen, P., Nielsen, L. S., and Skriver, L. (1985). Plasminogen activators, tissue degradation and cancer. *Adv. Cancer Res.* **44**, 139–266.

38. Saksela, O., and Rifkin, D. B. (1988). Cell-associated plasminogen activation: Regulation and physiological functions. *Annu. Rev. Cell Biol.* **4**, 93–126.

39. Ellis, V., Behrendt, N., and Dano, K. (1991). Plasminogen activation by receptor-bound urokinase: A kinetic study with both cell-associated and isolated receptor. *J. Biol. Chem.* **266**, 12752–12758.

40. Andreasen, P. A., Georg, B., Lund, L. R., Riccio, A., and Stacey, S. N. (1990). Plasminogen activator inhibitors: Hormonally regulated serpins. *Mol. Cell. Endocrinol.* **68**, 1–19.

41. Blasi, F., Vassalli, J.-D., and Dano, K. (1987). Urokinase-type plasminogen activator: Proenzyme, receptor and inhibitors. *J. Cell Biol.* **104**, 801–804.

42. Chapman, H. A., and Stone, O. L. (1985). Characterisation of a macrophage-derived plasminogen-activator inhibitor. Similarities with placental urokinase inhibitor. *Biochem. J.* **230**, 109–116.

43. Kruithof, E. K. O. (1988). Plasminogen activator inhibitors—a review. *Enzyme* **40**, 113–121.

44. Conese, M., Olson, D., and Blasi, F. (1994). Protease nexin-1-urokinase complexes are internalised and degraded through a mechanism that requires both urokinase receptor and α_2-macroglobulin receptor. *J. Biol. Chem.* **269**, 17886–17892.

45. Belcher, C., Fawthrop, F., Bunning, R., and Doherty, M. (1996). Plasminogen activators and their inhibitors in synovial fluids from normal, osteoarthritis, and rheumatoid arthritis knees. *Ann. Rheum. Dis.* **55**, 230–236.

46. Ronday, H. K., Smits, H. H., Van Muijen, G. N. P., Pruszczynski, M. S. M., Van Langelaan, E. J., Breedveld, F. C., and Verheijen, J. H. (1996). Difference in expression of the plasminogen activator system in synovial tissue of patients with rheumatoid arthritis and osteoarthritis. *Br. J. Rheumatol.* **35**, 416–423.

47. Busso, N., Peclat, V., So, A., and Sappino, A. P. (1997). Plasminogen activation in synovial tissues: Differences between normal, osteoarthritis, and rheumatoid arthritis joints. *Ann. Rheum. Dis.* **56**, 550–557.

48. Oleksyszyn, J., and Augustine, A. J. (1996). Plasminogen modulation of IL-1-stimulated degradation in bovine and human articular cartilage explants—the role of the endogenous inhibitors PAI-1, α_2-antiplasmin, α_1-PI, α_2-macroglobulin and TIMP. *Inflammation Res.* **45**, 464–472.

49. Saito, S., Katoh, M., Matsumoto, M., Matsumoto, S., and Masuho, Y. (1997). Collagen degradation induced by the combination of IL-1α and plasminogen in rabbit articular cartilage explant culture. *J. Biochem.* **122**, 49–54.

50. Vignon, E., Mathieu, P., Ejui, J., Descotes, J., Hartmann, D., Patricot, L. M., and Richard, M. (1991). Study of an inhibitor of plasminogen activator (tranexamic acid) in the treatment of experimental osteoarthritis. *J. Rheumatol.* **18** (Suppl. 27), 131–133.

51. Ronday, H. K., Tekoppele, J. M., Deroos, J. A. D. M., Verheijen, J. H., Dijkmans, B. A. C., Breedveld, F. C., Moak, S. A., and Greenwald, R. A. (1996). Tranexamic acid (TEA), an inhibitor of plasminogen activation, reduces collagen cross-link excretion in arthritis. *Arthritis Rheum.* **39** (Suppl.), 1541.

52. Martin, T. J., Allan, E. H., and Fukumoto, S. (1993). The plasminogen activator and inhibitor system in bone remodeling. *Growth Regul.* **3**, 209–214.

53. Hoekman, K., Lowik, C. W. G. M., Van Derruit, M., Bijvoet, O. L. M., Verheijen, J. H., and Papapoulos, S. E. (1991). Regulation of the production of plasminogen activators by bone resorption-enhancing and inhibiting factors in 3 types of osteoblast-like cells. *Bone Miner.* **14**, 189–204.

54. Leloup, G., Lemoine, P., Carmeliet, P., and Vaes, G. (1996). Bone resorption and response to calcium regulating hormones in the absence of tissue or urokinase plasminogen activator or of their type 1 inhibitor. *J. Bone Miner. Res.* **11**, 1146–1157.

55. Suzuki, K., Lees, M., Newlands, G. F. J., Nagase, H., and Woolley, D. E. (1995). Activation of precursors for matrix metalloproteinases 1

(interstitial collagenase) and 3 (stromelysin) by rat mast cell proteinases I and II. *Biochem. J.* **305**, 301–306.

56. Tetlow, L. C., and Woolley, D. E. (1995). Distribution, activation and tryptase chymase phenotype of mast cells in the rheumatoid lesion. *Ann. Rheum. Dis.* **54**, 549–555.

57. Froelich, C. J., Zhang, X. L., Turbov, J., Hudig, D., Winkler, U., and Hanna, W. L. (1993). Human granzyme B degrades aggrecan proteoglycan in matrix synthesized by chondrocytes. *J. Immunol.* **151**, 7161–7171.

58. Tak, P. P., Kumer, J. A., Hack, C. E., Daha, M. R., Smeets, T. J. M., and Erkelens, G. W. (1994). Granzyme-positive cytotoxic cells are specifically increased in early rheumatoid synovial tissue. *Arthritis Rheum.* **12**, 1735–1743.

59. Werb, Z. (1997). ECM and cell surface proteolysis: Regulating cellular ecology. *Cell* **91**, 439–442.

60. McKie, N., Edwards, T., Dallas, D. J., Houghton, A., Stringer, B., Graham, R., Russell, G., and Croucher, P. I. (1997). Expression of members of a novel membrane linked metalloproteinase family (ADAM) in human articular chondrocytes. *Biochem. Biophys. Res. Commun.* **230**, 335–339.

61. Inoue, D., Reid, M., Lum, L., Kratzschmar, J., Weskamp, G., Myung, Y. M., Baron, R., and Blobel, C. P. (1998). Cloning and initial characterization of mouse meltrin beta and analysis of the expression of four metalloprotease-disintegrins in bone cells. *J. Biol. Chem.* **273**, 4180–4187.

62. Wolfsberg, T. G., Primakoff, P., Myles, D. G., and White, J. M. (1995). ADAMs, membrane proteins containing a disintegrin and metalloprotease domain—multipotential roles in cell-cell and cell-matrix interaction. *J. Cell Biol.* **131**, 275–278.

63. Flannery, C. R., Lark, M. W., and Sandy, J. D. (1992). Identification of a stromelysin cleavage site within the interglobular domain of human aggrecan—evidence for proteolysis at this site in vivo in human articular cartilage. *J. Biol. Chem.* **267**, 1008–1014.

64. Sandy, J. D., Neame, P. J., Boynton, R. E., and Flannery, C. R. (1991). Catabolism of aggrecan in cartilage explants—identification of a major cleavage site within the interglobular domain. *J. Biol. Chem.* **266**, 8683–8685.

65. Fosang, A. J., Last, K., Knäuper, V., Neame, P. J., Murphy, G., Hardingham, T. E., Tschesche, H., and Hamilton, J. A. (1993). Fibroblast and neutrophil collagenases cleave at 2 sites in the cartilage aggrecan interglobular domain. *Biochem. J.* **295**, 273–276.

66. Billington, C. J., Clark, I. M., and Cawston, T. E. (1998). An aggrecandegrading activity associated with chondrocyte membranes *Biochem. J.* **336**, 207–212.

67. Arner, E., Burn, T., Pratta, M., Liu, R., Trzaskos, J., Newton, R., Decicco, C., Rockwell, A., Copeland, R., Yang, F., *et al.* (1999). Isolation and identification of "aggrecanase": A novel cartilage aggrecandegrading-metalloprotease (ADMP). *Trans. 45th Annu. Meet. Orthop. Res. Soc.* Abstr. 0038.

68. Kessler, E., Takahara, K., Biniaminov, L., Brusel, M., and Greenspan, D. S. (1996). Bone morphogenetic protein-1: The type I procollagen C-proteinase. *Science* **271**, 360–362.

69. Sarras, M. P., Jr. (1996). BMP-1 and the astacin family of metalloproteinases: A potential link between the extracellular matrix, growth factors and pattern formation. *BioEssays* **18**, 439–442.

70. Eble, J. A., Ries, A., Lichy, A., Mann, K., Stanton, H., Gavrilovic, J., Murphy, G., and Kühn, K. (1996). The recognition sites of the integrins $\alpha_1\beta_1$ and $\alpha_2\beta_1$ within collagen IV are protected against gelatinase A attack in the native protein. *J. Biol. Chem.* **271**, 30964–30970.

71. Nagase, H. (1995). Human stromelysins 1 and 2. *In* "Methods in Enzymology" (A. J. Barrett, ed.), Vol. 248, pp. 449–470. Academic Press, San Diego, CA.

72. Borkakoti, N., Winkler, F. K., Williams, D. H., D'Arcy, A., Broadhurst, M. J., Brown, P. S., Johnson, W. H., and Murray, E. J. (1994). Structure of the catalytic domain of human fibroblast collagenase complexed with an inhibitor. *Nat. Struct. Biol.* **1**, 106–110.

73. Spurlino, J. C., Smallwood, A. M., Carlton, D. D., Banks, T. M., Vavra, K. J., Johnson, J. S., Cook, E. R., Falvo, J., Wahl, R. C., Pulvino, T. A., Wendoloski, J. J., and Smith, D. L. (1994). 1.56 A structure of mature truncated human fibroblast collagenase. *Proteins* **19**, 98–109.

74. Lovejoy, B., Cleasby, A., Hassell, A. M., Longley, K., Luther, M. A., Weigl, D., McGeehan, G., McElroy, A. B., Drewry, D., Lambert, M. H., and Jordan, S. R. (1994). Structure of the catalytic domain of fibroblast collagenase complexed with an inhibitor. *Science* **263**, 375–377.

75. Dhanaraj, V., Ye, Q. Z., Johnson, L. L., Hupe, D. J., Ortwine, D. F., Dubar, J. B., Jr., Rubin, J. R., Pavlovsky, A., Humblet, C., and Blundell, T. L. (1996). X-ray structure of a hydroxamate inhibitor complex of stromelysin catalytic domain and its comparison with members of the zinc metalloproteinase superfamily. *Structure* **4**, 375–386.

76. Stams, T., Spurlino, J. C., Smith, D. L., Wahl, R. C., Ho, T. F., Qoronfleh, M. W., Banks, T. M., and Rubin, B. (1994). Structure of human neutrophil collagenase reveals large S1′ specificity pocket. *Nat. Struct. Biol.* **1**, 119–123.

77. Bode, W., Reinemer, P., Huber, R., Kleine, T., Schnierer, S., and Tschesche, H. (1994). The X-ray crystal structure of the catalytic domain of human neutrophil collagenase inhibited by a substrate analogue reveals the essentials for catalysis and specificity. *EMBO J.* **13**, 1263–1269.

78. Grams, F., Reinemer, P., Powers, J. C., Kleine, T., Pieper, M., Tschesche, H., Huber, R., and Bode, W. (1995). X-ray structures of human neutrophil collagenase complexed with peptide hydroxamate and peptide thiol inhibitors. Implications for substrate binding and rational drug design. *Eur. J. Biochem.* **228**, 830–841.

79. Lovejoy, B., Hassell, A. M., Luther, M. A., Weigl, D., and Jordan, S. R. (1994). Crystal structures of recombinant 19-kDa human fibroblast collagenase complexed to itself. *Biochemistry* **33**, 8207–8217.

80. Gooley, P. R., Johnson, B. A., Marcy, A. I., Cuca, G. C., Salowe, S. P., Hagmann, W. K., Esser, C. K., and Springer, J. P. (1993). Secondary structure and zinc ligation of human recombinant short-form stromelysin by multidimensional heteronuclear NMR. *Biochemistry* **32**, 13098–13108.

81. Gooley, P. R., O'Connell, J. F., Marcy, A. I., Cuca, G. C., Salowe, S. P., Bush, B. L., Hermes, J. D., Esser, C. K., Hagmann, W. K., Springer, J. P., and Johnson, B. A. (1994). The NMR structure of the inhibited catalytic domain of human stromelysin-1. *Nat. Struct. Biol.* **1**, 111–118.

82. Van Doren, S. R., Kurochkin, A. V., Ye, Q.-Z., Johnson, L. L., Hupe, D. J., and Zuiderweg, E. R. P. (1993). Assignments for the main-chain nuclear magnetic resonances and delineation of the secondary structure of the catalytic domain of human stromelysin-1 as obtained from tripleresonance 3D NMR experiments. *Biochemistry* **32**, 13109–13122.

83. Li, J., Brick, P., O'Hare, M. C., Skarzynski, T., Lloyd, L. F., Curry, V. A., Clark, I. M., Bigg, H. F., Hazleman, B. L., Cawston, T. E., and Blow, D. M. (1995). Structure of full-length porcine synovial collagenase reveals a C-terminal domain containing a calcium-linked, four-bladed β-propeller. *Structure* **3**, 541–549.

84. De Souza, S. J., and Brentani, R. R. (1994). On the structure/function relationship of polymorphonuclear-leucocyte collagenase. *Biochem. J.* **300**, 605.

85. Bode, W. (1995). A helping hand for collagenases: The haemopexinlike domain. *Structure* **3**, 527–530.

86. Gomis-Rüth, F. X., Gohlke, U., Betz, M., Knäuper, V., Murphy, G., López-Otín, C., and Bode, W. (1996). The helping hand of collagenase-3 (MMP-13): 2.7 Å crystal structure of its C-terminal haemopexin-like domain. *J. Mol. Biol.* **264**, 556–566.

87. Gohlke, U., Gomis-Rüth, F. X., Crabbe, T., Murphy, G., Docherty, A. J. P., and Bode, W. (1996). The C-terminal (haemopexin-like) domain structure of human gelatinase A (MMP2): Structural implications for its function. *FEBS Lett.* **378**, 126–130.

88. Clark, I. M., and Cawston, T. E. (1989). Fragments of human fibroblast collagenase: Purification and characterisation. *Biochem. J.* **263** 201–206.

89. Murphy, G., Allan, J. A., Willenbrock, F., Cockett, M. I., O'Connell, J. P., and Docherty, A. J. P. (1992). The role of the C-terminal domain in collagenase and stromelysin specificity. *J. Biol. Chem.* **267**, 9612–9618.

90. Hirose, T., Patterson, C., Pourmotabbed, T., Mainardi, C. L., and Hasty, K. A. (1993). Structure-function relationship of human neutrophil collagenase: Identification of regions responsible for substrate specificity and general proteinase activity. *Proc. Natl. Acad. Sci. U.S.A.* **90**, 2569–2573.

91. Murphy, G., Willenbrock, F., Ward, R. V., Cockett, M. I., Eaton, D., and Docherty, A. J. P. (1992). The C-terminal domain of 72 kDa gelatinase A is not required for catalysis, but is essential for membrane activation and modulates interactions with tissue inhibitors of metalloproteinases. *Biochem. J.* **283**, 637–641.

92. Baragi, V. M., Fliszar, C. J., Conroy, M. C., Ye, Q.-Z., Shipley, J. M., and Welgus, H. G. (1994). Contribution of the C-terminal domain of metalloproteinases to binding by tissue inhibitor of metalloproteinases. C-terminal truncated stromelysin and matrilysin exhibit equally compromised binding affinities as compared to full-length stromelysin. *J. Biol. Chem.* **269**, 12692–12697.

93. Knäuper, V., Osthues, A., DeClerck, Y. A., Langley, K. E., Blaser, J., and Tschesche, H. (1993). Fragmentation of human polymorphonuclear leukocyte collagenase. *Biochem. J.* **291**, 847–854.

94. Frisch, S. M., and Morisaki, J. H. (1990). Positive and negative transcriptional elements of the type IV collagenase gene. *Mol. Cell. Biol.* **10**, 6524–6532.

95. Jonat, C., Rahmsdorf, H. J., Park, K. K., Cato, A. C. B., Gebel, S., Ponta, H., and Herrlich, P. (1990). Anti-tumor promotion and anti-inflammation—down modulation of AP-1 (Fos, Jun) activity by glucocorticoid hormone. *Cell* **62**, 1189–1204.

96. Nicholson, R. C., Mader, S., Nagpal, S., Leid, M., Rochette-Egly, C., and Chambon, P. (1990). Negative regulation of the rat stromelysin gene promoter by retinoic acid is mediated by an AP1 binding site. *EMBO J.* **9**, 4443–4454.

97. Springman, E. B., Angleton, E. L., Birkedal-Hansen, H., and Van Wart, H. E. (1990). Multiple modes of activation of latent human fibroblast collagenase—evidence for the role of a cys-73 active site zinc complex in latency and a cysteine switch mechanism for activation. *Proc. Natl. Acad. Sci. U.S.A.* **87**, 364–368.

98. Pei, D., and Weiss, S. J. (1995). Furin-dependent intracellular activation of the human stromelysin-3 zymogen. *Nature* **375**, 244–247.

99. Crabbé, T., Ioannou, C., and Docherty, A. J. P. (1993). Human progelatinase A can be activated by autolysis at a rate that is concentration-dependent and enhanced by heparin bound to the C-terminal domain. *Eur. J. Biochem.* **218**, 431–438.

100. Murphy, G., and Knäuper, V. (1997). Relating matrix metalloproteinase structure to function: Why the "hemopexin" domain. *Matrix Biol.* **15**, 511–518.

101. Okada, Y., Morodomi, T., Enghild, J. J., Suzuki, K., Yasui, A., Nakanishi, I., Salvesen, G., and Nagase, H. (1990). Matrix metalloproteinase 2 from human rheumatoid synovial fibroblasts. Purification and activation of the precursor and enzymic properties. *Eur. J. Biochem.* **194**, 721–730.

102. Hipps, D. S., Hembry, R. M., Docherty, A. J. P., Reynolds, J. J., and Murphy, G. (1991). Purification and characterisation of human 72-kDa gelatinase (type IV) collagenase. Use of immunolocalisation to demonstrate the non-coordinated regulation of the 72-kDa and 95-kDa gelatinases by human fibroblasts. *Biol. Chem. Hoppe-Seyler* **372**, 287–296.

103. Cowell, S., Knäuper, V., Stewart, M. L., d'Ortho, M. P., Stanton, H., Hembry, R. M., Lopez-Otin, C., Reynolds, J. J., and Murphy, G. (1998). Induction of matrix metalloproteinase activation cascades based on membrane-type 1 matrix metalloproteinase: Associated activation of gelatinase A, gelatinase B and collagenase 3. *Biochem. J.* **331**, 453–458.

104. Docherty, A. J. P., Lyons, A., Smith, B. J., Wright, E. M., Stephens, P. E., Harris, T. J. R., Murphy, G., and Reynolds, J. J. (1985). Sequence of human tissue inhibitor of metalloproteinases and its identity to erythroid-potentiating activity. *Nature* **318**, 66–69.

105. Boone, T. C., Johnson, M. J., De Clerck, Y. A., and Langley, K. E. (1990). cDNA cloning and expression of a metalloproteinase inhibitor related to tissue inhibitor of metalloproteinases. *Proc. Natl. Acad. Sci. U.S.A.* **87**, 2800–2804.

106. Pavloff, N., Staskus, P. W., Kishnani, N. S., and Hawkes, S. P. (1992). A new inhibitor of metalloproteinases from chicken—ChIMP-3—a 3rd member of the TIMP family. *J. Biol. Chem.* **267**, 17321–17326.

107. Apte, S. S., Hayashi, K., Seldin, M. F., Mattei, M.-G., Hayashi, M., and Olsen, B. R. (1994). Gene encoding a novel murine tissue inhibitor of metalloproteinases (TIMP), TIMP-3, is expressed in developing mouse epithelia, cartilage, and muscle, and is located on mouse chromosome 10. *Dev. Dyn.* **200**, 177–197.

108. Apte, S. S., Mattei, M.-G., and Olsen, B. R. (1994). Cloning of the cDNA encoding human tissue inhibitor of metalloproteinases-3 (TIMP-3) and mapping of the TIMP3 gene to chromosome 22. *Genomics* **19**, 86–90.

109. Apte, S. S., Olsen, B. R., and Murphy, G. (1995). The gene structure of tissue inhibitor of metalloproteinases (TIMP)-3 and its inhibitory activities define the distinct TIMP gene family. *J. Biol. Chem.* **270**, 14313–14318.

110. Leco, K. J., Khokha, R., Pavloff, N., Hawkes, S. P., and Edwards, D. R. (1994). Tissue inhibitor of metalloproteinases-3 (TIMP-3) is an extracellular matrix-associated protein with a distinctive pattern of expression in mouse cells and tissues. *J. Biol. Chem.* **269**, 9352–9360.

111. Silbiger, S. M., Jacobsen, V. L., Cupples, R. L., and Koski, R. A. (1994). Cloning of cDNAs encoding human TIMP-3, a novel member of the tissue inhibitor of metalloproteinase family. *Gene* **141**, 293–297.

112. Uria, J. A., Ferrando, A. A., Velasco, G., Freije, J. M. P., and Lopez-Otin, C. (1994). Structure and expression in breast tumors of human TIMP-3, a new member of the metalloproteinase inhibitor family. *Cancer Res.* **54**, 2091–2094.

113. Greene, J., Wang, M., Liu, Y. E., Raymond, L. A., Rosen, C., and Shi, Y. E. (1996). Molecular cloning and characterization of human tissue inhibitor of metalloproteinase 4. *J. Biol. Chem.* **271**, 30375–30380.

114. Leco, K. J., Apte, S. S., Taniguchi, G. T., Hawkes, S. P., Khokha, R., Schultz, G. A., and Edwards, D. R. (1997). Murine tissue inhibitor of metalloproteinases-4 (*Timp-4*): cDNA isolation and expression in adult mouse tissues. *FEBS Lett.* **401**, 213–217.

115. Gomis-Ruth, F. X., Maskos, K., Betz, M., Bergner, A., Huber, R., Suzuki, K., Yoshida, N., Nagase, H., Brew, K., Bourenkov, G. P., Bartunik, H., and Bode, W. (1997). Mechanism of inhibition of the human matrix metalloproteinase stromelysin-1 by TIMP-1. *Nature* **389**, 77–81.

116. Wilhelm, S. M., Collier, I. E., Marmer, B. L., Eisen, A. Z., Grant, G. A. and Goldberg, G. I. (1989). SV40-transformed human lung fibroblasts secrete a 92-kDa type IV collagenase which is identical to that secreted by normal human macrophages. *J. Biol. Chem.* **264**, 17213–17221.

117. Goldberg, G. I., Strongin, A., Collier, I. E., Genrich, L. T., and Marmer, B. L. (1992). Interaction of 92-kDa type IV collagenase with the tissue inhibitor of metalloproteinases prevents dimerization, complex formation with interstitial collagenase, and activation of the proenzyme with stromelysin. *J. Biol. Chem.* **267**, 4583–4591.

118. Goldberg, G. I., Marmer, B. L., Grant, G. A., Eisen, A. Z., Wilhelm, S., and He, C. (1989). Human 72-kilodalton type IV collagenase forms a complex with a tissue inhibitor of metalloproteases designated TIMP-2. *Proc. Natl. Acad. Sci. U.S.A.* **86**, 8207–8211.

119. Stetler-Stevenson, W. G., Krutzsch, H. C., Wacher, M. P., Margulies, I. M. K., and Liotta, L. A. (1989). The activation of human type IV collagenase proenzyme. Sequence identification of the major conversion product following organomercurial activation. *J. Biol. Chem.* **264**, 1353–1356.

120. Howard, E. W., Bullen, E. C., and Banda, M. J. (1991). Regulation of the autoactivation of human 72-kDa progelatinase by tissue inhibitor of metalloproteinases-2. *J. Biol. Chem.* **266**, 13064–13069.

121. Murphy, G., Houbrechts, A., Cockett, M. I., Williamson, R. A., O'Shea, M., and Docherty, A. J. P. (1991). The N-terminal domain of tissue inhibitor of metalloproteinases retains metalloproteinase inhibitory activity. *Biochemistry* **30**, 8097–8101.

122. Fridman, R., Fuerst, R. R., Bird, R. E., Hoyhtya, M., Oelkuct, M., Kraus, S., Komarek, D., Liotta, L. A., Berman, M. L., and Stetler-Stevenson, W. G. (1992). Domain structure of human 72-kDa gelatinase/ type IV collagenase. Characterization of proteolytic activity and identification of the tissue inhibitor of metalloproteinases-2 (TIMP-2) binding regions. *J. Biol. Chem.* **267**, 15398–15405.

123. Willenbrock, F., Crabbé, T., Slocombe, P. M., Sutton, C. W., Docherty, A. J. P., Cockett, M. I., O'Shea, M., Brocklehurst, K., Phillips, I. R., and Murphy, G. (1993). The activity of the tissue inhibitors of metalloproteinases is regulated by C-terminal domain interactions: A kinetic analysis of the inhibition of gelatinase A. *Biochemistry* **32**, 4330–4337.

124. Howard, E. W., Bullen, E. C., and Banda, M. (1991). Preferential inhibition of 72-kDa and 92-kDa gelatinases by tissue inhibitor of metalloproteinases-2. *J. Biol. Chem.* **266**, 13070–13075.

125. Howard, E. W., and Banda, M. J. (1991). Binding of tissue inhibitor of metalloproteinases 2 to two distinct sites on human 72-kDa gelatinase. Identification of a stabilization site. *J. Biol. Chem.* **266**, 17972–17977.

126. Kleiner, D. E., Tuuttila, A., Tryggvason, K., and Stetler-Stevenson, W. G. (1993). Stability analysis of latent and active 72-kDa type IV collagenase: The role of tissue inhibitor of metalloproteinases-2 (TIMP-2). *Biochemistry* **32**, 1583–1592.

127. Strongin, A. Y., Collier, I., Bannikov, G., Marmer, B. L., Grant, G. A., and Goldberg, G. I. (1995). Mechanism of cell surface activation of 72-kDa type IV collagenase. Isolation of the activated form of the membrane metalloprotease. *J. Biol. Chem.* **270**, 5331–5338.

128. Butler, G. S., Butler, M. J., Atkinson, S. J., Will, H., Tamura, T., van Westrum, S. S., Crabbe, T., Clements, J., D'Ortho, M.-P., and Murphy, G. (1998). The TIMP2 membrane type 1 metalloproteinase "receptor" regulates the concentration and efficient activation of progelatinase A. *J. Biol. Chem.* **273**, 871–880.

129. Murphy, G., Ward, R., Hembry, R. M., Reynolds, J. J., Kühn, K., and Tryggvason, K. (1989). Characterization of gelatinase from pig polymorphonuclear leucocytes. A metalloproteinase resembling tumour type IV collagenase. *Biochem. J.* **258**, 463–472.

130. Ward, R. V., Hembry, R. M., Reynolds, J. J., and Murphy, G. (1991). The purification of tissue inhibitor of metalloproteinases-2 from its 72 kDa progelatinase complex—demonstration of the biochemical similarities of tissue inhibitor of metalloproteinases-2 and tissue inhibitor of metalloproteinases-1. *Biochem. J.* **278**, 179–187.

131. Edwards, D. R., Leco, K. J., Leco, P. A., Lim, M. S., Phillips, B. W., Raja, J., and Sharma, R. (1999). Regulation of TIMP gene expression *In* "Inhibitors of Metalloproteinases in Development and Disease" (S. P. Hawkes, D. R. Edwards, and R. Khokha, eds.). Harwood Academic Press, Lausanne, Switzerland (in press).

132. Sottrup-Jensen, L., and Birkedal-Hansen, H. (1989). Human fibroblast collagenase-α_2-macroglobulin interactions. Localization of cleavage sites in the bait regions of five mammalian α-macroglobulins. *J. Biol. Chem.* **264**, 393–401.

133. Borth, W. (1992). α_2-macroglobulin, a multifunctional binding protein with targeting characteristics. *FASEB J.* **6**, 3345–3353.

134. Borth, W. (1994). α_2-macroglobulin, a multifunctional binding and targeting protein with possible roles in immunity and autoimmunity. *Ann. N.Y. Acad. Sci.* **737**, 267–272.

135. Stephens, R. W., Tapiovaara, H., Reisberg, T., Bizik, J., and Vaheri, A. (1991). Alpha-2-macroglobulin restricts plasminogen activation to the surface of RC2A leukemia cells. *Cell Regul.* **2**, 1057–1065.

136. Dean, D. D., Martel-Pelletier, J., Pelletier, J.-P., Howell, D. S., and Woessner, J. F. (1989). Evidence for metalloproteinase and metalloproteinase inhibitor imbalance in human osteoarthritic cartilage. *J. Clin. Invest.* **84**, 678–685.

137. Martel-Pelletier, J., McCollum, R., Fujimoto, N., Obata, K., Cloutier, J.-M., and Pelletier, J.-P. (1994). Excess of metalloproteases over tissue inhibitor of metalloproteases may contribute to cartilage degradation in osteoarthritis and rheumatoid arthritis. *Lab. Invest.* **70**, 807–815.

138. Cawston, T., McLaughlan, P., Coughlan, R., Kyle, V., and Hazleman, B. (1990). Synovial fluids from infected joints contain metalloproteinase-tissue inhibitor of metalloproteinase (TIMP) complexes. *Biochim. Biophys. Acta* **1033**, 96–102.

139. Jubb, R. W., and Fell, H. B. (1980). The breakdown of collagen by chondrocytes. *J. Pathol.* **130**, 159–162.

140. Ellis A. J., Powell, L. K., Curry, V. A., and Cawston, T. E. (1994). TIMP-1 and TIMP-2 prevent the release of collagen fragments in cartilage stimulated with IL-1. *Biochem. Biophys. Res. Commun.* **201**, 94–101.

141. Bottomley, K. M., Borkakoti, N., Bradshaw, D., Brown, P. A., Broadhurst, M. J., Budd, J. M., Elliot, L., Eyers, P., Hallam, T., Handa, B. K., Hill, C. H., James, M., Lahm, H.-W., Lawton, G., Merritt, J. E., Nixon, J. S., Röthlisberger, U., Whittle, A., and Johnson, W. H. (1997). Inhibition of bovine nasal cartilage degradation by selective matrix metalloproteinase inhibitors. *Biochem. J.* **323**, 483–488.

142. Partridge, N. C., Walling, H. W., Bloch, S. R., Omura, T. H., Chan, P. T., Pearman, A. T., and Chou, W.-Y. (1996). The regulation and regulatory role of collagenase in bone. *Crit. Rev. Eukaryotic Gene Expression* **6**, 15–27.

143. Bord, S., Horner, A., Hembry, R. M., Reynolds, J. J., and Compston, J. E. (1997). Distribution of matrix metalloproteinases and their inhibitor, TIMP-1, in developing human osteophytic bone. *J. Anat.* **191**, 39–48.

144. Hill, P. A., Docherty, A. J. P., Bottomley, K. M., O'Connell, J. P., Morphy, J. R., Reynolds, J. J., and Meikle, M. C. (1995). Inhibition of bone resorption in vitro by selective inhibitors of gelatinase and collagenase. *Biochem. J.* **308**, 167–175.

145. Stahle-Backdahl, M., Sandstedt, B., Bruce, K., Lindahl, A., Jimenez, M. G., Vega, J. A., and Lopez-Otin, C. (1997). Collagenase-3 (MMP-13) is expressed during human fetal ossification and re-expressed in postnatal bone remodeling and in rheumatoid arthritis. *Lab. Invest.* **76**, 717–728.

146. Okada, Y., Naka, K., Kawamura, K., Matsumoto, T., Nakanishi, I., Fujimoto, N., Sato, H., and Seiki, M. (1995). Localization of matrix metalloproteinase-9 (92-kilodalton gelatinase/type IV collagenase, gelatinase B) in osteoclasts—implications for bone resorption. *Lab. Invest.* **72**, 311–322.

PART II

Structure and Metabolism of the Extracellular Matrix of Bone and Cartilage

CHAPTER 11

Mineralization, Structure, and Function of Bone

ADELE L. BOSKEY   Hospital for Special Surgery, New York, New York 10021; and Cornell University Medical College and Cornell University Graduate School of Medical Sciences, New York, New York 10021

I. ABSTRACT

The development of bone is a complex process that involves cellular, extracellular, and physicochemical events. Here, the overall process of bone formation is reviewed from a biological and chemical viewpoint. The factors regulating the initial mineralization of osteoid and those regulating the entire process of mineralization are the main subjects of this chapter. Attention is paid to new data on the role of matrix proteins in these processes and to the interaction between collagen and matrix proteins and matrix proteins and cells in regulating bone mineralization.

II. THE STRUCTURE AND FUNCTION OF BONE

Bones are dynamic tissues, replaced with newly deposited bone as they age or are damaged. These dynamic tissues serve numerous essential functions. Bone provides mechanical protection for internal organs, allows the direction of motion, and facilitates the locomotion process. In addition to these mechanical functions, bone provides a protective housing for blood-forming marrow and serves as a reservoir for mineral ions (Ca^{2+}, Mg^{2+}, PO_4^{3-}).

There are two histologically or radiologically defined bone types [1]: dense bone (also known as compact bone), and spongy or cancellous bone (also known as trabecular bone). When bone is newly formed, as during development or fracture healing, the matrix is "loose" or "woven." With maturation, the bone becomes denser, better organized, and better able to serve its mechanical function. Mature bone is described as compact (dense) or trabecular (meaning composed of little beams). The general features of both compact and trabecular bones are similar. Both are solid mineralized matrices with small canals (canaliculi), spaces (lacunae), and bone cells (for discussion of bone cells, see Chapter 12). In cancellous bone, the matrix, lacunae, and mineral-encased cells (osteocytes) are organized in the form of thin interconnecting spicules. In cortical bone, the tissue is organized in Haversian systems, or osteons. The Haversian systems consist of a canal containing a blood vessel surrounded by concentric and interstitial lamellae.

In addition to descriptions based on architecture (spicules or lamellae), bone may also be described based on its mechanism of formation during development. Bones that develop by the replacement of a cartilage model (endochondral

153

ossification) are often distinguished from those that form directly (intramembranous ossification). Details of these events will be presented later in the chapter.

A. The Composition of Bone

Bone is a composite material consisting, in decreasing proportions, of mineral, collagen, water, noncollagenous proteins, lipids, vascular elements, and cells. The absolute amounts of these constituents vary with animal age, tissue site, health, and dietary status. The arrangement of the bone tissues, as described by Wolff [2], is such that bones are organized optimally to resist loads imposed by functional activities. Thus with growth and development, the tissue must be constantly reshaped and remodeled to maintain this maximization and to maintain a form appropriate to its mechanical function. As used here, "modeling" refers to formation of bone on sites where it has not been before, whereas "remodeling" refers to its formation on surfaces previously containing bone. Both these processes are required to shape bone.

The mineral found in bone is an analog of the geologic mineral hydroxyapatite, $Ca_{10}(PO_4)_6(OH)_2$ [3]. Bone apatite is a calcium- [4] and hydroxide- [5] deficient apatite containing numerous impurities, the most abundant of which is carbonate [6]. Magnesium, potassium, fluoride, acid, phosphate, and citrate are also common substituents [3–7]. In general, in animals of the same age, the proportion of mineral is greatest in the bones of the ear and lowest in the ribs. Woven and lamellar bones have a lower mineral content than compact bone. These bone types will be discussed below.

Bone mineral apatite crystals are relatively small (200–400 Å in largest dimension) compared to the apatite found in tooth enamel or the geologic apatites. It is this small size that facilitates the incorporation and adsorption of foreign ions and enables bone mineral to dissolve in the acidic mileu created by the osteoclast during bone remodeling. This small size also enables the crystals to provide the flexible collagen fibrils of the mineral-collagen composite with structural rigidity. Bone mineral crystals, while appearing like needles, have been shown to be thin curved plates [8] which agglomerate, or fuse, as the bone matures [9].

The variation in the amount of mineral with maturation (e.g., in an osteon) was first appreciated from the examination of backscattered electron images [10] and has been quantified by Fourier transform infrared microspectroscopy (FTIRM), a technique in which an infrared spectrophotometer, coupled to a light microscope, is used to measure mineral content, composition, and parameters related to mineral crystal size and perfection at 10–20 μm resolution [11]. Figure 1A shows a light micrograph of one such osteon from healthy adult bone and Figure 1B shows typical FTIR spectral maps from this osteon. Figure 1C shows the mineral content, calculated from these spectra as the ratio of absorptions of the phosphate

(900–1200 cm^{-1}) and amide I (1585–1720 cm^{-1}) peaks, respectively, in four lines orthogonal to the center of the Haversian canal. Figure 1D shows the variation in carbonate-to-phosphate ratio along these same directions, and Figure 1E shows the changes in crystal maturity estimated from analyses of the underlying subbands in the complex phosphate spectra. These data, which show a progression of mineral content from the area of new mineral deposition adjacent to the Haversian canal to the oldest mineral on the periphery of the osteon, are presented to illustrate that significant changes in mineral properties occur as the tissue ages, and to emphasize that bone is a dynamic tissue.

The carbonate content of bone mineral increases with maturity [6] and there are also variations in the nature of the carbonate substitution. Carbonate can replace hydroxide ions (A-type carbonate) or phosphate ions (B-type carbonate), or it can adsorb onto the surface of the apatite (labile carbonate). With increasing bone age, the proportion of labile carbonate decreases, and in the most mature bone apatites there is a preponderance of B-substituted carbonate [6]. Less is known about the age and site variation of the other ions that accumulate in bone, and there is some debate as to whether ions such as magnesium are incorporated into the apatite lattice or only reside on the surface of the mineral crystals [3, 7].

The second most abundant component of bone is collagen, predominantly type I (for discussion of collagen structure and function see Chapters 1 and 2). Collagen provides bone with elasticity and flexibility and directs the organization of the matrix. The collagen fibers in bone are organized in sheets (periosteal bone) or circumferentially (osteonal bone). They are oriented spirally in the lamellae and all lie in the same direction in a single lamellae, but in adjacent lamellae they are oriented in different directions. In physiologically mineralized tissues, the long axes of the apatite crystals are always aligned parallel to the axis of the collagen fibrils [9]. This orientation allows the crystals to contribute to the strength of bone. Illustrations of the importance of collagen for the mechanical integrity of bone can be seen from a comparison of the stress-strain curves of similarly aged bone of comparable mineral content and mineral crystallite size but with altered collagen cross-linking induced by vitamin B_6 deficiency (Fig. 2). These data demonstrate that the plastic deformation for the collagen lacking cross-links is limited [12]. A second illustration is the observation that when bone is decalcified (by soaking in acid or decalcifying agents) it becomes soft and rubber-like.

Water accounts for 5–10% of the weight of bone tissue. Tissue hydration is needed both for nutrition and function of cells, and also for mechanical function of the mineral-collagen composite. Hydrogen bonds between water and collagen contribute to the stabilization of the collagen fibril, and there have been suggestions that dehydration of the bone collagen (i.e., replacement of water by mineral, as is seen in the mineralizing turkey tendon [13]) may take place during the mineralization of bone. However, the change in water content during bone mineralization is not sufficient to account for the space occupied by mineral.

Noncollagenous proteins, reviewed in Chapters 3–5, make up approximately 5% of the dry weight of bone. They are important for a variety of processes described elsewhere [14] as well as in this book. The functions of noncollagenous proteins in mineralization will be discussed in detail below. Lipids, which account for 2–8% of the organic matrix of bone, are components of cell membranes, and as such are essential for cell function. They also appear to play an important role in initial mineralization and bone [15].

B. The Cell Biology of Bone Formation

The matrix of bone changes with growth and development. To appreciate these changes, it is useful to briefly review the embryological stages of development. More details can be found in the review by Raisz and Rodan [16]. Initial long bone development begins by the vascular invasion of a cartilaginous model. During embryogenesis, a cartilage matrix formed in the center of the bone is surrounded by the periosteum/perichondrium, which throughout development defines the boundary between the bone and the soft connective tissues. As the cartilage cells become enlarged, the matrix calcifies, while the cells in the periosteum form a thin layer of bone. The calcified cartilage is removed as a vascular bud, along with tissue from the periosteum, invades. Concurrently, the cartilage cells on either side of this cavity continue to proliferate, causing the bone to grow in length and width. The periosteum continues to form, the cartilage cells closest to the cavity hypertrophy, and the calcified matrix forms. Bone forms on the spicules of calcified cartilage (endochondral bone) and eventually is remodeled, as marrow cells fill in the cavity. As bone starts to form surrounding the marrow cavity, growth continues as the proximal and distal epiphyses move further and further apart. The role of growth factors, cytokines, hormones, and gene regulatory elements that regulate these processes has been discussed elsewhere in this book (Chapters 6 and 7). For this review, it is only important to note that during development, calcification of cartilage occurs first, and calcified cartilage is replaced by bone. The calcifying cartilage matrix is distinct from the noncalcified matrix. It is enriched in type X collagen [17] and in extracellular matrix vesicles [18], both of which are important for mineralization. The matrix vesicles contain Ca-transport proteins known as annexins [19], complexed acidic phospholipids [15, 20], and other associated proteins, as part of their "nucleational core" [21]. As endochondral ossification starts, the calcifying cartilage matrix is depleted to some extent of the large aggregating proteoglycans [22]. All of these changes in the cartilage matrix are important for the calcification process.

TABLE I.   The Extracellular Proteins of Bone

Collagens	Phosphoproteins
Type I	Bone sialoprotein
Type XI	Osteopontin
Type V	Osteonectin
Type III	BAG-75
Proteoglycans	Gamma carboxy glutamate
Versican	containing proteins
Syndecan	Osteocalcin
CS-Decorin	Matrix gla protein
CS-Biglycan	
Lumican	Other
	Thrombospondin
Serum Proteins	Fibromodulin
Albumin	Proteolipids
Fetuin (α 2HS-glycoprotein)	
IgE	
IgG	

During intramembranous ossification, as in endochondral ossification, bone is first laid down as a network of spicules. Similar to the accumulation of osteoblasts on the calcified cartilage spicules, osteoblasts aggregate on these spicules and deposit osteoid, which then becomes mineralized. Like calcifying and uncalcified cartilage, the unmineralized (osteoid) and mineralized bone matrices have different compositions. During initial osteoid formation, the matrix is rich in cellbinding proteins such as laminin and fibronectin, and later, bone sialoprotein and osteopontin, also cell-binding proteins, are added [23]. Type I collagen and the small proteoglycans decorin and biglycan, which regulate collagen fibrollogenesis [24], are laid down upon this initial network. As the tissue matures, the collagen fibrils form inter- and intra-fibrillar cross-links and the number of such cross-links increases with tissue age [25, 26]. Osteocalcin, the most abundant of the noncollagenous matrix proteins in humans [27], does not accumulate in the osteoid, but is only expressed and appears in the bones as they mineralize [23, 28]. Several other proteins that are found in the mineralized matrix are listed in Table I. Some of these are synthesized by osteoblasts, but some found in serum accumulate in bone because of their affinity for the mineral [14].

As reviewed elsewhere in this volume, the factors regulating the expression and posttranslational modification of most of these proteins are known. But how their expression and posttranslational modification are linked with the onset of mineralization is less clear.

III. BONE MINERALIZATION

Physiologic bone mineralization in mammals refers to the ordered deposition of apatite on a type I collagen matrix. The mature bone apatite crystals are always deposited such that

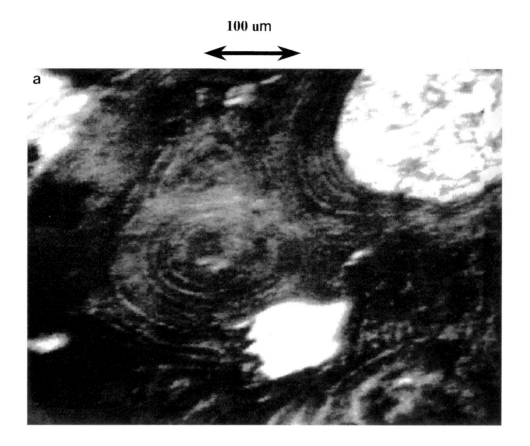

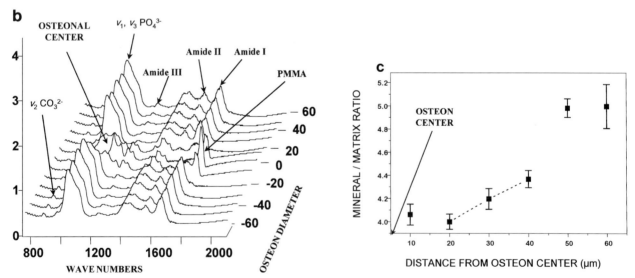

FIGURE 1   Mineral density changes in osteonal bone. (A) Light micrograph of an osteon in adult human bone. (B) Fourier transform infrared spectra going from the center of the osteon (0) to 60 μm from the origin at 10 μm resolution. (C) Mineral-to-matrix ratio in the osteon calculated from the spectra obtained in four orthogonal directions increases gradually from the center of the Haversian Canal. (D) Carbonate-to-phosphate ratio calculated from the spectra increases as mineral content increases in the four directions orthogonal to the center of the Haversian Canal. (E) The mineral crystal maturity (size and perfection) as calculated from curve-fit spectra increases with distance from the center of the Haversian Canal. Reprinted from Paschalis *et al.* [11] "FTIR microspectroscopic analysis of human osteonal bone," *Calcif. Tissue Int.* **59**, 480–487, with permission.

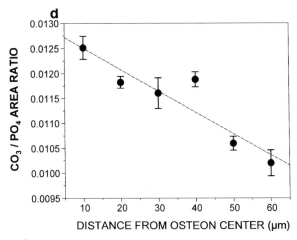

FIGURE 1 *(continued)*

their longest dimension lies parallel to the axis of the collagen fibril (Fig. 3). The cascade of events therefore must include the formation of that collagenous matrix and the oriented deposition of the apatite crystals.

Our knowledge of the process of bone mineralization is derived from a combination of cell and organ culture studies, analyses of bones from normal and mutant or diseased animals, analogies drawn from biomineralization in other species, and cell-free solution studies [14]. While phases other than apatite have been proposed to be formed as precursors, X-ray diffraction [3], NMR [3, 29], and other studies of newly formed bone [30–33] have failed to show the presence of other calcium phosphate phases. This does not exclude the possibility that such phases may form transiently during the initial steps of bone formation, and there are reports in some experiments using isolated matrix vesicles that such transient phases are formed prior to apatite deposition [34, 35].

Calcium phosphate mineral deposition in bone is, in part, a physical chemical process. Precipitation, in general, takes place from solution when the ion activity product in the solution exceeds the solubility product of the precipitating phase. As a first approximation, in the case of hydroxyapatite

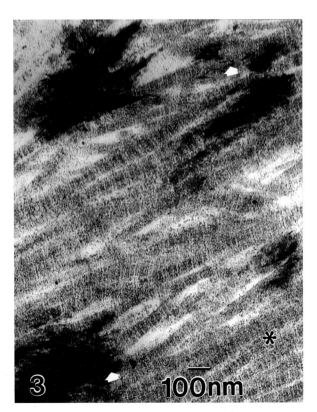

FIGURE 3 Electron micrograph of the newly formed mineral in a developing rat bone showing the alignment of the long axis of electron-dense mineral crystals along the collagen fibrils. Solid arrows, mineral crystals aligned along collagen fibrils; *, collagen fibrils without mineral. Courtesy of Dr. S. B. Doty.

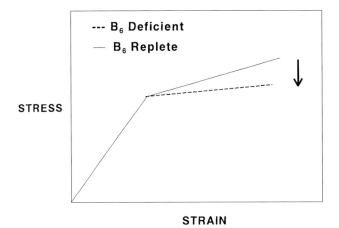

FIGURE 2 Four-point bend testing of vitamin B_6-deficient and control bones as illustrated by stress–strain curves shows the decreased plasticity of the bones with decreased collagen cross-links.

crystals, that would mean $[Ca^{+2}]^{10}[PO_4^{-3}]^6[OH]^2 \geq 10^{-117}$ [36], and most body fluids would be undersaturated. When the concentration of any of these ions is increased, as may be the case during the formation of urinary or salivary stones, crystal deposition may occur. However, even in such cases, an energy-requiring nucleation process must occur. During nucleation, ions or ion clusters must associate to form a stable configuration containing the building block(s) of the crystal in question. Once this structure (the "critical nucleus") is large enough to persist in solution, it requires less energy to continue to add ions or ion clusters during the crystal growth process. Secondary nucleation occurs as new crystals start to form on the initial crystal in a fashion analogous to glycogen branching. The new crystal branches separate and provide additional nuclei.

Nucleation, as described above, may occur *de novo,* or may occur on foreign substances (heterogenous nucleation). If the foreign substance's surface resembles the surface of the nucleus, the process of "epitaxial nucleation" occurs, as one crystal grows on the surface of another. In biological systems, there are thought to be numerous heterogenous and a few possible epitaxial nucleators that facilitate mineralization in a variety of ways. Furthermore, in bone, it is apparent that there are many nucleation sites, because initial crystals start to form at numerous separated loci [3]. Examination of newly mineralized collagen shows the first crystals forming in the "e-bands" throughout the collagen fiber [37].

There are two not necessarily mutually exclusive theories concerning how mineral deposition starts at these discrete sites. During endochondral ossification, cartilage calcification is widely believed to begin within extracellular membrane-bound bodies known as matrix vesicles (ECMVs) [18, 38]. ECMVs (Fig. 4), probably produced during apoptosis of chondrocytes, are seen as the site where mineral first appears in the extraterritorial matrix adjacent to the hypertrophic cells of the calcifying cartilage. ECMVs provide protected areas for the accumulation of mineral ions away from the space-filling proteoglycan aggregates which keep the cartilage matrix hydrated, and which by virtue of their negative charge and bulk are effective inhibitors of mineral nucleation and growth [39–42]. ECMVs contains a nucleational core [21] consisting of acidic phospholipids, calcium, inorganic phosphate, and a Ca-transport protein, annexin. This nucleational core is believed to be responsible for mineral formation within the ECMVs. The ECMVs also contain enzymes [43] that can modulate inhibitors of mineral formation found in the extracellular matrix [44].

Isolated ECMVs often have cartilage matrix proteins such as type X collagen associated with them [20]. Despite early suggestions that type X collagen might, by itself, act as an apatite nucleator, cell-free solution studies [14] failed to show any such ability. In culture, type X expression occurred after mineralization [17], supporting the solution data. It appears that type X collagen is most important for organizing the

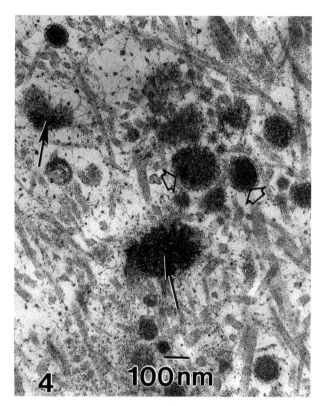

FIGURE 4   Electron micrograph showing extracellular matrix vesicles in calcifying cartilage of a young rat. Solid arrows, matrix vesicles containing mineral crystals; open arrows, matrix vesicles without mineral. Courtesy of Dr. S. B. Doty.

matrix during endochondral bone formation, facilitating the transition from type II to type I collagen.

The ECMVs are always adjacent to collagen during endochondral bone formation (Fig. 4). The controversy concerns how the mineral formed within the ECMVs gets to the collagenous matrix upon which the bone mineral is deposited. High-resolution 3-D tomographic imaging of the mineralizing turkey tendon, a highly organized model system frequently used to study mineral formation processes in bone [13], has demonstrated mineral crystals forming concurrently in ECMVs and on the collagen fibers [45].

Osteoid, as opposed to cartilage and tendon mineral deposition, is rarely reported to be associated with ECMVs; however, where mineralization is impaired, e.g., due to vitamin D-deficiency in rickets and osteomalacia, ECMVs are seen [38]. It is not known whether the delayed mineralization of the osteoid enables this observation, or whether ECMVs are formed specifically to promote mineral formation when other mechanism are hindered.

It has long been known that purified type I collagen aggregated into fibrils can support apatite formation from metastable calcium phosphate solutions [46, 47]. The rate of nucleation and the number of nucleation sites were measurable [47]. However, when extracted collagen was implanted in an animal, although mineral deposition occurred, the process was relatively slow [48]. Termine showed that when noncollagenous proteins were extracted from bone collagen with chaotropic agents, the collagen could not be remineralized *in vitro* [49]. Likewise, Endo [50] and Glimcher [51] found that progressive dephosphorylation of bone collagen retarded its *in vitro* mineralization in a dose-dependent manner. From this and other evidence it has become apparent that there are noncollagenous proteins associated with the collagen that can serve as nucleators of the initial mineral [3, 14].

The challenge has been determining which proteins are involved in apatite nucleation [52]. The approach to this question has included identifying which proteins are expressed at the boundary between mineralized bone and osteoid (the mineralization front) using molecular [23, 53] and histochemical [23, 54] techniques. These studies have indicated, *inter alia*, that osteopontin, osteonectin, and bone sialoprotein appear concurrent with matrix mineralization. Other studies have demonstrated the presence of enzymes that can phosphorylate or dephosphorylate each of these proteins at the mineralization front [55].

Even though a protein may have an altered distribution or composition at the mineralization front, it may not be directly involved in causing minerals to deposit. It may simply be there because it has a high affinity for apatite. To determine which proteins can act as nucleators, investigators [52] have studied the effects of individual proteins, either isolated from bone or prepared using recombinant technology, on *in vitro* mineralization. Studies of solution-mediated mineralization have included analyses done in media containing only calcium and phosphate ions, media made to mimic the composition of body fluids (synthetic lymph), media in which the calcium, phosphate, and hydroxide ion concentrations are kept fixed, and others in which these concentrations are allowed to vary. Some studies examine growth of calcium phosphates added as "seed crystals" to these solutions, others evaluate nucleators in solutions free of dust and other potential heterogenous nucleators, while still others look for these effects in agar, silica, or gelatin gels containing the proteins in question. Despite the variation in these conditions, there is consistency as to which proteins are nucleators and which can bind to nucleii or crystals and inhibit or regulate crystal proliferation and growth.

Only a few bone matrix proteins, and the constituents of the nucleational core discussed above [21], have acted as nucleators. The most effective of the proteins analyzed is bone sialoprotein, BSP [56]. This bone-specific protein causes apatite formation in a variety of *in vitro* conditions [14, 56]. Both the native and the recombinant forms of BSP can also inhibit mineral crystal growth [57]. Bone sialoprotein is distinguished from the other phosphorylated sialoproteins made by osteoblasts in that it is rich in polyglutamate repeats, whereas osteopontin contains polyaspartate sequences, and bone acidic glycoprotein (BAG-75) has a mixture of polyglutamate and polyaspartate repeats [14]. It has been suggested, based on studies with synthetic polypeptides, that the polyglutamate repeat stabilizes the apatite nuclei [58, 59]. This would explain why BSP at high concentrations could coat apatite crystals and retard their growth.

A variety of other bone and dentin matrix constituents seem to have this bifunctional ability, serving as nucleators at low concentrations and regulating the extent of proliferation of mineral crystals at higher concentration (Fig. 5). These constituents include the lipids of the "nucleational core" of ECMVs [60], biglycan, the small CS-containing leucine-rich proteoglycan of bone [61], and several bone and dentin phosphoproteins [14, 52, 62]. Although the precise mechanisms of action of these proteins may differ, it is likely that they can interact with specific faces on the apatite crystal, stabilizing the critical nucleus and blocking growth in certain directions [59, 63]. Other isolated matrix proteins, such as osteonectin, osteocalcin, and osteopontin, which bind to apatite with high affinities, have not been shown to act as nucleators but are effective inhibitors of apatite crystal proliferation [14, 53, 64–66].

Solution studies of isolated proteins are limited because *in situ* these proteins interact with one other, and with collagen. Although it is known that the proteins shown to be nucleators in solution are associated with collagen [14], to determine their action *in situ* investigators have used *in vitro* studies of cell and organ systems [14, 23, 53]. Most of these studies have focused on the expression and synthesis of these proteins and not on the mineralization process per se. These studies, however, provide data on the sequence of expression of the proteins [23, 27]. A few studies have attempted to alter the properties of the matrix proteins expressed in culture, often verifying the results of cell-free *in vitro* systems. For example, blocking the synthesis of large proteoglycans, preventing the sulfation of these proteoglycans, and accelerating the degradation of large proteoglycans each enhanced the rate of mineralization in high density calcifying cartilage cultures [67]. Blocking phosphoprotein phosphorylation in the same high density cultures blocked mineralization [68]. These studies support the postulated role of large proteoglycans as mineralization inhibitors and phosphoproteins as nucleators.

The development of embryonic stem cell technology by which proteins synthesized *in ovo* could be modified or "knocked out" provided an additional tool to probe the functions of the matrix proteins. Knocking out noncollagenous matrix proteins has not consistently produced a bone phenotype, perhaps because many essential processes, such as mineralization, are regulated in redundant ways. However, proof of function of several bone matrix proteins has become available through studies of both transgenic (expressing an altered protein) and knockout (null mutation) animals. The first example of a transgenic mouse relevant to bone disease was the model of human osteogenesis imperfecta (brittle bone disease) produced by the random insertion of a viral gene

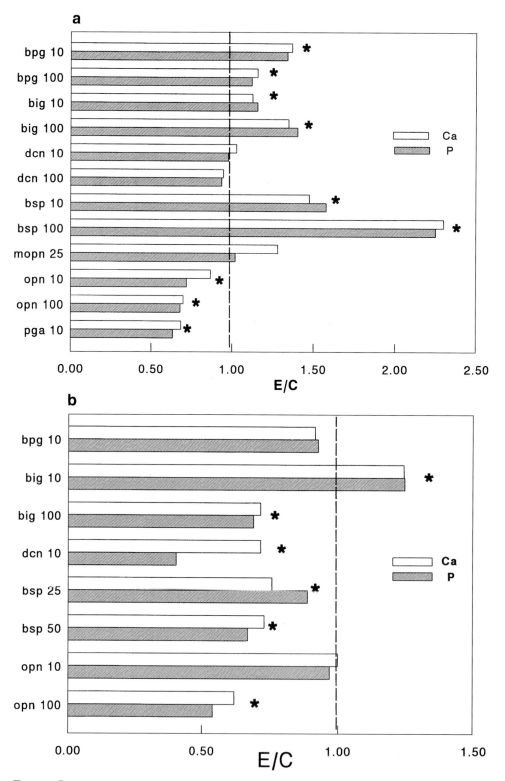

FIGURE 5   Matrix proteins may be multifunctional, nucleating apatite at low concentrations and inhibiting crystal growth at higher concentrations. Yields of mineral are presented as experimental (E) with protein (P) over control (C). (A) The relative yield of mineral ions in a gel system containing 10, 25, or 100 μg/ml matrix protein. The proteins shown are bone proteoglycans (bpg), biglycan (big), decorin (dcn), bone sialoprotein (bsp), milk osteopontin (mopn), bone osteopontin (opn), and proteoglycan aggregate (pga). ∗, values are significantly different from the control (dashed line). (B) Similar data for experiments with apatite seed crystals.

sequence into the mouse collagen genome [69]. These transgenic mice showed the typical bone fragility of the human disease [70]. Similarly, the expression of a minigene within the type X collagen sequence resulted in a phenotype characteristic of several human diseases typified by spinal deformities resulting in lung collapse [71], and mice lacking the type IX collagen gene developed osteoarthritis [72].

A few of the noncollagenous bone matrix proteins have also been knocked out, including osteocalcin [73], matrix gla protein [74], and biglycan [75]. The osteocalcin-deficient mice had an increased rate of bone formation and thickened bones, implicating osteocalcin in the regulation of osteoid formation. FTIRM analysis of the bones of 4-week, 6-month, and 9-month-old knockout animals and their age-matched wild-type controls demonstrated that the knockout mice bones had a higher proportion of mineral (mineral to matrix ratio) with crystals of smaller size and lesser maturity than the wild-type animals [76]. Further, the mineral properties in the knockout animals' cancellous and cortical bones were comparable, whereas in the wild-type animals, the cortical bone contained crystals that were larger and more perfect than those in the trabeculae. These data demonstrated a role for osteocalcin in regulating the maturation of mineral crystals. While in solution, osteocalcin inhibited crystal growth [14, 28] and by binding to apatite-recruited osteoclasts [14, 28] in the mice, the absence of osteocalcin caused crystals to be smaller and osteoclast numbers to be enhanced [73]. This is an example where studies in the mutant animals did not verify predictions from solution and cell culture studies.

In contrast, the biglycan knockout animals developed by Tainshun Xu and Marian Young [75] confirm the biglycan functions predicted by *in vitro* studies. Solution studies indicated that biglycan could both nucleate and inhibit apatite formation and growth [61], and that biglycan, similar to decorin, another leucine-rich proteoglycan found in bone, could regulate collagen fibrillogenesis [24]. The biglycan knockout mice overexpressed decorin and had thinned collagen fibrils, in agreement with the *in vitro* function of these small proteoglycans. As the animals aged, their bones thinned and their mechanical strength diminished relative to age-matched wild-type mice [75]. FTIRM analyses of the bones of these animals at 3 weeks, 3 months, and 6 months showed the knockouts had a decreased mineral-to-matrix ratio and larger, more perfect crystals. This is consistent with a decreased number of nucleation sites and the growth of these decreased numbers of nuclei at the expense of new crystal formation. It is also consistent with the shortened stature seen in patients with Turner's syndrome in whom biglycan expression is decreased [77].

The study of animals with null mutations in matrix protein has also enabled elucidation of functions of proteins which have not been isolated in pure form. Thus the matrix gla protein knockout mice [74] had calcifications throughout their trachea and blood vessels, along with shortened stature and decreased growth plate height, demonstrating, as could be predicted from studies of vitamin K-deficient animals [28], that matrix gla protein is a calcification inhibitor.

Combining results of the *in vitro* and *in vivo* studies, it is apparent that matrix proteins not only can act as nucleators and regulators of crystal growth, but also can control interactions with other proteins and with cells. All of these interactions are important for bone formation and bone mineralization. Greater insight into the mechanisms controlling these processes should come from *in vitro* studies in which these interactions are modulated, and from cross matings of knockout and transgenic animals with different protein mutations.

IV. BONE MODELING AND REMODELING

Following initial mineralization of calcified cartilage or osteoid, the mineralized matrix remains in a dynamic state. It is reshaped as the bones grow and as the loads applied to the bone vary. The periosteum, where new bone formation starts, is very responsive to mechanical load [1], enabling the modelling to occur. Mineral crystals grow, agglomerate, and change in composition [3, 8, 9, 11].

During endochondral ossification, the calcified cartilage matrix serves as a site for the deposition of mineral in the form of the primary spongiosa. Mineral crystals in the woven bone are smaller and contain more impurities than those in compact bone [30, 76] and larger than those in calcified cartilage. This combination of calcified cartilage and woven bone is removed and replaced by woven bone alone. As the epiphyses move further apart and the bone grows longer, the proportions of the bone also change. This modeling is accomplished by the resorption of bone on the endosteal surface and by the formation of periosteal bone. Modeling of the structures formed by intramembranous ossification is similarly governed by the periosteum.

Remodeling, in contrast to modeling, refers to the continuous shaping of the bones in response to repair in which the events of endochondral ossification are recapitulated. Remodeling is the skeletal process that allows mineral ion homeostasis. It is regulated by a number of hormones such as parathyroid hormone, calcitonin, vitamin D, and estrogen. The remodeling process in the healthy bone involves the coupled actions of bone forming and bone resorbing cells. Sequentially, the remodeling process involves recruitment of osteoclasts to a site on the bone surface and the removal of bone mineral and matrix, creating a resorption pit. As the osteoclast moves away, osteoblasts move in and fill in the pit with osteoid, which is then mineralized, presumably by the same processes involved initially. It is this coupling that is thought to be defective in osteoporosis; thus with age, the bones become more and more porous and less able to perform their mechanical function. These processes are regulated by growth factors, hormones, and cytokines [78, 79]. The ways in which the signals are conveyed to the osteoclast and osteoblast and between these cells are still being probed. As with other matrix proteins, the growth factors can bind to the mineral and to other proteins. It is likely that as these signals become better understood, more will also be learned about the fundamental aspects of all stages of bone mineralization.

Acknowledgments

Dr. Boskey's data described in this review was supported by NIH grants DE 04141 and AR 37661, and AR 41325. Special thanks to Dr. S. B. Doty for providing the electron micrographs.

References

1. Reith, E. J., and Ross, M. J. (1970). "Atlas of Descriptive Histology," 2nd ed., pp. 23–40. Harper & Row, Hagerstown, MD.

2. Wolff, J. (1986). "The Law of Bone Remodelling," (translated from the original 1892 edition by P. Maquet and R. Furlong). Springer-Verlag, Berlin.

3. Glimcher, M. J. (1998). The nature of the mineral phase in bone: Biological and clinical implications. In "Metabolic Bone Disease and Clinically Related Disorders" (L. V. Avioli and S. M. Krane, eds.), pp. 23–50. Academic Press, San Diego, CA.

4. Posner, A. S. (1985). The mineral of bone. Clin. Orthop. 200, 87–99.

5. Rey, C. Miguel, J. L., Facchini, L., Legrand, A. P., and Glimcher, M. J. (1995). Hydroxyl groups in bone mineral. Bone 16, 583–586.

6. Rey, C., Renugopalakrishnan, V., Collins, B., and Glimcher, M. J. (1991). Fourier transform infrared spectroscopic study of the carbonate ions in bone mineral during aging. Calcif. Tissue Int. 49, 251–258.

7. Elliot, J. C. (1994). "Structure and Chemistry of the Apatites and Other Calcium Orthophosphates," Studies in Inorganic Chemistry 18. Elsevier, Amsterdam.

8. Kim, H.-M., Rey, C., and Glimcher, M. J. (1995). Isolation of calcium-phosphate crystals of bone by nonaqueous methods of low temperature. J. Bone Miner. Res. 10, 1589–1660.

9. Landis, W. J., Hodgens, K. J., Arena, J., Song, M. J., and McEwen, B. F. (1996). Structural relations between collagen and mineral in bone as determined by high voltage electron microscopic tomography. Microsc. Res. Tech. 33, 192–202.

10. Boyde, A., and Jones, S. J. (1996). Scanning electron microscopy of bone: Instrument, specimen, and issues. Microsc. Res. Tech. 33, 92–120.

11. Paschalis, E. P., DiCarlo, E., Betts, F., Sherman, P., Mendelsohn, R., and Boskey, A. L. (1996). FTIR microspectroscopic analysis of human osteonal bone. Calcif. Tissue Int. 59, 480–487.

12. Masse, P. G., Rimnac, C., Yamauchi, M., Coburn, P., Rucker, R. B., and Boskey, A. L. (1996). Pyridoxine deficiency affects biomechanical properties of chick tibial bone. Bone 18, 567–575.

13. Lees, S., and Page, E. A. (1992). A study of some properties of mineralized turkey leg tendon. Connect. Tissue Res. 28, 263–287.

14. Robey, P. G., and Boskey, A. L. (1996). Mineral and matrix In "Osteoporosis" (D. Feldman and J. Jowsey, eds.), pp. 95–184. Academic Press, San Diego, CA.

15. Goldberg, M., and Boskey, A. L. (1997). Lipids and biomineralizations. Prog. Histochem. Cytochem. 31, 1–187.

16. Raisz, L. G., and Rodan, G. A. (1998). Embryology and cellular biology of bone. In "Metabolic Bone Disease and Clinically Related Disorders" (L. V. Avioli and S. M. Krane, eds.), pp. 1–22. Academic Press, San Diego, CA.

17. Schmid, T. M., Bonen, D. K., Luchene, L., and Linsenmayer, T. F. (1991). Late events in chondrocyte differentiation: Hypertrophy, type X collagen synthesis and matrix calcification. In Vivo 5, 533–540.

18. Wuthier, R. E. (1993). Involvement of cellular metabolism of calcium and phosphate in calcification of avian growth plate cartilage. J. Nutr. 123S, 301–309.

19. Arispe, N., Rojas, E., Genge, B. R., Wu, L. N., and Wuthier, R. E. (1996). Similarity in calcium channel activity of annexin V and matrix vesicles in planar lipid bilayers. Biophys. J. 71, 1764–1775.

20. Wuthier, R. E., Wu, L. N., Sauer, G. R., Genge, B. R., Yoshimori, T., and Ishikawa, Y. (1992). Mechanism of matrix vesicle calcification: Characterization of ion channels and the nucleational core of growth plate vesicles. Bone Miner. 17, 290–295.

21. Wu, L. N., Genge, B. R., Dunkelberger, D. G., LeGeros, R. Z., Concannon, B., and Wuthier, R. E. (1997). Physicochemical characterization of the nucleational core of matrix vesicles. J. Biol. Chem. 272, 4404–4411.

22. Buckwalter, J. A., and Rosenberg, L. C. (1983). Structural changes during development in bovine fetal epiphyseal cartilage. Collagen Relat. Res. 3, 489–504.

23. Cowles, E. A., DeRome, M. E., Pastizzo, G., Brailey, L. L., and Gronowicz, G. A. (1998). Mineralization and the expression of matrix proteins during in vivo bone development. Calif. Tissue Int. 62, 74–82.

24. Vogel, K. G., Paulsson, M., and Heinegard, D. (1984). Specific inhibition of type I and type II collagen fibrillogenesis by the small proteoglycan of tendon. Biochem. J. 223, 587–597.

25. Kuboki, Y., Kudo, A., Mizuno, M., and Kawamura, M. (1992). Time-dependent changes of collagen cross-links and their precursors in culture of osteogeneic cells. Calcif. Tissue Int. 50, 473–480.

26. Eyre, D. R., Dickson, I. R., and Van Ness, K. (1988). Collagen cross-linking in human bone and articular cartilage. Age-related changes in the content of mature hydroxypyridinium residues. Biochem. J. 252, 495–500.

27. Gerstenfeld, L. C., Chipman, S. D., Glowacki, J., and Lian, J. B. (1986). Expression to differentiate function by mineralizing cultures of chicken osteoblasts. Dev. Biol. 122, 49–60.

28. Hauschka, P. V., and Wians, F. H., Jr. (1989). Osteocalcin-hydroxyapatite Interaction in the extracellular organic matrix of bone. Anat. Rec. 224, 180–188.

29. Wu, Y., Glimcher, M. J., Rey, C., and Ackerman, J. L. (1994). A unique protonated phosphate group in bone mineral not present in synthetic calcium phosphates: Identification by phosphorus-31 solid state NMR spectroscopy. J. Mol. Biol. 244, 423–435.

30. Mbuyi-Muamba, J. M., Dequeker, J., and Gevers, G. (1989). Collagen and non-collagenous proteins in different mineralization stages of human femur. Acta Anat. 134, 265–268.

31. Lane, J. M., Betts, F., Posner, A. S., and Yue, D. W. (1984). Mineral parameters in early fracture repair. J. Bone Jt. Surg., Am. Vol. 66, 1289–1293.

32. Boskey, A. L., and Marks, S. C. (1985). Mineral and matrix alterations in the bones of incisors-absent (ia/ia). Osteopetrotic rat. Calcif. Tissue Int. 37, 287–292.

33. Mendelsohn, R., Hassenkhani, A., DiCarlo, E., and Boskey A. L. (1989). FT-IR microscopy of endochondral ossification at 20μ spatial resolution. Calcif. Tissue Int. 44, 20–24.

34. Sauer, G. R., and Wuthier, R. E. (1988). Fourier transform infrared characterization of mineral phases formed during induction of mineralization by collagenase-released matrix vesicles in vitro. J. Biol. Chem. 263, 13718–13724.

35. Wuthier, R. E., Rice, G. S., Wallace, J. E., Jr., Weaver, R. L., LeGeros, R. Z., and Eanes, E. D. (1985). In vitro precipitation of calcium phos-

phate under intracellular conditions: Formation of brushite from an amorphous precursor in the absence of ATP. *Calcif. Tissue Int.* **37**, 401–410.

36. Driessens, F. C. M., and Verbeeck, R. M. H. (1990). "Biominerals," Chapter 3, pp. 37–61. CRC Press, Boca Raton, FL.

37. Traub, W., Arad, T., and Weiner, S. (1992). Origin of mineral crystal growth in collagen fibrils. *Matrix* **12**, 251–255.

38. Anderson, H. C. (1989). Mechanism of mineral formation in bone. *Lab. Invest.* **60**, 320–330.

39. Eanes, E. D., Hailer, A. W., Midura, R. J., and Hascall, V. C. (1992). Proteoglycan inhibition of calcium phosphate precipitation in liposomal suspensions. *Glycobiology* **2**, 571–578.

40. Boskey, A. L., Maresca, M., Armstrong, A. L., and Ehrlich, M. G. (1992). Treatment of proteoglycan aggregates with growth plate neutral metalloprotease reduces their ability to inhibit hydroxyapatite proliferation in a gelatin gel. *J. Orthop. Res.* **10**, 313–319.

41. Yasuda, T., Shimizu, K., Nakagawa, Y., Yamamoto, S., Niibayashi, H., and Yamamuro, T. (1995). m-Calpain in rat growth plate chondrocyte cultures: Its involvement in the matrix mineralization process. *Dev. Biol.* **170**, 159–168.

42. Cornelissen, M., and de Ridder, L. (1993). Electron microscopic study of proteoglycan aggregates synthesized by embryonic chick sternal chondrocytes in vitro. *Eur. J. Morphol.* **31**, 17–20.

43. Dean, D. D., Boyan, B. D., Muniz, O. E., Howell, D. S., and Schwartz, Z. (1996). Vitamin D metabolites regulate matrix vesicle metalloproteinase content in a cell maturation-dependent manner. *Calcif. Tissue Int.* **59**, 109–116.

44. Boskey, A. L., Boyan, B. D., and Schwartz, Z. (1997). Matrix vesicles promote mineralization in a gelatin gel. *Calcif. Tissue Int.* **60**, 309–315.

45. Landis, W. J., Hodgens, K. J., McKee, M. D., Nanci, A., Song, M. J., Kiyonaga, S., Arena, J., and McEwen, B. (1992). Extracellular vesicles of calcifying turkey leg tendon characterized by immunocytochemistry and high voltage electron microscopic tomography and 3-D graphic image reconstruction. *Bone Miner.* **17**, 237–241.

46. Glimcher, M. J., Hodge, A. J., and Schmitt, F. O. (1957). Macromolecular aggregation states in relation to mineralization: The collagen hydroxyapatite system as studied in vitro. *Proc. Natl. Acad. Sci. U.S.A.* **43**, 860–967.

47. Katz, E. P. (1969). The kinetics of mineralization in vitro. I. The nucleation properties of 640-angstrom collagen at 25 degrees. *Biochim. Biophys. Acta* **194**, 121–129.

48. Mergenhagen, S. E., Martin, G. R., Rizzo, A., Wright, D. N., and Scott, D. B. (1960). Calcification in vivo of implanted collagens. *Biochim. Biophys. Acta* **43**, 563–565.

49. Termine, J. D., Kleinman, H. K., Whitson, S. W., Conn, K. M., McGarvey, M. L., and Martin, G. R. (1981). Osteonectin, a bone-specific protein linking mineral to collagen. *Cell* **26**, 99–105.

50. Endo, A. (1987). Potential role of phosphoprotein in collagen mineralization—an experimental study in vitro. *J. Orthop. Assoc.* **61**, 563–569.

51. Glimcher, M. J. (1989). Mechanism of calcification: Role of collagen fibrils and collagen-phosphoprotein complexes in vitro and in vivo. *Anat. Rec.* **224**, 139–153.

52. Boskey, A. L. (1996). Matrix proteins and mineralization: An overview. *Connect. Tissue Res.* **35**, 357–363.

53. Stein, G. S., and Lian, J. B. (1993). Molecular mechanisms mediating proliferation/differentiation interrelationships during progressive development of the osteoblast phenotype. *Endocr. Rev.* **14**, 424–442.

54. McKee, M. D., and Nanci, A. (1995). Postembedding colloidal-gold immunocytochemistry of noncollagenous extracellular matrix proteins in mineralized tissues. *Microsc. Res. Tech.* **31**, 44–62.

55. Mikuni-Takagaki, Y., and Glimcher, M. J. (1990). Post-translational processing of chicken bone phosphoproteins. Identification of bone (phospho)protein kinase. *Biochem. J.* **268**, 593–597.

56. Hunter, G. K., and Goldberg, H. A. (1993). Nucleation of hydroxyapatite by bone sialoprotein. *Proc. Natl. Acad. Sci. U.S.A.* **90**, 8562–8565.

57. Stubbs, J. T., 3rd, Mintz, K. P., Eanes, E. D., Torchia, D. A., and Fisher, L. W. (1997). Characterization of native and recombinant bone sialoprotein: Delineation of the mineral-binding and cell adhesion domains and structural analysis of the RGD domain. *J. Bone Miner. Res.* **12**, 1210–1222.

58. Fujisawa, R., Wada, Y., Nodasaka, Y., and Kuboki, Y. (1996). Acidic amino acid-rich sequences as binding sites of osteonectin to hydroxyapatite crystals. *Biochim. Biophys. Acta* **1292**, 53–60.

59. Fujisawa, R., and Kuboki, Y. (1991). Preferential absorption of dentin and bone acidic proteins on the (100) face of hydroxyapatite crystals. *Biochim. Biophys. Acta* **1075**, 56–60.

60. Boskey, A. L., Ullrich, W., Spevak, L., and Gilder, H. (1996). Persistence of complexed acidic phospholipids in rapidly mineralizing tissues is due to affinity for mineral and resistance to hydrolytic attack: In vitro data. *Calcif. Tissue Int.* **58**, 45–51.

61. Boskey, A. L., Spevak, L., Doty, S. B., and Rosenberg, L. (1997). Effects of bone CS-proteoglycans, DS-decorin, and DS-biglycan on hydroxyapatite formation in a gelatin Gel. *Calcif. Tissue Int.* **61**, 298–305.

62. Boskey, A. L., Maresca, M, Doty, S., Sabsay, B., and Veis, A. (1990). Concentration dependent effects of dentin-phosphophoryn in the regulation of *in vitro* hydroxyapatite formation and growth. *Bone Miner.* **11**, 55–65.

63. Moradian-Oldak, J., Frolow, F., Addadi, L., and Weiner, S. (1992). Interactions between acidic matrix macromolecules and calcium phosphate ester crystals: Relevance to carbonate apatite formation in biomineralization. *Proc. R. Soc. London, Ser. B* **247**, 47–55.

64. Doi, Y., Horiguchi, T., Kim, S. H., Moriwaki, Y., Wakamatsu, N., Adachi, M., Ibaraki, K., Moriyama, K., Sasaki, S., and Shimokawa, H. (1992). Effects of non-collagenous proteins on the formation of apatite in calcium beta-glycerophosphate solutions. *Arch. Oral Biol.* **37**, 15–21.

65. Boskey, A. L., Maresca, M., Ulrich, W., Doty, S. B., Butler, W. T., and Prince, C. W. (1993). Osteopontin-hydroxyapatite interactions in vitro: Inhibition of hydroxyapatite formation and growth in a gelatin-gel. *Bone Miner.* **22**, 147–159.

66. Hunter, G. K., Kyle, C. L., and Goldberg, H. A. (1994). Modulation of crystal formation by bone phosphoproteins: Structural specificity of the osteopontin-mediated inhibition of hydroxyapatite formation. *Biochem. J.* **300**, 723–728.

67. Boskey, A. L., Stiner, D., Binderman, I., and Doty, S. B. (1997). Effects of proteoglycan modification on mineral formation in a differentiating chick limb-bud mesenchymal cell culture system. *J. Cell. Biochem.* **64**, 632–643.

68. Boskey, A. L., Guidon, P., Doty, S. B., Stiner, D., Leboy, P., and Binderman, I. (1996). The mechanism of β-glycerophosphate action in mineralizing chick limb-bud mesenchymal cells. *J. Bone Miner. Res.* **11**, 1694–1702.

69. Stacey, A., Bateman, J., Choi, T., Mascara, T., Cole, W., and Jaenisch, R. (1988). Perinatal lethal osteogenesis imperfecta in transgenic mice bearing an engineered mutant pro-alpha 1(i). Collagen gene. *Nature* **332**, 131–136.

70. Bonadio, J., Jepsen, K. J., Mansoura, M. K., Jaenisch, R., Kuhn, J. L., and Goldstein, S. A. (1993). A murine skeletal adaptation that significantly increases cortical bone mechanical properties. Implications for human skeletal fragility. *J. Clin. Invest.* **92**, 1697–1705.

71. Jacenko, O., LuValle, P., Solum, K., and Olsen, B. R. (1993). A dominant negative mutation in the alpha 1 (X). Collagen gene produces spondylometaphyseal defects in mice. *Prog. Clin. Biol. Res.* **383B**, 427–436.

72. Fassler, R., Schnegelsberg, P. N., Dausman, J., Shinya, T., Muragaki, Y., McCarthy, M. T., Olsen, B. R., and Jaenisch, R. (1994). Mice lacking alpha 1 (IX). Collagen develop noninflammatory degenerative joint disease. *Proc. Natl. Acad. Sci. U.S.A.* **91**, 5070–5074.

73. Ducy, P., Desbois, C., Boyce, B., Pinero, G., Story, B., Dunstan, C.,

Smith, E., Bonadio, J., Goldstein, S., Gundberg, C., Bradley, A., and Karsenty, G. (1996). Increased bone formation in osteocalcin-deficient mice. *Nature* **382**, 448–452.

74. Luo, G., Ducy, P., McKee, M. D., Pinero, G. J., Loyer, E., Behringer, R. R., and Karsenty, G. (1997). Spontaneous calcification of arteries and cartilage in mice lacking matrix GLA protein. *Nature* **386**, 78–81.

75. Zu, T., Fisher, L., Bianco, P., Longnecker, G., Boskey, A. L., Smith, E., Bonadio, J., Goldsteins, S., Zhao, C., Dominguez, P., Heegaard, A. M., Satomura, K., Gehron-Robey, P., Kulkarni, A., Sommer, B., and Young, M. (1998). Targeted disruption of the biglycan gene leads to Osteoporosis in mice. *Nature Genet.* **20**, 78–86.

76. Boskey, A. L., Gadaleta, S., Gundberg, C., Doty, S. B., Ducy, P., and Karsenty, G. (1998). FT-IR microspectroscopic analysis of bones of osteocalcin-deficient mice provides insight into the function of osteocalcin. *Bone* **23**, 187–196.

77. Geerkens, C., Vetter, U., Just, W., Fedarko, N. S., Fisher, L. W., Young, M. F., Termine, J. D., Robey, P. G., Wohrle, D., and Vogel, W. (1995). The X-chromosomal human biglycan gene BGN is subject to X inactivation but is transcribed like an X-Y homologous gene. *Hum. Genet.* **96**, 44–52.

78. Dequeker, J., and Mundy, G. R. (1998). Bone structure and function. *In* "Rheumatology" (J. H. Klippel and P. A. Dieppe, eds.), 2nd ed., pp. 34.1–34.12. Mosby, London.

79. Parfitt, A. M. (1998). Osteomalacia and related disorders. *In* "Metabolic Bone Disease and Clinically Related Disorders" (L. V. Avioli and S. M. Krane, eds.), pp. 327–386. Academic Press, San Diego, CA.

CHAPTER 12

The Cells of Bone

JANE B. LIAN AND GARY S. STEIN

Department of Cell Biology, University of Massachusetts Medical School, Worcester, Massachusetts 01655

I. ABSTRACT

In this chapter, the properties of osteoblast and osteoclast lineage cells are described. Emphasis is placed on the functional aspects of subpopulations of cells contributing to bone formation and bone resorption as well as on responsiveness of the cells to physiological regulators of bone metabolism. Advances in understanding molecular and cellular mechanisms regulating the progression of osteoblast and osteoclast differentiation are presented. Characterized markers of each cell population at progressive stages of maturation provide a basis for understanding skeletal development and improving diagnosis and treatment of the skeletal diseases.

II. INTRODUCTION

Bone is a dynamic connective tissue, composed of an exquisite assembly of functionally distinct cell populations that are required to support both the structural, biochemical, and mechanical integrity of this mineralized tissue and its central role in mineral homeostasis. The responsiveness of bone to mechanical forces and metabolic regulatory signals that accommodate requirements for maintaining serum calcium and phosphate are operative throughout life. As such, bone tissue undergoes remodeling, a continual process of resorption and renewal (see Chapter 18). The principal cells that mediate these structural and functional properties of the mammalian skeleton are: *osteoblasts*, which synthesize the bone matrix on bone forming surfaces; *osteocytes*, which support bone structure and are organized throughout the mineralized bone matrix; the protective bone surface *lining cells*; and the multinucleated *osteoclasts*, which are responsible for the resorption of bone matrix. Fidelity of bone formation and remodeling necessitates exchange of regulatory signals among these cell populations and their progenitors. The basis for our current understanding of bone development and homeostasis has been and continues to be principally derived from the properties of skeletal cells and their progenitors and the characterization of gene expression (genes and their regulatory factors) that controls bone formation andresorption.

Osteoblasts and osteoclasts are derived from two distinct cell lineages. It is becoming increasingly evident that both osteoblast and osteoclast differentiation require a multistep series of events modulated by an integrated cascade of gene expression that initially supports proliferation and the sequential expression of genes associated with each component of bone formation and resorption. Equally significant are the growth factor and steroid hormone responsive regulatory signals which mediate developmental competency for expression of genes associated with skeletal cell proliferation and differentiation. In this chapter, current concepts in understanding molecular and cellular mechanisms regulating the progression of osteoblast and osteoclast differentiation and functional activities of distinct cell populations will be explored. Within this context, a basis can be provided for improved diagnosis of skeletal disease and treatment that is targeted to specific cells in bone tissue.

III. EMBRYONIC ORIGINS OF BONE

The differentiation of osteoblast lineage cells must be considered within the context of embryologic development, bone formation during growth, and bone tissue remodeling in the adult skeleton. Under these circumstances, progenitor cells must be responsive to a broad spectrum of regulatory signals that mediate commitment to osteoblast differentiation and progression of phenotype development, as well as sustaining structural and functional properties of differentiated bone cells. Progenitors of the bone-forming cells are considered to be of mesenchymal origin derived from the mesodermal germ cell layer. The dorsal paraxial mesoderm gives rise to somites and the sclerotome, which is a source of cells for most of the axial skeleton; the lateral plate mesoderm gives rise to the appendicular skeleton and the cephalic mesoderm gives rise to the neural crest which provides progenitor cells for cranial-facial skeletal structures. Thus, different regions of the skeleton have distinct embryonic lineages reflecting origins from these specific primordial structures. Considering these different embryonic developmental programs of the mesoderm to form membranous bone (e.g., calvarium) and subtypes of endochondral bone (e.g., limbs and vertebrae), an early osteoprogenitor may divert from a stem cell at these skeletal sites. It has been well documented that axial and appendicular bone exhibit selective responsiveness to hormones [1, 2]. It remains to be determined whether this reflects the tissue environment or inherent properties of the cells selected at an early stage during osteoblast differentiation. The extent to which skeletal stem cell populations undergo expansion has yet to be established.

IV. BONE-FORMING CELLS

A. From Stem Cell To Osteoprogenitor

It would be particularly instructive to characterize the stem cells that give rise to progeny for bone formation and tissue renewal. The presumptive stem cell can only be identified by biological consequence. For example, one assay of stem cell activity is by transplantation to a recipient animal and examination of the differentiated cell in long-term animals (e.g., after a year) [3]. The progression of the most primitive pluripotent cell to the undifferentiated multipotential mesenchymal cell is not understood. Several factors have been identified in mediating induction of a pluripotent cell to an immature osteoprogenitor (Fig. 1). The osteoprogenitor appears to have limited self-renewal capacity and, in contrast to the stem cell, has a capacity for extensive proliferation. Stem cells by their nature are generally in a noncycling (G_0) stage of the cell cycle. Presently, a key obstacle in understanding the osteoblast lineage is the inability to identify an osteoprogenitor cell prior to expression of bone phenotypic properties. Using characterization of hematopoietic stem cells as a paradigm, several groups have developed antibodies to cell surface proteins using presumptive marrow stromal cell populations (Fig. 1). These reagents have the potential for both recognition and purification of skeletal stem cells [4–15]. As indicated in Figure 1, the antigens for some of these antibodies have been characterized.

An important source of the putative stem cell, the multipotential mesenchymal progenitor, and the osteoprogenitor cell is the marrow. The marrow and its stromal "bedding" give rise to cells of both the hematopoietic lineage (origin of osteoclasts) and nonhematopoietic lineage cells from which many tissue-specific cells derive (e.g., chondrocytes, myoblasts, adipocytes). When suspensions of marrow cells are plated *in vitro*, clonal colonies of adherent fibroblasts are formed; each is derived from the single cell which has been designated as the colony forming fibroblastic unit, or CFU/F [16] formation. Formation of CFUs requires the presence of hematopoietic cells [17]. A proportion of these cells have high proliferative and differentiation capacity and exhibit characteristics of stem cells when transplanted in the closed environment of a diffusion chamber [18].

Several signaling molecules, including cytokines, growth factors, and hormones, that influence commitment to osteoblastic colony forming units and osteoprogenitor growth and differentiation have been characterized (Fig. 1). Leukemia inhibitory factor (LIF), which maintains stem cell populations by inhibiting their differentiation, has also been reported to have osteogenic activity by enhancing differentiation of preosteoblasts [19]. Platelet-derived growth factor and epidermal growth factor [20] have been identified as important in stimulating expansion of the CFU/F [17]. The fibroblast growth factor (bFGF) and transforming growth factor $\beta 1$ (TGF-$\beta 1$) are potent mitogens for periosteal osteoprogenitors and marrow stromal cells [21–23] and are expressed and produced by osteoblast lineage cells. These growth factors are stored in the bone extracellular matrix and thus provide a local mechanism for stimulating proliferation of progenitors in the bone microenvironment [24, 25]. The osteoinductive effects of the bone morphogenetic proteins (BMPs) are complex (reviewed by Onishi *et al.* [26]) and depend on the specific BMP, concentration dependency, and the progenitor

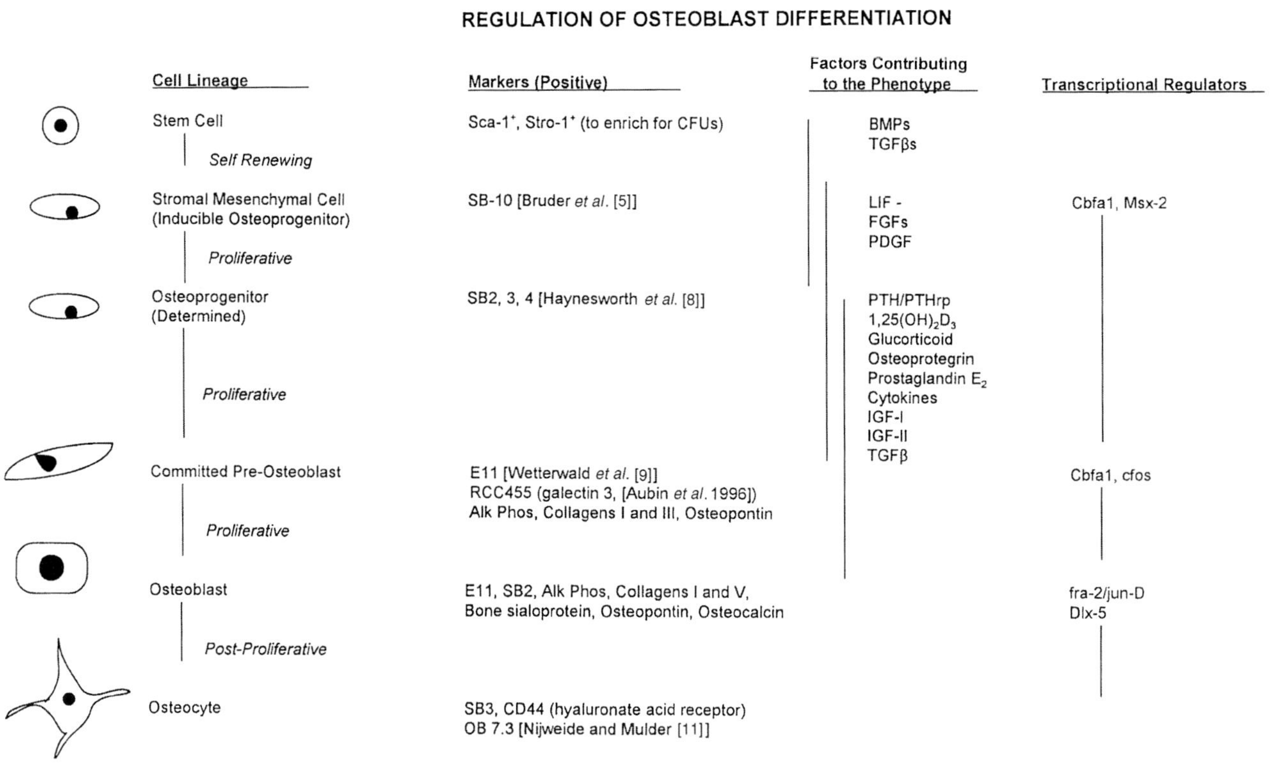

REGULATION OF OSTEOBLAST DIFFERENTIATION

Cell Lineage	Markers (Positive)	Factors Contributing to the Phenotype	Transcriptional Regulators
Stem Cell	Sca-1+, Stro-1+ (to enrich for CFUs)	BMPs TGFβs	
Self Renewing			
Stromal Mesenchymal Cell (Inducible Osteoprogenitor)	SB-10 [Bruder *et al.* [5]]	LIF - FGFs PDGF	Cbfa1, Msx-2
Proliferative			
Osteoprogenitor (Determined)	SB2, 3, 4 [Haynesworth *et al.* [8]]	PTH/PTHrp 1,25(OH)$_2$D$_3$ Glucorticoid Osteoprotegrin Prostaglandin E$_2$ Cytokines IGF-I IGF-II TGFβ	
Proliferative			
Committed Pre-Osteoblast	E11 [Wetterwald *et al.* [9]] RCC455 (galectin 3, [Aubin *et al.* 1996]) Alk Phos, Collagens I and III, Osteopontin		Cbfa1, cfos
Proliferative			
Osteoblast	E11, SB2, Alk Phos, Collagens I and V, Bone sialoprotein, Osteopontin, Osteocalcin		fra-2/jun-D Dlx-5
Post-Proliferative			
Osteocyte	SB3, CD44 (hyaluronate acid receptor) OB 7.3 [Nijweide and Mulder [11]]		

FIGURE 1   Phenotypic properties of cells of the osteoblast lineage. Column 1 illustrates the morphologic features of osteoblast lineage cells at each stage from stem cell to osteocyte, the final stage of the differentiated osteoblast. The mature osteoblast on the quiescent bone surface, the bone lining cell, is not shown. Column 2 describes either cell surface markers or proteins that are highly expressed at the indicated stage of maturation. Column 3 lists those factors which promote differentiation of the precursor cell populations. In column 4, those transcription factors which have been identified as key regulators of bone formation or expression of osteoblast specific genes are indicated.

cell phenotype. BMP-2, BMP-4, and BMP-7 (also designated OP-1) are potent inducers of osteogenesis *in vivo* and *in vitro* [27–30]. BMP-2 rapidly induces osteoblast differentiation in marrow stromal cells [31] and in a number of pluripotent cell lines [32]. BMP-2 is also competent to transdifferentiate the mouse myogenic cell line C2C12 into osteoblasts [33]. Systemic factors also influence early stages of bone formation. Parathyroid hormone (PTH) stimulates growth of osteoprogenitor populations [34], while parathyroid hormone related peptide (PTHrP) functions as a cellular cytokine regulating cell growth for differentiation in development (reviewed in Moseley and Martin [35]). The significance of many of these growth factors and morphogens in regulating progression of the pluripotent stem cell and multipotential mesenchymal cell to the committed osteoprogenitor and finally to recognizable osteoblasts is appreciated from mouse models in which these genes or receptors for these proteins have been ablated with consequences on formation of the skeleton (reviewed by Erlebacher *et al.* [36]). Most notable are the mouse "knockout" of PTHrP and the PTH/PTHrP receptor [37, 38] and the FGF receptors [39–41]. Glucocorticoids have been shown to stimulate the growth and differentiation of CFUs and osteoprogenitors

from human and rat, but not from mouse-derived marrow stromal cells, towards the osteogenic lineage ([42] and references therein).

B. Osteoblast Differentiation: From Osteoprogenitor To Osteoblast

The final stages of osteoblast ontogeny are defined by the biosynthesis and organization of the bone extracellular matrix. When the preosteoblast ceases to proliferate, a key signaling event occurs for development of the large cuboidal surface osteoblast from the spindle shaped osteoprogenitor. The osteoblast vectorially secretes type I collagen and specialized bone matrix proteins towards the mineralizing front of the tissue (Table I). Osteoblast differentiation and function are regulated by interaction of the cell with matrix proteins [43, 44]. Functional studies establishing requirement of the type I collagen and other ECM components in promoting osteoblast/osteocyte differentiation have been carried out by modifying production of osteoblast-secreted products or by culturing osteoblasts on various matrices [45–48]. The molecular mechanisms guiding these transitions are

TABLE I. Representative Osteoblast Products Supporting Structural Properties of Bone

	Properties
Collagens	
Type III	Significant levels in preosteoblasts
Type I	Principle bone protein; 90% of the organic matrix
Type V	Present in low levels; may regulate fiber diameter
Noncollagenous Proteins	
Osteonectin	~40 kDa; expressed constitutively during osteoblast differentiation; binds calcium and growth factors
BAG-75	75 kDa; binds calcium; sequence homology with bone and dentin phosphoproteins
Decorin	~130 kDa intact protein with one chondroitin sulfate chain; binds to collagen and TGFβ; may regulate fibril diameter; inhibits cell attachment to fibronectin
Biglycan	~270 kDa intact protein having 2 CS chains; localized in the pericellular environment
Osteocalcin	~6 kDa characterized by three vitamin K dependently synthesized γ-carboxyglutamic acid residues which bind calcium; abundant bone-specific matrix protein
Cell Adhesion Proteins	
Thrombospondins	~450 kDa; binds to heparin, platelets, types I and V collagens, thrombin, fibrinogen, laminin, plasminogen, and plasminogen activator inhibitor; histidine rich glycoprotein
Fibronectin	~400 kDa; binds to cells, collagen
Vitronectin	~70 kDa; binds to collagen, heparin, plasminogen, and plasminogen activator inhibitor
Osteopontin	~44–75 kDa; glycosylated; phosphorylated; RGD sequences; facilitates osteoclast/ECM interactions; may contribute to growth control
Bone sialoprotein	~46–75 kDa; polyglutamyl stretches; 50% carbohydrate; RGD sequence; may initiate mineralization and "ahome" cancer cells to bone

poorly understood. However, cell–matrix and cell–cell interactions are presumed to be important for the maturation of osteoblasts.

A spectrum of integrins has been shown to be expressed by osteoblasts. Osteoblasts appear to use β1 integrins to adhere to the full range of RGD-containing bone matrix proteins, although the precise role of integrins and other adhesion molecules in the regulation of osteoprogenitor differentiation and functional maturation is not clear [49]. Several members of the cadherin family of cell–cell adhesion proteins are expressed in osteoblasts; these include cadherin-11, cadherin-4, N-cadherin, and OB-cadherin [50]. N-cadherin is present on proliferative preosteoblastic cells but is lost as they become osteocytic [51]. In contrast, OB-cadherin is barely detected in osteoprogenitor cells and is upregulated in alkaline phosphatase expressing cells [52]. Interestingly, the antigens to a cell surface marker antibody (SB-10) produced in response to mesenchymal stem cells is the activated leukocyte cell adhesion molecule ALCAM [5]. Expression of ALCAM becomes downregulated in concert with changes in morphology and detection of alkaline phosphatase activity of the periosteal osteoprogenitors as it migrates and develops

into an osteoblast. In addition, ICAM-1 and VCAM-1 have been found on the osteoblast surface, thereby providing a potential mechanism for T cell interactions that contribute to regulation of bone turnover [53]. Signaling pathways from the extracellular matrix through the cytoskeleton and finally to the nucleus, which allow expression and upregulation of bone-specific and bone-related genes, need to be investigated. For example, β-catenin, which colocalizes and coprecipitates with cadherins [50], is a potential candidate. CD44, the hyaluronate receptor, is a nonintegrin adhesion receptor which is linked to the cytoskeleton. It is a useful marker for osteocyte differentiation [13, 14] and is also expressed in osteoclasts [54].

The *in vitro* study of primary osteoblasts from several species has allowed molecular analysis of expressed genes and transcription factors that regulate proliferation and differentiation of osteoblasts in relation to progressive formation of the bone matrix [55]. These studies, carried out over a period of several weeks, provide a definition of discrete stages of maturation of the osteoblasts (Fig. 2). Proliferating preosteoblast stage cells are engaged in synthesis of growth factors and matrix components of woven bone. The

A

Pre-osteoblast > Osteoblast > Pre-osteocyte > Osteocyte

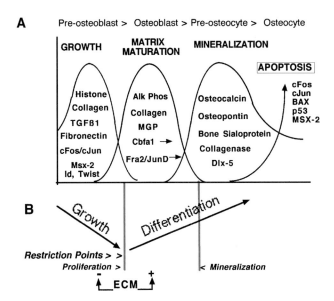

B

FIGURE 2 *In vitro* development of the osteoblast phenotype. (A) Illustration of the temporal expression of cell growth and osteoblast phenotype related genes during 35 days of culture of fetal rat calvarial-derived osteoblasts. Peak mRNA levels, which were determined in total cellular RNA prepared at 3 day intervals, define the growth period, the postproliferative matrix maturation stage, and the mineralization stage. Experimental conditions and origin of the probes are detailed in Stein *et al.* [55]. During the proliferation period marked by (H4) histone, growth factors (TGF-β1), adhesion proteins (fibronectin), collagen, and low levels of osteopontin (not shown) are expressed. Peak levels of alkaline phosphatase mRNA (AP) represent the matrix maturation period. In the mineralization period, an increase in mRNA transcripts of osteocalcin and osteopontin bone sialoprotein reflects calcium (Ca^{++}) deposition. Increased levels of collagenase are related to remodeling or editing of the extracellular matrix. Apoptotic cells are observed during the mineralization period associated with the bone forming nodule. The expression of transcription factors during osteoblast differentiation is based on either mRNA levels (Msx-2, Dlx-5, Id, Twist) or functional protein levels determined by Western blot or gel shift analyses of nuclear extracts (c-fos, c-jun, c-fra-2, jun D, Cbfa1). See text for references. (B) Reciprocal and functionally coupled relationship between cell growth and differentiation-related gene expression in osteoblasts. These relationships are schematically illustrated as arrows representing changes in expression of cell cycle- and cell growth-related genes as well as genes associated with regulated and regulatory events associated with onset and progression of differentiation. Three principal periods of osteoblast developmental sequence are designated within broken vertical lines (proliferation, matrix maturation, and mineralization). These broken lines indicate two experimentally established transition points exhibited by normal diploid osteoblasts during sequential acquisition of bone cell phenotype: (1) at completion of proliferation when genes associated with extracellular matrix development and maturation of the phenotype are upregulated and (2) at onset of extracellular matrix mineralization. Formation of the extracellular matrix contributes to cessation of cell growth and induction of genes rendering the matrix competent for mineralization.

bone extracellular matrix changes in composition as tissue organization and mineralization develop. Initially, the large proteoglycans versican and hyaluronan are produced by pre-osteoblasts and then are replaced by the small chondroitin sulfate proteoglycans decorin and biglycan [56]. The matrix maturation stage marks the postproliferative osteoblast expressing maximal levels of alkaline phosphatase to render

the matrix competent for mineralization. Type I collagen accumulates, together with the specialized classes of calcium binding proteins (osteopontin, bone sialoprotein, and osteocalcin), which are upregulated when extracellular matrix mineralization initiates. An apoptotic stage is indicated in Fig. 2. The *in vitro* characterization of some osteoblasts undergoing apoptosis within the mineralized nodule may reflect an *in vivo* mechanism for triaging those osteoblasts recruited to produce matrix but that can not all be accommodated in the mineralized matrix as osteocytes.

It is apparent that important intracellular proteins which are expressed in the proliferating osteoblasts are permissive for the expression of phenotypic genes in the postproliferative period. For example, expression of Msh homeodomain proteins, oncogenic proteins, and cell cycle factors regulating progression through the cell cycle must become downregulated for osteoblast differentiation to proceed (reviewed in Stein *et al.* [57]). A reciprocal relationship between growth and expression of many genes reflecting the mature osteoblast phenotype has been established. The temporal expression of proteins and enzymes involved in cell adherence, initial production of the extracellular matrix, and modification of the extracellular matrix, providing competency for mineralization and the final stage of osteocyte development in the mineralization period, demonstrates the various subpopulations of osteoblasts. Thus, the expression of subclasses of osteoblastic genes (Fig. 2) can also be used as markers of the stages of osteoblast maturation and may reflect selective functions of osteoblasts dependent on their location in bone. This concept is supported by the analysis of expressed genes and protein levels at the single cell level in osteoblast cultures developing a tissue organization (the bone nodule) and in bone sections [58–61]. The variations in levels of expressed gene products reveal subtle yet important differences in functional properties that relate to the establishment and maintenance of bone structure.

Based on this model, we can better understand the properties and physiologic responses of the cells at their individual stages of differentiation. This is best exemplified by selective responses to growth factors [62–64] and hormones [42, 65–68]. It is established that TGFβ stimulates the replication of progenitor cells and directly stimulates collagen synthesis. The mitogenic effects of TGFβ are not apparent on mature postproliferative osteoblasts. The fibroblast growth factors (FGF-1, FGF-2) also stimulate bone cell replication in cells capable of collagen synthesis. However, FGF does not directly effect the differentiated functions and indeed, in mature osteoblasts, FGF both inhibits type I collagen synthesis and increases collagenase expression. The steroid hormones, glucocorticoid [42], 1,25(OH)$_2$D$_3$ [65, 66], and estrogen [67], also have selective effects, either promoting differentiation of the cells at early stages of maturation or inhibiting anabolic activities and promoting resorptive properties of the osteoblast at later stages.

C. The Osteocyte: Differentiation Supports Bone Structure and Viability

As mineralization of the matrix envelopes the osteoblast, morphologic changes are induced in the cell when the osteoblast progresses to the final differentiated stage, the osteocyte. *In vitro*, the distinct morphology characteristic of an osteocyte can be distinguished in cross-sections of a bone nodule. Cellular extensions of the plasma membrane can be observed [61]. The osteocyte is a terminally differentiated cell and when isolated directly from bone tissue, it retains its morphologic features *in vitro*. In culture, the cell does not divide and upon attachment to surface, it forms characteristic cytoplasmic extrusions in all directions [11, 69, 70]. Osteocytes have the capacity to synthesize certain matrix molecules (as abundantly as osteoblasts) that have been visualized by *in situ* studies. The detection of osteocalcin, for example, is particularly robust, supporting the relevance of *in vitro* models for osteoblast differentiation which show maximal levels of osteocalcin in mineralized nodules (reviewed in Nijweide *et al.* [71]). In bone [72, 73] and matrix, *in vitro* [74, 75] apoptosis of osteoblasts and osteocytes has been reported. *In vitro*, we observe apoptosis of cells associated with the mineralized nodule [75], a finding which may be analogous to *in vivo* bone formation, where osteoblasts at bone forming surfaces may not all mature to an osteocyte [76]. The increase in collagenase detected in cells at the mineralization stage *in vitro* may reflect the reorganization of the extracellular matrix necessary for maturation of osteoblasts to osteocytes. Alternatively, *in vitro*, osteocytes may lack requisite factors for survival, as observed *in vivo* [77].

The influence of the mineralized extracellular matrix in modifying the phenotype of the cell, with respect to the induction of genes that have functional consequences, is illustrated by hypertrophic chondrocytes and cells associated with pathological calcifications. Hypertrophic chondrocytes have unique properties defined morphologically, functionally, and by the expression of proteins restricted to this cell, for example by the type X collagen molecule. Hypertrophic chondrocytes have a limited life span, yet there is evidence that a subset of these cells produce products characteristic of osteoblasts, such as osteocalcin [78, 79]. Thus, the mineralized calcified cartilage matrix may mediate a "transdifferentiation" of some hypertrophic chondrocytes to become osteoblasts [79–82]. This may be necessitated by the requirements for tissue organization where the mineralized matrix at the growth plate eventually recruits the cells which produce the cortical and trabecular bone to accommodate lengthening of the bone during growth. Other examples of transition of a nonosseous cell to an osteoblast-like cell are pericytes, which can be directed to osteoblast differentiation [83, 84], and cells associated with calcifying vascular tissues [83, 85] that express bone-related proteins. The sequence of events is not clear, although one might presume that the initial calcified plaque may provide similar signals to those produced by a mineralized bone extracellular matrix (ECM). A mineralized ECM may transduce signals to the local cell resulting in induction of bone-related proteins that function in regulating (to inhibit or control) mineral deposition. One could then propose a cascade of events which eventually results in a cell with some osteoblastic properties. The ability of smooth muscle cells to be induced to produce a mineralizing matrix (*in vitro*) and express bone-related genes supports this concept [85].

V. THE FUNCTIONAL PROPERTIES AND REGULATED ACTIVITY OF BONE CELLS EVOLVE DURING PROGRESSION ALONG THE OSTEOBLAST LINEAGE

Osteoblasts on active bone-forming surfaces produce bone matrix, contributing to expansion of bone volume by laying down osteoid and secreting factors that facilitate mineral deposition (Table I). The insulin-like growth factors (IGFs) are key regulators of osteoblast anabolic activities [86]. IGF-1 and IGF-2, which are synthesized by osteoblasts [87, 88], directly increase type I collagen synthesis and complementarily decrease the activity of collagenase 3 or MMP-13 enzyme, reflecting the role of IGFs in maintenance of the bone matrix. Anabolic effects of IGF-1 and IGF-2 in bone remodeling are further underscored by regulation of these proteins by growth factors (reviewed in Delany [89]). Notably, parathyroid hormone stimulates IGF-1 synthesis, whereas glucocorticoids inhibit skeletal IGF-1 expression [90, 91]. An equally important function of osteoblasts and the preosteoblasts which lie in close proximity is their response to endocrine factors and the production of paracrine and autocrine factors for the recruitment of osteoprogenitors, the growth of preosteoblasts, and the regulation of osteoclastic resorption of the mineralized bone matrix. Osteoblasts and osteocytes have receptors for cytokines [92, 93], parathyroid hormone, $1,25(OH)_2D_3$ [69, 94], and estrogen [95], which are key regulators of bone turnover. These features provide mechanisms for mediating the coupling of osteoblast and osteoclast activities (Fig. 3 and see Section VII).

On quiescent bone surfaces, the osteoblast develops into a flattened bone-lining cell of a single layer forming the endosteum against the marrow and underlying the periosteum directly on the mineralized surfaces. The lining cell layer protects the bone from the extracellular fluid space. These osteoblasts are in direct communication with the osteocytes within the mineralized matrix through cellular processes that lie within the canaliculi. Thus, the osteocytes and surface lining cells form a continuum, or syncytium, by connection of their cell processes through gap junctions.

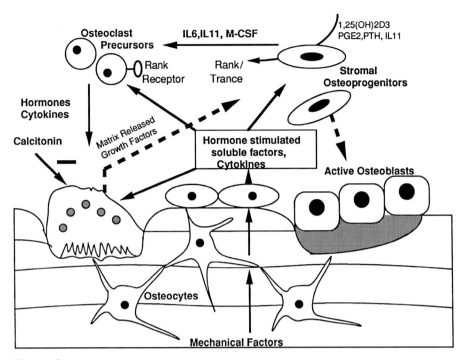

FIGURE 3   Interactions among the cell populations of bone. The figure summarizes regulatory signaling pathways between cells of the osteoblast and osteoclast lineage that are coupled for the regulation of bone turnover. Osteoclast differentiation is influenced by cytokines produced by osteoblasts and osteoprogenitor cells. Interaction between the RANK receptor on mononuclear pre-osteoclasts and the RANK ligand (TRANCE) on the stromal osteoblastic cell facilitates differentiation to the multinucleated osteoclasts. This coupling is influenced by the indicated hormones and cytokines. Physical forces stimulate osteocyte signalling pathways to surface osteoblasts. In response to calciotrophic hormones and mechanical stimuli, osteoblasts secrete cytokines and soluble factors which regulate growth and differentiation of osteoclast and osteoblast progenitors, as well as activities of the differentiated cells. Resorption of the bone matrix by osteoclasts releases active growth factors that stimulate proliferation and differentiation of stromal/mesenchymal cells to osteoblasts.

Osteoblasts and osteocytes are metabolically and electrically coupled through different gap junction proteins called connexins [96–98]. Rapid fluxes of bone calcium across these junctions are thought to facilitate transmission of information between osteoblasts on the bone surface and osteocytes within the structure of bone itself [99]. This structural organization and the direct contact of active osteoblast or surface lining cells with the osteocytes is consistent with the concept that bone cells, responding to varying physiological signals, can communicate their responses. Osteoblasts receive the majority of systemic and local signals and can transmit these to osteocytes. Reciprocally, mechanical forces on the bone produce stress-generated signals that are perceived by osteocytes, which then transmit the regulatory information to surface osteoblasts. Stress-generated electric potentials experienced by bone are either produced by strain in the organic components (piezo electric potential) or result from electrolyte fluid flow produced by deformation of the bone (streaming potential) ([100], and reviewed by Einhorn [101]). Thus, the ability of bone to act as a tissue responding to physiological homeostatic demands and to function as a structural connective tissue organ to meet physical demands depends on communication among its resident cells.

The ability to carry out studies in bone tissue and isolated cells following applied stress has advanced our understanding of osteocyte functions and responses. Osteocytes produce IGF-1 and release prostaglandins in response to stress [102]. Direct evidence that osteocytes sense mechanical loading [103] has been demonstrated by rapid changes in metabolic activity by ^{3}H-uridine uptake [104], increased glucose-6-phosphate dehydrogenase activity [105], and increased IGF-1 expression [106]. Signals induced by fluid flow that have been reported include prostaglandin PGE-2, cAMP, and nitrous oxide [107, 108]. In addition, extracellular matrix receptors, such as integrins and CD44 receptors, are also thought to mediate cellular sensing of mechanical loads [109]. The disruption of cell matrix interactions by loading could induce a mechanical twisting of the integrins. Integrins are tightly coupled to the cytoskeleton [110], and together the integrin–cytoskeleton complex facilitates the transduction of mechanical signals that may ultimately lead to modifications in gene expression.

VI. MOLECULAR MECHANISMS MEDIATING EXPRESSION OF THE OSTEOBLAST PHENOTYPE

The progression of osteoblast differentiation requires the sequential activation and suppression of genes that encode phenotypic and regulatory proteins. In addition to signaling molecules like BMPs and TGFβs that indirectly result in a cascade of gene expression, regulatory factors that directly engage in protein–DNA as well as protein–protein interactions are important [55]. Several classes of transcription factors have been implicated in key roles during the commitment and progressive differentiation of osteoblasts through specific stages of maturation. These include, for example, members of the protooncogene family, the helix-loop-helix (HLH) proteins (Twist, Id, Scleraxis), leucine zipper proteins (hXBP-1), zinc finger proteins (zif268), homeodomain proteins (Msx-2, Dlx-5), steroid receptors, and *runt* domain transcription factors (Cbfa/AML/PEBP2α). Modifications in the representation and activities of family members of these classes of transcription factors during osteoblast differentiation reflect linkage to transcriptional control of bone phenotype development. Id (inhibitor of differentiation), twist, and scleraxis are expressed in mesoderm of the developing embryo [111, 112]. Scleraxis is expressed in cells that form the skeleton and is not detected at the onset of ossification [112]. Several *in vitro* studies have established expression of these factors during osteoblast differentiation [113]. Id and Twist expression must be downregulated for osteoblast differentiation to proceed [114]; overexpression of these factors inhibits osteogenesis *in vitro* [115].

Msx-2 and Dlx-5 are members of the homeodomain gene family of transcription factors [116]. Both factors are expressed in mesenchymal cells at sites that will undergo skeletogenesis [117–119]. Their importance for normal bone formation is realized by skeletal abnormalities that result from mutations or misexpression of these factors [120, 121]. During osteoblast differentiation *in vitro*, Msx-2 is expressed maximally in the preosteoblast and is subsequently downregulated [122]. In a reciprocal fashion, Dlx-5 appears in the postproliferative osteoblast and increases during mineralization [123]. It appears that there is selectivity for expression of homeodomain factors as well as developmental variations in activities during osteoblast differentiation. These activities may in part reflect the sequence content of homedomain responsive promoter elements in genes that are developmentally expressed in osteoblasts [122–126]. Protein–protein interactions may also be determinants for developmental activities of these factors, as demonstrated by Zhang *et al.* [127].

The fos (c-fos, fra1, fra2) and jun (c-jun, jun-D, jun-B) oncogene-encoded families of transcription factors form homo- or heterodimeric complexes that regulate gene expression at AP-1 motifs. These factors exhibit developmental stage-specific expression and activities during osteoblast differentiation *in vivo* [128] and *in vitro* [129]. Studies of c-fos expression in transgenic mouse models reveal the importance of c-fos in establishing the osteoblast phenotype [130]. *In vivo* immunohistochemical staining revealed that c-fos was expressed in osteoprogenitor cells and in the perichondrium and periosteal tissues, but not in mature osteoblasts [128]. During osteoblast differentiation *in vitro*, we observed c-fos and jun expression maximally in proliferating preosteoblasts. However, retention and upregulation of fra2 and jun-D protein levels and mRNA expression was observed postproliferatively in differentiated osteoblasts [131]. Confirmation of the functional activities of these factors in regulating progressive maturation of the osteoblast phenotype has been demonstrated by several experimental approaches including specific repressor and enhancer activities of c-fos/c-jun and fra2/jun-D, respectively, on the osteocalcin promoter, as well as inhibition of osteoblast differentiation resulting from antisense inhibition of fra2 expression [131].

The *runt* homology domain-related core binding factors (CBFα) have been shown to play key roles in regulating bone-specific expression of the osteocalcin gene [132, 133]. In humans, these factors were also designated as AML because they are encoded by gene loci that are rearranfed in acute myelogenous leukemia (AML) [134]. The family of Cbf/AML transcription factors support the differentiation of both hematopoietic cells and osteoprogenitor cells. There are three related genes that each encode numerous splice variants having different functional activities [134–137]. Cbfa2 (AML-1B/PEBP2αB) is critical for T- and B-cell differentiation, Cbfa3 (AML-2/PEBP2αC) exhibits more restricted expression, and Cbfa1 (AML-3/PEBP2αA) is specifically required for bone formation, as demonstrated by the inhibition of bone tissue formation in the Cbfa1 null mutation mouse model [138, 139]. Although the skeleton forms through the chondrogenic stage, mineralization is blocked. The transient expression of Cbfa1 in early embryogenesis [138, 139], followed by an upregulation in late stages of bone development [140, 141], suggests that the factor may be important in early specification of the phenotype but may play a sustained role in the final stages of osteoblast differentiation. Some studies suggest that the Cbfa factors may be necessary, but not sufficient, for induction of osteogenesis. Preliminary findings [142] show that both TGFβ and BMP-2 induce Cbfa1 expression in the myogenic C2C12 line, but only BMP-2 transdifferentiates the cells to osteoblasts. We do not yet understand if Cbfa1 can provide to a cell the cascade of signals induced by the bone morphogenic proteins that leads both to commitment and to osteogenic differentiation, which is ultimately defined by extracellular matrix mineralization. In addition, the specific isoform of Cbfa1 necessary for commitment to osteoblast differentiation remains to be established.

The isoforms arise from alternative usage of two promoters and multiple ATGs, resulting in proteins with different N-terminal sequences [135, 136, 141]. Because all functionally active Cbfa/AML factors can transactivate the osteocalcin gene equally well in transient transfection assays and in nonosseous cells [133, 140], the biological significance and activities of the osteoblast-represented Cbfa1 splice variants must be further clarified [143, 144]. High levels of expression of one Cbfa1 RNA splice variant (til-1 isoform) was reported in osteosarcoma cells [135] and in osteoblasts (unpublished observations of this laboratory; [144]). It was also reported that a unique N-terminal extension, upstream of the til-1 isoform, encoded a putative bone-specific protein, Osf2 [141]. However, a high titer antibody directed against the initial 22 amino acids of Osf2 [144] did not recognize the Cbfa-containing osteoblast-specific DNA binding complex in gel shift immunoassays. In contrast, using an antibody recognizing the C terminus of Cbfa1 [136, 145], protein is detected by Western blot analysis, and osteoblast-specific binding activity is completely supershifted. These findings indicate that proteins translated from downstream ATGs [135, 136] are expressed at high levels in osteoblasts and that the putative Osf2 protein is not a major translation product of Cbfa1 mRNAs.

Important concepts are emerging regarding the transcriptional control of osteoblast phenotype development. First, factors that have roles in specifying spatial differentiation and pattern formation during embryogenesis are reexpressed at selective stages of osteoblast maturation in the postnatal animal. Their target genes are phenotypic markers of the mature osteoblast, such as osteocalcin. Because bone remodels, there is a continuing requirement to reestablish and sustain a complex tissue organization. Second, it is apparent that expression of many transcription factors is requisite in the undifferentiated mesenchymal cell or early osteoprogenitor; however, downregulation of the factor (e.g., Msx-2) is required for further maturation of the osteoblast. This observation suggests that transient expression of other factors (e.g., Cbfa1) in the early stages of development of the phenotype dictates the final commitment of a progenitor to the osteoblast lineage. Last, related family members of specific classes of proteins may be expressed reciprocally during osteoblast differentiation to ensure maintenance of the osteoblast phenotype. Alternatively, their activities may be regulated through interactions with a partner protein. A typical molecular mechanism may involve a change in heterodimerization proteins to form a transactivating complex rather than one that suppresses transcription of the gene at specific stages of osteoblast maturation. Research results suggest that partner proteins acetylate or deacetylate histones to modify chromatin organization. A basis is thereby provided for controlling accessibility of promoter elements to cognate transcription factors and supporting integration of activities at independent promoter domains. The osteocalcin gene serves as a prime example for these types of mechanisms; notably, the c-fos and c-jun heterodimers downregulate osteocalcin expression in proliferating osteoblasts through their interaction at AP-1 sites and in differentiated osteoblasts, the higher levels of fra2 and jun-D mediate enhancement of osteocalcin gene expression. The Cbfa1–Cbfβ heterodimer complex transactivates the osteocalcin gene [132]; in contrast, Cbfa1 interaction with Groucho proteins [146] leads to suppression of osteocalcin promoter activity [147]. The repertoire of transcription factors that control either bone development or the expression of bone phenotypic genes is expanding. Screens such as differential display, expression cloning, and two hybrid assays are providing additional regulators of osteoblast differentiation.

VII. THE OSTEOCLAST: A FUNCTIONALLY UNIQUE CELL FOR PHYSIOLOGICALLY REGULATED RESORPTION OF BONE MINERAL

The osteoclast is a multinucleated cell; its ability to degrade mineralized tissues depends on cellular attachment to the bone substratum. Osteoclasts are large cells (~100 μm) and appear in histologic sections of bone generally in resorption pits called Howships lacunae. Nuclei numbers are variable and in normal human osteoclasts 4–10 can be seen. Nuclei numbers appear to reflect osteoclast activity; as many as 20–50 nuclei can be found in Paget's disease [148]. It remains to be determined if specific nuclei in osteoclasts express subsets of housekeeping or phenotypic genes or whether all are equivalently transcriptionally active.

The highly specialized morphological features of the osteoclast are recognized only when the osteoclast is activated, a process which requires attachment to the mineralized bone surface. Characteristic features that are highly correlated to resorbing activity are: (1) the extent of convolution of the plasma membrane at the apical surface (on the bone) and projections of the basal lateral membrane; (2) the distinct organization of the cytoskeleton; and (3) polarization of the osteoclast nuclei at the basolateral surface. Osteoclast attachment is mediated by the classical integrin receptors, the vitronectin receptor, $\alpha_V\beta3$ (which interacts with RGD-containing extracellular proteins expressed by osteoblasts [149–152], such as osteopontin, fibronectin, or bone sialoprotein), and the collagen receptor $\alpha2\beta1$ [151]. Disruption of integrin-mediated adhesion results in inhibition of bone resorption [153, 154]. Interaction of the attached osteoclast to integrin receptors results in cytoskeletal changes [155] leading to cell spreading and polarization of the nuclei in the activated osteoclast as the sealing zone forms, separating the apical and basal lateral membranes. The podosome, or focal adhesion complex [156], is the specialized cell-extracellular matrix adhesion structure that allows the osteoclast to form a tight seal against the bone surface [157]. Podosomes completely surrounding the ruffled membrane are rich in F-actin filaments that are oriented perpendicular to the bone surface and form a ring. Focal adhesion kinase (P^{125FAK}) plays a central role in organizing the cytoskeleton at focal adhesions where signaling molecules such as phosphotidylinositol $(PI)^{-3}$ kinase can bind [158, 159]. Several signaling molecules have been identified in the polarization of osteoclasts, including rhoprotein (rho p21) [160], which regulates cytoskeletal organization [161], $P60^{c-src}$, and proteins c-Cbl [162] and $p130^{Cas}$ [163] that associate with oncogene products ($p60^{r-src}$) [92]. The actin rings can be used to differentiate resorbing osteoclasts and nonresorbing cells [155]. Calcitonin and other agents that inhibit osteoclast function also induce rapid disappearance of the actin rings [156, 164, 165].

Attachment of the osteoclast to bone also results in tubulin polymerization for the movement of intracellular vesicles along the microtubules to be targeted to ruffled membrane. Insertion of the proton pump-bearing vesicles into the apical membrane leads to formation of the ruffled membrane, the actual resorbing component facing the resorption lacunae [166, 167]. The tight seal of the surrounding plasma membrane to the bone surface is necessary to form a proton impermeable acidic environment in the lacunae [168] for degradation of mineralized bone. Acidification of the resorption lacunae is accomplished by the activities of carbonic anhydrase II and the proton pump enzyme (the vacuolar H^+-ATPase), both regarded as osteoclast associated [169, 170]. Various ion channels (chloride/carbonate and sodium/proton antiporters) maintain cellular electroneutrality (reviewed in Teitelbaum *et al.* [171]). Unlike foreign body giant cells, the osteoclast has numerous mitochondria for these energy requiring functions (reviewed in Athanasou [172]). Osteoclasts are rich in matrix-degrading enzymes [173–175], particularly cathespins [174] and collagenases [176–178]. Some enzymes provide histochemical markers commonly used to identify osteoclast activity, including the tartrate-resistant acid phosphatase isoenzyme [175] (although this is not an osteoclast-specific enzyme) and a related tartrate-resistant trinucleotide phosphatase; both are regarded as osteoclast associated. Transcytotic vesicles containing degraded bone proteins and inorganic matrix components transport products of bone resorption from the ruffled border to the basolateral surface. Resorption activity of the osteoclast can be rapidly terminated by the binding of calcitonin [179]. The calcitonin receptor of the osteoclast is also a characteristic marker [180].

A. Osteoclast Ontogeny

It is generally accepted that the multinucleated osteoclast forms only through the fusion of mononuclear precursors.

Proliferation of osteoclasts has never been documented. Numerous lines of evidence from naturally occurring animal models of osteopetroses [181], null mutation mouse models, bone marrow transplants or splenic parabiosis studies, and studies determining phenotypic markers of pre-osteoclast lineage cells, have firmly established the hematopoietic origin of the mononuclear precursors (reviewed in Walker [182], and [92, 93, 183]). Thus, the lineage of the osteoclast is distinct from that of the connective tissue cells of bone arising from the marrow stroma. Classical studies have included, for example, a healing fracture produced in an irradiated rat demonstrating that the cells which fused to form osteoclasts had to have been derived from the nonirradiated rat through the circulation [184]. In quail-chick chimera experiments, it was possible to determine the origin of different types of cells present in developing bone based on the morphologic difference between chick and quail nuclei [185, 186]. *In vitro* experiments using cocultures of hematopoietic cells and fetal bone ligaments or mouse osteoblastic cells and spleen cells provided evidence that osteoclast progenitors were present in the marrow [187].

Osteoclasts can be formed from isolated hematopoietic cells differentiated to the colony forming unit for granulocytes (CFU-GM). The CFU-GM is the earliest recognized precursor. Generation of multinucleated cells from isolated macrophage and monocyte cell populations provides substantial proof that the osteoclast is a member of the mononuclear phagocyte system ([92, 188–190], and reviewed in [92, 93, 172]). The process of osteoclast differentiation involves a number of steps associated with the proliferation and commitment of mononuclear osteoclast precursor cells into mature functional osteoclasts (Fig. 4). Expression of cell surface antigens has been used to identify osteoclast precursors and delineate their maturation to osteoclasts. Osteoclasts express a limited number of antigenic markers associated with macrophages (e.g., CD45 and CD51, and the α chain of the vitronectin receptor). However, other macrophage markers, such as CD-11a, CD-11b, CD-14, CD-18, HLA-TR, and receptors for FC and complement components are not expressed [191, 192]. Mononuclear cells containing nonspecific esterase macrophage markers appear at sites of bone resorption before mononuclear cells with nonspecific esterase and/or tartrate-resistant acid phosphatase (TRAP) [193]. At one stage of differentiation, osteoclast precursors expressed macrophage markers, nonspecific esterase, Mac-1 and Mac-2, as well as osteoclast markers, such as TRAP and calcitonin receptors. Unlike osteoclasts, monocytes, macrophages, mononuclear osteoclast precursors, and macrophage polykaryons do not respond to calcitonin or express calcitonin receptors. However, they can solubilize mineralized tissues, but this property is not associated with the ability to carry out lacuna bone resorption, as only the osteoclast can. Demonstration of expression of the calcitonin receptor is considered a reliable and highly specific marker of

REGULATION OF OSTEOCLAST DIFFERENTIATION

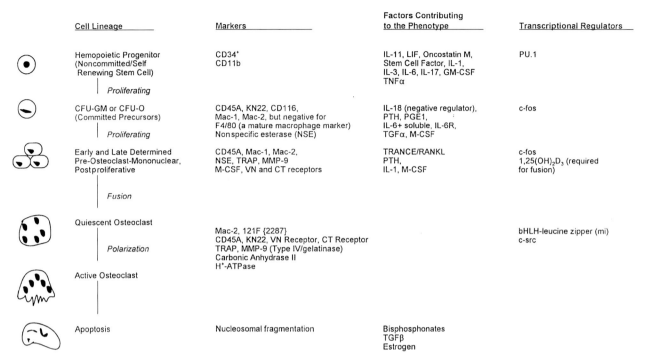

Cell Lineage	Markers	Factors Contributing to the Phenotype	Transcriptional Regulators
Hemopoietic Progenitor (Noncommitted/Self Renewing Stem Cell) *Proliferating*	CD34⁺ CD11b	IL-11, LIF, Oncostatin M, Stem Cell Factor, IL-1, IL-3, IL-6, IL-17, GM-CSF TNFα	PU.1
CFU-GM or CFU-O (Committed Precursors) *Proliferating*	CD45A, KN22, CD116, Mac-1, Mac-2, but negative for F4/80 (a mature macrophage marker) Nonspecific esterase (NSE)	IL-18 (negative regulator), PTH, PGE1, IL-6+ soluble, IL-6R, TGFα, M-CSF	c-fos
Early and Late Determined Pre-Osteoclast-Mononuclear, Postproliferative *Fusion*	CD45A, Mac-1, Mac-2, NSE, TRAP, MMP-9 M-CSF, VN and CT receptors	TRANCE/RANKL PTH, IL-1, M-CSF	c-fos 1,25(OH)₂D₃ (required for fusion)
Quiescent Osteoclast *Polarization* Active Osteoclast	Mac-2, 121F {2287} CD45A, KN22, VN Receptor, CT Receptor TRAP, MMP-9 (Type IV/gelatinase) Carbonic Anhydrase II H⁺-ATPase		bHLH-leucine zipper (mi) c-src
Apoptosis	Nucleosomal fragmentation	Bisphosphonates TGFβ Estrogen	

FIGURE 4   Phenotypic properties of cells of the osteoclast lineage. Column 1 illustrates the morphologic features of osteoblast lineage cells at each stage from stem cell to multinucleated active osteoclast, the final stage of differentiation. Column 2 describes either cell surface markers or proteins that are highly expressed at the indicated stage of maturation. Column 3 lists those factors which promote differentiation of the precursor cell populations. In column 4, those transcription factors that have been identified as key regulators of osteoclast differentiation are indicated.

a mammalian osteoclast, although this has been problematic for avian osteoclasts [194].

Questions that are currently being resolved relate to the properties of the mononuclear osteoclast precursor as an osteoclast-specific cell line formed at some point in time after formation of the colony forming unit for granulocytes and macrophages (CFU-GM, Fig. 4). Alternatively, when the peripheral blood monocytes leave the circulation to become macrophages, this cell would be induced to differentiate into a specialized mononuclear cell type competent for fusion to osteoclast (CFU-O), under the influence of local cellular and immuno factors present in the bone microenvironment.

B. Requirement of Osteoblast Lineage Cells for Osteoclast Differentiation from Hematopoietic Precursors: Role in Mediating Endocrine Responses and Production of Cytokines

The bone microenvironment appears to be essential for two components of osteoclastogenesis: (1) maturation and fusion of the mononuclear precursor to the multinucleated osteoclast and (2) activation and regulation of the activity of the functional osteoclast. The requirement for stromal os-

teoprogenitors or osteoblasts in mediating osteoclast differentiation is linked to the role of osteotrophic hormones and cytokines in regulating development of pre-osteoclasts and the multinucleated phenotype. $1\alpha,25(OH)_2D_3$ and parathyroid hormone (PTH) influence osteoclastogenesis at multiple stages of differentiation and activation [195, 196]. Receptors for these hormones are located preferentially in the osteoblastic lineage cells and these hormones modulate the synthesis of cytokines that have mitogenic effects on osteoclast progenitors.

Although the primary activity of these hormones in promoting osteoclastic resorption of bone is mediated through the osteoblast, there is growing evidence that these hormones may affect osteoclasts directly. For example, the C-terminal peptide of PTHrP can directly inhibit bone resorption of osteoclasts [197]. Sensitive methods of detection have also revealed that osteoclasts express PTH receptors [198–200]. It is well established that $1,\alpha25(OH)_2D_3$ induces differentiation of mouse myeloid leukemia cells into mature macrophages and promotes activation and fusion of the macrophages mediated by steroid hormone ([195], and references therein). Thus, vitamin D has direct effects on osteoclast progenitors. However, these cells can not form resorption pits on dentin slices. Only in the presence of osteoblastic cells [201–203] could the steroid promote differentiation of the macrophage lineage cells into osteoclast-like cells.

Osteoclasts undergo dramatic changes when exposed to PTH. The number of multinucleated cells increases proportionately to PTH concentration and the hormone stimulates ruffled membrane formation, a characteristic of active osteoclasts [204]. The majority of evidence supports an indirect activity of PTH, mediated through osteoblasts and marrow stromal cells, on osteoclastic bone resorption [205]. The studies of Uy *et al.* [196] suggest that PTH and PTHrP increase the number of committed osteoclast progenitors and multinucleated osteoclasts *in vivo*. *In vitro* PTH does not influence isolated osteoclasts to resorb bone [206]. That PTH induces c-fos expression in osteoclasts [207] and that c-fos promotes precursor differentiation along the osteoclast pathway [208], provides further support for the role of PTH in the early stages of osteoclast recruitment. Although the effects of PTH are dramatic, the mechanisms are still unclear. Osteoclast cell formation is mediated by cAMP signalling induced by parathyroid hormone (PTH) and PTHrP [209].

Stromal osteoblastic cells are the major source of the colony stimulating factors (CSFs) and IL-6 family of cytokines which are also potent stimulators of bone resorption and participate in osteoclastogenesis at early and later stages. TNFα and IL-1, which are predominantly derived from monocytes, have mitogenic effects on the mononuclear osteoclast precursor. However, IL-1 and TNFα feed back on stromal cells to regulate their production of M-CSF (CSF-1) and IL-11 (reviewed in Teitelbaum [171]), which are key regulators of osteoclast formation. IL-11 also appears to function at early stages of osteoclastogenesis when hematopoietic cells are cocultured with osteoblastic cells [210–212]. IL-18, initially described as a T-cell cytokine that promotes interferon production by lymphocytes, was shown to be an important negative regulator of osteoclast formation expressed in osteoblasts [213, 214].

PTH and vitamin D stimulate osteoblast production of IL-6, as do IL-1, TNFα, and TGFβ [215, 216]. The mechanisms by which IL-6 affects the generation of early osteoclast precursors from CFU-GM colonies has been documented. Membrane-bound IL-6 receptors on osteoblasts are essential for IL-6-mediated osteoclast formation [215, 217]. IL-6 and related cytokines that include (but are not limited to) IL-11, oncostatin M, and leukemia inhibitory factors, which can enhance osteoclast differentiation, exert their selective effects through the same signal transduction pathway [92, 171]. Their cell surface receptor consists of two components, a specific ligand binding subunit and a second subunit (which can bind some ligands) that participates in the signaling cascade and is the transducing protein gp130 [211, 218]. The signal transduction cascade includes the nonreceptor tyrosine kinases known as Janus kinases (JAKs), which in turn phosphorylate components of the receptor kinases, and a series of cytoplasmic proteins designated signal transducers and activators of transcription (STATs). Notably, 1,25(OH)2D3 upregulates, whereas estrogen downregulates, expression of the IL-6 receptor and gp130 [219], thereby modulating stromal cell responsiveness to IL-6. Interestingly, IL-6 transgenic mice do not show increased bone resorption [220] and the gp130 -/- null mouse has a normal marrow cavity and normal osteoclast numbers [221]. Thus, it is likely that redundant proteins may mediate the signalling of these important cytokines.

Several lines of evidence support the essential role of M-CSF (also designated CSF-1) in mediating the proliferation and differentiation of osteoclast precursors [222, 223]. For example, neutralizing antibodies against M-CSF can completely inhibit multinucleated cell formation in mouse bone marrow cultures. Recombinant M-CSF injections cure osteopetrosis in the OP/OP mouse which is characterized by production of a nonfunctional M-CSF [223, 224]. Coculture experiments using either spleen cells or osteoblastic cells from OP/OP and normal mice demonstrated that the osteoclast deficiency is due to a defect in the osteoblast cells and not in the hematopoietic precursors, but M-CSF plays a critical role in osteoclast phenotype development [225]. Because the M-CSF mutation in the OP/OP mouse targets stromal cells and osteoblasts that normally express the cytokine, it is postulated that this factor initiates signaling cascades that affect osteoclast progenitors prior to macrophage differentiation, but later than early hematopoietic stem cell involvement [171]. Secretion of M-CSF from stromal or osteoblastic cells is stimulated by 1,25(OH)$_2$D$_3$ and parathyroid hormone, as well as by the cytokines IL-1 and TNFα [93, 183, 195].

Two discoveries provide insight into mechanisms for the essential role of osteoblasts in mediating osteoclastogenesis. Osteoprotegerin (OPG), also designated osteoclastogenesis inhibitory factor, is a protein with strong homology to known TNF receptors. OPG is expressed in several tissues including bone, cartilage, kidney, blood vessels, and osteoblast lineage cells [226]. Overexpression of OPG in transgenic mice resulted in severe osteopetrosis [226]. The presence of F4/80-positive osteoclast precursors in these mice suggests that OPG inhibits terminal stages of osteoclast differentiation. In search of the specific ligand for OPG, several groups cloned a novel member of the transmembrane TNF ligand family [227, 228]. This OPG ligand is identical to a TNF cytokine family member designated TRANCE (TNF-related activation induced cytokine) [229], a cytokine that regulates T-cell dependent immune responses. Also identical to the TRANCE/OPG-ligand is the ligand for RANK (receptor activation of NF-$\kappa\beta$), a TNF receptor family member cloned from T cells [230]. Yasuda and co-workers [231] directly demonstrated that TRANCE produced by osteoblasts blocks

OPG inhibition of osteoclast formation by binding OPG. In other cell types (dendritic cells) [230], TRANCE has been shown to inhibit apoptosis [229] and may also function in bone to promote the survival of osteoclasts. Importantly, the TRANCE/OPG ligand was demonstrated to have competency for inducing osteoclast formation from hematopoietic cells in the absence of stromal cells. Furthermore, expression of the OPG ligand in osteoblasts is upregulated by $1,25(OH)_3D_3$, IL-11, and PGE-2, all stimulators of bone resorption [231]. In summary, the TRANCE/RANK/OPG ligand, together with M-CSF, may represent factors required for coupling stromal/osteoblastic cells to the formation of osteoclasts.

VIII. MOLECULAR MECHANISMS MEDIATING OSTEOCLAST DIFFERENTIATION

The fusion of circulating mononuclear precursors to the multinucleated osteoclasts is not only regulated by hormones and cytokine-induced signal transduction pathways, but also by transcriptional targets that control commitment, proliferation, and differentiation of the mononuclear precursors. Our understanding of the transcriptional mediators that drive osteoclast differentiation and regulate their activation derives largely from characterization of murine animal models that manifest the osteopetrotic disorders of bone resorption (reviewed by Popoff and Marks [181]).

The first transcription factor implicated in osteoclastogenesis, c-fos, was revealed by a marked osteopetrosis disorder in the null mutant mouse [232]. Bone sections revealed an abundance of macrophages but an absence of osteoclasts, suggesting that c-fos promotes proliferation and differentiation of a specific mononuclear precursor committed to the osteoclast pathway [208, 233]. Mice deficient in both subunits (p50 and p52) of Nf-kB, a transcription factor regulating expression of GM-CSF, TNFa, Il-1, and Il-6, results in osteopetrosis [234]. Transgenic mice in which the myeloid and B lymphoid transcription factor PU.1 is ablated also fail to generate macrophages or osteoclasts and develop osteopetrosis [235]. The mutant mice are successfully rescued by marrow transplantation, supporting the concept of the common lineage of osteoclasts and macrophages and that the PU.1 factor is involved in establishing one of the early myeloid cells. Additionally, the macrophage transcription factor PU.1 directs expression of M-CSF [236]. Thus, a temporal sequence of the involvement of these two factors in ontogeny of the osteoclast is likely, as proposed by Teitelbaum *et al.* [183].

Several animal models have revealed defects at later stages of maturation in the multinucleated osteoclast, expanding our knowledge of the repertoire of mechanisms required for re-sorbing activity of the cell. The proto oncogene c-src, having a nonreceptor tyrosinase kinase enzyme activity, has a key role in activating quiescent osteoclasts to become resorbing cells. The c-src-/- mutants have many multinucleated cells present in bone with some properties of the osteoclast, but they lack function because they are incapable of forming a ruffled border [237]. The basis for this defect is that c-src associates with tubulin when osteoclasts adhere to bone [238]. Thus, c-src represents an important signalling pathway for formation of the ruffled membrane and polarization of the osteoclast [239]. MI/MI mice develop osteopetrosis, although many TRAP-positive osteoclasts are present in trabecular bones of these mice. However, the osteoclasts fail to form ruffled borders, suggesting that the MI gene product, which encodes a member of the basic helix-loop-helix leucine zipper protein family, also appears to be involved at the late stage of differentiation in osteoclast function [240].

IX. PERSPECTIVES

Our understanding of the biological properties of bone cells is rapidly evolving. Complex regulatory mechanisms that are operative in establishment of skeletal stem cell populations as well as in commitment to the osteoblast or osteoclast phenotypes are being clarified. Although systemic and local factors that promote and regulate differentiation of lineage-specific phenotypes are being identified, a goal for the future is a better understanding of the mechanisms that facilitate interactions between subpopulations of osteoblasts and osteoclasts to support maintenance of bone mass and mineral homeostasis. Pursuing the identity of cell type-specific proteins and transcription factors that regulate their expression has been instructive. As the signalling pathways that mediate expression of genes controlling proliferation and differentiation of bone cells are further clarified, a new generation of options for diagnosis and treatment of skeletal disorders will emerge.

References

1. Suwanwalaikorn, S., van Auken, M., Kang, M. I., Alex, S., Braverman, L. E., and Baran, D. T. (1997). Site selectivity of osteoblast gene expression response to thyroid hormone localized by in situ hybridization. *Am. J. Physiol.* **272**, E212–217.

2. Kasperk, C., Wergedal, J., Strong, D., Farley, J., Wangerin, K., Gropp, H., Ziegler, R., and Baylink, D. J. (1995). Human bone cell phenotypes differ depending on their skeletal site of origin. *J. Clin. Endocrinol. Metab.* **80**, 2511–2517.

3. Dunbar, C. E., Tisdale, J., Yu, J. M., Soma, T., Zujewski, J., Bodine, D., Sellers, S., Cowan, K., Donahue, R., and Emmons, R. (1997). Transduction of hematopoietic stem cells in humans and in nonhuman primates. *Stem Cells* **15**, 135–139.

4. Bruder, S. P., Fink, D. J., and Caplan, A. I. (1994). Mesenchymal stem cells in bone development, bone repair, and skeletal regeneration therapy. *J. Cell. Biochem.* **56**, 283–294.

5. Bruder, S. P., Ricalton, N. S., Boynton, R. E., Connolly, T. J., Jaiswal, N., Zaia, J., and Barry, F. P. (1998). Mesenchymal stem cell surface antigen SB-10 corresponds to activated leukocyte cell adhesion molecule and is involved in osteogenic differentiation. *J. Bone Miner. Res.* **13**, 655–663.

6. Gronthos, S., Graves, S. E., Ohta, S., and Simmons, P. J. (1994). The STRO-1+ fraction of adult human bone marrow contains the osteogenic precursors. *Blood* **84**, 4164–4173.

7. Gronthos, S., Stewart, K., Graves, S. E., Hay, S., and Simmons, P. J. (1997). Integrin expression and function on human osteoblast-like cells. *J. Bone Miner. Res.* **12**, 1189–1197.

8. Haynesworth, S. E., Baber, M. A., and Caplan, A. I. (1992). Cell surface antigens on human marrow-derived mesenchymal cells are detected by monoclonal antibodies. *Bone* **13**, 69–80.

9. Wetterwald, A., Hoffstetter, W., Cecchini, M. G., Lanske, B., Wagner, C., Fleisch, H., and Atkinson, M. (1996). Characterization and cloning of the E11 antigen, a marker expressed by rat osteoblasts and osteocytes. *Bone* **18**, 125–132.

10. Joyner, C. J., Bennett, A., and Triffitt, J. T. (1997). Identification and enrichment of human osteoprogenitor cells by using differentiation stage-specific monoclonal antibodies. *Bone* **21**, 1–6.

11. Nijweide, P. J., and Mulder, R. J. (1986). Identification of osteocytes in osteoblast-like cell cultures using a monoclonal antibody specifically directed against osteocytes. *Histochemistry* **84**, 342–347.

12. Malaval, L., Modrowski, D., Gupta, A. K., and Aubin, J. E. (1994). Cellular expression of bone-related proteins during in vitro osteogenesis in rat bone marrow stromal cell cultures. *J. Cell. Physiol.* **158**, 555–572.

13. Hughes, D. E., Salter, D. M., and Simpson, R. (1994). CD44 expression in human bone: A novel marker of osteocytic differentiation. *J. Bone Miner. Res.* **9**, 39–44.

14. Jamal, H. H., and Aubin, J. E. (1996). CD44 expression in fetal rat bone: *In vivo* and *in vitro* analysis. *Exp. Cell Res.* **223**, 467–477.

15. Turksen, K., and Aubin, J. E. (1991). Positive and negative immunoselection for enrichment of two classes of osteoprogenitor cells. *J. Cell Biol.* **114**, 373–384.

16. Friedenstein, A. J., Chailakhjan, R. K., and Lalykina, K. S. (1970). The development of fibroblast colonies in monolayer cultures of guinea-pig bone marrow and spleen cells. *Cell Tissue Kinet.* **3**, 393–403.

17. Friedenstein, A. J., Latzinik, N. V., Gorskaya, Yu. F., Luria, E. A., and Moskvina, I. L. (1992). Bone marrow stromal colony formation requires stimulation by haemopoietic cells. *Bone Miner.* **18**, 199–213.

18. Friedenstein, A. J., Chailakhyan, R. K., and Gerasimov, U. V. (1987). Bone marrow osteogenic stem cells: In vitro cultivation and transplantation in diffusion chambers. *Cell Tissue Kinet.* **20**, 263–272.

19. Cornish, J., Callon, K., King, A., Edgar, S., and Reid, I. R. (1993). The effect of leukemia inhibitory factor on bone in vivo. *Endocrinology* **132**, 1359–1366.

20. Owen, M. E., Cave, J., and Joyner, C. J. (1987). Clonal analysis in vitro of osteogenic differentiation of marrow CFU-F. *J. Cell. Sci.* **87**, 731–738.

21. Nakamura, T., Hanada, K., Tamura, M., Shibanushi, T., Nigi, H., Tagawa, M., Fukumoto, S., and Matsumoto, T. (1995). Stimulation of endosteal bone formation by systemic injections of recombinant basic fibroblast growth factor in rats. *Endocrinology* **136**, 1276–1284.

22. Noda, M., and Camilliere, J. J. (1989). In vivo stimulation of bone formation by transforming growth factor-beta. *Endocrinology* **124**, 2991–2994.

23. Hock, J. M., Canalis, E., and Centrella, M. (1990). Transforming growth factor-beta stimulates bone matrix apposition and bone cell replication in cultured fetal rat calvariae. *Endocrinology* **126**, 421–426.

24. Hauschka, P. V., Mavrakos, A. E., Iafrati, M. D., Doleman, S. E., and Klagsbrun, M. (1986). Growth factors in bone matrix. *J. Biol. Chem.* **261**, 12665–12674.

25. Long, M. W., Robinson, J. A., Ashcraft, E. A., and Mann, K. G. (1995). Regulation of human bone marrow-derived osteoprogenitor cells by osteogenic growth factors. *Ibid.* **96** (5), 2541. *J. Clin. Invest.* **95**, 881–887; erratum: (1995).

26. Onishi, T., Ishidou, Y., Nagamine, T., Yone, K., Imamura, T., Kato, M., Sampath, T. K., Dijke, P. T., and Sakou, T. (1998). Distinct and overlapping patterns of localization of bone morphogenetic protein (BMP) family members and a BMP type II receptor during fracture healing in rats. *Bone* **22**, 605–612.

27. Wang, E. A., Rosen, V., D'Alessandro, J. S., Bauduy, M., Cordes, P., Harada, T., Israel, D. I., Hewick, R. M., Kerns, K. M., LaPan, P., Luxenberg, D. P., McQuaid, D., Moutsatsos, I. K., Nove, J., and Wozney, J. M. (1990). Recombinant human bone morphogenetic protein induces bone formation. *Proc. Natl. Acad. Sci. U.S.A.* **87**, 2220–2224.

28. Sampath, T. K., Maliakal, J. C., Hauschka, P. V., Jones, W. K., Sasak, H., Tucker, R. F., White, K. H., Coughlin, J. E., Tucker, M. M., and Pang, R. H. (1992). Recombinant human osteogenic protein-1 (hOP-1) induces new bone formation in vivo with a specific activity comparable with natural bovine osteogenic protein and stimulates osteoblast proliferation and differentiation in vitro. *J. Biol. Chem.* **267**, 20352–20362.

29. Rosen, V., and Thies, R. S. (1992). The BMP proteins in bone formation and repair. *Trends Genet.* **8**, 97–102.

30. Asahina, I., Sampath, T. K., Nishimura, I., and Hauschka, P. V. (1993). Human osteogenic protein-1 induces both chondroblastic and osteoblastic differentiation of osteoprogenitor cells derived from newborn rat calvaria. *J. Cell Biol.* **123**, 921–933.

31. Thies, R. S., Bauduy, M., Ashton, B. A., Kurtzberg, L., Wozney, J. M., and Rosen, V. (1992). Recombinant human bone morphogenetic protein-2 induces osteoblastic differentiation in W-20–17 stromal cells. *Endocrinology* **130**, 1318–1324.

32. Wang, E. A., Israel, D. I., Kelly, S., and Luxenberg, D. P. (1993). Bone morphogenetic protein-2 causes commitment and differentiation in C3H10T1/2 and 3T3 cells. *Growth Factors* **9**, 57–71.

33. Katagiri, T., Yamaguchi, A., Komaki, M., Abe, E., Takahashi, N., Ikeda, T., Rosen, V., Wozney, J. M., Fujisawa-Sehara, A., and Suda, T. (1994). Bone morphogenetic protein-2 converts the differentiation pathway of C2C12 myoblasts into the osteoblast lineage. *J. Cell Biol.* **127**, 1755–1766.

34. Hock, J. M., Fonseca, J., Gunness-Hey, M., Kemp, B. E., and Martin, T. J. (1989). Comparison of the anabolic effects of synthetic parathyroid hormone-related protein (PTHrP) 1-34 and PTH 1-34 on bone in rats. *Endocrinology* **125**, 2022–2027.

35. Moseley, J. M., and Martin, T. J. (1996). Parathyroid hormone-related protein: Physiological actions. *In* "Principles of Bone Biology" (J. P. Bilezikian, L. G. Raisz, and G. A. Rodan, eds.), pp. 363–376. Academic Press, San Diego, CA.

36. Erlebacher, A., Filvaroff, E. H., Gitelman, S. E., and Derynck, R. (1995). Toward a molecular understanding of skeletal development. *Cell* **80**, 371–378.

37. Karaplis, A. C., Luz, A., Glowacki, J., Bronson, R. T., Tybulewicz, V. L., Kronenberg, H. M., and Mulligan, R. C. (1994). Lethal skeletal dysplasia from targeted disruption of the parathyroid hormone-related peptide gene. *Genes Dev.* **8**, 277–289.

38. Lanske, B., Karaplis, A. C., Lee, K., Luz, A., Vortkamp, A., Pirro, A., Karperien, M., Defize, L. H. K., Ho, C., Mulligan, R. C., Abou-Samra, A. B., Juppner, H., Segré, G. V., and Kronenberg, H. M. (1996). PTH/PTHrP receptor in early development and Indian hedgehog-regulated bone growth. *Science* **273**, 663–666.

39. Muenke, M., Schell, U., Hehr, A., Robin, N. H., Losken, H. W., Schinzel, A., Pulleyn, L. J., Rutland, P., Reardon, W., and Malcolm, S. (1994). A common mutation in the fibroblast growth factor receptor 1 gene in Pfeiffer syndrome. *Nat. Genet.* **8**, 269–274.

40. Jabs, E. W., Li, X., Scott, A. F., Meyers, G., Chen, W., Eccles, M., Mao, J. I., Charnas, L. R., Jackson, C. E., and Jaye, M. (1994). Jackson-Weiss and Crouzon syndromes are allelic with mutations in fibroblast growth factor receptor 2. *Nat. Genet.* **8**, 275–279.

41. Shiang, R., Thompson, L. M., Zhu, Y. Z., Church, D. M., Fielder, T. J., Bocian, M., Winokur, S. T., and Wasmuth, J. J. (1994). Mutations in the transmembrane domain of FGFR3 cause the most common genetic form of dwarfism, achondroplasia. *Cell* **78**, 335–342.

42. Shalhoub, V., Aslam, F., Breen, E., Bortell, R., Stein, G. S., Stein, J. L., and Lian, J. B. (1998). Multiple levels of steroid hormone-dependent control of osteocalcin during osteoblast differentiation: Glucocorticoid regulation of basal and vitamin D stimulated gene expression. *J. Cell. Biochem.* **69**, 154–168.

43. Grzesik, W. J. and Robey, P. G. (1994). Bone matrix RGD glycoproteins: Immunolocalization and interaction with human primary osteoblastic bone cells in vitro. *J. Bone Miner. Res.* **9**, 487–496.

44. Majeska, R. J., Port, M., and Einhorn, T. A. (1993). Attachment to extracellular matrix molecules by cells differing in the expression of osteoblastic traits. *J. Bone Miner. Res.* **8**, 277–289.

45. Lynch, M. P., Stein, J. L., Stein, G. S., and Lian, J. B. (1995). The influence of type I collagen on the development and maintenance of the osteoblast phenotype in primary and passaged rat calvarial osteoblasts: Modification of expression of genes supporting cell growth, adhesion, and extracellular matrix mineralization. *Exp. Cell Res.* **216**, 35–45.

46. Vukicevic, S., Luyten, F. P., Kleinman, H. K., and Reddi, A. H. (1990). Differentiation of canalicular cell processes in bone cells by basement membrane matrix components: Regulation by discrete domains of laminin. *Cell* **63**, 437–445.

47. Andrianarivo, A. G., Robinson, J. A., Mann, K. G., and Tracy, R. P. (1992). Growth on type I collagen promotes expression of the osteoblastic phenotype in human osteosarcoma MG-63 cells. *J. Cell. Physiol.* **153**, 256–265.

48. Franceschi, R. T., and Iyer, B. S. (1992). Relationship between collagen synthesis and expression of the osteoblast phenotype in MC3T3-E1 cells. *J. Bone Miner. Res.* **7**, 235–246.

49. Gronowicz, G. A., and Derome, M. E. (1994). Synthetic peptide containing Arg-Gly-Asp inhibits bone formation and resorption in a mineralizing organ culture system of fetal rat parietal bones. *J. Bone Miner. Res.* **9**, 193–201.

50. Cheng, S. L., Lecanda, F., Davidson, M. K., Warlow, P. M., Zhang, S. F., Zhang, L., Suzuki, S., St. John, T., and Civitelli, R. (1998). Human osteoblasts express a repertoire of cadherins, which are critical for BMP-2-induced osteogenic differentiation. *J. Bone Miner. Res.* **13**, 633–644.

51. Lee, Y. S., and Chuong, C. M. (1992). Adhesion molecules in skeletogenesis: I. Transient expression of neural cell adhesion molecules (NCAM) in osteoblasts during endochondral and intramembranous ossification. *J. Bone Miner. Res.* **7**, 1435–1446.

52. Okazaki, M., Takeshita, S., Kawai, S., Kikuno, R., Tsujimura, A., Kudo, A., and Amann, E. (1994). Molecular cloning and characterization of OB-cadherin, a new member of cadherin family expressed in osteoblasts. *J. Biol. Chem.* **269**, 12092–12098.

53. Tanaka, Y., Morimoto, I., Nakano, Y., Okada, Y., Hirota, S., Nomura, S., Nakamura, T., and Eto, S. (1995). Osteoblasts are regulated by the cellular adhesion through ICAM-1 and VCAM-1. *J. Bone Miner. Res.* **10**, 1462–1469.

54. Nakamura, H., Kenmotsu, S., Sakai, H., and Ozawa, H. (1995). Localization of CD44, the hyaluronate receptor, on the plasma membrane of osteocytes and osteoclasts in rat tibiae. *Cell Tissue Res.* **280**, 225–233.

55. Stein, G. S., Lian, J. B., Stein, J. L., van Wijnen, A. J., and Montecino, M. (1996). Transcriptional control of osteoblast growth and differentiation. *Physiol. Rev.* **76**, 593–629.

56. Robey, P. G. (1996). Bone matrix proteoglycans and glycoproteins. *In* "Principles of Bone Biology" (J. P. Bilezikian, L. G. Raisz, and G. A. Rodan, eds.), pp. 155–165. Academic Press, San Diego, CA.

57. Stein, G. S., Lian, J. B., Stein, J. S., van Wijnen, A. J., Frenkel, B., and Montecino, M. (1996). Mechanisms regulating osteoblast proliferation and differentiation. *In* "Principles of Bone Biology" (J. P. Bilezikian, L. G. Raisz, and G. A. Rodan, eds.), pp. 69–86. Academic Press, San Diego, CA.

58. Liu, F., Malaval, L., Gupta, A. K., and Aubin, J. E. (1994). Simultaneous detection of multiple bone-related mRNAs and protein expression during osteoblast differentiation: Polymerase chain reaction and immunocytochemical studies at the single cell level. *Dev. Biol.* **166**, 220–234.

59. Pockwinse, S. M., Lawrence, J. B., Singer, R. H., Stein, J. L., Lian, J. B., and Stein, G. S. (1993). Gene expression at single cell resolution associated with development of the bone cell phenotype: Ultrastructural and in situ hybridization analysis. *Bone* **14**, 347–352.

60. Pockwinse, S. M., Stein, J. L., Lian, J. B., and Stein, G. S. (1995). Developmental stage-specific cellular responses to vitamin D and glucocorticoids during differentiation of the osteoblast phenotype: Interrelationship of morphology and gene expression by in situ hybridization. *Exp. Cell Res.* **216**, 244–260.

61. Pockwinse, S. M., Wilming, L. G., Conlon, D. M., Stein, G. S., and Lian, J. B. (1992). Expression of cell growth and bone specific genes at single cell resolution during development of bone tissue-like organization in primary osteoblast cultures. *J. Cell. Biochem.* **49**, 310–323.

62. Breen, E. C., Ignotz, R. A., McCabe, L., Stein, J. L., Stein, G. S., and Lian, J. B. (1994). TGF beta alters growth and differentiation related gene expression in proliferating osteoblasts in vitro, preventing development of the mature bone phenotype. *J. Cell. Physiol.* **160**, 323–335.

63. Tang, K.-T., Capparelli, C., Stein, J. L., Stein, G. S., Lian, J. B., Huber, A. C., Braverman, L. E., and DeVito, W. J. (1996). Acidic fibroblast growth factor inhibits osteoblast differentiation in vitro: Altered expression of collagenase, cell growth-related and mineralization-associated genes. *J. Cell. Biochem.* **61**, 152–166.

64. Debiais, F., Hott, M., Graulet, A. M., and Marie, P. J. (1998). The effects of fibroblast growth factor-2 on human neonatal calvaria osteoblastic cells are differentiation stage specific. *J. Bone Miner. Res.* **13**, 645–654.

65. Gerstenfeld, L. C., Zurakowski, D., Schaffer, J. L., Nichols, D. P., Toma, C. D., Broess, M., Bruder, S. P., and Caplan, A. I. (1996). Variable hormone responsiveness of osteoblast populations isolated at different stages of embryogenesis and its relationship to the osteogenic lineage. *Endocrinology* **137**, 3957–3968.

66. Owen, T. A., Aronow, M. S., Barone, L. M., Bettencourt, B., Stein, G. S., and Lian, J. B. (1991). Pleiotropic effects of vitamin D on osteoblast gene expression are related to the proliferative and differentiated state of the bone cell phenotype: Dependency upon basal levels of gene expression, duration of exposure, and bone matrix competency in normal rat osteoblast cultures. *Endocrinology* **128**, 1496–1504.

67. Bodine, P. V. N., Henderson, R. A., Green, J., Aronow, M., Owen, T., Stein, G. S., Lian, J. B., and Komm, B. S. (1998). Estrogen receptor-α is developmentally regulated during osteoblast differentiation and contributes to selective responsiveness of gene expression. *Endocrinology* **139**, 2048–2057.

68. Ishizuya, T., Yokose, S., Hori, M., Noda, T., Suda, T., Yoshiki, S., and Yamaguchi, A. (1997). Parathyroid hormone exerts disparate effects on osteoblast differentiation depending on exposure time in rat osteoblastic cells. *J. Clin. Invest.* **99**, 2961–2970.

69. van der Plas, A., Aarden, E. M., Feijen, J. H., de Boer, A. H., Wiltink, A., Alblas, M. J., de Leij, L., and Nijweide, P. J. (1994). Characteristics and properties of osteocytes in culture. *J. Bone Miner. Res.* **9**, 1697–1704.

70. Mikuni-Takagaki, Y., Kakai, Y., Satoyoshi, M., Kawano, E., Suzuki, Y., Kawase, T., and Saito, S. (1995). Matrix mineralization and the differentiation of osteocyte-like cells in culture. *J. Bone Miner. Res.* **10**, 231–242.

71. Nijweide, P. J., Burger, E. H., Klein-Nulend, J., and van der Plas, A. (1996). The osteocyte. *In* "Principles of Bone Biology" (J. P. Bilezikian, L. G. Raisz, and G. A. Rodan, eds.), pp. 115–126. Academic Press, San Diego, CA.

72. Hughes, D. E., and Boyce, B. F. (1997). Apoptosis in bone physiology and disease. *Mol. Pathol.* **50**, 132–137.

73. Noble, B. S., Stevens, H., Loveridge, N., and Reeve, J. (1997). Identification of apoptotic changes in osteocytes in normal and pathological human bone. *Bone* **20**, 273–282.

74. Jilka, R. L., Weinstein, R. S., Bellido, T., Parfitt, A. M., and Manolagas, S. C. (1998). Osteoblast programmed cell death (apoptosis): Modulation by growth factors and cytokines. *J. Bone Miner. Res.* **13**, 793–802.

75. Lynch, M. P., Capparelli, C., Stein, J. L., Lian, J. B., and Stein, G. S. (1997). Apoptosis during bone-like tissue development in vitro. *J. Cell. Biochem.* **68**, 31–49.

76. Parfitt, A. M., Villanueva, A. R., Foldes, J., and Rao, D. S. (1995). Relations between histologic indices of bone formation: Implications for the pathogenesis of spinal osteoporosis. *J. Bone Miner. Res.* **10**, 466–473.

77. Tomkinson, A., Reeve, J., Shaw, R. W., and Noble, B. S. (1997). The death of osteocytes via apoptosis accompanies estrogen withdrawal in human bone. *J. Clin. Endocrinol. Metab.* **82**, 3128–3135.

78. Gerstenfeld, L. C., Kelly, C. M., Von Deck, M., and Lian, J. B. (1990). Effect of 1,25-dihydroxyvitamin D3 on induction of chondrocyte maturation in culture: Extracellular matrix gene expression and morphology. *Endocrinology* **126**, 1599–1609.

79. Ishizeki, K., Hiraki, Y., Kubo, M., and Nawa, T. (1997). Sequential synthesis of cartilage and bone marker proteins during transdifferentiation of mouse Meckel's cartilage chondrocytes in vitro. *Int. J. Dev. Biol.* **41**, 83–89.

80. Erenpreisa, J., and Roach, H. I. (1996). Epigenetic selection as a possible component of transdifferentiation. Further study of the commitment of hypertrophic chondrocytes to become osteocytes. *Mech. Ageing Dev.* **87**, 165–182.

81. Thesingh, C. W., Groot, C. G., and Wassenaar, A. M. (1991). Transdifferentiation of hypertrophic chondrocytes into osteoblasts in murine fetal metatarsal bones, induced by co-cultured cerebrum. *Bone Miner.* **12**, 25–40.

82. Roach, H. I., Erenpreisa, J., and Aigner, T. (1995). Osteogenic differentiation of hypertrophic chondrocytes involves asymmetric cell divisions and apoptosis. *J. Cell Biol.* **131**, 483–494.

83. Canfield, A., Sutton, A., Hoyland, J., and Schor, A. (1996). Association of thrombospondin-1 with osteogenic differentiation of retinal pericytes in vitro. *J. Cell Sci.* **109**, 343–353.

84. Schor, A. M., Allen, T. D., Canfield, A. E., Sloan, P., and Schor, S. L. (1990). Pericytes derived from the retinal microvasculature undergo calcification in vitro. *J. Cell Sci.* **97**, 449–461.

85. Balica, M., Bostrom, K., Shin, V., Tillisch, K., and Demer, L. L. (1997). Calcifying subpopulation of bovine aortic smooth muscle cells is responsive to 17 beta-estradiol. *Circulation* **95**, 1954–1960.

86. Ebeling, P. R., Jones, J. D., O'Fallon, W. M., Janes, C. H., and Riggs, B. L. (1993). Short-term effects of recombinant human insulin-like growth factor I on bone turnover in normal women. *J. Clin. Endocrinol. Metab.* **77**, 1384–1387.

87. Canalis, E., Pash, J., Gabbitas, B., Rydziel, S., and Varghese, S. (1993). Growth factors regulate the synthesis of insulin-like growth factor-I in bone cell cultures. *Endocrinology* **133**, 33–38.

88. McCarthy, T. L., Centrella, M., and Canalis, E. (1992). Constitutive synthesis of insulin-like growth factor-II by primary osteoblast-enriched cultures from fetal rat calvariae. *Endocrinology* **130**, 1303–1308.

89. Delany, A. M., Pash, J. M., and Canalis, E. (1994). Cellular and clinical perspectives on skeletal insulin-like growth factor I. *J. Cell. Biochem.* **55**, 328–333.

90. McCarthy, T. L., Centrella, M., and Canalis, E. (1990). Cortisol inhibits the synthesis of insulin-like growth factor-I in skeletal cells. *Endocrinology* **126**, 1569–1575.

91. McCarthy, T. L., Centrella, M., and Canalis, E. (1989). Parathyroid hormone enhances the transcript and polypeptide levels of insulin-like growth factor I in osteoblast-enriched cultures from fetal rat bone. *Endocrinology* **124**, 1247–1253.

92. Suda, T., Nakamura, I., Jimi, E., and Takahashi, N. (1997). Regulation of osteoclast function. *J. Bone Miner. Res.* **12**, 869–879.

93. Roodman, G. D. (1996). Advances in bone biology: The osteoclast. *Endocr. Rev.* **17**, 308–332.

94. Boivin, G., Mesguish, P., Pike, J. W., Bouillon, R., Meunier, P. J., Haussler, M. R., Dubois, P. M., and Morel, G. (1987). Ultrastructural immunolocalization of endogenous 1,25-dihydroxyvitamin D3 and its receptor in osteoblasts and osteocytes from neonatal mouse and rat calvaria. *Bone Miner.* **3**, 125–136.

95. Eriksen, E. F., Colvard, D. S., Berg, N. J., Graham, M. L., Mann, K. G., Spelsberg, T. C., and Riggs, B. L. (1988). Evidence of estrogen receptors in normal human osteoblast-like cells. *Science* **241**, 84–86.

96. Civitelli, R., Beyer, E. C., Warlow, P. M., Robertson, A. J., Geist, S. T., and Steinberg, T. H. (1993). Connexin43 mediates direct intercellular communication in human osteoblastic cell networks. *J. Clin. Invest.* **91**, 1888–1896.

97. Yamaguchi, D. T., Ma, D., Lee, A., Huang, J., and Gruber, H. E. (1994). Isolation and characterization of gap junctions in the osteoblastic MC3T3-E1 cell line. *J. Bone Miner. Res.* **9**, 791–803.

98. Donahue, H. J., McLeod, K. J., Rubin, C. T., Andersen, J., Grine, E. A., Hertzberg, E. L., and Brink, P. R. (1995). Cell-to-cell communication in osteoblastic networks: Cell line-dependent hormonal regulation of gap junction function. *J. Bone Miner. Res.* **10**, 881–889.

99. Rubin, C. T., and Lanyon, L. E. (1987). Osteoregulatory nature of mechanical stimuli: Function as a determinant for adaptive bone remodeling. *J. Orthop. Res.* **5**, 300–310.

100. Weinbaum, S., Cowin, S. C., and Zeng, Y. (1994). A model for the excitation of osteocytes by mechanical loading-induced bone fluid shear stresses. *J. Biomech.* **27**, 339–360.

101. Einhorn, T. A. (1996). Biomechanics of bone. *In* "Principles of Bone Biology" (J. P. Bilezikian, L. G. Raisz, and G. A. Rodan, eds.), pp. 25–38. Academic Press, San Diego, CA.

102. Klein-Nulend, J., van der Plas, A., Semeins, C. M., Ajubi, N. E., Frangos, J. A., Nijweide, P. J., and Burger, E. H. (1995). Sensitivity of osteocytes to biomechanical stress in vitro. *FASEB J.* **9**, 441–445.

103. Turner, C. H., Forwood, M. R., and Otter, M. W. (1994). Mechanotransduction in bone: Do bone cells act as sensors of fluid flow? *FASEB J.* **8**, 875–878.

104. el Haj, A. J., Minter, S. L., Rawlinson, S. C., Suswillo, R., and Lanyon, L. E. (1990). Cellular responses to mechanical loading in vitro. *J. Bone Miner. Res.* **5**, 923–932.

105. Skerry, T. M., Bitensky, L., Chayen, J., and Lanyon, L. E. (1989). Early strain-related changes in enzyme activity in osteocytes following bone loading in vivo. *J. Bone Miner. Res.* **4**, 783–788.

106. Lean, J. M., Jagger, C. J., Chambers, T. J., and Chow, J. W. (1995). Increased insulin-like growth factor I mRNA expression in rat osteocytes in response to mechanical stimulation. *Am. J. Physiol.* **268**, E318–E327.

107. Fox, S. W., Chambers, T. J., and Chow, J. W. M. (1995). Nitric oxide

is an early mediator of the induction of bone formation by mechanical stimulation. *J. Bone Miner. Res.* **10**, S201 (abstr.).

108. Burger, E. H., Klein-Nulend, J., Semeins, C. M., Ajubi, N. E., and Nijweide, P. J. (1996). Osteocytes but not periosteal fibroblasts produce nitric oxide (NO) in response to pulsatile fluid flow. *Trans. Orthop. Res. Soc.* **21**, 531 (abstr.).

109. Wang, N., Butler, J. P., and Ingber, D. E. (1993). Mechanotransduction across the cell surface and through the cytoskeleton. *Science* **260**, 1124–1127.

110. Hitt, A. L., and Luna, E. J. (1994). Membrane interactions with the actin cytoskeleton. *Curr. Opin. Cell Biol.* **6**, 120–130.

111. Chen, Z. F., and Behringer, R. R. (1995). Twist is required in head mesenchyme for cranial neural tube morphogenesis. *Genes Dev.* **9**, 686–699.

112. Cserjesi, P., Brown, D., Ligon, K. L., Lyons, G. E., Copeland, N. G., Gilbert, D. J., Jenkins, N. A., and Olson, E. N. (1995). Scleraxis: A basic helix-loop-helix protein that prefigures skeletal formation during mouse embryogenesis. *Development* **121**, 1099–1110.

113. Murray, S. S., Glackin, C. A., Winters, K. A., Gazit, D., Kahn, A. J., and Murray, E. J. (1992). Expression of helix-loop-helix regulatory genes during differentiation of mouse osteoblastic cells. *J. Bone Miner. Res.* **7**, 1131–1138.

114. Ogata, T., and Noda, M. (1991). Expression of Id, a negative regulator of helix-loop-helix DNA binding proteins, is down-regulated at confluence and enhanced by dexamethasone in a mouse osteoblastic cell line, MC3T3E1. *Biochem. Biophys. Res. Commun.* **180**, 1194–1199.

115. Glackin, C. A., Lee, M., Lowe, G., Morales, S., Wergedal, J., and Strong, D. (1997). Overexpressing human TWIST in high SaOS (HSaOS) cells results in major differences in cellular morphology, proliferation rates, and ALP activities. Knocking out human Id-2 greatly reduces the expression of all TWIST family members, indicating that Id-2 may regulate TWIST during osteoblast differentiation. *J. Bone Miner. Res.* **12**, S154 (abstr.).

116. Gehring, W. J., Affolter, M., and Burglin, T. (1994). Homeodomain proteins. *Annu. Rev. Biochem.* **63**, 487–526.

117. Mina, M., Gluhak, J., Upholt, W. B., Kollar, E. J., and Rogers, B. (1995). Experimental analysis of Msx-1 and Msx-2 gene expression during chick mandibular morphogenesis. *Dev. Dyn.* **202**, 195–214.

118. Zhao, G. Q., Zhao, S., Zhou, X., Eberspaecher, H., Solursh, M., and de Crombrugghe, B. (1994). rDlx, a novel distal-less-like homeoprotein is expressed in developing cartilages and discrete neuronal tissues. *Dev. Biol.* **164**, 37–51.

119. Ferrari, D., Sumoy, L., Gannon, J., Sun, H., Brown, A. M., Upholt, W. B., and Kosher, R. A. (1995). The expression pattern of the Distal-less homeobox-containing gene Dlx-5 in the developing chick limb bud suggests its involvement in apical ectodermal ridge activity, pattern formation, and cartilage differentiation. *Mech. Dev.* **52**, 257–264.

120. Lufkin, T., Mark, M., Hart, C. P., Dolle, P., LeMeur, M., and Chambon, P. (1992). Homeotic transformation of the occipital bones of the skull by ectopic expression of a homeobox gene. *Nature* **359**, 835–841.

121. Jabs, E. W., Muller, U., Li, X., Ma, L., Luo, W., Haworth, I. S., Klisak, I., Sparkes, R., Warman, M. L., Mulliken, J. B., Snead, M. L., and Maxson, R. (1993). A mutation in the homeodomain of the human MSX2 gene in a family affected with autosomal dominant craniosynostosis. *Cell* **75**, 443–450.

122. Hoffmann, H. M., Catron, K. M., van Wijnen, A. J., McCabe, L. R., Lian, J. B., Stein, G. S., and Stein, J. L. (1994). Transcriptional control of the tissue-specific, developmentally regulated osteocalcin gene requires a binding motif for the Msx family of homeodomain proteins. *Proc. Natl. Acad. Sci. U.S.A.* **91**, 12887–12891.

123. Ryoo, H.-M., Hoffmann, H. M., Beumer, T. L., Frenkel, B., Towler, D. A., Stein, G. S., Stein, J. L., van Wijnen, A. J., and Lian, J. B.

124. Rossert, J., Eberspaecher, H., and de Crombrugghe, B. (1995). Separate cis-acting DNA elements of the mouse pro-alpha 1 (I) collagen promoter direct expression of reporter genes to different type I collagen-producing cells in transgenic mice. *J. Cell Biol.* **129**, 1421–1432.

125. Dodig, M., Kronenberg, M. S., Bedalov, A., Kream, B. E., Gronowicz, G., Clark, S. H., Mack, K., Liu, Y. H., Maxon, R., Pan, Z. Z., Upholt, W. B., Rowe, D. W., and Lichtler, A. C. (1996). Identification of a TAAT-containing motif required for high level expression of the COL1A1 promoter in differentiated osteoblasts of transgenic mice. *J. Biol. Chem.* **271**, 16422–16429.

126. Towler, D. A., Bennett, C. D., and Rodan, G. A. (1994). Activity of the rat osteocalcin basal promoter in osteoblastic cells is dependent upon homeodomain and CP1 binding motifs. *Mol. Endocrinol.* **8**, 614–624.

127. Zhang, H., Hu, G., Wang, H., Sciavolino, P., Iler, N., Shen, M. M., and Abate-Shen, C. (1997). Heterodimerization of Msx and Dlx homeoproteins results in functional antagonism. *Mol. Cell. Biol.* **17**, 2920–2932.

128. Machwate, M., Jullienne, A., Moukhtar, M., and Marie, P. J. (1995). Temporal variation of c-fos proto-oncogene expression during osteoblast differentiation and osteogenesis in developing bone. *J. Cell. Biochem.* **57**, 62–70.

129. McCabe, L. R., Kockx, M., Lian, J., Stein, J., and Stein, G. (1995). Selective expression of fos- and jun-related genes during osteoblast proliferation and differentiation. *Exp. Cell Res.* **218**, 255–262.

130. Grigoriadis, A. E., Schellander, K., Wang, Z.-Q., and Wagner, E. F. (1993). Osteoblasts are target cells for transformation in c-fos transgenic mice. *J. Cell Biol.* **122**, 685–701.

131. McCabe, L. R., Banerjee, C., Kundu, R., Harrison, R. J., Dobner, P. R., Stein, J. L., Lian, J. B., and Stein, G. S. (1996). Developmental expression and activities of specific fos and jun proteins are funtionally related to osteoblast maturation: Role of fra-2 and jun D during differentiation. *Endocrinology* **137**, 4398–4408.

132. Merriman, H. L., van Wijnen, A. J., Hiebert, S., Bidwell, J. P., Fey, E., Lian, J., Stein, J., and Stein, G. S. (1995). The tissue-specific nuclear matrix protein, NMP-2, is a member of the AML/CBF/PEBP2/runt domain transcription factor family: Interactions with the osteocalcin gene promoter. *Biochemistry* **34**, 13125–13132.

133. Banerjee, C., Hiebert, S. W., Stein, J. L., Lian, J. B., and Stein, G. S. (1996). An AML-1 consensus sequence binds an osteoblast-specific complex and transcriptionally activates the osteocalcin gene. *Proc. Natl. Acad. Sci. U.S.A.* **93**, 4968–4973.

134. Speck, N. A., and Stacy, T. (1995). A new transcription factor family associated with human leukemias. *Crit. Rev. Eukaryotic Gene Expression* **5**, 337–364.

135. Stewart, M., Terry, A., Hu, M., O'Hara, M., Blyth, K., Baxter, E., Cameron, E., Onions, D. E., and Neil, J. C. (1997). Proviral insertions induce the expression of bone-specific isoforms of PEBP2alphaA (CBFA1): Evidence for a new myc collaborating oncogene. *Proc. Natl. Acad. Sci. U.S.A.* **94**, 8646–8651.

136. Ogawa, E., Maruyama, M., Kagoshima, H., Inuzuka, M., Lu, J., Satake, M., Shigesada, K., and Ito, Y. (1993). PEBP2/PEA2 represents a family of transcription factors homologous to the products of the Drosophila runt gene and the human AML1 gene. *Proc. Natl. Acad. Sci. U.S.A.* **90**, 6859–6863.

137. Lenny, N., Westendorf, J. J., and Hiebert, S. W. (1997). Transcriptional regulation during myelopoiesis. *Mol. Biol. Rep.* **24**, 157–168.

138. Komori, T., Yagi, H., Nomura, S., Yamaguchi, A., Sasaki, K., Deguchi, K., Shimizu, Y., Bronson, R. T., Gao, Y.-H., Inada, M., Sato, M., Okamoto, R., Kitamura, Y., Yoshiki, S., and Kishimoto, T. (1997). Targeted disruption of Cbfa1 results in a complete lack of bone formation owing to maturational arrest of osteoblasts. *Cell* **89**, 755–764.

(1997). Stage-specific expression of Dlx-5 during osteoblast differentiation: Involvement in regulation of osteocalcin gene expression. *Mol. Endocrinol.* **11**, 1681–1694.

139. Otto, F., Thornell, A. P., Crompton, T., Denzel, A., Gilmour, K. C., Rosewell, I. R., Stamp, G. W. H., Beddington, R. S. P., Mundlos, S., Olsen, B. R., Selby, P. B., and Owen, M. J. (1997). Cbfa1, a candidate gene for cleidocranial dysplasia syndrome, is essential for osteoblast differentiation and bone development. *Cell* **89**, 765–771.

140. Banerjee, C., McCabe, L. R., Choi, J.-Y., Hiebert, S. W., Stein, J. L., Stein, G. S., and Lian, J. B. (1997). Runt homology domain proteins in osteoblast differentiation: AML-3/CBFA1 is a major component of a bone specific complex. *J. Cell. Biochem.* **66**, 1–8.

141. Ducy, P., Zhang, R., Geoffroy, V., Ridall, A. L., and Karsenty, G. (1997). Osf2/Cbfa1: A transcriptional activator of osteoblast differentiation. *Cell* **89**, 747–754.

142. Ryoo, H.-M., Lee, M. H., Javed, A., Kim, H. J., Shin, H. I., Choi, J.-Y., Rosen, V., Stein, J. L., van Wijnen, A. J., Stein, G. S., and Lian, J. B. (1998). Transient expression of Cbfa1 in response to bone morphogenetic protein-2 and transforming growth factor-beta1 in C2C12 myogenic cells: A necessary milestone but not sufficient for osteoblast. *J. Bone Miner. Res.* (abstr.).

143. Geoffroy, V., Corral, D. A., Zhou, L., Lee, B., and Karsenty, G. (1998). Genomic organization, expression of the human CBFA1 gene, and evidence for an alternative splicing event affecting protein function. *Mamm. Genome* **9**, 54–57.

144. Banerjee, C., Javed, A., Choi, J., Green, J., van Wijnen, A., Stein, J., Stein, G., and Lian, J. (1998). Representation and activities of multiple Cbfa transcription factors in osteoblasts. *J. Bone Miner. Res.* (abstr.).

145. Meyers, S., Lenny, N., Sun, W.-H., and Hiebert, S. W. (1996). AML-2 is a potential target for transcriptional regulation by the t (8; 21) and t (12; 21) fusion proteins in acute leukemia. *Oncogene* **13**, 303–312.

146. Fisher, A. L. and Caudy, M. (1998). Groucho proteins: Transcriptional corepressors for specific subsets of DNA-binding transcription factors in vertebrates and invertebrates. *Genes Dev.* **12**, 1931–1940.

147. Guo, B., Javed, A., Green, J., Stein, J. L., Lian, J. B., van Wijnen, A. J., and Stein, G. S. (1998). Groucho/TLE proteins associate with the nuclear matrix and repress Cbfa/AML mediated transactivation on osteocalcin promoter. *J. Bone Miner. Res.* (abstr.).

148. Roodman, G. D. (1995). Osteoclast function in Paget's disease and multiple myeloma. *Bone* **17**, 57S–61S.

149. Reinholt, F. P., Hultenby, K., Oldberg, A., and Heinegard, D. (1990). Osteopontin—a possible anchor of osteoclasts to bone. *Proc. Natl. Acad. Sci. U.S.A.* **87**, 4473–4475.

150. Helfrich, M. H., Nesbitt, S. A., Dorey, E. L., and Horton, M. A. (1992). Rat osteoclasts adhere to a wide range of RGD (Arg-Gly-Asp) peptide-containing proteins, including the bone sialoproteins and fibronectin, via a beta 3 integrin. *J. Bone Miner. Res.* **7**, 335–343.

151. Nesbitt, S., Nesbit, A., Helfrich, M., and Horton, M. (1993). Biochemical characterization of human osteoclast integrins. Osteoclasts express alpha v beta 3, alpha 2 beta 1, and alpha v beta 1 integrins. *J. Biol. Chem.* **268**, 16737–16745.

152. Ross, F. P., Chappel, J., Alvarez, J. I., Sander, D., Butler, W. T., Farach-Carson, M. C., Mintz, K. A., Robey, P. G., Teitelbaum, S. L., and Cheresh, D.A. (1993). Interactions between the bone matrix proteins osteopontin and bone sialoprotein and the osteoclast integrin alpha v beta 3 potentiate bone resorption. *J. Biol. Chem.* **268**, 9901–9907.

153. Fisher, J. E., Caulfield, M. P., Sato, M., Quartuccio, H. A., Gould, R. J., Garsky, V. M., Rodan, G. A., and Rosenblatt, M. (1993). Inhibition of osteoclastic bone resorption in vivo by echistatin, an "arginyl-glycyl-aspartyl" (RGD)-containing protein. *Endocrinology* **132**, 1411–1413.

154. Engleman, V. W., Nickols, G. A., Ross, F. P., Horton, M. A., Griggs, D. W., Settle, S. L., Ruminski, P. G., and Teitelbaum, S. L. (1997). A peptidomimetic antagonist of the alpha(v)beta3 integrin inhibits bone resorption in vitro and prevents osteoporosis in vivo. *J. Clin. Invest.* **99**, 2284–2292.

155. Lakkakorpi, P. T., and Vaananen, H. K. (1991). Kinetics of the osteoclast cytoskeleton during the resorption cycle in vitro. *J. Bone Miner. Res.* **6**, 817–826.

156. Tanaka, S., Takahashi, N., Udagawa, N., Murakami, H., Nakamura, I., Kurokawa, T., and Suda, T. (1995). Possible involvement of focal adhesion kinase, p125FAK, in osteoclastic bone resorption. *J. Cell. Biochem.* **58**, 424–435.

157. Vaananen, H. K., and Horton, M. (1995). The osteoclast clear zone is a specialized cell-extracellular matrix adhesion structure. *J. Cell Sci.* **108**, 2729–2732.

158. Schaller, M. D., Borgman, C. A., Cobb, B. S., Vines, R. R., Reynolds, A. B., and Parsons, J. T. (1992). pp125FAK, a structurally distinctive protein-tyrosine kinase associated with focal adhesions. *Proc. Natl. Acad. Sci. U.S.A.* **89**, 5192–5196.

159. Nakamura, I., Sasaki, T., Tanaka, S., Takahashi, N., Jimi, E., Kurokawa, T., Kita, Y., Ihara, S., Suda, T., and Fukui, Y. (1997). Phosphatidylinositol-3 kinase is involved in ruffled border formation in osteoclasts. *J. Cell. Physiol.* **172**, 230–239.

160. Zhang, D., Udagawa, N., Nakamura, I., Murakami, H., Saito, S., Yamasaki, K., Shibasaki, Y., Morii, N., Narumiya, S., and Takahashi, N. (1995). The small GTP-binding protein, rho p21, is involved in bone resorption by regulating cytoskeletal organization in osteoclasts. *J. Cell Sci.* **108**, 2285–2292.

161. Hall, A. (1990). The cellular functions of small GTP-binding proteins. *Science* **249**, 635–640.

162. Tanaka, S., Amling, M., Neff, L., Peyman, A., Uhlmann, E., Levy, J. B., and Baron, R. (1996). c-Cbl is downstream of c-Src in a signalling pathway necessary for bone resorption. *Nature* **383**, 528–531.

163. Nakamura, I., Jimi, E., Sasaki, T., Kurokawa, T., Takahashi, N., and Suda, T. (1996). p130^Cas is involved in actin ring formation in osteoclasts. *J. Bone Miner. Res.* **11**, S188 (abstr.).

164. Nakamura, I., Takahashi, N., Sasaki, T., Tanaka, S., Udagawa, N., Murakami, H., Kimura, K., Kabuyama, Y., Kurokawa, T., and Suda, T. (1995). Wortmannin, a specific inhibitor of phosphatidylinositol-3 kinase, blocks osteoclastic bone resorption. *FEBS Lett.* **361**, 79–84.

165. Lakkakorpi, P. T., and Vaananen, H. K. (1990). Calcitonin, prostaglandin E2, and dibutyryl cyclic adenosine 3′, 5′-monophosphate disperse the specific microfilament structure in resorbing osteoclasts. *J. Histochem. Cytochem.* **38**, 1487–1493.

166. Blair, H. C., Teitelbaum, S. L., Ghiselli, R., and Gluck, S. (1989). Osteoclastic bone resorption by a polarized vacuolar proton pump. *Science* **245**, 855–857.

167. Kallio, D. M., Garant, P. R., and Minkin, C. (1971). Evidence of coated membranes in the ruffled border of the osteoclast. *J Ultrastruct. Res.* **37**, 169–177.

168. Fallon, M. D. (1984). Bone resorbing fluid from osteoclasts is acidic: An in vitro micropuncture study. *In* "Endocrine Control of Bone and Calcium Metabolism" (C. V. Conn, J. R. Fujita, J. R. Potts *et al.*, eds.), pp. 144–146. Elsevier/North-Holland, Amsterdam.

169. Chatterjee, D., Chakraborty, M., Leit, M., Neff, L., Jamsa-Kellokumpu, S., Fuchs, R., and Baron, R. (1992). Sensitivity to vanadate and isoforms of subunits A and B distinguish the osteoclast proton pump from other vacuolar H$^+$ ATPases. *Proc. Natl. Acad. Sci. U.S.A.* **89**, 6257–6261.

170. Toyosawa, S., Ogawa, Y., Chang, C. K., Hong, S. S., Yagi, T., Kuwahara, H., Wakasa, K., and Sakurai, M. (1991). Histochemistry of tartrate-resistant acid phosphatase and carbonic anhydrase isoenzyme II in osteoclast-like giant cells in bone tumours. *Virchows Arch. A: Pathol. Anat. Histopathol.* **418**, 255–261.

171. Teitelbaum, S. L., Tondravi, M. M., and Ross, F. P. (1996). Osteoclast biology. *In* "Osteoporosis" (R. Marcus, D. Feldman, J. Kelsey, eds.), pp. 61–94. Academic Press, San Diego, CA.

172. Athanasou, N. A. (1996). Cellular biology of bone-resorbing cells. *J. Bone Jt. Surg., Am. Vol.* **78**, 1096–1112.

173. Sasaki, T., and Ueno-Matsuda, E. (1993). Cysteine-proteinase localization in osteoclasts: An immunocytochemical study. *Cell Tissue Res.* **271**, 177–179.

174. Goto, T., Kiyoshima, T., Moroi, R., Tsukuba, T., Nishimura, Y., Himeno, M., Yamamoto, K., and Tanaka, T. (1994). Localization of cathepsins B, D, and L in the rat osteoclast by immuno-light and electron microscopy. *Histochemistry* **101**, 33–40.

175. Ek-Rylander, B., Barkhem, T., Ljusberg, J., Ohman, L., Andersson, K. K., and Andersson, G. (1997). Comparative studies of rat recombinant purple acid phosphatase and bone tartrate-resistant acid phosphatase. *Biochem. J.* **321**, 305–311.

176. Delaisse, J. M., Eeckhout, Y., Neff, L., François-Gillet, C., Henriet, P., Su, Y., Vaes, G., and Baron, R. (1993). (Pro) collagenase (matrix metalloproteinase-1) is present in rodent osteoclasts and in the underlying bone-resorbing compartment. *J. Cell Sci.* **106**, 1071–1082.

177. Okada, Y., Naka, K., Kawamura, K., Matsumoto, T., Nakanishi, I., Fujimoto, N., Sato, H., and Seiki, M. (1995). Localization of matrix metalloproteinase 9 (92-kilodalton gelatinase/type IV collagenase = gelatinase B) in osteoclasts: Implications for bone resorption. *Lab. Invest.* **72**, 311–322.

178. Chambers, T. J., Darby, J. A., and Fuller, K. (1985). Mammalian collagenase predisposes bone surfaces to osteoclastic resorption. *Cell Tissue Res.* **241**, 671–675.

179. Hattersley, G., and Chambers, T. J. (1989). Calcitonin receptors as markers for osteoclastic differentiation: Correlation between generation of bone-resorptive cells and cells that express calcitonin receptors in mouse bone marrow cultures. *Endocrinology* **125**, 1606–1612.

180. Lee, S. K., Goldring, S. R., and Lorenzo, J. A. (1995). Expression of the calcitonin receptor in bone marrow cell cultures and in bone: a specific marker of the differentiated osteoclast that is regulated by calcitonin. *Endocrinology* **136**, 4572–4581.

181. Popoff, S. N., and Marks, S. C. J. (1995). The heterogeneity of the osteopetroses reflects the diversity of cellular influences during skeletal development. *Bone* **17**, 437–445.

182. Walker, D. G. (1975). Bone resorption restored in osteopetrotic mice by transplants of normal bone marrow and spleen cells. *Science* **190**, 784–785.

183. Teitelbaum, S. L., Tondravi, M. M., and Ross, F. P. (1997). Osteoclasts, macrophages, and the molecular mechanisms of bone resorption. *J. Leukocyte Biol.* **61**, 381–388.

184. Gothlin, G., and Ericsson, J. L. (1973). On the histogenesis of the cells in fracture callus. Electron microscopic autoradiographic observations in parabiotic rats and studies on labeled monocytes. *Virchows Arch. B: Cell Pathol.* **12**, 318–329.

185. Jotereau, F. V., and Le Douarin, N. M. (1978). The development relationship between osteocytes and osteoclasts: A study using the quail-chick nuclear marker in endochondral ossification. *Dev. Biol.* **63**, 253–265.

186. Kahn, A. J., and Simmons, D. J. (1975). Investigation of cell lineage in bone using a chimaera of chick and quail embryonic tissue. *Nature* **258**, 325–327.

187. Takahashi, N., Akatsu, T., Udagawa, N., Sasaki, T., Yamaguchi, A., Moseley, J. M., Martin, T. J., and Suda, T. (1988). Osteoblastic cells are involved in osteoclast formation. *Endocrinology* **123**, 2600–2602.

188. Abe, Y., Yonemura, K., Nishida, K., and Takagi, K. (1994). Giant cell tumor of bone: Analysis of proliferative cells by double-labeling immunohistochemistry with anti-proliferating cell nuclear antigen antibody and culture procedure. *Nippon Seikeigeka Gakkai Zasshi* **68**, 407–414.

189. Zambonin Zallone, A., Teti, A., and Primavera, M. V. (1984). Monocytes from circulating blood fuse in vitro with purified osteoclasts in primary culture. *J. Cell Sci.* **66**, 335–342.

190. Burger, E. H., Van der Meer, J. W., van de Gevel, J. S., Gribnau, J. C., Thesingh, G. W., and van Furth, R. (1982). In vitro formation of osteoclasts from long-term cultures of bone marrow mononuclear phagocytes. *J. Exp. Med.* **156**, 1604–1614.

191. Athanasou, N. A., and Quinn, J. (1990). Immunophenotypic differences between osteoclasts and macrophage polykaryons: immunohistological distinction and implications for osteoclast ontogeny and function. *J. Clin. Pathol.* **43**, 997–1003.

192. Shapiro, I. M., Jones, S. J., Hogg, N. M., Slusarenko, M., and Boyde, A. (1979). Use of SEM for the study of the surface receptors of osteoclasts in situ. *Scanning Electron Microsc.*, pp. 539–545.

193. Baron, R., Neff, L., Tran Van, P., Nefussi, J. R., and Vignery, A. (1986). Kinetic and cytochemical identification of osteoclast precursors and their differentiation into multinucleated osteoclasts. *Am. J Pathol.* **122**, 363–378.

194. Nicholson, G. C., Moseley, J. M., Sexton, P. M., and Martin, T. J. (1987). Chicken osteoclasts do not possess calcitonin receptors. *J. Bone Miner. Res.* **2**, 53–59.

195. Suda, T., Takahashi, N., and Etsuko, A. (1992). Role of vitamin D in bone resorption. *J. Cell. Biochem.* **49**, 53–58.

196. Uy, H. L., Guise, T. A., De La Mata, J., Taylor, S. D., Story, B. M., Dallas, M. R., Boyce, B. F., Mundy, G. R., and Roodman, G. D. (1995). Effects of parathyroid hormone (PTH)-related protein and PTH on osteoclasts and osteoclast precursors in vivo. *Endocrinology* **136**, 3207–3212.

197. Fenton, A. J., Martin, T. J., and Nicholson, G. C. (1994). Carboxyl-terminal parathyroid hormone-related protein inhibits bone resorption by isolated chicken osteoclasts. *J. Bone Miner. Res.* **9**, 515–519.

198. Agarwala, N., and Gay, C. V. (1992). Specific binding of parathyroid hormone to living osteoclasts. *J. Bone Miner. Res.* **7**, 531–539.

199. Tong, H., Lin, H., Wang, H., Sakai, D., and Minkin, C. (1995). Osteoclasts respond to parathyroid hormone and express mRNA for its receptor. *J. Bone Miner. Res.* **10**, S322 (abstr.).

200. Teti, A., Rizzoli, R., and Zambonin Zallone, A. (1991). Parathyroid hormone binding to cultured avian osteoclasts. *Biochem. Biophys. Res. Commun.* **174**, 1217–1222.

201. Udagawa, N., Takahashi, N., Akatsu, T., Tanaka, H., Sasaki, T., Nishihara, T., Koga, T., Martin, T. J., and Suda, T. (1990). Origin of osteoclasts: Mature monocytes and macrophages are capable of differentiating into osteoclasts under a suitable microenvironment prepared by bone marrow-derived stromal cells. *Proc. Natl. Acad. Sci. U.S.A.* **87**, 7260–7264.

202. Owens, J. M., Gallagher, A. C., and Chambers, T. J. (1996). Bone cells required for osteoclastic resorption but not for osteoclastic differentiation. *Biochem. Biophys. Res. Commun.* **222**, 225–229.

203. Kukita, A., Kukita, T., Shin, J. H., and Kohashi, O. (1993). Induction of mononuclear precursor cells with osteoclastic phenotypes in a rat bone marrow culture system depleted of stromal cells. *Biochem. Biophys. Res. Commun.* **196**, 1383–1389.

204. Holtrop, M. E. and Raisz, L. G. (1979). Comparison of the effects of 1,25-dihydroxycholecalciferol, prostaglandin E2, and osteoclast-activating factor with parathyroid hormone on the ultrastructure of osteoclasts in cultured long bones of fetal rats. *Calcif. Tissue Int.* **29**, 201–205.

205. Shevde, N., Anklesaria, P., Greenberger, J. S., Bleiberg, I., and Glowacki, J. (1994). Stromal cell-mediated stimulation of osteoclastogenesis. *Proc. Soc. Exp. Biol. Med.* **205**, 306–315.

206. McSheehy, P. M., and Chambers, T. J. (1986). Osteoblastic cells mediate osteoclastic responsiveness to parathyroid hormone. *Endocrinology* **118**, 824–828.

207. Lee, K., Deeds, J. D., Chiba, S., Un-No, M., Bond, A. T., and Segré, G. V. (1994). Parathyroid hormone induces sequential c-fos expression in bone cells in vivo: In situ localization of its receptor and c-fos messenger ribonucleic acids. *Endocrinology* **134**, 441–450.

208. Grigoriadis, A. E., Wang, Z.-Q., Cecchini, M. G., Hofstetter, W., Felix, R., Fleisch, H. A., and Wagner, E. F. (1994). c-Fos: A key regulator of osteoclast-macrophage lineage determination and bone remodeling. *Science* **266**, 443–448.

209. Greenfield, E. M., Horowitz, M. C., and Lavish, S. A. (1996). Stimulation by parathyroid hormone of interleukin-6 and leukemia inhibitory factor expression in osteoblasts is an immediate-early gene response induced by cAMP signal transduction. *J. Biol. Chem.* **271**, 10984–10989.

210. Girasole, G., Passeri, G., Jilka, R. L., and Manolagas, S. C. (1994). Interleukin-11: A new cytokine critical for osteoclast development. *J. Clin. Invest.* **93**, 1516–1524.

211. Romas, E., Udagawa, N., Zhou, H., Tamura, T., Saito, M., Taga, T., Hilton, D. J., Suda, T., Ng, K. W., and Martin, T. J. (1996). The role of gp130-mediated signals in osteoclast development: Regulation of interleukin 11 production by osteoblasts and distribution of its receptor in bone marrow cultures. *J. Exp. Med.* **183**, 2581–2591.

212. Elias, J. A., Tang, W., and Horowitz, M. C. (1995). Cytokine and hormonal stimulation of human osteosarcoma interleukin-11 production. *Endocrinology* **136**, 489–498.

213. Udagawa, N., Horwood, N. J., Elliott, J., Mackay, A., Owens, J., Okamura, H., Kurimoto, M., Chambers, T. J., Martin, T. J., and Gillespie, M. T. (1997). Interleukin-18 (interferon-gamma-inducing factor) is produced by osteoblasts and acts via granulocyte/macrophage colony-stimulating factor and not via interferon-gamma to inhibit osteoclast formation. *J Exp. Med.* **185**, 1005–1012.

214. Horwood, N. J., Udagawa, N., Elliott, J., Grail, D., Okamura, H., Kurimoto, M., Dunn, A. R., Martin, T., and Gillespie, M. T. (1998). Interleukin 18 inhibits osteoclast formation via T cell production of granulocyte macrophage colony-stimulating factor. *J. Clin. Invest.* **101**, 595–603.

215. Suda, T., Udagawa, N., Nakamura, I., Miyaura, C., and Takahashi, N. (1995). Modulation of osteoclast differentiation by local factors. *Bone* **17**, 87S–91S.

216. Roodman, G. D. (1996). Advances in bone biology: The osteoclast. *Endocr. Rev.* **17**, 308–332.

217. Devlin, R. D., Reddy, S. V., Savino, R., Ciliberto, G., and Roodman, G. D. (1998). IL-6 mediates the effects of IL-1 or TNF, but not PTHrP or 1, 25(OH)2D3, on osteoclast-like cell formation in normal human bone marrow cultures. *J. Bone Miner. Res.* **13**, 393–399.

218. Kishimoto, T., Akira, S., Narazaki, M., and Taga, T. (1995). Interleukin-6 family of cytokines and gp130. *Blood* **86**, 1243–1254.

219. Lin, S. C., Yamate, T., Taguchi, Y., Borba, V. Z., Girasole, G., O'Brien, C. A., Bellido, T., Abe, E., and Manolagas, S. C. (1997). Regulation of the gp80 and gp130 subunits of the IL-6 receptor by sex steroids in the murine bone marrow. *J. Clin. Invest.* **100**, 1980–1990.

220. Woodroofe, C., Muller, W., and Ruther, U. (1992). Long-term consequences of interleukin-6 overexpression in transgenic mice. *DNA Cell Biol.* **11**, 587–592.

221. Kawasaki, K., Gao, Y. H., Yokose, S., Kaji, Y., Nakamura, T., Suda, T., Yoshida, K., Taga, T., Kishimoto, T., Kataoka, H., Yuasa, T., Norimatsu, H., and Yamaguchi, A. (1997). Osteoclasts are present in gp130-deficient mice. *Endocrinology* **138**, 4959–4965.

222. Tanaka, S., Takahashi, N., Udagawa, N., Tamura, T., Akatsu, T., Stanley, E. R., Kurokawa, T., and Suda, T. (1993). Macrophage colony-stimulating factor is indispensable for both proliferation and differentiation of osteoclast progenitors. *J. Clin. Invest.* **91**, 257–263.

223. Felix, R., Cecchini, M. G., and Fleisch, H. (1990). Macrophage colony-stimulating factor restores in vivo bone resorption in the op/op osteopetrotic mouse. *Endocrinology* **127**, 2592–2594.

224. Yoshida, H., Hayashi, S., Kunisada, T., Ogawa, M., Nishikawa, S., Okamura, H., Sudo, T., and Shultz, L. D. (1990). The murine mutation osteopetrosis is in the coding region of the macrophage colony stimulating factor gene. *Nature* **345**, 442–444.

225. Takahashi, N., Udagawa, N., Akatsu, T., Tanaka, H., Isogai, Y., and Suda, T. (1991). Deficiency of osteoclasts in osteopetrotic mice is due to a defect in the local microenvironment provided by osteoblastic cells. *Endocrinology* **128**, 1792–1796.

226. Simonet, W. S., Lacey, D. L., Dunstan, C. R., Kelley, M., Chang, M. S., Luthy, R., Nguyen, H. Q., Wooden, S., Bennett, L., Boone, T., Shimamoto, G., DeRose, M., Elliott, R., Colombero, A., Tan, H. L., Trail, G., Sullivan, J., Davy, E., Bucay, N., Renshaw-Gegg, L., Hughes, T. M., Hill, D., Pattison, W., Campbell, P., and Boyle, W. J. (1997). Osteoprotegerin: A novel secreted protein involved in the regulation of bone density. *Cell* **89**, 309–319.

227. Yasuda, H., Shima, N., Nakagawa, N., Yamaguchi, K., Kinosaki, M., Mochizuki, S., Tomoyasu, A., Yano, K., Goto, M., Murakami, A., Tsuda, E., Morinaga, T., Higashio, K., Udagawa, N., Takahashi, N., and Suda, T. (1998). Osteoclast differentiation factor is a ligand for osteoprotegerin/osteoclastogenesis-inhibitory factor and is identical to TRANCE/RANKL. *Proc. Natl. Acad. Sci. U.S.A.* **95**, 3597–3602.

228. Lacey, D. L., Timms, E., Tan, H. L., Kelley, M. J., Dunstan, C. R., Burgess, T., Elliott, R., Colombero, A., Elliott, G., Scully, S., Hsu, H., Sullivan, J., Hawkins, N., Davy, E., Capparelli, C., Eli, A., Qian, Y. X., Kaufman, S., Sarosi, I., Shalhoub, V., Senaldi, G., Guo, J., Delaney, J., and Boyle, W. J. (1998). Osteoprotegerin ligand is a cytokine that regulates osteoclast differentiation and activation. *Cell* **93**, 165–176.

229. Wong, B. R., Josien, R., Lee, S. Y., Sauter, B., Li, H. L., Steinman, R. M., and Choi, Y. (1997). TRANCE (tumor necrosis factor [TNF]-related activation-induced cytokine), a new TNF family member predominantly expressed in T cells, is a dendritic cell-specific survival factor. *J. Exp. Med.* **186**, 2075–2080.

230. Anderson, D. M., Maraskovsky, E., Billingsley, W. L., Dougall, W. C., Tometsko, M. E., Roux, E. R., Teepe, M. C., DuBose, R. F., Cosman, D., and Galibert, L. (1997). A homologue of the TNF receptor and its ligand enhance T-cell growth and dendritic-cell function. *Nature* **390**, 175–179.

231. Yasuda, H., Shima, N., Nakagawa, N., Mochizuki, S. I., Yano, K., Fujise, N., Sato, Y., Goto, M., Yamaguchi, K., Kuriyama, M., Kanno, T., Murakami, A., Tsuda, E., Morinaga, T., and Higashio, K. (1998). Identity of osteoclastogenesis inhibitory factor (OCIF) and osteoprotegerin (OPG): A mechanism by which OPG/OCIF inhibits osteoclastogenesis in vitro. *Endocrinology* **139**, 1329–1337.

232. Johnson, R. S., Spiegelman, B. M., and Papaioannou, V. (1992). Pleiotropic effects of a null mutation in the c-fos proto-oncogene. *Cell* **71**, 577–586.

233. Wang, Z.-Q., Ovitt, C., Grigoriadis, A. E., Mohle-Steinlein, U., Ruther, U., and Wagner, E. F. (1992). Bone and haematopoietic defects in mice lacking c-fos. *Nature* **360**, 741–745.

234. Xing, L., Franzoso, G., Siebenlist, U., and Boyce, B. (1997). Targeted disruption of the p50 and p52 subunits of NF-kB transcription factor leads to failure of osteoclast formation and osteopetrosis. *J. Bone Miner. Res.* **12**, S136 (abstr.).

235. Tondravi, M. M., McKercher, S. R., Anderson, K., Erdmann, J. M., Quiroz, M., Maki, R., and Teitelbaum, S. L. (1997). Osteopetrosis in mice lacking haematopoietic transcription factor PU.1. *Nature* **386**, 81–84.

236. Zhang, D. E., Hetherington, C. J., Chen, H. M., and Tenen, D. G. (1994). The macrophage transcription factor PU.1 directs tissue-specific expression of the macrophage colony-stimulating factor receptor. *Mol. Cell. Biol.* **14**, 373–381.

237. Soriano, P., Montgomery, C., Geske, R., and Bradley, A. (1991). Targeted disruption of the c-src proto-oncogene leads to osteopetrosis in mice. *Cell* **64**, 693–702.

238. Abu-Amer, Y., Ross, F. P., Schlesinger, P., Tondravi, M. M., and Teitelbaum, S. L. (1997). Substrate recognition by osteoclast precursors induces C-src/microtubule association. *J. Cell Biol.* **137**, 247–258.

239. Boyce, B. F., Yoneda, T., Lowe, C., Soriano, P., and Mundy, G. R. (1992). Requirement of pp60c-src expression for osteoclasts to form ruffled borders and resorb bone in mice. *J. Clin. Invest.* **90**, 1622–1627.

240. Hodgkinson, C. A., Moore, K. J., Nakayama, A., Steingrimsson, E., Copeland, N. G., Jenkins, N. A., and Arnheiter, H. (1993). Mutations at the mouse microphthalmia locus are associated with defects in a gene encoding a novel basic-helix-loop-helix-zipper protein. *Cell* **74**, 395–404.

CHAPTER 13

Parathyroid Hormone: Structure, Function, and Dynamic Actions

LORRAINE A. FITZPATRICK   Endocrine Research Unit, Mayo Clinic and Mayo Foundation, Rochester, Minnesota 55905

JOHN P. BILEZIKIAN   Departments of Medicine and Pharmacology, College of Physicians and Surgeons, Columbia University, New York, New York 10032

I. INTRODUCTION

Parathyroid hormone (PTH) regulates calcium homeostasis via its actions on target tissues. It maintains serum calcium concentrations within a narrow physiological range by direct actions on bone and kidney tissue and indirect action on the intestinal tract. Parathyroid hormone release and gene expression, in turn, are regulated by serum calcium concentrations. Hypocalcemia stimulates the release of PTH from the parathyroid gland. By reabsorption of calcium in the kidney tubule or by osteoclast-mediated bone resorption, serum calcium concentrations increase. PTH also stimulates renal 1-α-hydroxylase activity. These actions of PTH are mediated through a G-protein-coupled receptor system in the cells of target tissues. A rise in extracellular calcium inhibits further secretion of parathyroid hormone.

II. STRUCTURE OF THE PTH GENE

The gene that encodes parathyroid hormone is representative of typical eukaryotic genes with consensus sequences for initiation of RNA synthesis, RNA splicing, and polyadenylation. Restriction enzyme analysis of the human PTH gene has indicated polymorphism in the cleavage products in different individuals, and the polymorphisms are useful for genetic

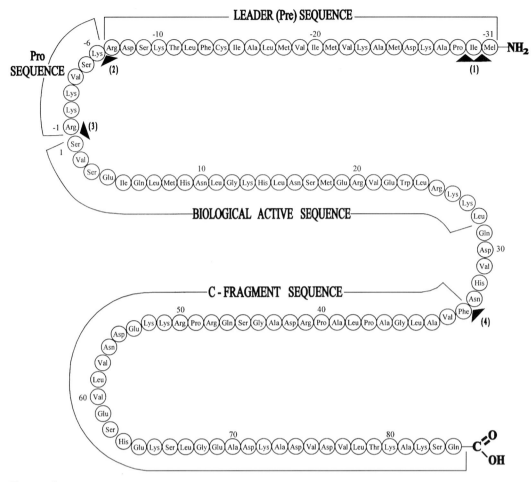

FIGURE 1   Primary structure of human preparathyroid hormone. The arrows indicate sites of specific cleavages which occur in the sequence of biosynthesis and peripheral metabolism. The biologically active sequence is noted. Reprinted from Choren and Rosenblatt [2a], with permission.

analysis [1]. Complementary DNAs encoding for human, rat, chicken, bovine, and dog PTH have been cloned. These genes have several structural features in common: all contain two introns (or intervening sequences) and three exons (Fig. 1) [2, 2a]. The introns vary in size among species. The first intron is large; the second intron is smaller (about 100 base pairs) in human, bovine, and rat genes. The first intron encodes the 5′-noncoding sequences; the second exon encodes most of the "prepro" sequence. The mature PTH sequence and the 3′-noncoding region are contained within the third exon. RNA is transcribed from the sequences in both the introns and exons. Subsequently, RNA sequences derived from the introns are spliced. The product, resulting from transcription of the exons, is mature PTH mRNA, which is then translated into preproPTH.

Considerable homology among the mammalian PTH genes is seen between human and bovine proteins (85%) and between human and rat proteins (75%). Identity is less in the 3′-noncoding region. In contrast, human and bovine PTH genes contain two functional TATA transcription start sites whereas the rat and chicken genes have only one. Both initiation sites of transcription are utilized in the bovine and human genes.

Tissue specificity of PTH gene expression is determined by coding regions upstream of the structural gene. Analysis of these regulatory sequences has been difficult due to the lack of a well-defined cell line to express the gene. A cAMP-response element has been identified and other sequences that bind 1,25 $(OH)_2 D_3$ receptors have been recognized [3].

III. CHROMOSOME LOCATION

The human PTH gene has been localized to the short arm of chromosome 11 and is close to the calcitonin gene [4, 5]. Additional localization studies have indicated that the human PTH gene is located at band 11p15 [6]. Restriction fragment length polymorphisms indicate that the human PTH gene is linked to genes encoding calcitonin, catalase, insulin, H-ras, and B-globin [1].

IV. CONTROL OF GENE EXPRESSION

A. The Role of Extracellular Calcium

Minute-to-minute regulation of serum calcium levels depends on the regulation of secretion of PTH by calcium. Long-term homeostasis depends on several regulatory mechanisms. Expression of the PTH gene occurs almost exclusively in the parathyroid chief cells. Early studies indicated that increased levels of extracellular calcium resulted in a reversible fall in PTH mRNA in cultured parathyroid cells (Fig. 2) [7]. Suppression was most pronounced after 72 hours of incubation. The rate of PTH gene transcription was also reduced in the presence of high concentrations of calcium.

In vivo studies in intact rats revealed rapid changes in PTH mRNA in response to changes in serum calcium concentrations (Fig. 3) [8]. The largest effects were noted in response to lowered levels of calcium (2.6 to 2.1 mmol/liter). Increased levels of serum calcium, whether induced by infusion of calcium or by transplantation of Walker carcinosarcoma 256 cells, had little effect on PTH mRNA levels. One major difference in the *in vivo* studies in comparison to the *in vitro* work is in the time course of response to calcium. *In vivo*, high calcium levels lead to a rapid fall in PTH mRNA within a few hours; *in vitro*, a longer time frame is required to detect changes in PTH mRNA in the models tested. Another major difference is that *in vivo*, hypercalcemia does not alter PTH mRNA levels, suggesting that at the molecular level, the parathyroid gland is responsive to the signal of hypocalcemia.

Many studies to evaluate the genetic mechanism of the action of calcium and to search for DNA sequences responsible for the transcriptional effects of calcium have been hampered by the lack of a well-differentiated parathyroid cell line that produces PTH in response to changes in extracellular cal-

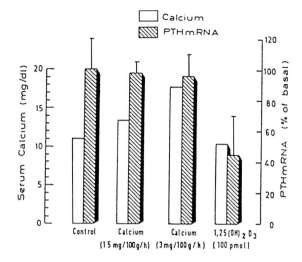

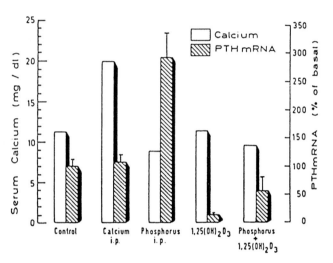

FIGURE 3   The effect of calcium, phosphorus, 1,25(OH)₂D₃, and phosphorus with 1,25(OH)₂D₃ on serum calcium and PTH mRNA of rat parathyroid glands at 6 h. Rats were injected with calcium gluconate ip (2 ml at 0 and 3 h) or sodium phosphate ip (0.6 mmol/100 g body weight at 0 and 3 h) or 1,25(OH)₂D₃ ip (100 pmol/100 g body weight at 0 h) or phosphorus (at 0 and 3 h) with 1,25(OH)₂D₃ (at 0 h). Total parathyroid-thyroid RNA was determined by dot blot hybridization. Reprinted with permission from Naveh-Many, T., *et al.* [8] (1989). Calcium regulates parathyroid hormone messenger ribonucleic acid (mRNA), but not calcitonin mRNA in vivo in the rat. *Endocrinology* **125**, 275–280, © The Endocrine Society.

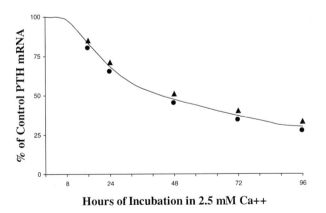

FIGURE 2   Bovine parathyroid cells were exposed to 2.5 mM calcium for 0 to 96 hours. PTH mRNA was quantified by solution hybridization (triangles) and dot blot hybridization (circles). Hybridizable PTH mRNA declined over time. Reprinted from Russell, J., *et al.* [7]. *J. Clin. Invest.* **72**, 1851–1855 (1983), with permission.

cium. Several short sequences located several thousand base pairs upstream from the start site of PTH gene transcription may be involved in the regulation of PTH by calcium. A negative calcium regulatory element (nCaRE) has been identified in the PTH gene. It is also present in the atrial natriuretic peptide gene [9]. Further studies by the same investigators revealed the identity of a redox factor protein (ref1) that activates several transcription factors and binds nCaRE. The levels of ref1 mRNA and protein were elevated by an increase in extracellular calcium concentration. Unfortunately, these studies had to be performed in a nonparathyroid cell line, so the role of the protein in the regulation of PTH expression remains to be determined.

The *in vivo* effects of calcium also may be due to post-transcriptional mechanisms. Preliminary evidence indicates that regions in the 3′ UTR of PTH mRNA bind specifically to cytosolic proteins and may be involved in the posttranscriptional increase in PTH gene expression induced by decreased calcium concentration [10]. Bovine parathyroid cells were incubated in the presence of low extracellular calcium (0.4 mM) and resulted in a posttranscriptional increase in the membrane-bound polysomal content of PTH mRNA [11] Using a cell-free assay system, Vadher et al [12] presented preliminary evidence that the 3′ untranslated region is important in the translational regulation of PTH synthesis by cytosolic regulatory proteins. These *in vitro* studies add support for a posttranslational role of calcium on PTH gene expression. Taken together, these studies suggest that posttranslational regulation of PTH mRNA may involve calcium-sensitive proteins binding to the 3′-UTR region.

B. The Role of 1,25 Dihydroxyvitamin D

In vivo and *in vitro* studies support the significant role of 1,25 dihydroxyvitamin D in the regulation of PTH gene expression via a well-defined feedback loop between PTH and $1,25(OH)_2D_3$. The renal synthesis of $1,25(OH)_2D_3$ is increased by PTH; in turn, $1,25(OH)_2D_3$ increases serum calcium concentrations by enhancing intestinal absorption of calcium. $1,25(OH)_2D_3$ reduces transcription of the PTH gene. In bovine parathyroid cells in primary culture, $1,25(OH)_2D_3$ exposure resulted in reduced levels of PTH mRNA and PTH gene transcription rates [13, 14]. *In vitro* studies in rats confirmed the regulatory role of $1,25(OH)_2D_3$ in PTH gene expression. Rats received injections of $1,25(OH)_2D_3$ at levels that did not alter serum calcium levels but resulted in a decrease in the transcription of the PTH gene and reduced levels of PTH mRNA [15].

Transfection assays and DNA binding studies have attempted to identify specifically the sequences responsible for modulation of PTH gene transcription by $1,25(OH)_2D_3$. Utilizing a rat pituitary cell line (GH4), Okazaki *et al.* [16] linked 684 base pairs of the 5′-flanking region of the human PTH gene to a reporter gene. Transfection of the rat pituitary cell line resulted in responsiveness of gene expression to $1,25(OH)_2D_3$. DNA binding studies identified DNA sequences upstream of the PTH gene that bind to $1,25(OH)_2D_3$ receptors *in vitro*. A specific 26 bp sequence located 125 base pairs upstream from the transcription start site on the PTH gene binds to $1,25(OH)_2D_3$ receptors. Confirmation of this activity was performed by transfection of a pituitary cell line with the sequence linked to a reporter gene, with the result that $1,25(OH)_2D_3$ suppressed the reporter gene [3]. In contrast, the human PTH DNA sequence does not mediate repression

of transcription in the osteoblast cell line ROS 17/2.8, in spite of the fact that the vitamin D response elements (VDRE) are active in these cells. One difference is that the human PTH DNA sequence contains a single copy of a hexameric motif homologous to those repeated in the upregulatory vitamin D response elements. When the nuclear extracts from bovine parathyroid cells are incubated with the vitamin D receptor, the receptor binds the downregulatory human PTH DNA sequence independent of the presence of the retinoid X receptor (RXR). In the nuclear extracts from GH4CI pituitary cells, two vitamin D-containing complexes are present, one of which contains RXR. In nuclear extracts derived from the ROS 17/2.8 osteoblasts, a single VDR-dependent complex containing RXR is present. The negative $1,25(OH)_2D_3$ response element contains one copy of a motif that is duplicated in the mouse osteopontin gene, a gene that is upregulated by $1,25(OH)_2D_3$. When the osteocalcin vitamin D response element is utilized as a probe, only VDR-RXR-containing complexes are generated from the nuclear extracts of all three cell types. This series of experiments indicates that transcriptional repression in response to $1,25(OH)_2D_3$ differs from the upregulatory response elements in sequence composition and in the ability to bind VDR independent of RXR [17].

An additional mechanism by which $1,25(OH)_2D_3$ may regulate PTH gene expression is through alterations in the $1,25(OH)_2D_3$ receptor. Modulation of the concentration of the $1,25(OH)_2D_3$ receptor may alter the effect of $1,25(OH)_2D_3$ at its target sites. The administration of $1,25(OH)_2D_3$ to rats resulted in an increase in $1,25(OH)_2D_3$ receptors in parathyroid tissue with a concomitant decrease in PTH mRNA [18]. In another study, weanling rats fed a calcium-deficient diet became markedly hypocalcemic and had high serum levels of $1,25(OH)_2D_3$. There was no change in $1,25(OH)_2D_3$ receptor mRNA levels in spite of the high levels of $1,25(OH)_2D_3$ and, furthermore, PTH mRNA levels were increased [19]. The low serum calcium levels may prevent the increase in parathyroid $1,25(OH)_2D_3$ receptor levels and the suppression of PTH mRNA levels. These finding have been confirmed in an avian model [20] and in vitamin D-deficient rats [21].

The use of calcitriol analogs that are biologically active but result in less hypercalcemia also helped to separate the effects of calcium from the actions of vitamin D on PTH gene expression. Detailed dose response curves suggest that $1,25(OH)_2D_3$ is the most effective analog to inhibit PTH levels *in vivo*. The ability of $1,25(OH)_2D_3$ to decrease PTH gene expression is a significant therapeutic management tool for patients at risk of developing secondary hyperparathyroidism.

C. Phosphate as a Modulator of PTH Gene Expression

PTH has a potent effect on the tubular reabsorption of phosphate by the kidney. This observation has been utilized as a clinical test to evaluate target organ resistance to parathyroid hormone. In severe renal failure, the hyperphosphatemia that occurs results in secondary hyperparathyroidism. Clinically, the effects of the associated hypocalcemia and the decrease in serum levels of $1,25(OH)_2D_3$ have complicated our understanding of the role of phosphate on PTH secretion. Slatopolsky and Bricker [22] showed that in experimental renal failure, restriction of dietary phosphate prevented secondary hyperparathyroidism. Clinical studies confirmed the utility of restricting oral phosphate intake. These initial *in vitro* and *in vivo* studies suggested that phosphate directly alters the production of $1,25(OH)_2D_3$. A series of elegant, carefully designed studies revealed that the effect of phosphate on PTH was independent of serum calcium and $1,25(OH)_2D_3$ levels. Uremic dogs were placed on diets deficient in both calcium and phosphate, resulting in lower levels of serum phosphate and calcium and no change in the concentration of $1,25(OH)_2D_3$ (Fig. 4) [23]. In hypophosphatemic rats, phosphate regulated the PTH gene independent of the effects of phosphate on calcium and $1,25(OH)_2D_3$ [18]. This series of elegant studies indicated that phosphate regulated expression of PTH in a hypophosphatemic, normocalcemic model in the presence of normal levels of $1,25(OH)_2D_3$. Nuclear transcript run-on assays showed that the decrease in PTH mRNA due to low phosphate was posttranscriptional, in contrast to the transcriptional effects of $1,25(OH)_2D_3$ on the PTH gene. Protein-mRNA binding studies in hypophosphatemic rats have revealed decreased binding of PTH cytosolic proteins. Confirmation of the functional role was provided with an *in vitro* degradation assay. The length of time that an intact transcript was present was reduced from 40 minutes in parathyroid proteins obtained from control rats to 5 minutes in the proteins from hypophosphatemic animals. In contrast, parathyroid proteins from hypocalcemic rats had increased binding, and intact transcripts were present for a longer time (180 minutes). The study also indicated that degradation of PTH mRNA depends on sequences in the $3'$-UTR region [24]. In human parathyroid tissue, high phosphate directly stimulated PTH secretion and PTH mRNA levels [25].

D. Other Regulators of PTH Gene Expression

Other circulating factors besides calcium, $1,25(OH)_2D_3$, and phosphate may modulate PTH gene transcription. A cAMP response element on the PTH gene suggests that hormones that stimulate adenylate cyclase activity may increase PTH gene transcription. Another potential regulator are glucocorticoids; they increase mRNA levels in dispersed, hyperplastic human parathyroid cells [26] and they attenuate the decrease in PTH mRNA in response to $1,25(OH)_2D_3$ in dispersed bovine parathyroid cells [27].

Other intracellular signaling mechanisms are capable of PTH gene regulation. Protein kinases A and C regulate PTH mRNA *in vitro* in dispersed bovine parathyroid cells [28, 29]. Inhibition of levels of protein kinase C by the addition of staurosporine or a phorbol ester resulted in decreased levels of PTH mRNA; stimulators of protein kinase A increased PTH mRNA levels. The physiological relevance of the role of intracellular second messengers in the minute-to-minute control of calcium homeostasis remains to be resolved.

Estrogen is thought to play a role in the regulation of PTH gene expression due to the proposed roles of PTH in the pathophysiology of postmenopausal osteoporosis. In primary cultures of bovine parathyroid cells, estrogen increases the secretion of PTH. Rat parathyroid glands contain receptors for estrogen and in ovariectomized rats, estradiol administration increases PTH mRNA [30]. Progesterone has also been demonstrated to enhance secretion of PTH and synthesis of PTH mRNA in cell culture. The addition of 19-nor progestin R5020 to ovariectomized rats resulted in a two-fold increase in PTH mRNA [31]. In the rat, PTH mRNA levels were increased in the proestrus and estrus phase, suggesting alteration of PTH gene expression in response to the rat estrus cycle.

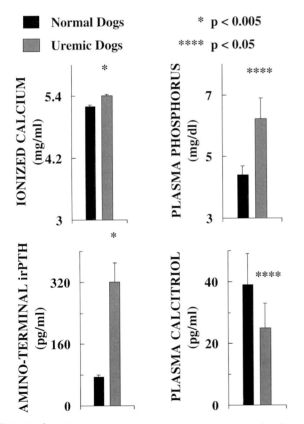

FIGURE 4 Effects of uremia on plasma ionized calcium, phosphorus, NH_2-terminal immunoreactive parathyroid hormone, and calcitriol. Dogs were rendered uremic by ligation of all but one of the terminal branches of the left renal artery followed by right contralateral nephrectomy. Paired t-test was used to quantitative statistical differences. Reprinted from Lopez-Hilker *et al.* [23], with permission.

V. BIOSYNTHESIS OF PARATHYROID HORMONE

Parathyroid hormone is synthesized in the parathyroid cell as a 115-amino acid single-chain polypeptide termed "pre-proparathyroid hormone." The "pre" sequence is the "leader" or "signal" sequence and is identical to signal sequences associated with other polypeptide hormones. The "preproPTH" sequences are known for human, rat, bovine, pig, and chicken. All have in common the 25-residue "pre" and 6-residue "pro" sequences. The pre sequence contains a hydrophobic stretch of amino acids preceded by a positively charged residue. The signal sequence is cleaved from the amino terminus during the process of synthesis. The signal sequence binds to a signal recognition particle (SRP), which is an intracellular RNA–protein complex that recognizes the signal sequence. The SRP binds to a receptor on the rough endoplasmic reticulum and directs preproPTH to a protein-lined channel, thereby "docking" the protein. A signal peptidase on the inner surface of the endoplasmic reticulum cleaves the signal sequence. The resultant peptide, "proparathyroid hormone," is left in the cisternae of the endoplasmic reticulum. The pro region is a highly positively charged hexapeptide and its cleavage is necessary to initiate biological activity of the hormone [32]. Packaged into vesicles, proPTH progresses to the Golgi apparatus where the amino-terminal pro sequences are removed by the proprotein convertase furin [33]. PTH is concentrated into dense core secretory vesicles which fuse with the plasma membrane to release the contents in response to a decrease in extracellular calcium concentration.

VI. METABOLISM OF PARATHYROID HORMONE

Proteolysis of newly synthesized PTH is influenced by extracellular calcium [34, 35]. Most of the hormone secreted under conditions of hypercalcemia is already fragmented, whereas in the case of hypocalcemia, the secreted molecule tends to be intact and active. Variable extracellular calcium provides a dynamic regulatory mechanism which is similar to mechanisms in proteolytic cleavage of the stored hormone.

Intact PTH is rapidly cleared from the circulation with a half-life of approximately two minutes [36]. The liver plays the dominant role in PTH metabolism, removing 60–70% of the hormone. The kidney removes 20–30% by glomerular filtration. Uptake by other cells (such as bone cells) accounts for a minor component. Clearance by the liver is under the direction of the high capacity, nonsaturable Kupffer cells when PTH undergoes extensive proteolysis [37].

PTH is not only rapidly cleared from the circulation, but it is also rapidly cleaved by endoproteases, resulting in a series of carboxy-terminal fragments that are in the circula-

tion. Carboxy-terminal fragments make up 50–90% of the total circulating PTH immunoactivity in spite of the fact that quantitatively, only 10–20% of secreted intact PTH is converted to circulating carboxy-terminal fragments. This is because clearance of these fragments is limited by glomerular filtration mechanisms in the kidney. In renal insufficiency, large amounts of carboxy-terminal fragments are found in the circulation. The major secretory form of PTH is the 84-amino acid peptide.

VII. RECEPTOR INTERACTIONS OF PARATHYROID HORMONE AND PARATHYROID HORMONE-RELATED PROTEIN

The discovery that PTH and PTHrP share a common receptor has generated additional information about the structure-function relationship of these two peptides. The gene for PTHrP is located on chromosome 12, but it is thought that PTH and PTHrP share a common ancestral gene [38]. There is strong homology in the first half of the active amino-terminal core of PTH and PTHrP in that eight of the first 13 amino acid residues are identical. The remainder of the first 34 amino acids differs in sequence and in spite of limited homology between the two peptides, PTH and PTHrP share a common receptor in various tissues. In the nonhomologous 14–34 portions, substantial three-dimensional structure is shared between the two peptides and may explain the ability to bind to a common receptor [39–41]. PTHrP is synthesized in adult and fetal tissue and mediates several paracrine/autocrine functions (see Chapter 14).

The physicochemical properties of PTH receptors have been partially characterized with affinity cross-linking PTH ligands and solubilization of the receptor [42]. Biological properties of PTH and PTHrP have further defined the important residues in the ligand and allowed creation of analogs that can modify the activity of the receptor. Comparisons of the binding affinity for PTH(1–34) and PTHrP (1–36) revealed that the same receptor bound both ligands with equal affinity in opposum kidney cells [43]. The human PTH receptor binds both PTH and PTHrP but binds PTH preferentially [44]. Diversity exists in the receptor mRNAs of different lengths that encode the PTH receptor in several tissues and organs, suggesting that certain receptors may specifically bind the carboxy-terminal portions of the PTH molecule.

VIII. STRUCTURE OF THE PTH/PTHrP (PTH1R) RECEPTOR

cDNAs encoding the PTH/PTHrP receptors predicted that they would have topographical features in common with other G-protein-coupled receptors. The PTH/PTHrP receptors have an amino-terminal extracellular sequence, three extracellular loops, three intracellular loops, and a carboxy-terminal cytoplasmic region. The hydrophilic regions are linked by seven relatively hydrophobic membrane-spanning helices. The PTH/PTHrP receptors from different species are highly homologous; rat and mouse PTH/PTHrP receptors are 99% identical at the amino acid level and human and rat PTH/PTHrP receptors are 91% identical. The greatest amino acid differences are limited to discrete areas in the first extracellular loop and to the carboxy-terminal sequences. Renal and bone receptors are identical within each species suggesting that the same receptor transcript is present in the two traditional target tissues [44].

In all G-protein-coupled receptors, the following cascade is initiated by the binding of agonist to the receptor. The agonist-occupied receptor activates a G coupling protein. Guanosine diphosphate (GDP) bound in the inactive state to the alpha subunit of the G protein is exchanged for guanosine triphosphate (GTP). The alpha subunit dissociates from the beta-gamma subunits and activation of an effector system by the GTP-occupied Gα-subunit occurs. The classical actions of PTH are mediated by the activation of the stimulatory G protein which enhances the action of adenylyl cyclase. Stimulation of the PTH/PTHrP receptor results in activation of other intracellular mechanisms including phospholipase C and acceleration of inositol phosphate hydrolysis. PTH promotes calcium entry into cells by direct stimulation of phospholipase A2.

The membrane-spanning helices of the PTH/PTHrP receptors are strongly conserved across species and serve a vital role in the signal transduction across the membrane. Studies that utilized mutant or chimeric receptors have generated information about the importance of several domains in the PTH/PTHrP receptors responsible for ligand binding, G-protein binding, and receptor activation. The PTH/PTHrP receptor is capable of stimulating multiple second messenger pathways. In stably transfected LLC-PK1 porcine cells expressing rat or oppossum PTH/PTHrP, receptors exhibited high affinity binding of PTH, dose-dependent activation of cyclic AMP, and release of intracellular calcium. The EC_{50} of the cyclic AMP response was 20- to 50-fold lower than the intracellular calcium response. PTH also altered cell proliferation which was mimicked by the addition of forskolin, phorbol esters, calcium ionophores, and cAMP analogs. The effect on phosphate transport was only seen when a phorbol ester was added [45]. These data suggest that activation of multiple intracellular pathways is possible with a single ligand. Scanning mutagenetic techniques of the intracellular regions of the receptor have provided evidence for the roles of various intracellular regions critical for receptor activation, receptor-ligand binding, and activation of various second messengers. For example, activation of phospholipase C requires one of the intracellular loops. Mutation of residues in the N-terminal region of the third intracellular loop of the opossum PTH/PTHrP receptor and expression in COS-7 cells results in normal binding of ligand but impaired adenylyl cyclase and phospholipase C activation. These data suggest that the N-terminal region of the third intracellular loop plays a critical role in the coupling of G_s- and G_q-mediated second messenger systems [46].

One of the most interesting and provocative studies regarding the structure-function relationship between receptors and ligands is evaluation of the cavity formed by the receptor into which the ligands fit. Specific amino acids residues are responsible for optimal ligand binding and signal transduction. The polypeptides secretin and parathyroid hormone were used as models of two ligands with no sequence homology and no cross reactivity with the other's receptor. Mutation of a single amino acid in the second transmembrane domain of the secretin receptor to the corresponding amino acid in the PTH receptor resulted in a receptor that could bind and transmit the intracellular signals effected by PTH. The reciprocal mutation in the PTH receptor conferred responsiveness to secretin in a similar manner. Thus, the transmembrane residues on receptors recognize a specific ligand and restrict the access and activation of inappropriate ligands [47].

IX. ACTIVATION OF THE CYCLIC ADENOSINE MONOPHOSPHATE SECOND MESSENGER SYSTEM BY PARATHYROID HORMONE

Parathyroid hormone was one of the first hormones shown to utilize the cAMP second messenger system. In the kidney, cAMP is involved in PTH-mediated effects to reduce calcium excretion, enhance tubular reabsorption of phosphate, and stimulate $1,25(OH)_2D_3$ formation. Cyclic AMP is also believed to be the mediator of many of the actions of PTH on bone (Fig. 5) [48, 49]. Clinical evidence indicates the important role of cAMP in the mediation of the effects of PTH. Patients suffering from a hereditary syndrome of PTH resistance, pseudohypoparathyroidism type 1, do not respond to exogenously administered PTH with an increase in urinary cAMP [50].

The full length 84-amino acid polypeptide is not required for activation of adenylyl cyclase. PTH(1–34) is as potent as the intact molecule. Carboxy-terminal fragments are inactive and progressive loss in adenylyl cyclase-stimulating activity occurs with the stepwise deletion of amino acids from the amino-terminal end of PTH(1–34) [51]. PTH(1–25) is also inactive, suggesting that the 25–34 positions are important for the binding of PTH to its receptor. Stepwise removal of the amino acids from the amino-terminal end of the molecule rapidly reduces the adenylyl cyclase-stimulating properties such that PTH(2–34) is a very weak stimulator. Further truncation leads to analogs that are competitively inhibitory, such as PTH(7–34).

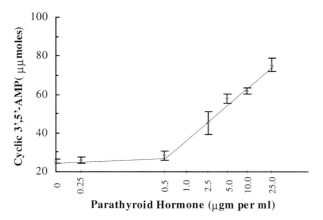

FIGURE 5   Calvaria were removed from fetal Sprague-Dawley rats and particulate suspension prepared. PTH was added at the concentrations noted and adenyl cyclase assayed by measuring the conversion of ATP-α-^{32}P to 3',5'-AM^{32}P. Reprinted with permission from Chase, L. R., *et al.* [49] (1969). Activation of skeletal adenyl cyclase by parathyroid hormone in vitro. *Endocrinology* **84**, 761–768, © The Endocrine Society.

X. ACTIVATION OF CALCIUM AND INOSITOL PHOSPHATES BY PARATHYROID HORMONE

Studies indicating that PTH can increase intracellular calcium levels without changing levels of intracellular cAMP have produced evidence for the activation of messenger systems that alter cytosolic calcium concentrations. Phosphatidylinositols are present in minute quantities in the plasma membrane of cells. Phosphatidylinositol (PI) kinases phosphorylate PI to phosphatidylinositol 4-phosphate and then to phosphatidylinositol 4,5-phosphate (PIP2). These PIs are substrates for a family of enzymes, designated phospholipase C, which hydrolyze PIs, resulting in a series of products known as inositol phosphates (IPs). For each IP formed, diacyglycerol and its metabolites also act as second messengers within the cell.

Although PIP2 is present in low concentrations within the cell, it is preferentially hydrolyzed to Ins(1,4,5)P$_3$ by phospholipase C in response to agonists such as PTH. Ins(1,4,5)P$_3$ binds to specific receptors and mediates the release of calcium from intracellular stores [52, 53].

XI. IDENTIFICATION OF A SECOND PTH RECEPTOR

Another PTH receptor, designated PTH2R, has been identified (Fig. 6). This receptor differs substantially from the PTH/PTHrP receptor (also designated PTH1R) in that the PTH2R responds only to PTH as a ligand. Selectivity of the receptors for PTH and PTH/PTHrP has been explored.

In order to determine the domains of the PTH receptor responsible for binding PTHrP, PTH1R, and PTH2R, chimeras were generated in which the extracellular amino-terminal domains were exchanged. In cells expressing the PTH2R with the PTH1R amino terminus, the cAMP response to PTH or PTHrP was identical. Mutations to the PTH1R sequence were made in each of the seven transmembrane spanning domains. Mutations in the transmembrane domains 3 and 7 resulted in receptors unable to respond to PTHrP [54]. In the ligand itself, position 23 (Trp in PTH and Phe in PTHrP) determines binding selectivity and position 5 (Ile in PTH and His in PTHrP) is responsible for signaling selectivity. To determine the site in the PTH2R that discriminates between the two residues at site 5, PTH2R and PTH1R chimeras were constructed, expressed in COS-7 cells, and tested for their response to cAMP. Two single residues in the membrane spanning/loop region of the receptor determine signaling selectively: Ile244 at the extracellular end of the transmembrane helix 3 and Try318 at the carboxy-terminal portion of extracellular loop 2 [55].

XII. PHYSIOLOGICAL ACTIONS OF PTH

A. Catabolic Actions of PTH at the Cellular Level

The complexity of the skeleton with its many components has made evaluation of the cellular effects of PTH a challenge to understand. Both *in vivo* and *in vitro* approaches have been utilized. With *in vitro* studies, the usual physiological milieu is lacking and potentially important intercommunication among various cells as well as cytokines/growth factor interactions in response to PTH may be missed. With *in vivo* experiments, such interactions among cell types can be appreciated but it is difficult to assign a particular event with a specific cell. Thus, both kinds of studies are needed for optimal insight into the mechanism of PTH action in bone.

Because PTH can be catabolic to bone, it is reasonable to focus on the osteoclast. However, the osteoclast is relatively inaccessible for direct studies. Our understanding of the catabolic actions of PTH is further diminished by the fact that osteoclasts do not respond directly to PTH. They do not contain receptors for PTH, and hence, all interactions appear to be the result of direct effects on the osteoblast [56]. When osteoblasts are stimulated by PTH, it is believed that the subsequent generation of factor or factors results in stimulation of osteoclast function and numbers [57, 58].

The initial rapid response to PTH involves the cells lining the endosteal surface of bone [59]. This rapid response (less than 1 hour), which results in the release of calcium into the circulation, is an important regulatory mechanism for the

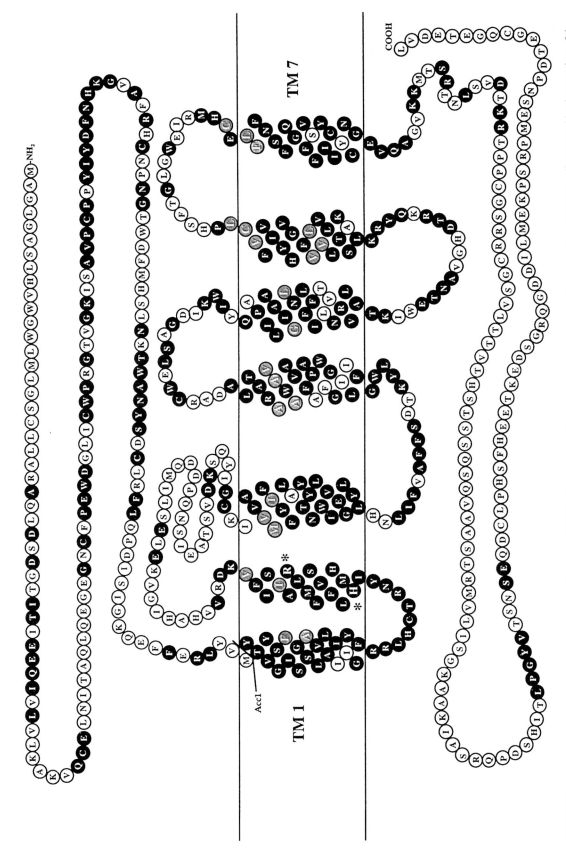

FIGURE 6 Primary sequence and typological structure of the human PTH2R. The seven putative transmembrane-spanning regions are indicated based on alignment with other members of the secretin/PTH receptor subfamily. Conserved residues with the opossum kidney PTH1R are indicated by the black circles. Reprinted from Turner *et al.* [54], with permission.

quick correction of hypocalcemia. This initial phase of PTH activity is associated with increased metabolic activity of the osteoclast. This process does not require new protein synthesis. A second phase of calcium mobilization which is dependent on protein synthesis occurs approximately 24 hours later. This second phase results in an increase in the number and activity of osteoclasts.

Current concepts attribute such indirect actions on the osteoclast to direct effects on the osteoblast. Incubation of osteoclasts with osteoblast-like cells results in osteoclast activation. Osteoblasts and adjacent bone marrow stromal cells contain PTH/PTHrP receptors. The increased number and activity of osteoclasts [60] may also be mediated through cells of the osteoblast lineage such as lining cells [56]. Several clonal, conditionally immortalized PTH-responsive, bone marrow stromal cell lines derived from mouse marrow were shown to support formation of tartrate-resistant acid phosphatase-positive multinucleated cells in response to PTH. These multinucleated cells contained calcitonin receptors and formed resorption lacunae on dentine slices, which are characteristics consistent with the osteoclast pheno type [61].

The precise mechanism by which PTH stimulates the osteoclast to activate bone resorption remains unknown. Many different enzymes or other factors are released by PTH. They include collagenase, lysosomal hydroxylase, acid phosphatases, carbonic anhydrase, H^+-K^+-ATPases, Na^+-Ca^{2+} exchange systems, cathepsin B, and cysteine proteases. An acidic environment, essential for the protonation of the alkaline salt hydroxyapatite, is formed by the osteoclast when it seals by podosomes the area between the osteoclast membrane and the mineralized surface. Several enzymes are present at this site, such as H^+, K^+-ATPase. Omeprozole blocks this proton pump resulting in inhibition of PTH-mediated bone resorption [62]. Carbonic anhydrase, also activated by PTH, generates hydrogen ion for H^+-K^+-ATPase activity. PTH-mediated bone resorption is attenuated by inhibition of carbonic anhydrase [63]. Amiloride and its analog, $3'4'$-dichlorobenzamil (DCB), affect calcium transport systems such as ATP-dependent calcium pumps. These compounds inhibit PTH-induced bone resorption in neonatal mouse calvaria [64]. The mechanism of bone resorption remains controversial, however, as other studies suggest that PTH is not required for the buffering of protons in neonatal mouse calvaria [65].

The hypothetical construct suggests that PTH induces catabolic activation in the osteoblast that in turn influences the osteoclast. PTH induces the production of plasmin-metalloproteinases such as tissue-type plasminogen activator (tPA) which may initiate bone resorption via breakdown of the extracellular matrix. In neonatal rat osteoblast cell cultures, bovine PTH (1–34) increases tPA by approximately 6- to 8-fold. After induction of osteoblast differentiation with 1,25-dihydroxyvitamin D3, PTH has no effect on tPA

[66]. Other catabolic actions of PTH in the osteoblast include stimulation of hyaluronase synthesis [67] and induction of collagenase-3 gene transcription [68].

B. Anabolic Actions of PTH at the Cellular Level

The multiple anabolic actions of PTH on the skeleton are due directly to its effects on osteoblasts which contain receptors for PTH.

PTH induces the retraction of preosteoblasts from the bone surface through a calcium-dependent, proteolytic modification of the cytoskeleton. Regulation of cell attachment via regulation of E-cadherins [69] might be a mechanism by which PTH leads to an increase in osteoblast number. PTH may also be mitogenic for bone cells *in vivo* [70]. The role of PTH in the differentiation of osteoblasts was evaluated in a bone morphogeneic protein (BMP)-dependent system using a mesenchymal progenitor cell (C3H10T1/2). Constitutive expression of the PTH/PTHrP receptor resulted in stimulation of osteogenic development. PTH(1–34) stimulated the early and suppressed the late stages of osteogenic development. The effect appeared to be mediated by a cAMP signaling cascade. Other PTH peptides such as PTH(28–48) or PTH(53–84) did not result in significant responses.

Parathyroid hormone enhances collagenase synthesis, inhibits type I collagen synthesis, and reduces alkaline phosphatase activity in the osteoblast [71–73]. Studies have defined better the roles of carboxy-terminal fragments of PTH versus amino-terminal fragments in these effects. In the osteoblast-like cell line UMR-106, PTH(1–84) and PTH(1–34) inhibited cell proliferation and stimulated alkaline phosphatase activity; C-terminal fragments had no effect. Expression of type I procollagen was stimulated by PTH(35–84), PTH(53–84), and PTH(69–84), inhibited by PTH(1–34), and unaffected by PTH(1–84). These results suggest that the carboxy-terminal region of PTH may contain information in its sequence that influences bone formation [74].

The effects of PTH on 24-hydroxylase in osteoblasts in opposite to that in the kidney. In combination with 1,25-dihydroxyvitamin D3, PTH enhances mRNA levels of the 24-hydroxylase cytochrome P450 components. This synergism is in marked contrast to regulation of 24-hydroxylase in the kidney where PTH and 1,25-dihydroxyvitamin D have antagonistic effects [75].

Parathyroid hormone alters the nuclear matrix in osteoblasts. The rat type I collagen alpha 1(I) polypeptide chain (COL1A1) promoter confirmation is linked to cell structure via the nuclear matrix. Parathyroid hormone increased the binding of a soluble nuclear protein (NMP4) and decreased COL1A1 mRNA in osteosarcoma cells [76]. The same laboratory demonstrated that PTH can alter osteoblast gene expression via changes in the organization of the nuclear structural proteins [77].

XIII. CELL-TO-CELL COMMUNICATION: OSTEOBLASTS AND OSTEOCLASTS

Cell-to-cell communication is enhanced by parathyroid hormone. PTH enhances the formation of gap junctions in calvarial osteoblasts [78]. The enhancement of gap junctions, primarily composed of connexin 43 (Cx43), is due to an increased rate of Cx43 gene transcription caused by PTH. These results, shown for UMR-106 cells, vary when other osteoblast-like cells are studied. The differences may be due to the stage of differentiation of the particular cell model studied. PTH changes the level of Cx43 gene expression in proliferating and maturing osteoblasts but has little effect on nondividing, differentiated osteoblasts [79, 80].

The factors responsible for communication between cells of the osteoblast lineage and those that are osteoclast in nature are the subject of much interest and speculation. Utilizing a human osteosarcoma cell line, SaOS-2, Elias *et al.* [81] demonstrated that PTH stimulates production of IL-11 protein and mRNA. They proposed this cytokine as the link between the osteoblast and osteoclast. Other investigators have evaluated the effect of IGF-1 in mediating cell signaling between these two bone cells. In newborn rat calvaria, PTH stimulated the production of IGF-1 and IGFBP-3 at the message and peptide levels [82, 83]. Other studies have implicated PTH-induced production of prostaglandins by the osteoblast to induce bone resorption by the osteoclast. In primary cultures of human osteoblast-like cells, PTH has been shown to induce cyclooxygenase-2 gene expression resulting in prostaglandin E_2 production [84].

At the molecular level, the influence of PTH on c-fos gene expression in UMR-106 cells was explored [85]. Both PTH(1–34) and PTHrP(1–34) induced c-fos gene expression. Antisense oligonucleotides inhibited PTH-mediated cell proliferation in the osteoblast-like cells and also inhibited PTH-enhanced osteoclast-like cell formation. Those results suggest PTH might regulate bone formation and bone resorption by effects on c-fos gene expression.

XIV. PREFERENTIAL ACTIONS OF PTH AT SELECTED SKELETAL SITES

A. Animal Models

Many studies in animals and in humans have attempted to understand the basis of a selective effect of PTH on cortical bone for catabolic events and on cancellous bone for anabolic events. The effects of PTH on indices of bone formation such as bone mineral density are significantly increased after only 10 days, and biomechanical properties improved after 15 days in a rat model [86]. In another study, Wistar rats were given parathyroid hormone after ovariectomy. The entire skeleton showed an increase in bone mineral content during the period of administration of PTH and no effect of withdrawal was noted. The metaphysis was highly sensitive to PTH. The lumbar vertebrae and diaphysis had moderate changes in bone mass in response to PTH whereas the skull and caudal vertebral bodies were not responsive to PTH. After withdrawal of PTH, BMD decreased markedly at the sites that were initially responsive to PTH; readministration of PTH resulted in accretion of BMD at PTH sensitive sites [87]. Weekly administration of PTH to ovariectomized rats effectively stimulated bone formation in both the cancellous and cortical compartments, suggesting that administration may not have to be as frequent as originally planned in the initial studies in humans [88].

An ovariectomized rat model was utilized to test the effect of analogs of human PTH(1–34) that differ from the native sequence in their receptor-activating properties on promoting bone formation. Single substitutions for serine in the 3-position resulted in peptides that were partial agonists in the kidney. Cancellous bone volume was significantly lower in the vehicle-treated group of animals and none of the compounds altered cancellous bone volume. All three peptides produced marked dose-related increases in bone formation rates but the two analogs were less potent than hPTH(1–34). All three peptides produced dose-related increases in osteocalcin. Bone resorption markers had variable effects: pyridinoline cross-link excretion was altered by treatment with hPTH(1–34), but the analog [His]hPTH(1–34) caused a dose-dependent decrease in this parameter of bone resorption [89].

Evidence exists for the role of PTH in the responsiveness of the skeleton to mechanical stress [90]. PTH increased the mechanical strength of the femur diaphysis in aged rats. In normal rats, mechanical stimulation of the caudal vertebra induced an osteogenic response. In the absence of PTH, this response was attenuated but was restored by a single injection of PTH before loading. The expression of c-fos in the osteocytes was detectable only in rats receiving both PTH and mechanical stimulation [91].

One of the most informative models regarding the effect of PTH on the skeleton is a mouse model in which the genes encoding the PTH/PTH-receptor peptide have been ablated by homologous recombination. These mice have skeletal dysplasia due to accelerated endochondral bone formation and die at birth or in utero. The targeted expression of constitutively active PTH/PTHrP receptors result in delayed mineralization, decelerated conversion of proliferative chondrocytes into hypertrophic cells, and delayed vascular invasion [92].

B. Human Studies

Several informative studies that address the effect of PTH on bone markers in human subjects were performed in patients with primary or secondary hyperparathyroidism. For a complete description of studies in patients with primary hyperparathyroidism, see Chapter 41. In a group of patients with secondary hyperparathyroidism and hypovitaminosis D, treatment with either cholecalciferol or calcitriol resulted in a lowering of N-telopeptide excretion [93]. In a small group of patients with prostate cancer, the excessive bone formation that can occur in metastatic disease results in hypocalcemia and subsequent stimulation of PTH in response to the calcium demand. In these patients, serum bone alkaline phosphatase and urinary levels of bone collagen are markedly elevated. Infusion of the bisphosphonate pamidronate significantly decreased serum levels of calcium, phosphate, bone alkaline phosphatase, and urinary markers of bone resorption [94]. In patients with primary hyperparathyroidism, or in normal volunteers receiving infusions of PTH(1–38), serum ICTP (C-terminal of type I collagen) was elevated and serum PICP (the carboxy-terminal propeptide of type I collagen) was decreased [95].

Baseline values of bone turnover, which included osteocalcin and urinary deoxypyridinoline and pyridinoline cross-link excretion, were higher in a group of postmenopausal osteoporotic women in spite of decreased serum PTH levels as compared to normal postmenopausal women. Calcium deprivation resulted in similar changes in serum levels of calcium, PTH, $1,25(OH)_2D_3$, and pyridinoline and deoxypyridinoline cross-link excretion. Serum osteocalcin increased and serum procollagen carboxy-terminal propeptide decreased in normal women who were calcium deprived, but marker levels were not altered in the postmenopausal osteoporotic group. These data suggest that there is not a difference in the skeletal responsiveness to PTH in patients with osteoporosis [96].

To determine the role of PTH in age-related and nocturnal increases in bone resorption, calcium infusion was utilized to suppress endogenous PTH secretion in young and elderly normal women. Serum PTH and urinary cross-linked N-telopeptide of type I collagen (NTX) were circadian in pattern. Peak levels of PTH occurred in the midafternoon and at night, and a rise in urinary NTX was found at night. At baseline, levels of urinary NTX were higher in the elderly compared to the young women. Calcium infusion reduced the PTH peaks but did not alter the nocturnal increase in urinary NTX excretion. The authors suggest that PTH is responsible for the age-related increase in bone resorption but that it does not mediate the circadian pattern of bone resorption [97]. In contrast, administration of recombinant PTH(1–84) to healthy postmenopausal women resulted in no change in urinary deoxypyrridinoline although urinary cAMP excretion was appropriately elevated in response to PTH administration [98].

Racial differences exist in the incidence of hip and vertebral fractures: Afro-American women have a lower incidence of fracture at these sites compared to Caucasian women. One possible mechanism is a difference in the sensitivity of the skeleton to PTH. Cosman and colleagues [99] infused PTH(1–34) in healthy premenopausal black and white women and measured indices of bone turnover. Baseline levels of $1,25(OH)_2D_3$ were significantly lower in black women. There were trends toward higher PTH and lower urinary calcium and pyridinoline levels in this group. No differences in serum calcium or endogenous levels of PTH were noted among the groups during PTH infusion. Black women had lower levels of urinary calcium during the PTH infusion and no differences were detected in bone formation markers among black and white women. Marked differences were noted in markers of bone resorption. Cross-linked N-telopeptide, cross-linked C-telopeptide, and free pyridinoline were much more elevated in white subjects as compared to blacks. These findings suggest that black women have decreased sensitivity to PTH and may be an explanation for the relative preservation of skeletal tissue in black women [99].

In postmenopausal women receiving estrogen replacement therapy, daily administration of PTH(1–34) (400 units/d) over a 3 year period resulted in a continuous increase in bone mineral density compared to no increase in the estrogen-treatment only control group (Fig. 7). The increase in vertebral BMD was 13% while the increase at the hip was less at 2.7%; no loss of bone was noted at any skeletal site tested. Serum osteocalcin measurements were increased 55% during the first six months of treatment while a marker of bone resorption, excretion of crosslinked N-telopeptide, increased by only 20% [101]. These changes were interpreted to be due to an uncoupling of the bone formation-resorption cycle and the differences fell toward baseline during the study progression.

Using a somewhat different experimental design, Hodsman *et al.* studied a group of 30 osteoporotic postmenopausal women with cyclical parathyroid hormone [101]. Over a 2-year period, 800 units of PTH(1–34) was administered 1 month out of 3. Immediately following each cycle of PTH, patients received either calcitonin or placebo. There was a highly significant 10.2% increase in vertebral bone density after 2 years with or without the additional use of calcitonin. In the PTH only arm, there was a 2.4% increase in femoral neck bone mass (Fig. 7). These data suggest that PTH has potent anabolic effects on the human skeleton.

In a randomized, double-blind, placebo controlled trial of idiopathic osteoporosis in men, the effect of administration of parathyroid hormone was evaluated on markers of bone turnover. Bone formation markers, which included osteocalcin, carboxy-terminal propeptide of type I collagen, and bone-specific alkaline phosphatase, increased in the PTH-treated group. The carboxy-terminal propeptide of type I collagen peaked at 67% above baseline at 6 months and bone-specific alkaline phosphatase peaked at 169% above baseline at 9 months. Osteocalcin was highest (230%) at 1 year. PTH administration also dramatically altered bone resorption markers. Pyridinoline was 131% above baseline at 9 months

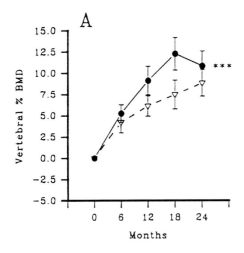

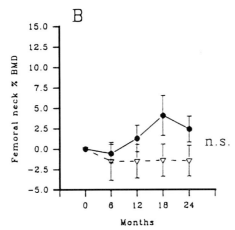

FIGURE 7   Randomized study of cyclical PTH in postmenopausal women with osteoporosis. The results are shown for vertebral (A) or femoral neck (B) bone density. PTH was administered 1 month every 3 months for 2 years. Calcitonin (open symbols) or placebo (closed symbols) followed PTH each cycle for 42 days. The two arms PTH with or without calcitonin were not different from each other. The asterisks indicate a significant change from baseline, $p < 0.001$. Reproduced with permission [101].

and urinary N-telopeptide was 375% above baseline at 1 year. The relationship between pyridinoline and markers of bone formation were highly correlated in the PTH-treated group but not in the control group. Elevations in bone formation markers were consistent with a 13.5% increase in bone mass in the PTH-treated group at 18 months. Pyridinoline was the best predictor of response to treatment. Parathyroid hormone is the potent stimulator of bone turnover even in men with idiopathic low turnover osteoporosis [102].

References

1. Miric, A., and Levine, M. A. (1992). Analysis of the preproPTH gene by denaturing gradient gel electrophoresis in familial isolated hypoparathyroidism. *J. Clin. Endocrinol. Metab.* **74**, 509–516.

2. Kronenberg, H. M., Igarashi, T., Freeman, M. W., Okazaki, T., Brand, S. J., Wiren, K. M., and Potts, J. T., Jr. (1986). Structure and expression of the human parathyroid hormone gene. *Recent Prog. Horm. Res.* **42**, 641–663.

2a. Chorev, M., and Rosenblatt, M. (1996). "Principles of Bone Biology," (J. Bilezikian, ed.), p.1411. Academic Press, New York.

3. Demay, M. B., Kiernan, M. S., DeLuca, H. F., and Kronenberg, H. M. (1992). Sequences in the human parathyroid hormone gene that bind the 1,25-dihydroxyvitamin D3 receptor and mediate transcriptional repression in response to 1,25-dihydroxyvitamin D3. *Proc. Natl. Acad. Sci. U.S.A.* **89**, 8097–8101.

4. Antonarakis, S. E., Phillips, J. A., Mallonee, R. L., Kazazian, H. H. J., Fearon, E. R., Waber, P. G., Kronenberg, H. M., Ullrich, A., and Meyers, D. A. (1983). Beta-globin locus is linked to the parathyroid hormone (PTH) locus and lies between the insulin and PTH loci in man. *Proc. Natl. Acad. Sci. U.S.A.* **80**, 6615–6619.

5. Mayer, H., Breyel, E., Bostock, C., and Schmidtke, J. (1983). Assignment of the human parathyroid hormone gene to chromosome 11. *Hum. Genet.* **64**, 283–285.

6. Zabel, B. U., Kronenberg, H. M., Bell, G. I., and Shows, T. B. (1985). Chromosome mapping of genes on the short arm of human chromosome 11: Parathyroid hormone gene is at 11p15 together with the genes for insulin, c-Harvey-*ras* 1, and beta-hemoglobin. *Cytogenet. Cell Genet.* **39**, 200–205.

7. Russell, J., Lettieri, D., and Sherwood, L. M. (1983). Direct regulation of calcium of cytoplasmic messenger ribonucleic acid coding for pre-proparathyroid hormone in isolated bovine parathyroid cells. *J. Clin. Invest.* **72**, 1851–1855.

8. Naveh-Many, T., Friedlander, M. M., Mayer, H., and Silver, J. (1989). Calcium regulates parathyroid hormone messenger ribonucleic acid (mRNA), but not calcitonin mRNA in vivo in the rat. Dominant role of 1,25-dihydroxyvitamin D. *Endocrinology* **125**, 275–280.

9. Okazaki, T., Zajac, J. D., Igarashi, T., Ogata, E., and Kronenberg, H. M. (1991). Negative regulatory elements in the human parathyroid hormone gene. *J. Biol. Chem.* **266**, 21903–21910.

10. Moallem, E., Kilav, R., Silver, J., and Naveh-Many, T. (1998). RNA-protein binding and post-transcriptional regulation of parathyroid hormone gene expression by calcium and phosphatase. *J. Biol. Chem.* **273**, 5253–5259.

11. Hawa, N. S., O'Riordan, J. L., and Farrow, S. M. (1993). Post-transcriptional regulation of bovine parathyroid hormone synthesis. *J. Mol. Endocrinol.* **10**, 43–49.

12. Vadher, S., Hawa, N. S., O'Riordan, J. L., and Farrow, S. M. (1996). Translational regulation of parathyroid hormone gene expression and RNA: Protein interactions. *J. Bone Miner. Res.* **11**, 746–753.

13. Silver, J., Russell, J., and Sherwood, L. M. (1985). Regulation by vitamin D metabolites of messenger ribonucleic acid for preproparathyroid hormone in isolated bovine parathyroid cells. *Proc. Natl. Acad. Sci. U.S.A.* **82**, 4270–4273.

14. Russell, J., Lettieri, D., and Sherwood, L. M. (1986). Suppression by 1,25-(OH)2D3 of transcription of the pre-proparathyroid hormone gene. *Endocrinology* **119**, 2864–2866.

15. Silver, J., Naveh-Many, T., Mayer, H., Schmelzer, H. J., and Popovtzer, M. M. (1986). Regulation by vitamin D metabolites of parathyroid hormone gene transcription *in vivo* in the rat. *J. Clin. Invest.* **78**, 1296–1301.

16. Okazaki, T., Igarashi, T., and Kronenberg, H. M. (1988). 5'-flanking region of the parathyroid hormone gene mediates negative regulation by 1,25-(OH)2 vitamin D3. *J. Biol. Chem.* **263**, 2203–2208.

17. Mackey, S. L., Heymont, J. L., Kronenberg, H. M., and Demay, M. B. (1996). Vitamin D receptor binding to the negative human parathyroid hormone vitamin D response element does not require the retinoid x receptor. *Mol. Endocrinol.* **10**, 298–305.

18. Kilav, R., Silver, J., Biber, J., Murer, H., and Naveh-Many, T. (1995). Coordinate regulation of the rat renal parathyroid hormone receptor mRNA and the Na-Pi cotransporter mRNA and protein. *Am. J. Physiol.* **268**, F1017-F1022.

19. Naveh-Many, T., Marx, R., Keshet, E., Pike, J. W., and Silver, J. (1990). Regulation of 1,25-dihydroxyvitamin D$_3$ receptor gene expression by 1,25-dihydroxyvitamin D$_3$ in the parathyroid in vivo. *J. Clin. Invest.* **86**, 1968–1975.

20. Russell, J., Bar, A., Sherwood, L. M., and Hurwitz, S. (1993). Interaction between calcium and 1,25-dihydroxyvitamin D3 in the regulation of preproparathyroid hormone and vitamin D receptor messenger ribonucleic acid in avian parathyroids. *Endocrinology* **132**, 2639–2644.

21. Brown, A. J., Zhong, M., Finch, J., Ritter, C., and Slatopolsky, E. (1995). The roles of calcium and 1,25-dihydroxyvitamin D3 in the regulation of vitamin D receptor expression by rat parathyroid glands. *Endocrinology* **136**, 1419–1425.

22. Slatopolsky, E., and Bricker, N. S. (1973). The role of phosphorus restriction in the prevention of secondary hyperparathyroidism in chronic renal disease. *Kidney Int.* **4**, 141–145.

23. Lopez-Hilker, S., Dusso, A. S., Rapp, N. S., Martin, K. J., and Slatopolsky, E. (1990). Phosphorus restriction reverses hyperparathyroidism in uremia independent of changes in calcium and calcitriol. *Am. J. Physiol.* **259**, F432–F437.

24. Moallem, E., Kilav, R., Silver, J., and Naveh-Many, T. (1998). RNA-Protein binding and post-transcriptional regulation of parathyroid hormone gene expression by calcium and phosphate. *J. Biol. Chem.* **273**, 5253–5259.

25. Almaden, Y., Hernandez, A., Torregrosa, V., Campistol, J., Torres, A., and Rodriguez, M. S. (1995). High phosphorous directly stimulates PTH secretion by human parathyroid tissue. *J. Am. Soc. Nephrol.* **6**, 957.

26. Peraldi, M. N., Rondeau, E., Jousset, V., el M'Selmi, A., Lacave, R., Delarue, F., Garel, J. M., and Sraer, J. D. (1990). Dexamethasone increases preproparathyroid hormone messenger RNA in human hyperplastic parathyroid cell in vitro. *Eur. J. Clin. Invest.* **20**, 392–397.

27. Karmali, R., Farrow, S., Hewison, M., Barker, S., and O'Riordan, J. L. H. (1989). Effects of 1,25-dihydroxyvitamin D$_3$ and cortisol on bovine and human parathyroid cells. *J. Endocrinol.* **123**, 137–142.

28. Moallem, E., Silver, J., and Naveh-Many, T. (1995). Regulation of parathyroid hormone messenger RNA levels by protein kinase A and C in bovine parathyroid cells. *J. Bone Miner. Res.* **10**, 447–452.

29. Clarke, B. L., Hassager, C., and Fitzpatrick, L. A. (1993). Regulation of parathyroid hormone release by protein kinase-C is dependent on extracellular calcium in bovine parathyroid cells. *Endocrinology* **132**, 1168–1175.

30. Naveh-Many, T., Almogi, G., Livni, N., and Silver, J. (1992). Estrogen receptors and biologic response in rat parathyroid tissue and C cells. *J. Clin. Invest.* **90**, 2434–2438.

31. Epstein, E., Silver, J., Almogi, G., Livni, N., and Naveh-Many, T. (1996). Parathryoid hormone mRNA levels are increased by progestins and vary during the rat estrous cycle. *Am. J. Physiol.* **33**, E158–E163.

32. Kronenberg, H. M., Bringhurst, F. R., Segré, G. V., and Potts, J. T., Jr. (1994). Parathyroid hormone biosynthesis and metabolism. *In* "The Parathyroids: Basic and Clinical Concepts" (J. P. Bilezikian, R. Marcus, and M. A. Levine, eds.), pp. 125–137. Raven Press, New York.

33. Lazure, C., Gauthier, D., Jean, F., Boudreault, A., Seidah, N. G., Bennett, H. P., and Hendy, G. N. (1998). In vitro cleavage of internally quenched fluorogenic human proparathyroid hormone and proparathyroid-related peptide substrates by furin. Generation of a potent inhibitor. *J. Biol. Chem.* **273**, 8572–8580.

34. Habener, J. F., Kemper, B., and Potts, J. T., Jr. (1975). Calcium-dependent intracellular degradation of parathyroid hormone: A possible mechanism for the regulation of hormone stores. *Endocrinology* **97**, 431–441.

35. Chu, L. L. H., MacGregor, R. R., Anast, C. S., Hamilton, J. W., and Cohn, D. V. (1973). Studies on the biosynthesis of rat parathyroid hormone and proparathyroid hormone: Adaptation of the parathyroid gland to dietary restriction of calcium. *Endocrinology* **93**, 915–924.

36. Bringhurst, F. R., Stern, A. M., Yotts, M., Mizrahi, N., Segré, G. V., and Potts, J. T., Jr. (1988). Peripheral metabolism of PTH: Fate of biologically active amino terminus in vivo. *Am. J. Physiol.* **255**, E886–E893.

37. Bringhurst, F. R., Segré, G. V., Lampman, G. W., and Potts, J. T., Jr. (1982). Metabolism of parathyroid hormone by Kupffer cells: Analysis by reverse-phase high-performance liquid chromatography. *Biochemistry* **21**, 4252–4258.

38. Yasuda, T., Banville, D., Hendy, G. N., and Goltzman, D. (1989). Characterization of the human parathyroid hormone-like peptide gene: Functional and evolutionary aspects. *J. Biol. Chem.* **264**, 7720–7725.

39. Caulfield, M. P., McKee, R. L., Goldman, M. E., Duong, L. T., Fisher, J. E., Gay, C. T., DeHaven, P. A., Levy, J. J., Roubini, E., Nutt, R. F., et al. (1990). The bovine renal parathyroid hormone (PTH) receptor has equal affinity for two different amino acid sequences: the receptor binding domains of PTH and PTH-related protein are located within the 14–34 region. *Endocrinology* **127**, 83–87.

40. Strewler, G. J., Stern, P. H., Jacobs, J. W., Eveloff, J., Klein, R. F., Leung, S. C., Rosenblatt, M., and Nissenson, R. A. (1987). Parathyroid hormone-like protein from human renal carcinoma cells. Structural and functional homology with parathyroid hormone. *J. Clin. Invest.* **80**, 1803–1807.

41. Suva, L. J., Winslow, G. A., Wettenhall, R. E., et al. (1987). A parathyroid hormone-related protein implicated in malignant hypercalcemia: Cloning and expression. *Science* **237**, 893–896.

42. Karpf, D. B., Arnaud, C. D., Bambino, T., Duffy, D., King, K. L., Winer, J., and Nissenson, R. A. (1988). Structure properties of the renal parathyroid hormone receptor: hydrodynamic analysis and protease sensitivity. *Endocrinology* **123**, 2611–2619.

43. Jüppner, H., Abou-Samra, A. B., Freeman, M., Kong, X. F., Schipani, E., Richards, J., Kolakowski, L. F., Jr., Hock, J., Potts, J. T., Jr., Kronenberg, H. M., et al. (1991). A G protein-linked receptor for parathyroid hormone and parathyroid hormone-related peptide. *Science* **254**, 1024–1026.

44. Schipani, E., Karga, H., Karaplis, A. C., Potts, J. T., Jr., Kronenberg, H. M., Segre, G. V., Abou-Samra, A. B., and Juppner, H. (1993). Identical cDNAs encode a human renal and bone parathyroid hormone/parathyroid hormone-related peptide receptor. *Endocrinology* **132**, 2157–2165.

45. Bringhurst, F. R., Juppner, H., Guo, J. Urena, P., Potts, J. T., Jr., Kronenberg, H. M., Abou-Samra, A. B., and Segré, G. V. (1993). Cloned, stably expressed parathyroid hormone (PTH)/PTH-related peptide receptors activate multiple messenger signals and biological responses in LLC-PK1 kidney cells. *Endocrinology* **132**, 2090–2098.

46. Huang, Z., Chen, Y., Pratt, S., Chen, T. H., Bambino, T., Nissenson, R. A., and Shoback, D. M. (1996). The N-terminal region of the third intracellular loop of the parathyroid hormone (PTH)/PTH-related peptide receptor is critical for coupling to cAMP and inositol phosphate/Ca2+ signal transduction pathways. *J. Biol. Chem.* **271**, 33382–33389.

47. Turner, P. R., Bambino, T., and Nissenson, R. A. (1996). A putative selectivity filter in the G-protein-coupled receptors for parathyroid hormone and secretion. *J. Biol. Chem.* **271**, 9205–9208.

48. Majesca, R. J., Rodan, S., B., and Rodan, G. A. (1980). Parathyroid hormone-responsive clonal cell lines from rat osteosarcoma. *Endocrinology* **107**, 1494–1503.

49. Chase, L. R., Fedak, S. A., and Aurbach, G. D. (1969). Activation of skeletal adenyl cyclase by parathyroid hormone in vitro. *Endocrinology* **84**, 761–768.

50. Chase, L. R., Melson, G. L., and Aurbach, G. D. (1969). Pseudohypoparathyroidism: Defective excretion of 3′, 5′-AMP in response to parathyroid hormone. *J. Clin. Invest.* **48**, 1832–1844.

51. Tregear, G. W., Van Rietschoten J., Greene, E., Keutmann, H. T., Niall, H. D., Reit, B., Parsons, J. A., and Potts, J. T., Jr. (1973). Bovine parathyroid hormone: Minimum chain length of synthetic peptide required for biological activity. *Endocrinology* **93**, 1349–1353.

52. Rasmussen, H. (1986). The calcium messenger system (first of two parts). *N. Engl. J. Med.* **314**, 1094–1101.

53. Rasmussen, H. (1986). The calcium messenger system (second of two parts). *N. Engl. J. Med.* **314**, 1164–1170.

54. Turner, P. R., Mefford, S., Bambino, T., and Nissenson, R. A. (1998). Transmembrane residues together with the amino terminus limit the response of the parathyroid hormone (PTH) 2 receptor to PTH-related peptide. *J. Biol. Chem.* **273**, 3830–3837.

55. Bergwitz, C., Jusseaume, S. A., Luck, M. D., Juppner, H., and Gardella, T. J. (1997). Residues in the membrane-spanning and extracellular loop regions of the parathyroid hormone (PTH)−2 receptor determine signaling selectivity for PTH and PTH-related peptide. *J. Biol. Chem.* **272**, 28861–28868.

56. McSheehy, P. M. J., and Chambers, T. J. (1986). Osteoblastic cells mediate osteoclastic responsiveness to parathyroid hormone. *Endocrinology* **118**, 824–828.

57. Martin, T. J., and Udagawa, N. (1998). Hormonal regulation of osteoclast function. *Trends Endocrinol. Metab.* **9**, 6–12.

58. Roodman, G. D. (1998). Osteoclast differentiation and activity. *Biochem. Soc. Trans.* **26**, 7–13.

59. Talmage, R. V., *et al.* (1978). The demand for bone calcium in maintenance of plasma calcium concentration. *In* "Mechanisms of Localized Bone Loss" (J. E. Horton, T. M., Tarplay, and W. F., Davis, eds.), pp. 73–91. Information Retrieval, Washington, DC.

60. Rodan, G. A., and Martin, T. J. (1981). Role of osteoblasts in hormonal control of bone resorption—a hypothesis. *Calcif. Tissue Int.* **33**, 349.

61. Liu, B. Y., Guo, J., Lanske, B., Divieti, P., Kronenberg, H. M., and Bringhurst, F. R. (1998). Conditionally immortalized murine bone marrow stromal cells mediate parathyroid hormone-dependent osteoclastogenesis in vitro. *Endocrinology* **139**, 1952–1964.

62. Tuukkanen, J., and Vaananen, H. K. (1986). Omeprazole, a specific inhibitor of H^+-K^+-ATPase, inhibits bone resorption in vitro. *Calcif. Tissue Int.* **38**, 123–125.

63. Hall, G. E., and Kenny, A. D. (1986). Bone resorption induced by parathyroid hormone and dibutyryl cyclic AMP: Role of carbonic anhydrase. *J. Pharmacol. Exp. Ther.* **223**, 778–782.

64. Krieger, N. S., and Kim, S. G. (1988). Dichlorobenzamil inhibits stimulated bone resorption in vitro. *Endocrinology* **122**, 415–420.

65. Bushinsky, D. A. (1987). Effects of parathyroid hormone on net proton flux from neonatal mouse calvariae. *Am. J. Physiol.* **252** (4, Part 2), F585–F589.

66. Catherwood, B. D., Titus, L., Evans, C. O., Rubin, J., Boden, S. D., and Nanes, M. S. (1994). Increased expression of tissue plasminogen activator messenger ribonucleic acid is an immediate response to parathyroid hormone in neonatal rat osteoblasts. *Endocrinology* **134**, 1429–1436.

67. Midura, R. J., Evanko, S. P., and Hascall, V. C. (1994). Parathyroid hormone stimulates hyaluronan synthesis in an osteoblast-like cell line. *J. Biol. Chem.* **269**, 13200–13206.

68. Selvamurugan, N., Chou, W. Y., Pearman, A. T., Pulumati, M. R., and Partridge, N. C. (1998). Parathyroid hormone regulates the rat collagenase-3 promoter in osteoblastic cells through the cooperative interaction of the activator protein-1 site and the runt domain binding sequence. *J. Biol. Chem.* **273**, 10647–10657.

69. Babich, M., and Foti, L. R. (1994). E-cadherins identified in osteoblastic cells: Effects of parathyroid hormone and extracellular calcium on localization. *Life Sci.* **54**, 201–208.

70. Schlüter, K. D., Hellstern, H., Wingender, E., and Mayer, H. (1989). The central part of parathyroid hormone stimulates thymidine incorporation of chondrocytes. *J. Biol. Chem.* **264**, 11087–11092.

71. Hall, A. K., and Dickson, I. R. (1985). The effects of parathyroid hormone on osteoblast-like cells from embryonic chick calcaria. *Acta Endocrinol.* **108**, 217–233.

72. Heath, J. K., Atkinson, S. J., Meikle, M. C., and Reynolds, J. J. (1984). Mouse osteoblasts synthesize collagenase in response to bone resorbing agents. *Biochim. Biophys. Acta* **802**, 151–154.

73. Simon, L. S., Slovik, S. M., Neer, R. M., and Krane, S. M. (1988). Changes in serum levels of type I and III procollagen extension peptides during infusion of human parathyroid hormone fragment (1–34). *J. Bone Miner. Res.* **3**, 241–246.

74. Nasu, M., Sugimoto, T., Kaji, H., *et al.* (1998). Carboxyl-terminal parathyroid hormone fragments stimulate type-1 procollagen and insulin-like growth factor-binding protein-5 mRNA expression in osteoblastic UMR-106 cells. *Endocr. J.* **45**, 229–234.

75. Armbrecht, J. H., and Hodam, T. L. (1994). Parathyroid hormone and 1,25-dihydroxyvitamin D synergistically induce the 1,25-dihydroxyvitamin D-24-hydroxylase in rat UMR-106 osteoblast-like cells. *Biochem. Biophys. Res. Commun.* **205**, 674–679.

76. Alvarez, M., Thunyakitpisal, P., Morrison, P., Onyia, J., Hock, J., and Bidwell, J. P. (1998). PTH-responsive osteoblast nuclear matrix architectural transcription factor binds to the rat type I collagen promoter. *J. Cell. Biochem.* **69**, 336–352.

77. Torrungruang, K., Feister, H., Swartz, D., *et al.* (1998). Parathyroid hormone regulates the expression of the nuclear mitotic apparatus protein in the osteoblast-like cells. *Bone* **22**, 317–324.

78. Massas, R., and Benayahu, D. (1998). Parathyroid hormone effect on cell-to-cell communication in stromal and osteoblastic cells. *J. Cell. Biochem.* **69**, 81–86.

79. Schiller, P. C., Roos, B. A., and Howard, G. A. (1997). Parathyroid hormone upregulation of connexin 43 gene expression in osteoblasts depends on cell phenotype. *J. Bone Miner. Res.* **12**, 2005–2013.

80. Civitelli, R., Ziambaras, K., Warlow, P. M., Lecanda, R., Nelson, T., Harley, J., Atal, N., Beyer, E. C., and Steinberg, T. H. (1998). Regulation of connexin43 expression and function by prostaglandin E2 (PGE2) and parathyroid hormone (PTH) in osteoblastic cells. *J. Cell. Biochem.* **68**, 8–21.

81. Elias, J. A., Tang, W., and Horowitz, M. C. (1995). Cytokine and hormonal stimulation of human osteosarcoma interleukin-11 production. *Endocrinology* **136**, 489–498.

82. Schmid, C., Schlapfer, I., Peter, M., Boni-Schnetzler, M., and Schwander, J. (1994). Growth hormone and parathyroid hormone stimulate IGFBP-3 in rat osteoblasts. *Am. J. Physiol.* **267**, E226–E233.

83. Conover, C. A. (1995). Insulin-like growth factor binding protein proteolysis in bone cell models. *Prog. Growth Factor Res.* **6**, 301–309.

84. Maciel, F. M., Sarrazin, P., Morisset, S., Lora, M., Patry, C., Dumais, R., and de Brum-Fernandes, A. J. (1997). Induction of cyclooxygenase-2 by parathyroid hormone in human osteoblasts in culture. *J. Rheumatol.* **24**, 2429–2435.

85. Kano, J., Sugimoto, T., Kanatani, M., Kuroki, Y., Tsukamoto, T., Fukase, M., and Chinara, K. (1994). Second messenger signaling of c-fos gene induction by parathyroid hormone (PTH) and PTH-related peptide in osteoblastic osteosarcoma cells: Its role in osteoblast proliferation and osteoclast-like cell formation. *J. Cell. Physiol.* **161**, 358–366.

86. Toromanoff, A., Ammann, P., and Riond, J. L. (1998). Early effects of short-term parathyroid hormone administration on bone mass, mineral content, and strength in female rats. *Bone* **22**, 217–223.

87. Kishi, T., Hagino, H., Kishimoto, H., and Nagashima, H. (1998). Bone responses at various skeletal sites to human parathyroid hormone in ovariectomized rats: Effects of long-term administration, withdrawal, and readministration. *Bone* **22**, 515–522.

88. Okimoto, N., Tsurukami, H., Okazaki, Y., Nishida, S., Sakai, A., Ohnishi, H., Hori, M., Yasukawa, K., and Nakamura, T. (1998). Effects of a weekly injection of human parathyroid hormone (1–34) and withdrawal on bone mass, strength, and turnover in mature ovariectomized rats. *Bone* **22**, 523–531.

89. Lane, N. E., Kimmel, D. B., Nilsson, M. H., Cohen, F. E., Newton, S., Nissenson, R. A., and Strewler, G. J. (1996). Bone-selective analogs of human PTH (1–34) increase bone formation in an ovariectomized rat model. *J. Bone Miner. Res.* **11**, 614–625.

90. Ejersted, C., Oxlund, H., Eriksen, E. F., and Andreassen, T. T. (1998). Withdrawal of parathyroid hormone treatment causes rapid resorption of newly formed vertebral cancellous and endocortical bone in old rats. *Bone* **23**, 43–52.

91. Chow, J. W. M., Fox, S., Jagger, C. J., and Chambers, T. J. (1998). Role for parathyroid hormone in mechanical responsiveness of rat bone. *Am. J. Physiol.- Endoc. M.* **37**, E146–E154.

92. Schipani, E., Lanske, B., Hunzelman, J., Luz, A., Kovacs, C. S., Lee, K., Pirro, A., Kronenberg, H. M., and Juppner, H. (1997). Targeted expression of constitutively active receptors for parathyroid hormone and parathyroid hormone-related peptide delays endochondral bone formation and rescues mice that lack parathyroid hormone-related peptide. *Proc. Natl. Acad. Sci. U.S.A.* **94**, 13689–13694.

93. Theiler, R., Bischoff, H., Tyndall, A., and Stahelin, H. B. (1998). Elevated PTH levels in hypovitaminosis D are more rapidly suppressed by the administration of 1,25-dihydroxy-vitamin D3 than by vitamin D3. *Int. J. Vitam. Nutr. Res.* **68**, 36–41.

94. Berruti, A., Sperone, P., Fasolis, G., Torta, M., Fontana, D., Dogliotti, L., and Angeli, A. (1997). Pamidronate administration improves the secondary hyperparathyroidism due to "Bone Hunger Syndrome" in a patient with osteoblastic metastases from prostate cancer. *Prostate* **33**, 252–255.

95. Brahm, H., Ljunggren, O., Larsson, K., Lindh, E., and Ljunghall, S. (1994). Effects of infusion of parathyroid hormone and primary hyperparathyroidism on formation and breakdown of type I collagen. *Calcif. Tissue Int.* **55**, 412–416.

96. Ebeling, P. R., Jones, J. D., Burritt, M. F., Duerson, C. R., Lane, A. W., Hassager, C., Kumar, R., and Riggs, B. L. (1992). Skeletal responsiveness to endogenous parathyroid hormone in postmenopausal osteoporosis. *J. Clin. Endocrinol. Metab.* **75**, 1033–1038.

97. Ledger, G. A., Burritt, M. F., Kao, P. C., O'Fallon, W. M., Riggs, B. L., and Khosla, S. (1995). Role of parathyroid hormone in mediating nocturnal and age-related increases in bone resorption. *J. Clin. Endocrinol. Metab.* **80**, 3304–3310.

98. Schwietert, H. R., Groen, E. W., Sollie, F. A., and Jonkman, J. H. (1997). Single-dose subcutaneous administration of recombinant human parathyroid hormone [rhPTH(1–84)] in healthy postmenopausal volunteers. *Clin. Pharmacol. Ther.* **61**, 360–376.

99. Cosman, F., Morgan, D. C., Nieves, J. W., Shen, V., Luckey, M. M., Dempster, D. W., Lindsay, R., and Parisien, M. (1997). Resistance to bone resorbing effects of PTH in black women. *J. Bone Miner. Res.* **12**, 958–966.

100. Lindsay, R., Nieves, J., Formica, C., Henneman, E., Woelfert, L., Shen, V., Dempster, D., and Cosman, F. (1997). Randomised controlled study of effect of parathyroid hormone on vertebral-bone mass and fracture incidence among postmenopausal women on oestrogen with osteoporosis. *Lancet* **350**, 550–555.

101. Hodsman, A. B., Fraher, L. J., Watson, P. H., Ostbye, T., Stitt, L. W., Adachi, J. D., Taves, D. H., and Drost, D. (1997). A randomized controlled trial to compare the efficacy of cyclical parathyroid hormone versus cyclical parathyroid hormone and sequential calcitonin to improve bone mass in postmenopausal women with osteoporosis. *J. Clin. Endocrinol. Metab.* **82**, 620–628.

102. Kurland, E. S., Cosman, F., McMahon, D. J., Shen, V., Lindsay, R., Rosen, C. J., and Bilezikian, J. P. (1998). Changes in bone markers predict bone accural in osteoporotic men treated with parathyroid hormone. *Bone* (Suppl. 5) **23**, 1040 (abstr.).

CHAPTER 14

PTHrP: Of Molecules, Mice, and Men

ANDREW C. KARAPLIS Division of Endocrinology, Department of Medicine, and Lady Davis Institute for Medical Research, Sir Mortimer B. Davis-Jewish General Hospital, McGill University, Montréal, H3T 1E2 Canada

DAVID GOLTZMAN Calcium Research Laboratory, Department of Medicine, Royal Victoria Hospital, McGill University, Montréal, H3A 1A1 Canada

I. ABSTRACT

Parathyroid hormone-related peptide (PTHrP) was discovered as a mediator of hypercalcemia associated with malignancy but is now known to be expressed by a large number of normal fetal and adult tissues. The amino-terminal region of PTHrP reveals limited but significant homology with parathyroid hormone (PTH), resulting in the interaction of the first 34 to 36 residues of either peptide with a single seven-transmembrane spanning G-protein linked receptor termed the PTH/PTHrP receptor or the PTH-1 receptor. Targeted inactivation of the PTHrP gene in mice has established the critical role that PTHrP plays in chondrocyte biology and in endochondral bone formation. Animals homozygous for PTHrP gene deletion demonstrate impaired chondrocyte proliferation, premature differentiation, and accelerated apoptosis. These alterations result in a distorted epiphyseal growth plate and marked skeletal deformity with ensuing neonatal death due to respiratory compromise. Other alterations in skin, tooth, and breast development also occur. The complex processes resulting in normal endochondral bone development involve additional factors such as the hedgehog signaling pathway with which PTHrP interacts. PTHrP, like PTH, binds to receptors on cells of the osteoblast lineage resulting in enhanced bone formation and also, indirectly, in augmented osteoclastic bone resorption. Overall, these findings point to a critical role for PTHrP in normal skeletal development and in its maintenance. Further elucidation of the molecular role and interactions of PTHrP may therefore reveal new facets of the pathogenesis of a variety of metabolic bone diseases and potentially point to new directions for therapeutic interventions.

II. INTRODUCTION

The association of malignancies and hypercalcemia was first reported in 1936 [1] and the production and secretion by tumors of a circulating factor causing hypercalcemia was postulated by Fuller Albright in 1941 [2]. The hypercalcemia of malignancy syndrome is characterized by hypercalcemia and hypophosphatemia, biochemical features that are usually

203

indicative of oversecretion of parathyroid hormone (PTH), the major regulator of calcium homeostasis. Initial studies that searched for immunoreactive PTH within the tumors, however, were equivocal or negative. However, PTH-like activity in tumor extracts was evident in assays that measured renal glucose-6-phosphate dehydrogenase (G6PD) activity by a cytochemical technique [3] and adenylate cyclase activity in osteoblast cell lines and in renal membranes. The latter assay proved to be critical for monitoring the purification and the final isolation of the PTH-like peptide from human lung [4], breast [5], and kidney [6] cancer cell lines. The finding of structural similarity of the amino-terminal region of this peptide (PTHrP, for PTH-related peptide) with the corresponding domain of PTH, and the resultant capacity of both molecules to interact with the same G protein-coupled cell surface receptor (PTH/PTHrP or PTH-1 receptor) via this region [7, 8], appear to account for the ability of circulating, tumor-derived PTHrP to inappropriately activate receptors in classic PTH target organs such as bone and kidney and to elicit PTH-like bioactivity. By the same mechanism, PTHrP may also enhance osteoclastic activity when released locally by tumor cells that have already metastasized to bone [9]. Further studies, however, have demonstrated the importance of PTHrP not only as an osteolytic factor in malignancy but also as a paracrine/autocrine regulator of many physiologic pro-

cesses, most notably of bone and cartilage metabolism. The pivotal role of the PTHrP signaling pathway in endochondral bone development and in adult skeletal homeostasis will be the focus of this review.

III. MOLECULAR BIOLOGY AND MECHANISM OF ACTION

A. Organization of the *PTHrP* Gene

The human gene for *PTHrP* has been mapped to the short arm of chromosome 12 [10], whereas the *PTH* gene is assigned to human chromosome 11. An evolutionary relationship between the *PTHrP* and *PTH* genes has been suggested, because human chromosomes 11 and 12 are thought to have arisen by a tetraploidization event of a common ancestral chromosome. Indeed, the *PTHrP* and *PTH* genes and their respective gene clusters have been maintained as syntenic groups in human, rat, and mouse genomes [11].

Considerably more complex than the *PTH* gene, however, the human *PTHrP* gene comprises at least seven exons, spans more than 15 kb of genomic DNA (Fig. 1), and utilizes at least three distinct promoters, two containing a classical TATA box and one including a GC-rich region [12–15]. Exon I,

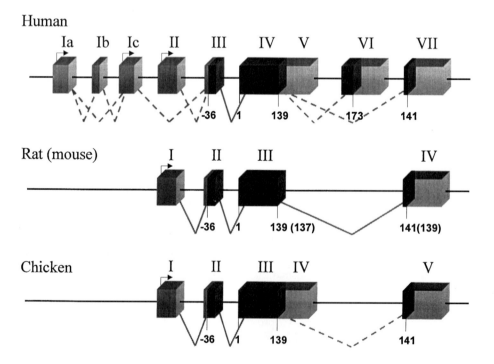

FIGURE 1   Organization of the human, rat, mouse, and chicken *PTHrP* gene. Roman numerals depict numbering of exons. Arabic numbers depict amino acid positions in the precursor (denoted by − symbols) or in the mature peptide. Arrows indicates promoter. Open boxes (□) denote exons encoding 5′ untranslated regions, closed boxes (■) denote coding exons, and stippled boxes (▨) denote exons encoding 3′ untranslated sequences. Exons joined by solid Vs indicate obligatory splicing, whereas exons joined by broken Vs denote alternative splicing.

subdivided into Ia, Ib, and Ic, and exon II encode different 5′ untranslated regions. Exon III encodes the prepro coding region, and exon IV encodes most of the mature peptide sequence. At the end of exon IV, the splice site interrupts codon 139 of the mature peptide. Exon V, which is contiguous with exon IV, encodes a stop codon and a 3′ noncoding sequence. Exon VI encodes 36 additional amino acids, a stop codon, and a second 3′ noncoding region. Exon VII encodes two extra amino acids, a stop codon, and a third noncoding region. Hence, by the use of alternative splicing of exons, a multitude of human PTHrP RNA transcripts can occur, giving rise to three different isoforms of 139, 141, and 173 amino acids in length which are identical as far as amino acid 139.

In contrast with this complexity, the rat [16], mouse [17], and chicken [18] PTHrP genes are considerably simpler in organization and consist of four or five exons and only a single promoter, corresponding to the downstream promoter in the human gene. Overall, this simpler organization predicts that in most species, a single promoter will be found and the 141-amino-acid isoform of the peptide will predominate. In the mouse, the mature peptide is 139 amino acids rather than 141 amino acids because of a 6-base pair deletion (corresponding to amino acids 130 and 131 of human and rat protein). Moreover, the chicken gene can encode two isoforms, one of 139 amino acids arising by read-through of exon III into exon IV, and one of 141 amino acids, which is the predominant form, arising from splicing to exon V. Human, rat, mouse, dog [19], and chicken peptides are virtually identical in the amino terminal and midregion of the molecule but diverge beyond residue 112. This striking conservation throughout this large evolutionary range suggested early on that PTHrP is of essential biological importance.

B. Regulation of PTHrP Production

In view of the fact that PTHrP secretion is generally constitutive, regulation of gene expression and intracellular processing appear to be critical mechanisms for determining the rate of PTHrP production and secretion.

1. Regulation of Gene Expression

Several factors have been shown to regulate PTHrP gene expression in normal tissues or cells, at least in part, at the transcriptional level. For example, PTHrP mRNA in lactating mammary tissue is stimulated by prolactin [20], although the precise mechanism of this effect is unknown. Estrogen administration causes increased PTHrP expression in the uterus as does intrauterine occupancy in preterm myometrium [21]. In cultured vascular smooth muscle cells, glucocorticoids decrease PTHrP levels [22]. However, in most cells, including for example cultured keratinocytes, breast epithelial cells, and smooth muscle cells, growth factors stimulate PTHrP expression, whereas $1,25(OH)_2$vitamin D_3

inhibits this production [23]. Both stimulation and inhibition occur predominantly at the transcriptional level. These regulatory agents appear particularly important in modulating PTHrP production in a variety of tissues and in tumors arising from these tissues. Consequently, novel approaches are being applied to reduce PTHrP overproduction by cancer cells based on employing nonhypercalcemic vitamin D analogs that impede the growth factor signaling pathway [24, 25].

2. Posttranslational Processing

With the availability of the PTHrP cDNA-based amino acid sequence, it became evident that the mature form of the protein is preceded by a 36-residue prepro sequence. This sequence has all the classic feature of a signal peptide that would target the nascent protein to the rough endoplasmic reticulum. While the precise site of cleavage by signal peptidase has yet to be determined, it is likely that it occurs at position −9, thereby generating a nascent propeptide extending from position −8. The evidence that the pro sequence is subsequently cleaved to generate the mature form of the protein at position Ala +1 is based primarily on (1) direct sequencing of the secreted PTHrP form by three independent laboratories, (2) the presence of an endoproteolytic site for prohormone convertases of the furin and PC1/3 family proximal to it [26], and (3) the homology of this region with that of PTH.

Closer examination of the mature PTHrP sequence reveals additional clusters of basic amino acids that could potentially serve as endoproteolytic processing sites (Fig. 2). Hence, cleavage appears to occur carboxy-terminal to arginine at position 37, most likely yielding the secretory form, PTHrP (1–36). A midregion fragment that begins at amino acid 38 and terminates in the 80–100 region has also been identified, both within cells and outside cells following secretion [27]. An additional carboxy-terminal PTHrP fragment may exist that encompasses the highly conserved pentapeptide 107–111. It would seem, therefore, that PTHrP could function as a polyhormone precursor of a number of biologically active fragments with distinct biological actions.

C. Receptors and Signal Transduction Pathways

In view of the extensive posttranslational processing that PTHrP undergoes, it would not be surprising if multiple receptors for the various forms of the protein exist. These can be divided primarily into four categories that recognize determinants in (1) the amino-terminal region of the protein, (2) the midregion form, (3) the nuclear localization sequence, and (4) the carboxyl-terminal form.

The amino-terminal domain of PTHrP binds to the classical PTH-1 receptor in bone and kidney and activates both the adenylyl cyclase/protein kinase A pathway as well as the

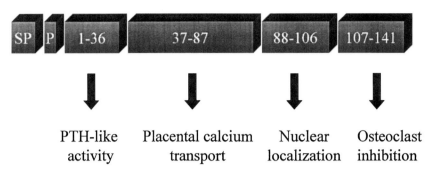

FIGURE 2   Posttranslational processing of PTHrP. PTHrP could function as a polyhormone precursor to a number of active fragments with distinct biological actions, as shown. Numbers denote amino acid positions where endoproteolytic processing of the nascent PTHrP protein takes place. SP, signal peptide; P, propeptide.

calcium/inositol phosphate/protein kinase C pathway (Fig. 3). In fact, most of the well-characterized actions of PTHrP appear to be mediated by this receptor for the NH$_2$-terminal domain of PTHrP since its expression has been observed in a variety of tissues that might well be PTHrP targets. In addition, a novel splice variant of the PTH-1 receptor has been reported, primarily found intracellularly, and may represent a form of the receptor used to bind the intracellularly targeted PTHrP ligand [28].

The existence of a "receptor" that recognizes the N-terminal domain of PTHrP but is distinct from the classic type 1 receptor has also been suggested [29, 30]. This high-capacity, low-affinity receptor was identified in keratinocytes and pancreatic β-cells and signals only through the protein kinase C pathway. Cloning and molecular characterization of this receptor, however, have not been accomplished.

Even less is known about the putative receptor that binds the midregion form of PTHrP. The existence of such a

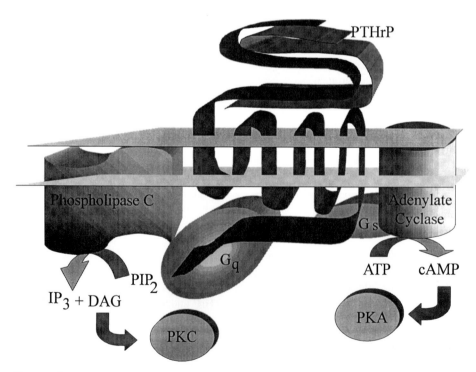

FIGURE 3   Interaction of PTHrP with the PTH-1 receptor. The amino-terminal domain of PTHrP (and PTH) binds to the seven-transmembrane spanning receptor, causing the guanyl nucleotide binding proteins Gs and Gq to activate adenylate cyclase or phospholipase C, respectively. Therefore, cAMP or inositol triphosphate (IP3) and diacylglycerol (DAG) are produced. Cyclic AMP and DAG will respectively stimulate protein kinase A (PKA) and protein kinase C (PKC).

receptor, likely linked to the protein kinase C pathway, is circumstantial and is based primarily on the finding that residues 67–86 of PTHrP are critical for the control of placental calcium transport [31]. While the receptor has not yet been identified, support for its existence has come from work with the PTHrP gene knockout mouse in which placental calcium transport is severely impaired and can only be restored by administration of PTHrP (1–86) and PTHrP (67–86) peptides. PTHrP (1–34) and PTH (1–84) have no effect [32].

Amino acids 87–107 of the mature form of PTHrP encode a putative bipartite nuclear localization signal (NLS) consisting of two basic clusters separated by a spacer region, analogous to the prototypical nucleoplasmin NLS [33]. Studies have shown that elimination of the NLS from pre-proPTHrP effectively abolished intranuclear localization of the recombinant protein. Moreover, the NLS alone was capable of translocating a heterologous cytoplasmic protein, β-galactosidase, to the nucleolus when expressed as a fusion protein in COS-7 cells. Selective protein import into the nucleus proceeds through the nuclear pore complex and requires the interaction between the NLS and an importin-like NLS receptor complex [34]. The absolute requirement for the NLS in targeting PTHrP to the nucleus argues strongly for the classic nuclear pore route as being operative in this process.

Receptors for the carboxyl-terminal form of PTHrP have been inferred from studies reporting that picomolar concentrations of this peptide can profoundly inhibit resorption in an isolated osteoclast bone resorption assay [35, 36]. In addition, the C-terminal peptide PTHrP (107–139) has been shown to elicit a rise in cytosolic calcium in cultured hyppocampal neurons [37]. It is likely, therefore, that novel receptors for carboxyl-terminal fragments might be expected in osteoclasts and neurons. The cloning and characterization of these receptors will be necessary in order to establish the physiological relevance associated with their activation.

D. Endocrine, Autocrine/Paracrine, and Intracrine Actions

Although PTHrP was initially discovered through its "endocrine" effects (i.e., it is released from tumors into the circulation and it acts at distant sites such as the skeleton and kidneys), this mechanism of action is generally considered to be the exception rather than the rule. In fact, under normal circumstances, the only other endocrine effect ascribed to PTHrP is its influence on placental calcium transport following release from the fetal parathyroids.

This scenario notwithstanding, PTHrP, unlike PTH, does not circulate in appreciable amounts in normal subjects [38]; rather, it is thought to exert its biological effects locally in a paracrine/autocrine fashion. For example, in some tissues

such as mammary tissue, PTHrP is an epithelial-derived factor that acts on mesenchymal cells expressing the PTH-1 receptor to influence mammary gland development [39]. Similarly, PTHrP derived from the endothelium can act on vascular smooth muscle cells to regulate vascular tone and blood pressure. Alternatively, PTHrP can be secreted by vascular smooth muscle cells, and in turn, feed back to alter the contractility of these cells. Likewise, keratinocytes, pancreatic β cells, and uterine smooth muscle cells can both secrete and respond to PTHrP.

In addition to the autocrine/paracrine effects, experimental evidence has been presented suggesting that PTHrP may also have an intracrine site of action. This conclusion is based on the following observations: (1) endogenous PTHrP localizes to the nucleus of murine bone cells *in vitro* as well as *in situ* [33], (2) immunogold labeling for the endogenous peptide *in situ* was observed over the dense fibrillar component of nucleoli, a subnucleolar structure thought to represent the major site of transcription of genes coding for rRNA, and (3) the nuclear actions of PTHrP have been subsequently confirmed in a human keratinocyte cell line (HaCaT) [40] and in cultured vascular smooth muscle cells [41]. While providing unequivocal evidence for the nucleus being an intracrine site of action of PTHrP, these findings have also raised a number of important issues. For example, how does PTHrP, a secretory protein, gain access to the cytoplasm? Once in the cytoplasm, how is its transport to the cell nucleus regulated? How does nuclear/nucleolar PTHrP modulate cellular function? What are the consequences of nuclear signaling by PTHrP? Preliminary data suggest that nuclear translocation of PTHrP is cell-cycle dependent. Hence, in the human keratinocyte cell line HaCaT, PTHrP localizes to the nucleolus at G_1 and is excluded from the nucleus from the start of the S phase to mitosis. In vascular smooth muscle cells, nuclear PTHrP has been observed in cells that are dividing or in the process of completing cell division, suggesting that nuclear translocation is associated with activation of the cell cycle. Whether these differences are a reflection of the methodology employed or whether they reflect truly distinct nuclear actions of PTHrP remains to be defined. Other studies have suggested that nuclear translocation of PTHrP is involved in the regulation of programmed cell death such as that which may occur at the distal end of the hypertrophic zone of the cartilaginous growth plate in the course of endochondral bone development.

It would appear, therefore, that PTHrP influences a spectrum of cellular functions by exerting its effects near or at its site of synthesis. Expressed in a remarkable variety of normal adult and fetal tissues, this protein has been reported to have a number of diverse actions such as relaxation of smooth muscle in the uterus, bladder, and blood vessels, neurotransmission, regulation of cellular proliferation and differentiation in skin, mammary tissue, and the fetal and adult skeleton. The remaining part of this review will explore our understanding of PTHrP and its amino terminal PTH-1 receptor function in endochondral bone development and in the maintenance of the adult skeleton.

IV. THE SKELETAL ACTIONS OF PTHrP

Endochondral ossification is a complex, multistep process involving the formation of cartilaginous skeleton from aggregated mesenchymal cells and its subsequent replacement by bone. The cellular and molecular events that regulate the highly ordered progression of chondrocytes within the growth plate through the stages of proliferation and differentiation must be under precise spatial and temporal control. Ultimately, these events determine the extent and rate of skeletal growth.

A. PTHrP Signaling and Chondrocyte Biology

1. CHONDROCYTE PROLIFERATION AND DIFFERENTIATION

The generation of mice homozygous for a disrupted PTHrP gene provided the first direct evidence of a physiological role for this protein in chondrocyte biology [42]. PTHrP-null mice die in the immediate postnatal period, likely from respiratory failure because of widespread abnormalities of endochondral bone development. Characterized by diminished proliferation, accelerated differentiation, and premature apoptotic death of chondrocytes, this form of osteochondrodysplasia results in the untimely and rapid maturation of the skeleton [43–45].

The critical role of PTHrP as an inhibitor of the chondrocyte differentiation program has been further substantiated by the targeted overexpression of PTHrP in chondrocytes by means of the mouse collagen type II promoter [46]. This targeting induces a novel form of chondrodysplasia that is the antithesis of the PTHrP-null phenotype and is characterized by a delay in endochondral ossification so profound that mice are born with cartilaginous endochondral skeletons. However, by 7 weeks of age, this delay in chondrocyte differentiation and ossification has been largely corrected, leaving foreshortened and misshapen but histologically near-normal bones. This ultimate histological healing and the sequence by which it proceeds are reminiscent of those seen in patients with Jansen's metaphyseal chondrodysplasia, a condition arising from constitutive activation of the PTH-1 receptor [47–49]. Similar effects on the chondrocyte maturation program have been observed in transgenic mice in which expression of a constitutively active PTH-1 receptor was targeted to the growth plate [50]. Therefore, overexpression of PTHrP or the presence of a constitutively active PTH-1 receptor in the growth plate, either naturally or by transgenic technology, ultimately results in a similar pattern of abnormalities in endochondral bone formation.

2. PTHrP AND CHONDROCYTE APOPTOSIS

The mechanism by which PTHrP delays the process of chondrocyte differentiation is only now beginning to unravel. Hypertrophic chondrocytes in the growth plate are thought to undergo apoptosis immediately prior to ossification [51] and, therefore, represent the terminal stage of differentiation in the chondrogenic lineage. PTHrP expression might be expected to delay, or even prevent, the progression to terminal differentiation and eventual programmed cell death. Studies with the chondrocytic cell line CFK2 overexpressing PTHrP demonstrated enhanced cell survival under conditions that promote apoptotic death [33]. In addition, quantitative analysis of the growth plate of PTHrP-null mice revealed significantly more apoptotic chondrocytes near the chondroosseous junction compared to wild-type littermates [44, 45]. Thus, PTHrP influences not only chondrocyte proliferation and differentiation, but also programmed cell death.

In several cell types, apoptosis is regulated by the ratio of expression of the cell death inhibitor, Bcl-2, and the cell death inducer, Bax. Bcl-2 is expressed in growth plate chondrocytes in a pattern similar to that of PTHrP [52], with the highest levels detected in late proliferative and prehypertrophic chondrocytes. Both *in vitro* and in transgenic mice, PTHrP overexpression causes a marked increase in Bcl-2 with no detectable change in Bax levels. A shift of the Bcl-2/Bax ratio in favor of Bcl-2 delays terminal differentiation, prolongs chondrocyte survival, and leads to the accumulation of cells in their prehypertrophic stage. These observations place Bcl-2 downstream of PTHrP in the pathway that controls chondrocyte maturation and endochondral skeletal development.

3. THE HEDGEHOG PROTEINS

A most interesting development has been the observation that PTHrP may mediate the actions of Indian hedgehog (Ihh) on chondrocyte differentiation. Ihh is a member of a family of proteins, the most notable of which is Sonic hedgehog (Shh). Shh is the vertebrate homolog of the *Drosophila* segment polarity gene product, hedgehog (*hh*), which regulates a variety of patterning events during embryonic development. The mouse Hedgehog (Hh) gene family consists of *Sonic* (*Shh*), *Desert* (*Dhh*), and *Indian* (*Ihh*) *hedgehog*, and all encode secreted proteins implicated in cell–cell interactions. Upon secretion, they undergo autocatalytic internal cleavage, generating a ~20 kDa amino-terminal domain and a ~25 kDa carboxyl-terminus domain. While the amino domain possesses all known signaling activity of these proteins, the carboxyl terminus is responsible for the autocatalytic processing [53]. In addition to cleavage, this processing causes the covalent attachment of a cholesterol moiety in ester linkage to the carboxylate of the terminal residue of the amino-terminal fragment [54]. This modification may set constraints on the diffusion of Hh by tethering it to the plasma membrane, thereby spatially restricting the localization of the Hh signal. Local effects, based on a requirement for a high concentration of amino-terminal Hh, can be easily envisioned for cells in close proximity to Hh-expressing cells. While long-range signaling also appears to function via diffusion of the amino-terminal fragment, indirect effects have also been reported. Both local- and long-range signaling of Hh proteins on target cells are mediated by a receptor that consists of two subunits, Patched (Ptc), a twelve transmembrane protein which is the binding subunit [55, 56], and Smoothened (Smo), a seven transmembrane protein which is the signaling subunit. In the absence of Hh, Ptc associates with Smo and inhibits its activities. In contrast, binding of Hh to Ptc relieves the Ptc-dependent inhibition of Smo [57]. Signaling then ensues and includes downstream components such as the Gli family of transcriptional activators. The three cloned *Gli* genes (*Gli*, *Gli-2*, and *Gli-3*) encode a family of DNA-binding zinc finger proteins with related target sequence specificities. Expression of the three mouse genes has been observed in both ectoderm- and mesoderm-derived tissues, suggesting that the *Gli* genes play multiple roles during postimplantation development [58].

The importance of the Hh inductive signaling in skeletal patterning has been underscored by a number of observations: (1) the effects of Shh in the differentiation of somites into sclerotome [59] and in the growth and patterning of the developing limb [60, 61], (2) the skeletal abnormalities arising from targeted disruption in mice [62] and from natural mutations in mice [62, 63] and humans [64] of the *Gli* genes, and (3) the demonstration that Ihh, produced by growth plate chondrocytes making the transition to the hypertrophic stage of differentiation, attenuates this programmed process [65]. Studies have indicated that Ihh action within the vertebrate growth plate is indirect and mediated primarily by the PTHrP signaling pathway [65, 66]. It has been postulated that Ihh acts on cells in the perichondrium, signaling via Ptc and Gli, to induce, directly or indirectly, the release of PTHrP from the periarticular perichondrium. In turn, PTHrP exerts influence upon the growth plate chondrocytes by activating their receptors and thereby attenuating their propensity to differentiate.

While attractive, this paracrine negative feedback loop within the growth plate requires further clarification. At present it remains unclear how the *Hh* signaling pathway functioning on the perichondrium would lead to increased PTHrP expression by periarticular cells. In other studies, both PTHrP and PTH-1 receptor expression were reported in resting, proliferating, and prehypertrophic chondrocytes. Moreover, *Ptc*, *Smo*, and *Gli* expression has been observed in chondrocytes within the murine growth plate and in clonal mouse ATDC5 cells undergoing chondrogenesis and cartilage differentiation [67, 68]. Such localization would therefore predict an alternative molecular regulation of cartilage differentiation. We proposed that Ihh acts directly as a morphogen on growth plate

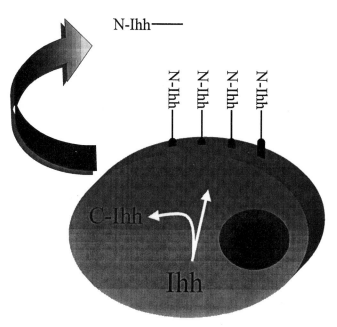

FIGURE 4   Proposed molecular regulation of cartilage differentiation in the growth plate. Prehypertrophic chondrocytes express *Ihh*, which undergoes autocatalytic internal cleavage generating an amino- and a carboxyl-terminal domain (N-Ihh and C-Ihh, respectively). In addition to cleavage, this processing causes the covalent attachment of a cholesterol moiety to the amino-terminal fragment (■). This modification sets constraints on the diffusion of N-Ihh by tethering it to the plasma membrane. Local effects arising from high concentrations of amino-terminal Ihh promote terminal chondrocyte differentiation independent of PTHrP. In contrast, long-range signaling via diffusion of the amino-terminal fragment (arrow) activates the PTHrP signaling pathway and delays the differentiation of proliferating chondrocytes. These inductive short- and long-range signals, therefore, act in a concentration-dependent manner to determine differential cell fate within the growth plate.

chondrocytes in a concentration-dependent fashion and exerts both short and long-range effects (Fig. 4) [69]. Thus, local effects arising from high concentrations of amino-terminal Ihh could be envisioned as promoting terminal chondrocyte differentiation independent of PTHrP. Long-range signaling would occur via diffusion of the Ihh amino-terminal fragment, would activate the PTHrP signaling pathway, and would thus delay the differentiation of proliferating chondrocytes. Additional evidence substantiating the local direct effects of Ihh has been provided by *in vitro* studies. For example, *Ihh* mRNA expression parallels that of *Col-X* mRNA in ATDC5 cells undergoing chondrogenesis, and subsequent cartilage differentiation and ectopic expression of *Hh* in limb bud micromass cultures promotes alkaline phosphatase and *Col-X* expression, i.e., differentiation of hypertrophic chondrocytes, in a mechanism independent of the PTHrP system [70]. This apparent dual action of Ihh on the program of chondrocyte maturation will likely require the use of powerful genetic tools for further substantiation in the *in vivo* setting.

4. THE ROLE OF OTHER HUMORAL REGULATORS

While a number of other signaling molecules produced within the growth plate, such as FGF and the FGF receptor, exert important effects on chondrocyte proliferation and differentiation, their interactions with PTHrP are at present unknown. Other factors appear to influence growth plate development, likely by modulating the Ihh/PTHrP pathway. Signaling by bone morphogenetic proteins (BMPs) has been implicated in the development of the vertebrate limb. Studies have reported that BMP receptor-IA is specifically expressed in prehypertrophic chondrocytes and modulates the program of chondrocyte maturation [71]. Consequently, misexpression of a constitutively active form of BMP receptor-IA delayed chondrocyte differentiation and was associated with decreased *Col-X* and *Ihh* expression, while *PTHrP* expression was increased. Analysis of this model suggests that BMP signals are downstream mediators of Ihh function in both a local signaling loop and a longer-range relay system that may involve PTHrP.

In other studies, the overexpression of a truncated type II TGF-β receptor (a dominant-negative mutant) in skeletal tissue of transgenic mice resulted in degenerative joint disease resembling human osteoarthritis and in growth plate abnormalities characterized by increased *Col-X* and *Ihh* expression [72]. Thus, loss of responsiveness to TGF-β promotes chondrocyte terminal differentiation through a pathway that likely involves Ihh/PTHrP signaling. Mechanistic details, however, are presently lacking.

5. DEFINING THE ROLE OF THE PTH-1 RECEPTOR

There is abundant evidence that the PTH-1 receptor mediates most PTHrP actions in the cartilaginous growth plate, both from the natural receptor mutations that cause Jansen's metaphyseal chondrodysplasia and from targeted overexpression of constitutively active PTH-1 receptor to the growth plate that delays endochondral bone formation [50]. It was, however, the generation of PTH-1 receptor knockout mice that provided unequivocal proof that this receptor mediates the cartilaginous effects of PTHrP [66]. The small number of homozygous mice that do survive to the peripartum period exhibit a phenotype similar to that observed in the PTHrP-negative mutants, although they are proportionally smaller. Skeletal alterations are characterized by accelerated differentiation of chondrocytes leading to a severe and lethal form of osteochondrodysplasia.

Of note, however, is the observation that most receptor-negative animals exhibit a more severe phenotype than the PTHrP-null mice characterized by early embryonic lethality (embryonic day E14.5). It was originally speculated that PTHrP synthesized by maternal decidual cells could complement the absence of fetal PTHrP but not that of its receptor. Another possibility may be that circulating PTH can partly compensate for the absence of PTHrP but not for the recep-

tor deficiency. Alternatively, the more severe phenotype may implicate the presence of another member of the PTH/PTHrP ligand family that interacts with the common receptor. The existence of such a protein, however, remains speculative at present.

Perhaps the most intriguing explanation for the early demise of these animals stems from the apparent dual mechanism of action of PTHrP on cellular function, i.e., the amino-terminal end of the protein acting on the cell surface receptor promoting proliferation and the nucleolar form modulating differentiation [73]. In the absence of the amino-terminal receptor, the unopposed nucleolar effects of PTHrP would lead to severe imbalance of cellular proliferation/differentiation and hence, to early lethality of the receptor-negative mutants. In contrast, ablation of the ligand would eliminate both receptor- and nucleolar-mediated activities, leading to a more "coordinated" impairment and a less severe phenotype. At present, however, it is reasonable to conclude that the small size and early death of the PTH-1 receptor-null mice remains unexplained.

B. PTHrP Signaling and Osteoblast Biology

1. PTHrP HAPLOINSUFFICIENCY LEADS TO OSTEOPENIA

Accumulating evidence indicates that PTHrP also regulates osteogenic cell differentiation and/or function. The evidence can be summarized as follows. First, PTHrP and PTH-1 receptors are expressed in cells of the osteogenic lineage [43, 45, 74–80]. Second, in the PTHrP-null mouse, osteoblastic progenitor cells contain inappropriate accumulations of glycogen [43]. This finding, also observed in PTHrP-null chondrocytes, is indicative of a defect, metabolic or otherwise, in cells of the osteogenic lineage arising as a consequence of PTHrP deficiency. Third, heterozygous PTHrP-null mice, while phenotypically normal at birth, by three months of age exhibit a form of osteopenia characterized by a marked decrease in trabecular thickness and connectivity [81]. Moreover, their bone marrow contains an abnormally high number of adipocytes. Since the same pluripotent stromal cells in the bone marrow compartment can give rise to adipocytes and osteoprogenitor cells [82], the increased number of adipocytes and osteopenia in these mice could be attributed to altered stem cell differentiation as a consequence of PTHrP haploinsufficiency (Fig. 5). Taken together, these findings suggest that PTHrP is important for the orderly commitment of pluripotential bone marrow stromal cells toward the osteogenic lineage and for their subsequent maturation and/or function.

In these animals, a physiological concentration of PTH is unable to compensate for PTHrP haploinsufficiency. One possible explanation is that a defect in skeletal progenitor cells was caused by PTHrP deficiency *in utero* and was only

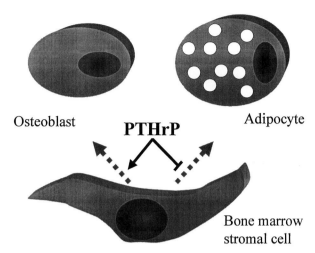

Osteoblast **PTHrP** Adipocyte

Bone marrow
stromal cell

FIGURE 5   Proposed regulation of mesenchymal bone marrow stromal cell differentiation by PTHrP. Produced within the skeletal microenvironment, PTHrP promotes the transition of these pluripotent stem cells toward the osteogenic lineage while inhibiting their differentiation to adipocytes. Decreased local concentrations, as in the PTHrP-null heterozygous state, would favor the formation of adipocytes and a correspondent osteopenic state. Dashed arrows indicate the unknown number of transitional steps required for these differentiation processes.

manifest in the postnatal state. Alternatively, domains of PTHrP not shared with the PTH molecule may subserve unique functions that are important for normal adult skeletal development. PTHrP was shown to translocate to the nucleolus of bone cells *in vitro* and *in situ* and to modulate programmed cell death. Cell death by apoptosis is necessary for maintenance of homeostatic growth in many adult tissues, including bone. Alterations in this mechanism may also have important implications in the development of the osteopenic state.

2. PTHrP AND THE BONE REMODELING PROCESS

With increasing evidence that PTHrP plays an important role in osteoblast biology, it becomes necessary to understand the regulation of its expression and the mechanisms by which it exerts its effects within the skeletal microenvironment. While a number of factors have been reported to influence PTHrP gene expression in nonskeletal tissues [83], its regulation in bone remains poorly defined. The effect of glucocorticoids on PTHrP gene expression in bone is of interest in view of the severe bone loss associated with their prolonged use. Glucocorticoid administration inhibits PTHrP mRNA expression in human osteogenic cells [84].

Studies have shown that members of the Hh family of proteins (Shh and Ihh) can stimulate the osteogenic differentiation of mouse preosteoblastic MC3T3-E1 and fibroblastic C3H10T1/2 cell lines [85, 86]. While this stimulatory effect was synergistically enhanced by BMP-2, Hh proteins did not induce *Bmp* gene expression. These cells, however, express *Ptc*, indicating that the effects of Hh proteins on the osteoblast

differentiation program are direct. What the role of Hh proteins is in modulating the expression of *PTHrP* and its receptor in cells of the osteogenic lineage remains to be defined.

In common with PTH, PTHrP in the postnatal skeleton appears to regulate both bone formation and bone resorption and both actions occur after binding to cells of the osteoblast phenotype (Fig. 6) [87]. The anabolic effects of the NH_2-terminal region of both PTHrP and PTH occur via their action on the PTH-1 receptor; however, at least some of the effects of PTHrP and PTH on bone formation may be partly mediated through cytokines. Thus, PTHrP-stimulated IGF-1 production may stimulate collagen synthesis [88], and PTHrP-stimulated leukemia inhibitory factor (LIF) [89], may promote osteoblast differentiation and mediate some of the anabolic actions of PTHrP in bone.

The effects of PTHrP (and PTH) on osteoclastic bone resorption also appear to be mediated by interaction with PTH-1 receptors. Multinucleated osteoclasts are of hematogenous origin and are formed by fusion of mononuclear osteoclasts, which are derived by differentiation of mononuclear precursors presumably of the monocyte/macrophage lineage. The interaction of PTHrP with its receptor on the osteoblast appears to increase soluble or cell-bound cytokines, which in turn enhance differentiation and fusion of osteoclast precursors to augment the numbers of active multinucleated osteoclasts. Several cytokines, such as interleukin-6 (IL-6) [89] and colony stimulating factor-1 (CSF-1) [90], have been implicated as intermediaries in the process, however, the likeliest candidate is the TNF family molecule, osteoprotegerin ligand also known as osteoclast differentiation factor [91].

Several important steroid modulators may influence the action of PTHrP and of PTH on bone anabolism and catabolism. Thus, glucocorticoids may increase PTH-1 mRNA receptor expression [92], PTH binding, and PTH-stimulated cAMP production, effects which could lead to a net increase in PTHrP-mediated bone resorption. Estrogen, on the other hand, may inhibit PTHrP- and PTH-stimulated adenylate cyclase stimulation in osteoblasts [93, 94], and estrogen deficiency in postmenopausal women leads to increased skeletal catabolic effects of continuous PTH administration [95].

It is important to note that in view of the fact that osteoblastic cells produce PTHrP as well as the PTH-1 receptor, the capacity either of circulating PTH or of circulating or locally released PTHrP to exert anabolic or catabolic effects will be determined not only by ambient levels of these two peptides but also by the state of occupancy of the receptors by either of these ligands.

3. POTENTIAL THERAPEUTIC ROLE IN OSTEOPOROSIS

The anabolic effects of intermittent PTH administration on bone and its therapeutic potential in osteoporosis have been extensively explored [96]. With the recognition that PTHrP is the endogenous ligand for the PTH/PTHrP receptor in osteoblasts, its use as an anabolic agent has also been

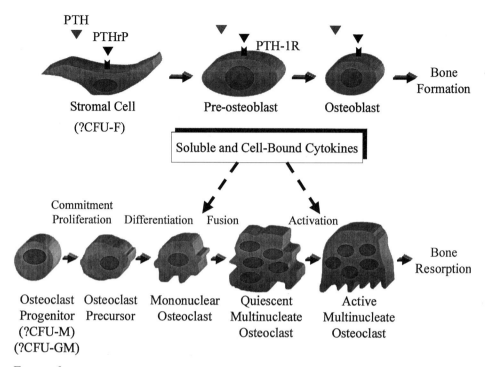

FIGURE 6   Effects of PTHrP on bone formation and bone resorption. PTHrP, circulating or locally released from osteoblastic cells, acts on PTH-1 receptors that are expressed on cells of the osteoblastic phenotype. This may elicit bone formation. Alternatively, this action may result, via stimulation of soluble or cell-bound cytokines, in the production of active multinucleated osteoclasts that resorb bone. Circulating PTH may compete with PTHrP for receptor occupancy.

investigated. PTHrP (1–74) was shown to increase bone mass in rats [97]. PTHrP (1–36) has been reported to have equivalent potency to PTH (1–34) in its actions [98], yet its anabolic effects on bone remain to be defined. PTHrP (1–34) was less potent than PTH (1–34) in producing an anabolic response in bone [99], although that could be partly attributed to its higher clearance rate [100].

Analogs of PTHrP (1–34) have been developed in an attempt to improve its anabolic efficacy. One such analog, RS-66271, has received much attention because of its pronounced bone anabolic activity *in vivo*. It markedly increased trabecular and cortical bone formation when given intermittently to ovariectomized, osteopenic rats [101]. The anabolic benefits of RS-66271 have been confirmed in a nonhuman primate model of estrogen deprivation osteopenia [102] and in glucocorticoid-induced bone loss [103]. A rapid increase in size and number of osteoblasts on trabecular surfaces was observed following initiation of treatment [104]. The rapidity with which these changes occurred suggests that the lining cells on trabecular surfaces were induced to differentiate into osteoblasts. With cessation of the drug, the osteoblasts reverted to lining cells.

While promising, there are nonetheless some potential concerns arising from the use of PTHrP and its analogs for the treatment of osteoporosis [105], such as induction of hypercalcemia. Clearly, more studies using these peptides are needed to verify their safety and efficacy as therapeutic agents.

V. SUMMARY

The discovery of PTHrP has led to improved understanding of the pathogenesis of hypercalcemia of malignancy and may also be relevant for understanding malignancy-induced bone resorption even in the absence of hypercalcemia. Unexpectedly, and of equal importance, this humoral factor has been found to play a role in a number of normal developmental processes and in the differentiated function of a variety of normal tissues. Most notable is its crucial role in the development of the cartilaginous growth plate as demonstrated by gene disruption technology. Analyses of knockout mice have also emphasized the function of PTHrP in normal osteoblastic bone formation. Powerful new *in vitro* and *in vivo* molecular technologies are also providing insights into detailed intracellular signaling mechanisms of PTHrP and its interaction with other regulatory factors. Continued advances in this field should provide important new understanding of the pathophysiology of osteochondrodysplasias, osteopetrosis, hyperparathyroidism, and osteoporosis and should facilitate the development of new therapeutic tools for these disorders.

Acknowledgments

Work on PTHrP in our laboratories was supported in part by the Medical Research Council of Canada and the National Cancer Institute of Canada.

References

1. Gutman, A. B., Tyson, T. L., and Gutman, E. B. (1936). Inorganic phosphorus and phosphatase activity in hyperparathyroidism, Paget's disease, multiple myeloma and neoplastic disease of the bones. *Arch. Intern. Med.* **57**, 379–413.
2. Albright, F. (1941). Case records of the Massachusetts General Hospital: Case 27461. *N. Engl. J. Med.* **225**, 789–791.
3. Goltzman, D., Stewart, A. F., and Broadus, A. E. (1981). Malignancy-associated hypercalcemia: Evaluation with a cytochemical bioassay for parathyroid hormone. *J. Clin. Endocrinol. Metab.* **53**, 899–904.
4. Moseley, J. M., Kubota, M., Diefenbach-Jagger, H., Wettenhall, R. E. H., Kemp, B. E., Suva, L. J., Rodda, C. P., Ebeling, P. R., Hudson, P. J., Zajac, J. D., and Martin, T. J. (1987). Parathyroid hormone-related protein purified from a human lung cancer cell line. *Proc. Natl. Acad. Sci. U.S.A.* **84**, 5048–5052.
5. Stewart, A. F., Wu, T., Goumas, D., Burtis, W. J., and Broadus, A. E. (1987). N-terminal amino acid sequence of two novel tumor-derived adenylate cyclase-stimulating proteins: Identification of parathyroid hormone-like and parathyroid hormone-unlike domains. *Biochem. Biophys. Res. Commun.* **146**, 672–678.
6. Strewler, G. J., Stern, P. H., Jacobs, J. W., Eveloff, J., Klein, R. F., Leung, S. C., Rosenblatt, M., and Nissenson, R. A. (1987). Parathyroid hormone-like protein from human renal carcinoma cells. Structural and functional homology with parathyroid hormone. *J. Clin. Invest.* **80**, 1803–1807.
7. Jüppner, H., Abou-Samra, A.-B., Freeman, M., Kong, X.-F., Schipani, E., Richards, J., Kolakowski, L. F., Jr., Hock, J., Potts, J. T., Jr., Kronenberg, H. M., and Segré, G. V. (1991). A G protein-linked receptor for parathyroid hormone and parathyroid hormone-related peptide. *Science* **254**, 1024–1026.
8. Abou-Samra, A.-B., Jüppner, H., Force, T., Freeman, M. W., Kong, X. F., Schipani, E., Urena, P., Richards, J., Bonventre, J. V., Potts, J. T., Jr., Kronenberg, H. M., and Segré, G. V. (1992). Expression cloning of a common receptor for parathyroid hormone and parathyroid hormone-related peptide from rat osteoblast-like cells: A single receptor stimulates intracellular accumulation of both cAMP and inositol trisphosphates and increases intracellular free calcium. *Proc. Natl. Acad. Sci. U.S.A.* **89**, 2732–2736.
9. Guise, T. A., Yin, J. J., Taylor, S. D., Kumagai, Y., Dallas, M., Boyce, B. F., Yoneda, T., and Mundy, G. R. (1996). Evidence for a causal role of parathyroid hormone-related protein in the pathogenesis of human breast cancer-mediated osteolysis. *J. Clin. Invest.* **98**, 1544–1549.
10. Mangin, M., Webb, A. C., Dreyer, B. E., Posillico, J. T., Ikeda, K., Weir, E. C., Stewart, A. F., Bander, N. H., Milstone, L., Barton, D. E., Francke, U., and Broadus, A. E. (1988). Identification of a cDNA encoding a parathyroid hormone-like peptide from a human tumor associated with hypercalcemia of malignancy. *Proc. Natl. Acad. Sci. U.S.A.* **85**, 597.
11. Hendy, G. N., Sakaguchi, A. Y., Yasuda, T., Weber, D. K., Wang, L.-M., Yoshida, M. C., Banville, D., and Goltzman, D. (1988). Gene for parathyroid hormone-like peptide is on rat chromosome 2. *Biochem. Biophys. Res. Commun.* **157**, 558–562.
12. Mangin, M., Ikeda, K., Dreyer, B. E., and Broadus, A. E. (1989). Isolation and characterization of the human parathyroid hormone-like peptide gene. *Proc. Natl. Acad. Sci. U.S.A.* **86**, 2408–2412.
13. Yasuda, T., Banville, D., Hendy, G. N., and Goltzman, D. (1989). Characterization of the human parathyroid hormone-like peptide gene. *J. Biol. Chem.* **264**, 7720–7725.
14. Mangin, M., Ikeda, K., Dreyer, B. E., and Broadus, A. E. (1990). Identification of an up-stream promoter of the human parathyroid hormone-related peptide gene. *Mol. Endocrinol.* **4**, 851–858.
15. Vasavada, R. C., Wysolmerski, J. J., Broadus, A. E., and Philbrick, W. M. (1993). Identification and characterization of a GC-rich promoter of the human parathyroid hormone-related peptide gene. *Mol. Endocrinol.* **7**, 273–282.
16. Karaplis, A. C., Yasuda, T., Hendy, G. N., Goltzman, D., and Banville, D. (1990). Gene encoding parathyroid hormone-like peptide: Nucleotide sequences of the rat gene and comparison with the human homologue. *Mol. Endocrinol.* **4**, 441–446.
17. Mangin, M., Ikeda, K., and Broadus, A. E. (1990). Structure of the mouse gene encoding parathyroid hormone-related peptide. *Gene* **95**, 195–202.
18. Thiede, M. A., and Rutledge, S. J. (1990). Nucleotide sequence of a parathyroid hormone-related peptide expressed by the 10 day chicken embryo. *Nucleic Acids Res.* **18**, 3062.
19. Rosol, T. J., Steinmeyer, C. L., McCauley, L. K., Grone, A., DeWille, J. W., and Capen, C. C. (1995). Sequence of the cDNAs encoding canine parathyroid hormone-related protein and parathyroid hormone. *Gene* **160**, 241–243.
20. Thiede, M. A. (1989). The mRNA encoding a parathyroid hormone-like peptide is produced in mammary tissue in response to elevations in serum prolactin. *Mol. Endocrinol.* **3**, 1443–1447.
21. Thiede, M. A., Daifotis, A. G., Weir, E. C., Brines, M. L., Burtis, W. J., Ikeda, K., Dreyer, B. E., Garfield, R. E., and Broadus, A. E. (1990). Intrauterine occupancy controls expression of the parathyroid hormone-related peptide gene in preterm rat myometrium. *Proc. Natl. Acad. Sci. U.S.A.* **87**, 6969–6973.
22. Hongo, T., Kupfer, J., Enomoto, H., Sharifi, B., Giannella-Neto, D., Forrester, J. S., Singer, F. R., Goltzman, D., Hendy, G. N., Fagin, J. A., and Clemens, T. L. (1991). Abundant expression of parathyroid hormone-related protein in primary rat aortic smooth muscle cells accompanies serum-induced proliferation. *J. Clin. Invest.* **88**, 1841.
23. Kremer, R., Karaplis, A. C., Henderson, J., Gulliver, W., Banville, D., Hendy, G. N., and Goltzman, D. (1991). Regulation of parathyroid-like peptide in cultured normal human keratinocytes: Effect of growth factors and 1,25 dihydroxyvitamin D$_3$ on gene expression and secretion. *J. Clin. Invest.* **87**, 884–893.
24. Haq, M., Kremer, R., Goltzman, D., and Rabbani, S. A. (1993). A vitamin D analogue (EB1089) inhibits parathyroid hormone related protein production and prevents the development of malignancy-associated hypercalcemia *in vivo*. *J. Clin. Invest.* **91**, 2416–2422.
25. Aklilu, F., Park, M., Goltzman, D., and Rabbani, S. A. (1997). Induction of parathyroid hormone-related peptide by the Ras oncogene: Role of Ras farnesylation inhibitors as potential therapeutic agents for hypercalcemia of malignancy. *Cancer Res.* **57**, 4515–4522.
26. Liu, B., Goltzman, D., and Rabbani, S. A. (1995). Processing of parathyroid hormone-related peptide (pro-PTHrP) by the prohormone convertase furin: Effect on biological activity. *Am. J. Physiol.* **268**, E832–E838.
27. Soifer, N. E., Dee, K. E., Insogna, K. L., Burtis, W. J., Matovcik, L. M., Wu, T. L., Milstone, L. M., Broadus, A. E., Philbrick, W. M., and Stewart, A. F. (1992). Secretion of a novel mid-region fragment of parathyroid hormone-related protein by three different cell lines in culture. *J. Biol. Chem.* **267**, 18236–18243.

28. Joun, H., Lanske, B., Karperien, M., Qian, F., Defize, L., and Abou-Samra, A.-B. (1997). Tissue-specific transcription start sites and alternative splicing of the parathyroid hormone (PTH)/PTH-Related Peptide (PTHrP) receptor gene: A new PTH/PTHrP receptor splice variant that lacks the signal peptide. *Endocrinology* **138**, 1742–1749.

29. Orloff, J. J., Ganz, M. B., Ribaudo, A. E., Burtis, W. J., Reiss, M., Milstone, L. M., and Stewart, A. F. (1992). Analysis of PTHRP binding and signal transduction mechanisms in benign and malignant squamous cells. *Am. J. Physiol.* **262**, E599–607.

30. Orloff, J. J., Kats, Y., Urena, P., Schipani, E., Vasavada, R. C., Philbrick, W. M., Behal, A., Abou-Samra, A.-B., Segré, G. V., and Jüppner, H. (1995). Further evidence for a novel receptor for amino-terminal parathyroid hormone-related protein on keratinocytes and squamous carcinoma cell lines. *Endocrinology* **136**, 3016–3023.

31. Care, A. D., Abbas, S. K., Pickard, D. W., Barri, M., Drinkhill, M., Findlay, J. B. C., White, I. R., and Caple, I. W. (1990). Stimulation of ovine placental transport of calcium and magnesium by mid-molecule fragments of human PTHrP. *Exp. Physiol.* **75**, 605–608.

32. Kovacs, C. S., Lanske, B., Hunzelman, J. L., Guo, J., Karaplis, A. C., and Kronenberg, H. M. (1996). Parathyroid hormone-related peptide (PTHrP) regulated fetal-placental calcium transport through a receptor distinct from the PTH/PTHrP receptor. *Proc. Natl. Acad. Sci. U.S.A.* **93**, 15233–15238.

33. Henderson, J. E., Amikuza, N., Warshawsky, H., Biasotto, D., Lanske, B. M. K., Goltzman, D., and Karaplis, A. C. (1995). Nucleolar localization of parathyroid hormone-related peptide enhances survival of chondrocytes under conditions that promote apoptotic cell death. *Mol. Cell. Biol.* **15**, 4064–4075.

34. Gorlich, D., and Mattaj, I. (1996). Nucleocytoplasmic transport. *Science* **271**, 1513–1518.

35. Fenton, A. J., Kemp, B. E., Kent, G. N., Moseley, J. M., Zheng, M.-H., Rowe, D. J., Britto, J. M., Martin, T. J., and Nicholson, G. C. (1991). A carboxyl-terminal peptide from the parathyroid hormone-related protein inhibits bone resorption by osteoclasts. *Endocrinology* **129**, 1762–1768.

36. Fenton, A. J., Kemp, B. E., R. G. Hammonds, J., Mitchelhill, K., Moseley, J. M., Martin, T. J., and Nicholson, G. C. (1991). A potent inhibitor of osteoclastic bone resorption within a highly conserved pentapeptide region of parathyroid hormone-related protein; PTHrP [107–111]. *Endocrinology* **129**, 3424–3426.

37. Fukayama, S., Tashjian, Jr., A., Davis, J. N., and Chisholm, J. C. (1995). Signaling by N- and C-terminal sequences of parathyroid hormone-related protein in hippocampal neurons. *Proc. Natl. Acad. Sci. U.S.A.* **92**, 10182–10186.

38. Henderson, J., Shustik, C., Kremer, R., Rabbani, S. A., Hendy, G. N., and Goltzman, D. (1990). Circulating concentrations of parathyroid hormone-like peptide in malignancy and in hyperparathyroidism. *J. Bone Miner. Res.* **5**, 105–113.

39. Wysolmerski, J. J., Philbrick, W. M., Dunbar, M. E., Lanske, B., Kronenberg, H., Karaplis, A., and Broadus, A. E. (1998). Rescue of the parathyroid hormone-related protein knockout mouse demonstrates that parathyroid hormone-related protein is essential for mammary gland development. *Development* **125**, 1285–1294.

40. Lam, M. H., Olsen, S. L., Rankin, W. A., Ho, P. W., Martin, T. J., Gillespie, M. T., and Moseley, J. M. (1997). PTHrP and cell division: Expression and localization of PTHrP in a keratinocyte cell line (HaCaT) during the cell cycle. *J. Cell. Physiol.* **173**, 433–446.

41. Massfelder, T., Dann, P., Wu, T. L., Vasavada, R., Helwig, J. J., and Stewart, A. F. (1997). Opposing mitogenic and anti-mitogenic actions of parathyroid hormone-related protein in vascular smooth muscle cells: A critical role for nuclear targeting. *Proc. Natl. Acad. Sci. U.S.A.* **94**, 13630–13635.

42. Karaplis, A. C., Luz, A., Glowacki, J., Bronson, R. T., Tybulewicz, V. L. J., Kronenberg, H. M., and Mulligan, R. C. (1994). Lethal skeletal dysplasia from targeted disruption of the parathyroid hormone-related peptide (PTHrP) gene. *Genes Dev.* **8**, 277–289.

43. Amizuka, N., Henderson, J. E., Warshawsky, H., Goltzman, D., and Karaplis, A. C. (1994). Parathyroid hormone-related peptide (PTHrP)-depleted mice show abnormal epiphyseal cartilage development and altered endochondral bone formation. *J. Cell Biol.* **126**, 1611–1623.

44. Lee, K., Lanske, B., Karaplis, A. C., Deeds, J. D., Kohno, H., Nissenson, R. A., Kronenberg, H. M., and Segré, G. V. (1996). Parathyroid hormone-related peptide delays terminal differentiation of chondrocytes during endochondral bone development. *Endocrinology* **137**, 5109–5118.

45. Amizuka, N., Henderson, J. E., Hoshi, K., Warshawsky, H., Ozawa, H., Goltzman, D., and Karaplis, A. C. (1996). Programmed cell death of chondrocytes and aberrant chondrogenesis in mice homozygous for parathyroid hormone-related peptide gene deletion. *Endocrinology* **137**, 5055–5067.

46. Weir, E. C., Philbrick, W. M., Amling, M., Neff, L. A., Baron, R., and Broadus, A. E. (1996). Targeted overexpression of parathyroid hormone-related peptide in chondrocytes causes chondrodysplasia and delayed endochondral bone formation. *Proc. Natl. Acad. Sci. U.S.A.* **93**, 10240–10245.

47. Kruse, K. (1993). Calcium metabolism in the Jansen type of metaphyseal dysplasia. *Eur. J. Pediatr.* **152**, 912–915.

48. Schipani, E., Kruse, K., and Jüppner, H. (1995). A constitutively active mutant PTH-PTHrP receptor in Jansen-type metaphyseal chondrodysplasia. *Science* **268**, 98–100.

49. Schipani, E., Langman, C. B., Parfitt, A. M., Jensen, G. S., Kikuchi, S., Kooh, S. W., Cole, W. G., and Jüppner, H. (1996). Constitutively activated receptors for parathyroid hormone-related peptide in Jansens metaphyseal chondrodysplasia. *N. Engl. J. Med.* **335**, 708–714.

50. Schipani, E., Lanske, B., Hunzelman, J., Luz, A., Kovacs, C. S., Lee, K., Pirro, A., Kronenberg, H. M., and Jüppner, H. (1997). Targeted expression of constitutively active receptors for parathyroid hormone and parathyroid hormone-related peptide delays endochondral bone formation and rescues mice that lack parathyroid hormone-related peptide. *Proc. Natl. Acad. Sci. U.S.A.* **94**, 13689–13694.

51. Farnum, C. E., and Wilsman, N. J. (1989). Condensation of hypertrophic chondrocytes at the chondro-osseous junction of growth plate cartilage in Yucatan swine: relationship to long bone growth. *Am. J. Anat.* **186**, 346–358.

52. Amling, M., Neff, L., Tanaka, S., Inoue, D., Kuida, K., Weir, E., Philbrick, W. M., Broadus, A. E., and Baron, R. (1997). Bcl-2 lies downstream of parathyroid hormone-related peptide in a signaling pathway that regulates chondrocyte maturation during skeletal development. *J. Cell Biol.* **136**, 205–213.

53. Porter, J. A., Ekker, S. C., Park, W. J., von Kessler, D. P., Young, K. E., Chen, C. H., Ma, Y., Woods, A. S., Cotter, R. J., Koonin, E. V., and Beachy, P. A. (1996). Hedgehog patterning activity: role of a lipophilic modification mediated by the carboxy-terminal autoprocessing domain. *Cell* **86**, 21–34.

54. Porter, J. A., Young, K. E., and Beachy, P. A. (1996). Cholesterol modification of hedgehog signaling proteins in animal development. *Science* **274**, 255–259.

55. Marigo, V., Davey, R. A., Zuo, Y., Cunningham, J. M., and Tabin, C. J. (1996). Biochemical evidence that Patched is the Hedgehog receptor. *Nature* **384**, 176–179.

56. Stone, D. M., Hynes, M., Armanini, M., Swanson, T. A., Gu, Q., Johnson, R. L., Scott, M. P., Pennica, D., Goddard, A., Phillips, H., Noll, M., Hooper, J. E., Sauvage, F. D., and Rosenthal, A. (1996). The tumour-suppressor gene *patched* encodes a candidate receptor for Sonic hedgehog. *Nature* **384**, 129–134.

57. Nusse, R. (1996). Patching up Hedgehog. *Nature* **384**, 119–120.

58. Hui, C.-C., Slusarski, D., Platt, K. A., Holmgren, R., and Joyner, A. L. (1994). Expression of three mouse homologs of the *Drosophila* segment polarity gene cubitus interruptus, *Gli*, *Gli-2*, and *Gli-3*, in

ectoderm- and mesoderm-derived tissues suggests multiple roles during postimplantation development. *Dev. Biol.* **162**, 402–413.

59. Johnson, R. L., Laufer, E., Riddle, R. D., and Tabin, C. (1994). Ectopic expression of Sonic hedgehog alters dorsal-ventral patterning of somites. *Cell* **79**, 1165–1173.

60. Cohn, M. J., and Tickle, C. (1996). Limbs: A model for pattern formation within the vertebrate body plan. *Trends Genet.* **12**, 253–257.

61. Chiang, C., Litingtung, Y., Lee, E., Young, K. E., Corden, J. L., Westphal, H., and Beachy, P. A. (1996). Cyclopia and defective axial patterning in mice lacking *Sonic hedgehog* gene function. *Nature* **383**, 407–413.

62. Mo, R., Freer, A. M., Zinyk, D. L., Crackower, M. A., Michaud, J., Heng, H. H. Q., Chik, K. W., Shi, X.-M., Tsui, L.-C., Cheng, S. H., Joyner, A. L., and Hui, C.-C. (1997). Specific and redundant functions of *Gli2* and *Gli3* zinc finger genes in skeletal patterning and development. *Development* **124**, 113–123.

63. Hui, C.-C., and Joyner, A. L. (1993). A mouse model of Greig cephalopolysyndactyly syndrome: The *extra-toes*[j] mutation contains an intragenic deletion of the *Gli3* gene. *Nat. Genet.* **3**, 241–246.

64. Vortkamp, A., Gessler, M., and Grzeschik, K.-H. (1991). GLI3 zinc-finger gene interrupted by translocations in Greig syndrome families. *Nature* **352**, 539–540.

65. Vortkamp, A., Lee, K., Lanske, B., Segré, G. V., Kronenberg, H. M., and Tabin, C. J. (1996). Regulation of rate of cartilage differentiation by indian hedgehog and PTH-related protein. *Science* **273**, 613–622.

66. Lanske, B., Karaplis, A. C., Lee, K., Luz, A., Vortkamp, A., Pirro, A., Karperien, M., Defize, L. H. K., Ho, C., Mulligan, R. C., Abou-Samra, A.-B., Jüppner, H., Segré, G. V., and Kronenberg, H. M. (1996). PTH/PTHrP receptor in early development and indian hedgehog-regulated bone growth. *Science* **273**, 663–666.

67. Helms, J., Iwasai, M., and Lee, A. (1997). Expression of hedgehog, BMP and GLI genes during cartilage and bone development. *Annu. Meet. Orthop. Res. Soc. Abstr.*, p. 34.

68. Akiyama, H., Shigeno, C., Hiraki, Y., Shukunami, C., Kohno, H., Akagi, M., Konishi, J., and Nakamura, T. (1997). Cloning of a mouse smoothened cDNA and expression patterns of hedgehog signalling molecules during chondrogenesis and cartilage differentiation in clonal mouse EC cells, ATDC5. *Biochem. Biophys. Res. Commun.* **235**, 142–147.

69. Karaplis, A. C., and Vautour, L. (1997). Parathyroid hormone-related peptide and the parathyroid hormone/parathyroid hormone-related peptide receptor in skeletal development. *Curr. Opin. Nephrol. Hyperten.* **6**, 308–313.

70. Stott, N. S., and Chuong, C.-M. (1997). Dual action of sonic hedgehog on chondrocyte hypertrophy: retrovirus mediated ectopic sonic hedgehog expression in limb bud micromass culture induces novel cartilage nodules that are positive for alkaline phosphatase and type X collagen. *J. Cell Sci.* **110**, 2691–2701.

71. Zou, H., Wieser, R., Massagué, J., and Niswander, L. (1997). Distinct roles of type I bone morphogenetic protein receptors in the formation and differentiation of cartilage. *Genes Dev.* **11**, 2191–2203.

72. Serra, R., Johnson, M., Filvaroff, E. H., Laborde, J., Sheehan, D. M., Derynck, R., and Moses, H. L. (1997). Expression of a truncated, kinase-defective TGF-beta type II receptor in mouse skeletal tissue promotes terminal chondrocyte differentiation and osteoarthritis. *J. Cell Biol.* **139**, 541–552.

73. Nguyen, M. T. A., and Karaplis, A. C. (1998). The nucleus: A target site for parathyroid hormone-related peptide (PTHrP) action. *J. Cell. Biochem.* **70**, 193–199.

74. Lee, K., Deeds, J. D., Bond, A. T., Jüppner, H., Abou-Samra, A.-B., and Segré, G. V. (1993). In situ localization of PTH/PTHrP receptor mRNA in the bone of fetal and young rats. *Bone* **14**, 341–345.

75. Lee, K., Deeds, J. D., Chiba, S., Un-No, M., Bond, A. T., and Segré, G. V. (1994). Parathyroid hormone induces sequential c-fos expression in bone cells in vivo: In situ localization of its receptor and c-fos messenger ribonucleic acids. *Endocrinology* **134**, 441–450.

76. Lee, K., Deeds, J. D., and Segré, G. V. (1995). Expression of parathyroid hormone related-peptide and its receptor messenger ribonucleic acids during fetal development of rats. *Endocrinology* **136**, 453–463.

77. Fermor, B., and Skerry, T. M. (1995). PTH/PTHrP receptor expression on osteoblasts and osteocytes but not resorbing bone surfaces in growing rats. *J. Bone Miner. Res.* **10**, 1935–1943.

78. Celic, S., Chilco, P. J., Zajac, J. D., Martin, T. J., and Findley, D. M. (1996). A type 1 collagen substrate increases PTH/PTHrP receptor mRNA expression and suppresses PTHrP mRNA expression in UMR106-06 osteoblast-like cells. *J. Endocrinol.* **150**, 299–308.

79. Suda, N., Gillespie, M. T., Traianedes, K., Zhou, H., Ho, P. W. M., Hards, D. K., Allan, E. H., Martin, T. J., and Moseley, J. M. (1996). Expression of parathyroid hormone-related protein in cells of osteoblast lineage. *J. Cell. Physiol.* **166**, 94–104.

80. McCauley, L. K., Koh, A. J., Beecher, C. A., Cui, Y., Rosol, T. J., and Franceschi, R. T. (1996). PTH/PTHrP receptor is temporally regulated during osteoblast differentiation and is associated with collagen synthesis. *J. Cell. Biochem.* **61**, 638–647.

81. Amizuka, N., Karaplis, A. C., Henderson, J. E., Warshawsky, H., Lipman, M. l., Matsuki, Y., Ejiri, S., Tanaka, M., Izumi, N., Ozawa, H., and Goltzman, D. (1996). Haploinsufficiency of parathyroid hormone-related peptide (PTHrP) results in abnormal postnatal bone development. *Dev. Biol.* **175**, 166–176.

82. Owen, M., and Friedenstein, A. J. (1988). Stromal stem cells: marrow-derived osteogenic precursors. *Ciba Found. Symp.* **136**, 42–60.

83. Philbrick, W. M., Wysolmerski, J. J., Galbraith, S., Holt, E., Orloff, J. J., Yang, K. H., Vasavada, R. C., Weir, E. C., Broadus, A. E., and Stewart, A. F. (1996). Defining the roles of parathyroid hormone-related protein in normal physiology. *Physiol. Rev.* **76**, 127–173.

84. Walsh, C. A., Birch, M. A., Fraser, W. D., Laton, R., Dorgan, J., Walsh, S., Sansom, D., Beresford, J. N., and Gallagher, J. A. (1995). Expression and secretion of parathyroid hormone-related protein by human bone-derived cells in vitro: Effects of glucocorticoids. *J. Bone Miner. Res.* **10**, 17–25.

85. Kinto, N., Iwamoto, M., Enomoto-Iwamoto, M., Noji, S., Ohuchi, H., Yoshioka, H., Kataoka, H., Wada, Y., Yuhao, G., Takahashi, H. E., Yoshiki, S., and Yamaguchi, A. (1997). Fibroblasts expressing sonic hedgehog induce osteoblast differentiation and ectopic bone formation. *FEBS Lett.* **404**, 319–323.

86. Nakamura, T., Aikawa, T., Iwamoto-Enomoto, M., Iwamoto, M., Higuchi, Y., Maurizio, P., Kinto, N., Yamaguchi, A., Noji, S., Kurisu, K., and Matsuta, T. (1997). Induction of osteogenic differentiation by hedgehog proteins. *Biochem. Biophys. Res. Commun.* **237**, 465–469.

87. Rouleau, M. F., Mitchell, J., and Goltzman, D. (1990). Characterization of the major parathyroid hormone target cell in the endosteal metaphysis of rat long bones. *J. Bone Miner. Res.* **5**, 1043–1053.

88. Canalis, E., McCarthy, T. L., and Centrella, M. (1990). Differential effects of continuous and transient treatment with parathyroid hormone related peptide (PTHrP) on bone collagen synthesis. *Endocrinology* **126**, 1806–1812.

89. Pollock, J. H., Blaha, M. J., Lavish, S. A., Stevenson, S., and Greenfield, E. M. (1996). In vivo demonstration that parathyroid hormone and parathyroid hormone-related protein stimulate expression by osteoblasts of interleukin-6 and leukemia inhibitory factor. *J. Bone Miner. Res.* **11**, 754–759.

90. Weir, E. C., Lowik, C. W. G. M., Paliwal, I., and Insogna, K. L. (1996). Colony stimulating factor-1 plays a role in osteoclast formation and function in bone resorption induced by parathyroid hormone and parathyroid hormone-related peptide. *J. Bone Miner. Res.* **11**, 1474–1481.

91. Yasuda, H., Shima, N., Nakagawa, N., Yamaguchi, K., Kinosaki, M., Mochizuki, S., Tomoyasu, A., Yano, K., Goto, M., Murakami,

A., Tsuda, E., Morinaga, T., Higashio, K., Udagawa, N., Takahashi, N., and Suda, T. (1998). Osteoclast differentiation factor is a ligand for osteoprotegerin/osteoclastogenesis-inhibitory factor and is identical to TRANCE/RANKL. *Proc. Natl. Acad. Sci. USA* **95**, 3597–3602.

92. Urena, P., Iida-Klein, A., Kong, X.-F., Jüppner, H., Kronenberg, H. M., Abou-Samra, A.-B, and Segré, G. V. (1994). Regulation of parathyroid (PTH)/PTH-related peptide receptor messenger ribonucleic acid by glucocorticoids and PTH in ROS 17/2.8 and OK Cells. *Endocrinology* **134**, 451–456.

93. Ernst, M., Heath, J. K., and Rodan, G. A. (1989). Estradiol effects on proliferation, messenger ribonucleic acid for collagen and insulin-like growth factor-I, and parathyroid hormone-stimulated adenylate cyclase activity in osteoblastic cells from calvariae and long bones. *Endocrinology* **125**, 825–833.

94. Fukayama, S., and Tashjian, A. H. (1989). Direct modulation by estradiol of the response of human bone cells (SaOS-2) to human parathyroid hormone (PTH) and PTH-related protein. *Endocrinology* **124**, 397–401.

95. Joborn, C., Ljunghall, S., Larsson, K., Lindh, E., Naessen, T., Wide, L., Akerstrom, G., and Rastad, J. (1991). Skeletal responsiveness to parathyroid hormone in healthy females: Relationship to menopause and estrogen replacement. *Clin. Endocrinol.* **34**, 335–339.

96. Reeve, J. (1996). PTH: A future role in the management of osteoporosis? *J. Bone Miner. Res.* **11**, 440–445.

97. Weir, E. C., Terwilliger, G., Sartori, L., and Insogna, K. L. (1992). Synthetic parathyroid hormone-like protein (1-74) is anabolic for bone *in vivo*. *Calcif. Tissue Int.* **51**, 30–34.

98. Evenhart-Caye, M., Inzucchi, S. E., Guinness-Henry, J., Mitnick, M. A., and Stewart, A. F. (1996). Parathyroid hormone (PTH)-related protein(1-36) is equipotent to PTH(1-34) in humans. *J. Clin. Endocrinol. Metab.* **81**, 199–208.

99. Hock, J. M., Fonseca, J., Gunness-Hey, M., Kemp, B. E., and Martin, T. J. (1989). Comparison of the anabolic effects of synthetic parathyroid hormone-related protein (PTHrP) 1-34 and PTH 1-34 on bone in rats. *Endocrinology* **125**, 2022–2027.

100. Fraher, L. J., Klein, K., Marier, R., Freeman, D., Hendy, G. N., Goltzman, D., and Hodsman, A. B. (1995). Comparison of the pharmacokinetics of parenteral parathyroid hormone-(1-34) [PTH-(1-34)] and PTH-related peptide-(1-34) in healthy young humans. *J. Clin. Endocrinol. Metab.* **80**, 60–64.

101. Vickery, B. H., Avnur, Z., Cheng, Y., Chiou, S., Leaffer, D., Caulfield, J. P., Kimmel, D. B., Ho, T., and Krstenansky, J. L. (1996). RS-66271, a C-terminally substituted analog of human parathyroid hormone-related protein (1-34), increases trabecular and cortical bone in ovariectomized, osteopenic rats. *J. Bone Miner. Res.* **11**, 1943–1951.

102. Avnur, Z., McRae, G. I., Tallentire, D., and Vickery, B. H. (1995). RS66271 rapidly increases bone mineral density at spine, hip and forearm in ovariectomized cynomolgus macaques. *J. Bone Miner. Res.* **10** (S1), S196.

103. Vickery, B. H., Bergstrom, K., DeRosier, A., Katigbak, L., and Waters, R. V. (1995). RS66271 very rapidly reverses bone loss induced by prednisone in rabbits. *J. Bone Miner. Res.* **10** (S1), S257.

104. Leaffer, D., Sweeney, M., Kellerman, L. A., Avnur, Z., Krśtenansky, J. L., Vickery, B. H., and Caulfield, J. P. (1995). Modulation of osteogenic cell ultrastructure by RS-23581, an analog of human parathyroid hormone (PTH)-related peptide-(1-34), and bovine PTH-(1-34). *Endocrinology* **136**, 3624–3631.

105. Stewart, A. F. (1996). PTHrP(1-36) as a skeletal anabolic agent for the treatment of osteoporosis. *Bone* **19**, 303–306.

CHAPTER 15

The Vitamin D Hormone and Its Nuclear Receptor: Genomic Mechanisms Involved in Bone Biology

GEERT CARMELIET, ANNEMIEKE VERSTUYF, EVIS DACI, AND ROGER BOUILLON

Laboratorium for Experimental Medicine and Endocrinology, K. U. Leuven, 3000 Leuven, Belgium

I. ABSTRACT

The active metabolite of vitamin D, 1α,25 dihydroxyvitamin D$_3$ [1,25(OH)$_2$D$_3$], has multiple actions but its major role is related to bone metabolism and mineral homeostasis. Vitamin D is metabolized to its active form by two sequential hydroxylations on the carbon-25 and carbon-1 atoms. The genomic action of 1,25(OH)$_2$D$_3$ is mediated by the nuclear vitamin D receptor (VDR) that binds its ligand with high affinity. VDR is a phosphoprotein that regulates gene expression by heterodimerizing with the retinoid X receptor and associating specifically with vitamin D responsive elements (VDREs) in target genes. VDREs consisting of direct hexanucleotide repeats with a spacer of three nucleotides have been identified in the promoter regions of positively controlled genes expressed in bone, such as osteocalcin, osteopontin, 25-hydroxyvitamin D-24-hydroxylase, and β_3 integrin. Negatively regulated genes such as parathyroid hormone often contain not-classical VDREs. However, additional protein–protein interaction of the VDR is necessary for transactivation. VDR can bind to the basal transcription factor TFIIB and the AF-2 domain of the VDR, positioned at the extreme C terminus, may associate with coactivators. At the cellular level, 1,25(OH)$_2$D$_3$ treatment inhibits or induces osteoblast differentiation depending on whether it is given at proliferation or differentiation stages, respectively. It also can promote osteoclast differentiation. However, the effects of 1,25(OH)$_2$D$_3$ on bone metabolism *in vivo* are until now not well defined. Vitamin D deficiency or mutations in the 25-hydroxyvitamin D-1α-hydroxylase gene or VDR gene lead to rickets and osteomalacia. A similar phenotype is observed in VDR-deficient mice, while mice deficient in 25-hydroxyvitamin D-24-hydroxylase show abnormal intramembranous mineralization. The exact roles of $1,25(OH)_2D_3$ in bone mineralization remain to be determined.

II. SYNTHESIS AND METABOLISM OF $1,25(OH)_2D_3$

A. Skin and Dietary Sources

The secosteroid vitamin D_3 can be produced endogenously in the skin by the action of UV light (290–300 nm), converting 7-dehydrocholesterol into previtamin D_3 that is in thermoequilibrium with vitamin D_3 (Fig. 1). Prolonged exposure to sunlight does not produce toxic amounts of vitamin D_3 because of photoconversion of previtamin D_3 via alternative pathways into lumisterol or tachysterol. A second source of vitamin D_3 is dietary intake. Approximately 50% of dietary vitamin D_3 is absorbed by enterocytes and transported via chylomicrons to the general circulation. In blood, vitamin D_3 and its active metabolites are transported by a specific plasma binding protein, vitamin D binding protein (DBP).

B. 25-Hydroxylase and 25-Hydroxyvitamin D-1α-hydroxylase

A first step in the activation pathway of vitamin D_3 is the hydroxylation at carbon 25 in the liver by the enzyme 25-hydroxylase to produce 25-hydroxyvitamin D_3 [$25(OH)D_3$], the major circulating form of vitamin D_3. This enzyme is present in mitochondria or microsomes depending on the species. In humans, only the mitochondrial form of the enzyme has been detected, namely the liver sterol 27-hydroxylase (CYP27) [1]. CYP27 is a multifunctional enzyme that can also hydroxylate a variety of other steroid substrates [2]. Its expression in several tissues, including bone, has been reported [3]. $25(OH)D_3$ is biologically inactive and requires further hydroxylation in the kidney to the active hormone 1,25-dihydroxyvitamin D_3 [$1,25(OH)_2D_3$] by 25-hydroxyvitamin D-1α-hydroxylase (P450$_{1α}$). The production of $1,25(OH)_2D_3$ is regulated primarily at the second hydroxylation step by several factors, including calcium and parathyroid hormone (PTH). Rat, mouse, and human P450$_{1α}$

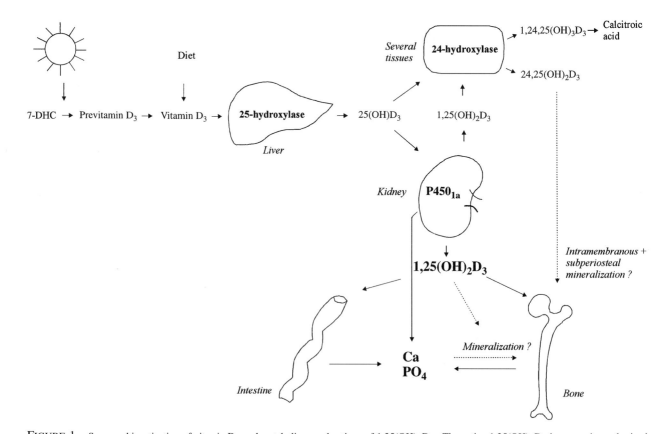

FIGURE 1 Sources, bioactivation of vitamin D_3 and metabolism, and actions of $1,25(OH)_2D_3$. The active $1,25(OH)_2D_3$ hormone is synthesized from the vitamin D precursor by two successive enzymatic hydroxylations on carbon-25 and carbon-1 in liver and kidney, respectively. $1,25(OH)_2D_3$ acts principally on intestine, kidney, and bone in order to keep serum calcium constant. The major pathway in catabolism is via 24-hydroxylase that has a broad tissue distribution. Whether $1,25(OH)_2D_3$ and $24,25(OH)_2D_3$ have a direct effect on mineralization is still a subject of investigation.

have recently been cloned by several groups [4–8]; the human P450$_{1\alpha}$ has been mapped to chromosome 12q13.3. The proximal renal tubule is the principal site of 1α-hydroxylation, but high levels of 1α-hydroxylase mRNA have been found in human keratinocytes [8] and gene expression is also observed in mouse macrophages [C. Mathieu and R. Bouillon, unpublished results].

In the genetic disorder pseudovitamin D-deficiency rickets (PDDR), also known as vitamin D-dependency rickets type I, this renal enzyme is defective, leading to low serum 1,25(OH)$_2$D$_3$ concentrations [9]. Mutations in the P450$_{1\alpha}$ gene in patients with PDDR provide the molecular genetic basis for this disease [8, 10].

C. 24-Hydroxylase: Catabolism or Specific Function?

An alternative hydroxylation pathway of 25(OH)D$_3$ occurs on carbon 24 by the multifunctional enzyme 24-hydroxylase, mapped to human chromosome 20q13 [11]. This enzyme not only initiates the catabolic cascade of 25(OH)D$_3$ and 1α,25(OH)$_2$D$_3$ [12, 13] by 24-hydroxylation, but it also catalyzes the dehydrogenation of the 24-OH group and performs 23-hydroxylation resulting in 24-oxo-1,23,25-(OH)$_3$D$_3$ [14]. This C24 oxidation pathway leads finally to calcitroic acid, which is the major end product of 1,25(OH)$_2$D$_3$. 1,25(OH)$_2$D$_3$ itself is one of the factors that regulates this pathway. 24-hydroxylase activity may play an important role in regulating the functions of 1,25(OH)$_2$D$_3$ in the target cells.

The physiological function of 24R,25(OH)$_2$D$_3$ is not yet fully clarified since a genetic disorder of 24-hydroxylase is unknown in man. Mutant mice, homozygous for defective 24-hydroxylase activity and born from heterozygous mothers, show normal prenatal development and normal bone histology [15]. However, high mortality (50%) is observed early in life that is probably related to 1,25(OH)$_2$D$_3$ toxicity. Interestingly, the skeletal development of homozygous mice born from homozygous mutant mice shows abnormal intramembranous and subperiosteal ossification [16]. This phenotype is partially rescued by treating gestating homozygote mutant females with 24,25(OH)$_2$D$_3$, indicating a key role for 24,25(OH)$_2$D$_3$ in the developmental regulation of intramembranous ossification. This physiological role for 24,25(OH)$_2$D$_3$ has already been suggested by more classical experiments on chondrocyte development [17, 18] or bone fracture repair [19, 20].

III. NUCLEAR VITAMIN D RECEPTOR

A. General Characteristics of the Protein and Gene

The actions of 1,25(OH)$_2$D$_3$ are mediated by the nuclear vitamin D receptor (VDR), a member of the superfamily of steroid/thyroid hormone receptors [21]. The VDR has been cloned from several species (*Xenopus*, chick, quail, mouse, rat, and human [22–27]. It is a 55 kDa protein made up of 427 amino acids. The VDR is present at a low concentration (10–100 fmol/mg protein), consistent with the fact that it is a potent transcription regulatory molecule.

The human VDR is encoded by a single gene mapped to chromosome 12q13. The gene is comprised of 11 exons that, together with intervening introns, span approximately 75 kb (Fig. 2) [28]. The noncoding 5′ end of the gene includes exons 1A, 1B, and 1C. Eight additional exons (exons 2–9) encode the structural portion of the VDR gene product. Three human kidney mRNA species have been found due to differential splicing of the noncoding exons 1B and 1C. The functional relevance of this finding is not yet established.

B. Structure–Function Analysis

Using site-directed mutation experiments, knowledge of the structural and functional properties of the VDR protein has increased dramatically. However, X-ray crystallography of the three-dimensional structure is not yet available. The structural organization of VDR includes a highly conserved amino-terminal DNA-binding domain and a carboxy-terminal ligand-binding domain (Fig. 2).

1. LIGAND BINDING DOMAIN

a. Ligand Binding Function The VDR binds its ligand with extremely high affinity, in the range of 10^{-10} M. The three-dimensional binding pocket comprises many segments spanning the entire carboxy-terminal domain of 300 amino acids [29]. The exact amino acid residues in the region in contact with the ligand remain unknown. Using deletion mapping, Jin *et al.* [30] narrowed the critical region to a region between amino acids 232 and 382. Site-directed mutagenesis of cysteine 288 and, to a lesser extent, cysteine 337 impairs ligand binding, without affecting heterodimerization and DNA binding [31].

b. Dimerization The ligand binding domain is multifunctional in that it not only binds 1,25(OH)$_2$D$_3$ but also possesses a dimerization surface as well as the ligand-dependent transactivation function, AF-2. VDR forms homo- or heterodimers that can interact with specific DNA segments. Part of the dimerization function of the receptor maps to two regions (239–269 and 317–401) in the ligand binding domain that are highly conserved across the steroid hormone receptor family [30]. In addition, regions in the DNA binding domain are also involved in dimerization (see Section III.B.2).

c. Transcriptional Activation The precise molecular details through which VDR affects the rate of RNA polymerase II-directed transcription are currently under intensive investigation. As with other transcriptional regulatory proteins,

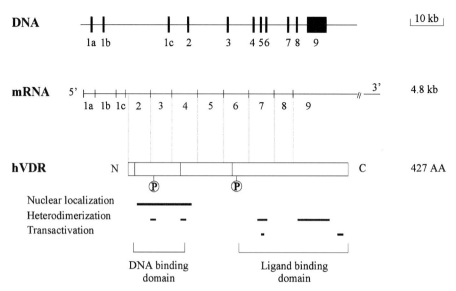

FIGURE 2   Gene and protein structure of human vitamin D receptor (hVDR). The hVDR gene is composed of 11 exons spanning approximately 75 kb of DNA. The location of exons relative to the mRNA transcript of ~4800 nucleotides and the encoded VDR protein of 427 amino acids is illustrated. Indicated are the general functional domains for DNA and ligand binding, nuclear localization, heterodimerization, and transactivation, as well as the two major phosphorylation sites.

this mechanism is likely to involve selective interaction of VDR with general transcription factors, including TFIIB, either directly or indirectly through the action of bridging proteins such as the TATA-binding protein-associated factors or various coactivator/corepressor proteins. The carboxy terminus of the VDR was shown to interact directly with a 43 residue amino-terminal region of TFIIB [32, 33] (Fig. 3). The structural integrity of the amino-terminal zinc finger of TFIIB is essential for VDR–TFIIB complex formation [34]. Interestingly, both *in vitro* and *in vivo* protein interaction assays showed that hVDR-TFIIB association is not dependent upon $1,25(OH)_2D_3$ and that the VDR–TFIIB protein complex is disrupted by the $1,25(OH)_2D_3$ ligand. Based on these data, a model is proposed in which unliganded VDR recruits TFIIB to the promoter regions of vitamin D-responsive target genes, concentrating these limiting transcription factors for enhanced transcription induced by the ligand. When $1,25(OH)_2D_3$ binds to VDR, the sequestered TFIIB is released to the assembling transcription preinitiation complex.

As already mentioned, transcriptional activation may also involve interactions with coactivators/repressors that are promoter- and tissue-specific. The subdomain of VDR that is required for transcriptional activation is the extreme C terminus (helix 12) [35] that shares the ligand-dependent activation function (AF-2) with other nuclear receptors [36–39]. Concurrently, mutations of Leu-417 and Glu-420 in this region of hVDR [40] abolish $1,25(OH)_2D_3$ stimulated transcription without effect on ligand binding, heterodimerization, and association with VDRE. In addition, the interaction

with TFIIB is not impaired, indicating that the domain of VDR that interfaces with TFIIB lies elsewhere. These experiments also suggest that the AF-2 domain of VDR functions to recruit coactivators. Several transcriptional coactivators (mSUG1, hTAF$_{II}$135, mGRIP1, RAC3, and SRC-1) [41–45] have been shown to interact with the AF-2 domain of the VDR and/or to potentiate transcriptional activation. Taken together, the AF-2 domain plays an important role in ligand activated transcription that is further supported by the large homology in this region with mRAR-γ, rTRα, and hRXR-α [37, 46, 47], whose three-dimensional crystal structure was determined. Based on these data, a proposed model postulates that ligand binding induces a conformational change so that helix 12 essentially covers the opening of the ligand binding pocket and locks the lipophilic ligand in the internal binding pocket ("mouse trap"). This conformational change facilitates the interaction of helix 12 with coactivator/transcription factors.

2. DNA BINDING

The DNA binding domain, the most highly conserved region among the nuclear receptors, consists of two similar modules, each comprising a zinc-coordinated finger structure. Whereas the amino-terminal module functions to direct specific DNA binding in the major groove of the DNA binding site [48], the carboxy-terminal module serves as a dimerization interface for interaction with a partner protein [49] which is enhanced by residues within the ligand binding domain.

Despite evidence that VDR is a nuclear protein, little is known about the nature of nuclear localization signals within

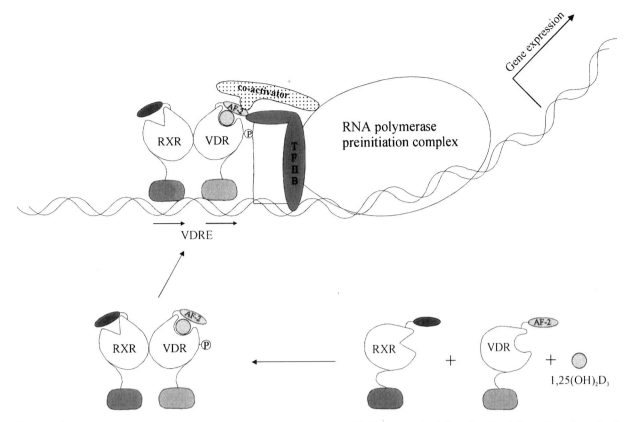

FIGURE 3   General model of transactivation by VDR. 1,25(OH)$_2$D$_3$ binding to VDR is proposed to induce phosphorylation and a conformational change of VDR, promoting heterodimerization with RXR. This RXR/VDR complex will bind to the 5' and 3' half-sites respectively of the VDRE upstream of a regulated gene. In addition, transactivation requires interaction of the AF-2 domain of VDR with both coactivators and TFIIB promoting the assembly of the RNA polymerase II preinitiation complex.

the VDR. The presence of basic residues at both ends of the VDR region 79–105 was shown to be necessary for nuclear accumulation [50].

C. Dimer Formation and DNA Interaction

The VDR forms either homo- or heterodimers, most often with the retinoid X receptor (RXR) [51–53]. The interaction with other nuclear receptors, and consequently the interplay between the different ligand signaling pathways, is discussed in some excellent reviews [54, 55]. The general concept is that upon 1,25(OH)$_2$D$_3$ binding, VDR recruits RXR into a heterodimeric complex and RXR and VDR bind to the 5'- and 3' half-sites of VDRE, respectively [56, 57]. The consensus high affinity VDRE comprises two hexameric half-sites (PuG(G/T)-TCA) arranged as a direct repeat with spacing of 3 bp (DR3) [58]. Most of the genes carrying DR3-type VDREs are positively regulated and associated with the hormone's classical function, which is the regulation of calcium homeostasis (osteocalcin, osteopontin, 24-hydroxylase, β_3 integrin) [59–62]. Interestingly, VDR/RXR heterodimers bound to osteocalcin or osteopontin VDRE differ in their

conformation, as shown by immunological assays; these data suggest the possibility of different interactions with coactivators or repressor proteins [63].

D. Modulation of Vitamin D Receptor

1. PHOSPHORYLATION AND RECEPTOR ACTIVITY

Upon addition of ligand, rapid phosphorylation of the VDR occurs [64], although the exact functional consequences of this phosphorylation have been difficult to determine. External factors may modulate the phosphorylation of VDR [65]. The phosphorylated residues have been localized to the ligand binding domain of the protein. Recently, Jurutka *et al.* [66] showed that although phosphorylation of hVDR at Ser-208 is not obligatory for 1,25(OH)$_2$D$_3$ action, phosphorylation of this residue by casein kinase II specifically modulates transcriptional capacity. In relation to this, the region of hVDR reported to participate in the association with TFIIB includes Ser-208 [33]. In contrast, PKC-mediated phosphorylation of Ser-51 [67] decreased DNA binding of the receptor [68]. Less is known about PKA-dependent phosphorylation of VDR, but it may be involved in the PTH-signaling pathway that negatively regulates VDR activity [69]. Taken together, VDR activity is both positively and negatively regulated depending on the type of phosphorylation, and this might represent a mechanism whereby other cell signaling systems influence the genomic (or nongenomic) actions of $1,25(OH)_2D_3$ [54].

2. REGULATION OF VITAMIN D RECEPTOR ABUNDANCE

a. Heterologous Regulation of VDR Several studies have demonstrated that there is a strong correlation between the VDR level and the biological response in target cells [70]. PTH [71], pharmacological activators of the protein kinase A pathway [72], TGF-β [73], estrogens [74], thyroid hormone [75], glucocorticoids [76], and retinoic acid [77] all can alter VDR mRNA levels in a tissue-specific pattern. Interestingly, both cell cycle [78] and the differentiation state of cells in culture [79] influence the extent of VDR mRNA expression. However, the underlying mechanisms regulating VDR gene expression are not yet completely understood [28, 80].

b. Homologous Regulation of VDR Autoregulation of VDR expression has been demonstrated both *in vitro* and *in vivo*, again in a very tissue-specific fashion. It is well established that $1,25(OH)_2D_3$ increases the VDR content by stabilizing the receptor [81, 82]. The role of $1,25(OH)_2D_3$ in the transcriptional regulation of the VDR gene is less evident. $1,25(OH)_2D_3$-inducibility of the hVDR gene has not been found with the part of the promoter that has been characterized [28, 80]. One possible explanation is that the autoregulatory actions of $1,25(OH)_2D_3$ are indirect. For example, one study suggests that $1,25(OH)_2D_3$ can stimulate the expression of c-fos in osteoblastic cells that might in turn stimulate hVDR gene expression [83]. Other possibilities for the $1,25(OH)_2D_3$-responsive region of the gene may, however, remain to be defined.

IV. $1,25(OH)_2D_3$-REGULATED GENE EXPRESSION RELATED TO BONE PHYSIOLOGY

Although over 50 genes have been reported to be regulated by $1,25(OH)_2D_3$, only a small number have been reported to contain VDREs [84].

A. Osteocalcin

Osteocalcin, a noncollagenous protein of bone extracellular matrix that regulates bone formation [85], is synthesized only by mature postproliferative cells in which the osteocalcin gene is transcriptionally activated at the onset of extra-cellular matrix mineralization [86]. At this stage of differentiation, osteocalcin expression in rat and human osteoblasts becomes responsive to $1,25(OH)_2D_3$. The VDRE of the rat osteocalcin gene has been characterized as a DR3 element (-465 to -437). The mechanism underlying $1,25(OH)_2D_3$ unresponsiveness during proliferation has been partially clarified. The multifunctional regulator YY1 represses $1,25(OH)_2D_3$-induced transactivation of the osteocalcin gene by two pathways [87]. First, YY1 recognition sequences are present within the osteocalcin VDRE, and YY1 competes with the VDR/RXR heterodimer for binding to this site. Second, YY1 can interact directly with TFIIB and thereby inhibit the interaction between DNA-bound VDR/RXR and TFIIB. In addition, $1,25(OH)_2D_3$ responsiveness of the rat osteocalcin gene is more complex than occupied receptor binding to its response element. The DNA sequence lying 3' to the VDRE (-420 to -414) has been identified as critical for maximal transactivation by $1,25(OH)_2D_3$ [88], suggesting that a transcription factor bound to this site facilitates the interaction between the receptor-occupied VDRE and the basal transcription apparatus.

In contrast to the rat and human model, $1,25(OH)_2D_3$ inhibits mouse osteocalcin expression by abolishing the binding of osteoblast nuclear extracts to OSE2, a critical osteoblast-specific *cis*-acting element present in the osteocalcin promoter [89]. The nuclear factor has been identified as Osf2, an osteoblast-specific activator of transcription. Consistent with this observation, treatment of primary mouse osteoblasts with $1,25(OH)_2D_3$ abolished Osf2 expression [90]. This illustrates that $1,25(OH)_2D_3$ can play different roles in the expression of the same gene in various species and indicates that this regulation in mouse occurs through an indirect mechanism.

B. PTH–PTHrP

Parathyroid hormone (PTH) is an important regulator of mineral homeostasis and acts to increase serum calcium. As part of an endocrinological feedback loop, $1,25(OH)_2D_3$ suppresses prepro PTH mRNA and PTH secretion in rats [91]. A single motif (-113 to -107) has been identified in the 5'-regulatory region of the human PTH gene that binds the VDR and mediates transcriptional repression in response to $1,25(OH)_2D_3$ in a cell-specific way [92]. The hPTH sequence differs from the upregulatory VDREs in two ways: it contains a single copy of a hexameric motif (AGGTTC) homologous to those repeated in the upregulatory VDREs and this sequence can bind VDR independently of RXR [93]. In contrast, RXR is necessary for binding of the VDR complex to the VDRE of the chicken PTH gene [94]. In the bovine PTH gene, two DNA sequences were identified (-485 to -452 and -451 to -348) that bind VDR [95], but this interaction is not inhibited with the osteocalcin VDRE suggesting that interactions of VDR with the PTH and osteocalcin genes require different accessory factors [96].

The PTHrP gene is widely expressed and has been suggested to play an autocrine or paracrine role in growth and development. PTHrP gene expression is inhibited by 1,25(OH)$_2$D$_3$ [97], and two sequence motifs that mediate this repression were identified. One element consists of two hexanucleotide motifs separated by three nucleotides, and the second element consists of a single hexanucleotide motif. Both motifs interact with the VDR [98].

C. 24-Hydroxylase

The role of the 24-hydroxylase enzyme (CYP24) in 1,25(OH)$_2$D$_3$ is discussed in Section II.C. This enzyme displays a broad tissue distribution, and 1,25(OH)$_2$D$_3$ is its strongest inducer. Three groups have independently identified two functional VDREs (-258 to -244 and -150 to -136) [99–101] separated by a stretch of approximately 93 bp in an antisense orientation in the human and rat CYP24 promoter. Both of these VDREs are necessary to confer full transcriptional expression in the presence of 1,25(OH)$_2$D$_3$, and the interaction between the two VDREs is additive [102] or synergistic [103]. The type of interaction probably depends on the promoter context used. Studies suggested that the proximal VDRE, or VDRE-1, is a stronger mediator of 1,25(OH)$_2$D$_3$ function than the distal VDRE, or VDRE-2 [104], although VDRE-2 exhibits a smaller dissociation constant for the VDR/RXR complex than VDRE-1. This difference is most likely due to the presence of the accessory element located adjacent to VDRE-1 (-169 to -155) [102].

D. $\alpha_v\beta_3$ Integrin

The vitronectin receptor $\alpha_v\beta_3$ is highly expressed in mature osteoclasts that adhere via this protein to bone matrix proteins containing the RGD sequence (such as osteopontin, fibronectin, vitronectin), an event critical in the process of bone resorption [105, 106]. Treatment of avian osteoclast precursors with 1,25(OH)$_2$D$_3$ increases $\alpha_v\beta_3$ expression [107]. The promoter sequence comprises three hexameric direct repeat half-sites separated by three and nine nucleotides, to which VDR/RXR and RAR/RXR heterodimers bind respectively [108]. Coaddition of the steroids produces neither synergy nor an additive effect; rather, the result equals that for retinoic acid alone. Scatchard analysis demonstrates that RAR–RXR has greater affinity than VDR–RXR for the composite element. These results identify a novel mechanism by which one steroid hormone can modulate the activity of a second, by competing for a shared half-site in a composite response element [109].

V. EFFECTS OF 1,25(OH)$_2$D$_3$ ON OSTEOBLASTS

The general concept is that 1,25(OH)$_2$D$_3$ has a biphasic effect on osteoblasts; it abrogates or stimulates the normal developmental pathway or gene expression profiles depending on whether it is present during the proliferation or differentiation stage respectively (Fig. 4). 1,25(OH)$_2$D$_3$ given during the proliferative period of rat calvaria osteoblast cultures inhibits proliferation and downregulates collagen synthesis and alkaline phosphatase activity. No increase in osteocalcin

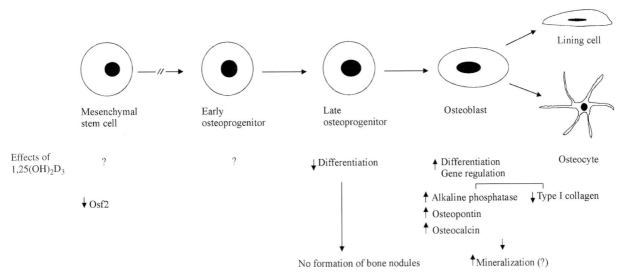

FIGURE 4   Effect of 1,25(OH)$_2$D$_3$ treatment on osteoblast differentiation and gene expression. Depending on the stage of differentiation of the osteoblasts, 1,25(OH)$_2$D$_3$ will inhibit or induce differentiation and concurrent gene expression. Osf2, osteoblast specific factor 2.

expression is observed [110] and nodule formation is blocked [111], suggesting an inhibitory effect on osteoblast differentiation. In contrast, 1,25(OH)$_2$D$_3$ treatment of mature osteoblast cultures results in upregulation of some osteoblast-associated genes, such as osteopontin and osteocalcin, and in stimulation of calcium accumulation [112]. At this stage of differentiation 1,25(OH)$_2$D$_3$ appears to "push" osteoblasts toward an even more mature state. A comparable result was found in a conditionally transformed adult human osteoblast cell line [113]. The *in vivo* consequence of these *in vitro* observations is difficult to ascertain at this time, mainly because of the paucity of detailed information. Local factors involved in bone remodeling are also modulated by 1,25(OH)$_2$D$_3$, but again different responses have been observed depending on the system used and on the stage of cell differentiation. As an example, the effect on IGF-I production is either stimulatory or inhibitory, whereas on TGFβ it is mainly stimulatory [114]; on vascular endothelial growth factor it is always stimulatory [115].

VI. EFFECTS OF 1,25(OH)$_2$D$_3$ ON OSTEOCLASTS

Osteoclast-like cell formation in coculture systems, consisting of bone marrow, spleen, or peripheral blood and osteoblastic stromal cells, is 1,25(OH)$_2$D$_3$ dependent. Osteoblastic stromal cells are critical in this process. The proposed mechanism is that 1,25(OH)$_2$D$_3$ acts directly on stromal cells in order to induce the production of a factor(s) responsible for osteoclast differentiation [116]. This hypothesis was confirmed by coculture experiments with VDR-deficient mice; no osteoclasts were formed in response to 1,25(OH)$_2$D$_3$ when VDR-/-osteoblastic cells were cocultured with WT (wild-type) spleen cells, whereas normal osteoclasts were present

when WT osteoblastic cells and VDR-/-spleen cells were cocultured [117]. Treatment of murine cocultures with 1,25(OH)$_2$D$_3$ during the last 2 days of the 6-day culture period is sufficient to induce significant numbers of osteoclasts [118], suggesting that 1,25(OH)$_2$D$_3$ stimulates mainly the differentiation process of osteoclast precursors and acts as a fusigen for committed osteoclast precursors. Interestingly, the action of 1,25(OH)$_2$D$_3$ is not essential for osteoclast formation *in vivo* since VDR deficient mice have normal number of osteoclasts [119]. The osteoblastic factor induced by 1,25(OH)$_2$D$_3$ and required for osteoclast differentiation is not yet identified, but several candidate proteins have been described. Antibody-inhibition studies have shown that osteopontin, macrophage stimulating factor (M-CSF), and the third component of complement (C3) [120–122] are involved in 1,25(OH)$_2$D$_3$-induced osteoclast formation. However, adding this factor alone, as tested with C3, was not sufficient to stimulate osteoclast formation, indicating that several 1,25(OH)$_2$D$_3$-dependent factors act in concert.

Osteoclast precursors contain a VDR, whereas no VDR is detected in mature osteoclasts. In addition, several markers of the osteoclast phenotype are induced by 1,25(OH)$_2$D$_3$ in cultures of osteoclast precursors (Fig. 5). One of them, the $\alpha_v\beta_3$ integrin, was already discussed in Section IV.D. Another 1,25(OH)$_2$D$_3$-regulated protein is the nonreceptor tyrosine kinase pp60$^{c\text{-}src}$ [123] that probably plays an important role in bone resorption, since c-src-/-mice develop osteopetrosis [124]. Chappel *et al.* [125] showed that 1,25(OH)$_2$D$_3$ accelerates pp60$^{c\text{-}src}$ kinase-specific activity without affecting its expression. 1,25(OH)$_2$D$_3$ also increases mRNA levels of carbonic anhydrase-II (CA-II) that produces hydrogen protons necessary to acidify the resorption lacuna. A VDRE consensus sequence has been identified in the promoter of the chicken CA-II gene [126], but the VDR/RXR complex binds to it with an inverse polarity compared to the classical

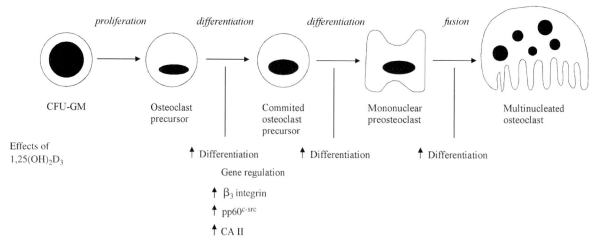

FIGURE 5   Effect of 1,25(OH)$_2$D$_3$ treatment on osteoclast differentiation and gene expression. 1,25(OH)$_2$D$_3$ has its major effect on osteoclast precursors and modulates at this stage the expression of osteoclast specific genes. CAII, carbonic anhydrase II.

TABLE I. Pathology: Vitamin D-Related Calcium/Bone Diseases

	Mechanism	Pathology
1. Substrate availability	↓intake ↓sun exposure	rickets/osteomalacia
2. Metabolism		
genetic	CYP24: KO mice human -chr20q13	defect in intramembranous ossification
	P450$_{1\alpha}$: human -chr12q13	HVDRR I
acquired	chronic renal failure oncogenic osteomalacia	renal osteodystrophy osteomalacia and hypophosphatemia
3. Vitamin D action		
genetic	VDR: KO mice human -chr12q13	rickets HVDRR II

VDRE. In contrast, the 1,25(OH)$_2$D$_3$-induced CA-II expression in murine marrow cultures is thought not to be the result of increased transcription but rather a part of the differentiation process [127].

VII. PATHOLOGY AND THERAPY RELATED TO VITAMIN D AVAILABILITY, METABOLISM, AND FUNCTION

A. Pathology

Vitamin D is either primarily or secondarily involved in many metabolic bone diseases. Rickets or osteomalacia are characterized by deficient mineralization of the cartilaginous (growth plate) and bone matrix. Depending on the major pathogenic mechanism involved, calciopenic or phosphopenic subtypes can be distinguished from primary mineralization defects [128]. Abnormalities in vitamin D availability, metabolism, or action are responsible for calciopenic rickets/osteomalacia, whereas the exact role or contribution in hypophosphatemic rickets is largely unknown since both families and cases with low (usual) or high (exceptional) 1,25(OH)$_2$D$_3$ levels have been described. Moreover, 1,25(OH)$_2$D$_3$ therapy alone fails to correct the biochemical or morphological defects [129]. Vitamin D is not a primary cause of osteoporosis but it can be secondarily involved. Indeed reduced vitamin D levels are quite common in the elderly, and inducing secondary hyperparathyroidism may accelerate the negative balance of bone turnover [130]. Moreover, vitamin D metabolism or action is frequently disturbed in secondary forms of osteoporosis (e.g., low 1,25(OH)$_2$D$_3$ levels in hyperthyroidism).

The mode of action of vitamin D on calcium and bone homeostasis is probably a mixture of indirect effects on calcium and phosphate availability for hydroxyapatite forma-tion and deposition and direct effects on bone cells. Indeed 1,25(OH)$_2$D$_3$ stimulates intestinal absorption, bone resorption, and renal reabsorption of the essential minerals calcium and phosphate.

1. 1,25(OH)$_2$D$_3$ DEFICIENCY

Classic nutritional rickets is caused by the simultaneous deprivation of sunlight exposure and dietary vitamin D [131] (Table I). The bioactivation of 25-(OH) D$_3$ in the kidney to 1,25(OH)$_2$D$_3$ as catalyzed by the 25-hydroxyvitamin D-1α-hydroxylase can be inadequate by genetic or acquired disorders. Mutations in this gene are the cause of PDDR (see Section II.B). The activity of P450$_{1\alpha}$ is reduced in acquired chronic renal failure due to compromised renal mass, resulting in renal rickets and hyperphosphatemia. Low 1,25(OH)$_2$D$_3$ production can also be found in oncogenic osteomalacia by the tumoral production of an unknown factor causing inhibition of renal phosphate reabsorption and 1,25(OH)$_2$D$_3$ production.

2. MUTATIONS IN THE VDR GENE

A total of 13 mutations causing hereditary hypocalcemic vitamin D-resistant rickets (HVDRR), also known as vitamin D-resistant rickets type II (HVDRR), has been characterized. The HVDRR syndrome is inherited as a recessive trait. Most of these mutations are localized to the DNA binding zinc finger region [132], whereas a smaller number of mutations are limited to the hormone binding domain [133, 134]. Whitfield et al. [135] demonstrated two novel hormone binding domain mutations affecting the heterodimerization of VDR with RXR. HVDRR results in a phenotype characterized by early onset rickets, hypocalcemia, secondary hyperparathyroidism, and markedly increased 1,25(OH)$_2$D$_3$ levels. The alopecia observed in some kindreds with mutant VDRs has not been observed in vitamin D deficiency, suggesting that VDR not only mediates the bone mineral homeostatic actions of vitamin D but plays also a role in the differentiation of hair follicles. Recently, VDR knockout mice have been created by two different groups [119, 136]. Although the VDR is widely expressed early during embryonic development, no major developmental abnormalities are observed in VDR-/- mice. Homozygous mice are phenotypically normal at birth and show normal growth until weaning. Demay, however, describes an expansion in the zone of hypertrophic chondrocytes in the growth plate by day 15. By day 21, they become hypocalcemic and PTH levels begin to rise. Rickets develops progressively; surviving mice possess 10-fold elevated levels of $1,25(OH)_2D_3$ together with very low $24,25(OH)_2D_3$ levels. These mice show marked growth retardation and decreased survival rates (15 weeks and 6 months for Kato's and Demay's groups, respectively). The development of alopecia, although not to the same extent, is observed in the two groups, but uterine hypoplasia is only present in Kato's animals reported by Yoshisewa et al. Thus, the phenotype of these mice mimics the features of patients with HVDRR, confirming the critical role of VDR in bone metabolism and mineral homeostasis.

B. Polymorphism

A polymorphism associated with exon 2 has been identified that leads to the synthesis of two different hVDR mRNAs [28], a normal and an abbreviated protein of only 424 amino acids. Two studies have reported the distribution of these alleles in the human population [137, 138]. The ATG to ACG allele, which can be detected by the presence of a FokI site, represents the more common form. Interestingly, the frequency of this allele correlates with an increase in bone density in two different human female populations; the corresponding smaller protein exhibits greater transcriptional activity [138]. Additional polymorphisms have been identified within the VDR gene and reported to be associated with reduced bone mineral density [139]. This finding has not been widely reproduced, suggesting a relatively weak linkage, and remains highly controversial [140].

C. $1,25(OH)_2D_3$ and Analogs as Therapeutics in Bone Pathology

The role of $1,25(OH)_2D_3$ in the treatment of bone disorders characterized by defective mineralization, such as rickets and renal osteodystrophy, is well established. Moreover, prevention or correction of subclinical $1,25(OH)_2D_3$ deficiency can substantially reduce the incidence of hip and other fractures in age-related osteoporosis, at least when given in combination with oral calcium supplementation [141]. The rationale for $1,25(OH)_2D_3$ as a therapeutic for osteoporosis is based on the finding of decreased bone formation or at least an imbalance between bone formation and resorption in many

patients with osteoporosis [142]. Tilyard et al. [143] demonstrated a major reduction in the number of new vertebral fractures during $1,25(OH)_2D_3$ therapy. However, the optimal therapeutic range for $1,25(OH)_2D_3$ appears to be quite narrow and may vary among patients. An alternative therapy employs the vitamin D_3 analog $1\alpha(OH)D_3$ (alfacalcidiol). $1\alpha(OH)D_3$ is less effective on intestinal calcium absorption compared with its effect on bone because it must first be hydroxylated at the 25 position to become fully active [144]. Like $1,25(OH)_2D_3$, therapeutic dose monitoring is needed to avoid side effects such as hypercalcemia and hypercalciuria. Efforts to develop new synthetic analogs for bone diseases have been modest. Other developmental initiatives have found analogs with potent antiproliferative and prodifferentiating effects on normal cells (keratinocytes, immune cells) and malignant cells (breast, prostate) [145] with minimal effects on bone. Nonsteroidal analogs with increased noncalcemic biological properties and low calcemic activity have been developed [146]. In relation to skeletal disorders, the compounds 22-oxa-$1,25(OH)_2D_3$ (OCT) and 2β-(3-hydroxypropoxy)-$1,25(OH)_2D_3$ (ED-71) have been proposed as therapeutic agents for secondary hyperparathyroidism and osteoporosis, respectively. OCT is equally as active as $1,25(OH)_2D_3$ in suppressing PTH secretion [147] but it does not induce hypercalcemia [148]. Single administration of ED-71 has greater effects than $1,25(OH)_2D_3$ on growth plate thickness in rachitic rats (15- to 20-fold) and increases the bone mineral density of the femurs, but it has less effect on serum calcium [149]. In studies employing either normal or ovariectomized rats, ED-71 stimulates bone mass and bone formation rates [150]. Both OCT and ED-71 are being tested in clinical trials. It is possible that these and other vitamin D analogs that are superior to native compounds will be developed.

VIII. CONCLUSIONS

Insight into the molecular mechanisms of $1,25(OH)_2D_3$ action via binding to VDR and interacting with VDRE has grown considerably since the mid-1990s. Many elements of this complex machinery are not yet fully identified. The mechanism of negatively regulated genes by $1,25(OH)_2D_3$ is still an open question. Certainly the participation of coactivators or corepressors remains to be established and their functional significance elucidated. In addition, knowledge of the three-dimensional structure of the VDR will provide valuable information for more complete understanding of ligand–protein and protein–protein interactions. Identification of the 25-hydroxyvitamin D-1α-hydroxylase and the development of knockout mice (VDR and 24-hydroxylase) strengthen our knowledge of the importance of vitamin D and its metabolites in mineral and bone homeostasis. The exact function of

1,25$(OH)_2D_3$ in bone metabolism awaits new physiological *in vivo* models.

References

1. Calli, J. J., and Russell, D. W. (1991). Characterization of human sterol 27-hydroxylase. A mitochondrial cytochrome P-450 that catalyzes multiple oxidation reaction in bile acid biosynthesis. *J. Biol. Chem.* **266**, 7774–7778.

2. Okuda, K. I (1994). Liver mitochondrial P450 involved in cholesterol catabolism and vitamin D activation. *J. Lipid Res.* **35**, 361–372.

3. Ichikawa, F., Sato, K., Nanjo, M., Nishii, Y., Shinki, T., Takahashi, N., and Suda, T. (1995). Mouse primary osteoblasts express vitamin D_3 25-hydroxylase mRNA and convert 1alpha-hydroxyvitamin D_3 into 1alpha,25-dihydroxyvitamin D_3. *Bone* **16**, 129–135.

4. St-Arnaud, R., Messerlian, S., Moir, J. M., Omdahl, J. L., and Glorieux, F. H. (1997). The 25-hydroxyvitamin D 1-alpha-hydroxylase gene maps to the pseudovitamin D-deficiency rickets (PDDR) disease locus. *J. Bone Miner. Res.* **12**, 1552–1559.

5. Takeyama, K., Kitanaka, S., Sato, T., Kobori, M., Yanagisawa, J., and Kato, S. (1997). 25-hydroxyvitamin D_3 1α-hydroxylase and vitamin D synthesis. *Science* **277**, 1827–1830.

6. Monkawa, T., Yoshida, T., Wakino, S., Shinki, T., Anazawa, H., DeLuca, H. F., Suda, T., Hayashi, M., and Saruta, T. (1997). Molecular cloning of cDNA and genomic DNA for human 25-hydroxyvitamin D_3 1α-hydroxylase. *Biochem. Biophys. Res. Commun.* **239**, 527–533.

7. Shinki, T., Shimada, H., Wakino, S., Anazawa, H., Hayashi, M., Saruta, T., DeLuca, H. F., and Suda, T. (1997). Cloning and expression of rat 25-hydroxyvitamin D_3-1α-hydroxylase cDNA. *Proc. Natl. Acad. Sci. U.S.A.* **94**, 1290–1295.

8. Fu, G. K., Lin, D., Zhang, M. Y., Bikle, D. D., Shackleton, C. H. L., Miller, W. L., and Portale, A. A. (1997). Cloning of human 25-hydroxyvitamin D-1α-hydoxylase and mutations causing vitamin D-dependent rickets type 1. *Mol. Endocrinol.* **11**, 1961–1970.

9. Fraser, D., Kooh, S. W., Kind, H. P., Holick, M. F., Tanaka, Y., and DeLuca, H. F. (1973). Pathogenesis of hereditary vitamin D-dependent rickets. An inborn error of vitamin D metabolism involving defective conversion of 25-hydroxyvitamin D to 1alpha,25-dihydroxyvitamin D. *N. Engl. J. Med.* **289**, 817–822.

10. Kitanaka, S., Takeyama, K., Murayama, A., Sato, T., Okumura, K., Nogami, M., Hasegawa, Y., Niimi, H., Yanagisawa, J., Tanaka, T., and Kato, S. (1998). Inactivating mutations in the 25-hydroxyvitamin D_3 1α-hydroxylase gene in patients with pseudovitamin D-deficiency rickets. *N. Engl. J. Med.* **338**, 653–661.

11. Ohyama, Y., Noshiro, M., Eggertsen, G., Gotoh, O., Kato, Y., Bjorkhem, I., and Okuda, K. (1993). Structural characterization of the gene encoding rat 25-hydroxyvitamin D_3 24-hydoxylase. *Biochemistry* **32**, 76–82.

12. Lohnes, D., and Jones, G. (1987). Side chain metabolism of vitamin D_3 in osteosarcoma cell line UMR-106. Characterization of products. *J. Biol. Chem.* **262**, 14394–14401.

13. Reddy, G. S., and Tserng, K. Y. (1989). Calcitroic acid, end product of renal metabolism of 1,25-dihydroxyvitamin D_3 through C24 oxidation pathway. *Biochemistry* **28**, 1763–1769.

14. Akiyoshi-Shibata, M., Sakaki, T., Ohyama, Y., Noshiro, M., Okuda, K., and Yabusaki, Y. (1994). Further oxidation of hydroxycalcidiol by calcidiol 24-hydroxylase. A study with the mature enzyme expressed in *Escherichia coli*. *Eur. J. Biochem.* **224**, 335–343.

15. St.-Arnaud, R., Arabian, A., and Glorieux, F. H. (1996). Abnormal bone development in mice deficient for the vitamin D 24-hydroxylase gene. *J. Bone Miner. Res.* **11**, S126.

16. St.-Arnaud, R., Arabian, A., Travers, R., and Glorieux, F. H. (1997). Partial rescue of abnormal bone formation in 24-hydroxylase knock-out mice supports a role for 24,25$(OH)_2D_3$ in intramembranous ossification. *J. Bone Miner. Res.* **12**, S110.

17. Yamaura, M., Nakamura, T., Nagai, Y., Yoshishara, A., and Suzuki, K. (1993). Reduced mechanical competence of bone by ovariectomy and its prevention with 24R,25-dihydroxyvitamin D_3 administration in beagles. *Calcif. Tissue Int.* **25**, 49–56.

18. Shwartz, Z., Bonewald, L. F., Caulfield, K., Brooks, B., and Boyan, B. D. (1993). Direct effects of transforming growth factor-beta on chondrocytes are modulated by vitamin D metabolites in a cell maturation-specific manner. *Endocrinology* **132**, 1544–1552.

19. Kato, A., Seo, E., Einhorn, T. A., and Norman, A. W. (1997). 24R,25-dihydroxyvitamin D_3 is essential for the fracture healing process and has receptor in the fracture healing callus. *In* "Vitamin D: Chemistry, Biology and Clinical Applications of the Steroid Hormone" (A. W. Norman, R. Bouillon, and M. Thomasset, eds.), pp. 645–646. University of California, Riverside.

20. Seo, E., Einhorn, T. A., and Norman, A. W. (1997). 24R,25-dihydroxyvitamin D_3: An essential vitamin D_3 metabolite for both normal bone integrity an healing of tibial fracture in chicks. *Endocrinology* **138**, 3864–3872.

21. Mangelsdorf, D. J., Thummel, C., Beato, M., Herrlich, P., Schütz, G., Umesono, K., Blumberg, B., Kastner, P., Mark, M., Chambon, P., and Evans, R. M. (1995). The nuclear receptor superfamily: The second decade. *Cell* **83**, 835–839.

22. Li, Y. C., Bergwitz, C., Jüppner, H., and Demay, M. B. (1997). Cloning and characterization of the vitamin D receptor from *Xenopus laevis*. *Endocrinology* **138**, 2347–2353.

23. McDonnell D. P., Mangelsdorf, D. J., Pike, J. W., Haussler, M. R., and O'Malley, B. W. (1987). Molecular cloning of complementary DNA encoding the avian receptor for vitamin D. *Science* **235**, 1214–1217.

24. Elaroussi, M. A., Prahl, J. M., and DeLuca, H. F. (1994). The avian vitamin D receptors: Primary structures and their origins. *Proc. Natl. Acad. Sci. U.S.A.* **91**, 11596–11600.

25. Kamei, Y., Kawada, T., Fukuwatari, T., Ono, T., Kato, S., and Sugimoto, E. (1995). Cloning and sequencing of the gene encoding the mouse vitamin D receptor. *Gene* **152**, 281–282.

26. Burmester, J., Wiese, R., Maeda, N., and DeLuca, H. F. (1988). Structure and regulation of the rat 1,25-dihydroxyvitamin D_3 receptor. *Proc. Natl. Acad. Sci. U.S.A.* **85**, 9499–9502.

27. Baker, A. R., McDonnell, D. P., Hughes, M., Crisp, T. M., Mangelsdorf, D. J., Haussler, M. R., Pike, J. W., Shine, J., and O'Malley, B. W. (1988). Cloning and expression of full-length cDNA encoding human vitamin D receptor. *Proc. Natl. Acad. Sci. U.S.A.* **85**, 3294–3298.

28. Miyamoto, K., Kesterson, R. A., Yamamoto, H., Taketani, Y., Nishiwaki, E., Tatsumi, S., Inoue, Y., Morita, K., Takeda, E., and Pike, J. W. (1997). Structural organization of the human vitamin D receptor chromosomal gene and its promoter. *Mol. Endocrinol.* **11**, 1165–1179.

29. Allegretto, E. A., Pike, J. W., and Haussler, M. R. (1987). C-terminal proteolysis of the avian 1,25-dihydroxyvitamin D_3 receptor. *Biochem. Biophys. Res. Commun.* **147**, 479–485.

30. Jin, C. H., Kerner, S. A., Hong, M. H., and Pike, J. W. (1996). Transcriptional activation and dimerization functions in the human vitamin D receptor. *Mol. Endocrinol.* **10**, 945–957.

31. Nakajima, S., Hsieh, J.-C., Jurutka, P. W., Galligan, M. A., Haussler, C. A., Whitfield, G. K., and Haussler, M. R. (1996). Examination of the potential functional role of conserved cysteine residues in the hormone binding domain of the human 1,25-dihydroxyvitamin D_3 receptor. *J. Biol. Chem.* **271**, 5143–5149.

32. Macdonald, P. N., Sherman, D. R., Dowd, D. R., Jefcoat, S. C., Jr., and DeLisle, R. K. (1995). The vitamin D receptor interacts with general transcription factor IIB. *J. Biol. Chem.* **270**, 4748–4752.

33. Blanco, J. C. G., Wang, I. M., Tsai, S. Y., Tsai, M. J., O'Malley, B. W., Jurutka, P. W., Haussler, M. R., and Ozato, K. (1995). Transcription factor TFIIB and the vitamin D receptor cooperatively activate ligand-dependent transcription. *Proc. Natl. Acad. Sci. U.S.A.* **92**, 1535–1539.

34. Masuyama, H., Jefcoat, S. C., Jr., and MacDonald, P. N. (1997). The N-terminal domain of trancription Factor IIB is required for direct interaction with the vitamin D receptor and participates in vitamin D-mediated transcription. *Mol. Endocrinol.* **11**, 218–228.

35. Nakajima, S., Hsieh, J.-C., MacDonald, P. N., Galligan, M. A., Haussler, C. A., Whitfield, G. K., and Haussler, M. R. (1994). The C-terminal region of the vitamin D receptor is essential to form a complex with a receptor auxiliary factor required for high affinity binding to the vitamin D responsive element. *Mol. Endocrinol.* **8**, 159–172.

36. Barettino, D., Vivanco-Kviz, M. M., and Stunnenberg, H. G. (1994). Characterization of the ligand-dependent transactivation domain of thyroid hormone receptor. *EMBO J.* **13**, 3039–3049.

37. Renaud, J-P., Rochel, N., Ruff, M., Vivat, V., Chambon, P., Gronemeyer, H., and Moras, D. (1995). Crystal structure of the RAR-γ ligand-binding domain bound to all-*trans* retinoic acid. *Nature* **378**, 681–689.

38. Leng, X., Blanco, J., Tsai, S. Y., Ozato, K., O'Malley, B. W., and Tsai, M.-J. (1995). Mouse retinoid X receptor contains a separable ligand-binding and transactivation domain in its E region. *Mol. Cell. Biol.* **15**, 255–263.

39. Danielian, P. S., White, R., Lees, J. A., and Parker, M. G. (1992). Identification of a conserved region required for hormone dependent transcriptional activation by steroid hormone receptors. *EMBO J.* **11**, 1025–1033.

40. Jurutka, P. W., Hsieh, J-C., Remus, L. S., Whitfield, G. K., Thompson, P. D., Haussler, C. A., Blanco, J. C. G., Ozato, K., and Haussler, M. R. (1997). Mutations in the 1,25-dihydroxyvitamin D_3 receptor identifying C-terminal amino acids required for transcriptional activation that are functionally dissociated from hormone binding, heterodimeric DNA binding, and interaction with basal transcription factor IIB, in vitro. *J. Biol. Chem.* **272**, 14592–14599.

41. vom Baur, E., Zechel, C., Heery, D., Heine, M. J. S., Garnier, J. M., Vivat, V., Le Douarin, B., Gronemeyer, H., Chambon, P., and Losson, R. (1996). Differential ligand-dependent interactions between the AF-2 activating domain of nuclear receptors and the putative transcriptional intermediary factors mSUG1 and TIF1. *EMBO J.* **15**, 110–124.

42. Mengus, G., May, M., Carré, L., Chambon, P., and Davidson, I. (1997). Human $TAF_{II}135$ potentiates transcriptional activation by the AF-2s of the retinoic acid, vitamin D_3, and thyroid hormone receptors in mammalian cells. *Genes Dev.* **11**, 1381–1395.

43. Hong, H., Kohli, K., Garabedian, M. J., and Stallcup, M. R. (1997). GRIP1, a transcriptional coactivator for the AF-2 transactivation domain of steroid, thyroid, retinoid, and vitamin D receptors. *Mol. Cell. Biol.* **17**, 2735–2744.

44. Li, H., Gomes, P. J., and Chen, J. D. (1997). RAC3, a steroid/nuclear receptor-associated coactivator that is related to SRC-1 and TIF2. *Proc. Natl. Acad. Sci. U.S.A.* **94**, 8479–8484.

45. Gill, R. K., Atkins, L. M., Hollis, B. W., and Bell, N. H. (1998). Mapping the domains of the interaction of the vitamin D receptor and steroid receptor coactivator-1. *Mol. Endocrinol.* **12**, 57–65.

46. Bourguet, W., Ruff, M., Chambon, P., Gronemeyer, H., and Moras, D. (1995). Crystal structure of the ligand-binding domain of the human nuclear receptor RXR-α. *Nature* **375**, 377–382.

47. Wagner, R. L., Apriletti, J. W., McGrath, M. E., West, B. L., Baxter, J. D., and Fletterick, R. J. (1995). A structural role for hormone in the thyroid hormone receptor. *Nature* **378**, 690–697.

48. Freedman, L. P. (1992). Anatomy of the steroid receptor zinc finger region. *Endocr. Rev.* **13**, 129–145.

49. Rastinejad, F., Perlmann, T., Evans, R. M., and Sigler, P. B. (1995). Structural determinants of nuclear receptor assembly on DNA direct repeats. *Nature* **375**, 203–211.

50. Luo, Z., Rouvinen, J., and Maenpaa, P. H. (1994). A peptide C-terminal to the second Zn finger of human vitamin D receptor is able to specify nuclear localization. *Eur. J. Biochem.* **223**, 381–387.

51. Sone, T., Ozono, K., and Pike, J. W. (1991). A 55-kilodalton accessory factor facilitates vitamin D receptor DNA binding. *Mol. Endocrinol.* **5**, 1578–1586.

52. Kliewer, S. A., Umesono, K., Mangelsdorf, D. J., and Evans, R. M. (1992). Retinoid X receptor interacts with nuclear receptors in retinoic acid, thyroid hormone and vitamin D_3 signaling. *Nature* **355**, 446–449.

53. Carlberg, C., Bendik, I., Wyss, A., Meier, E., Sturzenbecker, L. J., Grippo, J. F., and Hunziker, W. (1993). Two nuclear signalling pathways for vitamin D. *Nature* **361**, 657–660.

54. Christakos, S., Raval-Pandya, M., Werny, J., and Yang, W. (1996). Genomic mechanisms involved in the pleiotropic actions of 1,25-dihydroxyvitamin D_3. *Biochem. J.* **316**, 361–371.

55. Carlberg, C. (1995). Mechanisms of nuclear signalling by vitamin D_3. Interplay with retinoid and thyroid hormone signalling. *Eur. J. Biochem.* **231**, 517–527.

56. Schrader, M., Nayeri, S., Kahlen, J. P., Muller, K. M., and Carlberg, C. (1995). Natural vitamin D_3 response elements formed by inverted palindromes: Polarity-directed ligand sensitivity of vitamin D_3 receptor-retinoid X receptor heterodimer-mediated transactivation. *Mol. Cell. Biol.* **15**, 1154–1161.

57. Jin, C. H., and Pike, J. W. (1996). Human vitamin D receptor-dependent transactivation in *Saccharomyces cerevisiae* requires retinoid X receptor. *Mol. Endocrinol.* **10**, 196–205.

58. Umesono, K., Murakami, K. K., Thompson, C. C., and Evans, R. M. (1991). Direct repeats as selective response elements for the thyroid hormone, retinoic acid, and vitamin D_3 receptors. *Cell* **65**, 1255–1266.

59. Demay, M. B., Gerardi, J. M., Deluca, H. F., and Kronenberg, H. M. (1990). DNA sequences in the rat osteocalcin gene that bind the 1,25-dihydroxyvitamin D_3 receptor and confer responsiveness to 1,25-dihydroxyvitamin D_3. *Proc. Natl. Acad. Sci. U.S.A.* **87**, 369–373.

60. Noda, M., Vogel, R. L., Craig, A. M., Prahl, J., Deluca, H. F., and Denhardt, D. T. (1990). Identification of a DNA sequence responsible for binding of the 1,25-dihydroxyvitamin D_3 receptor and 1,25-dihydroxyvitamin D_3 enhancement of mouse secreted phophoprotein 1 (*Spp-1* or osteopontin) gene expression. *Proc. Natl. Acad. Sci. U.S.A.* **87**, 9995–9999.

61. Ohyama, Y., Ozono, K., Uchida, M., Shinki, T., Kato, S., Suda, T., Yamamoto, O., Noshiro, M., and Kato, Y. (1994). Identification of a Vitamin D-responsive element in the 5′-flanking region of the rat 25-hydroxyvitamin D_3 24-hydroxylase gene. *J. Biol. Chem.* **269**, 10545–10550.

62. Cao, X., Ross, F. P., Zhang, L., MacDonald, P. N., Chappel, J., and Teitelbaum, S. L. (1993). Cloning of the promoter for the avian integrin β3 subunit gene and its regulation by 1,25-dihydroxyvitamin D_3. *J. Biol. Chem.* **268**, 27371–27380.

63. Staal, A., van Wijnen, A. J., Birkenhäger, J. C., Pols, H. A. P., Prahl, J., DeLuca, H., Gaub, M.-P., Lian, J. B., Stein, G. S., van Leeuwen, J. P. T. M., and Stein, J. L. (1996). Distinct conformations of vitamin D receptor/retinoid X receptor -α heterodimers are specified in the vitamin D-responsive elements of the osteocalcin and osteopontin genes. *Mol. Endocrinol.* **10**, 1444–1456.

64. Brown, T. A., and DeLuca, H. F. (1990). Phosphorylation of the 1,25-dihydroxyvitamin D_3 receptor. A primary event in 1,25-dihydroxyvitamin D_3 action. *J. Biol. Chem.* **265**, 10025–10029.

65. Krishnan, A. V., and Feldman, D. (1991). Activation of protein kinase-C inhibits vitamin D receptor gene expression. *Mol. Endocrinol.* **5**, 605–612.

66. Jurutka, P. W., Hsieh, J-C., Nakajima, S., Haussler, C. A., Whitfield, G. K., and Haussler, M. R. (1996). Human vitamin D receptor phosphorylation by casein kinase II at Ser-208 potentiates transcriptional activation. *Proc. Natl. Acad. Sci. U.S.A.* **93**, 3519–3524.

67. Hsieh, J.-C., Jurutka, P. W., Galligan, M. A., Terpening, C. M., Haussler, C. A., Samuels, D. S., Shimizu, Y., Shimizu, N., and Haussler, M. R. (1991). Human vitamin D receptor is selectively phosphorylated by protein kinase C on serine 51, a residue crucial to its trans-activation function. *Proc. Natl. Acad. Sci. U.S.A.* **88**, 9315–9319.

68. Hsieh, J. C., Jurutka, P. W., Nakajima, S., Galligan, M. A., Haussler, C. A., Shimizu, Y., Shimizu, N., Whitfield, G. K., and Haussler, M. R. (1993). Phosphorylation of the human vitamin D receptor by protein kinase C. Biochemical and functional evaluation of the serine 51 recognition site. *J. Biol. Chem.* **268**, 15118–15126.

69. Reinhardt, T. A., and Horst, R. L. (1990). Parathyroid hormone downregulates 1,25-dihydroxyvitamin D receptors (VDR) and VDR messenger ribonucleic acid *in vitro* and blocks homologous up-regulation of VDR *in vivo*. *Endocrinology* **127**, 942–948.

70. Chen, T. L., and Feldman, D. (1981). Regulation of 1,25-dihydroxyvitamin D_3 receptors in cultured mouse bone cells. Correlation of receptor concentration with the rate of cell division. *J. Biol. Chem.* **256**, 5561–5566.

71. Pols, H. A. P., van Leeuwen, J. P. T. M., Schilte, J. P., Visser, T. J., and Birkenhager, J. C. (1988). Heterologous up-regulation of the 1,25-dihydroxyvitamin D_3 receptor by parathyroid hormone (PTH) and PTH-like peptide in osteoblast-like cells. *Biochem. Biophys. Res. Commun.* **156**, 588–594.

72. van Leeuwen, J. P. T. M., Birkenhager, J. C., Wijngaarden, T. V. V., van den Bemd, G. J. C. M., and Pols, H. A. P. (1992). Regulation of 1,25-dihydroxyvitamin D_3 receptor gene expression by parathyroid hormone and cAMP-agonists. *Biochem. Biophys. Res. Commun.* **185**, 881–886.

73. Staal, A., Van Wijnen, A. J., Desai, R. K., Pols, H. A., Birkenhager, J. C., DeLuca, H. F., Denhardt, D. T., Stein, J. L., van Leeuwen, J. P., Stein, G. S., and Lian, J. B. (1996). Antagonistic effects of transforming growth factor-beta on vitamin D_3 enhancement of osteocalcin and osteopontin transcription: Reduced interactions of vitamin D receptor/retinoid X receptor complexes with vitamin D response elements. *Endocrinology* **137**, 2001–2011.

74. Walters, M. R. (1981). An estrogen-stimulated 1,25-dihydroxyvitamin D_3 receptor in rat uterus. *Biochem. Biophys. Res. Commun.* **103**, 721–726.

75. Mahonen, A., Pirskanen, A., and Maenpaa, P. H. (1991). Homologous and heterlologous regulation of 1,25-dihydroxyvitmain D-3 receptor mRNA levels in human osteosarcoma cells. *Biochim. Biophys. Acta* **188**, 111–118.

76. Chen, T. L., Cone, C. M., Morey-Holton, E., and Feldman, D. (1983). 1,25-Dihydroxyvitamin D_3 receptors in cultured rat osteoblasts-like cells. Glucocorticoid treatment increases receptor content. *J. Biol. Chem.* **258**, 4350–4355.

77. Petkovitch, P. M., Heersche, J. N. M., Tinker, D. O., and Jones, G. (1984). Retinoic acid stimulates 1,25-dihydroxyvitamin D_3 binding in rat osteosarcoma cells. *J. Biol. Chem.* **259**, 8274–8290.

78. Krishnan, A. V., and Feldman, D. (1991). Stimulation of 1,25-dihydroxyvitamin D_3 receptor gene expression in cultured cells by serum and growth factors. *J. Bone Miner. Res.* **6**, 1099–1107.

79. Zhao, X., and Feldman, D. (1993). Regulation of vitamin D receptor abundance and responsiveness during differentiation of HT-29 human colon cancer cells. *Endocrinology* **132**, 1808–1814.

80. Jehan, F., and DeLuca, H. F. (1997). Cloning and characterization of the mouse vitamin D receptor promoter. *Proc. Natl. Acad. Sci. U.S.A.* **94**, 10138–10143.

81. Wiese, R. J., Uhland-Smith, A., Ross, T. K., Prahl, J. M., and DeLuca, H. F. (1992). Up-regulation of the vitamin D receptor in response to 1,25-dihydroxyvitamin D_3 results from ligand-induced stabilization. *J. Biol. Chem.* **267**, 20082–20086.

82. Arbour, N. C., Prahl, J. M., and DeLuca, H. F. (1993). Stabilization of the vitamin D receptor in rat osteosarcoma cells through the action of 1,25$(OH)_2D_3$. *Mol. Endocrinol.* **7**, 1307–1312.

83. Candeliere, G. A., Jurutka, P. W., Haussler, M. R., and St-Arnaud, R. (1996). A composite element binding the vitamin D receptor, retinoid X receptor α, and a member of teh CTF/NF-1 family of transcription factors mediates the vitamin D responsiveness of the c-*fos* promoter. *Mol. Cell. Biol.* **16**, 584–592.

84. Darwish, H., and DeLuca, H. F. (1993) Vitamin D-regulated gene expression. *Crit. Rev. Eukaryotic Gene Expression.* **3**, 89–116.

85. Ducy, P., Desbois, C., Boyce, B., Pinero, G., Story, B., Dunstan, C., Smith, E., Bonadio, J., Goldstein, S., Gundberg, C., Bradley, A., and Karsenty, G. (1996). Increased bone formation in osteocalcin-deficient mice. *Nature* **382**, 448–452.

86. Stein, G. S., Lian, J. B., Stein, J. L., van Wijnen, A. J., and Montecino, M. (1996). Transcriptional control of osteoblast growth and differentiation. *Physiol. Rev.* **76**, 593–629.

87. Guo, B., Aslam, F., van Wijnen, A. J., Robers, S. G. E., Frenkel, B., Green, M. R., DeLuca, H., Lian, J. B., Stein, G. S., and Stein, J. L. (1997). YY1 regulates vitamin D receptor/retinoid X receptor mediated transactivation of the vitamin D responsive osteocalcin gene. *Proc. Natl. Acad. Sci. U.S.A.* **94**, 121–126.

88. Sneddon, W. B., Bogado, C. E., Kiernan, M. S., and Demay, M. B. (1997). DNA sequences downstream from the vitamin D response element of the rat osteocalcin gene are required for ligand-dependent transactivation. *Mol. Endocrinol.* **11**, 210–217.

89. Zhang, R., Ducy, P., and Karsenty, G. (1997). 1,25-dihydroxyvitamin D_3 inhibits osteocalcin expression in mouse through an indirect mechanism. *J. Biol. Chem.* **272**, 110–116.

90. Ducy, P., Zhang, R., Geoffroy, V., Ridall, A. L., and Karsenty, G. (1997). Osf2/Cbfa1: A transcriptional activator of osteoblast differentiation. *Cell* **89**, 747–754.

91. Russell, J., Lettieri, D., and Sherwood, L. M. (1986). Suppression by 1,25$(OH)_2D_3$ of transcription of the pre-proparathyroid hormone gene. *Endocrinology* **119**, 2864–2866.

92. Demay, M. B., Kiernan, M. S., DeLuca, H. F., and Kronenberg, H. M. (1992). Sequences in the human parthyroid hormone gene that bind the 1,25-dihydroxyvitamin D_3 receptor and mediate transcriptional repression in response to 1,25-dihydroxyvitamin D_3. *Proc. Natl. Acad. Sci. U.S.A.* **89**, 8097–8101.

93. Mackey, S. L., Heymont, J. L., Kronenberg, H. M., and Demay, M. B. (1996). Vitamin D receptor binding to the negative human parathyroid hormone vitamin D response element does not require the retinoid X receptor. *Mol. Endocrinol.* **10**, 298–305.

94. Liu, S. M., Koszewski, N., Lupez, M., Malluche, H. H., Olivera, A., and Russell, J. (1996). Characterization of a response element in the 5′-flanking region of the avian (chicken) parathyroid hormone gene that mediates negative regulation of gene transcription by 1,25-dihydroxyvitamin D_3 and binds the vitamin D_3 receptor. *Mol. Endocrinol.* **10**, 206–215.

95. Hawa, N. S., O'Riordan, J. L. H., and Farrow, S. M. (1994). Binding of 1,25-dihydroxyvitamin D_3 receptors to the 5′-flanking region of the bovine parathyroid hormone gene. *J. Endocrinol.* **142**, 53–60.

96. Hawa, N. S., O'Riordan, J. L. H., and Farrow, S. M. (1996). Functional analysis of vitamin D response elements in the parathyroid hormone gene and a comparison with the osteocalcin gene. *Biochem. Biophys. Res. Commun.* **228**, 352–357.

97. Kremer, R., Karaplis, A. C., Henderson, J., Gulliver, W., Banville, D., Hendy, G. N., and Goltzman, D. (1991). Regulation of parathyroid hormone-like peptide in cultured normal human keratinocytes. Effect of growth factors and 1,25-dihydroxyvitamain D_3 on gene expression and secretion. *J. Clin. Invest.* **87**, 884–893.

98. Falzon, M. (1996). DNA sequences in the rat parathyroid hormone-related peptide gene responsible for 1,25-dicydroxyvitamin D$_3$-mediated transcriptional repression. *Mol. Endocrinol.* **10**, 672–681.

99. Zierold, C., Darwish, H. M., and DeLuca, H. F. (1994). Identification of a vitamin D-response element in the rat calcidiol (25-hydroxyvitamin D$_3$) 24-hydroxylase gene. *Proc. Natl. Acad. Sci. U.S.A.* **91**, 900–902.

100. Ohyama, Y., Ozono, K., Uchida, M., Shinki, T., Kato, S., Suda, T., Yamamoto, O., Noshiro, M., and Kato, Y. (1994). Identification of a vitamin D-responsive element in the 5'-flanking region of the rat 25-hydroxyvitamin D$_3$ 24-hydroxylase gene. *J. Biol. Chem.* **269**, 10545–10550.

101. Hahn, C. N., Kerry, D. M., Omdahl, J. L., and May, B. K. (1994). Identification of a vitamin D responsive element in the promoter of the rat cytochrome P450$_{24}$ gene. *Nucleic Acids Res.* **22**, 2410–2416.

102. Ohyama, Y., Ozono, K., Uchida, M., Yoshimura, M., Shinki, T., Suda, T., and Yamamoto, O. (1996). Functional assessment of two vitamin D-responsive elements in the rat 25-hydroxyvitamin D$_3$ 24-hydroxylase gene. *J. Biol. Chem.* **271**, 30381–30385.

103. Zierold, C., Darwish, H. M., and DeLuca, H. F. (1995). Two vitamin D response elements function in the rat 1,25-dihydroxyvitamin D 24-hydroxylase promoter. *J. Biol. Chem.* **270**, 1675–1678.

104. Ozono, K., Ohyama, Y., Nakajima, S., Uchida, M., Yoshimura, M., Shinki, T., Suda, T., and Yamamoto, O. (1995). Characterization of two vitamin D-responsive elements in the rat 25-hydroxyvitamin D$_3$ 24-hydroxylase gene. *J. Bone Miner. Res.* **10**, S288.

105. Roodman, G. D. (1996). Advances in bone biology: The osteoclast. *Endocr. Rev.* **17**, 308–332.

106. Rodan, S. B., and Rodan, G. A. (1997). Integrin function in osteoclasts. *J. Endocrinol.* **154**, S47–S56.

107. Mimura, H., Cao, X., Ross, F. P., Chiba, M., and Teitelbaum, S. L. (1994). 1,25-dihydroxyvitamin D$_3$ transcriptionally activates the β_3-integrin subunit gene in avian osteoclast precursors. *Endocrinology*. **134**, 1061–1066.

108. Cao, X., Ross, F. P., Zhang, L., MacDonald, P. N., Chappel, J., and Teitelbaum, S. L. (1993). Cloning of the promoter for the avian integrin β_3 subunit gene and its regulation by 1,25-dihydroxyvitamin D$_3$. *J. Biol. Chem.* **268**, 27371–27380.

109. Cao, X., Teitelbaum, S. L., Zhu, H.-J., Zhang, L., Feng, X., and Ross, F. P. (1996). Competition for a unique response element mediates retinoic acid inhibition of vitamin D$_3$-stimulated transcription. *J. Biol. Chem.* **271**, 20650–20654.

110. Ishida, H., Bellows, C. G., Aubin, J. E., and Heersche, J. N. M. (1993). Characterization of the 1,25(OH)$_2$D$_3$-induced inhibition of bone nodule formation in long-term cultures of fetal rat calvaria cells *Endocrinology* **132**, 61–66.

111. Owen, T. A., Aronow, M. S., Barone, L. M., Bettencourt, B., Stein, G. S., and Lian, J. B. (1991). Pleiotropic effects of vitamin D on osteoblast gene expression are related to the proliferative and differentiated state of the bone cell phenotype: Dependency upon basal levels of gene expression, duration of exposure and bone matrix competency in normal rat osteoblast cultures. *Endocrinology* **128**, 1496–1504.

112. Matsumoto, T., Igarashi, C., Taksuchi, Y., Harada, S., Kikuchi, T., Yamamoto, H., and Ogata, E. (1991). Stimulation by 1,25-dihydroxyvitamin D$_3$ of in vitro mineralization induced by osteoblast-like MC3T3-E1 cells. *Bone* **12**, 27–32.

113. Bodine, P., Henderson, R., Green, J., Lian, J. B., Stein, G. S., and Komm, B. (1997). 1,25(OH)$_2$D$_3$ promotes osteoblast differentiation and matrix mineralization of a conditionally transformed adult human osteoblast cell line. *In* "Vitamin D: Chemistry, Biology and Clinical Applications of the Steroid Hormone" (A. W. Norman, R. Bouillon, and M. Thomasset, eds.) pp. 665–666. University of California, Riverside.

114. Stern, P. H. (1997). 1,25-dihydroxyvitamin D$_3$ interactions with local factors in bone remodeling. *In* "Vitamin D" (D. Feldman, F. H.

115. Wang, D. S., Miura, M., Demura, H., and Sato, K. (1997). Anabolic effects of 1,25-dihydroxyvitamin D$_3$ on osteoblasts are enhanced by vascular endothelial growth factor produced by osteoblasts and by growth factors produced by endothelial cells. *Endocrinology* **138**, 2953–2962.

116. Suda, T., Udagawa, N., and Takahashi, N. (1996). Cells of bone: Osteoclast generation. *In* "Principles of Bone Biology" (J. P. Bilezikian, L. G. Raisz, and G. A. Rodan, eds.), pp.87–102. Academic Press, San Diego, CA.

117. Takeda, S., Yoshizawa, T., Fukumoto, S., Nagai, Y., Murayama, H., Matsumoto, T., Kato, S., and Fujita, J. (1997). Bone metabolism and in vitro osteoclast formation in VDR knock-out mice. *J. Bone Miner. Res.* **12**, S110.

118. Takahashi, N., Udagawa, N., Tanaka, S., Murakami, H., Owan, I., Tamura, T., and Suda, T. (1993). Postmitotic osteoclast precursors are mononuclear cells which express macrophage-associated phenotypes. *Dev. Biol.* **163**, 212–221.

119. Yoshizawa, T., Handa, Y., Uematsu, Y., Takesa, S., Sekine, K., Yoshihara, Y., Kawakami, T., Arioka, K., Sato, H., Uchiyama, Y., Masushige, S., Fukamizu, A., Matsumoto, T., and Kato, S. (1997). Mice lacking the vitamin D receptor exhibit impaired bone formation, uterine hypoplasia and growth retardation after weaning. *Nat. Genet.* **16**, 391–396.

120. Yamate, T., Mocharla, H., Taguchi, Y., Igietseme, J. U., Manolagas, S. C., and Abe, E. (1997). Osteopontin expression by osteoclast and osteoblast progenitors in the murine bone marrow: Demonstration of its requirements for osteoclastogenesis and its increase after ovariectomy. *Endocrinology* **138**, 3047–3055.

121. Rubin, J., Fan, X., Thornton, D., Bryant, R., and Biskobing, D. (1996). Regulation of murine osteoblast macrophage colony-stimulating factor production by 1,25(OH)$_2$D$_3$. *Calcif. Tissue Int.* **59**, 291–296.

122. Sato, T., Abe, E., Jin, C. H., Hong, M. H., Katagiri, T., Kinoshita, T., Amizuka, N., Ozawa, H., and Suda, T. (1993). The biological roles of the third component of complement in osteoclast formation. *Endocrinology* **133**, 397–404.

123. Yoneda, T., Niewolna, M., Lowe, C., Izbicka, E., and Mundy, G. R. (1993). Hormonal regulation of pp60^{c-src} expression during osteoclast formation in vitro. *Mol. Endocrinol.* **7**, 1313–1318.

124. Soriano, P., Montgomery, C., Geske, R., and Bradley, A. (1991). Targeted disruption of the c-src proto-oncogene leads to osteopetrosis in mice. *Cell* **64**, 693–702.

125. Chappel, J., Ross, F. P., Abu-Amer, Y., Shaw, A., and Teitelbaum, S. L. (1997). 1,25-dihydroxyvitamin D$_3$ regulates pp60^{c-src} activity and expression of a pp60^{c-src} activating phosphatase. *J. Cell. Biochem.* **67**, 432–438.

126. Quelo, I., Kahlen, J. P., Rascle, A., Jurdic, P., and Carlberg, C. (1994). Identification and characterization of a vitamin D$_3$ response element of chicken carbonic anhydrase-II. *DNA Cell Biol.* **13**, 1181–1187.

127. Biskobing, D. M., Fan, D., Fan, X., and Rubin, J. (1997). Induction of carbonic anhydrase II expression in osteoclast progenitors requires physical contact with stromal cells. *Endocrinology* **138**, 4852–4857.

128. Bouillon, R. (1998). The many faces of rickets. Editorial. *N. Engl. J. Med.* **388**, 681–682.

129. Drezner, M. K. (1996). Phosphorus homeostasis and related disorders. *In* "Principles of Bone Biology" (J. P. Bilezikian, L. G. Raisz, and G. A. Rodan, eds.), pp. 263–276. Academic Press, San Diego, CA.

130. Bouillon, R., Carmeliet, G., and Boonen, S. (1997). Ageing and calcium metabolism. *Baillière's Clin. Endocrinol. Metab.* **11**, 341–365.

131. Schmidt-Gayk, H., Bouillon, R., and Roth, H. J. (1997). The determination of vitamin D metabolites (calcidiol and calcitriol) and their clinical significance. *Scand. J. Clin. Lab. Invest.* **57**, 35–45.

Glorieux, and J. W. Pike, eds.), pp. 341–352. Academic Press, San Diego, CA.

132. Hughes, M. R., Malloy, P. J., Kieback, D. G., Kesterson, R. A., Pike, J. W., Feldman, D., and O'Malley, B. W. (1988). Point mutations in the human vitamin D receptor gene associated with hypocalcemic rickets. *Science* **242**, 1702–1705.

133. Kristjannson, K., Rut, A. R., Hewison, M., O'Riordan, J. L. H., and Hughes, M. R. (1993). Two mutations in the hormone binding domain of the vitamin D receptor cause tissue resistance to 1,25-dihydroxyvitamin D$_3$. *J. Clin. Invest.* **92**, 12–16.

134. Malloy, P. J., Eccleshall, T. R., Van Maldergem, L., Bouillon, R., and Feldman, D. (1995). A vitamin D receptor gene mutation that results in decreased 1,25(OH)$_2$D$_3$ binding affinity and cellular hyporesponsiveness. *J. Bone Miner. Res.* **10**, S167.

135. Whitfield, G. K., Selznick, S. H., Haussler, C. A., Hsieh, J. C., Callligan, M. A., Jurutka, P. W., Thompson, P. D., Lee, S. M., Zerwekh, J. E., and Haussler, M. R. (1996). Vitamin D receptors from patients with resistance to 1,25-dihydroxyvitamin D$_3$: Point mutations confer reduced transactivation in response to ligand and impaired interaction with the retinoid X receptor heterodimeric partner. *Mol. Endocrinol.* **10**, 1617–1631.

136. Li, Y. C., Pirro, A. E., Amling, M., Delling, G., Baron, R., Bronsons, R., and Demay, M. (1997). Targeted ablation of the vitamin D receptor: An animal model of vitamin D-dependent rickets type II with alopecia. *Proc. Natl. Acad. Sci. U.S.A.* **94**, 9831–9835.

137. Gross, C., Eccleshall, T. R., Mallow, P. J., Vill, M. L., Marcus, R., and Feldman, D. (1996). The presence of a polymorphism at the translation initiation site of the vitamin D receptor gene is associated with low bone mineral density in postmenopausal Mexican-American women. *J. Bone Miner. Res.* **11**, 1850–1855.

138. Arai, H., Miyamoto, K.-I., Taketani, Y., Yamamoto, H., Iemori, Y., Morita, K., Tonai, T., Nishisho, T., Mori, S., and Takeda, E. (1997). A vitamin D receptor gene polymorphism in the translation initiation codon: Effect on protein activity and relation to bone mineral density in Japanese women. *J. Bone Miner. Res.* **12**, 915–921.

139. Morrison, N. A., Qi, J. C., Tokita, A., Kelly, P. J., Crofts, L., Nguyen, T. V., Sambrook, P. N., and Eisman, J. A. (1994). Prediction of bone density from vitamin D receptor alleles. *Nature* **367**, 284–287.

140. Cooper, G. S., and Umbach, D. M. (1996). Are vitamin D receptor poly-morphisms associated with bone mineral density? A meta-analysis. *J. Bone Miner. Res.* **11**, 1841–1849.

141. Chapuy, M., Arlot, M., Duboeuf, F., Brun, J., Crouzet, B., Arnaud, S., Delmas, P. D., and Meunier, P. J. (1992). Vitamin D$_3$ and calcium to prevent hip fractures in elderly women. *N. Engl. J. Med.* **327**, 1637–1642.

142. Civitelli, R. (1995). The role of vitamin D metabolism in the treatment of osteoporosis. *Calcif. Tissue Int.* **57**, 409–414.

143. Tilyard, M. W., Spears, G. F., Thomson, J., and Dovey, S. (1992). Treatment of postmenopausal osteoporosis with calcitriol or calcium. *N. Engl. J. Med.* **326**, 357–362.

144. Akesson, K., Lau, K.-H. W., and Baylink, D. J. (1997). Rationale for active vitamin D analog therapy in senile osteoporosis. *Calcif. Tissue Int.* **60**, 100–105.

145. Bouillon, R., Okamura, W. H., and Norman, A. W. (1995). Structure-function relationships in the vitamin D endocrine system. *Endocr. Rev.* **16**, 200–257.

146. Verstuyf, A., Verlinden, L., Van Baelen, H., Sabbe, K., D'Halleweyn, C., De Clercq, P., Vandewalle, M., and Bouillon, R. (1998). The biological activity of nonsteroidal vitamin D hormone analogs lacking both the C- and D-rings. *J. Bone Miner. Res.* **13**, 549–558.

147. Brown, A. J., Ritter, C. R., Finish, J. L., Morrincy, J., Martin, K. J., Murayama, E., Nishii, Y., and Slatopolski, E. (1989). The noncalcemic analogue of vitamin D, 22-oxacalcitriol, suppresses parathyroid hormone synthesis and secretion. *J. Clin. Invest.* **84**, 728–732.

148. Fukagawa, M., Kaname, S., Igarashi, T., Ogata, E., and Kurokawa, K. (1991). Regulation of parathyroid hormone synthesis in chronic renal failure in rats. *Kidney Int.* **39**, 874–881.

149. Kubodera, N., Sato, K., and Nishii, Y. (1997). Characteristics of 22-oxacalcitriol (OCT) and 2β-(3-hydroxypropoxy)-calcitriol (ED-71). *In* "Vitamin D" (D. Feldman, F. H. Glorieux, and J. W. Pike, eds.), pp. 1071–1086. Academic Press, San Diego, CA.

150. Tsurukami, H., Nakamura, T., Suzuki, K., Sato, K., Higuchi, Y., and Nishii, Y. (1994). A novel synthetic vitamin D analogue 2β-(3-hydroxypropoxy) 1α,25-dihydroxyvitamin D$_3$ (ED-71), increases bone mass by stimulating the bone formation in normal and ovariectomized rats. *Calcif. Tissue Int.* **54**, 142–149.

CHAPTER 16

Sex Steroid Effects on Bone Metabolism

S. KHOSLA Division of Endocrinology, Metabolism, and Internal Medicine, Mayo Clinic and Foundation, Mayo Medical School, Rochester, Minnesota 55905

THOMAS C. SPELSBERG Mayo Medical and Graduate School, Rochester, Minnesota 55905

B. LAWRENCE RIGGS Division of Endocrinology, Metabolism, and Internal Medicine, Mayo Clinic and Foundation, Mayo Medical School, Rochester, Minnesota 55905

I. ABSTRACT

Sex steroids clearly have major effects on bone and calcium metabolism. Thus, hypogonadism in either sex is associated with rapid bone loss, which is preventable with gonadal steroid replacement. In this chapter, we review the molecular structures, biosynthesis, and mechanism of action of the major clinically relevant sex steroids. The identification of estrogen and androgen receptors in bone cells was followed by an explosion of studies on the effects of sex steroids and, in particular, estrogen on osteoblasts and osteoclasts. This has led to the identification of candidate autocrine and paracrine mediators of estrogen and androgen action in bone, although important gaps remain in our understanding of the direct effects of sex steroids on bone cell function. Sex steroids also have important indirect effects on bone metabolism, via their effects on intestinal calcium absorption and renal calcium handling, and perhaps direct effects on parathyroid hormone secretion. Finally, genetic and epidemiologic evidence has challenged traditional notions of the relative importance of estrogen on bone metabolism in men. While androgens clearly have significant effects on the male skeleton, estrogen may also play a key role in males, and conversely, androgens have important skeletal effects in women. These dual roles for estrogen and androgens have long been known in reproductive tissues and now also appear to be true for the skeleton. Thus, while much already has been learned about sex steroid effects on bone, this is a rapidly evolving area and future studies are likely to reveal new insights both into the mechanism of sex steroid action on bone as well as the relative contributions of estrogens versus androgens towards bone metabolism in both sexes.

II. INTRODUCTION

Estrogens and androgens play major roles in skeletal homeostasis. Estrogen deficiency following menopause is recognized as the major cause of postmenopausal osteoporosis. Thus, the effects of estrogen on bone and on overall calcium homeostasis have been the subject of intensive investigation. It is clear that androgens also have important effects on bone, although the relative contributions of estrogens and androgens towards bone metabolism in both sexes remain unclear at present. In this chapter, we review the molecular structures, synthesis, and role of the major sex steroids in bone and calcium metabolism.

III. MOLECULAR STRUCTURES, SYNTHESIS, AND MECHANISM OF ACTION OF MAJOR SEX STEROIDS

A. Sex Steroid Structure and Synthesis

Figure 1 provides an overview of the major steps in the biosynthetic pathway for the sex steroids [1]. In the ovary, estrone and estradiol are formed from androstenedione and testosterone, respectively. This reaction is mediated by the enzyme, aromatase, which is a cytochrome P-450 enzyme (P-450 aromatase) present in the ovary [2]. This enzyme is also present in numerous other tissues, including the testes, fat cells, and bone cells [3]. In ovulating women and during pregnancy, progesterone is also secreted by the ovaries,

although the role of progesterone in bone metabolism is not as well defined as that of estrogens or androgens. Individual cell types in these tissues/organs are often responsible for the synthesis of each of the species of steroids.

The steroidogenic pathway is essentially similar in the testes except that testosterone is the major secretory product, although there is some conversion of both androstenedione and testosterone to estrone and estradiol, respectively (Fig. 1). In target tissues, including bone [4], testosterone is further converted to dihydrotestosterone (DHT). Unlike testosterone, DHT can not be aromatized to estrogens.

The adrenal glands are a significant source of weak androgens, principally dehydroepiandrosterone (DHEA) and androstenedione (Fig. 1). DHEA is further converted by the enzyme steroid sulfotransferase to dehydroepiandrosterone sulfate (DHEAS), and DHEA and DHEAS represent the major circulating adrenal androgens. In peripheral tissues, these can be further converted to more potent sex steroids, such as testosterone and estradiol, although there is increasing evidence that adrenal androgens may have independent direct effects on certain tissues, including bone cells [5].

In the circulation, the major sex steroids, testosterone and estrogens (estradiol and estrone), are mostly bound to serum-binding proteins, and only 1–3% of the total circulating sex steroids are free. Approximately 35–55% of the sex steroids are bound to albumin, which constitutes a high-capacity, low-affinity reservoir of the steroids. Both the free fraction as well

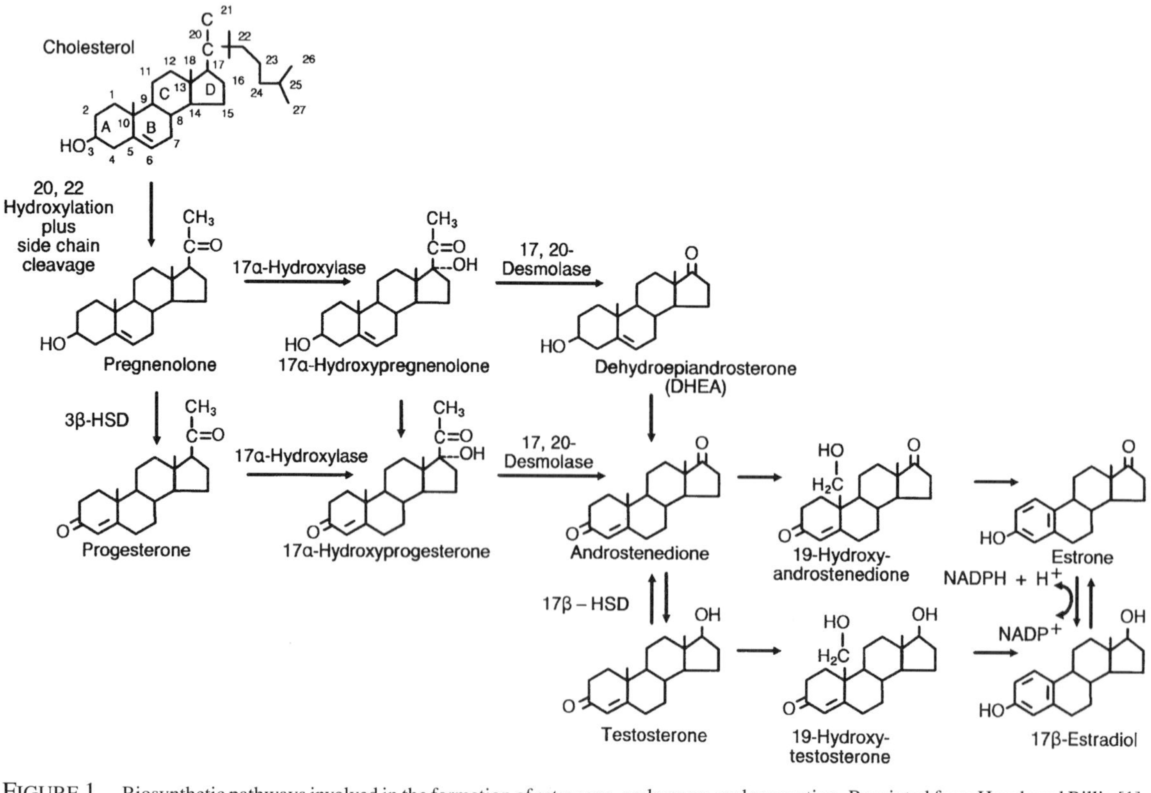

FIGURE 1   Biosynthetic pathways involved in the formation of estrogens, androgens, and progestins. Reprinted from Hseuh and Billig [1], with permission.

as the fraction bound to albumin appear to have access to target tissues [6] and thus represent the "bioavailable" sex steroid fraction. The fraction bound to sex hormone-binding globulin (SHBG), which has a high affinity but much lower capacity for the sex steroids than albumin, is unavailable to target tissues. In contrast to testosterone and estrogens, adrenal androgens do not bind SHBG to a significant degree, and more than 90% of adrenal androgens circulate loosely bound to albumin [7].

B. Mechanism of Action of Steroids

Considerable work has defined the mechanism of action of sex steroids in target tissues, and Figure 2 [7a] summarizes

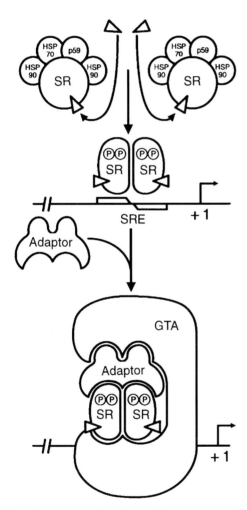

FIGURE 2   The classical pathway for steroid hormone action. The steroid hormones interact with their cognate receptors (SR), resulting in activation of the latent receptor. Following this, the receptor dissociates from heat-shock proteins (HSPs), dimerizes, undergoes phosphorylation, and binds specific steroid response elements (SRE) located within the regulatory regions of target promoters. The SR complex then interacts with the general transcription apparatus (GTA), directly or indirectly through adapter proteins. From McDonnell and Norris [7a], © European Foundation for Osteoporosis and National Osteoporosis Foundation. Reprinted with permission.

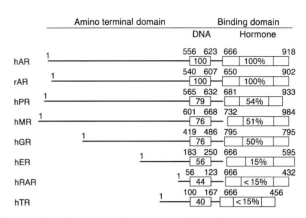

FIGURE 3   Comparison of the structures of the various steroid receptors. Numbers above refer to amino acid positions of the receptors. Numbers within rectangles are the percent identity of the amino acid sequence of the particular receptor domain in comparison to the same domain in the human androgen receptor. h, human; r, rat; AR, PR, MR, GR, ER, RAR, TR: androgen, progestin, mineralocorticoid, glucocorticoid, estrogen, retinoic acid, and thyroid hormone receptors, respectively. Reprinted from Hiipakka and Shutsung [10a], with permission.

what is generally accepted as the classical pathway for sex steroid action. Sex steroids rapidly diffuse into cells through the plasma membrane lipid bilayer. Once in the cell, they bind their cognate receptors, which are proteins of high molecular weight present in low concentrations (approximately 5000 to 40,000 molecules per cell) found primarily in the nucleus. The primary role of the steroid hormones is to bind the receptor and to modify the conformation of the receptor, thus exposing a DNA binding site on the receptor protein. Concomitant with this conformational change, the receptor dissociates from receptor-associated proteins [8], dimerizes as a homo- or heterodimer [9], and undergoes phosphorylation [10].

All of the sex steroid receptors have been shown to be structurally related, constituting a family of nuclear transcription factors (Fig. 3) [10a]. The hormone–receptor complex interacts with DNA enhancer elements (steroid response elements [SRE]) of steroid-dependent genes, leading to a stimulation of transcription (Fig. 2).

Only a single form of the androgen receptor has been identified. Two forms of the progesterone receptor (A and B) have been characterized [11]. A novel molecular species of the estrogen receptor, termed ER-β, was discovered in humans and rats and was found to have partial homology to the first described and extensively studied ER (ER-α) [12]. While the DNA binding domains of ER-α and ER-β are similar, their transactivation domains, tissue distribution, and molecular sizes differ. The β species is found in high levels in prostate, ovary, brain, and bladder, but is found in low levels or is absent in the uterus, kidney, pituitary, and epididymis; these tissues contain high levels of the α species [12]. Studies also indicate that bone cells express both α and β forms of the ER [13].

IV. EFFECTS OF SEX STEROIDS ON BONE CELLS AND BONE TURNOVER

A. Estrogen

Estrogen deficiency is recognized as the most important factor in the pathogenesis of postmenopausal bone loss [14]. Bone resorption increases in the absence of estrogen, although the precise local mediator(s) of the effects of estrogen deficiency on bone resorption remains controversial. Moreover, estrogen replacement therapy has been shown in numerous studies to be effective in preventing and treating osteoporosis [15]. The identification of estrogen receptors on human osteoblasts [16] (Fig. 4) led to the notion that estrogen likely had direct skeletal effects, as opposed to the concept that changes in calcitropic hormones mediate the skeletal effects of estrogen deficiency.

ERs have been identified on osteoclasts [17] and estrogen can inhibit osteoclastic bone resorption *in vitro*, suggesting that the effects of estrogen in inhibiting bone resorption may be mediated directly through osteoclasts. In addition, estrogen can increase the production of TGF-β by osteoclasts [18] and osteoblasts [19], which may then inhibit osteoclastic activity in an autocrine or paracrine fashion, respectively. Moreover, studies indicate that estrogen promotes apoptosis (i.e., programmed cell death) of osteoclasts and that this effect may also be mediated by TGF-β [20].

In addition to possible direct effects of estrogen on osteoclasts, estrogen may also regulate the production of cytokines by osteoblasts or bone marrow mononuclear cells, thus modulating osteoclastic activity in a paracrine fashion [21]. Studies suggest that bone-resorbing cytokines, such as interleukin (IL)-1, tumor necrosis factor α (TNF-α), macrophage-colony stimulating factor (M-CSF), IL-6, and prostaglandins may be potential candidates for mediating bone loss following estrogen deficiency.

Pacifici *et al.* [22] initially reported that IL-1 production by peripheral blood monocytes increased in oophorectomized women, and this was suppressed by estrogen replacement therapy. Subsequently, Kimble *et al.* [23] reported that the administration of IL-1 receptor antagonist (IL-1ra), a specific competitive inhibitor of IL-1, to ovariectomized rats decreased bone resorption and bone loss. In similar studies, Kitazawa *et al.* [24] demonstrated that administration of a soluble type I TNF receptor that binds to TNF-α and inhibits TNF action prevented the increase in bone resorption and bone loss following ovariectomy in rats. Moreover, Ammann *et al.* [25] demonstrated that transgenic mice expressing soluble TNF receptor were protected against bone loss following ovariectomy. Thus, these data indicate that both IL-1 and TNF-α play important roles in mediating the bone loss following estrogen deficiency.

Another potential cytokine involved in mediating the effects of estrogen deficiency on the skeleton is M-CSF, which is a potent stimulator of the proliferation and differentiation of osteoclast precursors [26]. Stromal cells from ovariectomized mice produce greater amounts of M-CSF than cells from control mice. Moreover, *in vivo* treatment with either estrogen or a combination of IL-1 receptor antagonist and TNF-binding protein abolished the *in vitro* increase in M-CSF production by stromal cells from the ovariectomized mice [27]. These data suggest that enhanced production of IL-1 and TNF from bone marrow mononuclear cells following ovariectomy leads to expansion of a high M-CSF-secreting bone marrow stromal cell population.

Other studies indicate, however, that IL-6 may also play a key role in mediating bone loss following estrogen deficiency. Girasole *et al.* [28] initially reported that estrogen suppressed IL-1- or TNF-α-induced IL-6 production by murine bone marrow stromal and osteoblastic cells. Subsequently, Jilka *et al.* [29] reported that an IL-6 neutralizing antibody could prevent the increase in osteoclastogenesis induced by ovariectomy in rats. Kassem *et al.* [30] showed that estrogen inhibited the production of IL-6 mRNA and protein induced by IL-1 and TNF-α in human osteoblastic cells stably transfected with the human ER-α gene. Finally, Poli *et al.* [31] found that IL-6-knockout mice were protected against ovariectomy-induced bone loss.

There are, then, a number of candidate cytokines that could mediate the effects of estrogen deficiency on the skeleton. It appears, however, that multiple cytokines may act cooperatively in inducing bone resorption following estrogen deficiency and that a single cytokine may only partially account for the effects of estrogen deficiency on the skeleton. In support of this, Miyaura *et al.* [32] found that IL-6 neutralizing antibody only partially inhibited the bone resorbing activity of bone marrow supernatants from ovariectomized mice. Moreover, the bone resorbing activity was also decreased by indomethacin, indicating that prostaglandins may also mediate, in part, the bone resorption induced by estrogen

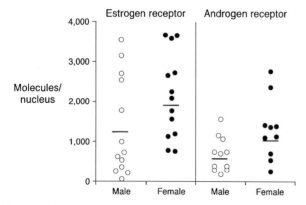

FIGURE 4   Demonstration of the presence of estrogen receptors (ERs, left) and androgen receptors (ARs, right) in human bone cells. Reprinted from Colvard *et al.* [65], with permission.

deficiency. In addition, Kawaguchi *et al.* [33] found that marrow supernatants from ovariectomized mice stimulated cyclooxygenase (COX)-2 mRNA expression and prostaglandin E synthesis in mouse calvarial cultures. Simultaneous treatment with submaximal doses of IL-1α, IL-6, and soluble IL-6 receptor (which enhances IL-6 action) resulted in a marked induction *in vitro* of osteoclast formation and COX-2 mediated PGE synthesis. Taken together, these data are consistent with the hypothesis that several bone-resorbing cytokines, such as IL-1, TNF-α, IL-6, prostaglandins, and probably others, act cooperatively in inducing bone resorption following estrogen deficiency. This may account for the fact that clinical investigative studies comparing either peripheral serum [34] or marrow plasma [35] concentrations of these cytokines in estrogen-deplete or estrogen-replaced postmenopausal women have failed to detect any consistent differences in any of these cytokines. It is likely that, *in vivo*, multiple cytokines are involved, and the changes in individual cytokines are of a magnitude that are difficult to detect in clinical-investigative studies.

In contrast to the inhibitory effects of estrogen on bone resorption, the effects of estrogen on bone formation and on osteoblast proliferation and differentiation are less clear. Because estrogen deficiency is associated with both increased bone resorption and impaired compensatory bone formation [36], it is likely that estrogen has significant effects on bone formation. In support of this, estrogen has been shown to increase production of IGF-I [37] and transforming growth factor-β [19] by osteoblastic cells *in vitro*. Estrogen also has been reported to stimulate fibroblast [38] and osteoblast [37] type I collagen synthesis, which represents >90% of the biosynthetic capacity of these cells. However, estrogen treatment has been reported both to stimulate [33] and to inhibit [39] bone formation in experimental animals, so this issue is far from resolved.

In vitro, estrogen effects on osteoblast proliferation and differentiation markers have likewise been variable, depending on the model system used. Gray *et al.* [40, 41], for example, found that estrogen treatment transiently inhibited proliferation and increased alkaline phosphatase activity in a rat osteogenic sarcoma cell line, UMR-106. In contrast, Ernst *et al.* [37] found that estrogen treatment of cultured osteoblast-like cells derived from fetal rat calvaria increased cell proliferation, mRNA for type I procollagen, and synthesis of collagenase-digestable protein. Studies using a conditionally immortalized human fetal osteoblast cell line (hFOB/ER9) that expresses high levels of ER-α, however, have found a consistent inhibitory effect of estrogen on proliferation [42, 43]. This has been associated with an increase in insulin-like growth factor (IGF) binding protein (IGFBP)-4 levels, which is inhibitory to IGF action [42]. Estrogen treatment of these cells also resulted in an increase in alkaline phosphatase mRNA and activity, a decrease in osteocalcin mRNA, and no effects on type I collagen protein levels or osteonectin steady-

state mRNA levels [43]. In addition, estrogen also induced the mRNA for bone morphogenetic protein-6 (BMP-6) in these cells, but did not induce mRNA for other BMPs [44]. Because BMP-6 is expressed in the hypertrophic cartilage in the developing fetal skeleton [45], these data suggest that estrogen may regulate skeletal development, at least in part, through BMP-6. Taken together, then, these data indicate that estrogen does directly regulate osteoblast proliferation and differentiation, although the net effect of estrogen on osteoblasts likely depends on a number of factors, including species differences, cellular heterogeneity, incomplete differentiation, and/or low or variable ER content among the various cell lines and primary cultures.

Preliminary evidence also suggests that, in addition to the osteoblast, the osteocyte may also be a target for estrogen action. Estrogen withdrawal associated with GnRH therapy has, for example, been shown to induce apoptosis of osteocytes in iliac bone [46]. Since osteocytes may be involved in mechanosensing and transducing loading responses [47], these effects of estrogen deficiency could impair the skeletal response to loading.

As summarized in Figure 5, all of the major cells in bone (osteoclasts, osteoblasts, and osteocytes) are potential targets for estrogen action. More studies clearly need to be performed, however, to fully define the effects of estrogen on each of these cell types, as well as the potential role of ER-α versus ER-β in mediating estrogen effects on these cells.

In addition to effects on bone resorption and possibly on bone formation in the adult skeleton, estrogen clearly also has major effects on skeletal development. Thus, the increase in estrogen levels at the onset of puberty in girls is associated with the pubertal increase in growth velocity as well as the ultimate closure of the epiphyseal growth plate and cessation of linear growth [48]. The pubertal growth spurt in girls is also associated with an increase in bone mass through a combination of increases in bone length, bone diameter, cortical bone width, and cancellous bone mass.

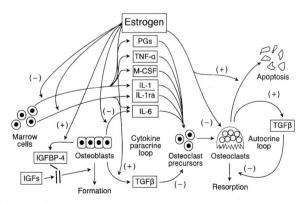

FIGURE 5   Summary of estrogen effects on osteoblasts, osteoclasts, and osteocytes.

The mechanism of action of estrogen on growth plate cartilage is at present poorly understood. It appears, however, that estrogen stimulates maturation of cartilage without increasing the growth rate [49, 50]. In addition, the effects of estrogen on cartilage growth and maturation are likely mediated by interactions with growth hormone and insulin-like growth factor-I; thus, although estrogen stimulates growth hormone secretion, it also inhibits IGF-I synthesis in the growth plate [51]. Therefore, the longitudinal growth rate may be influenced by the relative actions of estrogen and growth hormone on the growth plate.

Finally, studies on selective estrogen receptor modulators (SERMs), such as raloxifene, are providing new insights into possible alternate pathways for estrogen action in bone. These compounds have tissue-specific actions and can serve as either estrogen antagonists or agonists. For example, they can affect the skeleton without stimulating breast or endometrial tissue [52]. Although they bind the ER, they induce conformational changes in the ER that are different from estradiol [53]. The SERM-ER complex then, rather than activating estrogen responsive genes via the classical steroid pathway shown in Figure 2, may modulate the expression of genes via alternate, nonclassical pathways. For example, estrogen regulates the expression of the IL-6 gene not by direct interaction of the estrogen/ER complex with DNA, but by binding and inhibiting the activity of transcription factors, such as NF-kβ and C/EBPβ, which are required for IL-6 gene transcription [54, 55] (Fig. 6). It is possible that SERMs may also activate this pathway in bone cells but not the classical steroid pathway in bone cells or in reproductive tissue. Similarly, raloxifene has been shown to activate the gene for transforming growth factor-β3 even in human osteosarcoma MG63 cells transfected with a mutated ER-α that lacked the DNA binding domain of ER-α, and this effect may be mediated by a raloxifene response element in DNA that is distinct from the estrogen response element [56]. Finally, both ER-α and β interact with AP-1 sites in DNA (which are bound by the transcription factors, fos and jun) [57]. However, ER-α and β have different affinities for different estrogen analogs [58]. Moreover, when estradiol is present, ER-α activates transcription from the AP-1 site, whereas ER-β inhibits transcription. In contrast, in the presence of SERMs such as raloxifene, ER-β stimulates transcription from the AP-1 site, whereas ER-α inhibits transcription [57]. Thus, the elucidation of the mechanism of action of these SERMs is likely to provide new insights into estrogen action in bone and in other tissues.

B. Progesterone

The effects of progesterone on bone metabolism are much less clear than those of estrogen. However, progesterone receptors have been identified in primary human osteoblastic cells, human osteosarcoma cells, and immortalized fetal osteoblast cells [59, 60], although estrogen is generally required to induce progesterone receptors in these cells. In addition, progesterone has been shown to increase the proliferation and differentiation of human osteoblastic cells and also to stimulate IGF-II production by these cells [61]. Clinical studies using progesterone to prevent bone loss, however, report variable results; some studies show an effect of progesterone in prevention of spinal [62] or cortical [63] bone loss, whereas other studies report no significant benefit of progesterone treatment on postmenopausal bone loss [64]. Prior *et al.* [64] found that treatment of postmenopausal women with estrogen resulted, as expected, in a decrease in markers of bone resorption, whereas progesterone treatment did not decrease markers of bone resorption and, in contrast, increased markers of bone formation. Thus, the effects of progesterone on the skeleton likely differ significantly from those of estrogen. Indeed, since progesterone is a known antagonist of estrogen in certain cell processes and an agonist in others, it is possible that the major role of progesterone in bone metabolism is as a modulator of estrogen action. However, more work clearly needs to be done to address this possibility.

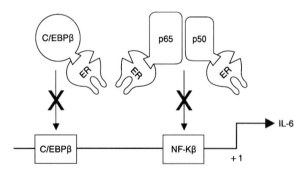

FIGURE 6   Estrogen mediated regulation of the interleukin-6 (IL-6) promotor: a model for estrogen response element (ERE)-independent regulation of gene transcription. According to this model, the activated ER can physically interact with either or both C/EBPβ or NF$\kappa\beta$ (p65/p50 complex) and inhibit their stimulation of the IL-6 promotor. This activity does not require a direct interaction of ER with DNA and may be one of the mechanisms by which SERMs protect against bone loss. From McDonnell and Norris [7a], © European Foundation for Osteoporosis and National Osteoporosis Foundation. Reprinted with permission.

C. Androgens

Human bone cells have been demonstrated to have specific androgen binding sites [65], and the androgen receptor concentrations found have been similar to estrogen receptor concentrations in these cells (Fig. 4). Moreover, the number of specific androgen binding sites in osteoblasts (1000–3000 sites/cell) is similar to the number of binding sites present in other androgen-responsive tissues, such as the prostate [66]. In addition to the androgen receptor, bone cells have also been shown to have 5α-reductase activity [67], which is responsible for the conversion of testosterone to DHT, the major biologically active metabolite of testosterone in most tissues. Testosterone may also be aromatized to estrogens in various tissues by the microsomal enzyme, aromatase, and there is also evidence that bone cells possess an aromatase activity [68].

As in the case of estrogen, there is evidence that androgens inhibit bone resorption. Thus, orchiectomy, like ovariectomy, is associated with increased bone resorption and rapid bone loss [69]. In addition, Tenover [70] has shown that 3 months of testosterone treatment of men with borderline serum testosterone levels resulted in a 28% reduction in urinary hydroxyproline excretion, an index of bone resorption. In another study of eugonadal men with osteoporosis who were treated with 6 months of intramuscular testosterone, testosterone therapy was associated with significant reductions in bone resorption markers [71]. Finally, Riggs *et al.* [72] performed bone biopsies in 29 women with postmenopausal osteoporosis before and after either estrogen or oxandrolone (a synthetic androgen) treatment and found similar decreases in resorption surfaces and comparable changes in bone resorption rate, as assessed by calcium kinetics.

Androgen receptors have been identified on osteoclasts, and androgens, like estrogen, have been shown to directly decrease bone resorption *in vitro* by avian and human osteoclast-like cells [73]. In addition to these direct effects on osteoclasts, androgens have also been shown to regulate the production of a number of bone-resorbing factors by osteoblasts or marrow stromal cells. Thus, both DHT and testosterone have been shown to reduce PGE_2 production in calvarial organ cultures exposed to stimulation with parathyroid hormone or IL-1 [74]. Similarly, androgens have been shown to inhibit IL-6 production by stromal cells as well to inhibit the increase in osteoclastogenesis following orchidectomy [75].

While androgens have generally been considered anabolic for bone, the evidence for this in adults is relatively sparse. Tenover [70] found that testosterone treatment had no effect on the bone formation marker, serum osteocalcin. In contrast, Raisz *et al.* [76] found that postmenopausal women treated with estrogen plus 2.5 mg of methyltestosterone had a 24% higher serum osteocalcin level after 3 months of treatment, as compared to a 40% lower osteocalcin level in the women treated with estrogen alone. In addition, Baran *et al.* [77] performed bone biopsies in a hypogonadal man before and after 6 months of testosterone treatment and noted increases in relative osteoid volume, total osteoid surface, linear extent of bone formation, and bone mineralization. Similarly, Cantatore *et al.* [78] administered synthetic androgens in postmenopausal women and found increases in markers of bone formation, at least over the short term (3–6 months), and Morley *et al.* [79] also noted that 3 months of testosterone therapy in elderly hypogonadal men resulted in a significant increase in serum osteocalcin levels. At least over the short term, androgens may have an anabolic effect on

bone, although further studies are needed to address this issue.

As in the case of estrogen, *in vitro* studies of androgen effects on osteoblast proliferation and differentiation have yielded inconsistent results. Androgens have been shown to have mitogenic effects on normal and transformed osteoblast-like cells in most [80, 81], but not all, systems [82, 83]. With respect to osteoblast differentiation, androgens have been shown to increase alkaline phosphatase activity in primary cultures of osteoblast-like cells and to increase the percentage of alkaline phosphatase-positive cells, suggesting a shift towards a more differentiated phenotype [81, 84, 85]. On the other hand, studies using a fetal human osteoblast cell line stably transfected with the androgen receptor have found a decrease in alkaline phosphatase activity in these cells following DHT exposure [83]. Androgen effects on type I collagen synthesis have been variable, with some studies showing a stimulatory effect [80, 82, 84], others finding no effect [74], and others reporting a decrease [83] in collagen synthesis. Finally, studies using primary osteoblast cultures have suggested that some of the effects of androgens in these cells may be mediated, at least in part, by increased TGF-β production [86], or by alterations in the insulin-like growth factor/insulin-like growth factor binding protein system [86].

In addition to testosterone and DHT, there is some evidence that adrenal androgens may have significant effects on bone metabolism. Durbridge *et al.* [87] found that in rats, adrenalectomy alone resulted in loss of metaphyseal trabecular bone of an extent similar to that produced by oophorectomy. These investigators interpreted these data as being consistent with an important role for adrenal androgens in the maintenance of skeletal mass in rats. In addition, Turner *et al.* [88] have shown that in rats, treatment with DHEA reduced the loss of cancellous bone following oophorectomy, indicating that adrenal androgens may prevent bone loss induced by estrogen deficiency.

DHEA, which is essentially a prohormone, can be converted locally in various tissues to androstenedione and then into potent androgens and/or estrogens, and it has generally been assumed that the effects of adrenal androgens on target tissues are due to the effects of these androgens or estrogens [89]. However, the description of specific binding sites for DHEA [90] raises the possibility that DHEA or similar compounds may have direct effects on bone. In support of this, Bodine *et al.* [5] have shown that DHEA caused a rapid reduction (30 minutes posttreatment) in steady-state levels of c-*fos* mRNA in normal human osteoblastic cells, whereas testosterone or DHT had no effects on c-*fos* expression. However, all three agents resulted in significant increases in TGF-β activity in these cells. These studies demonstrate that bone cells have the ability to respond to DHEA, and that the effects of DHEA may or may not be identical to the effects of testosterone, depending on the specific metabolism and perhaps independent action of DHEA in bone cells.

The major role of androgens in bone metabolism may occur at puberty. As in females, adolescence in males is associated with rapid longitudinal growth and marked increases in axial and appendicular bone mass [91]. The increase in bone mass is associated with increases in markers of bone formation and is closely linked to pubertal stage and to testosterone levels [48, 92], suggesting that testicular androgen production plays a major role in mediating the pubertal increase in bone mass. In addition, however, the increase in adrenal androgens that occurs before the onset of puberty also likely affects the acquisition of bone mass. Thus, longitudinal growth rate increases during adrenarche [93] and bone mass has been shown to increase before the onset of sexual development; this is likely related to the rise in adrenal androgens [94].

Androgens are also clearly responsible for the sexual dimorphism of the skeleton that is evident during adolescence: the male skeleton is larger in most dimensions compared to the female skeleton, the diameter and cortical thickness of long bones is greater in men than in women, and vertebral size is larger in men [95]. Despite these unequivocal effects of androgens on skeletal growth, however, it remains unresolved which of these effects are due to direct androgen effects on bone and which are due to indirect effects. For example, like estrogen, testosterone can influence growth hormone secretion [96] or the local production of IGF-I or its binding proteins [97], and thus affect bone mass indirectly. It is likely, therefore, that androgen effects on bone during adolescence are due both to direct and indirect effects.

V. EFFECTS OF SEX STEROIDS ON EXTRASKELETAL CALCIUM HOMEOSTASIS

In addition to direct effects on bone cells and on bone remodeling, it is becoming clear that sex steroids may affect bone turnover indirectly through action on extraskeletal calcium homeostasis; this action may include effects on intestinal calcium absorption, renal calcium handling, and perhaps direct effects on PTH secretion. Thus, Gallagher *et al.* [98] found that estrogen treatment increased both serum total 1,25(OH)$_2$D levels and calcium absorption in postmenopausal osteoporotic women, although this effect may have been due to the increase in serum PTH in response to the estrogen-induced decrease in bone resorption. However, in perimenopausal women before and 6 months after oophorectomy, Gennari *et al.* [99] found that the increase in calcium absorption in response to treatment with 1,25(OH)$_2$D was blunted in the presence of estrogen deficiency, suggesting a direct effect of estrogen on intestinal calcium absorption. Of note, estrogen receptors have been found in an untransformed cell line from rat small intestinal crypts (IEC-6 cells) as well as from epithelial cells from rat intestine using both classical receptor binding techniques and reverse transcriptase polymerase chain reaction [100]. Thus, estrogen may affect

bone turnover both directly, by acting on bone cells, and indirectly, by altering intestinal calcium absorption and hence, serum PTH levels.

Estrogen receptors have also been found in renal tubules [101], and estrogen has been reported to increase adenylate cyclase activity of renal membranes from hens [102] and from cultured opossum kidney cells [103]. Using estimates based on regression analysis, Nordin *et al.* [104] found that early postmenopausal women had a "renal calcium leak" that they attributed to estrogen deficiency. McKane *et al.* [105] assessed renal calcium transport by direct measurements both at baseline and during administration of a saturating dose of PTH in early postmenopausal women before and after six months of estrogen treatment. They demonstrated a PTH-independent decrease in tubular calcium reabsorption in the estrogen-deficient women compared to the estrogen-replete women; this finding is consistent with a direct effect of estrogen on renal calcium conservation.

In addition to these indirect effects on serum PTH levels, there is evidence that estrogen may directly regulate PTH secretion. Some [106], but not other [107], investigators have demonstrated the presence of estrogen receptors in parathyroid glands. Cosman *et al.* [108] reported that estrogen replacement therapy in elderly women decreased maximal PTH secretory rate, as assessed by measurement of serum PTH during EDTA-induced hypocalcemia. In contrast, studies in experimental animals and parathyroid cells *in vitro* suggest that estrogen increases PTH secretion. Estrogen administration to oophorectomized rats increased PTH mRNA in the parathyroid glands by 4-fold [106], and *in vitro* estrogen treatment of surgically removed human hyperplastic parathyroid glands increased PTH secretion in a dose- and time-dependent manner [109]. Some of the contrasting effects of estrogen on PTH secretion may be related to acute versus chronic effects, although more work is needed to address this issue.

There are several lines of evidence suggesting that androgens may also have similar, indirect effects on bone metabolism. Some data indicate that androgens may significantly enhance intestinal calcium absorption. Hope *et al.* [110] reported that duodenal active calcium transport decreased in male rats following orchiectomy and that testosterone treatment reversed this effect. Lafferty *et al.* [111] found that calcium absorption increased following short-term (2–3 months) testosterone treatment in three subjects, although these changes did not persist with long-term therapy. Need *et al.* [112] studied 27 women with postmenopausal osteoporosis and found a significant increase in the hourly fractional rate of radiocalcium absorption from 0.79 ± 0.06 to 0.93 ± 0.05 (mean $\pm$ SEM) following 3 months of therapy with the anabolic steroid nandrolone decanoate.

Some evidence also suggests that androgens may affect renal calcium transport. The androgen receptor gene is expressed in kidney epithelial cells [113], and androgens have been shown to modulate calcium fluxes in mouse kidney cortex preparations [114]. Reifenstein and Albright [115] initially noted that testosterone propionate decreased the urinary excretion of calcium. Several studies using synthetic androgens have also suggested an effect of androgens on renal calcium handling. Chesnut et al. [116] noted a 32% decrease in urinary calcium excretion in 23 women with postmenopausal osteoporosis following 8–32 months of therapy with the anabolic steroid stanozolol. Similarly, Need et al. [112] indirectly estimated renal tubular calcium reabsorption and found that this increased significantly in 27 women with postmenopausal osteoporosis treated for 3 months with nandrolone decanoate. Finally, Mason and Morris [117] showed that DHT administration increased the tubular reabsorption of calcium in oophorectomized rats.

Thus, both estrogen and androgens may affect bone metabolism indirectly via alterations in overall calcium homeostasis and subsequent changes in serum PTH levels. Indeed, loss of these indirect effects of sex steroids in elderly women and in some men may account, in large part, for the age-related increase in serum PTH levels in both sexes [118]. This, in turn, results in an age-related increase in bone turnover and, in the setting of a concomitant defect in osteoblast function, in bone loss [118].

VI. EFFECTS OF ESTROGENS AND ANDROGENS ON BONE METABOLISM IN MEN VERSUS WOMEN

Based on the sexual dimorphism of the skeleton, it had generally been believed that estrogens were the major determinant of bone metabolism in women and androgens primarily affected bone metabolism in men. Evidence, however, indicates there is considerable overlap of the effects of sex steroids on bone in men and women. Data from several "experiments of nature" are consistent, for example, with the concept that estrogen plays a major role in bone metabolism in men. Smith et al. [119] described a male with homozygous mutations in the ER-α gene who, even in the presence of normal testosterone levels, had unfused epiphyses and marked osteopenia, along with elevated indices of bone turnover. Subsequently, Morishima et al. [120] and Carani et al. [121] reported clinical findings in two males with homozygous mutations in the aromatase gene. In both cases, bone mineral density was significantly reduced and bone turnover markers were markedly elevated despite normal testosterone levels. Treatment with testosterone did not significantly affect bone metabolism in one patient, whereas treatment with estrogen markedly increased bone mineral density in both patients [121, 122]. In addition to these findings in humans, Korach et al. [123] found that disruption of ER-α by homologous recombination in mice resulted in decreases in bone density in both male and female mice. Finally, four population-based, observational studies [124–127] have demonstrated by multivariate analysis that serum estrogen levels (partic-

ularly bioavailable estrogen levels) are better predictors of bone density in men at all measured sites, except at some cortical bone sites in the appendicular skeleton. Thus, estrogen clearly plays a major role in bone metabolism in males, although the relative contributions of estrogen versus androgens towards regulating bone turnover and bone density in males remain to be defined.

Similarly, several lines of evidence indicate that androgens may have important effects on bone in women. In premenopausal women, serum androgen levels are significantly related to bone mineral density [124, 128], suggesting that androgens may contribute to the development of peak bone mass in women. Moreover, hyperandrogenic women with hirsutism have increased bone mass relative to control women [129]. Finally, testosterone levels correlate with bone mass and rates of decrease in bone mass in perimenopausal women [128].

VII. SUMMARY

Sex steroids clearly have major effects on all aspects of bone metabolism. These include effects on longitudinal growth at the time of puberty, the acquisition of peak bone mass, and the regulation of bone turnover in adults. While there are several candidate factors for mediating the autocrine and paracrine effects of estrogen and, to a lessor extent, androgens, on osteoclasts and osteoblasts, the precise mechanism of direct sex steroid effects on the skeleton remains to be clearly defined. In addition, sex steroids affect bone turnover indirectly via extraskeletal effects on calcium homeostasis. Finally, estrogen likely has a significant effect on bone not just in females, but also in males. Androgens also have important skeletal effects in both sexes. The relative contributions of estrogens versus androgens towards bone metabolism in both sexes, however, remain unclear and warrant further investigation.

Acknowledgments

This work was supported by Research Grants AG-04875 and AR-30582 from the National Institutes of Health, U.S. Public Health Service.

References

1. Hsueh, A. J. W., and Billig, H. (1995). Ovarian hormone synthesis and mechanism of action. In "Endocrinology" (L. J. DeGroot, M. Besser, H. G. Burger, J. L. Jameon, D. L. Loriaux, J. C. Marshall, W. D. Odell, J. T. Potts, and A. H. Rubenstein, eds.), pp. 2019–2030. Saunders, Philadelphia.

2. Simpson, E. R., Mahendroo, M. S., Means, G. D., Kilgore, M. W., Hinshelwood, M. M., Graham-Lorence, S., Amarneh, B., Ito, Y., Fisher, C. R., Michael, M. D., Mendelson, C. R., and Bulun, S. E. (1994). Aromatase cytochrome P450, the enzyme responsible for estrogen biosynthesis. Endocr. Rev. 15, 342–355.

3. Nawata, H., Tanaka, S., Takayanagi, R., Sakai, Y., Yanase, T., Ikuyama, S., and Haji, M. (1995). Aromatase in bone cell: Association with osteoporosis in postmenopausal women. *J. Steroid Biochem. Mol. Biol.* **53**, 165–174.

4. Dinneen, S., Alzaid, A., Miles, J., and Rizza, R. A. (1993). Metabolic effects of the nocturnal rise in cortisol on carbohydrate metabolism in normal humans. *J. Clin. Invest.* **91**, 2283–2290.

5. Bodine, P. V., Riggs, B. L., and Spelsberg, T. C. (1995). Regulation of c-fos expression and TGF-β production by gonadal and adrenal androgens in normal human osteoblastic cells. *J. Steroid Biochem. Mol. Biol.* **52**, 149–158.

6. Manni, A., Pardridge, W. M., Cefalu, W., Nisula, B. C., Bardin, C. W., Santner, S. J., and Santen, R. J. (1985). Bioavailability of albumin-bound testosterone. *J. Clin. Endocrinol. Metab.* **61**, 705–710.

7. Cekan, S., Xing, S., and Ritzen, M. (1984). On the binding of steroid sulfates to albumin. *Experientia* **40**, 949–953.

7a. McDonnell, D. P., and Norris, J. D. (1997). Analysis of the molecular pharmacology of estrogen receptor agonists and antagonists provides insights into the mechanism of action of estrogen in bone. *Osteoporosis Int.* **7**(Suppl. 1), S29–S34.

8. Smith, D. F., and Toft, D. O. (1993). Steroid receptors and their associated proteins. *Mol. Endocrinol.* **7**, 4–11.

9. Tsai, S. Y., Carlstedt-Duke, J., Weigel, N. L. Dahlman, K.. Gustafsson, J. A., Tsai, M. J., and O'Malley, B. W. (1988). Molecular interactions of steroid hormone receptor with its enhancer element: Evidence for dimer formation. *Cell* **55**, 361–369.

10. Takimots, G. S., Tasset, D. M., Eppert, E. C., and Horwitz, K. B. (1992). Hormone induced progesterone receptor phosphorylation consists of sequential DNA-independent and DNA-dependent stages. Analysis with zinc-finger mutants and the progesterone antagonist ZK-98299. *Proc. Natl. Acad. Sci. U.S.A.* **89**, 3050–3052.

10a. Hiipakka, R. A., and Shutsung, L. (1995). Androgen receptors and action. *In* "Endocrinology" (L. J. DeGroot, M. Besser, H. G. Burger, J. L. Jameon, D. L. Loriaux, J. C. Marshall, W. D. Odell, J. T. Potts, and A. H. Rubenstein, eds.), pp. 2336–2361. Saunders, Philadelphia.

11. Horwitz, K. B. (1988). Purification, monoclonal antibody production and structural analyses of human progesterone receptors. *J. Steroid Biochem.* **31**, 573–578.

12. Kuiper, G. G., Enmark, M. J., Pelto-Huikko, M., Nilsson, S., and Gustafsson, J. A. (1996). Cloning of a novel estrogen receptor expressed in rat prostate and ovary. *Proc. Natl. Acad. Sci. U.S.A* **93**, 5925–5930.

13. Onoe, Y., Miyaura, C., Ohta, H., Nozawa, S., and Suda, T. (1997). Expression of estrogen receptor beta in rat bone. *Endocrinology* **138**, 4509–4512.

14. Riggs, B. L., and Melton, L. J., III (1986). Involutional osteoporosis. *N. Engl. J. Med.* **314**, 1676–1686.

15. Riggs, B. L., and Melton, L. J., III (1992). The prevention and treatment of osteoporosis. *N. Engl. J. Med.* **327**, 620–627; erratum: *Ibid.* **328** (1), 65 (1993).

16. Eriksen, E. F., Colvard, D. S., Berg, N. J., Graham, M. L., Mann, K. G., Spelsberg, T. C., and Riggs, B. L. (1988). Evidence of estrogen receptors in normal human osteoblast-like cells. *Science* **241**, 84–86.

17. Oursler, M. J., Pederson, L., Fitzpatrick, L., Riggs, B. L., and Spelsberg, T. (1994). Human giant cell tumors of the bone (osteoclastomas) are estrogen target cells. *Proc. Natl. Acad. Sci. U.S.A.* **91**, 5227–5231.

18. Robinson, J. A., Riggs, B. L., Spelsberg, T. C., and Oursler, M. J. (1996). Osteoclasts and transforming growth factor-beta: Estrogen-mediated isoform-specific regulation of production. *Endocrinology* **137**, 615–621.

19. Oursler, M. J., Cortese, C., Keeting, P., Anderson, M. A., Bonde, S. K., Riggs, B. L., and Spelsberg, T. C. (1991). Modulation of transforming growth factor-beta production in normal human osteoblast-like cells

by 17β-estradiol and parathyroid hormone. *Endocrinology* **129**, 3313–3320.

20. Hughes, D. E., Dai, A., Tiffee, J. C., Li, H. H., Mundy, G. R., and Boyce, B. F. (1996). Estrogen promotes apoptosis of murine osteoclasts mediated by TGF-β. *Nat. Med.* **2**, 1132–1136.

21. Manolagas, S. C., and Jilka, R. L. (1995). Bone marrow, cytokines, and bone remodeling. Emerging insights into the pathophysiology of osteoporosis. *N. Engl. J. Med.* **332**, 305–311.

22. Pacifici, R., Brown, C., Puscheck, E., Friedrick, E., Slatopolsky, E., Maggio, D., McCracken, R., and Avioli, L. V. (1991). Effect of surgical menopause and estrogen replacement on cytokine release from human blood mononuclear cells. *Proc. Natl. Acad. Sci. U.S.A.* **88**, 5134–5138.

23. Kimble, R. B., Vannice, J. L., Bloedow, D. C., Thompson, R. C., Hopfer, W., Kung, V. T., and Brownfield, C., and Pacifici, R. (1994). Interleukin-1 receptor antagonist decreases bone loss and bone resorption in ovariectomized rats. *J. Clin. Invest.* **93**, 1959–1967.

24. Kitazawa, R., Kimble, R. B., Vannice, J. L., Kung, V. T., and Pacifici, R. (1994). Interleukin-1 receptor antagonist and tumor necrosis factor binding protein decrease osteoclast formation and bone resorption in ovariectomized mice. *J. Clin. Invest.* **94**, 2397–2406.

25. Ammann, P., Rizzoli, R., Bonjour, J., Bourrin, S., Meyer, J., Vassaili, P., and Garcia, I. (1997). Transgenic mice expressing soluble tumor necrosis factor-receptor are protected against bone loss caused by estrogen deficiency. *J. Clin. Invest.* **99**, 1699–1703.

26. Tanaka, S., Takahashi, N., Udagawa, N., Tamura, T., Akatsu, T., Stanley, E. R., Kurokawa, T., and Suda, T. (1993). Macrophage colony stimulating factor is indispensible for both proliferation and differentiation of osteoclast progenitors. *J. Clin. Invest.* **91**, 257–263.

27. Kimble, R. B., Srivastava, S., Ross, P. F., Matayoshi, A., and Pacifici, R. (1996). Estrogen deficiency increases the ability of stromal cells to support murine osteoclastogenesis via an interleukin-1 and tumor necrosis factor-mediated stimulation of macrophage colony stimulating factor production. *J. Biol. Chem.* **271**, 28890–28897.

28. Girasole, G., Jilka, R. L., Passeri, G., Boswell, S., Boder, G., Williams, D. C., and Manolagas, S. C. (1992). 17β-estradiol inhibits interleukin-6 production by bone marrow-derived stromal cells and osteoblasts in vitro: A potential mechanism for the antiresorptive effect of estrogens. *J. Clin. Invest.* **9**, 883–891.

29. Jilka, R. L., Hangoc, G., Girasole, G., Passeri, G., Williams, D. C., Abrams, J. S., Boyce, B., Boxmeyer, H., and Manolagas, S. C. (1992). Increased osteoclast development after estrogen loss: Mediation by interleukin-6. *Science* **257**, 88–91.

30. Kassem, M., Harris, S. A., Spelsberg, T. C., and Riggs, B. L. (1996). Estrogen inhibits interleukin-6 production and gene expression in a human osteoblastic cell line with high levels of estrogen receptors. *J. Bone Miner. Res.* **11**, 193–199.

31. Poli, V., Balena, R., Fattori, E., Markatos, A., Yamamoto, A., Tanaka, H., Ciliberto, G., Rodan, G. A., and Costantini, F. (1994). Interleukin-6 deficient mice are protected from bone loss caused by estrogen depletion. *EMBO J.* **13**, 1189–1196.

32. Miyaura, C., Kusano, K., Masuzawa, T., Chaki, O., Onoe, Y., Aoyagi, M., Sasaki, T., Tamura, T., Koishihara, Y., and Ohsugi, Y. (1995). Endogenous bone- resorbing factors in estrogen deficiency: Cooperative effects of IL-1 and IL-6. *J. Bone Miner. Res.* **10**, 1365–1373.

33. Kawaguchi, H., Pilbeam, C. C., Vargas, S. J., Morse, E. E., Lorenzo, J. A., and Raisz, L. G. (1995). Ovariectomy enhances and estrogen replacement inhibits the activity of bone marrow factors that stimulate prostaglandin production in cultured mouse calvaria. *J. Clin. Invest.* **96**, 539–548.

34. McKane, W. R., Khosla, S., Peterson, J. M., Egan, K., and Riggs, B. L. (1994). Circulating levels of cytokines that modulate bone resorption: Effects of age and menopause in women. *J. Bone Miner. Res.* **9**, 1313–1318.

35. Kassem, M., Khosla, S., Spelsberg, T. C., and Riggs, B. L. (1996). Cytokine production in the bone marrow microenvironment: Failure to demonstrate estrogen regulation in early postmenopausal women. *J. Clin. Endocrinol. Metab.* **81**, 513–518.

36. Ivey, J. L., and Baylink, D. J. (1981). Postmenopausal osteoporosis: Proposed roles of defective coupling and estrogen deficiency. *Metab. Bone Dis. Relat. Res.* **3**, 3–8.

37. Ernst, M., Heath, J. K., and Rodan, G. A. (1989). Estradiol effects on proliferation, messenger ribonucleic acid for collagen and insulin-like growth factor-1, and parathyroid hormone-stimulated adenylate cyclase activity in osteoblastic cells from calvariae and long bones. *Endocrinology* **125**, 825–833.

38. Brincat, M., Moniz, C. F., Kabalan, S., Versi, E., O'Dowd, T., Magos, A. L., Montgomery, J., and Studd, J. W. W. (1987). Decline in skin collagen content and metacarpal index after the menopause and its prevention with sex hormone replacement. *Br. J. Obstet. Gynaecol.* **94**, 126–129.

39. Westerlind, K. C., Wakley, G. K., Evans, G. L., and Turner, R. T. (1993). Estrogen does not increase bone formation in growing rats. *Endocrinology* **133**, 2924–2934.

40. Gray, T. K., Flynn, T. C., Gray, K. M., and Nabell, L. M. (1987). 17β-estradiol acts directly on the clonal osteoblastic cell line UMR106. *Proc. Natl. Acad. Sci. U.S.A.* **84**, 6267–6271.

41. Gray, T. K., Mohan, S., Linkhart, T. A., and Baylink, D. J. (1989). Estradiol stimulates in vitro the secretion of insulin-like growth factors by the clonal osteoblastic cell line, UMR106. *Biochem. Biophys. Res. Commun.* **158**, 407–412.

42. Kassem, M., Okazaki, R., De Leon, D., Harris, S. A., Robinson, J. A., Spelsberg, T. C., Conover, C. A., and Riggs, B. L. (1996). Potential mechanism of estrogen-mediated decrease in bone formation: Estrogen increases production of inhibitory insulin-like growth factor-binding protein-4. *Proc. Natl. Acad. Sci. U.S.A.* **108**, 155–164.

43. Robinson, J. A., Harris, S. A., Riggs, B. L., and Spelsberg, T. C. (1997). Estrogen regulation of human osteoblastic cell proliferation and differentiation. *Endocrinology* **138**, 2919–2927.

44. Rickard, D. J., Hofbauer, L. C., Bonde, S. K., Gori, F., Spelsberg, T. C., and Riggs, B. L. (1998). Bone morphogenetic protein-6 production in human osteoblastic cell lines. Selective regulation by estrogen. *J. Clin. Invest.* **101**, 413–422.

45. Lyons, K. M., Pelton, R. W., and Hogan, B. L. (1989). Patterns of expression of murine Vgr-1 and BMP-2a RNA suggest that TGFβ-like genes co-ordinately regulate aspects of embryonic development. *Genes Dev.* **3**, 1657–1668.

46. Tomkinson, A., Reeve, J., Shaw, R. W., and Noble, B. S. (1997). The death of osteocytes via apoptosis accompanies estrogen withdrawal in human bone. *J. Clin. Endocrinol. Metab.* **82**, 3128–3135.

47. Pitsillides, A., Rawlinson, S., Suswillo, R., Bourrin, S., Zaman, G., and Lanyon, L. (1995). Mechanical strain-induced NO production by bone cells: A possible role in adaptive bone (re)modelling. *FASEB J.* **9**, 1614–1622.

48. Bonjour, J. P., Theintz, G., Buchs, B., Slosman, D., and Rizzoli, R. (1991). Critical years and states of puberty for spinal and femoral bone mass accumulation during adolescence. *J. Clin. Endocrinol. Metab.* **73**, 555–563.

49. Strickland, A. L., and Sprinz, H. (1973). Studies of the influence of estradiol and growth hormone on the hypophysectomized immature rat epiphyseal cartilage growth plate. *Am. J. Obstet. Gynecol.* **115**, 471–477.

50. Gustafsson, P. O., Kasstrom, H., Lindberg, L., and Olsson, S. E. (1975). Growth and mitotic rate of the proximal tibial epiphyseal plate in hypophysectomized rats given estradiol and growth hormone. *Acta Radiol. Suppl.* **344**, 69–74.

51. Ho, K. K., and Weissberger, A. J. (1992). Impact of short-term estrogen administration on growth hormone secretion and action: Distinct route-dependent effects on connective and bone tissue metabolism. *J. Bone Miner. Res.* **7**, 821–827.

52. Delmas, P. D., Bjarnason, N. H., Mitlak, B. H., Ravoux, A. C., Shah, A. S., Huster, W. J., Draper, M., and Christiansen, C. (1997). Effects of raloxifene on bone mineral density, serum cholesterol concentrations, and uterine endometrium in postmenopausal women. *N. Engl. J. Med.* **337**, 1641–1647.

53. Brzozowski, A. M., Pike, A.C.W., Dauter, Z., Hubbard, R. E., Bonn, T., Engstrom, O., Ohman, L., Greene, G. L., Gustafsson, J. A., and Carlquist, M. (1997). Molecular basis of agonism and antagonism in the oestrogen receptor. *Nature* **389**, 753–758.

54. Stein, B., and Yang, M. (1995). Repression of the interleukin-6 promotor by estrogen is mediated by NF-kB and C/EBPB. *Mol. Cell. Biol,* **15**, 4971–4979.

55. Ray, A., Prefontaine, K. E., and Ray, P. (1994). Down-regulation of interleukin-6 gene expression by 17beta-estradiol in the absence of high affinity DNA binding by the estrogen receptor. *J. Biol. Chem.* **269**, 12940–12946.

56. Yang, N. N., Venugopalan, M., Hardikar, S., and Glasebrook, A. (1996). Identification of an estrogen response element activated by metabolites of 17β- estradiol and raloxifene. *Science* **273**, 1222–1225.

57. Paech, K., Webb, P., Kuiper, G. G. J. M., Nilsson, S., Gustafsson, J. A., Kushner, P. J., and Scanlan, T. S. (1997). Differential ligand activation of estrogen receptors ERα and ERβ at AP1 sites. *Science* **277**, 1508–1510.

58. Kuiper, G. G., and Gustafsson, J. A. (1997). The novel estrogen receptor-beta subtype: potential role in the cell- and promoter-specific actions of estrogens and antiestrogens. *FEBS Lett.* **410**, 87–90.

59. Wei, L. L., Leach, M. W., Miner, R. S., and Demers, L. M. (1993). Evidence for progesterone receptors in human osteoblast-like cells. *Biochem. Biophys. Res. Commun.* **195**, 525–532.

60. MacNamara, P., O'Shaughnessy, C. O., Manduca, P., and Loughrey, H. C. (1995). Progesterone receptors are expressed in human osteoblast-like cell lines and in primary human osteoblast cultures. *Calcif. Tissue Int.* **57**, 436–441.

61. Tremollieres, F. A., Strong, D. D., Baylink, D. J., and Mohan, S. (1992). Progesterone and promestone stimulate human bone cell proliferation and insulin-like growth factor-II production. *Acta Endocrinol.* **126**, 329–337.

62. Caird, L. E., Reid-Thomas, V., Hannan, W. J., Gows, S., and Glasier, A. F. (1994). Oral progestogen-only contraception may protect against loss of bone mass in breast-feeding women. *Clin. Endocrinol.* **41**, 739–745.

63. Gallagher, J. C., Kable, W. T., and Goldgar, D. (1991). The effect of progestin therapy on cortical and trabecular bone: Comparison with estrogen. *Am. J. Med.* **90**, 171–178.

64. Prior, J. C., Vigna, Y. M., Wark, J. D., Eyre, D. R., Lentle, B. C., Li, D.K.B., Ebeling, P. R., and Atley, L. (1997). Premenopausal ovariectomy-related bone loss: A randomized, double-blind, one-year trial of conjugated estrogen or medroxyprogesterone acetate. *J. Bone Miner. Res.* **12**, 1851–1863.

65. Colvard, D. S., Eriksen, E. F., Keeting, P. E., Wilson, E. M., Lubahn, D. B., French, F. S., Riggs, B. L., and Spelsberg, T. C. (1989). Identification of androgen receptors in normal human osteoblast-like cells. *Proc. Natl. Acad. Sci. U.S.A.* **86**, 854–857.

66. Sanchez-Visconti, G., Herrero, L., Rabadan, M., Pereira, I., and Ruiz-Rorres, A. (1995). Ageing and prostate: Age-related changes in androgen receptors of epithelial cells from benign and hypertrophic glands compared with cancer. *Mech. Ageing Dev.* **82**, 19–29.

67. Schweikert, H. U., Rulf, W., Niederle, N., Schafer, H. E., Keck, E., and Kruck, F. (1980). Testosterone metabolism in human bone. *Acta Endocrinol.* **95**, 258–264.

68. Nakano, Y., Morimoto, I., Ishida, O., Fujihara, T., Mizokami, A., Tanimoto, A., Yanagihara, N., Izumi, F., and Eto, S. (1994). The receptror, metabolism and effects of androgen in osteoblastic MC3T3-E1 cells. *Bone Miner.* **26**, 245–259.

69. Stepan, J. J., Lachman, M., Zverina, J., Pacovsky, V., and Baylink, D. J. (1989). Castrated men exhibit bone loss: Effect of calcitonin treatment on biochemical indices of bone remodeling. *J. Clin. Endocrinol. Metab.* **69**, 523–527.

70. Tenover, J. S. (1992). Effects of testosterone supplementation in the aging male. *J. Clin. Endocrinol. Metab.* **75**, 1092–1098.

71. Anderson, F. H., Francis, R. M., Peaston, R. T., and Wastell, H. J. (1997). Androgen supplementation in eugonadal men with osteoporosis: Effects of six months' treatment on markers of bone formation and resorption. *J. Bone Miner. Res.* **12**, 472–478.

72. Riggs, B. L., Jowsey, J., Goldsmith, R. S., Kelly, P. J., Hoffman, D. L., and Arnaud, C. D. (1972). Short- and long-term effects of estrogen and synthetic anabolic hormone in postmenopausal osteoporosis. *J. Clin. Invest.* **51**, 1659–1663.

73. Pederson, L., Kremer, M., Judd, J., Pascoe, D., Spelsberg, T. C., Riggs, B. L., and Oursler, M. J. (1999). Androgens regulate bone resorption activity of isolated octeoclasts in vitro. *Proc. Natl. Acad. Sci.* (In press).

74. Pilbeam, C. C., and Raisz, L. G. (1990). Effects of androgens on parathyroid hormone and interleukin-1-stimulated prostaglandin production in cultured neonatal mouse clavariae. *J. Bone Miner. Res.* **5**, 1183–1188.

75. Bellido, T., Jilka, R. L., Boyce, B. F., Girasole, G., Broxmeyer, H., Dalrymple, S. A., Murray, R., and Manolagas, S. C. (1995). Regulation of interleukin-6, osteoclastogenesis, and bone mass by androgens. The role of the androgen receptor. *J. Clin. Invest.* **95**, 2886-2895.

76. Raisz, L. G., Wiita, B., Artis, A., Bowen, A., Schwartz, S., Trahiotis, M., Shoukri, K., and Smith, J. (1996). Comparison of the effects of estrogen alone and estrogen plus androgen on biochemical markers of bone formation and resorption in postmenopausal women. *J. Clin. Endocrinol. Metab.* **81**, 37–43.

77. Baran, D. T., Bergfeld, M. A., Teitelbaum, S. L., and Avioli, L. V. (1978). Effect of testosterone therapy on bone formation in an osteoporotic hypogonadal male. *Calcif. Tissue Res.* **25**, 103–106.

78. Cantatore, F. P., Carrozzo, M., Magli, D. M., D'Amore, M., and Pipitone, V. (1988). The action of anabolic steroids in increasing serum $1,25(OH)_2 D_3$ and Glaprotein in osteoporotic females. *Clin. Trials* **25**, 65–71.

79. Morley, J. E., Perry, H. M., III., Kaiser, F. E., Kraenzle, D., Jensen, J., Houston, R., Mattammal, M., and Perry, H. M., Jr. (1993). Effects of testosterone replacement therapy in old hypogonadal males: A preliminary study. *J. Am. Geriatr. Soc.* **41**, 149–152.

80. Gray, C., Colston, K. W., Mackay, A. G., Taylor, M. L., and Arnett, T. R. (1992). Interaction of androgen and 1,25-dihydroxyvitamin D_3: Effects on normal rat bone cells. *J. Bone Miner. Res.* **7**, 41–46.

81. Kasperk, C. H., Wergedal, J. E., Farley, J. R., Linkhart, T. A., Turner, R. T., and Baylink, D. J. (1989). Androgens directly stimulate proliferation of bone cells in vitro. *Endocrinology* **124**, 1576–1578.

82. Benz, D. J., Haussler, M. R., Thomas, M. A., Speelman, B., and Komm, B. S. (1991). High-affinity androgen binding and androgenic regulation of A1(I)- procollagen and transforming growth factor-beta steady state messenger ribonucleic acid levels in human osteoblast-like osteosarcoma cells. *Endocrinology* **128**, 2723–2730.

83. Hofbauer, L. C., Hicok, K. C., and Khosla, S. (1998). Effects of gonadal and adrenal androgens in a novel androgen-responsive human osteoblastic cell line. *J. Cell Biochem.* **71**, 96–108.

84. Kasperk, C. H., Faehling, K., Borcsok, I., and Ziegler, R. (1996). Effects of androgens on subpopulations of the human osteosarcoma cell line SaOS2. *Calcif. Tissue Int.* **58**, 376–382.

85. Kasperk, C. H., Wakley, G. K., Hierl, T., and Ziegler, R. (1997). Gonadal and adrenal androgens are potent regulators of human bone cell metabolism in vitro. *J. Bone Miner. Res.* **12**, 464–471.

86. Kasperk, C. H., Fitzsimmons, R., Strong, D., Mohan, S., Jennings, J., Wergedal, J. E., and Baylink, D. J. (1990). Studies of the mechanisms by which androgens enhance mitogenesis and differentiation in bone cells. *J. Clin. Endocrinol. Metab.* **71**, 1322–1329.

87. Durbridge, T. C., Morris, H. A., Parsons, A. M., Parkinson, L. H., Moore, L. J., Porter, S., Need, A. G., Nordin, B. E. C., and Vernon-Roberts, B. (1990). Progressive cancellous bone loss in rats after adrenalectomy and oophorectomy. *Calcif. Tissue Int.* **47**, 383–387.

88. Turner, R. T., Lifrak, E. T., Beckner, M., Wakley, G. K., Hannon, K. S., and Parker, L. N. (1990). Dehydroepiandrosterone reduces cancellous bone osteopenia in ovariectomized rats. *Am. J. Physiol.* **258**, E673–E677.

89. Labrie, F., Bélanger, A., Simard, J., Luu-The, V., and Labrie, C. (1995). DHEA and peripheral androgen and estrogen formation: Intracrinology. *Ann. N. Y. Acad. Sci.* **774**, 16–28.

90. Meikle, A. W., Dorchuck, R. W., Araneo, B. A., Stringham, J. D., Evans, T. G., Spruance, S. L., and Daynes, R. A. (1992). The presence of a dehydroepiandrosterone-specific receptor binding complex in murine T cells. *J. Steroid Biochem. Mol. Biol.* **42**, 293–304.

91. Lu, P. W., Briody, J. N., Ogle, G. D., Morley, K., Humphries, I. R., Allen, J., Howman-Giles, R., Sillence, D., and Cowell, C. T. (1994). Bone mineral density of total body, spine, and femoral neck in children and young adults: a cross-sectional and longitudinal study. *J. Bone Miner. Res.* **9**, 1451–1458.

92. Riis, B. J., Krabbe, S., Christiansen, C., Catherwood, B. D., and Deftos, L. J. (1985). Bone turnover in male puberty: A longitudinal study. *Calcif. Tissue Int.* **37**, 213–217.

93. Parker, L. N. (1991). Adrenarche. *Endocrinol. Metab. Clin. North Am.* **20**, 71–83.

94. Slemenda, C. W., Reister, T. K., Hui, S. L., Miller, J. Z., Christian, J. C., and Johnston, C. C., Jr. (1994). Influences on skeletal mineralization in children and adolescents: Evidence for varying effects of sexual maturation and physical activity. *J. Pediatr.* **125**, 201–207.

95. Fehily, A. M., Coles, R. J., Evans, W. D., and Elwood, P. C. (1992). Factors affecting bone density in young adults. *Am. J. Clin. Nutr.* **56**, 579–586.

96. Mauras, M., Haymond, M. W., Darmaun, D., Vieira, N. E., Abrams, S. A., and Yergey, A. L. (1994). Calcium and protein kinetics in prepubertal boys. Positive effects of testosterone. *J. Clin. Invest.* **93**, 1014–1019.

97. Hobbs, C. J., Plymate, S. R., Rosen, C. J., and Adler, R. A. (1993). Testosterone administration increases insulin-like growth factor-I levels in normal men. *J. Clin. Endocrinol. Metab.* **77**, 776–779.

98. Gallagher, J. C., Riggs, B. L., and DeLuca, H. F. (1980). Effect of estrogen on calcium absorption and serum vitamin D metabolites in postmenopausal osteoporosis. *J. Clin. Endocrinol. Metab.* **51**, 1359–1364.

99. Gennari, C., Agnusdei, D., Nardi, P., and Civitelli, R. (1990). Estrogen preserves a normal intestinal responsiveness to 1,25-dihydroxyvitamin D_3 in oophorectomized women. *J. Clin. Endocrinol. Metab.* **71**, 1288–1293.

100. Thomas, M. L., Xu, X., Norfleet, A. M., and Watson, C. S. (1993). The presence of functional estrogen receptors in intestinal epithelial cells. *Endocrinology* **132**, 426–430.

101. Hagenfeldt, Y., and Eriksson, H. A. (1988). The estrogen receptor in the rat kidney. Ontogeny, properties and effects of gonadectomy on its concentration. *J. Steroid Biochem.* **31**, 49–56.

102. Forte, L. R., Langeluttig, S. G., Biellier, H. V., Poelling, R. E., Magliola, L., and Thomas, M. L. (1983). Upregulation of kidney adenylate cyclase in the egg-laying hen: Role of estrogen. *Am. J. Physiol.* **45**, E273–E280.

103. Stock, J. L., Coderre, J., Burke, E. M., Danner, D. B., Chipman, S. D., and Shapiro, J. R. (1992). Identification of estrogen receptor mRNA and the estrogen modulation of parathyroid hormone-stimulated cyclic AMP accumulation in opossum kidney cells. *J. Cell. Physiol.* **150**, 517–525.

104. Nordin, B. E. C., Need, A. G., Morris, H. A., Horowitz, M., and Robertson, W. G. (1991). Evidence for a renal calcium leak in postmenopausal women. *J. Clin. Endocrinol. Metab.* **72**, 401–407.

105. McKane, W. R., Khosla, S., Burritt, M. F., Kao, P. C., Wilson, D. M., Ory, S. J., and Riggs, B. L. (1995). Mechanism of renal calcium conservation with estrogen replacement therapy in women in early postmenopause—a clinical research center study. *J. Clin. Endocrinol. Metab.* **80**, 3458–3464.

106. Naveh-Many, T., Almogi, G., Livni, N., and Silver, J. (1992). Estrogen receptors and biologic response in rat parathyroid tissue and C cells. *J. Clin. Invest.* **90**, 2434–2438.

107. Prince, R. L., MacLaughlin, D. T., Gaz, R. D., and Neer, R. M. (1991). Lack of evidence for estrogen receptors in human and bovine parathyroid tissue. *J. Clin. Endocrinol. Metab.* **72**, 1226–1228.

108. Cosman, F., Nieves, J., Horton, J., Shen, V., and Lindsay, R. (1994). Effects of estrogen on response to edetic acid infusion in postmenopausal women. *J. Clin. Endocrinol. Metab.* **78**, 939–943.

109. Duarte, B., Hargis, G. K., and Kukreja, S. C. (1988). Effects of estradiol and progesterone on parathyroid hormone secretion from human parathyroid tissue. *J. Clin. Endocrinol. Metab.* **66**, 584–587.

110. Hope, W. G., Ibarra, M. J., and Thomas, M. L. (1992). Testosterone alters duodenal calcium transport and longitudinal bone growth rate in parallel in the male rat. *Proc. Soc. Exp. Biol. Med.* **200**, 536–541.

111. Lafferty, F. W., Spencer, G. E., and Pearson, O. H. (1964). Effects of androgens, estrogens, and high calcium intakes on bone formation and resorption in osteoporosis. *Am. J. Med.* **36**, 514–528.

112. Need, A. G., Morris, H. A., Hartley, T. F., Horowitz, M., and Nordin, B. E. C. (1987). Effects of nandrolone decanoate on forearm mineral density and calcium metabolism in osteoporotic postmenopausal women. *Calcif. Tissue Int.* **41**, 7–10.

113. Stefani, S., Aquiari, G. L., Bozza, A., Maestri, I., Magri, E., Cavazzini, P., Piva, R., and Del Senno, L. (1994). Androgen responsiveness and androgen receptor gene expression in human kidney cells in continuous culture. *Biochem. Mol. Biol. Int.* **32**, 597–604.

114. Goldstone, A. D., Koenig, H., and Lu, C. Y. (1983). Androgenic stimulation of endocytosis, amino acid and hexose transport in mouse kidney cortex involves increased calcium fluxes. *Biochim. Biophys. Acta* **762**, 366–371.

115. Reifenstein, E. C., and Albright, F. (1946). The metabolic effects of steroid hormones in osteoporosis. *J. Clin. Invest.* **26**, 24–56.

116. Chesnut, C. H. I., Ivey, J. L., Gruber, H. E., Matthews, M., Nelp, W. B., Sisom, K., and Baylink, D. J. (1983). Stanozolol in postmenopausal osteoporosis: Therapeutic efficacy and possible mechanisms of action. *Metab. Clin. Exp.* **32**, 571–580.

117. Mason, R. A., and Morris, H. A. (1997). Effects of dihydrotestosterone on bone biochemical markers in sham and oophorectomized rats. *J. Bone Miner. Res.* **12**, 1431–1437.

118. Riggs, B. L., Khosla, S., and Melton, L. J. I. (1998). A unitary model for involutional osteoporosis: Estrogen deficiency causes both type I and type II osteoporosis in postmenopausal women and contributes to bone loss in aging men. *J. Bone Miner. Res.* **13**, 763–773.

119. Smith, E. P., Boyd, J., Frank, G. R., Takahashi, H., Cohen, R. M., Specker, B., Williams, T. C., Lubahn, D. B., and Korach, K. S. (1994). Estrogen resistance caused by a mutation in the estrogen receptor gene in a man. *N. Engl. J. Med.* **331**, 1056–1061.

120. Morishima, A., Grumbach, M. M., Simpson, E. R., Fisher, C., and Qin, K. (1995). Aromatase deficiency in male and female siblings caused by a novel mutation and the physiological role of estrogens. *J. Clin. Endocrinol. Metab.* **80**, 3689–3698.

121. Carani, C., Qin, K., Simoni, M., Faustini-Fustini, M., Serpente, S., Boyd, J., Korach, K. S., and Simpson, E. R. (1997). Effect of testosterone and estradiol in a man with aromatase deficiency. *N. Engl. J. Med.* **337**, 91–95.

122. Bilezikian, J. P., Morishima, A., Bell, J., and Grumbach, M. M. (1998). Increased bone mass as a result of estrogen therapy in a man with aromatase deficiency. *N. Engl. J. Med.* **339**, 599–603.

123. Korach, K. S., Couse, J. F., Curtis, S. W., Washburn, T. F., Lindzey, J., Kimbro, K. S., Eddy, E. M., Migliaccio, S., Snedeker, S. M., Lubahn, D. B., Schomberg, D. W., and Smith, E. P. (1996). Estrogen receptor gene disruption: Molecular characterization and experimental and clinical phenotypes. Recent *Prog. Horm. Res.* **51**, 159–186.

124. Khosla, S., Melton, L. J. I., Atkinson, E. J., Klee, G. G., O'Fallon, W. M., and Riggs, B. L. (1998). Relationship of serum sex steroid levels with bone mineral density in aging women and men: A key role for bioavailable estrogen. *J. Clin. Endocrinol. Metab.* **83**, 2266–2274.

125. Slemenda, C. W., Longcope, C., Zhou, L., Hui, S. L., Peacock, M., and Johnston, C. C. (1997). Sex steroids and bone mass in older men. Positive associations with serum estrogens and negative associations with androgens. *J. Clin. Invest.* **100**, 1755–1759.

126. Center, J. R., Nguyen, T. V., White, C. P., and Eisman, J. A. (1997). Male osteoporosis predictors: Sex hormones and calcitropic hormones. *J. Bone Miner. Res.* **12**, S368.

127. Greendale, G. A., Edelstein, S., and Barrett-Connor, E. (1997). Endogenous sex steroids and bone mineral density in older women and men: The Rancho Bernardo study. *J. Bone Miner. Res.* **12**, 1833–1843.

128. Slemenda, C. W., Hui, S. L., Longcope, C., and Johnston, C. C. (1987). Sex steroids and bone mass: A study of changes about the time of menopause. *J. Clin. Invest.* **80**, 1261–1269.

129. Buchanan, J. R., Hospodar, P., Myers, C., Leuenberger, P., and Demers, L. M. (1988). Effect of excess endogenous androgens on bone density in young women. *J. Clin. Endocrinol. Metab.* **67**, 937–943.

CHAPTER 17

Physiology of Calcium and Phosphate Homeostasis

RENÉ RIZZOLI AND JEAN-PHILIPPE BONJOUR

Division of Bone Diseases, WHO Collaborating Center for Osteoporosis and Bone Diseases, Department of Internal Medicine, University Hospital, 1211 Geneva, Switzerland

I. ABSTRACT

Calcium and phosphate homeostasis is controlled by bidirectional calcium and phosphate fluxes occurring at the levels of intestine, bone, and kidney. The kidney plays a central role in regulating the extracellular concentration of either ion. Sensitive and efficient regulatory mechanisms involving local calcium sensing are triggered by changes in calcium demand or supply. Similarly, the renal handling of phosphate can adjust its capacity to meet the need of the organism. Not only are calciotropic peptides or steroid hormones capable of modifying calcium and phosphate fluxes, but also a variety of local factors are implicated in the regulation of calcium and phosphate homeostasis. Finally, by directly influencing renal tubular calcium transport, or by releasing calcium from intracellular stores, calcium itself plays the role of effector.

II. INTRODUCTION

Calcium and phosphate play key roles in the regulation of cell function. In addition, both are tightly connected to the process of bone mineralization, in which they participate in the formation of hydroxyapatite salts. The hydroxyapatite crystal ensures the structural integrity of the skeleton in its primary functions to support the body, and to house the marrow. Calcium and phosphate homeostasis maintains extracellular calcium and phosphate concentration and balance as constant as possible. Extracellular calcium concentrations are remarkably stable because of the high sensitivity of a variety of cell systems or organs to small variations in extracellular calcium. In contrast, to fulfill the requirements of adequate mineral supply for osteoid mineralization, the level of extracellular inorganic phosphate is adjusted to meet the demand of the organism. Homeostasis of both ions is controlled by a series of hormones and factors that together are highly interrelated in complex regulatory systems. The production of some of these factors is regulated by the concentration of the solute they are controlling, through negative feedback mechanisms. In this chapter, basic concepts of physiology of calcium and phosphate homeostasis are reviewed.

III. BODY DISTRIBUTION OF CALCIUM

Calcium is the fifth most abundant inorganic element in the body. In a 70 kg subject, calcium mass represents about 1300 grams, 99% of which is in bone and teeth and in the form of hydroxyapatite [1]. A small component of bone calcium (approximately 1%) is rapidly exchangeable with extracellular fluid, contributing to the rapidly responsive regulation of extracellular calcium concentration [2]. During puberty, there is nearly a doubling of body mineral stores [3, 4]. By the end of the second decade, most of the body mineral is accrued, although a very small additional amount may be realized, particularly in males, during the third decade [5].

Approximately 1% of total body calcium is intracellular. At the intracellular level, calcium homeostasis is controlled by an influx mechanism following an electrical and chemical gradient through selective calcium channels [6–8]. As compared with the 1 mmol/l extracellular calcium concentration, a 10,000-fold lower concentration in the cytosol is maintained by the constant extrusion of calcium through calcium-magnesium ATPase and sodium-calcium exchange mechanisms [9, 10]. Intracellular calcium homeostasis is also maintained by a dynamic equilibrium between intracellular mitochondrial and microsomal stores [11]. The concentration of free cytosolic calcium is approximately 0.1 μmol/l. The free calcium concentration is critical in controlling cell membrane permeability, a large variety of enzymatic reactions, endocrine and exocrine hormone secretions, and in regulating cardiac and skeletal muscle contraction (Table I). Calcium is also implicated in the control of cell replication and apoptosis [12, 13]. Regulation of intracellular enzymatic functions is achieved through the interaction of calcium with various calcium-binding proteins such as calmodulin or troponin, or the actin-myosin system [2, 8].

About 0.1% of total body calcium is found in the extracellular compartment. The extracellular calcium concentration plays a major role in the integrity and stability of cell membranes, in intercellular adhesion, in blood clotting, and in neuromuscular excitability. Plasma calcium, particularly the ionized form, which comprises about 50% of total plasma calcium and which represents the physiologically active form, is tightly regulated within a narrow range. 40% of the extracellular calcium is bound to proteins, mostly albumin, and 10% is in the form of ultrafiltrable ion complexes. The binding equilibrium of calcium with albumin is determined by

TABLE I.   Physiological Roles of Calcium and Phosphate

	Calcium	Phosphate
Structural constituent	hydroxyapatite (99% body calcium) exchangeable pool (mineral storage)	hydroxyapatite (85% body phosphorus) nucleic acids carbohydrates lipids
Function	intracellular signal transduction cell adhesion membrane permeability (neuromuscular excitability, muscle contraction, neurotransmission) cytoskeleton (cell motility) exo-/endosecretion	energy storage and delivery intracellular signal transduction enzyme activity acid–base homeostasis

the pH. Indeed, acidosis is associated with decreased binding and, thereby, a higher proportion of the ionized form. In contrast, alkalosis is associated with a decrease in ionized calcium.

IV. DETERMINANTS OF EXTRACELLULAR CALCIUM CONCENTRATION

Extracellular calcium concentration is maintained in a dynamic equilibrium through fluxes occurring at the level of the intestine, kidney, and bone (Fig. 1). At steady state, when ionic balance is zero, as in nongrowing individuals, the amounts of solutes entering the extracellular space are matched by the amounts leaving it. By controlling calcium output, the kidney plays a central role in the maintenance of calcium homeostasis.

A. Intestinal Flux

Net intestinal absorption of calcium represents the difference between the amounts of calcium absorbed and secreted into the gastrointestinal tract lumen. In human subjects, under normal conditions, intestinal absorption of calcium constitutes approximately 20% of ingested calcium. Net intestinal absorption of calcium depends on dietary intake, on the capacity of the intestinal wall to transport calcium, on the bioavailability of calcium present in the intestinal lumen, and on secretory flux. Under normal conditions, secretory flux does not appear to vary markedly. However, it could be increased in pathological conditions such as coeliac disease. Intestinal calcium absorptive capacity is mainly controlled by 1,25-dihydroxyvitamin D (calcitriol), which stimulates

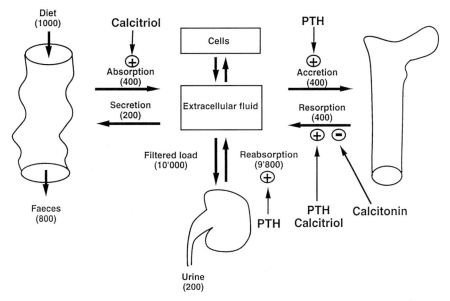

FIGURE 1   Main fluxes (mg/day) controlling calcium homeostasis.

transport through both genomic and nongenomic mechanisms [14–18]. The interaction of calcitriol with its specific nuclear receptor triggers the synthesis of a variety of proteins including its receptor itself, calbindins, and the calcium-magnesium ATPase pump, which is located in the enterocyte basolateral membrane. The duodenum, possessing the highest concentration of calcitriol receptors is the intestinal site most sensitive to calcitriol-mediated calcium absorption. However, the short length of the duodenal segment and its rapid transit time suggest that it does not play the major quantitative role in overall net intestinal calcium absorption. Thus, jejunal and ileal sites could quantitatively absorb more despite a less efficient calcium transport capacity. Parathyroid hormone does not exert any direct effect on intestinal cells [19]. The importance of bioavailability of calcium at absorptive sites is illustrated by impairment of calcium absorption by the formation of complexes with anions, such as phosphate, sulfate, phytate, or oxalate [20, 21]. Another example is provided by studies of calcium absorption in the large intestine. The colonic mucosa is equipped with a powerful vitamin D-sensitive mechanism of calcium transport. However, absorption is quantitatively little, since calcium in the large intestine lumen is in a form not accessible to absorption [22]. At steady state, the 24 hour urinary excretion of calcium is mainly the reflection of net intestinal calcium absorption.

B. Bone Fluxes

On average, about 1% of total bone calcium exchanges every month through a mechanism involving bidirectional fluxes. The main regulators of these fluxes are parathyroid hormone and calcitriol. Calcitonin is possibly an inhibitor of osteoclastic bone resorption under certain conditions [17, 18, 23, 24]. A large variety of substances, either circulating, produced locally, or present in the bone matrix, such as prostaglandins, thyroid hormones, glucocorticoids, sex hormones, growth factors, or interleukins, are capable of influencing bone remodeling, and thereby the bidirectional calcium fluxes [25–27]. In fasting urine, calcium excretion related to creatinine is a direct reflection of net bone resorption [28–30]. Indeed, after an overnight fast, provided there was no calcium supplement taken in the previous evening and the patient does not have a postprandial residue, calcium appearing in the urine originates mostly from bone.

C. Soft Tissues

A minute amount of body calcium is intracellular. Thus, any calcium shift from or into the intracellular compartment does not significantly influence extracellular calcium homeostasis, except maybe in response to parathyroid hormone. The transient decrease in plasma calcium observed in the minutes following parathyroid hormone injection has been attributed to a parathyroid hormone-mediated transfer of calcium into cells [31, 32].

D. Renal Fluxes

Approximately 75% of plasma calcium is ultrafiltrable. After filtration, more than 95% of calcium is reabsorbed. Thus, the amount of calcium appearing in the urine represents the difference between the amounts filtered and reabsorbed. At steady state, this amount is mainly a reflection of net

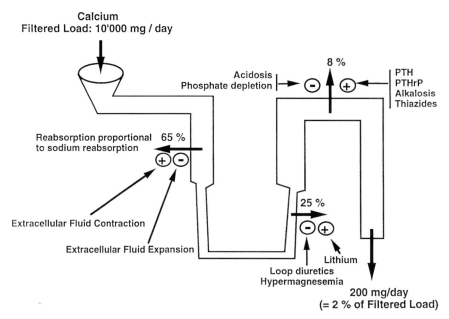

FIGURE 2   Central role of the kidney in controlling calcium homeostasis.

fluxes of calcium into the extracellular fluid compartment originating from intestine and bone. The proximal tubule reabsorbs 60 to 70% of calcium. This site of reabsorption is tightly connected to sodium reabsorption (Fig. 2). 20 to 30% of filtered calcium is reabsorbed along the ascending limb loop, and the remaining 10% is reabsorbed at the distal tubule. These two latter reabsorptive sites are influenced by parathyroid hormone. The renal tubular capacity to reabsorb calcium is the main determinant of extracellular calcium concentration. Any change of this capacity is able to induce variations of plasma calcium from 1.5 to 3.8 mmol/l [28, 29]. This concept has been established by the study of the relationship between urinary calcium excretion and plasma calcium in patients suffering from a lack or an excess of parathyroid hormone. Another example of the central control of extracellular calcium by the renal tubule is the syndrome of familial hypocalciuric hypercalcemia, the features of which include an increase in renal tubular reabsorption of calcium independent of parathyroid hormone [33, 34]. Various situations or pharmacological agents can modulate renal tubular reabsorption of calcium. Alkalosis stimulates renal tubular reabsorption of calcium, whereas acidosis decreases it. Thiazides and lithium salts increase reabsorption of calcium through mechanisms independent of parathyroid hormone [33–35]. Phosphate deficiency, pharmacological doses of calcitonin, and loop diuretics are associated with an increase in calcium clearance. Even large variations in the glomerular filtration rate do not cause major changes in extracellular calcium, because the renal tubule can easily regulate calcium excretion by modulating its reabsorptive capacity. However, the capacity of the kidney to excrete calcium is somewhat lim-

ited, particularly in the case of large calcium loads resulting from extensive bone destruction and/or very high net calcium absorption. Such situations lead to an increase in calcium levels.

V. RELATIVE IMPORTANCE OF THE VARIOUS CALCIUM FLUXES IN CONTROLLING EXTRACELLULAR CALCIUM HOMEOSTASIS

An important role in the regulation of calcium fluxes and balance between the various body compartments is played by the systemic hormones mentioned in the previous section. Other hormones such as insulin, growth hormone, insulin-like growth factors, parathyroid hormone-related protein [24, 36, 37], glucocorticoids, and sex hormones, as well as locally produced and acting interleukins [38], transforming growth factors, and colony-stimulating factors, could also modify target cell sensitivity to parathyroid hormone and/or calcitriol [25–27, 39–41]. However, the secretion of their potential modulators does not appear to be directly controlled by variations in extracellular calcium and/or calcium demand.

Any disturbance of calcium fluxes can result in an alteration of extracellular calcium homeostasis. For instance, an excess of vitamin D is associated with increased intestinal absorption of calcium and bone resorption, resulting in hypercalcemia when the renal excretion capacity is overwhelmed [42, 43]. On the other hand, when renal tubular reabsorption

TABLE II.   Hypercalcemic Disorders

	Increased bone resorption	Increased renal tubular reabsorption of calcium
Endocrine disorders		
Primary hyperparathyroidism	+	+
Hyperthyroidism	++	−
Malignancy	+ or ++	+ or −
Granulomatous disorders	++	−
Disuse	++	−
Drug-induced		
Vitamin D poisoning	++	−
Milk-alkali syndrome	−	+
Thiazide diuretics	−	+
Lithium salts	−	+
Benign familial hypocalciuric hypercalcemia	−	+

of calcium is stimulated, such as by parathyroid hormone or by parathyroid hormone-related protein, plasma calcium levels can also rise, despite very small changes of calcium influx into the extracellular fluid compartment. The relative and quantitative contribution of calcium mobilization from bone, and of renal tubular reabsorption of calcium, to hypercalcemia induced by parathyroid hormone-related protein has been investigated in the model of thyroparathyroidectomized rats chronically infused with parathyroid hormone-related protein [44]. Thyroparathyroidectomy prevents conterregulation of PTHrP-induced hypercalcemia by endogenous hormones. In this model, elevation of plasma calcium is determined both by increased bone resorption and by enhanced renal tubular reabsorption of calcium. However, complete inhibition of bone resorption by a bisphosphonate at a dose which fully normalized fasting urinary calcium excretion, was associated with an approximately 30% decrease, but not a correction of plasma calcium. Thus, the residual hypercalcemia can be attributed to a direct renal effect of PTHrP accounting for more than two-thirds of the elevated plasma calcium (Fig. 3A). Indeed, it is well established that bisphosphonates are devoid of any direct effect on the renal handling of calcium [45]. To influence renal tubular reabsorption, the administration of an agent (the free radical scavenger WR-2721), known to impair the tubular reabsorption of calcium through a parathyroid hormone independent mechanism [46,47] was able to acutely increase calcium excretion and to further reduce plasma calcium (Fig. 3B). The predominance of stimulated renal tubular reabsorption of calcium or of increased bone resorption in determining an altered extracellular calcium homeostasis can be demonstrated in a variety of clinical disorders associated with hypercalcemia [42] (Table II, Fig. 4).

VI. HOMEOSTATIC RESPONSES TO HYPOCALCEMIA

To maintain the extracellular calcium concentration as constant as possible, the response to acute variations implies changes in fluxes without major alteration in total body calcium stores. In contrast, when the organism is chronically challenged by calcium deficiency, its capacity to absorb calcium from the gut or to retain it in the kidney can be overwhelmed. It then has to mobilize skeletal mineral, leading to a progressive decrease in bone mineral mass. This mechanism might be implicated in the pathogenesis of senile osteoporosis. To recognize changes in extracellular calcium concentration, parathyroid cells have a sensitive sensor, capable of transmitting the information to the parathyroid hormone synthesizing and releasing machinery.

A. Extracellular Calcium-Sensing Receptor

A central role in the regulation of calcium homeostasis is played by parathyroid hormone produced by the parathyroid glands, which recognize alterations in plasma calcium [2, 24, 48]. Any change in plasma calcium is detected by a cell membrane-associated calcium-sensor/receptor, which can also be activated by other divalent cations [49–51]. This 1078 amino acid polypeptide belongs to the seven transmembrane domain guanine nucleotide binding protein-coupled receptor family. The calcium receptor is present in parathyroid cells, in C-cells of the thyroid, in renal epithelial cells, and in the central nervous system. A rise in extracellular calcium concentration stimulates protein kinase C and leads to an increase in cytosolic free calcium, thereby inhibiting parathyroid hormone synthesis and release. Conversely, a reduction in plasma calcium triggers the exocytosis of PTH within seconds, whereas it takes hours to increase PTH synthesis and days to stimulate parathyroid cell proliferation [2, 48]. Soon after the characterization of the calcium-sensing receptor, various mutations were reported which account for some syndromes of hyper- or hyposecretion of parathyroid hormone. In familial hypocalciuric hypercalcemia (FHH), circulating levels of parathyroid hormone are insufficiently suppressed for the degree of hypercalcemia, and the renal tubular reabsorption of calcium is increased through a parathyroid hormone-independent mechanism [33, 34, 52]. This disorder appears to be due to mutations associated with hypofunction of the cell membrane calcium-sensing mechanism [53]. A similar syndrome can be reproduced in transgenic mice by incorporation of transgenes displaying the same mutations [54]. Interestingly, the same biochemical pattern can be encountered in patients treated with lithium salts [55, 56]. Conversely, in certain cases of familial hypoparathyroidism, an activating mutation of the calcium-receptor is present [52].

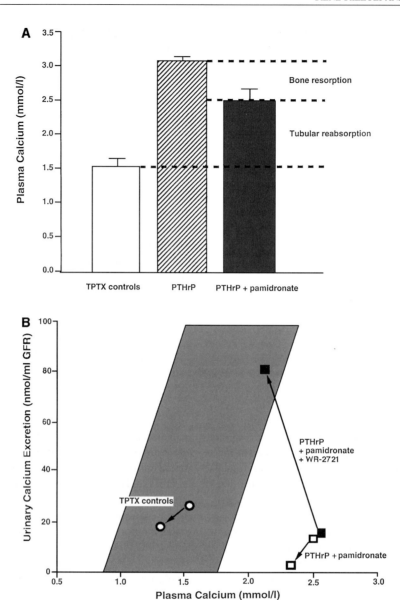

FIGURE 3   Relative contribution of net bone resorption and renal tubular reabsorption to parathyroid hormone-related protein-induced hypercalcemia in thyroparathyroidectomized rats. (A) Pair-fed animals were chronically infused by subcutaneous osmotic minipumps with synthetic parathyroid hormone-related protein (1–34) for 7 days. The bisphosphonate pamidronate was given subcutaneously at a dose which normalized bone resorption, as reflected by the correction of fasting urinary calcium excretion (adapted from Rizzoli *et al.* [44]). (B) The free radical scavenger WR-2721 was acutely administered to parathyroid hormone-related protein-infused and pamidronate-treated rats. The arrows connect the points before and after WR-2721 acute administration. WR-2721 acutely increased the clearance of calcium.

Under these conditions, parathyroid hormone production is not stimulated despite reduced calcium levels. Other receptor systems recognize changes in extracellular calcium concentration [57–59]. In osteoblasts, they are distinct from the receptor system present in parathyroid cells but have not yet been fully elucidated [60–62].

B. Effectors

A reduction in plasma calcium is corrected by stimulation of tubular reabsorption of calcium and mobilization of calcium from bone mineral (Fig. 5). Parathyroid hormone itself, as well as a decrease in calcium and/or phosphate

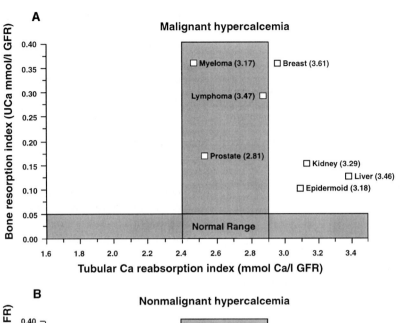

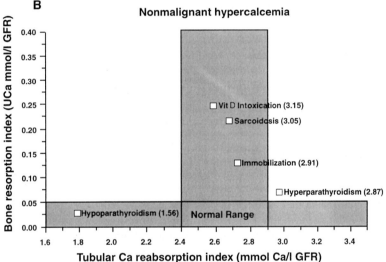

FIGURE 4   Relationship between bone resorption, as evaluated by the bone resorption index (BRI), and tubular reabsorption, as evaluated by the calcium index (TRCaI), in rehydrated patients with malignant (A) or nonmalignant (B) hypercalcemia. The mean plasma calcium concentration is in parentheses. Reprinted from [42] *Bone* **12**, Buchs *et al.*, Evaluation of bone resorption and renal tubular reabsorption of calcium and phosphate in malignant and nonmalignant hypercalcemia, pp. 47–56, Copyright 1991, with permission from Elsevier Science.

concentrations, directly stimulates the renal synthesis of calcitriol. In turn, calcitriol contributes to an increase of plasma calcium through mobilization of calcium from bone and stimulation of intestinal calcium absorption. Thus, calcitriol plays a central role in the intestinal adaptation to low calcium intake. This adaptative mechanism is blunted in the elderly, as a consequence of a decreased synthesis of and a lower responsiveness to calcitriol [63, 64]. It appears, therefore, that the integrated control of extracellular calcium homeostasis is governed by the requirement to maintain extracellular calcium concentration within a very narrow range. This system

is quite efficient in its capacity to respond to calcium needs. Conversely, prevention of hypercalcemia is ensured by a reversal of these regulatory mechanisms. Although calcitonin is able to inhibit bone resorption and to increase renal clearance of calcium, at pharmacological doses, it remains unclear whether this hormone significantly participates in the physiological defense against hypercalcemia.

During skeletal growth, or in the third trimester of pregnancy, when calcification of the fetus takes place, the need for additional calcium results in an increase in intestinal calcium absorption. Elevated levels of calcitriol are responsible

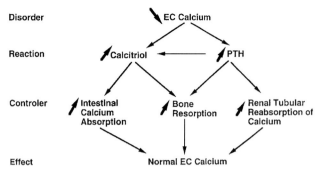

FIGURE 5   Homeostatic response to a decrease in extracellular (EC) calcium concentration.

for stimulating intestinal calcium absorption [15, 17, 18]. On the other hand, with estrogen deprivation at menopause bidirectional calcium fluxes in the skeleton are increased, with resorption overcoming accretion, resulting in a net negative skeletal balance. Under these conditions, reduced intestinal calcium absorption and/or higher urinary calcium excretion can be viewed as a homeostatic mechanism to prevent the extracellular calcium compartment from being overloaded. A similar mechanism accounts for net calcium loss with prolonged immobilization.

VII. CALCIUM AND BONE GROWTH

Several observational studies have suggested that increasing calcium intake promotes greater bone mass and thereby higher peak bone mass [65]. Furthermore, a few prospective randomized, double-blind, placebo-controlled intervention trials indicate that calcium supplementation can enhance bone mass, although the magnitude of the calcium effects appears to vary according to the skeletal sites examined, the stage of pubertal maturation, the ambient calcium intake [66–69], and its absorptive efficiency by [70]. The positive effects of calcium supplementation have essentially been ascribed to a reduction in bone remodeling. Indeed, in one study the plasma level of osteocalcin, a biochemical marker of bone remodeling in adults, was significantly reduced in calcium-supplemented children [66]. This interpretation is also in keeping with the currently-favored mechanism proposed to account for the inhibitory effect of calcium on age-related bone loss. In the elderly, the calcium effect on bone remodeling is usually ascribed to an inhibition of parathyroid hormone secretion, whose plasma level tends to increase with aging [71–75].

In a double-blind, placebo-controlled study on the effects of calcium supplementation in prepubertal girls, changes in bone area and in standing height suggest that calcium supplementation could affect bone *modeling* in addition to bone *remodeling* [69]. Indeed, milk and other calcium-enriched foods enhanced the gain of both mean bone area of several skeletal sites and statural height in the group of spontaneously low calcium consumers to the level achieved by the spontaneously high calcium consumers. Morphometric analysis of the changes observed in the lumbar spine and in femoral diaphysis suggests that calcium could enhance both the longitudinal and the cross-sectional growth of bones [69]. By which mechanisms calcium supplements can influence bone size are still unknown. Effects of calcium on secretion or action of growth factors, including the IGFs-IGF-binding proteins system, could be implicated [76, 77]. These effects go beyond an exclusive effect to reduce bone remodeling. Finally, because of a higher response to calcium supplements preferentially associated with a certain vitamin D receptor genotype [70], it remains to be determined whether the interaction between vitamin D receptor genotype and the influence of calcium supplementation on bone mass accrual affects modeling and/or remodeling.

VIII. BODY DISTRIBUTION OF PHOSPHORUS

Phosphorus is the sixth most abundant element in the body, mostly in the form of phosphate. Its mass represents about 1% of body weight (i.e., 700 g for an individual of 70 kg) [1]. More than 80% of phosphate is in bone; the remainder is in soft tissues in the cellular and extracellular compartments. Inside cells, phosphate can be either in an inorganic form or in an organic one, as a constituent of carbohydrates, lipids, or nucleic acids (Table I). It plays a crucial role in energy storage and delivery, in the regulation of a large variety of different enzymes, and in intracellular signal transduction mechanisms. It also helps to ensure intracellular and plasma membrane stability and is implicated in the modulation of hemoglobin affinity for oxygen. Phosphate enters cells through an active transport system, the energy for which is provided by the extra/intracellular sodium gradient [78, 79]. Extracellular phosphate represents 0.1% of body phosphate. In plasma, one-third of phosphate is inorganic, of which 90% is ultrafiltrable. Two-thirds are components of circulating phospholipids. At physiological pH, the divalent form of inorganic phosphate predominates. This anion contributes to the maintenance of extracellular acid-base homeostasis. Inorganic phosphate concentration varies in relation to age and body growth rate. In adults, its concentration ranges between 0.8 and 1.4 mmol/l, whereas it is 1.4 to 2.7 and 1.3 to 2.0 in the neonate and the adolescent, respectively. There is also a nyctohemeral rhythm in inorganic phosphate concentration, with highest values encountered in the late afternoon.

IX. DETERMINANTS OF EXTRACELLULAR PHOSPHATE CONCENTRATION

The levels of extracellular phosphate are determined by the balance between dynamic fluxes from and into the extracellular compartment. Sites of importance are intestine, bone, soft tissue, and kidney (Fig. 6).

A. Intestinal Fluxes

A normal balanced diet provides sufficient amounts of phosphate in most circumstances so that phosphate deficiency from dietary origin usually does not occur. In the intestinal lumen, phosphate can be complexed with various cations, including aluminum, which thereby prevents its absorption. This property used to be used to prevent phosphate overload in the context of advanced renal failure and phosphate retention. The jejunum exhibits the highest absorptive capacity for phosphate. Two mechanisms are involved. First, in the proximal small intestine, there is an active and saturable transport system activated by calcitriol [16, 80]. A second mechanism is passive and non-saturable and is the most important quantitative one. Indeed, an increase in phosphate intake is accompanied by a commensurate increase of net intestinal phosphate absorption. The saturable component becomes negligible at high phosphate intake. Under normal conditions, 60 to 70% of dietary phosphate is absorbed. At steady state, daily urinary phosphate excretion is mainly a reflection of phosphate absorbed in the intestine.

B. Bone Fluxes

The processes of bone formation and resorption implicate bidirectional fluxes of phosphate from and into bone mineral. Osteoclastic bone resorption releases phosphate into the extracellular fluid. The deposition of phosphate into newly formed osteoid tissue is dependent on its extracellular concentration. In addition, the plasma membrane of osteoblastic cells, as well as extracellular matrix vesicles found in epiphyseal cartilage and in woven bone, are endowed with a saturable, carrier-mediated phosphate transport system, modulated by various hormones and growth factors [81–83]. These extracellular matrix vesicles could play a role in the initiation of the calcification process. The plasma membrane-associated receptor for gibbon ape leukemia virus [84], which functions as a sodium-dependent phosphate transporter distinct from the renal type I and II sodium-dependent phosphate transporters, has been found in osteoblastic cells and is regulated by IGF-I [85]. Thus, this type III phosphate transporter could participate in the control of the flux of phosphate deposition into bone.

C. Renal Fluxes

Approximately 70% of the filtered inorganic phosphate is reabsorbed in the proximal tubule through saturable sodium

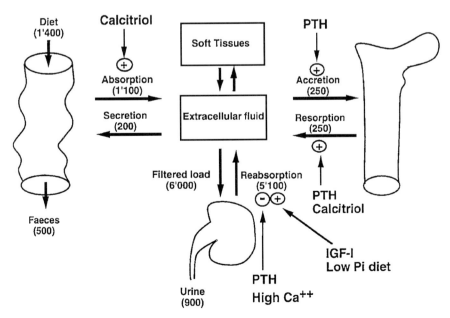

FIGURE 6   Main fluxes (mg/day) controlling phosphate homeostasis.

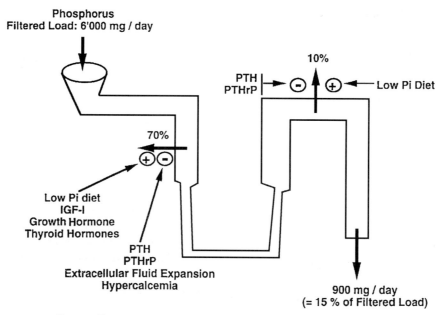

Phosphorus
Filtered Load: 6'000 mg / day

FIGURE 7   Central role of the kidney in controlling phosphate homeostasis.

cotransport mechanisms [86], whereas about 20% of the filtered load is excreted in the urine (Fig. 7). An important step in the transfer of phosphate from the lumen to peritubular capillaries takes place in the epithelial cell brush border membrane. At least two different sodium-dependent phosphate transporters have been identified in the renal tubule, and they share little homology in their amino acid sequence [78, 79]. The type I transporter appears to be constitutive, nonselective, and unregulated. The type II transporter is controlled by dietary phosphate intake or by parathyroid hormone/parathyroid hormone-related protein. Short term exposure to a low phosphate diet stimulates the insertion of type II phosphate transporters into the apical membrane, whereas parathyroid hormone decreases it. Prolonged low dietary phosphate intake increases the expression of the type II transporter. Its presence in the brush border membrane is markedly depressed in X-linked hypophosphatemic rachitic mice [78, 79]. However, this defect has been mapped to a gene other than that coding for the type II phosphate transporter. The gene mutated in the case of X-linked hypophosphatemia codes for an endopeptidase, for which the substrate is still not known [87–89].

The maximal tubular reabsorption capacity (TmPi/GFR) is the main determinant of plasma phosphate concentration [86]. Because tubular reabsorption is a saturable process, fractional reabsorption for a given TmPi/GFR varies according to the filtered load. Therefore, fractional excretion or reabsorption cannot be taken as a reliable reflection of the tubular reabsorptive capacity. This capacity is controlled by the phosphate supply and the need for phosphate by the organism through a hitherto unknown mechanism [90]. Not only

is the low dietary phosphate-mediated stimulation of phosphate transport independent of parathyroid hormone, but it prevents the phosphaturic response to the hormone [87]. During growth or during phosphate deficiency, TmPi/GFR is increased [86].

In proximal tubule kidney cells, phosphate transport is activated by IGF-I, whereas it is decreased by parathyroid hormone or parathyroid hormone-related protein [88, 89, 91]. Other factors could influence the sodium-dependent phosphate transport [41, 92]. However, their contribution to alterations observed in physiological or pathophysiological situations remains to be established. IGF-I, which plays a prominent role in the longitudinal growth of bone, also increases the renal synthesis of calcitriol [93], which in turn stimulates the intestinal absorption of phosphate [16, 80]. Thus, by acting indirectly on the intestine through calcitriol, and directly on the kidney, IGF-I favors a positive phosphate balance. Parathyroid hormone, parathyroid hormone-related protein, a state of phosphate overload, or elevated extracellular calcium concentration all reduce TmPi/GFR. Calcitriol appears to be devoid of any direct and significant effect on the renal tubular reabsorption of phosphate.

D. Soft Tissues

In constrast to calcium, phosphate fluxes from and into the intracellular compartment can alter extracellular phosphate concentration. During fasting, phosphate mobilization from soft tissues, such as the liver, can contribute to an increase in plasma phosphate. Inversely, during the postabsorptive phase, extracellular phosphate is transferred into soft tissues as a result of incorporation into carbohydrates or lipids under the influence of insulin [94]. Hyperphosphatemia, in the setting of a tumor lysis syndrome following the initiation of cytotoxic therapy of hematologic malignancies, or hypophosphatemia occurring during the treatment of diabetic ketoacidosis with insulin, are examples of the role played by soft tissues in phosphate homeostasis under pathological conditions [95, 96].

X. HOMEOSTATIC RESPONSES TO CHANGES IN PHOSPHATE SUPPLY OR DEMAND

Phosphate deficiency stimulates calcitriol production (Fig. 8). The renal synthesis and release of calcitriol are related to the phosphate supply and demand of the organism. On the other hand, low extracellular phosphate concentration is associated with higher calcium concentration through a physicochemical process. In turn, inhibition of parathyroid hormone release decreases urinary phosphate excretion. However, the most powerful mechanism for phosphate retention is certainly the system which allows the kidney to very tightly adapt its capacity to transport phosphate to dietary supplies and to the needs of the organism in a parathyroid hormone-independent manner [78, 79, 86, 87, 90, 97, 98]. Adaptation to low phosphate intake in terms of calcitriol production and changes in renal tubular phosphate reabsorption is missing in X-linked hypophosphatemic rickets [97]. This indicates that the homeostatic response to meet the phosphate supply and need is altered in this disorder, leading to a renal phosphate leak and inadequate calcitriol levels for the degree of hypophosphatemia, despite the phosphate required for bone growth and mineralization. Various mutations in the gene to which X-linked hypophosphatemic rickets has been mapped have been reported, both in humans and in mice [99–101]. The role played by this PEX (phosphate regulating gene with homology to endopeptidase on the X chromosome) gene product, which is a zinc binding endopeptidase, in the regulation of phosphate homeostasis is still not known.

The phosphate homeostatic mechanism could play a role in the increase of renal tubular reabsorption of phosphate observed during growth, possibly in association with IGF-I. It also could play a role in disorders characterized by an increased demand for phosphate, such as extensive osteoblastic metastases [102]. An inhibition of the same system could also be implicated to avoid phosphate overload in the frame of a decreased nephron mass, as for instance in progressive renal failure [103, 104]. There is also evidence that elevated extracellular phosphate concentration could directly increase parathyroid hormone production [105]. This mechanism is apparently less effective than the triggering of parathyroid hormone by hypocalcemia. Because of the phosphaturic effects of parathyroid hormone, such a regulatory system certainly represents an attempt to maintain the homeostasis of phosphate economy.

XI. CONCLUSIONS

The physiology of calcium and phosphate homeostasis is regulated by coordinated bidirectional calcium and phosphate fluxes occurring at the levels of intestine, bone, and kidney. These fluxes are influenced by calciotropic peptides or steroid hormones and by a variety of locally produced factors. By directly modifying renal tubular calcium and phosphate transport, or by releasing calcium from intracellular stores, calcium itself functions as a regulator. In the control of extracellular concentrations of either ion, the kidney tubule reabsorptive capacity plays a central role. Sensitive and efficient regulatory mechanisms involving local calcium sensing are triggered by changes in calcium demand or supply. Similarly, renal handling of phosphate can adjust its capacity to meet the need of the organism. The regulation of calcium and

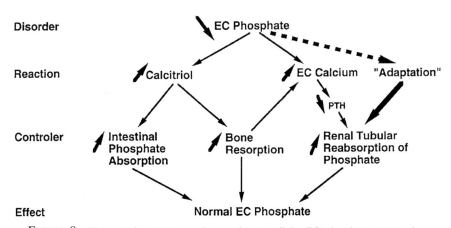

FIGURE 8   Homeostatic response to a decrease in extracellular (EC) phosphate concentration.

phosphate homeostasis counteracts a deficiency or an overload. In response to a variation of any regulatory flux, a series of homeostatic responses and adjustments is triggered, leading to a new steady state in which the initially altered variable has returned to normal.

Acknowledgments

We thank Dr. G. Palmer for reading the manuscript and Mrs. M. Perez for her expert secretarial assistance.

References

1. "William's Textbook of Endocrinology." (1992). (J. D. Wilson and D. W. Foster, eds.), pp. 1397–1536. Saunders, Philadelphia.

2. Brown, E. M. (1991). Extracellular Ca^{2+} sensing regulation of parathyroid cell function, and role of Ca^{2+} and other ions as extracellular (first) messengers. *Physiol. Rev.* **71**, 371–411.

3. Bonjour, J. P., Theintz, G., Buchs, B., Slosman, D., and Rizzoli, R. (1991). Critical years and stages of puberty for spinal and femoral bone mass accumulation during adolescence. *J. Clin. Endocrinol. Metab.* **73**, 555–563.

4. Theintz, G., Buchs, B., Rizzoli, R., Slosman, D., Clavien, H., Sizonenko, P. C., and Bonjour, J. P. (1992). Longitudinal monitoring of bone mass accumulation in healthy adolescents: Evidence for a marked reduction after 16 years of age at the levels of lumbar spine and femoral neck in female subjects. *J. Clin. Endocrinol. Metab.* **75**, 1060–1065.

5. Parsons, T. J., Prentice, A., Smith, E. A., Cole, T. J., and Compston, J. E. (1996). Bone mineral mass consolidation in young British adults. *J. Bone Miner. Res.* **11**, 264–274.

6. Malgaroli, A., Medolesi, J., Zambonin-Zallone, A., and Teti, A. (1989). Control of cytosolic free calcium in rat and chicken osteoclasts. The role of extracellular calcium and calcitonin. *J. Biol. Chem.* **264**, 14342–14347.

7. Ypey, D. L., Weidema, A. F., Hold, K. M., Vanderlaarse, A., Ravesloot, J. H., Vanderplas, A., and Nijweide, P. J. (1992). Voltage, calcium, and stretch activated ionic channels and intracellular calcium in bone cells. *J. Bone Miner. Res.* **7**, S377–S387.

8. Berridge, M. J. (1997). Elementary and global aspects of calcium signalling. *J. Physiol.* **499**, 290–306.

9. Pietrobon, D., Di Virgilio, F., and Pozzan, T. (1990). Structural and functional aspects of calcium homeostasis in eukaryotic cells. *Eur. J. Biochem.* **120**, 599–622.

10. Reeves, J. P., Condrescu, M., Chernaya, G., and Gardner, J. P. (1994). Na+/Ca2+ antiport in the mammalian heart. *J. Exp. Biol.* **196**, 375–388.

11. Krause, K. H. (1991). Ca(2+)-storage organelles. *FEBS Lett.* **285**, 225–229.

12. Berridge, M. J. (1995). Calcium signalling and cell proliferation. *BioEssays* **17**, 491–500.

13. McConkey, D. J., and Orrenius, S. (1996). The role of calcium in the regulation of apoptosis. *J. Leukocyte Biol.* **59**, 775–783.

14. Rizzoli, R., Fleisch, H., and Bonjour, J. P. (1977). Effect of thyroparathyroidectomy on calcium metabolism in rats: Role of 1,25-dihydroxyvitamin D3. *Am. J. Physiol.* **233**, E160–E164.

15. Reichel H., Koeffler, H. P., and Norman, A. W. (1989). The role of the vitamin D endocrine system in health and disease. *N. Engl. J. Med.* **320**, 981–991.

16. Johnson, J. A., and Kumar, R. (1994). Renal and intestinal calcium transport: Roles of vitamin D and vitamin D-dependent calcium binding proteins. *Semin. Nephrol.* **14**, 119–128.

17. Holick, M. F. (1995). Vitamin D: Photobiology, metabolism and clinical applications. *In* "Endocrinology" (L. DeGroot, M. Besser, H. G. Burger, J. L. Jameon, D. L. Loriaux, J. C. Marshall, W. D. Odell, J. T. Potts, and A. H. Rubenstein, eds.), 3rd ed., pp. 990–1013. Saunders, Philadelphia.

18. Feldman, D., Mallon, P. J., and Gross, C. (1996). Vitamin D: Metabolism and action. *In* "Osteoporosis" (R. Marcus, D. Feldman, and J. Kelsey, eds.), pp. 205–235. Academic Press, San Diego, CA.

19. Bonjour, J. P., Fleisch, H., and Trechsel, U. (1977). Calcium absorption in diphosphonate-treated rats: Effects of parathyroid function, dietary calcium and phosphorus. *J. Physiol.* **264**, 125–139.

20. Heaney, R. P., Weaver, C. M., and Recker, R. R. (1988). Calcium absorbability from spinach. *Am. J. Clin. Nutr.* **47**, 707–709.

21. Heaney, R. P., and Weaver, C. M. (1990). Calcium absorption from kale. *Am. J. Clin. Nutr.* **51**, 656–657.

22. Ammann, P., Rizzoli, R., and Fleisch, H. (1986). Calcium absorption in rat large intestine in vivo: Availability of dietary calcium. *Am. J. Physiol.* **251**, G14–G18.

23. Hefti, E., Trechsel, U., Fleisch, H., and Bonjour, J. P. (1983). Nature of calcemic effect of 1,25-dihydroxyvitamin D3 in experimental hypoparathyroidism. *Am. J. Physiol.* **244**, E313–E316.

24. Fitzpatrick, L. A., and Bilezikian, J. P. (1996). Actions of parathyroid hormone. *In* "Principles of Bone Biology" (J. P. Bilezikian, L. G. Raisz, and G. A. Rodan, eds.), pp. 339–346. Academic Press, San Diego, CA and London.

25. Mundy, G. R. (1993). Cytokines of bone. *In* "Handbook of Experimental Pharmacology" (G. R. Mundy, and T. J. Martin, eds.), Vol. 107, pp. 215–247. Springer-Verlag, Berlin, Heidelberg, and New York.

26. Gowen, M. (1994). Cytokines and cellular interactions in the control of bone remodeling. *In* "Bone and Mineral Research" (J. N. M. Heersche and J. A. Kanis, eds.), pp. 77–114. Elsevier, Amsterdam.

27. Martin, T. J., Findlay, D. M., and Moseley, J. M. (1996). Peptide hormones acting on bone. *In* "Osteoporosis" (R. Marcus, D. Feldman, and J. Kelsey, eds.), pp. 185–204. Academic Press, San Diego, CA.

28. Peacock, M., Robertson, W. G., and Nordin, B. E. C. (1969). Relation between serum and urinary calcium with particular reference to parathyroid hormone. *Lancet* **1**, 384–386.

29. Nordin, B. E. C., and Peacock, M. (1969). Role of kidney in regulation of plasma-calcium. *Lancet* **2**, 1280–1283.

30. Bonjour, J. P., Philippe, J., Guelpa, G., Bisetti, A., Rizzoli, R., Jung, A., Rosini, S., and Kanis, J. A. (1988). Bone and renal components in hypercalcemia of malignancy and responses to a single infusion of clodronate. *Bone* **9**, 123–130.

31. Parsons, J. A., Neer, R. M., and Potts, J. T., Jr. (1971). Initial fall of plasma calcium after intravenous injection of parathyroid hormone. *Endocrinology* **89**, 735–740.

32. Parsons, J. A., and Robinson, C. J. (1971). Calcium shift into bone causing transient hypocalcaemia after injection of parathyroid hormone. *Nature* **230**, 581–582.

33. Marx, S. J., Spiegel, A. M., Levine, M. A., Rizzoli, R. E., Lasker, R. D., Santora, A. C., Downs, R. W., Jr., and Aurbach, G. D. (1982). Familial hypocalciuric hypercalcemia. *N. Engl. J. Med.* **307**, 416–426.

34. Attie, M. F., Gill, J. R., Jr., Spiegel, A. M., Downs, R. W., Jr., Levine, M. A., and Marx, S. J. (1983). Urinary calcium excretion in familial hypocalciuric hypercalcemia. Persistence of relative hypocalciuria after induction of hypoparathyroidism. *J. Clin. Invest.* **72**, 667–676.

35. Rizzoli, R., Hugi, K., Fleisch, H., and Bonjour, J. P. (1981). Effect of hydrochlorothiazide on l,25-dihydroxyvitamin D3-induced changes in calcium metabolism in experimental hypoparathyroidism in rats. *Clin. Sci.* **60**, 101–107.

36. Rizzoli, R., Pizurki, L., and Bonjour, J. P. (1989). Tumoral parathyroid hormone-related protein: A new hormone affecting calcium and phosphate transport. *News Physiol. Sci.* **4**, 195–198.

37. Moseley, J. M., and Martin, T. J. (1996). Parathyroid hormone-related

protein: Physiological actions. *In* "Principles of Bone Biology" (J. P. Bilezikian, L. G. Raisz, and G. A. Rodan, eds.), pp. 363–376. Academic Press, San Diego, CA and London.

38. Caverzasio, J., Rizzoli, R., Vallotton, M. B., Dayer, J. M., and Bonjour, J. P. (1993). Stimulation by Interleukin-1 of renal calcium reabsorption in thyroparathyroidectomized rats. *J. Bone Miner. Res.* **8**, 1219–1225.

39. Pizurki, L., Rizzoli, R., Caverzasio, J., and Bonjour, J. P. (1990). Effect of transforming growth factor-α and parathyroid hormone-related protein on phosphate transport in renal cells. *Am. J. Physiol.* **259**, F929–F935.

40. Law, F., Rizzoli, R., and Bonjour, J. P. (1993). Transforming growth factor-β modulates the parathyroid hormone-related protein-induced responses in renal epithelial cells. *Endocrinology* **133**, 145–151.

41. Law, F., Bonjour, J. P., and Rizzoli, R. (1994). Transforming growth factor-β: A down-regulator of the parathyroid hormone-related protein receptor in renal epithelial cells. *Endocrinology* **134**, 2037–2043.

42. Buchs, B., Rizzoli, R., and Bonjour, J. P. (1991). Evaluation of bone resorption and renal tubular reabsorption of calcium and phosphate in malignant and nonmalignant hypercalcemia. *Bone* **12**, 47–56.

43. Rizzoli, R., Stoermann, C., Ammann, P., and Bonjour, J. P. (1994). Hypercalcemia and hyperosteolysis in vitamin D intoxication: Effects of clodronate therapy. *Bone* **15**, 193–198.

44. Rizzoli, R., Caverzasio, J., Chapuy, M. C., Martin, T. J., and Bonjour, J. P. (1989). Role of bone and kidney in parathyroid hormone-related peptide-induced hypercalcemia in rats. *J. Bone Miner. Res.* **4**, 759–765.

45. Rizzoli, R., Caverzasio, J., Bauss, F., and Bonjour, J. P. (1992). Inhibition of bone resorption by the bisphosphonate BM 21.0955 is not associated with an alteration of the renal handling of calcium in rats infused with parathyroid hormone-related protein. *Bone* **13**, 321–325.

46. Hirschel-Scholz, S., Caverzasio, J., and Bonjour, J. P. (1985). Inhibition of parathyroid hormone (PTH) secretion and PTH-independent diminution of tubular Ca reabsorption by WR-2721, a unique hypocalcemic agent. *J. Clin. Invest.* **76**, 1851–1856.

47. Hirschel-Scholz, S., Caverzasio, J., Rizzoli, R., and Bonjour, J. P. (1986). Normalization of hypercalcemia associated with a decrease in renal calcium reabsorption in Leydig cell tumor-bearing rats treated with WR-2721. *J. Clin. Invest.* **78**, 319–322.

48. Pocotte, S. L., Ehrenstein, G., and Fitzpatrick, L. A. (1991). Regulation of parathyroid hormone secretion. *Endocr. Rev.* **12**, 291–301.

49. Brown, E. M., Gamba, G., Riccardi, D., Lombardi, M., Butters, R., Kifor, O., Sun, A., Hediger, M. A., Lytton, J., and Hebert, S. C. (1993). Cloning and characterization of an extracellular Ca^{2+} sensing receptor from bovine parathyroid. *Nature* **366**, 575–580.

50. Nemeth, E. F. (1995). Ca^{2+} receptor-dependent regulation of cellular functions. *News Physiol. Sci.* **10**, 1–5.

51. Brown, E. M., and Hebert, S. C. (1997). Calcium-receptor-regulated parathyroid and renal function. *Bone* **20**, 303–309.

52. Brown, E. M. (1997). Mutations in the calcium-sensing receptor and their clinical implications. *Horm. Res.* **48**, 199–208.

53. Pollak, M. R., Brown, E. M., Chou, Y. H. W., Hebert, S. C., Marx, S. J., Steinmann, B., Levi, T., Seidman, C. E., and Seidman, J. G. (1993). Mutations in the human Ca^{2+} sensing receptor gene cause familial hypocalciuric hypercalcemia and neonatal severe hyperparathyroidism. *Cell* **75**, 1297–1303.

54. Ho, C., Conner, D. A., Pollak, M. R., Ladd, D. J., Kifor, O., Warren, H. B., Brown, E. M., Seidman, J. G., and Seidman C. E. (1995). A mouse model of human familial hypocalciuric hypercalcemia and neonatal hyperparathyroidism. *Nat. Genet.* **11**, 389–394.

55. Mallette, L. D., and Eichhorn, E. (1986). Effects of lithium carbonate on human calcium metabolism. *Arch. Intern. Med.* **146**, 770–776.

56. Larkins, R. G. (1991). Lithium and hypercalcaemia. *Aust. N. Z. J. Med.* **21**, 675–677.

57. House, M. G., Kohlmeier, L., Chattopadhyay, N., Kifor, O., Yamaguchi, T., Leboff, M. S., Glowacki, J., and Brown, E. M. (1997). Expression of an extracellular calcium-sensing receptor in human and mouse bone marrow cells. *J. Bone Miner. Res.* **12**, 1959–1970.

58. Sands, J. M., Naruse, M., Baum, M., Jo, I., Hebert, S. C., Brown, E. M., and Harris, H. W. (1997). Apical extracellular calcium/polyvalent cation-sensing receptor regulates vasopressin-elicited water permeability in rat kidney inner medullary collecting duct. *J. Clin. Invest.* **99**, 1399–1405.

59. Chattopadhyay, N., Cheng, I., Rogers, K., Riccardi, D., Hall, A., Diaz, R., Hebert, S. C., Soybel, D. I., and Brown, E. M. (1998). Identification and localization of extracellular Ca2+-sensing receptor in rat intestine. *Am. J. Physiol.—Gastrointestinal Liver Physiol.* **37**, G122–G130.

60. Mailland, M., Waelchli, R., Ruat, M., Boddeke, H. G. W. M., and Seuwen, K. (1997). Stimulation of cell proliferation by calcium and a calcimimetic compound. *Endocrinology* **138**, 3601–3605.

61. Quarles, L. D., Hartle, J. E., Siddhanti, S. R., Guo, R., and Hinson, T. K. (1997). A distinct cation-sensing mechanism in MC3T3-E1 osteoblasts functionally related to the calcium receptor. *J. Bone Miner. Res.* **12**, 393–402.

62. Yamaguchi, T., Kifor, O., Chattopadhyay, N., and Brown, E. M. (1998). Expression of extracellular calcium (Ca-o(2+))-sensing receptor in the clonal osteoblast-like cell lines, UMR-106 and SAOS-2. *Biochem. Biophys. Res. Commun.* **243**, 753–757.

63. Gallagher, J. C., Riggs, B. L., Eisman, J., Hamstra, A., Arnaud, S. B., and DeLuca, H. F. (1979). Intestinal calcium absorption and serum vitamin D metabolites in normal subjects and osteoporotic patients. *J. Clin. Invest.* **64**, 729–736.

64. Ebeling, P. R., Sandgren, M. E., DiMagno, E. P., Lane, A. W., DeLuca, H. F., and Riggs, B. L. (1992). Evidence of an age-related decrease in intestinal responsiveness to vitamin D: Relationship between serum 1,25-(OH)2D and intestinal vitamin D receptor concentrations in normal women. *J. Clin. Endocrinol. Metab.* **75**, 176–182.

65. Bonjour, J. P., and Rizzoli, R. (1996). Bone acquisition in adolescence. *In* "Osteoporosis" (R. Marcus, D. Feldman, and J. Kelsey, eds.), pp. 465–476. Academic Press, San Diego, CA.

66. Johnston, C. C., Miller, J. Z., Slemenda, C. W., Reister, T. K., Hui, S., Christian, J. C., and Peacock, M. (1992). Calcium supplementation and increases in bone mineral density in children. *N. Engl. J. Med.* **327**, 82–87.

67. Lloyd, T., Andon, M. B., Rollings, N., Martel, J. K., Landis, J. R., Demers, L. M., Eggli, D. F., Kieselhorst, K., and Kulin, H. E. (1993). Calcium supplementation and bone mineral density in adolescent girls. *J. Am. Med. Assoc.* **270**, 841–844.

68. Lee, W. T. K., Leung, S. S. F., Xu, Y. C., Wang, S. H., Zeng, W. P., Lau, J., and Fairweathertait, S. J. (1995). Effects of double-blind controlled calcium supplementation on calcium absorption in Chinese children measured with stable isotopes (Ca-42 and Ca-44). *Br. J. Nutr.* **73**, 311–321.

69. Bonjour, J. P., Carrié, A. L., Ferrari, S., Clavien, H., Slosman, D., Theintz, G., and Rizzoli, R. (1997). Calcium enriched foods and bone mass growth in prepubertal girls: A randomized, double-blind, placebo-controlled trial. *J. Clin. Invest.* **99**, 1287–1294.

70. Ferrari, S. L., Rizzoli, R., Slosman, D. O., and Bonjour, J. P. (1998). Do dietary calcium and age explain the controversy surrounding the relationship between bone mineral density and vitamin D receptor gene polymorphisms? *J. Bone Miner. Res.* **13**, 363–370.

71. Kanis, J. A. (1994). Calcium nutrition and its implications for osteoporosis. Part I. Children and healthy adults. *Eur. J. Clin. Nutr.* **48**, 757–767.

72. Kanis, J. A. (1994). Calcium nutrition and its implications for osteoporosis. Part II. After menopause. *Eur. J. Clin. Nutr.* **48**, 833–841.

73. Chapuy, M. C., Arlot, M. E., Duboeuf, F., Brun, J., Crouzet, B., Arnaud, S., Delmas, P. D., and Meunier, P. J. (1992). Vitamin-D3 and calcium

to prevent hip fractures in elderly women. *N. Engl. J. Med.* **327**, 1637–1642.

74. Chevalley, T., Rizzoli, R., Nydegger, V., Slosman, D., Rapin, C. H., Michel, J. P., Vasey, H., and Bonjour, J. P. (1994). Effects of calcium supplements on femoral bone mineral density and vertebral fracture rate in vitamin-D-replete elderly patients. *Osteoporosis Int.* **4**, 245–252.

75. Dawson-Hughes, B., Harris, S. S., Krall, E. A., and Dallal, G. E. (1997). Effect of calcium and vitamin D supplementation on bone density in men and women 65 years of age or older. *N. Engl. J. Med.* **337**, 670–676.

76. Honda, Y., Fitzsimmons, R. J., Baylink, D. J., and Mohan, S. (1995). Effects of extracellular calcium on insulin-like growth factor II in human bone cells. *J. Bone Miner. Res.* **10**, 1660–1665.

77. Yoo, A., Tanimoto, H., Akesson, K., Baylink, D. J., and Lau, K. H. (1998). Effects of calcium depletion and repletion on serum insulin-like growth factor I and binding protein levels in weanling rats. *Bone* **22**, 225–232.

78. Murer, H., and Biber, J. (1996). Molecular mechanisms of renal apical Na phosphate cotransport. *Annu. Rev. Physiol.* **58**, 607–618.

79. Murer, H., and Biber, J. (1997). A molecular view of proximal tubular inorganic phosphate (P-i) reabsorption and of its regulation. *Pfluegers Arch.* **433**, 379–389.

80. Rizzoli, R., Fleisch, H., and Bonjour, J. P. (1977). Role of 1,25-dihydroxyvitamin D3 on intestinal phosphate absorption in rats with a normal vitamin D supply. *J. Clin. Invest.* **60**, 639–647.

81. Pizurki, L., Rizzoli, R., Caverzasio, J., and Bonjour, J. P. (1991). Stimulation by parathyroid hormone-related protein and transforming growth factor-α of phosphate transport in osteoblast-like cells. *J. Bone Miner. Res.* **6**, 1235–1241.

82. Montessuit, C., Bonjour, J. P., and Caverzasio, J. (1995). Expression and regulation of Na-dependent Pi transport in matrix vesicles produced by osteoblast-like cells. *J. Bone Miner. Res.* **10**, 625–631.

83. Caverzasio, J., and Bonjour, J. P. (1996). Characteristics and regulation of Pi transport in osteogenic cells for bone metabolism. *Kidney Int.* **49**, 975–980.

84. Kavanaugh, M. P., Miller, D. G., Zhang, W., Law, W., Kozak, S. L., Kabat, D., and Miller, A. D. (1994). Cell-surface receptors for gibbon ape leukemia virus and amphotropic murine retrovirus are inducible sodium-dependent phosphate symporters. *Proc. Natl. Acad. Sci. U.S.A.* **91**, 7071–7075.

85. Palmer, G., Bonjour, J. P., and Caverzasio, J. (1997). Expression of a newly identified phosphate transporter/retrovirus receptor in human SaOS-2 osteoblast-like cells and its regulation by insulin-like growth factor I. *Endocrinology* **138**, 5202–5209.

86. Bonjour, J. P., and Caverzasio, J. (1984). Phosphate transport in the kidney. *Rev. Physiol. Biochem. Pharmacol.* **100**, 162–214.

87. Tröhler, U., Bonjour, J. P., and Fleisch, H. (1976). Renal tubular adaptation to dietary phosphorus. *Nature* **261**, 145–146.

88. Caverzasio, J., Rizzoli, R., and Bonjour, J. P. (1986). Sodium-dependent phosphate transport inhibited by parathyroid hormone and cyclic AMP stimulation in an opossum kidney cell line. *J. Biol. Chem.* **261**, 3233–3237.

89. Pizurki, L., Rizzoli, R., Moseley, J., Martin, T. J., Caverzasio, J., and Bonjour, J. P. (1988). Effect of synthetic tumoral PTH-related peptide on cAMP production and Na-dependent Pi transport. *Am. J. Physiol.* **255**, F957–F961.

90. Tröhler, U., Bonjour, J. P., and Fleisch, H. (1976). Inorganic phosphate homeostasis: Renal adaptation to the dietary intake in intact and thyroparathyroidectomized rats. *J. Clin. Invest.* **57**, 264–273.

91. Caverzasio, J., and Bonjour, J. P. (1989). Insulin-like growth factor I stimulates Na-dependent Pi transport in cultured kidney cells. *Am. J. Physiol.* **257**, F712–F717.

92. Law, F., Rizzoli, R., and Bonjour, J. P. (1993). Transforming growth factor-β inhibits phosphate transport in renal epithelial cells. *Am. J. Physiol.* **264**, 623–628.

93. Caverzasio, J., Montessuit, C., and Bonjour, J. P. (1990). Stimulatory effect of insulin-like growth factor-I on renal Pi transport and plasma 1,25-dihydroxyvitamin D3. *Endocrinology* **127**, 453–459.

94. Knochel, J. P. (1985). The clinical status of hypophosphatemia. *N. Engl. J. Med.* **313**, 447–449.

95. Bohannon, N. J. V. (1989). Large phosphate shifts with treatment for hyperglycemia. *Arch. Intern. Med.* **149**, 1423–1425.

96. Jones, D. P., Mahmoud, H., and Chesney, R. W. (1995). Tumor lysis syndrome: Pathogenesis and management. *Pediatr. Nephrol.* **9**, 206–212.

97. Hruska, K. A., Rifas, L., Cheng, S. L., Gupta, A., Halstead, L., and Avioli, L. (1995). X-linked hypophosphatemic rickets and the murine Hyp homologue. *Am. J. Physiol.* **37**, F357–F362.

98. Custer, M., Spindler, B., Verrey, F., Murer, H., and Biber, J. (1997). Identification of a new gene product (diphor-1) regulated by dietary phosphate. *Am. J. Physiol.—Renal Physiol.* **42**, F801–F806.

99. The Hyp Consortium. (1995). A gene (PEX) with homologies to endopeptidases is mutated in patients with X-linked hypophosphatemia rickets. *Nat. Genet.* **11**, 130–136.

100. Du, L., Desbarats, M., Viel, J., Glorieux, F. H., Cawthorn, C., and Ecarot, B. (1996). cDNA cloning of the murine *Pex* gene implicated in X-linked hypophosphatemia and evidence for expression in bone. *Genomics* **36**, 22–28.

101. Econs, M. J., and Francis, F. (1997). Positional cloning of the PEX gene: New insights into the pathophysiology of X-linked hypophosphatemic rickets. *Am. J. Physiol.—Renal Physiol.* **42**, F489–498.

102. Buchs, N., Bonjour, J. P., and Rizzoli, R. (1998). Renal tubular reabsorption of phosphate is positively related to the extent of bone metastatic load in patients with prostate cancer. *J. Clin. Endocrinol. Metab.* **83**, 1535–1541.

103. Caverzasio, J., Gloor, H. J., Fleisch, H., and Bonjour, J. P. (1982). Parathyroid hormone-independent adaptation of the renal handling of phosphate in response to renal mass reduction. *Kidney Int.* **21**, 471–476.

104. Bonjour, J. P., Caverzasio, J., and Rizzoli, R. (1992). Phosphate homeostasis, 1,25-dihydroxyvitamin D3, and hyperparathyroidism in early chronic renal failure. *Trends Endocrinol. Metab.* **3**, 301–305.

105. Slatopolsky, E., Finch, J., Denda, M., Ritter, C., Zhong, M., Dusso, A., Macdonald, P. N., and Brown, A. J. (1996). Phosphorus restriction prevents parathyroid gland growth—High phosphorus directly stimulates PTH secretion in vitro. *J. Clin. Invest.* **97**, 2534–2540.

CHAPTER 18

New Concepts in Bone Remodeling

DAVID W. DEMPSTER   College of Physicians and Surgeons, Columbia University, New York 10032; and
Regional Bone Center, Helen Hayes Hospital, West Haverstraw, New York 10993

I. INTRODUCTION

One of the many remarkable features of the mammalian skeleton is its ability to constantly renew itself throughout life. This is achieved by means of the concerted efforts of a diverse group of cells, collectively referred to as the bone remodeling unit (BRU), which includes osteoclasts, osteoblasts, osteocytes, and other accessory cells whose identity and function are still obscure. Our knowledge of the mechanics of bone remodeling has been reviewed in detail elsewhere [1–5] and will be considered only briefly here. The purpose of this chapter is to review some new concepts pertaining to the activation of BRUs, intercellular communication within the BRU, and the role of apoptosis in regulating the bone balance within each BRU and, ultimately, bone mass. We shall also consider why a reduction in remodeling activation frequency in osteoporotic patients may reduce the risk of fracture without substantial increases in bone mass.

II. AN OVERVIEW OF THE REMODELING CYCLE

There are four distinct phases in the remodeling cycle: activation, resorption, reversal, and formation (Figs. 1, 2). *Activation* refers to the initiating event that converts a previously quiescent bone surface into a remodeling one. The main processes involved are recruitment of mononucleated osteoclast precursors from the circulation, penetration of the bone lining cell layer, and fusion of the mononuclear cells to form multinucleated preosteoclasts. The extent to which the activation process is deterministic (purposeful) and the extent to which it is stochastic (random) is unclear [6]. However, as will be discussed below, there is now good experimental evidence for an increase in the activation frequency of remodeling units in response to local fatigue damage. The preosteoclasts bind tightly to the bone matrix, via interaction between integrin receptors in their membranes and RGD-containing peptides

261

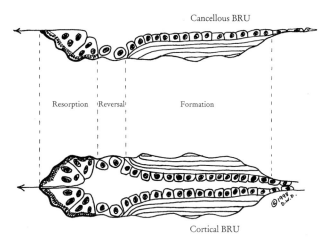

FIGURE 1   Cross-sectional diagrams of evolving BRU in cancellous bone (upper) and cortical bone (lower). The arrow indicates the direction of movement through space. Note that the cancellous BRU is essentially one half of the cortical BRU.

in the organic matrix, which creates an annular sealing zone. The *resorption* phase of the cycle begins when the fully differentiated osteoclasts create secrete protons and proteolytic enzymes into the hemivacuole created by the sealing zone (Fig. 3) [6a]. The proteolytic enzymes are primarily cathepsins, with the most recently implicated being cathepsin K [7]. Initially, the resorption is accomplished by multinucleated osteoclasts, but there is some evidence to suggest that the job is completed by mononucleated cells [8]. *In vitro* studies have confirmed that mononuclear cells derived from human bone marrow are capable of extensive resorption [9]. The resorption phase is followed by *reversal*. The resorption lacuna is occupied by mononuclear cells, including monocytes, by osteocytes that have been released from the bone, and by osteoblasts which are moving in to begin the formation phase of the cycle [10]. It is during the reversal phase that a coupling signal emanates from the resorption cavity to summon osteoblast progenitors into the area. The nature of this signal is not known, but osteoblast growth factors, such as transforming growth factor (TGF)-β and insulin-like growth factor II, that are released from the organic matrix by osteoclastic resorption are plausible candidates [11, 12]. One attractive feature of this hypothesis is that it provides a mechanism whereby the number of osteoblast precursors recruited could be quantitatively related to the amount of bone removed and, therefore, the amount that has to be replaced. Interestingly, TGF-β has also been shown to prolong osteoblast life span *in vitro* by inhibiting apoptosis. That TGF-β plays an important role in bone remodeling is supported by the demonstration that the concentration of TGF-β is positively correlated with histomorphometric indices of bone resorption and bone formation and with serum levels of osteocalcin and bone-specific alkaline phosphatase [13].

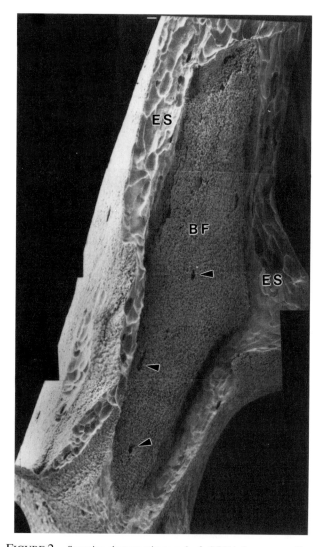

FIGURE 2   Scanning electron micrograph of a BRU in human cancellous bone. Note the eroded surface (ES) underlying an area of new bone formation (BF), and the forming osteocyte lacunae (arrowheads) in the area of new bone formation.

Formation is a two-step process in which the osteoblasts initially synthesize the organic matrix and then preside over its mineralization. As bone formation ensues, osteoblasts become incarcerated in the matrix as osteocytes. These cells, however, are not in "solitary confinement." They maintain close contact with each other and with the cells on the bone surface by means of a complex, three-dimensional web of cytoplasmic processes in the canalicular system (Fig. 4). It has been suggested that this arrangement puts the osteocytes in an ideal position to "sense" a change in the mechanical properties of the surrounding bone and to communicate this to the cells on the surface to initiate remodeling if it is necessary. There is certainly experimental evidence that osteocytes respond to a change in their mechanical environment [14–16]. The intercellular link could occur by wiring

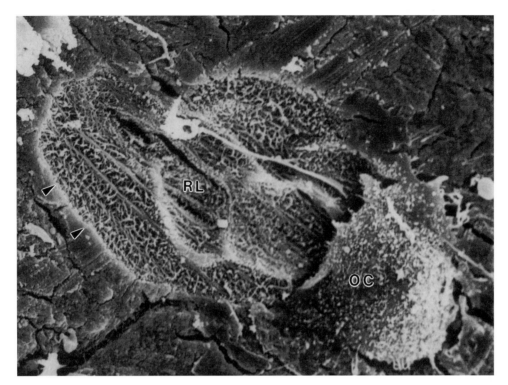

FIGURE 3   Human osteoclast (OC) fixed in the process of excavating a resorption lacuna (RL) *in vitro*. Note the sharpness of the edge (arrowheads) between unresorbed and resorbed areas indicating how tightly fitting the sealing zone must be. Reproduced with permission from Murrills *et al.* [6a].

transmission (WT) and/or volume transmission (VT), these being two mechanisms of communication that have been defined in the central nervous system [16]. WT refers to signaling through synapses, gap junctions, and cell–cell adhesion molecules, such as connexin 43 [17]. VT occurs by diffusion of soluble factors (hormones, cytokines, and growth factors) through the canalicular network.

When formation is completed, the bone surface returns to a resting state and is again covered by only a thin a layer of lining cells. The newly formed piece of bone is referred to as a "basic structural unit" (BSU) of bone (Fig. 5). In cancellous bone, it is generally called a "packet" or a "trabecular osteon"; in cortical bone it is an "Haversian system" or a "cortical osteon." Note that the process of bone remodeling is essentially identical in cancellous and cortical bone. The BRU in cortical bone is equivalent to two apposed cancellous BRUs (Fig. 1) [18]. The difference between the volume of bone removed by the osteoclasts and that replaced by the osteoblasts is referred to as the "bone balance." BRUs on the periosteal surface of cortical bone produce a slightly positive bone balance so that, with aging, the periosteal circumference increases as the effect of the small positive balance in each BRU accumulates. Remodeling units on the endosteal surface of cortical bone are in negative balance so that the marrow cavity enlarges with age. Furthermore, the balance is more negative on the endosteal surface than it is positive on

the periosteal surface and, as a result, cortical thickness decreases with age. The bone balance on cancellous surfaces is also negative, resulting in a gradual thinning of the trabecular plates with the passage of time [1].

III. FUNCTIONS OF BONE REMODELING

Two principal functions of bone remodeling are known, although some have argued convincingly that there must be other functions or other reasons why the human skeleton undergoes such extensive remodeling [19]. The main functions of bone remodeling are presumed to be maintenance of mechanical strength, by continuously replacing fatigued bone by new mechanically sound bone, and mineral homeostasis, by providing access to skeletal stores of calcium and phosphorus. While the turnover rate of 2–3% per year in cortical bone is consistent with maintenance of mechanical properties, the turnover rate in cancellous bone is much higher than would be required for this purpose, suggesting that this site is driven more by its role in mineral metabolism or other unknown functions [6]. In extreme situations, however, cortical bone can participate in the dynamics of mineral homeostasis. A striking example of this is the increase in cortical remodeling that occurs in Rocky Mountain deer during the antler forming

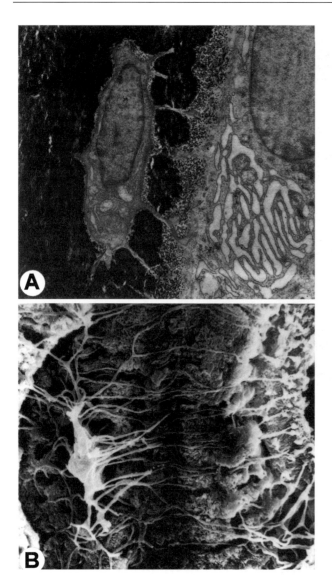

FIGURE 4   Transmission (A) and scanning (B) electron micrographs showing osteocyte processes communicating with cells on the bone surface. Reproduced from Marotti [16].

season [20]. Cortical porosity increases dramatically, but temporarily, during this time to provide the mineral necessary for antler growth. In less extreme situations, it has been proposed [6] that activation of new remodeling units is not required for short-term mineral homeostasis, but that this function may only require the presence of a minimum number of osteoclasts whose activity can be regulated. Continual remodeling activity therefore ensures the presence of this contingent of osteoclasts and a ready source of accessible skeletal calcium. Remodeling also ensures the continuous supply of young bone of low mineral density, which is necessary for ionic exchange at quiescent surfaces [6]. There are also a number of other postulated functions related to the skeleton's role as a depository. One of these is the skeleton's role in acid/base balance, with bone serving as a source of bicarbon-

ate buffer [21]. The skeleton is also a depot for growth factors and cytokines, some of which (e.g., transforming growth factor β) are activated by the acidic microenvironment created by the osteoclast. Remodeling may therefore function to supply hematopoietic marrow with these factors. This may account for some of the excess remodeling that occurs at cancellous sites where marrow and bone coexist in a symbiotic manner [6].

The best experimental evidence for a role of bone remodeling in the maintenance of the mechanical integrity of the skeleton has come from studies in dogs [22, 23]. When long bones were loaded to induce fatigue damage and then studied histologically, a statistical association between microcracks and resorption spaces was demonstrated, with as much as six times as many cracks associated with resorption spaces as predicted by chance alone (Fig. 6) [24]. This could be explained by a propensity of microcracks to form close to resorption spaces. However, further experiments showed that the activation of remodeling was *in response to* the appearance of microcracks [23]. This was demonstrated by loading the left forelimbs of dogs eight days prior to sacrifice and loading the right forelimbs immediately prior to sacrifice. If cracks simply localize at sites of resorption, then the number of cracks associated with resorption spaces should have been the same in each limb. The data showed that there were the same number of microcracks in each limb, but that the limb that was loaded first contained more resorption spaces and a greater association between microcracks and resorption than the limb that was loaded immediately prior to sacrifice. The conclusion from this observation is that microcracks cause the appearance of resorption spaces. One proposed mechanism for this deterministic remodeling is that microcracks may result in the debonding of a cortical osteon (Fig. 7) [25]. Consequently, there is a reduction in stress and strain in that aspect of the osteon, which may be "sensed" by the osteocytes and communicated to the surface lining cells by means of WT and/or VT. The lining cells may then initiate activation of a bone remodeling unit from the Haversian canal and this moves toward the damaged matrix. Once the crack is reached, the bone remodeling unit turns to move in a longitudinal direction, thus repairing the crack.

IV. THE ROLE OF APOPTOSIS IN REGULATING BONE BALANCE

One of the most interesting concepts to be applied to the study of bone biology is that of apoptosis, or programmed cell death. The biological significance of programmed cell death was first recognized by Kerr, Wyllie, and Currie, who also coined the term apoptosis to describe it [26, 27]. In contrast to necrosis, cells dying by apoptosis do so in a purposeful and orderly manner; they shrink rather than swell and do not spill their cytoplasmic contents, thus avoiding a local inflammatory response. Apoptosis plays a crucial role in the size and

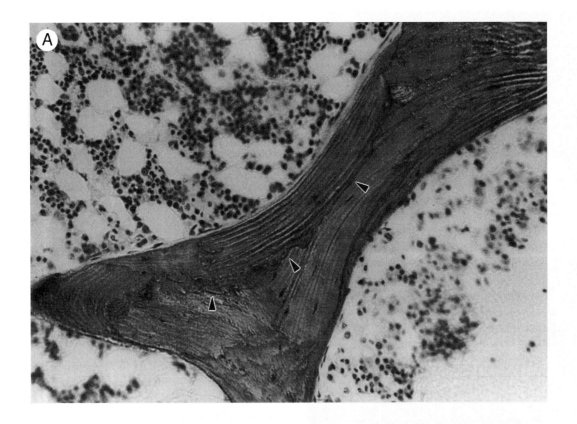

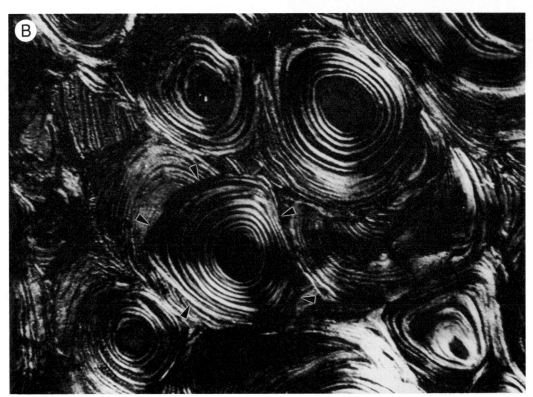

FIGURE 5   Basic structural units in cancellous bone (A) and cortical bone (B). The arrowheads delineate reversal lines. Reproduced with permission from Dempster [4].

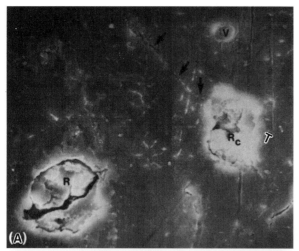

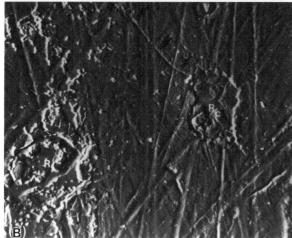

FIGURE 6   Images of a resorption space (Rc) associated with a microcrack (arrows) and another resorption space (R) that has no associated microcrack in dog long bones. A is a secondary electron image and B is backscattered electron image of the same sample. Reprinted from *J. Biomech.* **18**, Burr, D. B., Martin, R. B., Schaffler, M. B., and Radin, E. L. [22]. Bone remodeling in response to *in vivo* fatigue microdamage, pp. 189–200, Copyright 1985, with permission from Elsevier Science.

shape of organs and limbs during embryonic development, and a failure of apoptosis is responsible for the unbridled growth of solid tumors. By analogy, it has been proposed [28–30] that variations in the rate of apoptosis in osteoclasts and osteoblasts influence bone balance and, ultimately therefore, bone mass in adults. A note of caution is indicated, however, because almost all of the studies of apoptosis in bone to date have been performed in animals and the extent to which the observations can be extrapolated to humans is not known [30, 31].

One of the earliest descriptions of apoptosis in bone was in osteogenic cells involved in the formation of calvarial sutures [32]. The leading osteoblasts appeared to die by apoptosis in regions where there was a failure of the normal pattern of overlap between two approaching segments of bone. Apoptosis has also been observed in osteoclasts (Fig. 8) and

osteocytes. Because of its low frequency and transient nature, apoptosis is rarely observed in bone under normal conditions [28]. However, it is readily observed in the presence of agents that perturb the remodeling cycle. For example, osteoclast apoptosis is enhanced in the presence of estrogen [33, 34], selective estrogen receptor modulators (SERMs) [33, 35–37], bisphosphonates [38], and glucocorticoids [30], and it is suppressed in the presence of calcitonin [39] and macrophage colony stimulating factor [40].

Less work has been done on the factors regulating osteoblast apoptosis, but it has been shown to be increased in the presence of glucocorticoids [41], human T-cell leukemia virus Type I *tax* protein [42], and tumor necrosis factor [42, 43]. Osteoblast apoptosis is inhibited by various factors such as transforming growth factor-β and interleukin-6-type cytokines that are present in the bone/bone marrow environment [43].

Enhanced apoptosis of osteoclasts in response to estrogen, SERMs, and bisphosphonates may account for part of the therapeutic efficacy of these agents in the prevention and treatment of osteoporosis. With regard to estrogen, it has been suggested that a reduction in osteoclast apoptosis after menopause may contribute to the enhanced resorption and increased erosion depth that occurs at this time [28, 33]. Reducing apoptosis would extend the life span of individual osteoclasts, perhaps allowing them to penetrate deeper into the trabecular plates and thus shifting bone balance in a negative direction. A negative shift in bone balance would also occur in situations in which apoptosis is enhanced in osteoblasts, e.g., in the presence of glucocorticoid excess [41]. This could be an important component of the mechanism underlying the reduction in the wall thickness of trabecular packets that is observed in glucocorticoid-induced osteoporosis [44]. Osteocyte apoptosis is also enhanced by glucocorticoids [41], which may be a contributing factor to the aseptic or avascular osteonecrosis that is sometimes seen following high dose glucocorticoid therapy. The finding that glucocorticoids enhanced apoptosis in rat osteoclasts [30] initially appeared to be at odds with their well-known action of enhancing bone loss. However, studies have revealed that, in the rat, glucocorticoid excess actually inhibits bone resorption, increases bone mass, and protects against bone loss induced by ovariectomy, dietary calcium deficiency, and immobilization [45–47].

Apoptosis in osteocytes appears to be related to bone turnover rate. In a study of normal and pathological human bone, Noble *et al.* [48] found a high occurrence of osteocyte apoptosis in situations where either modeling or remodeling was rapid, e.g., pediatric calvariae, adult heterotopic bone, and osteophytes. Furthermore, reduced osteocyte apoptosis is associated with increased loading of bone, although whether this is related to the changes in bone formation and resorption that accompany loading or the loading itself is not clear [49, 50]. Bronckers *et al.* [50] observed enhanced osteocyte apoptosis in deeper layers of bone, i.e., in older cells. This was

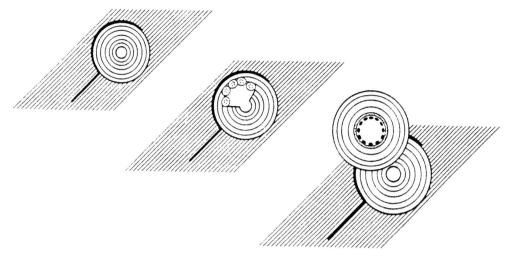

FIGURE 7   Possible mechanism whereby microcracks may initiate their own repair. Reproduced with permission from Martin and Burr [25].

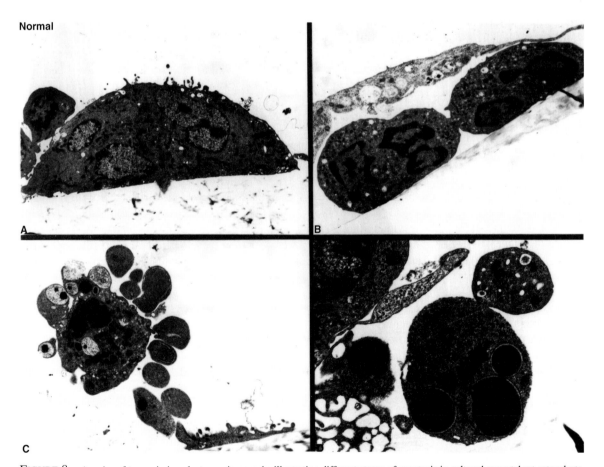

FIGURE 8   A series of transmission electron micrographs illustrating different stages of apoptosis in cultured neonatal rat osteoclasts. (A) Normal osteoclast. (B) Two osteoclasts in an early stage of apoptosis. Note cell shrinkage and compaction of nuclear chromatin against the nuclear membrane. (C) A later stage; the chromatin is condensed and fragmented and there is blebbing of the plasma membrane. These blebs contain recognizable cytoplasmic structures and are termed "apoptotic bodies." (D) Final stage; the cell has assumed a small spherical shape and chromatin is highly condensed. Original magnification: A, ×2925; B, ×5010; C, ×5000; D, ×11,000. Reproduced from Dempster *et al.* [30] by permission of the Journal of Endocrinology Ltd.

mainly seen in locations where intense bone resorption was occurring. Consequently, they have proposed that, while undergoing apoptosis, osteocytes may transmit signals that are conveyed through the lacuno-canalicular system to enhance osteoclast recruitment or activation.

V. POSSIBLE MECHANISMS WHEREBY A REDUCTION IN ACTIVATION FREQUENCY MAY PROTECT AGAINST FRACTURE

At first glance, the postulate that a reduction in remodeling rate may reduce fracture risk seems counterintuitive if, as discussed above, we believe that an important function of remodeling is to maintain bone strength. In fact there are relatively few data showing that reducing bone turnover results in an increase in fractures. The work that is most often cited is the study of Flora *et al.* [51] of the effects of etidronate in dogs, which showed an increase in spontaneous fractures at doses which severely depressed bone turnover. It should be noted, however, that this was a very dramatic inhibition of turnover, and at these high doses, etidronate may have adversely affected mineralization, which could also increase skeletal fragility.

In contrast to this finding, a growing body of data supports the view that high turnover rates are associated with increased fracture risk. Some of these data have come from two large prospective studies. The EPIDOS study [52] followed 7500 women for 22 months, and the Rotterdam study [53] followed 8000 men and women for almost 30 months. The EPIDOS study found an odds ratio (or risk of fracture) of 2.7 for patients with low bone mass and an odds ratio that was almost as high (2.2) for patients with normal bone mass who had high levels of urinary c-terminal telopeptide (CTx), a bone resorption marker [52]. Patients who had both low bone mass and high urinary CTx were at the highest risk of fracture (odds ratio of 4.8). Similar results were obtained in the Rotterdam study, with a significant association between a resorption marker level and fractures in women, even when adjusted for bone mineral density at the femur [53]. It has been known for many years that the degree of reduction in bone mass is a good predictor of fracture risk, but it is also true that the magnitude of the increase in bone mass upon treatment is not always a good predictor of the degree of fracture protection. One obvious example is sodium fluoride, which has been shown to produce significant increases in bone mass without affording fracture protection [54, 55]. This could be due to the fact that the matrix formed in the presence of sodium fluoride may be mechanically inferior [56]. From an analysis of the data from the Fracture Intervention Trial, Cummings *et al.* [57] found that the observed reduction in fracture incidence following treatment with alendronate was much greater than that predicted from the change in bone density alone. This was also the case for

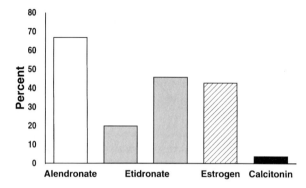

FIGURE 9   The increases in bone mass achieved by antiresorptive, or more correctly, antiremodeling, agents account for only a part, and in some cases a small part, of the degree of fracture protection observed. Drawn from data presented in Cummings *et al.* [57].

a number of other antiresorptive treatments in which the proportion of fracture protection that could be explained by the observed increase in bone mass ranged from about 70% in the case of alendronate to as low as 5% in the case of calcitonin (Fig. 9). Thus, there are now compelling data to support the hypothesis that a reduction in remodeling activation frequency reduces fracture risk by mechanisms other than those associated with an increase in bone mass. What are some of the possible mechanisms for this phenomenon?

First, reducing activation frequency has the effect of reducing the size of the remodeling space, which results in only a modest increase in bone mass [2]. Perhaps more important, however, it also reduces the number of resorptive sites that are active at any one time. In a trabecular network that is already compromised by bone loss, the resorptive phase of the remodeling cycle may weaken crucial, but unsupported, surviving trabeculae to the point of failure without causing a significant decrease in bone mass [58]. Furthermore, high turnover rates increase the probability that resorption will occur simultaneously at more than one point along the length of such trabeculae, rendering them vulnerable to buckling and failure (Figs. 10 [59] and 11). By analogy, a v-cut in the shaft of a thin walking stick has little effect on its mass but greatly reduces its ability to support a load, and several v-cuts have an even greater deleterious effect. In high turnover situations, the probability of trabecular plates being perforated is also increased. Loss of vital trabeculae in this manner could dramatically reduce bone strength, again with relatively little effect on bone mass. This is supported by histomorphometric studies [60] showing that when biopsies from fracture and nonfracture cases are matched for cancellous bone volume, the former show lower values for trabecular number. The importance of architecture in determining bone fragility has been confirmed by microcomputed tomography of the proximal femurs from hip fracture patients and controls [61]. Cancellous bone in specimens from fracture victims was found to have significantly greater anisotropy than bone in controls, even when the two groups were matched for bone mass. The greater anisotropy in the fracture cases was the

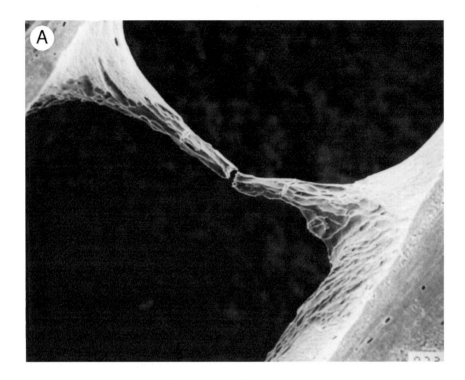

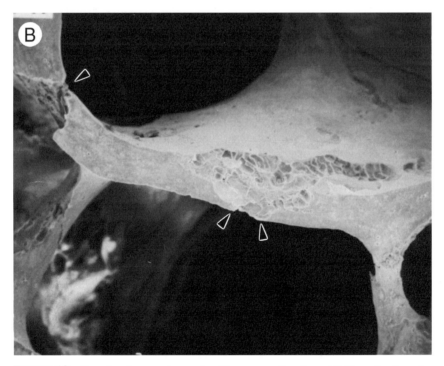

FIGURE 10   Scanning electron micrographs of human cancellous bone. (A) The entire circumference of a thinned trabecular rod in an osteoporotic patient rod is covered in resorption bays. Note that the rod has cracked at three points along its length. While this most likely occurred *ex vivo*, it nevertheless indicates how fragile the rod was. (B) A trabecular plate in a postmenopausal woman has been subjected to extensive osteoclastic resorption and has been perforated in the area between the arrowheads. A few millimeters to the left the plate has been breached by osteoclasts working from the other side (single arrowhead). Reproduced with permission from Dempster *et al.* [59] and Dempster [4], respectively.

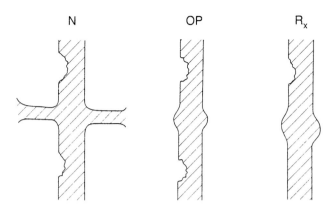

FIGURE 11 Theoretical explanation for the increase in bone fragility associated with enhanced remodeling and why treatment with an agent that reduces bone turnover may be beneficial without changing bone mass significantly. In a normal subject (N), the two resorption cavities do not represent a threat to the stability of the trabecula because it is buttressed by the two horizontal trabeculae. In an osteoporotic individual (OP), the same two cavities significantly increase the chance of failure because the horizontal trabeculae have disappeared and the trabecula is thinner. Reducing the number of resorption cavities by treatment (R_X) decreases the risk of failure. Reproduced with permission from Parfitt [58].

result of preferential loss of trabeculae in the medial-lateral plane.

Second, higher turnover rates are accompanied by a shorter bone formation period in each remodeling cycle and also a lower mean age of the matrix. Consequently, mineralization density of the matrix is decreased. This has been demonstrated by microradiography of bone samples from baboons which had been ovariectomized and either left untreated or treated with alendronate (Fig. 12) [62]. The degree of mineralization was reduced in the ovariectomized animals and this was partially reversed by alendronate treatment. Furthermore, Grynpas [63] has reported a shift towards lower mineral density in femoral heads from osteoporotic subjects compared to that in age-matched controls. It is also of interest to note that in a biopsy study of racial differences in bone structure and turnover [64], the most striking difference between black and white subjects was a longer bone formation period in the former, a factor that may contribute to the lower fracture incidence in this population.

It should be noted, however, that the relationship between the degree of mineralization and the mechanical properties of bone is complex and that the optimal mineralization density value for bone strength has not been determined [65]. Increasing mineralization density up to an ash content of 60% by weight increases the bending strength of cortical bone [66], but increasing it beyond that point decreases the ability of the bone to withstand impacts. Bone that is too highly mineralized is brittle and more prone to failure because microfractures propagate more easily through the highly mineralized matrix [67]. In contrast to the studies mentioned earlier in ovariectomized animals, Boyde *et al.* [65] found that estrogen withdrawal in young women treated with gonadotropin-

releasing hormone analogs was accompanied by an increase in mineralization density, which the authors felt could contribute to increased skeletal fragility. While it remains to be determined exactly how changes in mineralization density affect bone quality in humans, one can hypothesize that if the initial mineralization density is low, an increase due to a reduction in remodeling activation could have a beneficial effect on bone strength.

A third potential mechanism for a beneficial effect of decreasing bone turnover is a reduction of the probability of a positive feedback loop being established between damage and the porosity associated with repair. Excessive repair of any structure has the potential to be self-defeating. This is particularly true if, as in bone, the repair process initially involves removal of material. As noted above, there is now good evidence that fatigue damage stimulates a remodeling response. With this in mind, it has been hypothesized [68, 69] that the possibility exists for a positive feedback loop between damage and porosity. In this postulate it is suggested that each time bone repairs a microcrack, it creates additional porosity and reduces bone mass. This reduces bone strength, resulting in more microdamage, which in turn initiates another wave of remodeling, which will result in further microdamage. Martin has used a computer model to simulate this kind of scenario [68]. The model predicts that an increase in loading results in an increase in remodeling activation frequency to repair the increased damage. If loading is below a certain threshold the system is stable and reaches a new steady state. However, if the threshold is exceeded, the porosity associated with increased remodeling causes the system to become unstable, with damage, porosity, and strain all increasing at a very high rate and without limit. This instability has been suggested to be the theoretical equivalent of a stress fracture. One could propose, therefore, that a reduction in remodeling activation frequency would decrease the probability of this type of vicious cycle.

In conclusion, although the study of bone remodeling began in the late 1600s with the microscopical observations of Antonie van Leeuwenhoek [70], we still have much to learn about the intricacies and regulation of this fascinating process. Clinical studies have tended to focus on bone mass, partly because it can be measured noninvasively and with relative ease. It is clear, however, that bone mass gives us only part of the picture. In order to understand how drugs, both those currently available and those under development, prevent fractures, we must turn again to techniques, including the measurement of biochemical markers, that provide information on remodeling activity.

Acknowledgments

This work was supported in part by NIH grants AR 39191 and 41331. The author is grateful to Ms. Wendy Horbert, who prepared the sample and took the scanning electron micrograph shown in Figure 2.

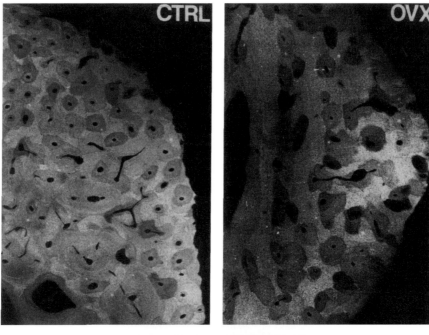

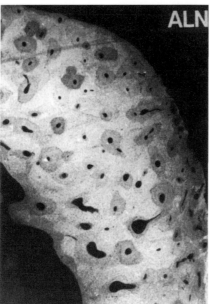

FIGURE 12   Microradiographs of cortical bone from control (CTRL), ovariectomized (OVX), and alendronate-treated (ALN) baboons. The darker osteons are of lower mineral density. Reprinted from *Bone* **21**, P. J. Meunier and G. Boivin [62]. Bone mineral density reflects bone mass but also the degree of mineralization of bone, pp. 373–377, Copyright 1997, with permission from Elsevier Science.

References

1. Frost, H. M. (1986). "Intermediary Organization of the Skeleton." CRC Press, Boca Raton, FL.
2. Parfitt, A. M. (1988). Bone remodeling: Relationship to the amount and structure of bone, and the pathogenesis and prevention of fractures. *In* "Osteoporosis: Etiology, Diagnosis and Management" (B. L. Riggs and L. J. Melton, III, eds.), 1st ed., Raven Press, New York.
3. Parfitt, A. M. (1992). The physiologic and pathogenetic significance of bone histomorphometric data. *In* "Disorders of Bone and Mineral Metabolism" (F. L. Coe and M. J. Favus, eds.), pp. 475–489. Raven Press, New York.
4. Dempster, D. W. (1992). Bone remodeling. *In* "Disorders of Bone and Mineral Metabolism" (F. L. Coe and M. J. Favus, eds.), pp. 355–380. Raven Press, New York.
5. Dempster, D. W. (1995). Bone remodeling. *In* "Osteoporosis: Etiology, Diagnosis, and Management" (B. L. Riggs and L. J. Melton, III, eds.), 2nd ed., pp. 67–91. Raven Press, New York.
6. Parfitt, A. M. (1995). Problems in the application of in vitro systems to

the study of human bone remodeling. *Calcif. Tissue Int.* **56** (Suppl. 1), S5–S7.

6a. Murrills, R. J., Shane, E., Lindsay, R., and Dempster, D. W. (1989). Bone resorption by isolated human osteoclasts in vitro: Effects of calcitonin. *J. Bone Miner. Res.* **4**, 259–268.

7. Littlewood-Evans, A., Kokubo, T., Ishibashi, O., Inaoka, T., Wlodarski, B., Gallagher, J. A., and Bilbe, G. (1997). Localization of cathepsin K in human osteoclasts by in situ hybridization and immunohistochemistry. *Bone* **20**, 81–86.

8. Eriksen, E. F. (1986). Normal and pathological remodeling of human trabecular bone: Three-dimensional reconstruction of the remodeling sequence in normals and in metabolic bone disease. *Endocr. Rev.* **7**, 379–408.

9. Sarma, U., and Flanagan, A. M. (1996). Macrophage-colony stimulating factor (M-CSF) induces substantial osteoclast generation and bone resorption in human marrow cultures. *Blood* **88**, 2531–2540.

10. Baron, R., Vignery, A., and Tran Van, P. (1980). The significance of lacunar erosion without osteoclasts: Studies on the reversal phase of the remodeling sequence. *Metab. Bone Dis. Relat. Res.* **2S**, 35–40.

11. Bonewald, L. F., and Mundy, G. R. (1990). Role of transforming growth factor beta in bone remodeling. *Clin. Orthop. Relat. Res.* **250**, 261–276.

12. Mohan, S., and Baylink, D. (1991). Bone growth factors. *Clin. Orthop. Relat. Res.* **263**, 30–48.

13. Pfeilschifter, J., Diel, I., Scheppach, B., Bretz, A., Krempien, R., Erdmann, J., Schmidd, G., Reske, N., Bismar, H., Seck, T., Krempien, B., and Ziegler, R. (1998). Concentration of transforming growth factor beta in human bone tissue: Relationship to age, menopause, bone turnover, and bone volume. *J. Bone Miner. Res.* **13**, 716–730.

14. Lanyon, L. E. (1993). Osteocytes, strain detection, bone modeling and remodeling. *Calcif. Tissue Int.* **53** (Suppl. 1), S102–S107.

15. Burger, E. H., KleinNulend, J., Van der Plas, A., and Nijwiede, P. J. (1995). Function of osteocytes in bone. *J. Nutr.* **125** (Suppl.), 2020S–2023S.

16. Marotti, G. (1996). The structure of bone tissues and the cellular control of their deposition. *Ital. J. Anat. Embryol.* **101**, 25–79.

17. Civitelli, R., Beyer, E. C., Warlow, P. M., Roberstson, A. J., Geist, S. T., and Steinberg, T. H. (1993). Connexin 43 mediates direct intercellular communication in human osteoblastic cell networks. *J. Clin. Invest.* **91**, 1888–1896.

18. Parfitt, A. M. (1994). Osteonal and hemiosteonal remodeling: The spatial and temporal framework for signal traffic in adult bone. *J. Cell. Biochem.* **55**, 273–286.

19. Currey, J. C. (1984). "The Mechanical Adaptation of Bones." Princeton University Press, Princeton, NJ.

20. Banks, W. J., Epling, G. P., Kainer, R. A., and Davio, R. W. (1968). Antler growth and osteoporosis. I. Morphological and morphometric changes in the costal compacta during the antler growth cycle. *Anat. Rec.* **162**, 387–398.

21. Barzel, U. S. (1995). The skeleton as an ion exchange system: Implications for the role of acid-base imbalance in the genesis of osteoporosis. *J. Bone Miner. Res.* **10**, 1431–1436.

22. Burr, D. B., Martin, R. B., Schaffler, M. B., and Radin, E. L. (1985). Bone remodeling in response to in vivo fatigue microdamage. *J. Biomech.* **18**, 189–200.

23. Mori, S., and Burr, D. B. (1993). Increased intracortical remodeling following fatigue damage. *Bone* **14**, 103–109.

24. Burr, D. B., Forwood, M. R., Fyhrie, D. P., Martin, R. B., Schaffler, M. B., and Turner, C. H. (1997). Perspective: Bone microdamage and skeletal fragility in osteoporotic and stress fractures. *J. Bone. Miner. Res.* **12**, 6–15.

25. Martin, R. B., and Burr, D. B. (1989). "Structure, Function, and Adaptation of Compact Bone." Raven Press, New York.

26. Kerr, J. F. R., Wyllie, A. H., and Currie, A. R. (1972). Apoptosis: A basic biological phenomenon with wide-ranging implications in tissue kinetics. *Br. J. Cancer* **26**, 239–257.

27. Wyllie, A. H., Kerr, J. F. R., and Currie, A. R. (1980). Cell death: The significance of apoptosis. *Int. Rev. Cytol.* **68**, 258–306.

28. Parfitt, A. M., Mundy, G. R., Roodman, G. D., Hughes, D. E., and Boyce, B. F. (1996). Theoretical perspective: A new model for the regulation of bone resorption, with particular reference to the effects of bisphosphonates. *J. Bone Miner. Res.* **11**, 150–159.

29. Boyce, B. F., Hughes, D. E., and Wright, K. R. (1997). Methods for studying cell death in bone. *In* "Methods in Bone Biology" (T. R. Arnett and B. Henderson, eds.), pp. 127–148. Chapman & Hall, London.

30. Dempster, D. W., Moonga, B. S., Stein, L. S., Horbert, W. R., and Antakly, T. (1997). Glucocorticoids inhibit bone resorption by isolated rat osteoclasts by enhancing apoptosis. *J. Endocrinol.* **154**, 397–406.

31. Hughes, D. E., and Boyce, B. F. (1997). Apoptosis in bone physiology and disease. *J. Clin. Pathol. Mol. Pathol.* **50**, 132–137.

32. Furtwangler, J. A., Hall, S. H., and Koskine-Moffett, L. K. (1985). Sutural morphogenesis in the mouse calvaria: The role of apoptosis. *Acta Anat.* **124**, 74–80.

33. Hughes, D. E., Dai, A., Tiffee, J. C., Li, H. H., Mundy, G. R., and Boyce, B. F. (1996). Estrogen promotes apoptosis of murine osteoclasts mediated by TGF-β. *Nat. Med.* **2**, 1132–1136.

34. Kameda, T., Mano, H., Yuasa, T., Mori, Y., Miyazawa, K., Shiokawa, M., Nakamura, Y., Hiroi, E., Hiura, K., Kameda, A., Yang, N. N., Hakeda, Y., and Kumegawa, M. (1997). Estrogen inhibits bone resorption by directly inducing apoptosis of the bone resorbing osteoclasts. *J. Exp. Med.* **186**, 489–495.

35. Arnett, T., Lindsay, R., Kilb, L., Moonga, B. S., Spowage, M., and Dempster, D. W. (1996). Selective toxic effects of tamoxifen on osteoclasts: Comparison with the effects of oestrogen. *J. Endocrinol.* **149**, 503–508.

36. Lutton, J. D., Moonga, B. S., and Dempster, D. W. (1996). Osteoclast demise: Physiological versus degenerative cell death. *Exp. Physiol.* **81**, 251–260.

37. Grasser, W. A., Pan, L. C., Thompson, D. D., and Paralkar, V. M. (1997). Common mechanism for the estrogen agonist and antagonist activities of droloxifene. *J. Cell. Biochem.* **65**, 159–171.

38. Hughes, D. E., Wright, K. R., Uy, H. L., Sasaki, A., Yoneda, T., Roodman, G. D., Mundy, G. R., and Boyce, B. F. (1995). Bisphosphonates promote apoptosis in murine osteoclasts in vitro and in vivo. *J. Bone Miner. Res.* **10**, 1478–1487.

39. Selander, K. S., Härkönen, P. L., Valve, E., Mönkkönen, J., Hannuniemi, R., and Väänänen, H. K. (1996). Calcitonin promotes osteoclast survival in vitro. *Mol. Cell. Endocrinol.* **122**, 119–129.

40. Fuller, K., Owens, J. M., Jagger, C. J., Wilson, A., Moss, R., and Chambers, T. J. (1993). Macrophage colony-stimulating factor stimulates survival and chemotactic behavior in isolated osteoclasts. *J. Exp. Med.* **178**, 1733–1744.

41. Weinstein, R. S., Jilka, R. L., Parfitt, A. M., and Manolagas, S. C. (1998). Inhibition of osteoblastogenesis and promotion of apoptosis of osteoblasts and osteocytes: Potential mechanisms of their deleterious effects on bone. *J. Clin. Invest.* **102**, 274–282.

42. Kitajima, I., Nakajima, T., Imamura, T., Takasaki, I., Kawahara, K., Okano, T., Tokioka, T., Soejima, Y., Abeyama, K., and Murayama, I. (1996). Induction of apoptosis in murine clonal osteoblasts expressed by human T-cell leukemia virus type I *tax* by NF-κB and TNF-α. *J. Bone Miner. Res.* **11**, 200–210.

43. Jilka, R. L., Weinstein, R. S., Bellido, A. M., Parfitt, A. M., and Manolagas, S. C. (1998). Osteoblast programmed cell death: Modulation by growth factors and cytokines. *J. Bone. Miner. Res.* **13**, 793–802.

44. Dempster, D. W. (1989). Bone histomorphometry in glucocorticoid-induced osteoporosis. *J. Bone Miner. Res.* **4**, 137–141.

45. King, C. S., Weir, C. E., Gundberg, C. W., Fox, J., and Insogna, K. L. (1996). Effects of continuous glucocorticoid infusion on bone metabolism in the rat. *Calcif. Tissue Int.* **59**, 184–191.

46. Li, M., Shen, Y., Halloran, B. P., Baumann, B. D., Miller, K., and

Wronski, T. J. (1996). Skeleton response to corticosteroid deficiency and excess in growing male rats. *Bone* **19**, 81–88.

47. Shen, V., Birchman, R., Liang, X. G., Wu, D. D., Lindsay, R., and Dempster, D. W. (1997). Prednisolone alone, or in combination with estrogen or dietary calcium deficiency or immobilization, inhibits bone formation but does not induce bone loss in mature rats. *Bone* **21**, 345–351.

48. Noble, B. S., Stevens, H., Loveridge, N., and Reeve, J. (1997). Identification of apoptotic changes in osteocytes in normal and pathological bone. *Bone* **20**, 273–282.

49. Noble, B. S., Stevens, H., Mosley, J. R., Pitsillides, A. A., Reeve, J., and Lanyon, L. (1997). Bone loading changes the number and distribution of apoptotic osteocytes in cortical bone. *J. Bone Miner. Res.* **12** (Suppl. 1), S111 (abstr.).

50. Bronckers, A. L. J. J., Goei, W., Luo, G., Karsenty, G., D'Sousa, R. N., Lyaruu, D. M., and Burger, E. H. (1996). DNA fragmentation during bone formation in neonatal rodents assessed by transferase-mediated end labeling. *J. Bone Miner. Res.* **11**, 1281–1291.

51. Flora, L., Hassing, G. S., Cloyd, G. G., Bevan, J. A., Parfitt, A. M., and Villanueva, A. R. (1981). The long term skeletal effects of EHDP in dogs. *Metab. Bone Dis. Relat. Res.* **3**, 289–300.

52. Garnero, P., Hausherr, E., Chapuy, M.-C., Marcelli, C., Grandjean, H., Muller, C., Cormier, C., Breart, G., Meunier, P. J., and Delmas, P. D. (1996). Markers of bone resorption predict hip fracture in elderly women: The EPIDOS prospective study. *J. Bone Miner. Res.* **11**, 1531–1538.

53. van Daele, P. L. A., Seibel, M. J., Burger, H., Hofman, A., Grobbee, D. E., van Leeuwen, J. P. T. M., Birkenhäger, J. C., and Pols, H. A. P. (1996). Case-control analysis of bone resorption markers, disability and hip fracture risk: The Rotterdam study. *Br. Med. J.* **312**, 482–483.

54. Riggs, B. L., Hodgson, S. F., O'Fallon, W. M., Chao, E. Y. S., Wahner, H. W., Muhs, J. M., Cedel, S. L., and Melton, L. J., III. (1990). Effect of fluoride treatment on the fracture rate in postmenopausal women with osteoporosis. *N. Engl. J. Med.* **322**, 802–809.

55. Kleerekoper, M., Peterson, E. L., Nelson, D. A., Phillips, E., Schork, M. A., Tilley, B. C., and Parfitt, A. M. (1991). A randomized trial of sodium fluoride as a treatment for postmenopausal osteoporosis. *Osteoporosis Int.* **1**, 155–161.

56. Sogaard, C. H., Mosekilde, L., Richards, A., and Mosekilde, L. (1994). Marked decrease in trabecular bone quality after five years of sodium fluoride therapy; assessed by biomechanical testing of iliac crest bone biopsies in osteoporotic patients. *Bone* **15**, 393–399.

57. Cummings, S. R., Black, D. M., and Vogt, T. M. (1996). Changes in BMD substantially underestimate the anti-fracture effects of alendronate other anti-resorptive drugs. *J. Bone Miner. Res.* **11** (Suppl. 1), S102 (abstr.).

58. Parfitt, A. M. (1991). Use of bisphosphonates in the prevention of bone loss and fractures. *Am. J. Med.* **91** (Suppl. 5B), 42S–46S.

59. Dempster, D. W., Shane, E. S., Horbert, W., and Lindsay, R. (1986). A simple method for correlative light and scanning electron microscopy of human iliac crest bone biopsies: Qualitative observations in normal and osteoporotic subjects. *J. Bone Miner. Res.* **1**, 15–21.

60. Kleerekoper, M., Villanueva, A. R., Stanciu, J., Rao, D. S., and Parfitt, A. M. (1985). The role of three dimensional trabecular microstructure in the pathogenesis of vertebral compression fractures. *Calcif. Tissue Int.* **37**, 594–597.

61. Wenzel, T., Fyhrie, D. P., Schaffler, M. B., and Goldstein, S. A. (1998). Variations in three-dimensional cancellous architecture of the proximal femur in hip fracture patients and controls. *Trans. Orthop. Res. Soc.* **25**, 86 (abstr.).

62. Meunier, P. J., and Boivin, G. (1997). Bone mineral density reflects bone mass but also the degree of mineralization of bone: Therapeutic implications. *Bone* **21**, 373–377.

63. Grynpas, M. (1993). Age and disease-related changes in the mineral of bone. *Calcif. Tissue Int.* **53** (Suppl. 1), S57–S64.

64. Parisien, M. P., Cosman, F., Morgan, D., Schnitzer, M., Liang, X., Nieves, J., Forese, L., Luckey, M., Meier, D., Shen, V., Lindsay, R., and Dempster, D. W. (1997). Histomorphometric assessment of bone mass, structure, and remodeling: A comparison between healthy black and white premenopausal women. *J. Bone Miner. Res.* **12**, 948–957.

65. Boyde, A., Compston, J. E., Reeve, J., Bell, K. L., Noble, B. S., Jones, S. J., and Loveridge, N. (1998). Effect of estrogen suppression on the mineralization density of iliac crest biopsies in young women as assessed by backscattered electron imaging. *Bone* **22**, 241–250.

66. Currey, J. D. (1969). The mechanical consequences of variation in the mineral content of bone. *J. Biomech.* **2**, 1–11.

67. Currey, J. D., Brear, K., and Zioupos, P. (1995). The effects of aging and changes in the mineral content in degrading the toughness of human femora. *J. Biomech.* **29**, 257–260.

68. Martin, B. (1995). Mathematical model for repair of fatigue damage and stress fracture in osteonal bone. *J. Orthop. Res.* **13**, 309–316.

69. Burr, D. B., Forwood, M. R., Fyhrie, D. P., Martin, R. B., Schaffler, M. B., and Turner, C. H. (1997). Perspective: Bone microdamage and skeletal fragility in osteoporosis and stress fractures. *J. Bone Miner. Res.* **12**, 6–15.

70. van Leeuwenhoek, A. (1678). Microscopical observations on the structure of teeth and other bones. *Philos. Trans. R. Soc. London* **12**, 1002–1003.

CHAPTER 19

Products of Bone Collagen Metabolism

JUHA RISTELI AND LEILA RISTELI

Department of Clinical Chemistry, University of Oulu, 90220 Oulu, Finland

I. INTRODUCTION

Most of the collagen in the organic matrix of bone is type I collagen, which provides a well-organized and insoluble scaffold for the deposition of the mineral. Although the mineral is even more abundant than collagen, it is difficult and tedious to reliably assess its metabolism. This leaves type I collagen as the best source for quantification of the metabolic turnover in the skeleton [1–3]. The synthesis of type I collagen involves the production of specific by-products that, among other things, provide the possibility of elegantly assessing the rate of the synthesis of this collagen. Another set of metabolic products is related to the degradation of this collagen, which can occur either together with the dissolution of the mineral phase or independently, e.g., in situations like rickets, when there is increased breakdown of a nonmineralized matrix [4, 5].

Although most of the type I collagen in the human body is located in the skeleton, this protein is also the most abundant collagen in soft tissues. Unfortunately, there are no good quantitative estimates for the distribution of type I collagen between these two pools, either in health or in disease. In all locations the protein is encoded by the same genes, the COL1A1 on chromosome 17 and the COL1A2 on chromosome 7. The basic pathways of collagen synthesis and degradation are shared by all tissues, but there are certain features that are more pronounced either in the hard or the soft tissues, allowing some relative distinction to be made between these two sources of type I collagen metabolites.

The main cells synthesizing type I collagen in soft tissues are fibroblasts, which also produce significant amounts of type III collagen. Bone collagen is synthesized by osteoblasts, which normally do not express type III collagen. However, certain established cell lines with an apparent osteoblastic nature (e.g., the human osteosarcoma line MG-63) produce large amounts of type III collagen [6]. Several other cell types (e.g., smooth muscle cells) also synthesize both type I and III collagens. They also produce several other collagens, the amounts of which are far less than those of the type I and III collagens.

The assembly of type I collagen molecules into fibrils differs between bones and skin and this arrangement affects the cross-linking of the collagen molecules in collagen fibers, in particular at their carboxytermini [7]. However, the fibrillar collagens of many soft tissues, such as tendons, fasciae, vessel walls, and internal organs, contain cross-links similar to those present in bone. The mineralization of bone also affects the maturation of bone collagen cross-links; more than half of them may remain immature, divalent in nature [8], and some of the α1-chains in the bone collagen molecules that contain potential cross-linking sites may even remain uncross-linked. Another difference between the soft tissues and bones is the fact that bone metabolites can be directly released into the circulation, whereas most soft tissues are first drained via lymphatics into larger vessels.

Because there is much microheterogeneity in type I collagen, it is not possible using only biochemical means to predict whether a certain metabolic product, present either in the blood or in the urine, will predominantly reflect bone metabolism. More well-focused studies are still needed, e.g., experimental work on the physiology of the collagens of various tissues, as well as clinical studies of different diseases.

Detection of most of the metabolic products of collagen metabolism depends on the use of well-characterized immunological reagents, and proper quantification, in principle, can be achieved with a number of techniques, including RIAs, ELISAs, IRMAs, etc. However, proper immunochemical and biological validation is always necessary; it is particularly relevant if the assay is just based on a linear synthetic peptide, as the natural collagen metabolites are relatively complex structures. Conclusions based on assays not properly validated may introduce confusion in the medical literature. An example of this [9] has led to confusion and uncertainty regarding procollagen propeptide assays.

II. PRODUCTS OF BONE COLLAGEN SYNTHESIS, THE PROCOLLAGEN PROPEPTIDES

A. Biochemical Basis

The biosynthesis of fibrillar collagens is a complex chain of events that includes the release of two additional proteins, known as the propeptides of the respective procollagen. These proteins seem to be largely removed from their sites of origin without further degradation and thus offer the potential of directly measuring the rate of collagen synthesis in a manner analogous to the use of the C-peptide of proinsulin as an indicator of endogenous insulin production. Interestingly, the two proteins removed from the two ends of the rod-like collagen molecule differ from each other profoundly in their chemical natures and their further metabolic fates. (Also see Chapter 2).

The type I collagen molecule is a long, thin, rigid rod—a shape necessary for its function as part of a collagen fiber in the tissue. The best known and most abundant form of this collagen, the "classical" type I collagen, is a heterotrimer of two α1(I) chains and one α2(I) chain, which are wrapped around each other into the triple helix. The original gene products, the proα1(I) and proα2(I) chains of type I procollagen, are about 50% longer than the corresponding final products. The two additional, bulky domains at both ends of the molecule are usually called the amino-terminal (abbreviation PINP) and the carboxy-terminal (PICP) propeptides of type I procollagen (Fig. 1) [10], despite their relatively large sizes, which are clearly outside the ordinary definition of a peptide (see Sections II.B and C). Once the molecule has reached the extracellular space, these parts are removed *en bloc* from procollagen by two specific endoproteinases, the N- and C-proteinase. The latter enzyme, which is identical to BMP-1 [11], requires a protein cofactor for maximal activity [12].

The propeptide domains have several functions in the procollagen molecule. The individual polypeptide chains are synthesized separately, with the most amino-terminal signal peptide and propeptide parts being assembled first, followed by the collagen molecule itself, and followed finally by the carboxy-terminal propeptide moiety. As the chains pass into the cisternae of the endoplasmic reticulum, they are, at the same time, being posttranslationally modified by several enzymes [10]. The carboxy-terminal propeptide sequences are needed for the proper selection and association of the three proα-chains of type I procollagen within the cisternae of the endoplasmic reticulum. The collagen helix is formed starting from the carboxy terminus and proceeding in the amino-terminal direction. The amino-terminal propeptide is thus the last part of the molecule to attain its native conformation, which includes an additional short collagenous triple helix in the middle of this domain.

During the further transit of the procollagen, its propeptide domains are believed to prevent premature fiber formation in

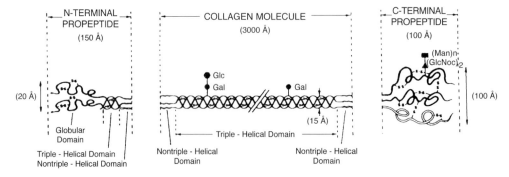

FIGURE 1   Schematic presentation of a procollagen molecule. Reproduced from Prockop *et al.* [10], Copyright ©1979 Massachusetts Medical Society. All rights reserved.

TABLE I. Comparison of the Amino-Terminal (PINP) and Carboxy-Terminal (PICP) Propeptides of the Classical Human Type I Procollagen

	PINP	PICP
Location	amino-terminal	carboxy-terminal
Molecular mass	35,000	100,000
Shape	elongated	globular
Chemical nature	phosphorylated, partially collagenous	glycoprotein, oligosaccharides of the high-mannose type
Related serum antigen		
Homogeneity	one major and one minor form	one form
Size	same as intact PINP (major) or Col1-like (minor)	same as PICP
Concentration (μg/L)	men: 20–76	38–202
	women: 19–84	50–170
Clearance from blood	scavenger receptor of liver endothelial cells	mannose receptor of liver endothelial cells
Blocked by	formaldehyde-treated albumin, acetylated LDL, PIIINP	ovalbumin, mannan

the cells and in the extracellular space, since there is a 1000-fold difference in solubility between procollagen and collagen. The carboxy-terminal propeptide can accomplish this on the basis of its bulky, globular form, whereas in the amino-terminal propeptide, a similar function is probably due to its negative charge, analogous to the situation in blood fibrinogen (see Section II.C). When the carboxy-terminal propeptide has been removed, the molecules still containing the amino-terminal propeptide (so-called type I pN-collagen) can be layered onto the collagen fibrils, but just on the surface of the fibril. A delayed cleavage of the amino-terminal propeptide is believed to regulate the lateral growth of the type I collagen fibers [13].

In addition to the classical type I collagen that is most abundant both in the skeleton and in the soft tissues, there is some evidence for the existence of two other molecular forms of type I collagen. A type I α1-trimer collagen, believed to be a homotrimer of three α1(I) chains, has been found in several situations [14, 15]. It is also the main collagen in the forms of osteogenesis imperfecta that are due to a genetic lack of the α2(I) chain [16]. A third variant, the so-called onco-fetal, laminin-binding collagen, has been described in several carcinomatous tissues by one group [17]. It has been difficult to elucidate the structure of this collagen; the present interpretation of the data suggests a combination of one α1(I) chain, one α2(I) chain, and one α1(III) chain, the last being possibly the same gene product as that found in type III collagen [18]. There is nothing to suggest the presence of this type I collagen variant in normal or pathological bone tissue at present.

B. Carboxy-Terminal Propeptide of Type I Procollagen (PICP)

The carboxy-terminal propeptide—both in free form and as part of the type I procollagen molecule—has a globular shape and the amino acid composition of a noncollagenous protein. The parts corresponding to the propeptide are encoded by exons 49 through 52 of the COL1A1 and COL1A2 genes. Its overall molecular mass is about 100,000 (Table I), and those of the subunits about 33,000 each.

All three component polypeptide chains contain an N-glycosylation site, which is normally occupied by an oligosaccharide of the high-mannose type [19]. For this reason, the propeptide is bound to an affinity column of immobilized Concanavalin A, a property that can be used in isolating the propeptide [20]. There are also interchain disulfide bridges between its three polypeptide chains; these are needed in the processes of chain selection and association. There also seems to be a free SH-group, since the propeptide can also be purified using an affinity column binding such groups [21]. It is relatively difficult to isolate the PICP antigen, but it has been purified from the culture media of human fibroblasts either in the form of type I procollagen, from which the PICP has been liberated by bacterial collagenase digestion [20, 22], or directly as a propeptide cleaved in cell culture, starting from a serum-free culture medium [21].

C. Amino-Terminal Propeptide of Type I Procollagen (PINP)

The amino-terminal propeptide contains a collagenous domain and thus has the shape of a short rod ending with a more globular part (Fig. 1). The subdomains of the propeptide have been named on the basis of their order of elution from a size-exclusion column after bacterial collagenase digestion. From the largest to the smallest, they are as follows: Col 1 (the globular amino-terminal end with intrachain disulfide bridges); Col 2 (the short noncollagenous part joining the propeptide to the most amino-terminal part of the collagen proper), and Col 3 (the central collagenous domain that is broken down by bacterial collagenase). The parts corresponding to the propeptide are encoded by exons 1 through 6 of the COL1A1 and COL1A2 genes.

The molecular mass of the propeptide is about 35,000 (Table I), and masses of the subunits are about 14,250 for the proα1 the chain and 5500 for the proα2 chain. The proα2 chain of the propeptide contains the collagenous domain (Col 3) and the short carboxy-terminal noncollagenous sequence (Col 2), but lacks the globular amino-terminal end (Col 1 domain). The mean length of the triple helix in the propeptide is 16 Gly-X-Y triplets, which is less than 5 percent of the length of the helical domain in the collagen molecule itself, which contains 338 such triplets.

The globular Col 1 domain is phosphorylated in the type I procollagens produced by both fibroblasts and osteoblasts, the phosphate being linked to serine as phosphoserine [23]. The acidic nature of the propeptide is advantageous when the protein is being isolated from various biological starting materials, such as pleural effusions or ascitic fluids, which often contain high concentrations of the propeptide [24]. Because the amino-terminal propeptide of the α1-trimer type I procollagen contains three globular Col 1 domains, it is more acidic that the propeptide of the classical type I procollagen with its two Col 1 domains and thus elutes later in anion exchange chromatography.

D. Clearances of the Circulating PICP and PINP

In comparison with the large amounts of the propeptides set free in the body, their circulating concentrations are surprisingly low, only 20–200 μg/L, which is in the nanomolar range (Table I). This fact suggests the existence of efficient removal mechanisms for this material. In fact, the further metabolic fates of both PICP and PINP are now known better than those of most other analytes used routinely in clinical medicine. The propeptides are not passively lost in the urine because they are either too large (PICP) or have such an elongated shape (PINP) that they cannot pass through the glomerular filter. In addition, the negative charge of the latter, due to the covalently attached phosphate groups, obviously repels the proteins from the negatively charged glomerular membrane.

The metabolic fates of the free propeptides have been clarified by several types of experiments, such as by following the disappearance of radioactively labeled or fluorescent propeptides from the circulation in rats, by feeding the proteins to cultured cells in the presence of known competing ligands for various membrane receptors, and by simultaneous measurement of the propeptide concentrations in different vascular beds. The propeptides are actively taken up and metabolized by a specialized part of the reticulo-endothelial system, the endothelial cells of the liver [25]. These cells bind and internalize the propeptides by receptor-mediated endocytosis

using two different receptor systems, the mannose receptor for PICP [26] and the scavenger receptor for PINP [27]. The clearance follows biphasic kinetics, with half-lives measured in minutes in the rat. The endocytosed material is delivered to the lysosomes and degraded, with the resulting amino acids most probably being passed to the hepatocytes.

The evolution of such a clearance mechanism could be related to the importance of having an effective recycling system for the large amounts of amino acids in the propeptides. The amount of type I collagen synthesized per year in adult humans has been estimated to be at least 1 kg [28], and for each kilogram of type I collagen, as much as 500 g of propeptide material is also produced. The oligosaccharides on PICP are of the high-mannose type that is considered relatively primitive; a special function related to such recycling could explain this feature, which has no effect on the functions or processing of the procollagen [29].

The two clearance systems, although present in the same cells, are independent of each other and also seem to be regulated separately. Some hormones, e.g., thyroxine, can affect the activities of these endocytotic systems and even sometimes can cause opposite changes in the circulating concentrations of the procollagen propeptides (Fig. 2) [30]. However, the effects of such endocrinological regulation are relatively small. In contrast, at least one family is known that has an obvious genetic defect in the uptake mechanism of PICP [31]. The circulating PICP concentrations of the affected family members tend to be several standard deviations above the upper limits of the age- and sex-adjusted reference intervals, with no other abnormalities in either type I collagen metabolites or other biochemical markers of bone metabolism. The feature is inherited in an autosomal dominant manner (Fig. 3) and is not associated with any obvious signs or symptoms. Interestingly, such grossly elevated PICP concentrations also react to factors known otherwise to increase or decrease this concentration, such as pregnancy [32] or glucocorticoid therapy [31]. Studies have shown also that the local PICP concentration in suction blisters of the skin (see Section II.E) is similarly elevated in these individuals, suggesting that there normally may be a local uptake of PICP, at least in the soft tissues, possibly by tissue macrophages carrying mannose receptors [A. Sorva, R. Sorva, J. Risteli, L. Risteli, P. Autio, unpublished].

E. Comparision of PICP and PINP in Physiological and Clinical Situations

The local synthesis of soft tissue type I procollagen can be assessed in human skin either by collecting the interstitial fluid in surgical wounds [33] or by a suction blister method [34]. Such studies have shown that the propeptides of type I procollagen are efficiently set free from the collagen in the extracellular fluid. Their concentrations increase

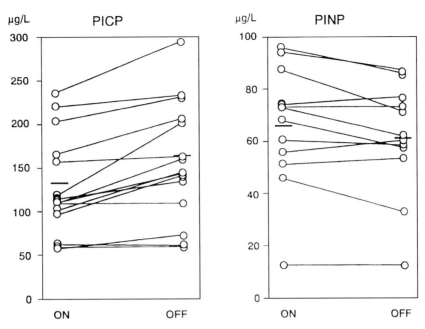

FIGURE 2   Effect of thyroid hormone on the circulating concentrations of the carboxy-terminal (PICP) and intact amino-terminal (PINP) propeptides of type I procollagen in 15 patients operated on for thyroid carcinoma and either using (ON) or not using (OFF) exogenous thyroxine. Reproduced from Toivonen *et al.* [30], with permission.

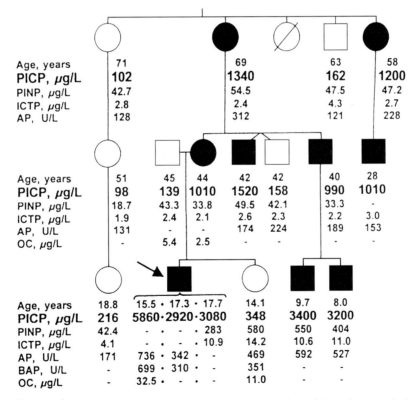

FIGURE 3   Family with inherited high circulating concentrations of the carboxy-terminal propeptide (PICP) of type I procollagen. The circles and squares indicate women and men, respectively. The open symbols show unaffected family members, whereas the solid symbols present individuals with high PICP concentrations. The arrow indicates the proband. AP, alkaline phosphatase; BAP, bone-specific alkaline phosphatase; OC, osteocalcin. Reproduced from Sorva *et al.* [31], with permission.

dramatically (up to 1000-fold within 1 week) during wound healing, when the expression of type I procollagen is induced [24, 33]. On the other hand, local treatment with glucocorticoids suppresses the synthesis of this collagen, leading to often dramatic decreases in the concentrations of the propeptides measured in the fluid in suction blisters that are made in the treated area of the skin [34]. Such experiments provide excellent means of testing the validity for any new test assumed to detect type I collagen synthesis reproducibly and practically noninvasively.

The relative contribution of soft tissue type I collagen synthesis to the circulating concentration of PICP has been studied in lymph flow experiments with conscious pigs [35]. There is a gradient of 10:1 from lymph to peripheral blood in the concentrations of the amino-terminal propeptide of type III procollagen (PIIINP; soft tissue origin), whereas there are no significant differences between the concentrations of PICP in lymph and blood. Stopping and restarting the lymph flow produces dramatic changes in the concentration of PIIINP in the blood, whereas there are no changes in the corresponding concentration of PICP. This study demonstrates that even large changes in the access of the products of soft tissue type I collagen synthesis into the circulation have little effect on the blood concentration of PICP. This is not surprising because we are, in fact, not measuring the absolute amounts of the proteins in any pool in the body, but just differences in the concentrations, and before mixing the lymph into the blood there is no gradient in this case. Because soft tissues have little effect on blood, bone formation rate is obviously the main determinant of the concentrations of the type I procollagen propeptides in the blood (Fig. 4). This view is also supported by histomorphometric and calcium kinetic studies in patients [36, 37].

In the blood, the carboxy-terminal propeptide (PICP) has always been found as the free antigen, with the size of the authentic propeptide [20] whereas the circulating antigenicity related to the amino-terminal propeptide (PINP) can be resolved into two peaks with different molecular sizes. The first is identical to the free, authentic trimeric antigen, and the second resembles part of a single polypeptide chain, probably containing at least the globular Col 1 domain of the proα1(I) chain of PINP [24]. PINP can be isolated as an intact, trimeric propeptide from pleural and ascitic fluids [24], whereas the corresponding propeptide isolated from amniotic fluid always seems to fall apart, into single, possibly truncated, chains [38]. The corresponding propeptide of type III procollagen, PIIINP, is also present in the blood as a series of antigens with partially different metabolic origins and differing metabolic fates [2, 3].

The origin of the smaller antigenic forms of PINP is most probably the tissue degradation of newly synthesized type I procollagen or of the type I pN-collagen with the retained propeptide (Section III.A). Thus the exclusive assay of the intact PINP seems to be more sensitive than that of total

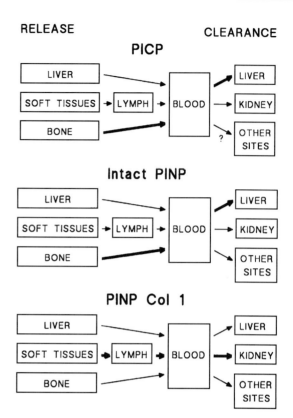

FIGURE 4   Schematic presentation of the distribution between various pools and of the clearances of the type I procollagen propeptides. PICP, the carboxy-terminal propeptide; Intact PINP, the intact triple helical amino-terminal propeptide of type I procollagen; PINP Col 1, the smaller, single chain antigen related to the Col 1 domain of the proα1 chain, recognized by some assays for PINP. Thick arrows indicate the major routes. Reproduced from Risteli et al. [2], with permission.

PINP for detecting changes in the rate of bone collagen synthesis (e.g., estrogen treatment in postmenopausal women leads to a 42% decrease in the circulating concentration of intact PINP, compared with the 30% decrease observed with an assay measuring both antigenic forms [39]). There is also an important difference in the elimination routes, since intact PINP is cleared by the liver (see Section II.D), whereas the small PINP Col 1-like peptides can also be filtered by the kidneys (Fig. 4) [3].

Because PICP and PINP are produced in equimolar amounts during the synthesis of type I procollagen, their molar concentrations in any relevant body fluids should, in principle, be almost identical. This is true, for example, in the fluid collected from a healing wound, where both the propeptides give similar estimates for the production rate of type I procollagen [24]. The ratio of PICP:PINP in adult blood is also approximately the expected 2–3:1, when the concentrations of both propeptides are expressed as protein concentrations, μg/L. However, there are both physiological and pathological situations in which this ratio differs from equimolarity.

In the blood of infants and children (up until puberty), the molar concentration of PINP is higher than that of PICP, the ratio of PICP:PINP (in μg/L) being even clearly lower than 1:1 [40a]. An even more dramatic discrepancy is found in patients with active Paget's disease of bone [41, 42] or with aggressive breast cancer [43]. In both cases, there can be an up to 6-fold molar excess of PINP in the blood. This finding may partially be explained by differences in the clearances of the two proteins, but it cannot be excluded that the result could be due to the synthesis of several variants of type I procollagen (e.g., the assay for intact PINP detects both the classical and the α1-trimer propeptides with equal avidity [24], whereas it is not known whether the PICP assays have a different specificity for the suggested variants [see Section II.A]).

III. DEGRADATION PRODUCTS OF TYPE I COLLAGEN

A. Biochemical Background

The rod-like collagen molecules possess a capacity for self-assembly and spontaneous formation of fibrils and fibers (see Chapter 2). The amino-terminal propeptide often remains transiently attached to some of the molecules and can be visualized on the surface of thin type I collagen fibers in tissues undergoing active collagen synthesis (see Section II.A) [13]. One characteristic location for such fibers is the epithelial-stromal junction below a metabolically active epithelium [44]. In the newly formed osteoid, some amino-terminal propeptides of type I procollagen (PINP) are retained for the time of matrix maturation, since the collagenous matrix can be stained with anti-PINP antibodies, but no substantial amounts of the propeptide are any longer present in the mineralized matrix [T. Taube, I. Elomaa, L. Risteli, J. Risteli, unpublished]. The amino-terminal propeptide has been isolated as a 24 kDa phosphoprotein from the organic matrix of fetal bone, but there is no propeptide left in the adult bone that has a much lower rate of synthesis of type I collagen [23]. In the case of type III collagen, a major collagen of soft tissues, pN collagen molecules seem to cover the surface of virtually all fibers, although they only represent a 5% fraction of the total amount of type III collagen [44a].

The biological function of a fibrillar collagen is to provide the tissue with tensile strength. This is due to covalent bonds, known as collagen cross-links, that form between the individual collagen molecules in a collagen fiber. The cross-links are formed in a complicated series of partially alternative chemical reactions that lead gradually through divalent cross-links, joining two polypeptide chains, to multivalent—tri- or even tetravalent—cross-links [45]. Continuing cross-linking also explains the fact that older collagen in soft tissues is progressively more insoluble when studied in various ways, e.g., by digestion with pepsin or bacterial collagenase. In addition to the intermolecular cross-links essential for tensile strength, intramolecular cross-links also exist.

In contrast to earlier beliefs, the collagen in many tissues and certainly that in the bones is actively turned over throughout the life of an individual, although the overall turnover rate is naturally at its highest in infants and children. A number of enzymes can degrade some form of type I collagen in the test tube. These enzymes include matrix metalloproteinases, cysteine proteinases, and serine proteinases [47]. However, it is more difficult to elucidate the real biological significance of such an activity because in the tissues, the collagen is not present as soluble single molecules but as a covalently cross-linked assembly of large numbers of molecules. In particular, the helical region of a collagen molecule can hardly be attacked by proteolytic enzymes before the cross-linking ends of the molecule are cleaved. In soft tissues, conditions associated with rapid remodeling of the tissue seem to involve a different route of collagen degradation than does the turnover under steady-state conditions [47]. In bones, collagenolytic enzymes seem to be produced by both the osteoblasts and osteoclasts.

Because of the complexity and the presence of alternative reaction pathways, the pattern of cross-linked peptides that arises from the degradation of a certain collagen type in a certain tissue is difficult to predict. The existence of different enzymes with differing cleaving specificities and functioning in different metabolic situations adds to this complexity. In addition, when new immunoassays for collagen telopeptides have been used in isolating the cross-linked telopeptides, it has become evident that all the possible mature cross-links in collagens are not yet known. There are also modifications associated with aging of collagen fibers, such as the cross-links derived from nonenzymatically attached sugar residues [48] and the β-isomerization of the aspartic acid residues in the carboxy-terminal telopeptide (see Section III.E). It is not known if these modifications proceed similarly in the soft tissues and in the skeleton.

B. Hydroxyproline and Glycosylated Hydroxylysines

4-Hydroxyproline, an imino acid formed from proline in a posttranslational enzyme reaction, is a necessary prerequisite for the triple-helical conformation of the collagen molecule at body temperature. It makes up about 12% of the weight of the collagen molecule and can thus be used as a measure of the collagen content of a tissue. The acid hydrolysis followed by a chemical color reaction used to assess this imino acid can be used both for tissue samples and for urine.

Once set free from the helical part of a collagen molecule, hydroxyproline can no longer be incorporated into new protein; however, exogenous hydroxyproline is absorbed from the diet. Most of the imino acid (up to 90%) is metabolized in the liver, leading to the formation of pyruvate and glyoxalate, but some is always passed into the urine. Excretion of hydroxyproline correlates with growth velocity in children and with the presence of bone degrading processes, e.g., bone metastases of cancers, in adults [29]. Also, a generally enhanced bone metabolic rate increases urinary hydroxyproline excretion. For this reason, hydroxyproline served as an indirect test of thyroid hormone action before the time of specific thyroid hormone assays. Some hydroxyproline is directly derived from collagen synthesis, since the helical domain of PINP contains it. A substantial part of the urinary hydroxyproline can also be derived from the C1q component of the complement, particularly in inflammatory conditions [49].

In contrast to the 4-hydroxyproline content, which is similar in all type I collagens, the extent of other posttranslational modifications varies from one situation and tissue to another. Such modifications include the hydroxylation of lysine, the subsequent glycosylation of hydroxylysine—first by galactose and then by glucose—and the hydroxylation of proline at position 3, leading to the formation of 3-hydroxyproline. The presence of a halfway glycosylated hydroxylysine, galactosylhydroxylysine, has been suggested to be characteristic of adult bone tissue, and the excretion of this amino acid in the urine has been used as a marker of bone collagen degradation [50].

C. Collagen Cross-Linking and the Stable Cross-Links

A characteristic approach in resolving the structures of collagen cross-links has been to isolate these compounds from hydrolyzed tissue samples, i.e., destroying the information of their original locations in the collagen molecules. Using this approach, the concentrations of either free or total cross-links—the latter after acid hydrolysis of the biological sample—can be measured in different body fluids, usually in the urine. This approach is more specific for assessing the breakdown of fibrillar collagen than the measurement of hydroxyproline, because the cross-links can only be derived from the degradation of those collagen molecules that have participated in collagen fibers. Furthermore, the pyridinoline cross-links are not absorbed from the diet, so their excretion is related only to their endogenous formation. Pyridinoline cross-links are abundant in the bone, but are even more so in the soft tissues where the maturation of the cross-links is mostly complete and occurs within a relatively short time after the assembly of the collagen fiber. At least in some tissues, the appearance of pyridinoline cross-links seems to be related to the development of an irreversible fibrosis, e.g., in the skin [51] and in the liver [52].

D. Cross-Link Immaturity in Bone Type I Collagen

Bone is the major connective tissue in which the collagen cross-links remain immature to a significant extent, the content of the divalent cross-links being about 2–4 times the concentration of the pyridinolines [53]. An obvious explanation for this finding is the fact that mineralization slows down the cross-linking process. The concentration of the divalent cross-links has been found to specifically decrease in osteoporosis [8, 53]. Unfortunately, analysis of the maturity of the cross-links in bones or other tissues suffers from the lack of easy, rapid, and reliable quantitative methods that would be suitable for a large number of small tissue samples. The development of immunoassays based either on synthetic peptides or on naturally cross-linked telopeptides may help in this respect, provided that the specificity of such assays is carefully tested. The application of such assays detecting the polypeptide chains involved in the cross-linked telopeptide structures has already revealed that in addition to the pyridinolines and the novel pyrrolic cross-links [54], there must still exist other uncharacterized mature cross-links [55].

Immaturely cross-linked collagens are, however, also transiently encountered during normal soft tissue collagen turnover and in the granulation tissues. Defective cross-linking can also be a major feature of the stroma of malignant tumor tissue [44a]. Interestingly, it has been found that lysyl oxidase, the only enzyme involved in the cross-link process, is identical to the tumor suppressor protein known as *rrg* [56], and that its synthesis is decreased in malignant breast tumor tissue [57].

E. The β-Isomerization of the Asp in the Carboxy-Terminal Telopeptide of Type I Collagen

At least one aspartic acid residue in the carboxy-terminal telopeptide of the α1-chain of type I collagen, located in the carboxy-terminal direction from the cross-link site, is subject to β-isomerization as the result of a nonenzymatic, physiological aging reaction [55]. This occurs via the formation of an unstable succinimide ring, which will spontaneously hydrolyze either back to a normal L-aspartyl or to an L-β-aspartyl residue (Fig. 5). The factors determining which Asp residues are susceptible to such isomerization are the nature of the adjacent amino acid residues and the constraints imposed by the surrounding secondary and tertiary structures [58].

On the basis of specific immunoassays, the ratio of the $\alpha : \beta$ forms has been reported to be 0.40 in cortical and 0.48 in trabecular bone collagen and as high as 1.33 in Pagetic bone [59]. Thus, even 70–80% of the L-Asp in this location in normal adult bone collagen could be isomerized into the

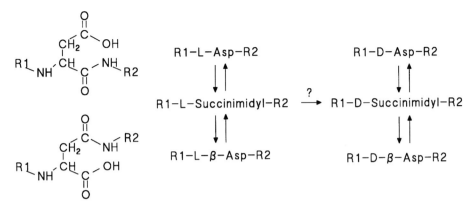

FIGURE 5   The β-isomerization and racemization reactions of aspartate residues in proteins. The former was recently found also in the amino-terminal telopeptide of type I collagen [77], whereas all the four variants (αL, βL, αD, and βD) can be found in the carboxy-terminal telopeptide [78].

β-configuration. Unfortunately, no corresponding data have been presented for the soft tissue type I collagen. It would also be interesting to know if the mineralization also affects the rate of β-isomerization, e.g., in the same way that mineralization decreases the maturation of the collagen cross-links. Several trivalently cross-linked peptides have been isolated from the urine that contain only two α or two β forms or one of both forms [55].

Theoretically, a racemization of the α-carbon of the aspartate to give the corresponding D-amino acid derivative is also possible (Fig. 5). Since only the L-Asp in the carboxy-terminal telopeptide region has been suggested to be subject to β-isomerization [55], such an additional modification seems likely. It has been found, at least, that D-Asp accumulates at a rate of about 0.1% per year during aging in the human bone fraction containing mostly collagen [60]; thus, at the age of 60 years, about 6% of the total amount of the L-Asp residues have been racemized into D-Asp.

F. Amino-Terminal Telopeptide of Type I Collagen

The amino-terminal telopeptide regions of both the α1(I) chain (17 amino acids) and the α2(I) chain (11 amino acids) of type I collagen contain lysine (or hydroxylysine) that can be oxidized to allysine (hydroxyallysine). The further events at this location can, in principle, lead to either intermolecular or intramolecular cross-links. The latter are formed from two aldehydes by aldol condensation and may, at least in the soft tissues, mature further to multivalent cross-links, e.g., five-atom ring structures known as pyrroles. Also, the bone type I collagen contains—in addition to pyridinoline cross-links and the divalent cross-links—many such pyrrolic cross-links. These structures are difficult to isolate for characterization because they easily aggregate when the constituent peptide chains are getting smaller (e.g., during enzymatic digestion). The dissolution of possible aggregates may be one of the reasons why the apparent concentration of the amino-terminal telopeptide, using an assay known as NTx [61], has been found to increase in urine samples when exposed to UV light [62]. The structure of the NTx peptide and its antigenic epitope is shown in Fig. 6.

G. Carboxy-Terminal Telopeptide of Type I Collagen

In the carboxy-terminal telopeptides of type I collagen, lysine/hydroxylysine is only present in the α1(I) chains (26 amino acids), making the number of possible alternative cross-linked structures smaller than the number at the amino terminus. Since the divalent cross-link formed first binds one telopeptide to the helical region of another collagen molecule, there is a possibility that the telopeptide of the second α1(I) chain remains free. Thus, several degradation products can be formed from the carboxy-terminal part of type I collagen that differ with respect to the α1-chain; this either has no cross-link or participates in a divalent or a trivalent cross-link. The latter may be hydroxylysyl pyridinoline, lysyl pyridinoline, pyrrole, or a noncharacterized nonfluorescent trivalent cross-link [55].

Several immunoassays have been developed for structures involving the carboxy-terminal telopeptides and they can give different results, depending on their immunochemical specificity with respect to size of the antigen and the maturity of the cross-link.

The ICTP antigen is a trivalently cross-linked structure that was originally isolated from human femoral bone after digestion with trypsin or bacterial collagenase and shown to contain the carboxy-terminal telopeptides of two α1(I) chains and material from the helical part of a third chain [63]. The

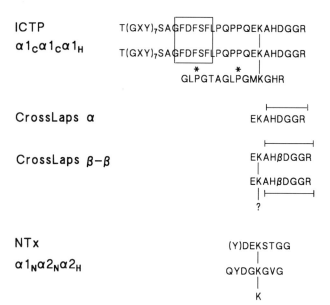

ICTP
α1$_c$α1$_c$α1$_H$

T(GXY)$_7$SAGFDFSFLPQPPQEKAHDGGR

T(GXY)$_7$SAGFDFSFLPQPPQEKAHDGGR
                    *   *
            GLPGTAGLPGMKGHR

CrossLaps α

EKAHDGGR

CrossLaps β–β

EKAHβDGGR

EKAHβDGGR
    ?

NTx
α1$_N$α2$_N$α2$_H$

(Y)DEKSTGG

QYDGKGVG

K

FIGURE 6   Antigenic epitopes in the carboxy-terminal (ICTP and Cross-Laps peptides) and the amino-terminal (NTx) telopeptide regions of the human type I collagen molecule. The ICTP assay detects only fragments having two phenylalanine-rich domains; to bring them together, a trivalent cross-link must be present. The CrossLaps assays detect linear, eight amino acid-long sequences where the Asp residue is either in an α- or a β-configuration. The epitope in the NTx assay demands the sequence QYDGKGVG, where K is embodied in a trivalent cross-link.

ICTP assay detects only large degradation products of mature type I collagen since the epitope demands two phenylalanine-rich regions [64], structures which are only formed when the cross-link is trivalent (Fig. 6). The original CrossLaps assay was developed for an eight amino acid-long synthetic peptide involving the cross-link site of the carboxy-terminal telopeptide of the α1(I) chain as an unmodified lysine [65]. Later, variants of the assay were introduced that can differentiate between the α- and β-forms of the Asp located in the epitope [66]. The CrossLaps α- or β-assays may detect both uncross-linked and di- or trivalently cross-linked species since the epitope is a linear sequence of only six amino acids (Fig. 5). However, the serum CrossLaps β-β-assay using a double antibody technique [67] may be less sensitive to the immature degradation products and measure better the peptides carrying trivalent cross-links (Fig. 6).

H. The Physiological Degradation Products of Type I Collagen

For the degradation of collagen in soft tissues, both an intracellular and an extracellular pathway have been suggested, the former functioning under metabolic steady-state conditions and the latter under conditions of rapid remodeling, e.g., in inflammation or during the involution of the uterus [47].

The extracellular route involves digestion of large amounts of collagen in the extracellular space and is initiated mainly by the action of matrix metalloproteinases. The intracellular route involves phagocytosis and lysosomal degradation of collagens; the enzymes responsible for this belong to cysteine and serine proteases [47].

The degradation of bone involves the specific attachment of osteoclasts to the mineralized surface, the dissolution of the inorganic mineral component (acidic microenvironment), and the degradation of matrix proteins (protease activity). Bone collagen degradation occurs mainly in the resorption lacuna and is analogous to the intracellular route of soft tissue collagen degradation. However, osteoclastic bone resorption seems to be initiated by the action of interstitial collagenase (one of the matrix metalloproteinases) derived from the stromal cells and osteoblasts adjacent to the osteoclasts [68]. Cathepsin K has been shown to be expressed selectively in osteoclasts [69] and to be the predominant cysteine protease in these cells [70].

Antigenic fragments reacting in assays for both the amino-terminal [71] and the carboxy-terminal [72] telopeptides of type I collagen have been found to be liberated when osteoclasts are cultured on bone slices, although the exact sizes of these degradation products have not been reported. Interestingly, no free hydroxylysyl pyridinoline or lysyl pyridinoline were found [71]. Unfortunately, neither the degradation products originating from the helical parts of the collagen molecules nor the liberation of hydroxyproline or galactosylhydroxylysine have been characterized in this system.

Although there are few studies on the mechanism of bone collagen degradation, studies on the urinary excretion of the degradation products abound. Both hydroxyproline and the pyridinoline cross-links are present partially in free form and partially in peptide-bound form in the urine; when the turnover rate of bone increases, there is typically a concomitant increase in the total excretion of the cross-links, but also a disproportionate increase in their peptide-bound fraction. The urinary antigens that are recognized either by the NTx or by the CrossLaps assay behave in a manner resembling the peptide-bound cross-links in this respect. Furthermore, different antiresorptive pharmaceuticals seem to affect the free and peptide-bound fractions differently. For example, estrogen therapy decreases the urinary excretion of both the free and peptide-bound cross-links in postmenopausal women, whereas bisphosphonate treatment of patients with Paget's disease has a marked effect only on the cross-linked peptides without a change in the free cross-links [73]. It can be speculated that the bisphosphonates would be specific for osteoclasts, which do not seem to produce free pyridinolines, whereas estrogen could have a more general effect on both bone and on nonmineralized tissues [71, 73]. This reasoning suggests that the free pyridinolines in the urine would largely be derived from the degradation of soft tissue collagens. While it is known that type III collagen contains a lot of hydroxylysyl pyridinoline, this most probably is not the whole explanation for the interesting finding, in particular because there is no significant difference between hydroxylysyl and lysyl pyridinolines in this respect.

Cathepsin K can generate the neoepitope of the amino-terminal NTx antigen *in vitro*, whereas in the same setting, no antigen was formed that would be recognized by the CrossLaps assay for the carboxy-terminal telopeptide [74]. Thus *in vivo*, either other enzymes in the osteoclasts or further degradation in the liver and/or the kidney tubuli must be involved, since the main urinary degradation products found by the CrossLaps assay only contain the core sequence EKAHDGGR [55]. Specificity tests of cathepsin K have indicated that the enzyme could cleave the carboxy-terminal telopeptide of the α1-chain of type I collagen within the sequence PQPPQE, which is located in the amino-terminal direction from the cross-link site, between it and the phenylalanine-rich region; thus, the degradation product resulting from the action of cathepsin K could not react in the ICTP assay (Fig. 6). This could be the main reason why the ICTP assay is not sensitive to situations where osteoclast-mediated normal turnover of bone collagen is taking place. On the other hand, as the circulating concentration of ICTP is elevated in clinical states involving enhanced pathological bone breakdown, such as in bone metastases of carcinomas, other pathways, possibly resembling the extracellular degradative pathway of collagen, must also exist.

The degradation of extraskeletal type I collagen and the further metabolism of the degradation products of bone collagen are not known in detail (Fig. 7). The majority of the hydroxyproline set free from collagens is metabolized in the liver. The endothelial cells of the liver possess specific gelatin receptors for the internalization of large collagenous peptides [25]. If such peptides still contain the cross-links, it is possible that the formation of free pyridinolines could partially take place in the liver.

Another site for further handling of the cross-linked peptides is the kidneys. In particular, the tubuli contain several exo- and endoproteinases, which digest small peptides to amino acids that can be reabsorbed. Accordingly, it has been shown by autogradiographic methods that the kidneys take part in the degradation of collagenous peptides [75]. The renal clearance of the free pyridinoline cross-links was shown to be 4-fold higher than that of the cross-links still present in peptides [76]. Since the fractional clearance of the former was greater than one and that of the latter less than one, some free pyridinolines excreted in urine are produced by the kidney (Fig. 7). The possible effects of pathological processes affecting the kidneys on cross-link excretion have not been studied.

IV. CLOSING REMARKS

The simultaneous analysis of the rates of both the formation and the degradation of bone collagen is a challenging goal for developing assays for collagen products. For assessing collagen formation there are two possibilities, and assays for both the carboxy-terminal (PICP) and the amino-terminal (PINP) propeptides of type I procollagen have been described. There is already a lot of clinical experience on their performance in different physiological and pathological situations, which suggests that the assay for the intact PINP is often superior to that for PICP. However, with respect to the analysis of type I collagen degradation, there is still a lot of confusion, and several methods measuring modified amino acids, collagen cross-links, or amino- or carboxy-terminal telopeptides have been described. Much experience has been gained using urine samples, but the present trend is to develop assays based on serum samples to allow more accurate quantification and a simultaneous analysis of collagen synthesis and degradation. A lot of work is still needed on the various metabolic processes that lead to collagen breakdown and on the further handling of the degradation products. The influence of the soft tissue collagen is also still largely unknown.

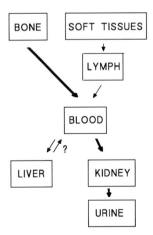

FIGURE 7   Schematic presentation of the distribution between various pools and of the clearances of type I collagen telopeptides.

References

1. Risteli, J., and Risteli, L. (1997). Assays of type I procollagen domains and collagen fragments: Problems to be solved and future trends. *Scand. J. Clin. Lab. Invest., Suppl.* **227**, 107–113.
2. Risteli, J., Niemi, S., Kauppila, S., Melkko, J., and Risteli, L. (1995). Collagen propeptides as indicators of collagen assembly. *Acta Orthop. Scand.* **66**(Suppl. 266), 183–188.
3. Risteli, J., and Risteli, L. (1995). Analysing connective tissue metabolites in human serum. Biochemical, physiological and methodological aspects. *J. Hepatol., Suppl.* **22**, 77–81.
4. Scariano, J. K., Walter, E. A., Glew, R. H., Hollis, B. W., Henry, A., Ocheke, I., and Isicei, C. O. (1995). Serum levels of pyridinoline crosslinked carboxy-terminal telopeptide of type I collagen (ICTP) and osteocalcin in rachitic children in Nigeria. *Clin. Biochem.* **28**, 541–545.
5. Sharp, C. A., Oginni, L. M., Worsfold, M., Oyelami, O. A., Risteli, L., Risteli, J., and Davie, M. W. J. (1997). Elevated collagen turnover in

Nigerian children with calcium-deficiency rickets. *Calcif. Tissue Int.* **61**, 87–94.

6. Jukkola, A., Risteli, L., Melkko, J., and Risteli, J. (1993). Procollagen synthesis and extracellular matrix deposition in MG-63 osteosarcoma cells. *J. Bone Miner. Res.* **8**, 651–657.

7. Mechanic, G. L., Katz, E. P., Henmi, M., Noyes, C., and Yamauchi, M. (1987). Locus of a histidine-based, stable trifunctional, helix to helix collagen cross-link: Stereospecific collagen structure of type I skin fibrils. *Biochemistry* **26**, 3500–3509.

8. Bailey, A. J., Wotton, S. F., Sims, T. J., and Thompson, P. W. (1993). Biochemical changes in the collagen of human osteoporotic bone matrix. *Connect. Tissue Res.* **29**, 119–132.

9. Ebeling, P. R., Peterson, J. M., and Riggs, B. L. (1992). Utility of type I procollagen propeptide assays for assessing abnormalities in metabolic bone diseases. *J. Bone Miner. Res.* **7**, 1243–1250.

10. Prockop, D. J., Kivirikko, K. I., Tuderman, L., and Guzman, N. A. (1979). The biosynthesis of collagen and its disorders. *N. Engl. J. Med.* **301**, 13–23, 77–85.

11. Kessler, E., Takahara, K., Biniaminov, L., Brusel, M., and Greenspan, D. S. (1996). Bone morphogenetic protein-1: The type I procollagen C-proteinase. *Science* **271**, 360–362.

12. Adar, R., Kessler, E., and Goldberg, B. (1986). Evidence for a protein that enhances the activity of type I procollagen C-proteinase. *Collagen Relat. Res.* **6**, 267–277.

13. Fleischmajer, R., Perlish, J. S., and Timpl, R. (1985). Collagen fibrillogenesis in human skin. *Ann. N.Y. Acad. Sci.* **460**, 246–257.

14. Jimenez, S. A., Bashey, R. I., Benditt, M., and Yankowski, R. (1977). Identification of collagen $\alpha 1$(I) trimer in embryonic chick tendons and calvaria. *Biochem. Biophys. Res. Commun.* **78**, 1354–1361.

15. Wohllebe, M., and Carmichael, D. J. (1978). Type-I trimer and type-I collagen in neutral-salt-soluble lathyritic-rat dentine. *Eur. J. Biochem.* **92**, 183–188.

16. Byers, P. H. (1993). Osteogenesis imperfecta. *In* "Connective Tissue and Its Heritable Disorders" (P. M. Royce and B. Steinmann, eds.), pp. 317–350. Wiley-Liss, New York.

17. Pucci-Minafra, I., Luparello, C., Andriolo, M., Basiricò, L., Aquino, A., and Minafra, S. (1993). A new form of tumor and fetal collagen that binds laminin. *Biochemistry* **32**, 7421–7427.

18. Pucci-Minafra, I., Andriolo, M., Basiricò, L., Aquino, A., Minafra, S., Boutillon, M. M., and van der Rest, M. (1995). Onco-fetal/laminin-binding collagen from colon carcinoma: Detection of new sequences. *Biochem. Biophys. Res. Commun.* **207**, 852–859.

19. Clark, C. C. (1979). The distributional initial characterization of oligosaccharide units on the COOH-terminal propeptide extensions of the pro-$\alpha 1$ and pro-$\alpha 2$ chains of type I procollagen. *J. Biol. Chem.* **254**, 10798–10802.

20. Melkko, J., Niemi, S., Risteli, L., and Risteli, J. (1990). Radioimmunoassay of the carboxy-terminal propeptide of human type I procollagen. *Clin. Chem.* **36**, 1328–1332.

21. Pedersen, B. J., and Bonde, M. (1994). Purification of human procollagen type I carboxyl-terminal propeptide cleaved as in vivo from procollagen and used to calibrate a radioimmunoassay of the propeptide. *Clin. Chem.* **40**, 811–816.

22. Taubman, M. B., Goldberg, B., and Sherr, C. J. (1974). Radioimmunoassay for human procollagen. *Science* **186**, 1115–1117.

23. Fischer, L. W., Robey, P. G., Tuross, N., Otsuka, A. S. O., Tepen, D. A., Esch, F. S., Shimasaki, S., and Termine, J. D. (1987). The M_r 24000 phosphoprotein from developing bone is the NH_2-terminal propeptide of the $\alpha 1$ chain of type I collagen. *J. Biol. Chem.* **37**, 13457–13463.

24. Melkko, J., Kauppila, S., Risteli, L., Niemi, S., Haukipuro, K., Jukkola, A., and Risteli, J. (1996). Immunoassay for intact amino-terminal propeptide of human type I procollagen. *Clin. Chem.* **42**, 947–954.

25. Smedsrød, B., Pertoft, H., Gustafsson, S., and Laurent, T. C. (1990). Scavenger functions of the liver endothelial cells. *Biochem. J.* **266**, 313–327.

26. Smedsrød, B., Melkko, J., Risteli, L., and Risteli, J. (1990). Circulating C-terminal propeptide of type I procollagen is cleared mainly via the mannose receptor in liver endothelial cells. *Biochem. J.* **271**, 345–350.

27. Melkko, J., Hellevik, T., Risteli, L., Risteli, J., and Smedsrød, B. (1994). Clearance of NH_2-terminal propeptides of types I and III procollagen is a physiological function of the scavenger receptor in liver endothelial cells. *J. Exp. Med.* **179**, 405–412.

28. Kivirikko, K. I. (1970). Urinary excretion of hydroxyproline in health and disease. *Int. Rev. Connect Tissue Res.* **5**, 93–163.

29. Lamandé, S. R., and Bateman, J. F. (1995). The type I collagen pro$\alpha 1$(I) COOH-terminal propeptide N-linked oligosaccharide. Functional analysis by site-directed mutagenesis. *J. Biol. Chem.* **270**, 17858–17865.

30. Toivonen, J., Tähtelä, R., Laitinen, K., Risteli, J., and Välimäki, M. J. (1998). Markers of bone turnover in patients with differentiated thyroid cancer on and off thyroxine suppressive therapy. *Eur. J. Endocrinol.* **138**, 667–673.

31. Sorva, A., Tähtelä, R., Risteli, J., Risteli, L., Laitinen, K., Juntunen-Backman, K., and Sorva, R. (1994). Familial high serum concentrations of the carboxyl-terminal propeptide of type I procollagen. *Clin. Chem.* **40**, 1591–1593.

32. Puistola, U., Risteli, L., Kauppila, A., Knip, M., and Risteli, J. (1993). Markers of type I and type III collagen synthesis in serum as indicators of tissue growth during pregnancy. *J. Clin. Endocrinol. Metab.* **77**, 178–182.

33. Haukipuro, K., Melkko, J., Risteli, L., Kairaluoma, M. I., and Risteli, J. (1991). Synthesis of type I collagen in healing wounds in humans. *Ann. Surg.* **213**, 75–80.

34. Oikarinen, A., Autio, P., Kiistala, U., Risteli, L., and Risteli, J. (1992). A new method to measure type I and III collagen synthesis in human skin in vivo: Demonstration of decreased collagen synthesis after topical glucocorticoid treatment. *J. Invest. Dermatol.* **98**, 220–225.

35. Jensen, L. T., Olesen, H. P., Risteli, J., and Lorenzen, I. (1990). External thoracic duct-venous shunt in conscious pigs for long term studies of connective tissue metabolism in lymph. *Lab. Anim. Sci.* **40**, 620–624.

36. Eriksen, E. F., Charles, P., Melsen, F., Mosekilde, L., Risteli, L., and Risteli, J. (1993). Serum markers of type I collagen formation and degradation in metabolic bone disease: Correlation to bone histomorphometry. *J. Bone Miner. Res.* **8**, 127–132.

37. Charles, P., Mosekilde, L., Risteli, L., Risteli, J., and Eriksen, E. F. (1994). Assessment of bone remodeling using biochemical indicators of type I collagen synthesis and degradation: Relation to calcium kinetics. *Bone Miner.* **24**, 81–94.

38. Price, K. M., Silman, R., Armstrong, P., and Grudzinskas, J. G. (1994). Development of a radioimmunoassay for fetal antigen 2. *Clin. Chim. Acta* **224**, 95–102.

39. Suvanto-Luukkonen, E., Risteli, L., Sundström, H., Penttinen, J., Kauppila, A., and Risteli, J. (1997). Comparison of three serum assays for bone collagen formation during postmenopausal estrogen-progestin therapy. *Clin. Chim. Acta* **266**, 105–116.

40. Linkhart, S. G., Linkhart, T. A., Taylor, A. K., Wergedahl, J. E., Bettica, P., and Baylink, D. J. (1993). Synthetic peptide-based immunoassay for amino-terminal propeptide of type I procollagen: Application for evaluation of bone formation. *Clin. Chem.* **39**, 2254–2258.

40a. Tähtelä, R., Turpeinen, M., Sorva, R., and Karonen, S.-L. (1997). The amino-terminal propeptide of type I procollagen: Evaluation of a commercial radioimmunoassay kit and values in healthy subjects. *Clin. Biochem.* **30**, 35–40.

41. Sharp, C. A., Davie, M. W. J., Worsfold, M., Risteli, L., and Risteli, J. (1996). Discrepant blood concentrations of type I procollagen propeptides in active Paget disease of bone. *Clin. Chem.* **42**, 1121–1122.

42. Sharp, C. A., Risteli, J., Risteli, L., and Davie, M. W. J. (1997). Type I procollagen propeptide ratio (PICP/PINP) responds rapidly to pamidronate in Paget's disease of bone. *J. Bone Miner. Res.* **12**(Suppl. 1), S269.

43. Jukkola, A., Tähtelä, R., Thölix, E., Vuorinen, K., Blanco, G.,

Risteli, L., and Risteli, J. (1997). Aggressive breast cancer leads to discrepant serum levels of the type I procollagen propeptides PINP and PICP. *Cancer Res.* **57**, 5517–5520.

44. Rasmussen, H. B., Teisner, B., Andersen, J. A., Brandrup, F., Purkis, T., and Leigh, I. (1991). Immunohistochemical studies on the localization of fetal antigen 2 (FA2), laminin and type IV collagen in basal cell carcinoma. *J. Cutaneous Pathol.* **18**, 215–219.

44a. Kauppila, S., Bode, M., Stenbäck, F., Risteli, L., and Risteli, J. (1999). Cross-linked telopeptides of type I and III collagens in malignant ovarian tumors *in vivo. Brit. J. Cancer*, in press.

45. Eyre, D. R., Paz, M. A., and Gallop, P. M. (1984). Cross-linking in collagen and elastin. *Annu. Rev. Biochem.* **53**, 717–748.

46. Doillon, C. J., Dunn, M. G., Bender, E., and Silver, D. H. (1985). Collagen fiber formation in repair tissue: development of strength and toughness. *Collagen Relat. Res.* **5**, 481–492.

47. Everts, V., van der Zee, E., Creemers, L., and Beertsen, W. (1996). Phagocytosis and intracellular digestion of collagen, its role in turnover and remodeling. *Histochem. J.* **28**, 229–245.

48. Sell, D. R., and Monnier, V. M. (1989). Structure elucidation of a senescence cross-link from human extracellular matrix. *J. Biol. Chem.* **264**, 21597–21602.

49. Robins, S. P. (1982). Turnover and cross-linking of collagen. *In* "Collagen in Health and Disease" (J. B. Weiss and M. I. V. Jayson, eds.), pp. 160–178. Churchill-Livingstone, Edinburgh.

50. Bettica, P., Taylor, A. K., Talbot, J., Moro, L., Talamini, R., and Baylink, D. J. (1996). Clinical performances of galactosyl hydroxylysine, pyridinoline, and deoxypyridinoline in postmenopausal osteoporosis. *J. Clin. Endocrinol. Metab.* **81**, 542–546.

51. Ricard-Blum, S., Esterre, P., and Grimaud, J. A. (1993). Collagen cross-linking by pyridinoline occurs in non-reversible skin fibrosis. *Cell. Mol. Biol.* **39**, 723–727.

52. Ricard-Blum, S., Bresson-Hadni, S., Guerret, S., Grenard, P., Volle, P.-J., Risteli, L., and Grimaud, J. A. (1996). Mechanism of collagen network stabilization in human irreversible granulomatous liver fibrosis. *Gastroenterology* **111**, 172–182.

53. Oxlund, H., Mosekilde, L., and Øxtoft, G. (1996). Reduced concentration of collagen reducible cross-links in human trabecular bone with respect to age and osteoporosis. *Bone* **19**, 479–484.

54. Hanson, D. A., and Eyre, D. R. (1996). Molecular site specificity of pyridinoline and pyrrole cross-linking in type I collagen in human bone. *J. Biol. Chem.* **271**, 26508–26516.

55. Fledelius, C., Johnsen, A. H., Cloos, P. A. C., Bonde, M., and Qvist, P. (1997). Characterization of urinary degradation products derived from type I collagen. Identification of a β-isomerized Asp-Gly sequence within the C-terminal telopeptide (α1) region. *J. Biol. Chem.* **272**, 9755–9763.

56. Kenyon, K., Contente, S., Trackman, P. C., Tang, J., Kagan, H. M., and Friedman, R. M. (1991). Lysyl oxidase and *rrg* messenger RNA? *Science* **253**, 802.

57. Peyrol, S., Raccurt, M., Gerard, F., Gleyzal, C., Grimaud, J. A., and Sommer, P. (1997). Lysyl oxidase gene expression in the stromal reactions to in situ and invasive ductal breast carcinoma. *Am. J. Pathol.* **150**, 497–507.

58. Lowenson, J., and Clarke, S. (1988). Does the chemical instability of aspartyl and asparaginyl residues in proteins contribute to erythrocyte aging. *Blood Cells* **14**, 103–117.

59. Garnero, P., Fledelius, C., Gineyts, E., Serre, C.-M., Vignot, E., and Delmas, P. D. (1997). Decreased β-isomerization of the C-terminal telopeptide of type I collagen α1 chain in Paget's disease of bone. *J. Bone Miner. Res.* **12**, 1407–1415.

60. Helfman, P. M., and Bada, J. L. (1976). Aspartic acid racemization in dentine as a measure of ageing. *Nature* **262**, 279–281.

61. Hanson, D. A., Weis, M. A. E., Bollen, A.-M., Maslan, S. L., Singer, F. R., and Eyre, D. R. (1992). A specific immunoassay for monitoring

human bone resorption: Quantitation of type I collagen cross-linked N-telopeptides in urine. *J. Bone Miner. Res.* **7**, 1251–1258.

62. Blumsohn, A. C., Naylor, K., and Eastell, R. (1995). Effect of light and γ-irradiation on pyridinolines and telopeptide of type I collagen in urine. *Clin. Chem.* **41**, 1195–1197.

63. Risteli, J., Elomaa, I., Niemi, S., Novamo, A., and Risteli, L. (1993). Radioimmunoassay for the pyridinoline cross-linked carboxy-terminal telopeptide of type I collagen: A new serum marker of bone collagen degradation. *Clin. Chem.* **39**, 635–640.

64. Risteli, J., Sassi, M.-L., Eriksen, H., Niemi, S., Mansell, J. P., and Risteli, L. (1997). Epitope of the assay for the carboxy-terminal telopeptide of human type I collagen (ICTP). *J. Bone Miner. Res.* **12**(Suppl. 1), S498.

65. Bonde, M., Qvist, P., Fledelius, C., Riis, B. J., and Christiansen, C. (1994). Immunoassay for quantifying type I collagen degradation products in urine. *Clin. Chem.* **40**, 2022–2025.

66. Bonde, M., Garnero, P., Fledelius, C., Qvist, P., Delmas, P. D., and Christiansen, C. (1997). Measurement of bone degradation products in serum using antibodies reactive with an isomerized form of an 8 amino acid sequence of the C-telopeptide of type I collagen. *J. Bone Miner. Res.* **12**, 1028–1034.

67. Christgau, S., Bonde, M., Qvist, P., and Christiansen, C. (1997). Measurement of serum CrossLaps^{TM} concentration for rapid assessment of the anti-resorptive effect of alendronate treatment. *J. Bone Miner. Res.* **12**(Suppl. 1), S137.

68. Holliday, L. S., Welgust, H. G., Fliszart, C. J., Veith, G. M., Jeffrey, J. J, and Gluck, S. L. (1997). Initiation of osteoblast bone resorption by interstitial collagenase. *J. Biol. Chem.* **272**, 22053–22058.

69. Inaoka, T., Bilbe, G., Ishibashi, O., Tezuka, K., Kumegawa, M., and Kokubo, T. (1995). Molecular cloning of human cDNA for cathepsin K: Novel cysteine proteinase predominantly expressed in bone. *Biochem. Biophys. Res. Commun.* **206**, 89–96.

70. Drake, F. H., Dodds, R. A., James, I. A., Connor, J. R., Debouck, C., Richardson, S., Lee-Rykaczewski, E., Coleman, L., Rieman, D., Barthlow, R., Hastings, G., and Gowen, M. (1996). Cathepsin K, but not cathepsins B, L, or S, is abundantly expressed in human osteoclasts. *J. Biol. Chem.* **271**, 12511–12516.

71. Apone, S., Lee, M. Y., and Eyre, D. R. (1997). Osteoclasts generate cross-linked collagen N-telopeptides (Ntx) but not free pyridinolines when cultured on human bone. *Bone* **21**, 129–136.

72. Foged, N. T., Delaissé, J.-M., Hou, P., Lou, H., Sato, T., Winding, B., and Bonde, M. (1996). Quantification of the collagenolytic activity of isolated osteoclasts by enzyme-linked immunosorbent assay. *J. Bone Miner. Res.* **11**, 226–237.

73. Garnero, P., Gineyts, E., Arbault, P., Christiansen, C., and Delmas, P. D. (1995). Different effects of bisphosphonate and estrogen therapy on free and peptide-bound bone cross-links excretion. *J. Bone Miner. Res.* **10**, 641–649.

74. Atley, L. M., Mort, J. S., Lalumiere, M., and Eyre, D. R. (1997). Quantitative release by cathepsin K of immunoreactive cross-linked N-telopeptides (NTX) from bone type I collagen. *J. Bone Miner. Res.* **12**(Suppl. 1), S417.

75. Ruckidge, G. J., Riddoch, G. I., Williams, L. M., and Robins, S. P. (1988). Autoradiographic studies of the renal clearance of circulating Type I collagen fragments in the rat. *Collagen Relat. Res.* **8**, 339–348.

76. Colwell, A., and Eastell, R. (1996). The renal clearance of free and conjugated pyridinium cross-links of collagen. *J. Bone Miner. Res.* **11**, 1976–1980.

77. Brady, J. D., Ju, J., and Robins, S. P. (1998). Isoaspartyl bonds in the N-terminal telopeptides of type I collagen and their use as urinary markers of collagen degradation. *Bone* **23**(5, Suppl.), S238.

78. Cloos, P., Fledelius, C., Qvist, P., and Garnero, P. (1998). Biological clocks of bone aging: Racemization and isomerization, potential tools to assess bone turnover. *Bone* **23**(5, Suppl.), S514.

CHAPTER 20

Supramolecular Structure of Cartilage Matrix

ERIC F. EIKENBERRY Department of Pathology, University of Medicine and Dentistry of New Jersey—Robert Wood Johnson Medical School, Piscataway, New Jersey 08854

PETER BRUCKNER Department of Physiological Chemistry and Pathobiochemistry, University of Münster, Germany

I. ABSTRACT

The extracellular matrix of hyaline cartilage comprises the great majority of the volume of this tissue and is responsible for its properties. The matrix consists of two basic suprastructural components: fibrils with a $D = 67$ nm periodic banding pattern and an electron-lucent extrafibrillar matrix with no conspicuous features. The structural properties of these matrix constituents and their functional implications are discussed in this chapter. The heterotypic fibrils contain not only several types of collagen but also noncollagenous macromolecules. These molecular components specifically self-assemble, either into distinct domains within the fibrils or, more attractively, into aggregates with characteristics of metal alloys in many respects. Thus, specific properties of the fibrils are indirectly determined by the mass proportions of their molecular components. Similar considerations apply to the extrafibrillar matrix which is rich in polyanionic carbohydrates and, thus, water. Implications of this concept are discussed for connective tissues other than cartilage and for extracellular matrices in general.

II. INTRODUCTION

Three types of cartilage have been distinguished on the basis of histological criteria and biomechanical properties: hyaline, elastic, and fibrous cartilages. The most prevalent type is hyaline cartilage which is a visually uniform, translucent tissue found in the skeleton of all vertebrates. Articular cartilage, the most familiar hyaline cartilage, forms the smooth gliding surfaces of joints, such as the knee and hip, that permit locomotion in animals. Injuries to this tissue and common diseases, such as osteoarthritis, impair joint mobility and constitute a major focus of modern medicine. Hyaline cartilage also comprises growth plate, the transient template required for endochondral bone formation in fetal development, skeletal growth, and repair. In addition, hyaline cartilage occurs as a permanent structural tissue in costal cartilages and tracheal reinforcing rings.

Elastic and fibrous cartilage are less widely distributed. Flexibility is the hallmark of elastic cartilage, found for example in the outer ear, and is a consequence of its large content of elastic fibers. Meniscus and annulus fibrosus are fibrous cartilages in which bundles of banded fibers, similar to those found in tendon, resist tensile forces generated by the load-bearing functions of these tissues. Elastic and fibrous cartilage will not be considered further in this review.

The biomechanical requirements of cartilage are met by the extracellular matrix that constitutes the predominant fraction of the tissue. In contrast, the cellular component, the chondrocytes, occupies a relatively small volume, with each cell embedded into extracellular matrix with no direct cell-to-cell contacts. The matrix properties are determined in turn by tissue-specific supramolecular structures, such as periodically banded fibrils, filaments, and proteoglycan aggregates. This review will outline the current frontiers of our knowledge in this field. Cartilage morphology has been studied by light microscopy, electron microscopy, and x-ray diffraction. These techniques have been complemented by biochemical investigation of isolated aggregates and their self-assembly *in vitro*, and by genetic studies of human diseases and transgenic animals.

III. LIGHT AND ELECTRON MICROSCOPY

At the level of light microscopy, articular cartilage matrix is an almost homogeneous mass of negatively charged material well stained by basic dyes such as alcian blue or toluidine blue. However, staining discontinuities do highlight specific matrix domains of adult articular cartilage. Such domains are much less conspicuous in immature cartilage, e.g., in fetal or neonatal epiphyseal cartilage. Territorial regions are seen near the cell surfaces that are distinct from the interterritorial matrix in the large intervening spaces. In his early investigations of adult articular cartilage by light microscopy, Benninghoff postulated a reinforcement of the tissue by fibers forming arcades with their bases in the subchondral bone and arches at the articular surface [1]. This arcade-like organization of the fibrils buttresses the tissue against shear forces in the superficial layers and secures the tissue to the underlying bone.

Near the osteochondral junction, a prominent light microscopic feature is the sharply defined limit of calcification of the tissue which is termed the tide-mark. Growth plate, the cartilage responsible for the longitudinal growth of long bones, does not show a tide-mark, but otherwise the salient features of its matrix structure are similar to those of adult articular cartilage.

Electron microscopy has been extensively used to visualize the supramolecular structures in hyaline cartilage matrix. General features include a network of banded fibrils and an extrafibrillar matrix with no conspicuous ultrastructure that was once referred to as "amorphous ground substance." In the immediate vicinity of the cells, there is a small space apparently lacking fibrils altogether. This region is known as the pericellular matrix and mainly contains a specialized extrafibrillar matrix that is easily extractable from the tissue during conventional histological fixation (see later in this section).

As apparent already by light microscopy, the matrix structure in immature cartilage is simpler than that in adult tissue. Fibrils in fetal or neonatal cartilage have a round cross section with a uniformly small diameter of about 20 nm which exhibits a faint longitudinal banding pattern [2]. Fibrils are almost randomly orientated throughout the tissue but tend to be parallel to tissue or cell surfaces near to those boundaries.

The architecture of adult hyaline cartilage is more complex. The fibril diameters are heterogeneous and depend on the precise anatomical location within the tissue. In articular cartilage, for example, the fibrils strongly align with joint surfaces, thereby forming conspicuous two-dimensional mats [2]. In the intermediate zones between joint surfaces and the junctions with the subchondral bone, fibrils are more randomly distributed in three dimensions. Reconstructions from thick sections show fibrils with a kinked morphology woven together in a three-dimensional knit [3]. In deep zones, fibrils are nearly parallel to the long bone axis. This distribution of fibril diameters and orientations corresponds well to the Benninghoff arcade model.

The structure of adult cartilage fibrils also varies between the territorial and interterritorial regions defined by light microscopy. As in immature cartilage, the immediate surrounding of the cell consists of an essentially fibril-free pericellular matrix. Further removed from the cell surface there is a weave of 20 nm fibrils forming a basket around the cells. Such basket structures can be isolated after mechanical disruption of the tissue and have been termed chondrons to designate a functional unit comprising a chondrocyte in its immediate extracellular environment [4]. Chondrons may contain more than one cell, in which case individual cells are separated by a thin septum of territorial matrix. Moving away from the cell surface, the territorial matrix gradually becomes the interterritorial region, in which fibrils progressively acquire diameters of 50–100 nm and have striking longitudinal cross-banding patterns. The period of the banding pattern is D, the characteristic periodicity of collagen fibrils which is typically about 65 nm in electron microscopy, but varies with the degree of shrinkage encountered in the preparation of the specimen (see Section IV).

With traditional chemical fixation and embedding in hydrophobic resins, a number of features are observed that are now thought to be artifacts. Among these is the formation of lacunae inside of the territorial matrix showing cells with apparent pseudopodia anchored in the fibril network [5]. This feature appears to be a consequence of shrinking of the cells and a loss of matrix macromolecules from the cellular environment. Also, in the extrafibrillar matrix, condensations of material into electron-dense globules result from the artifactual precipitation of polyanionic proteoglycans [6, 7].

The development of improved chemical fixation, cryopreservation, and freeze-substitution techniques appears to have overcome these problems and has allowed a more detailed analysis of cartilage matrix suprastructures. Using these techniques, the original round shape of chondrocytes is preserved and only small tube-like cell-surface projections are visible which may be part of the secretory machinery of the cells. Lacunae, however, are no longer observed. Further, filaments are seen in the pericellular matrix with a diameter of 10 to 15 nm and a very faint D-periodic banding pattern [7]. Because this feature is a hallmark of collagen-containing fibrils, the filaments may represent precursors of fibrils in the territorial matrix. Such filaments are also seen throughout the matrix, including in the interterritorial regions, where they are intermingled in random orientation with the large fibrils. In the interterritorial matrix, the thicker fibrils often fan out into smaller fibrils closely resembling those of the territorial matrix, giving the impression that the well-banded interterritorial fibrils arise by fusion of archetypal 20 nm fibrils [8]. This is supported by observations of fibrils in cross section; larger fibrils have an irregular outline and are surrounded by round fibrils that closely resemble the 20 nm fibrils. Verification that large fibrils are assembled by fusion of smaller ones rather than by accretion of individual molecules presents a challenge for future studies in cartilage structural biology.

Another detail visualized by the observation of unstained sections of cartilage vitrified at high pressure is the presence of a thin water-rich layer surrounding the fibrils [9]. This implies the existence of a previously unknown transition zone between the fibril surface and the extrafibrillar matrix, perhaps 5 nm in width, which has a lower density than either of these components. It will be of great interest to find the biochemical correlate of this zone.

IV. BIOCHEMISTRY OF CARTILAGE

A vast amount of information is available on cartilage matrix macromolecules. The extrafibrillar matrix is a complex of carbohydrates and proteins with a high negative charge density which leads to the binding of large amounts of water. Its main macromolecules are aggrecan, hyaluronan, and link protein (LP), which together form bottle-brush-like aggregates that have been reconstituted from the purified components and observed by electron microscopy of rotary-shadowed preparations [10–12]. Such complexes are known to bind matrilin-1 (also called cartilage matrix protein, CMP) as a further component [13]. Although a considerable degree of structural organization has thus been demonstrated for isolated extrafibrillar matrix components, electron microscopy has failed to visualize the ultrastructure of these components in tissues.

Cartilage fibrils are mostly proteinaceous, containing collagens II, IX, and XI, and also noncollagenous components, most notably decorin [14, 15]. Binding to collagens has also been reported for fibromodulin, biglycan, matrilin-1, and cartilage oligomeric matrix protein (COMP; also called thrombospondin-5), but their localization with respect to cartilage fibrils *in situ* remains to be documented. Other cartilage components described in Chapter 4 are likely to reside within the extrafibrillar matrix, but their localization also remains to be established.

The major collagenous component of hyaline cartilage is collagen II which comprises up to 50% of the dry weight of the tissue. Collagens II and XI are defined as fibril-forming collagens in that they can form fibrils as pure proteins. The other fibril-forming collagens, types I, III, and V, were conventionally thought to be absent from cartilage, but type I is reported to comprise as much as 10% of the collagenous component of normal hyaline cartilage [16]. Collagen III is a very minor component [17] of cartilage, while type V has not been detected. The levels of these three minor collagens are reported to increase in osteoarthritic cartilage [18–20].

Minor nonfibril-forming collagens that have been reported in cartilage include types VI [16, 21], XII, and XIV [22]. Collagen VI predominantly occurs in the territorial regions or in isolated chondrons [23]. The protein forms filamentous structures with a periodicity of 100 nm [24] that are independent of D-periodically banded fibrils. In contrast, collagens XII and XIV are likely to be constituents of D-periodic fibrils in skin [25] but their suprastructural organization in cartilage remains to be determined.

The polypeptides of fibril-forming collagens consist of uninterrupted long sequences (1017 amino acid residues in the case of collagen II) of repeating Gly-X-Y amino acid residue triplets, where X and Y are arbitrary but are frequently proline and hydroxyproline, respectively. Three chains of such a repeating primary sequence fold into a triple-helical collagen molecule with a length of 300 nm and a diameter of 1.5 nm [26]. Molecules of collagen pack laterally into "quarter-staggered" arrays as shown in Figure 1, in which adjacent molecules are staggered longitudinally by a multiple of $D = 67$ nm, which corresponds to 234 amino acid residues [27]. The molecules are about 4.4 D in length, which gives rise to the well-known gap-overlap longitudinal structure of collagen, where the gap, or hole zone, is about 0.6 D in length [28]. The longitudinal D period is the most obvious feature of

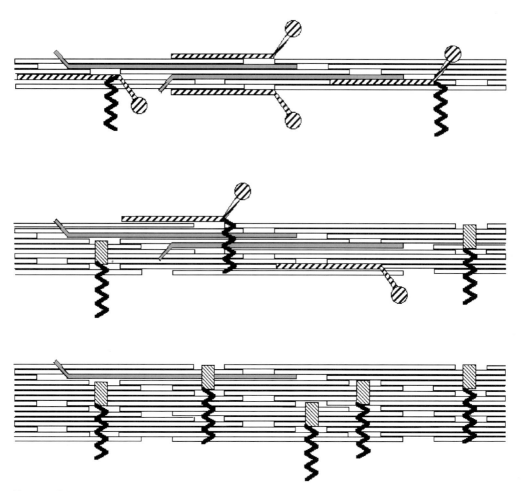

FIGURE 1   Changes in cartilage fibril structure with diameter. (Upper) Uniform diameter 20 nm fibrils of quarter-staggered collagen molecules illustrating the gap-overlap structure. Collagen XI molecules (gray) are shown with amino-terminal propeptides protruding from the surface of the fibril, which may act to control diameter. Collagen IX (hatched) is shown at the surface with the COL3 and NC4 (spherical) domains projecting from the fibril axis. The dark zig-zag represents the glycosaminoglycan (GAG) component covalently attached to the type IX molecules. (Center) Intermediate diameter fibril showing both collagen IX and decorin incorporated into the surface. GAG presented at the surface derives from both collagen IX and decorin. (Lower) Large diameter fibril showing only decorin and its attendant GAG on the surface. Collagen IX, perhaps processed, may remain in the interior of the fibril.

collagenous fibrils both in electron microscopy and in x-ray diffraction, the latter technique giving the precise value of D for fully hydrated native specimens.

Dermatan sulfate and keratan sulfate proteoglycans are important structural components of fibrils in cartilage and have been visualized in tissues and isolated fibrils by staining with the cationic dye cupromeronic blue under conditions of critical electrolyte concentration [29]. Filamentous chains of proteoglycan are seen with highly regular D-periodic distribution. These have been interpreted as integral components of cartilage fibrils that tether fibrils in position within the matrix.

Decorin has been shown to bind to individual collagen I and II molecules near the N-terminal end [30]. This location would place it at the "d" band within the gap of the fibril structure, a location to which proteoglycan has been mapped

by cupromeronic blue staining [31]. The proteinaceous part of decorin is a member of a large family of proteins containing leucine-rich repeating (LRR) sequences. The structure of ribonuclease inhibitor, another member of the LRR family, though not obviously related to decorin, has been solved by x-ray crystallography [32]. A detailed structural model of decorin binding based on similarity to the horseshoe-shaped ribonuclease inhibitor structure has been proposed [33]. Energy calculations of the model support the assignment of the binding to the "d" band of collagen fibrils, but other nearby sites are also possible.

Fibromodulin, another LRR proteoglycan, has been shown to bind specifically to collagen II [34]. Decorin and fibromodulin have one binding site each for collagen and do not compete with each other [35–37]; hence, they must occupy separate specific sites on the collagen molecule. Thus, proteoglycans, including decorin, fibromodulin, and collagen IX, appear to have important specific roles in establishing and maintaining the fibrils of cartilage.

V. STUDIES OF FIBRIL STRUCTURES BY X-RAY DIFFRACTION

X-ray diffraction has been used to determine the structure of collagen in rat tail tendon nearly to atomic resolution [38, 39]. For this reason and because of the biochemical similarities in fibril-forming collagens, the fibrils in rat tail tendon have often been considered as model structures of collagen-containing fibrils in general; however, this notion has now been revised [40]. Rat tail tendon is almost unique among connective tissues in that collagen molecules are packed in molecular crystals that diffract to high resolution. Analysis reveals a tissue composed of microfibrils of five triple helical collagen molecules twisted into left-handed strands distorted by crystal packing forces into a quasi-hexagonal array [41, 42]. These arrays exhibit coherently diffracting domains up to 100 nm in lateral size, which is considerably smaller than the size of the fibrils (up to 600 nm) in which they reside. Thus, the large fibrils seen by electron microscopy are not single crystals, but mosaics of smaller crystallites [43].

The average center-to-center intermolecular spacing in hydrated rat tail tendon is ca. 1.5 nm. Most other tendons do not give crystalline patterns, but x-ray diffraction can still be used in these specimens to evaluate the intermolecular spacing. In other fully hydrated collagen I-containing tissues, this spacing is also near 1.5 nm [44]. In the dry state, this distance collapses to about 1.1 nm, demonstrating that the collagen molecules in fibrils are separated from each other by substantial quantities of intrafibrillar water [45].

Cartilage fibrils have also been extensively studied by x-ray diffraction. In the sheath of the lamprey notochord, the collagen II-containing fibrils are apparently crystalline, but the uniform diameter fibrils are too small, ca. 20 nm, to give high resolution diffraction [46]. Both in this tissue and in mammalian cartilages, the average center-to-center intermolecular spacing in the fully hydrated state is ca. 1.7 nm, which is significantly higher than in collagen I-containing tissues [47]. This is consistent with a higher number of glucosyl-galactosyl-hydroxylysine residues found in collagen II; the levels of this posttranslational modification are 50–100% higher than in type I collagen. This results in a higher intrafibrillar water content in cartilage [48, 49]. Dried cartilage shows approximately the same intermolecular spacing (ca. 1.1 nm) as tendon, demonstrating that the collagen II molecular diameter is not significantly increased by the additional sugar content. The other fibril-forming collagen of cartilage, type XI, has an even higher degree of glycosylation than collagen II; however, there are no x-ray diffraction data specific for this collagen type.

Glycation, the nonenzymatic reaction by glucose with protein amino groups that occurs naturally in tissues with slow protein turnover, has shed light on the lateral organization of collagen in fibrils. Rat tail tendon was subjected to cross-linking by ribose as a model for the age-related effects of glycation [50]. It was found that the average intermolecular spacing increased with the degree of cross-linking. This was interpreted as showing that the separation of collagen molecules is a weakly constrained equilibrium such that there is little energetic cost involved in swelling or shrinking the structure by the exchange of water [46]. This supports the idea that collagen II has increased intrafibrillar water because of its increased posttranslational hydroxylysyl glycosylation. The biomechanical effects of age-related glycation in cartilage fibrils have also been modeled by ribosylation, but resulting changes in intrafibrillar water content were not reported [51].

VI. STRUCTURE OF FIBRIL FRAGMENTS OBTAINED BY MECHANICAL DISRUPTION OF TISSUE

Another approach to studying the structure of cartilage fibrils has been to prepare fragments of fibrils from cartilage or from chondrocyte cultures. Such fibril preparations, contrasted by negative or positive stain with or without immuno-gold labeling or by rotary shadowing, have yielded considerable information. Both cell cultures and tissues yield the thin fibrils characteristic of cartilage which have been shown by immunostaining to be heterotypic, in that individual fibrils contain collagens II, IX, and XI. Biochemical analysis of fragments isolated from chick embryo cartilage revealed a mass proportion of 8:1:1 for these collagen types, respectively [52]. Interestingly, collagen XI in fibril fragments from chick embryo sterna exhibited a strong immunochemical masking toward antibodies raised against the long triple helix of the protein. Upon disruption of the collagen packing by partial digestion with pepsin, however, this immunochemical masking was released [53]. Employing immuno-gold labeling with antibodies directed to the amino-terminal nonhelical domain, collagen XI was localized only to fibrils of small diameter in tissue sections of human rib and growth plate cartilage [54]. In contrast, undigested fibril fragments were readily labeled with antibodies to the pepsin treated forms of both collagens II and IX [53]. Taken together, these results raise the possibility that collagen XI is buried within the fibrillar body, and that, by forming a core structure, collagen XI regulates apposition of types II and IX onto the fibrils.

Rotary shadowed fibrils exhibit a D-periodic occurrence of collagen IX, with the amino-terminal domains NC4 and COL3 projecting from the fibril axis (see Chapter 1 for a discussion of these domains). This has been interpreted as showing collagen IX to be a surface component [52]. However, fibrils of older mammalian cartilage are biochemically heterogenous, with the detailed composition depending on which tissue layer is sampled. Small uniform fibrils characteristically have collagen IX at their surface, whereas large fibrils have decorin. Some intermediate diameter fibrils stain for both collagen IX and decorin [15] (Fig. 1). Since both of these molecules are glycoproteins carrying dermatan sulfate chains in cartilage, the fibrils are studded with anionic groups which could help to secure the extrafibrillar matrix to the fibrils.

VII. STUDIES OF COLLAGEN CROSS-LINKING IN CARTILAGE FIBRILS

Naturally occurring cross-links between collagen polypeptides in cartilage have been used as indicators for the fibrillar organization (the occurrence and chemistry of such cross-links are discussed in Chapter 2). Collagen IX purified from steer cartilage was found to have 1.7–2.3 mol of cross-linking residues to collagen II per mol of collagen, consistent with the heterotypic nature of cartilage fibrils [55]. If it is assumed that the collagen IX molecules lie parallel to the fibril axis, then the locations of these links indicate that the collagen IX is oriented antiparallel to the type II collagen and covers both the gap and the overlap region (Fig. 1). However, it is also possible to construct models in which the type IX collagen wraps around, or partially penetrates, the fibril, in which case the molecular configuration cannot be specified. Collagen IX is also cross-linked to other molecules of collagen IX. Collagen XI is cross-linked as well, largely to other type XI molecules, but also to a small degree to collagen II [56]. This observation has been interpreted as supporting the idea that collagen XI forms a core on which collagen II is deposited. Cross-links to other fibrillar and nonfibrillar components have not yet been described.

VIII. RECONSTITUTION OF CARTILAGE-LIKE FIBRILS FROM SOLUBLE COLLAGENS II, IX, AND XI

One of the fascinating questions concerning cartilage matrix structure is what mechanism controls the diameter of the thin, uniform fibrils. Fibril reconstitution experiments with purified components have been used to approach this question. In such experiments, collagens in solution are subjected to temperature and buffer conditions under which they spontaneously aggregate into fibrils. Chicken sternal chondrocytes from 17-day embryos grown in agarose maintain the cartilage phenotype and synthesize uniform 20 nm fibrils. Collagens II, IX, and XI have been purified from these cultures by salt fractionation and ion exchange chromatography. Fibrils

reconstituted from the mixture of the three collagen types directly extracted from the cultures gave uniform D-periodic fibrils closely resembling authentic 20 nm fibrils by their appearance in the electron microscope after negative contrasting. Collagen XI alone also formed small, uniform fibrils of about the same diameter [57].

The collagen purification technique has been greatly refined, yielding essentially pure components in fibrilcompetent form [U. K. Blaschke and P. Bruckner, unpublished]. The kinetics of in vitro fibrillogenesis was followed by turbidometry and by electron microscopy. In agreement with previous reports [58], collagen II alone developed turbidity only after a lag time of 90–120 min. After this lag phase, the protein formed wide tactoids which, in the electron microscope, appeared as relatively short, D-periodically banded aggregates with tapered ends and without apparent diameter control. Aggregation of collagen XI alone resulted in a hyperbolic increase in turbidity with no discernible lag phase at all. Immediately after initiation of in vitro fibrillogenesis, within the limits of time resolution of about 1 min, the protein assembled into long and flexible small diameter filaments. As turbidity developed to moderate amplitudes, the filaments turned into weakly cross-banded fibrils with tightly controlled diameters of ca. 20 nm. Mixtures of collagens II and XI, at mass proportions of up to 8:1, respectively, produced turbidity characteristics without lag phase similar to those of pure collagen XI, and the final fibrils also had a closely similar appearance. Therefore, the diameter control is inherent to these two components alone. Furthermore, the 8:1 limit of collagen proportions and the 20 nm diameter match the corresponding properties of authentic chick embryo sternal cartilage fibrils. At larger proportions of collagen II, two-phase turbidity curves were observed and 20 nm-fibrils and tactoids coexisted in the final reconstitution products. However, unlike the case of pure collagen II undergoing in vitro fibrillogenesis, tactoids formed in these supercritical mixtures of collagens II and XI were already present within the lag period of the second increase in turbidity. This means that such tactoids were heterotypic, in that they contained both collagen types, and that the decision on the shape of the final aggregate occurred during the early phase of assembly and was determined by the biochemical composition of the early aggregates. This conclusion is illustrated by the drawing in Figure 2. In addition, many tactoids were continuous with the 20 nm fibrils, suggesting that tactoid formation nucleated on fibrils.

IX. STUDIES OF TRANSGENIC MICE AND OF HUMAN GENETIC MATRIX DISEASES

Studies of mutations in genes encoding matrix macromolecules have also contributed to our understanding of cartilage matrix organization. A large repertoire of mutations

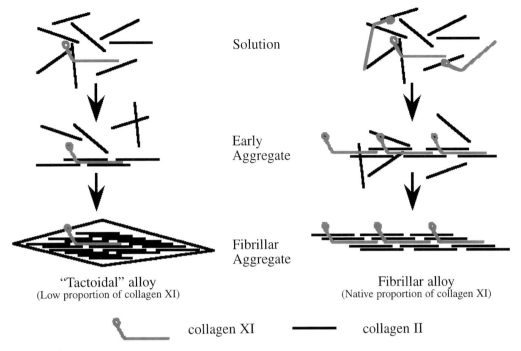

FIGURE 2   Illustration of the different aggregates resulting from fibril formation with different stoichiometries of collagens II and XI. (Left) Tactoids are formed in mixtures with an excess of collagen II (greater than 8:1), possibly as a result of separation of a collagen II-rich phase characterized by tight lateral packing of identical molecules. (Right) The native proportion of collagens II and XI result in uniform 20 nm fibrils.

in human and animal genes for almost all macromolecules discussed in the preceding sections has been reported. Information comes from experimentally induced mutations in transgenic mice as well as from naturally occurring mutations in human and animal diseases. Consequences of mutations in collagen genes to cartilage suprastructure will be discussed here. The mutations and their pathological consequences have been catalogued in other reviews [59, 60].

In-frame deletions resulting in a loss of peptide sequences within the triple helical domain in the collagen II gene (COL2A1 in man or Col2a1 in mice) lead to chondrodysplasia of variable severity depending on the extent and the location of the deletion within the gene. Such mutations result in shortened $\alpha 1$(II)-chains that are incorporated into homotrimeric collagen II molecules together with either normal or other mutated chains. This explains the dominant phenotype of the mutations. However, the penetrance of the mutations varies not only between mice with different genetic backgrounds but even between individual inbred animals. The ability of cells to eliminate mutated mRNA or polypeptide species may be subject to variation between individual animals, which may explain the heterogeneous severity of the consequences of a given mutation. Triple helix formation is impaired in affected molecules which, thereby, frequently have a lowered thermal stability and a compromised competence of incorporation into fibrillar aggregates. Due to the D-periodic regularity of collagen II molecules within the fibrils,

incorporation of shortened molecules, even though they are secreted by the cells in reduced amounts, will destroy the entire fibrillar organization. This translates into a generalized injury to the structure of the cartilage matrix and its functions. Point mutations, particularly those exchanging glycine residues in the Gly-X-Y repeats of the triple helical domain, have similar consequences. Such mutations have shown that the formation of cartilaginous tissue does not depend on the presence of collagen II; in patients with hypochondrogenesis or achondrogenesis, collagen II, though synthesized, was not secreted by chondrocytes, but an abnormal mixture of collagens I and III was present [61, 62]. The resulting cartilage even matured sufficiently to produce collagen X. Bone formation, however, was severely disrupted in these lethal mutations. In general, abnormalities within carboxyterminal regions of the triple helix tend to result in more severe phenotypes because collagen folding proceeds from the carboxyltowards the amino-terminal end in a zipper-like fashion [63].

Interestingly, transgenic mice harboring extra copies of the normal Col2a1 gene have a perinatally lethal phenotype. Although no gross abnormalities were found in their cartilages, wide and strongly banded fibrils occurred in the interterritorial regions. In these animals, the balance in the amounts of collagens II and XI is altered due to an overexpression of collagen II resulting from transcription and translation of the transgenes. This agrees well with the formation *in vitro* of tactoids rather than normal cartilage-like fibrils from solutions containing collagen II above physiological levels (see Section VIII).

Mice homozygous for a nonfunctional collagen II gene (type II knockout mice) also have been reported [64]. These animals show extensive abnormalities of their endoskeleton but, surprisingly, survive until birth. They extensively develop cartilage tissue in which collagen II is substituted, at least in part, by type I. Poorly organized fibrils occur in much smaller numbers than in normal cartilage and lack discernible longitudinal banding patterns as well as clearly defined lateral limits. The reasons for this fibrillar disorganization are not immediately clear. However, because the $\alpha 3(XI)$-chains are the same gene product as the $\alpha 1(II)$-chains (see Chapter 1), abnormal collagen XI molecules lacking $\alpha 3(XI)$ chains are assembled. The protein has a lowered thermal stability and, hence, occurs in lower quantities due to degradation in the tissue. In light of the results from *in vitro* reconstitution of mixtures of collagens II and XI, it is plausible that the absence of normal collagen XI accounts for the disarray of cartilage matrix to a greater extent than the lack of type II. Consistent with this notion, the abnormal collagen XI appears to be poorly incorporated into fibrillar arrays leading to a markedly increased extractability of the protein from cartilage [A. Aszódi, D. Chan, E. B. Hunziker, J. F. Bateman, and R. Fässler, unpublished].

A variety of mutations affecting the genes of collagen XI chains also have been discovered. A single base deletion in the gene encoding the $\alpha 1(XI)$ chain occurs naturally in the cho/cho mouse strain [65]. This represents a frameshift mutation leading to a prematurely terminated $\alpha 1(XI)$ polypeptide which either is not efficiently synthesized or is prematurely degraded. Collagen XI protein is absent in the cartilage of these mice and, again in keeping with *in vitro* fibrillogenesis of cartilage collagen mixtures, the cartilage of homozygous cho/cho mice contains disorganized fibrils with exceptionally large diameters. Analogous consequences are seen in patients with Stickler syndrome, where a splice-site mutation probably causes the production of shortened $\alpha 2(XI)$ chains [66]. Although neither histology at the suprastructural level nor protein data are available for cartilage affected by this mutation, it seems likely that collagen XI, at least in functionally intact form, is absent in these tissues since the macroscopic consequences are similar to those of other collagen XI abnormalities.

The deletion of collagen IX in mice [67] by inactivation of the Col9a1 gene [68] results in a remarkably mild phenotype. The mice show no extensive abnormality in skeletal development and the fibrils in cartilage of affected animals also are close to normal. Cartilage integrity appears to be impaired only in older animals that show premature onset of osteoarthritis-like cartilage degeneration. Again, this is consistent with *in vitro* fibrillogenesis and suggests that the main role of collagen IX is at the level of tissue organization of fibrils in cartilage. Nevertheless, it is surprising that bone development is almost normal in these animals in view of the fact that it is the thin fibrils arising in fetal and young cartilage that are rich in collagen IX [15]. However, collagen IX, like decorin, occurs at the surface of cartilage fibrils and carries a single dermatan sulfate chain. Therefore, decorin may well be functionally redundant, at least in part, with collagen IX and may generate the polyanionic charge density required during bone development at the cartilage fibril surface in collagen IX-deficient mice. Interestingly, decorin-deficient mice also do not exhibit gross cartilage abnormalities. This may well be since collagen IX is normal in these animals. It will be of interest to see whether thin fibrils in cartilage of immature collagen IX-deficient mice contain decorin, unlike the 20 nm fibrils in normal mammalian cartilage. In addition, mice deficient in both decorin and collagen IX may show more extensive skeletal abnormalities.

An exon skipping mutation in the COL9A2 gene of patients with multiple epiphyseal dysplasia [69] leads to the transcription of a shortened $\alpha 2(IX)$ mRNA, which is expected to result in $\alpha 2(IX)$ chains lacking 12 amino acids within the Col3 domain which protrudes from the fibril surface [52]. It still remains to be determined whether, in analogy to the Col9a1 knockout mice, the production of shortened $\alpha 2(IX)$ chains leads to an overall absence of collagen IX. However, fully functional protein is not likely to be synthesized in the affected tissues. Consistent with mice lacking collagen IX, the consequences of this mutation do not include severe skeletal abnormalities. Again, the genotype–phenotype correlation agrees with the notion that collagen IX is not essential for fibrillogenesis in cartilage but that the protein is required for long-term stability of the tissue. If an abnormal variant of collagen IX exists in the patient's cartilage, it will be interesting to determine the mode in which a shortened Col3 domain causes impairment of the interaction between fibrils and the extrafibrillar matrix.

X. CORRELATING STRUCTURE WITH THE BIOMECHANICAL ROLE OF ARTICULAR CARTILAGE

A major function of articular cartilage is to enable unhindered motion of joints by providing a smooth, low friction gliding surface and by cushioning the bone against stress and impact. These properties are achieved by prestressing the cartilagenous material through the interaction of the fibrils with their proteoglycan-rich matrix. The matrix has a high fixed-charge density, deriving from the negatively charged groups of its constituent glycosaminoglycans, chiefly those of aggrecan. This charge is responsible for the high degree of hydration of the tissue, which in turns causes the matrix component to swell strongly. Swelling is counteracted by the cartilage fibrils, which act to keep the glycosaminoglycans compressed and relatively dehydrated in comparison to their free, equilibrium hydration. The collagen fibril network is firmly attached to the extrafibrillar matrix by a high density of noncovalent interactions between proteins, such as between fibrils and decorin, and between glycosaminoglycans. In turn, some of the glycosaminoglycans are covalently bound to proteins. The arrangement of fibrils into arcades is precisely the architecture needed to counteract the stress.

The physical properties of cartilage have been extensively studied by mechanical testing, with the observed properties being modeled as a viscoelastic [70] or poroviscoelastic [71] material. The drawback of most of these investigations is that the tissue is regarded as a homogeneous substance, but Setton et al. [71] did investigate samples with the surface layer, the collagen-rich top of the arcades, removed. In this case it was found that exudation of fluid under pressure was more rapid than in intact tissue, demonstrating the role of the superficial zone in controlling interstitial movement of fluid.

The intratissue pressure in cartilage has been estimated by subjecting samples to various osmotic pressures and measuring changes in hydration [72]. Osmotic pressure was controlled by use of calibrated solutions of polyethylene glycol (PEG) at various concentrations. It was found that the unperturbed internal pressure of cartilage was ca. 3.9 bar. The mass of normal tissue varied surprisingly little with osmotic pressure changes; normal specimens transferred from 0.15 M NaCl to 0.015 M NaCl swelled by only 1–2%.

The collagen fibrils also respond to changes in osmotic pressure. Increases in osmotic pressure reduce the hydration, and thus the intermolecular spacing, of the collagen triple-helices [48]. The tension in the fibrils has been calculated and shown to be easily within the known tensile limits of collagen [73]. Very large increases in osmotic pressure by PEG, up to 10 bar with a concomitant 20% mass loss, were required to make the collagen fibrillar network go "limp" in normal cartilage [72].

The continuous tension to which cartilage fibrils are subjected is an unusual role for collagen. In other tissues, collagens are called on to resist tension only transiently. Further, the fibrils in cartilage must be synthesized and repaired while maintaining tension, requiring a mechanism that is not well understood. It is perhaps not surprising that a number of medically important conditions can develop in such a system. Ameliorating the biological problem of tissue maintenance is the exceptionally long life of cartilage components under normal circumstances. Collagen II has a half-life of more than 200 years in humans [51]. Consistent with this is the rate of accumulation of glycation-derived cross-links in cartilage collagen. Such cross-links increase linearly with age after 20 years, when the organism stops growing, and show no evidence of reaching a plateau level at advanced age [51]. By these measures, then, the collagen is never turned over. The rate of aspartic acid residue racemization has been used to show that the half-life of different species of aggrecan ranges from 3.4 to 25 years in man [74]. Thus, in the absence of disease or injury, cartilage is highly stable.

The mechanical properties of cartilage are drastically affected in osteoarthritis. An osteoarthritic specimen transferred from 0.15 M NaCl to 0.015 M NaCl swelled by more than 10%, demonstrating the effects of destruction of the fibrillar net in this disease [72]. In this condition, the tissue does not have the means to resist water uptake by the glycosaminoglycans. Thus, therapies that aim to make up the observed loss of glycosaminoglycans in osteoarthritis probably will not work as expected; the fibrillar network needs to be restored.

XI. MODELS OF CARTILAGE FIBRIL STRUCTURE

What models of fibril structure are compatible with these observations? The classical scheme has collagen XI forming a core or scaffold on which the collagen II is deposited. Collagen IX then serves to coat the structure and arrest the diametral growth. We now recognize that collagen IX is not necessary to achieve the morphology of the archetypal 20 nm cartilage fibril, but the model is still attractive. First, it appears to account for the observed greater difficulty in extracting type XI from cartilage as compared to type II. Second, the cross-link data showing that collagen XI is cross-linked mostly with other homologous molecules suggests that the protein forms a filamentous core of the fibrils. The core model for cartilage fibrils, unfortunately, does not easily provide a mechanism for diameter control in the absence of type IX; the fibrils should be indefinitely large.

The possible existence of a core filament has also been discussed in conjunction with the analogous collagen I–collagen V system in cornea tissue. Fibrils in cornea tissue also have tightly controlled diameters, a property that is responsible for corneal transparency. One suggestion for the control of diameter in these fibrils, and the relative inaccessibility of their collagen V component to antibody labeling, is the existence of a core fiber of type V [75]. As in the case of cartilage fibrils, this model does not easily provide a mechanism for diameter control in the absence of other components.

A different model is that of the biological alloy, in which collagens II and XI randomly commingle to form diameter-controlled fibrils as long as the ratio is 8:1 or less [76] (Fig. 3). This model is attractive because it explains why fibril diameter does not depend on composition. With the core model, one would expect mixed fibrils to be larger than the core material alone, which is not observed. Diameter control is an innate property of the alloy, mediated by collagen XI. It is known that most of the N-propeptides of type XI are retained in the tissue [77]. The requirement to accommodate these bulky moieties, probably on the exterior of the fibrils, could inhibit diametral growth [78, 79]. This class of alloys could incorporate a certain amount of collagen II up to approximately 8:1, the most favorable composition for the alloy, without structural modification. Beyond that ratio, the structure would not form and phase separation would take place. Collagen XI would be distributed throughout the fibril in this model. This

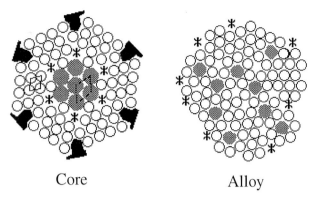

Core   Alloy

FIGURE 3   Illustration of the core model versus the alloy model of uniform cartilage fibrils. (Left) A cross section of the core model has collagen XI (gray) at its center, collagen II (open circles) apposed around it, and collagen IX (filled) capping the structure to limit diametral growth. It is now known that collagen IX is not required for diameter control. (Right) The alloy model posits a random commingling of collagen II and XI, with either molecule being able to occupy any lattice position. Diameter control could be achieved by the necessity to accommodate the collagen XI propeptides at the surface (cf. Figure 1). Lattice faults (*), arising from incommensurate packing of collagens II and XI, are important in both models, either providing a binding site for collagen IX in the core model or destabilizing large diameter fibrils in the alloy model.

is not necessarily contradicted by the type XI cross-link data because of the relatively great length and flexibility of the molecules. The resistance to extraction of type XI collagen in tissues can be a simple consequence of the cross-linking, rather than of any structural model.

What is the role of collagen IX? The fibril reconstitution experiments from purified types II and XI only worked with fresh material [U. K. Blaschke and P. Bruckner, unpublished]. After 1–2 weeks, the competency to form fibrils was lost by the pure proteins. However, competency could be rescued by the addition of collagen IX; restoring the 8:1:1 ternary mixture of collagens caused the mixture to continue to be fibril competent for a considerable time after the binary mixture had lost the ability. Thus, it appears that, in addition to directing the fibrillar tissue organization, collagen IX stabilizes characteristic cartilage fibrils *in vitro*, and may do so *in vivo* as well. This would be consistent with the results from the type IX-deficient mice, where early onset of osteoarthritis was the major finding; instability of cartilage fibrils is the major lesion in this disease.

XII. FUTURE PERSPECTIVES

A great deal of information has been accumulated on the identity and structure of cartilage matrix macromolecules. However, much remains to be learned about one of the quintessential characteristics of these components: their assembly into insoluble suprastructural aggregates. The fibrillar organization of cartilage collagens is gradually emerging and we are

beginning to understand the assembly of the bulk components of the extrafibrillar matrix, aggrecan and hyaluronan, but the aggregate structures of most of the other macromolecules identified as cartilage matrix components are either unknown or controversial. As is true for most extracellular matrices, even less is known about the formation of structure at the next hierarchic level, i.e., the principles directing the assembly of cartilage matrix from fibrils and the extrafibrillar matrix. As our knowledge about additional molecular components of fibrils or the extrafibrillar matrix increases, our chances to formulate viable working hypotheses will increase. For example, the definition of fibrillar components other than collagens, particularly those at surfaces, will be one of the challenges in the immediate future. Likewise, it will be interesting to learn about the identity of molecular components of the extrafibrillar matrix which occur in the immediate vicinity of fibrils. Methods will have to be devised to reconstitute matrix domains from suprastructural subunits to understand the forces driving matrix assembly. These efforts will be strongly supported by expanding our knowledge of the function of matrix macromolecules *in situ*. This goal will be achieved by defining in greater detail the connection between the genotype and the phenotype in human or animal genetic disorders or in transgenic animals. Concurrently, the refinement of techniques such as x-ray diffraction and electron and atomic force microscopy combined with specific labeling will provide additional opportunities to elucidate cartilage matrix structure at high resolution. The combined information will lay the groundwork for our understanding of the biomechanics of cartilage and its metabolic regulation through cell matrix interactions under normal conditions, as well as its abnormalities under pathological conditions.

Acknowledgments

The authors are grateful to Drs. Aszódi, Bateman, and Fässler for making available information on collagen II-knockout mice prior to publication and for helpful discussion.

References

1. Benninghoff, A. (1922). Über den funktionellen Bau des Knorpels. *Anat. Anz.* **55**, 250–267.
2. Hunziker, E. B. (1992). Articular cartilage structure in humans and experimental animals. *In* "Articular Cartilage and Osteoarthritis" (K. E. Kuettner, R. Schleyerbach, J. G. Peyron, and V. C. Hascall, eds.), pp. 183–199. Raven Press, New York.
3. Broom, N. D., and Silyn-Roberts, H. (1989). The 3-dimensional knit of collagen fibrils in articular cartilage. *Connect. Tissue Res.* **23**, 261–277.
4. Poole, C. A. (1997). Articular cartilage chondrons: Form, function and failure. *J. Anat.* **191**, 1–13.
5. Hunziker, E. B., Herrmann, W., and Schenk, R. K. (1983). Ruthenium hexamine trichloride (RHT)-mediated interaction between plasmalemmal components and pericellular matrix proteoglycans is responsible

for the preservation of chondrocyte plasma membranes in situ during cartilage fixation. *J. Histochem. Cytochem.* **31**, 717–727.

6. Studer, D., Michel, M., Wohlwend, M., Hunziker, E. B., and Buschmann, M. D. (1995). Vitrification of articular cartilage by high-pressure freezing. *J. Microsc.* **179**, 321–332.

7. Hunziker, E. B., Wagner, J., and Studer, D. (1996). Vitrified articular cartilage reveals novel ultra-structural features respecting extracellular matrix architecture. *Histochem. Cell Biol.* **106**, 375–382.

8. Hunziker, E. B., Michel, M., and Studer, D. (1997). Ultrastructure of adult human articular cartilage matrix after cryotechnical processing. *Microsc. Res. Tech.* **37**, 271–284.

9. Studer, D., Chiquet, M., and Hunziker, E. B. (1996). Evidence for a distinct water-rich layer surrounding collagen fibrils in articular cartilage extracellular matrix. *J. Struct. Biol.* **117**, 81–85.

10. Hascall, V. C., and Heinegård, D. (1974). Aggregation of cartilage proteoglycans. 1. The role of hyaluronic acid. *J. Biol. Chem.* **249**, 4232–4241.

11. Rosenberg, L., Hellmann, W., and Kleinschmidt, A. K. (1975). Electron microscopic studies of proteoglycan aggegates from bovine articular cartilage. *J. Biol. Chem.* **250**, 1877–1883.

12. Mörgelin, M., Paulsson, M., Heinegård, D., Aebi, U., and Engel, J. (1995). Evidence of a defined spatial arrangement of hyaluronate in the central filament of cartilage proteoglycan aggregates. *Biochem. J.* **307**, 595–601.

13. Hauser, N., Paulsson, M., Heinegård, D., and Mörgelin, M. (1996). Interaction of cartilage matrix protein with aggrecan. Increased covalent cross-linking with tissue maturation. *J. Biol. Chem.* **271**, 32247–32252.

14. Miosge, N., Flachsbart, K., Götz, W., Schultz, W., Kresse, H., and Herken, R. (1994). Light and electron microscopical immunohistochemical localization of the small proteoglycan core proteins decorin and biglycan in human knee joint cartilage. *Histochem. J.* **26**, 939–945.

15. Hagg, R., Bruckner, P., and Hedbom, E. (1998). Cartilage fibrils of mammals are biochemically heterogeneous: Differential distribution of decorin and collagen IX. *J. Cell Biol.* **142**, 285–294.

16. Wardale, R. J., and Duance, V. C. (1993). Quantification and immunolocalisation of porcine articular and growth plate cartilage collagens. *J. Cell Sci.* **105**, 975–984.

17. Young, R. D., Lawrence, P. A., Duance, V. C., Aigner, T., and Monaghan, P. (1995). Immunolocalization of type III collagen in human articular cartilage prepared by high-pressure cryofixation, freeze-substitution, and low-temperature embedding. *J. Histochem. Cytochem.* **43**, 421–427.

18. Adam, M., and Deyl, Z. (1983). Altered expression of collagen phenotype in osteoarthrosis. *Clin. Chim. Acta* **122**, 25–32.

19. Aigner, T., Bertling, W., Stöss, H., Weseloh, G., and von der Mark, K. (1993). Independent expression of fibril-forming collagens I, II, and III in chondrocytes of human osteoarthritic cartilage. *J. Clin. Invest.* **91**, 829–837.

20. Aigner, T., Glückert, K., and von der Mark, K. (1997). Activation of fibrillar collagen synthesis and phenotypic modulation of chondrocytes in early human osteoarthritic cartilage lesions. *Osteoarthritis Cartilage* **5**, 183–189.

21. Hagiwara, H., Schröter-Kermani, C., and Merker, H.-J. (1993). Localization of collagen type VI in articular cartilage of young and adult mice. *Cell Tissue Res.* **272**, 155–160.

22. Watt, S. L., Lunstrum, G. P., McDonough, A. M., Keene, D. R., Burgeson, R. E., and Morris, N. P. (1992). Characterization of collagen type XII and type XIV from fetal bovine cartilage. *J. Biol. Chem.* **267**, 20093–20099.

23. Poole, C. A., Ayad, S., and Gilbert, R. T. (1992). Chondrons from articular cartilage. V. Immunohistochemical evaluation of type VI collagen organisation in isolated chondrons by light, confocal and electron microscopy. *J. Cell Sci.* **103**, 1101–1110.

24. Furthmayr, H., Wiedemann, H., Timpl, R., Odermatt, E., and Engel, J.

(1983). Electron-microscopical approach to a structural model of intima collagen. *Biochem. J.* **211**, 303–311.

25. Keene, D. R., Lunstrum, G. P., Morris, N. P., Stoddard, D. W., and Burgeson, R. E. (1991). Two type XII-like collagens localize to the surface of banded collagen fibrils. *J. Cell Biol.* **113**, 971–978.

26. Rich, A., and Crick, F. H. C. (1961). The molecular structure of collagen. *J. Mol. Biol.* **3**, 483–506.

27. Hulmes, D. J. S., Miller, A., Parry, D. A. D., Piez, K. A., and Woodhead-Galloway, J. (1973). Analysis of the primary structure of collagen for the origins of molecular packing. *J. Mol. Biol.* **79**, 137–148.

28. Hodge, A. J., and Petruska, J. A. (1963). Recent studies with the electron microscope on ordered aggregates of the tropocollagen macromolecule. *In* "Aspects of Protein Structure" (G. N. Ramachandran, ed.), pp. 289–300. Academic Press, New York.

29. Scott, J. E. (1990). Proteoglycan-collagen interactions and subfibrillar structure in collagen fibrils. Implications in the development and ageing of connective tissues. *J. Anat.* **169**, 23–35.

30. Yu, L., Cummings, C., Sheehan, J. K., Kadler, K. E., Holmes, D. F., and Chapman, J. A. (1993). Visualization of individual proteoglycan-collagen interactions. *In* "Dermatan Sulfate Proteoglycans" (J. E. Scott, ed.), pp. 183–188. Portland Press, London.

31. Scott, J. E., and Orford, C. R. (1981). Dermatan sulphate-rich proteoglycan associates with rat tail-tendon collagen at the d band in the gap region. *Biochem. J.* **197**, 213–216.

32. Kobe, B., and Deisenhofer, J. (1993). Crystal structure of procine ribonuclease inhibitor, a protein with leucine-rich repeats. *Nature* **366**, 751–756.

33. Weber, I. T., Harrison, R. W., and Iozzo, R. V. (1996). Model structure of decorin and implications for collagen fibrillogenesis. *J. Biol. Chem.* **271**, 31767–31770.

34. Hedlund, H., Mengarelli-Widholm, S., Heinegård, D., Reinholt, F. P., and Svensson, O. (1994). Fibromodulin distribution and association with collagen. *Matrix Biol.* **14**, 227–232.

35. Hedbom, E., and Heinegård, D. (1993). Binding of fibromodulin and decorin to separate sites on fibrillar collagens. *J. Biol. Chem.* **268**, 27307–27312.

36. Schönherr, E., Hausser, H., Beavan, L., and Kresse, H. (1995). Decorin-type I collagen interaction. Presence of separate core protein-binding domains. *J. Biol. Chem.* **270**, 8877–8883.

37. Schönherr, E., Witsch-Prehm, P., Harrach, B., Robenek, H., Rauterberg, J., and Kresse, H. (1995). Interaction of biglycan with type I collagen. *J. Biol. Chem.* **270**, 2776–2783.

38. Fraser, R. D., and MacRae, T. P. (1979). The crystalline structure of collagen fibrils in tendon. *J. Mol. Biol.* **127**, 129–133.

39. Fraser, R. D., MacRae, T. P., Miller, A., and Suzuki, E. (1983). Molecular conformation and packing in collagen fibrils. *J. Mol. Biol.* **167**, 497–521.

40. Brodsky, B., and Eikenberry, E. F. (1985). Supramolecular collagen assemblies. *In* "Biology, Chemistry, and Pathology of Collagen" (R. Fleischmajer, B. R. Olsen, and K. Kühn, eds.), *Ann. N.Y. Acad. Sci.* Vol. 460, pp. 73–84. New York Academy of Sciences, New York.

41. Hulmes, D. J. S., and Miller, A. (1979). Quasi-hexagonal packing in collagen fibrils. *Nature* **282**, 878–880.

42. Wess, T. J., Hammersley, A. P., Wess, L., and Miller, A. (1998). Molecular packing of type I collagen in tendon. *J. Mol. Biol.* **275**, 255–267.

43. Hulmes, D. J. S., Holmes, D. F., and Cummings, C. (1985). Crystalline regions in collagen fibrils. *J. Mol. Biol.* **184**, 473–477.

44. Brodsky, B., and Eikenberry, E. F. (1982). Characterization of fibrous forms of collagen. *In* "Methods in Enzymology" (L. W. Cunningham and D. W. Frederiksen, eds.), Vol. 82, pp. 127–174. Academic Press, New York.

45. Katz, E. P., Wachtel, E. J., and Maroudas, A. (1986). Extrafibrillar proteoglycans osmotically regulate the molecular packing of collagen in cartilage. *Biochim. Biophys. Acta* **882**, 136–139.

46. Tanaka, S., Avigad, G., Eikenberry, E. F., and Brodsky, B. (1988).

Isolation and partial characterization of collagen chains dimerized by sugar-derived cross-links. *J. Biol. Chem.* **263**, 17650–17657.

47. Grynpas, M. D., Eyre, D. R., and Kirschner, D. A. (1980). Collagen type II differs from type I in native molecular packing. *Biochim. Biophys. Acta* **626**, 346–355.

48. Wachtel, E., Maroudas, A., and Schneiderman, R. (1995). Age-related changes in collagen packing of human articular cartilage. *Biochim. Biophys. Acta* **1243**, 239–243.

49. Price, R. I., Lees, S., and Kirschner, D. A. (1997). X-ray diffraction analysis of tendon collagen at ambient and cryogenic temperatures: Role of hydration. *Int. J. Biol. Macromol.* **20**, 23–33.

50. Tanaka, S., Avigad, G., Brodsky, B., and Eikenberry, E. F. (1988). Glycation induces expansion of the molecular packing of collagen. *J. Mol. Biol.* **203**, 495–505.

51. Bank, R. A., Bayliss, M. T., Lafeber, F. P. J. G., Maroudas, A., and Tekoppele, J. M. (1998). Ageing and zonal variation in post-translational modification of collagen in normal human articular cartilage. The age-related increase in non-enzymatic glycation affects biomechanical properties of cartilage. *Biochem. J.* **330**, 345–351.

52. Vaughan, L., Mendler, M., Huber, S., Bruckner, P., Winterhalter, K. H., Irwin, M. I., and Mayne, R. (1988). D-periodic distribution of collagen IX along cartilage fibrils. *J. Cell Biol.* **106**, 991–997.

53. Mendler, M., Eich-Bender, S. G., Vaughan, L., Winterhalter, K. H., and Bruckner, P. (1989). Cartilage contains mixed fibrils of collagen types II, IX, and XI. *J. Cell Biol.* **108**, 191–197.

54. Keene, D. R., Oxford, J. T., and Morris, N. P. (1995). Ultrastructural localization of collagen types II, IX, and XI in the growth plate of human rib and fetal bovine epiphyseal cartilage: Type XI collagen is restricted to thin fibrils. *J. Histochem. Cytochem.* **43**, 967–979.

55. Wu, J.-J., Woods, P. E., and Eyre, D. R. (1992). Identification of cross-linking sites in bovine cartilage type IX collagen reveals an antiparallel type II-type IX molecular relationship and type IX to type IX bonding. *J. Biol. Chem.* **267**, 23007–23014.

56. Wu, J.-J., and Eyre, D. R. (1995). Structural analysis of cross-linking domains in cartilage type XI collagen. Insights on polymeric assembly. *J. Biol. Chem.* **270**, 18865–18870.

57. Eikenberry, E. F., Mendler, M., Bürgin, R., Winterhalter, K. H., and Bruckner, P. (1992). Fibrillar organization in cartilage. *In* "Articular Cartilage and Osteoarthritis" (K. E. Kuettner, R. Schleyerbach, J. G. Peyron, and V. C. Hascall, eds.), pp. 133–149. Raven Press, New York.

58. Lee, S. L., and Piez, K. A. (1983). Type II collagen from lathyritic rat chondrosarcoma: Preparation and in vitro fibril formation. *Collagen Relat. Res.* **3**, 89–103.

59. Li, Y. F., and Olsen, B. R. (1997). Murine models of human genetic skeletal disorders. *Matrix Biol.* **16**, 49–52.

60. Aszódi, A., Pfeifer, A., Wendel, M., Hiripi, L., and Fässler, R. (1998). Mouse models for extracellular matrix diseases. *J. Mol. Med.* **76**, 238–252.

61. Chan, D., Cole, W. G., Chow, C. W., Mundlos, S., and Bateman, J. F. (1995). A COL2A1 mutation in achondrogenesis type II results in the replacement of type II collagen by type I and III collagens in cartilage. *J. Biol. Chem.* **270**, 1747–1753.

62. Mundlos, S., Chan, D., McGill, J., and Bateman, J. F. (1995). An $\alpha 1$(II) Gly913 to Cys substitution prevents the matrix incorporation of type II collagen which is replaced with type I and II collagens in cartilage from a patient with hypochondrogenesis. *Am. J. Med. Genet.* **63**, 129–136.

63. Bruckner, P., and Eikenberry, E. F. (1984). Formation of the triple helix of type I procollagen *in cellulo*. Temperature-dependent kinetics support a model based on *cis-trans* isomerization of peptide bonds. *Eur. J. Biochem.* **140**, 391–395.

64. Li, S. W., Prockop, D. J., Helminen, H., Fässler, R., Lapveteläinen, T., Kiraly, K., Peltarri, A., Arokoski, J., Lui, H., Arita, M., and Khillan, J. (1995). Transgenic mice with targeted inactivation of the COL2A1 gene for collagen II develop a skeleton with membranous and periosteal bone but no endochondral bone. *Genes Dev.* **9**, 2821–2830.

65. Li, Y., Lacerda, D. A., Warman, M. L., Beier, D. R., Yoshioka, H., Ninomiya, Y., Oxford, J. T., Morris, N. P., Andrikopoulos, K., Ramirez, F., Wardell, B. B., Lifferth, G. D., Teuscher, C., Woodward, S. R., Taylor, B. A., Seegmiller, R. E., and Olsen, B. R. (1995). A fibrillar collagen gene, Col11a1, is essential for skeletal morphogenesis. *Cell* **80**, 423–430.

66. Vikkula, M., Mariman, E. C. M., Lui, V. C. H., Zhidkova, N. I., Tiller, G. E., Goldring, M. B., Van Beersum, S. E. C., De Waal Malefijt, M. C., Van den Hoogen, F. H. J., Ropers, H.-H., Mayne, R., Cheah, K. S. E., Olsen, B. R., Warman, M. L., and Brunner, H. G. (1995). Autosomal dominant and recessive osteochondrodysplasias associated with the COL11A2 locus. *Cell* **80**, 431–438.

67. Hagg, R., Hedbom, E., Möllers, U., Aszódi, A., Fässler, R., and Bruckner, P. (1997). Absence of the $\alpha 1$(IX) chain leads to a functional knock-out of the entire collagen IX protein in mice. *J. Biol. Chem.* **272**, 20650–20654.

68. Fässler, R., Schnegelsberg, P. N. J., Dausman, J., Shinya, T., Muragaki, Y., McCarthy, M. T., Olsen, B. R., and Jaenisch, R. (1994). Mice lacking $\alpha 1$(IX) collagen develop noninflammatory degenerative joint disease. *Proc. Natl. Acad. Sci. U.S.A.* **91**, 5070–5074.

69. Muragaki, Y., Mariman, E. C. M., Van Beersum, S. E. C., Perälä, M., Van Mourik, J. B. A., Warman, M. L., Olsen, B. R., and Hamel, B. C. J. (1996). A mutation in the gene encoding the a2 chain of the fibril-associated collagen IX, COL9A2, causes multiple epiphyseal dysplasia (EDM2). *Nat. Genet.* **12**, 103–105.

70. Parsons, J. R., and Black, J. (1977). The viscoelastic shear behavior of normal rabbit articular cartilage. *J. Biomech.* **10**, 21–29.

71. Setton, L. A., Zhu, W., and Mow, V. C. (1993). The biphasic poroviscoelastic behavior of articular cartilage: Role of the surface zone in governing the compressive behavior. *J. Biomech.* **26**, 581–592.

72. Basser, P. J., Schneiderman, R., Bank, R. A., Wachtel, E., and Maroudas, A. (1998). Mechanical properties of the collagen network in human articular cartilage as measured by osmotic stress technique. *Arch. Biochem. Biophys.* **351**, 207–219.

73. Aspden, R. M., and Hukins, D. W. L. (1990). Stress in collagen fibrils of articular cartilage calculated from their measured orientations. *Matrix* **9**, 486–488.

74. Maroudas, A., Bayliss, M. T., Uchitel-Kaushansky, N., Schneiderman, R., and Gilav, E. (1998). Aggrecan turnover in human articular cartilage: Use of aspartic acid racemization as a marker of molecular age. *Arch. Biochem. Biophys.* **350**, 61–71.

75. Birk, D. E., Fitch, J. M., Babiarz, J. P., Doane, K. J., and Linsenmayer, T. F. (1990). Collagen fibrillogenesis *in vitro*—interaction of type I and type V collagen regulates fibril diameter. *J. Cell Sci.* **95**, 649–657.

76. Bruckner-Tuderman, L., and Bruckner, P. (1998). Genetic diseases of the extracellular matrix: More than just connective tissue disorders. *J. Mol. Med.* **76**, 226–237.

77. Rousseau, J. C., Farjanel, J., Boutillon, M. M., Hartmann, D. J., van der Rest, M., and Moradi-Améli, M. (1996). Processing of type XI collagen. Processing of the matrix forms of the $\alpha 1$(XI) chain. *J. Biol. Chem.* **271**, 23743–23748.

78. Chapman, J. A. (1989). The regulation of size and form in the assembly of collagen fibrils *in vivo*. *Biopolymers* **28**, 1367–1382; erratum: *Ibid.*, pp. 2201–2205.

79. Hulmes, D. J. S. (1983). A possible mechanism for the regulation of collagen fibril diameter *in vivo*. *Collagen Relat. Res.* **3**, 317–321.

CHAPTER 21

Products of Cartilage Metabolism

DANIEL-HENRI MANICOURT   Laboratoire de Chimie Physiologique (Metabolic Research Group), Christian de Duve Institute of Cellular Pathology and Department of Rheumatology, Saint Luc University Hospital, University of Louvain in Brussels, 1200 Brussels, Belgium

HAFIDA EL HAJJAJI   Laboratoire de Chimie Physiologique (Metabolic Research Group), Christian de Duve Institute of Cellular Pathology, 1200 Brussels, Belgium

JEAN-PIERRE DEVOGELAER   Department of Rheumatology, Saint Luc University Hospital, University of Louvain in Brussels, 1200 Brussels, Belgium

EUGENE J.-M. A. THONAR   Departments of Biochemistry, Internal Medicine, and Orthopedic Surgery, Rush Medical College, Rush-Presbyterian-St. Luke's Medical Center, Chicago, Illinois 60612

I. INTRODUCTION

Cartilage makes up approximately 1% of the body's dry weight [1]. Distributed throughout the body, this hard but resilient tissue performs a variety of functions. During development, it acts as a growing scaffold for limb elongation. Articular cartilage covering the ends of bone in diarthrodial joints as well as the softer and more compressible nucleus pulposus of the intervertebral discs allow the joints in the rigid skeleton to articulate smoothly. Cartilage is the supporting structure of the respiratory tract (nose, larynx, trachea) and, as costal cartilage, contributes to the protection of lungs, heart, liver, and spleen from external physical stresses. It is worth pointing out that articular cartilage in diarthrodial (synovial) joints makes up only approximately 10% of the total cartilage mass in the body [1].

Joint diseases and related conditions involving abnormalities in the metabolism of cartilaginous tissues cause widespread disability. While articular cartilage failure was first regarded as a passive degenerative process, modern studies have provided a large body of evidence that this is not so. In osteoarthritis (OA), for example, the destruction of the articular surface is now thought to result from an imbalance between dynamic anabolic and catabolic processes that normally proceed in a harmonized and strictly regulated manner. Current research on cartilage includes attempts to define the

301

mechanisms that regulate the expression of cartilage-specific genes, to shed light upon the structural and functional properties of individual matrix components, and to better understand how these matrix building blocks are turned over in both health and disease. This chapter discusses primarily the major products of articular cartilage metabolism with special emphasis upon those that are relevant as body fluid markers.

The structure and supramolecular organization of major cartilage components as well as the main regulatory pathways of chondrocyte metabolism have been described in previous chapters. The following section provides a brief review of the structure-function relationships of the major matrix building blocks.

II. THE CHONDROCYTE AND ITS EXTRACELLULAR MATRIX

The primary function of articular cartilage is physical, with water, ions, and anionic aggrecan molecules within the collagenous meshwork all playing key roles in endowing the tissue with its load-bearing properties. The collagenous meshwork rich in type II collagen molecules gives the tissue tensile strength and hinders the expansion of the viscoelastic underhydrated aggrecan molecules that provide compressive stiffness. The highly sulfated aggrecan molecules interact noncovalently with a single strand of hyaluronan (HA) and link protein (LP) molecules to form supramolecular aggregates of very large size, which become firmly entrapped within the collagenous meshwork (see Chapter 5) [2, 3]. The resulting high fixed negative charge density, balanced by mobile counterions, gives rise to high osmotic pressures (up to 2–3 atm) [4, 5]. These are counteracted by the constant tension that is developed within the meshwork of cross-linked collagenous fibrils [4–6]. Cartilage is thus made stiff by being swollen with water. As aggrecan molecules oppose the fluid loss and the redistribution of water within the tissue, cartilage shows compliance upon loading, with the tissue rapidly recovering its elasticity when the load is removed. During cyclical loading, the fluid flow through the fine pores of the tissue not only dissipates energy and absorbs shocks but also participates in joint lubrication and contributes to chondrocyte nutrition [6]. It is obvious, therefore, that the structural integrity of the collagenous meshwork and aggrecan molecules is critically important for the maintenance of the biomechanical properties of the tissue.

The extracellular matrix (ECM) of cartilage contains many additional components that contribute to the cohesiveness of the matrix and to the regulation of chondrocyte function. For example, types IX and XI collagens (see Chapters 1 and 20) are essential players in the organization and functions of the major collagenous fibrils, whereas type VI collagen forms distinct microfibrils that appear concentrated in the capsular matrix surrounding individual chondrocytes or groups of chondrocytes. This protective structure, termed the chondron, dampens the osmotic and physico-mechanical changes induced by joint loading [7]. By interacting with growth factors and other macromolecules of the ECM, including collagens and fibronectin, small nonaggregating proteoglycans (PGs) (including decorin, biglycan, and fibromodulin) contribute to the regulation of chondrocyte function and to the maintenance of the supramolecular organization of the matrix. An ill-defined number of noncollagenous proteins also participate in the complex interactions that together form a network in which chondrocytes and most molecules of the ECM are involved [8].

Cartilage matrix building blocks are synthesized, organized, and maintained by a sparse population of chondrocytes. These cells are protected from the potentially damaging forces of mechanical function by the ECM they produce. As the properties of cartilage are critically dependent upon the structure and integrity of the ECM, normal turnover is a conservative process in which the rate of degradation of each molecular species does not exceed the rate at which it is replaced by newly synthesized products. The degradation of matrix molecules involves primarily proteinases (see Chapter 10) but probably also free radicals secreted by chondrocytes. In disease states, the rate of degradation of matrix molecules often exceeds the rate of synthesis, and, as a consequence, the tissue becomes thin and mechanically weak.

As cartilage is avascular, chondrocyte nutrition in a diarthrodial joint has to rely upon the diffusion of nutrients from the synovial fluid that bathes the tissue and links the different components within the joint. The oxygen tension in cartilage may be as low as 1–3%, compared to 24% in normal atmosphere [9, 10]. Mitochondria are sparse in chondrocytes, and the cells are well adapted to the conditions prevailing in the tissue. They metabolize glucose, primarily by glycolysis, to produce lactate even under aerobic conditions [11]. Anaerobic glycolysis provides most of the energy needs; ATP levels are unaffected by incubation in the presence of azide or nitrogen treatment [11–13]. By inhibiting glycolysis, iodoacetate reduces ATP levels and lactate production markedly and, in so doing, leads to degenerative changes in articular cartilage.

Since aggrecan molecules are highly sulfated, the Donnan equilibrium ensures that chondrocytes *in vivo* also survive in a relatively acidic environment and at a higher osmolarity than other types of cells (350–450 mOsm compared with 280 mOsm) [14]. *In vitro*, chondrocytes respond readily to alterations in their ionic environment [14]. Changes in the rate of synthesis of matrix macromolecules also occur *in vivo* when PG concentrations are altered during fluid loss under load and when cartilage swells due to a decrease in the tensile stiffness of the collagenous meshwork, as observed in the initial stages of OA.

In vivo, chondrocytes constantly experience changing hydrostatic pressures that modulate their metabolic activities. Mechanisms of mechano-transduction are not yet fully understood, but they probably involve integrins and other adhesion molecules (see Chapter 8). Fluctuating loads stimulate matrix production, with the extent of the response being influenced by the frequency, amplitude, and waveforms, whereas static pressure causes a reduction in the rate of synthesis of both aggrecan and LP molecules without affecting HA synthesis [15–17]. Joint immobilization also causes a marked loss in PGs from articular cartilage [18, 19]. This depletion, reflecting both a decline in the rate of PG synthesis and an increase in PG catabolism, is however completely reversible when the joints are remobilized [18, 19]. The absence of motion appears more critical than the lack of loading, since even small amounts of motion of the unloaded joint reduce the severity of the PG depletion, a finding that justifies the clinical use of continuous passive motion [20].

It should be stressed that, with distance from the articular surface, chondrocytes exhibit heterogeneity with respect to shape, surface receptors, and metabolic activities [21, 22]. Chondrocytes from the deeper layers of articular cartilage exhibit a faster rate of PG synthesis and a slower rate of PG turnover than cells from the superficial layers, a finding that is consistent with the observation that net matrix accumulation is more pronounced around deep but superficial chondrocytes. On the other hand, chondrocytes from the superficial layers secrete greater amounts of matrix-degrading proteinases when stimulated with cytokines and are even more responsive to interleukin-1 [23]. The precise reasons for this type of heterogeneity among chondrocytes are not obvious. However, it is clear that the shape and magnitude of the biomechanical stresses are unevenly distributed throughout the cartilage matrix. It also is clear that chondrocytes in different layers are subjected to different concentrations of nutrients and metabolites.

III. PRODUCTS OF COLLAGEN METABOLISM

As stated in Chapter 1, the synthesis of type II collagen involves several unique posttranslational modifications. A large precursor molecule, termed procollagen (Fig. 1), is processed soon after its release extracellularly: its N- and C-terminal propeptides are cleaved by specific N- and C-propeptidases, allowing the resulting tropocollagen molecule to become incorporated into a fibril.

The C-propeptide of the pro [α(II)] chain, also referred to as chondrocalcin, contains 245 amino acids. Most C-propeptide molecules are thought to diffuse out of the cartilage matrix after they are produced: their concentration in body fluids can be measured by specific immunoassays [24]. Support for the contention that the level of this body fluid marker provides a measure of the rate of type II collagen synthesis in cartilage comes from the observation that the rate of synthesis of type II collagen in articular cartilage is directly proportional to the tissue content of C-propeptide: the latter was found to have a half-life of 15–20 hours [25]. Concentrations of the C-propeptide in synovial fluid were found to be higher in traumatic and primary OA than in rheumatoid arthritis (RA) or infectious arthritis [26], confirming the widely held view that the degradative events in OA are balanced, at least during the early stages, by an upregulation of the biosynthetic processes.

Once tropocollagen molecules have spontaneously aggregated into fibrils (Fig. 1), complex covalent cross-links form within and between the collagen molecules to enhance the cohesiveness of the collagenous meshwork (see Chapter 2). The only step of the cross-linking process that is known to be cell-controlled is the oxidative deamination (by lysyl oxidase) of the ε-amino group in telopeptidyl lysine and hydroxylysine residues to form the aldehydes termed allysine and hydroxyallysine, respectively [27]. The hydroxyallysine-derived cross-links predominate in cartilage and lead almost exclusively to the formation of the stable, nonreducible, and trivalent 3-hydroxypyridinium cross-link termed hydroxylysyl pyridinoline (also termed pyridinoline), whose concentrations change little during adulthood. It is worth noting that articular cartilage shows a marked age-related enrichment in a different type of cross-link produced by nonenzymatic means [28].

Since type II collagen is the most abundant component of the collagenous meshwork in cartilage (90–95% of the total collagen content), the proteolytic degradation of this fibrillar collagen is likely to be an important rate-limiting step in tissue remodeling both in health and disease. Proteinases can contribute to the extracellular degradation of type II collagen in several ways. First, by cleaving the telopeptides of collagen molecules, proteinases separate the intact triple helical domain from the telopeptide cross-links and thus depolymerize the collagen molecules without actually damaging the triple helix: the latter can be recognized by monoclonal antibodies that only react with the intact native triple helical molecule [29]. Second, proteinases can also cleave the triple helical domain of the native, fully wound collagen molecules. At physiologic temperature, the cleaved triple helix unwinds (Fig. 1) to yield denatured collagen or gelatin and exposes neoepitopes that are normally hidden and not recognized in the native triple helix but are recognizable on cyanogen bromide peptides of type II collagen [29, 30]. Third, proteinases can also degrade gelatin and/or activate zymogens, which thereby acquire the ability to cleave collagen molecules.

Neutrophil elastase and stromelysin-1 or metalloproteinase-3 (MMP-3) are the only mammalian proteinases known to cleave telopeptides *in vitro* [31, 32]. A recent study of cultured cartilage explants [33] has suggested that cleavage of the N-telopeptide by MMP-3 is not likely to be a major mechanism in the chondrocyte-mediated degradation of collagen. Nevertheless, MMP-3 could still contribute indirectly to collagen breakdown by activating collagenase-1 (MMP-1),

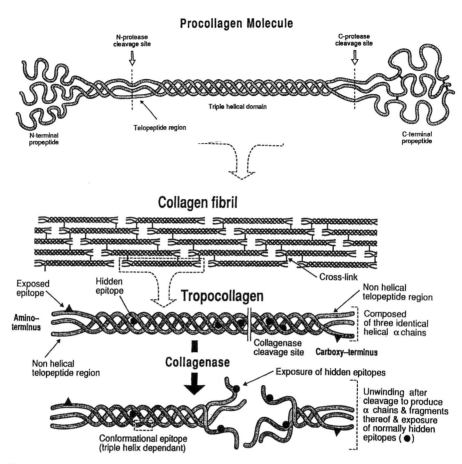

FIGURE 1   Type II collagen fibrils are made of tropocollagen molecules interconnected by cross-links between the nonhelical telopeptide regions of individual tropocollagen molecules and the helical region of adjacent molecules. Each tropocollagen molecule is composed of three identical α chains. After a first cleavage by any one of the three mammalian collagenases (MMP-1, MMP-8, and MMP-13), the cleaved triple helix unwinds at physiological temperature and exposes hidden epitopes on α chains that are not recognized on the native triple helix. Epitopes on nonhelical telopeptides and conformational triple helical dependent epitopes are also indicated. Adapted from Poole [29] with permission.

collagenase-3 (MMP-13), and gelatinase B (MMP-9) [34–36]. It also should be noted that neutrophil elastase can also activate MMP-3 and MMP-8 [36].

Thus far, MMP-1, MMP-8 (neutrophil collagenase), and MMP-13 are the only mammalian proteinases known to be capable of hydrolyzing the intrahelical domain of native fibrillar collagens at neutral pH [37–39]. The first cleavage occurs at a single site (Gly775–Leu/Ile776) through all three α chains, three quarters of the way from the N-terminal end (Fig. 1). This produces denatured α chain fragments with lengths approximately three-fourths (TC^A fragment) and one-fourth (TC^B fragment) of the native molecule. Immunohistochemical staining and immunoassays conducted with antibodies that react specifically with denatured but not with native type II α chains have established that adult normal human cartilage may contain up to 3% of its total collagen in the denatured form [30, 40] and that, although denaturation of type II collagen is enhanced in cartilage obtained from

joints with OA and RA, the topographical distribution of the collagen cleavages differs markedly between the two arthritides [41]. In OA cartilage, the earliest damage to collagen is detected in the superficial zone of the tissue, whereas in RA, denaturation of type II collagen is much more pronounced in the territorial matrix surrounding chondrocytes of the deeper layers. These findings strongly suggest that cytokines derived from subchondral bone might enhance chondrocyte-derived degradation of the collagen meshwork in RA.

After cleavage of the α chains by any one of the three collagenases (MMP-1, MMP-8, and MMP-13), unwinding of the triple helix exposes neoepitopes at the C terminus of the TC^A fragments and at the N terminus of the TC^B fragments (Fig. 2). Immunoassays conducted with antibodies reacting specifically with the C-terminal (COL2-3/4 short) and N-terminal (COL2-1/4 N1) neoepitopes have demonstrated that, in both normal and OA cartilages, the content of COL2-3/4 short neoepitope correlates strongly with the tissue content

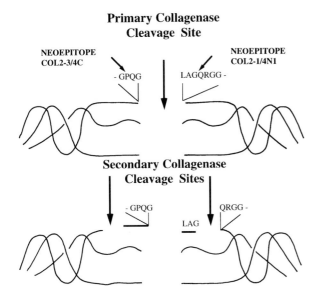

Primary Collagenase Cleavage Site

NEOEPITOPE COL2-3/4C

NEOEPITOPE COL2-1/4N1

- GPQG

LAGQRGG -

Secondary Collagenase Cleavage Sites

- GPQG

LAG

QRGG -

FIGURE 2   The three mammalian collagenases (MMP-1, MMP-8, and MMP-13) first cleave the triple helical domain of type II procollagen molecules at a site located three quarters of the way from the N terminus of the molecule. This cleavage unwinds the triple helix and exposes two neoepitopes, i.e., the C terminus of the N-terminal α chain fragment, termed COL2-3/4 C, and the N terminus of the C-terminal α chain fragment, termed COL2-1/4 N1. The N-terminal neoepitope COL2-1/4 N1 is rapidly destroyed by secondary cleavage sites of collagenases that also release the C-terminal neoepitope COL2-3/4 C that then diffuses out of the matrix to reach biological fluids where it can be detected. The amino acid sequence of the neoepitopes is also given. See Billinghurst *et al.* [42].

of denatured type II collagen. This finding supports the contention that collagenase activity is responsible for the cleavage of type II collagen in human articular cartilage [42].

In vitro, MMP-13 hydrolyzes type II collagen more readily than either MMP-1 or MMP-8 [35]. A study of cartilage explants exposed to synthetic inhibitors of collagenases has confirmed that MMP-13 might be the most important collagenase involved in type II collagen degradation [42]. However, other members of the MMP family, such as MMP-2 (gelatinase A), MMP-3, and MMP-9, are very efficient at cleaving denatured α chains and at removing damaged collagen from the extracellular matrix [43]. It is thought that this subsequent clearance of unwound α chains may be a necessary event to facilitate repair. On the other hand, it is possible the gelatinolytic enzymes cause additional damage to the cartilage matrix.

The COL2-3/4 short neoepitope seems to be a better marker of collagenase cleavage than the COL2-1/4 N1 neoepitope since the N-terminal neoepitope is readily destroyed by a secondary collagenase-mediated cleavage. As collagenases produce further cleavages at the C terminus of TC^A fragment [39, 42], albeit at a slower rate, the COL2-3/4 short neoepitope is released and can be readily detected in the culture medium of cartilage explants [42]. Quantification of the COL2-3/4 short neoepitope in body fluids might thus be of

great value for the assessment of type II collagen turnover *in vivo*.

Little is known about the degradation of other collagens in cartilage. By degrading type IX collagen [32], MMP-3 might decrease the tensile stiffness of cartilage, since this collagen is believed to function as a covalent bridge between collagenous fibrils. The degradation of type IX collagen also might allow the diameter of collagen fibrils to increase during growth and maturation, as the type IX molecules must be removed before fibril growth can occur, either by accretion of additional type II molecules or by lateral fusion of thin fibrils (see Chapter 20).

When cartilage collagens are degraded, fragments bearing pyridinoline cross-links are released into proximal fluids, i.e., synovial fluid in the case of a diarthrodial joint, and from there enter the systemic circulation. They have been shown to be most effectively cleared by filtration through the kidneys. Pyridinoline, but not deoxypyridinoline (the bone-specific cross-link), has been detected in OA and RA synovial fluids [44]. The urinary excretion of pyridinoline increases approximately two-fold in patients with OA and four-fold in patients with RA [45–48]. However, thus far it still is not clear how much of this increase can be attributed to degradative changes occurring in cartilaginous structures. Indeed, although urinary levels of pyridinoline correlate with the severity and the extent of joint involvement in patients with OA [47–50], the increase in urinary pyridinoline originating from cartilage is likely to be blurred by the concomitant increase in bone turnover associated with joint lesions. This is supported by the finding that the molar ratio of pyridinoline to deoxypyridinoline in urine from these patients is very similar to that in urine from healthy subjects and in normal human bone [51]. In RA patients, on the other hand, the increase in urinary pyridinoline levels exceeds that of deoxypyridinoline. Further, it correlates strongly with systemic and clinical parameters of disease activity [45, 48, 52], suggesting that diseased joints, including the inflamed synovium, contribute to the increase in urinary pyridinoline. Interpretation of analyses of pyridinium cross-links in body fluids, while difficult at this time, should become simpler once immunoassays capable of quantifying neoepitopes bound to the cross-links and generated by proteolytic cleavage of the telopeptides of α (II) chains become available. This approach, first used to quantify type I collagen-specific cross-links, is currently under development [53].

IV. PRODUCTS OF AGGRECAN METABOLISM

The numerous chondroitin sulfate (CS) and keratan sulfate (KS) chains carried by the long extended interglobular domain (IGD) of the aggrecan core protein give this PG a bottle-brush structure with viscoelastic properties (Fig. 3). This

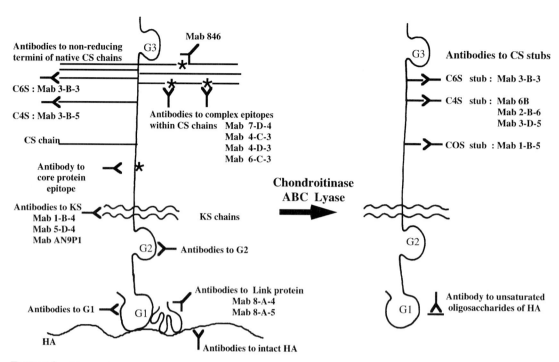

FIGURE 3 Through its globular domain G1, aggrecan interacts with hyaluronan (HA) and link protein (LP) to form supramolecular aggregates of a very large size. The function of G2 is unknown and G3 has a role in intracellular translocation. Some of the antibodies that react with the core protein and the chondroitin sulfate (CS) and keratan sulfate (KS) chains are indicated. Other monoclonal antibodies (Mabs) react with the chondroitin sulfate chain that remains attached to the core protein after chondroitinase ABC lyase digestion. Adapted from Poole [29] with permission.

elaborate architecture, however, leaves vulnerable to proteolytic attack the glycosaminoglycan (GAG)-poor N-terminal end of the molecule that separates the GAG attachment region from the first globular (G1) domain that interacts with HA and LP and thus anchors the aggrecan molecule in the matrix.

Newly secreted aggrecan molecules have low affinity for HA. Their maturation into the high-affinity form probably involves the formation of disulfide bonds in the G1 domain [54, 55]. This, coupled to an accelerated transport termed rapid polymer transport, may enable newly secreted molecules to diffuse away from the metabolically active pericellular environment and enter the metabolically inactive interterritorial matrix compartment before aggregating [56]. In contrast, LP molecules are fully capable of binding to both HA and aggrecan molecules when they are released extracellularly. Binding of LP to newly synthesized aggrecan molecules might provide the stability the latter need for interacting early with HA [8]. This may play a key role in determining what proportion of newly synthesized aggrecan molecules become established in the pericellular/cell-associated matrix.

While studies of the racemization of aspartic acid have suggested that aggrecan molecules turn over much more rapidly (average half-life of approximately 2 years) than collagen molecules within the fibrillar network [57, 58], the results of both *in vivo* [59, 60] and *in vitro* [61–63] studies have suggested that articular cartilage contains at least two pools

of aggrecan molecules with different rates of turnover. Recent studies have suggested that these two pools of aggrecan molecules reside in different compartments of the matrix: a cell-associated matrix compartment in which they turn over rapidly and a further removed, more abundant, interterritorial matrix compartment in which the PGs turn over much more slowly [56, 64].

GAG-rich fragments generated by proteolytic cleavage of the core protein of aggrecan molecules are lost relatively rapidly from the cartilage matrix. In the case of articular cartilage, they diffuse into the synovial fluid, where they can be quantified by chemical assays of their sulfated GAGs [65, 66] or by immunoassays capable of measuring specific protein [25, 67, 68] or carbohydrate epitopes [69, 70]. They also can be characterized by sequencing after isolation and deglycosylation [71–73]. The development of monospecific antibodies that recognize enzyme-generated neoepitopes has proved most useful for identifying and quantifying specific proteolytic cleavage products [74–80]. Proteinases of different classes and hydroxyl radicals [81] have the capacity to cleave the aggrecan core protein *in vitro*. Importantly, the use of antibodies against these types of neoepitopes has now provided strong evidence that several metalloproteinases and an as yet unidentified enzyme termed aggrecanase play major roles *in vivo* in the catabolism of aggrecan molecules both in health and disease.

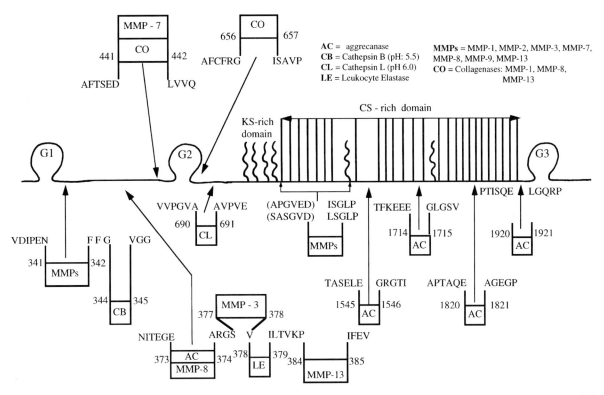

FIGURE 4   Sites of cleavage of aggrecan core protein by tissue proteinases. The two major sites of cleavage are located in the short extended interglobular domain between the globular domain G1 and the globular domain G2. The first one is generated by metalloproteinases (MMPs) and occurs between residues Asn 341 and Phe 342, whereas the second one generated by the so-termed aggrecanase is located between residues Glu 373 and Ala 374. Both cleavage sites separate the anchoring G1 domain from the bulk of the aggrecan molecule carrying the glycosaminoglycan side chains and thus deprive cartilage of its load-bearing properties. The N-terminal and C-terminal amino acid sequences of the neoepitopes resulting from the different cleavage sites as well as the nature of the proteinases acting at these sites are also indicated. The correct size of different domains is not respected.

The location of the sites of proteolytic attack upon the core protein of aggrecan is of critical importance (Fig. 4). When proteolytic processing is confined to the C terminus or the GAG-rich region, the aggrecan molecules retain some GAGs and thus are able to continue to exert their physicochemical properties. Cleavage of the aggrecan molecule near its G1 domain results in rapid loss of the whole GAG-attachment region and thus has more adverse consequences, at least from the functional standpoint [55]. The contention that progressive C-terminal trimming of aggrecan molecules occurs *in vivo* is supported by N-terminal sequencing of aggrecan fragments released into the conditioned medium of cartilage explants [55, 71, 82, 83] as well as by physiochemical and electron microscopic analysis of aggrecan molecules extracted from cartilage. These studies have identified in adult articular cartilage an abundance of polydisperse molecules lacking the G3 domain and exhibiting a great variability in the length of their CS-rich domain [84–87]. In contrast to MMP-2, MMP-3, and MMP-9, which apparently cleave at two sites within the CS domain, aggrecanase has at least three cleavage sites (Fig. 4) and, therefore, might be the most important enzyme responsible for the accumulation within the

vast interterritorial matrix of aggrecan molecules exhibiting a large variation in the length of their CS domain.

Two major cleavage sites have been identified in the short extended IGD that separates the G1 and G2 domains: one occurs between residues Asn 341 and Phe 342 and the other is located between residues Glu 373 and Ala 374 (Fig. 4). The first major cleavage site generates a G1-containing fragment with the C-terminal neoepitope VDIPEN-341 and a larger GAG-bearing fragment with the N-terminal neoepitope 342-FFGVGGE [78, 79, 88, 89]. It is the major cleavage site of several metalloproteinases, including stromelysin-1 (MMP-3), the three collagenases (MMP-1, MMP-8, and MMP-13), and the two gelatinases (MMP-2 and MMP-9). The results of many studies support the contention that MMPs are implicated in the breakdown of aggrecan molecules *in vivo*. First, cartilage and synovial fluid from patients with OA and other inflammatory arthritides contain enhanced levels of MMPs. Second, retinoic acid and pro-inflammatory cytokines (IL-1 and TNF-α) known to upregulate the expression of several MMPs promote aggrecan loss from cartilage explants [90–93]; this loss can be prevented by adding specific inhibitors of MMPs to the conditioned medium [94–96]. Third, the

N- and C-terminal neoepitope sequences specific for MMPs are present in both cartilage [88] and synovial fluid [77]. Finally, the demonstration that the concentration of the VDIPEN-341 neoepitope in normal human articular cartilage increases up to 25 years of age and then reaches an apparent steady state (representing 15–20% of the G1-containing molecules residing within the matrix) [80] suggests that MMP-generated G1 fragments might account, at least in part, for the increase in the cartilage content of aggrecan G1 domains with growth and maturation [97].

Although MMPs have the capacity to cleave at other sites within the IGD of aggrecan molecules, this requires higher enzyme concentrations. Thus, MMP-1, MMP-7, MMP-8, and MMP-13 all cleave the Asp 441–Leu 442 bond (Fig. 4), whereas MMP-3 also cleaves at Ser 377–Val 378, MMP-8 at Glu 373–Ala 374, and MMP-13 at Pro 384–Val 385 [98].

Aggrecanase cleaves the core protein of aggrecan at the second major cleavage site. This produces a large GAG-rich aggrecan fragment with the N-terminal neoepitope 374-ARGSVI and a G1 fragment with the C-terminal neoepitope NITEGE-373 (Fig. 4). Aggrecanase-mediated aggrecan cleavage occurs both *in vivo* and *in vitro*: the N-terminal neoepitope 374-ARGSVI has been found in the medium of cartilage explant cultures [71, 76, 82, 83] as well as in high density aggrecan fragments recovered from human synovial fluids [72–74].

The contention that MMPs and aggrecanase are both involved in the turnover of aggrecan molecules in normal and diseased cartilage is supported by the finding that MMP-generated G1 fragments terminating in VDIPEN-341 and aggrecanase-generated G1 fragments terminating in NITEGE-373 are both detected not only in cartilage from joints with OA and RA, two conditions exhibiting quite contrasting pathological and clinical features, but also in cartilage from normal adult joints (Fig. 5) [80]. The generation and/or turnover of these specific aggrecan fragments is not necessarily coordinated, since both the NITEGE-373 and VDIPEN-341 neoepitopes can be noncoincident within a single joint [78,

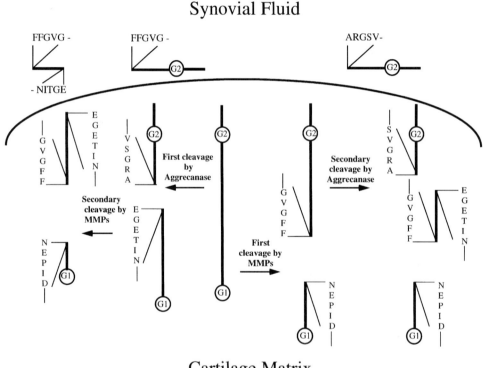

FIGURE 5   Hypothetical pathways for proteolytic cleavage of aggrecans in cartilage matrix. The VDIPEN neoepitope can be detected in the matrix after primary cleavage of the interglobular domain (IGD) between G1 and G2 by aggrecanase. After a secondary cleavage site by metalloproteinases (MMPs), the NITEGE neoepitope can also be detected in the matrix whereas large fragments with an N terminus of ARGVS and a small 30-amino-acid peptide with FFGVG- and -NITEGE termini can be detected in the synovial fluid. In contrast, only the VDIPEN neoepitope can be detected in the matrix after primary cleavage of aggrecan IGD by MMPs, which also allows large fragments with an N terminus of FFGVG to diffuse into the synovial fluid. Should secondary cleavage by aggrecanase occur, then large fragments with an N terminus of ARGVS and a small 30-amino-acid peptide with FFGVG- and -NITEGE termini would be detected in the synovial fluid depending on the efficacy of the second cleavage. Adapted from Lark *et al.* [80] with authors' permission.

80], and turnover of aggrecan by cultured rat chondrosarcoma cells and primary bovine chondrocytes can be mediated almost exclusively by aggrecanase [76]. It is interesting that immunostaining for both the VDIPEN-341 and NITEGE-373 neoepitopes is usually more marked in the pericellular/cell-associated matrix where aggrecan molecules are known to turn over more rapidly than in other matrix compartments.

Although the major cleavage site of MMPs is located in close proximity to that of aggrecanase, it is intriguing to note that the aggrecan fragments released from cartilage after MMP cleavage of the IGD are quite different from the aggrecan fragments released from the tissue after aggrecanase cleavage of the IGD. Aggrecanase-generated fragments are usually large and have a short N-terminal stretch of the IGD, a G2 domain, a KS-domain, and a CS-rich domain of variable length. MMP-generated fragments, however, lack CS chains and contain either no G2 domain or a G2 domain with or without a small part of the KS-rich region [55, 72]. The reason for this difference is not clear. It is possible that aggrecan molecules cleaved by MMPs at the Asn 341–Phe 342 bond are subject to further proteolysis by other proteinases or MMPs and/or that the aggrecan fragments that have undergone progressive C-terminal trimming over time represent preferred substrates for MMPs while longer aggrecan molecules are preferentially cleaved by aggrecanase. However, it is clear that even when the proteolysis of the core protein is extensive, aggrecan may be cleaved by MMPs or aggrecanase in the interglobular domain but not by both [79]. The observations that fragments bearing a G1 domain bearing a VDIPEN-341 neoepitope (rather than a NITEGE-373 neoepitope) are present in human synovial fluids [68, 80] and appear rapidly in rabbit knee joint fluid after an intra-articular injection of MMP-3 [100] suggest that there is further processing of the HA-G1 complex after the large interglobular domain has been cleaved off by aggrecanase and has diffused out of the matrix (Fig. 6). It should be noted that studies conducted in bovine cartilage explants have suggested that HA and aggrecan are catabolized at similar rates. It is probable, therefore, that part of the degradation involved internalization by the chondrocytes (Fig. 6) [100, 101]. Further work is clearly needed to clarify the fate of MMP- and aggrecanase-generated aggrecan fragments and to better evaluate the relative importance of both enzymatic activities in normal cartilage and in arthritis.

Measurement of GAG epitopes can also provide a measure of the turnover of PGs. Immunoassays that use monoclonal antibodies (Table I and Fig. 3) capable of recognizing KS epitopes in intact aggrecan molecules or fragments thereof [69, 102] have shown that levels of antigenic KS in blood circulation correlate well with the concentration of aggrecan core protein-related epitopes in serum, suggesting that the serum level of agKS offers a good measure of the level of aggrecan-derived fragments in this body fluid

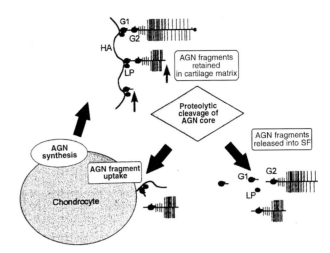

FIGURE 6 Diagram of metabolic pathways of G1-containing fragments of aggrecan (AGN) in cartilage matrix. By assuming that there is no further C-terminal processing of AGN fragments, the matrix content of G1 fragments containing the C terminus of VDIPEN or NITEGE results from (1) the rate of secretion of aggrecan by chondrocytes; (2) the rate of cleavage of the interglobular domain located between G1 and G2 by aggrecanase or matrix metalloproteinases; (3) the rate of chondrocyte uptake of free G1 or complexes made of hyaluronan (HA), link protein (LP), and G1; and (4) the rate of diffusion of the free G1 and HA–G1–LP complexes into the synovial fluid (SF). Reproduced from Lark *et al.* [80] with authors' permission.

(see Chapter 32). Although the function of KS is still unclear, its rate of synthesis is inversely related to the ambient oxygen tension [103], and, accordingly, the KS content of aggrecan increases with distance from the articular surface [104, 105]. Aggrecan exhibits an age-related increase in the number and size of their KS chains, and a decrease in its KS content in OA cartilage. Monoclonal antibodies have also been raised against unusual sequences on CS chains (Table I and Fig. 3). Two epitopes, 3-D-5 and 7-D-4, are present in normal mature articular cartilage [106]. The content of the 7-D-4 epitope in aggrecan increases markedly in diseased cartilage from different species [106]. The CS epitopes 846 and 3-B-3 are found at highest concentrations in fetal cartilage; they are barely detectable in adult cartilage, but both reappear in enhanced amounts in cartilage and synovial fluid from OA and RA joints [70, 106]. The 846 epitope does not contain unsaturated disaccharides of chondroitin-6-sulfate [29]. As it is present on intact CS chains located in close proximity to the G3 domain of the core protein of newly synthesized aggrecan molecules, it may be a useful marker of aggrecan synthesis during inflammation and disease processes. On the other hand, the emergence of the 3-B-3 epitope in articular cartilage showing progressive destructive changes after intra-articular injection of chymopapain suggests it may be a marker of irreversible changes, a contention strengthened by the finding that the 3-B-3 epitope is found in much lower amounts in joints whose articular surface repairs successfully [107].

TABLE I. Monoclonal Antibodies Commonly Used to Analyze Aggrecan and Other Components of Proteoglycan Aggregates

Monoclonal antibody	Antibody specificity
5-D-4 and 1-B-4	Skeletal and corneal keratan sulfate. Highly sulfated sequence of several repeats of 6-sulfated N-acetylglucosamine-β1,3-6-sulfated galactose-β1,4.
AN9P1	Keratan sulfate. Sulfated poly (N-acetyl lactosamine) sequences of hepta- or larger oligosaccharides of 6-sulfated galactose and N-acetylglucosamine.
2-B-4 (B) and 9-A-2 (B)	Generated by chondroitinase digestion of aggrecans. Delta-unsaturated disaccharides of chondroitin-4-sulfate, but not chondroitin-6-sulfate and unsulfated chondroitin.
846 (A)	Intact chondroitin-6-sulfate chains but not unsaturated disaccharides of chondroitin-6-sulfate
3-B-3 (C)	Nonreducing termini of native chondroitin sulfate chains containing a terminal hexuronate residue adjacent to a 6-sulfated N-acetylglucosamine residue. Delta-unsaturated or saturated oligosaccharides of chondroitin-6-sulfate generated by chondroitinase or testicular hyaluronidase digestion.
3-D-5 (C)	Nonreducing termini of native chondroitin sulfate chains containing a terminal hexuronate residue adjacent to a 4-sulfated N-acetylglucosamine residue. Delta-unsaturated or saturated oligosaccharides of chondroitin-4-sulfate generated by chondroitinase or testicular hyaluronidase digestion.
2-B-6 (B)	Delta-unsaturated or saturated oligosaccharides of chondroitin-4-sulfate generated by chondroitinase or testicular hyaluronidase digestion.
1-B-5 (B)	Delta-unsaturated or saturated oligosaccharides of unsulfated chondroitin generated by chondroitinase or testicular hyaluronidase digestion.
7-D-4 (A)	Chondroitin sulfate oligosaccharide containing 10–12 sugar residues. Probably contains several of the eight possible CS-isomer disaccharide combinations.
4-C-3 (A) 4-D-3 (A) 6-C-3 (A)	Complex epitopes residing within native chondroitin sulfate chains.
8-A-4	Determinant common to link protein (LP) isolated from aggregates recovered from cartilage of different species. Determinant present in the three molecular forms of LP (LP1, LP2, and LP3).
8-A-5	Similar to that of 8-A-4. Reduction and carboxymethylation of the link protein does not alter the epitope.

Note. The list is not exhaustive. Monoclonal antibodies directed against chondroitin sulfate epitopes can be divided into two categories: (1) those that recognize epitopes present on the native chondroitin sulfate glycosaminoglycan chains (A) and (2) those that require predigestion of the chondroitin sulfate glycosaminoglycan with endo- or exoglycosidases to generate their reducing terminal epitopes (B). Some antibodies (C) recognize epitopes that fall into both of these categories.

V. PRODUCTS OF THE METABOLISM OF LINK PROTEIN AND HYALURONAN

The synthesis of LP follows the biosynthetic pathway of other secretory proteins through the endoplasmic reticulum and the Golgi. HA, however, is synthesized on the inner side of the plasma membrane: the growing HA chain is extruded into the extracellular space [108]. This unusual mode of synthesis allows unconstrained polymer growth and explains why HA molecules can reach exceptionally large sizes. Three mammalian putative HA synthases have been identified (as reviewed in 109): they are the products of three different genes, but it is not clear which one is present at the surface of the chondrocyte.

Although chondrocytes synthesize two molecular forms of LP that differ in their degrees of glycosylation (LP1, $M_r = 48,000$; LP2, $M_r = 44,000$), PG aggregates contain an additional smaller form (LP3, $M_r = 41,000$) that results from the cleavage of the N-terminal region of the two larger forms [110]. Three major cleavage sites have been identified in this N-terminal region of intact LPs (Fig. 7). The first one occurs between residues 16 and 17 (His and Ile); it is the only one found in LP3 isolated from newborn cartilage and seems to be produced by MMP-3. LP3 from mature cartilage exhibits two additional amino termini: one is compatible with cleavage between residues 18 and 19 (Glu and Ala), a property of cathepsins B and G, whereas the other one occurs between residues 23 and 24 (Pro and His). The enzyme(s) responsible for this site of cleavage has not been identified. As the three forms of LP possess the three disulfide-bonded loops that are associated with LP function, LP3 generation is not likely to affect the stability of PG aggregates. *In vitro* studies have also shown that the N-terminal disulfide-bonded loop of LPs can be cleaved at one site by cathepsin L [110] and at two sites by hydroxyl radicals [81]; however, none of these corresponds to the sites of cleavage observed *in vivo*, i.e., between residues 65 and 66 (Lys and Tryp) and 72 and 73 (Asp and Tyr). Whether these native cleavage sites result

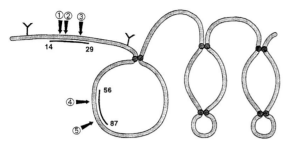

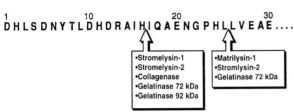

FIGURE 7   Sites of cleavage of link protein (LP) in human articular cartilage. *In vitro*, many proteolytic agents are able to cleave the LP within the N-terminal region between amino acid residues 14 and 29 to produce the LP3 forms of the molecule. In contrast, only a few proteolytic agents can cleave the LP *in vitro* within the disulfide-bonded loop between amino acid residues 56 and 87 to produce LP fragments upon reduction. The site for LP3 generation (1 between residues 16 and 17, 2 between residues 18 and 19, and 3 between residues 23 and 24) and LP fragment generation (4 between residues 65 and 66 and 5 between residues 72 and 73) *in vivo* occur within the same regions that are susceptible to *in vitro* proteolysis. The sites cleaved by metalloproteinases are also shown. Adapted from Roughley *et al.* [110] with permission.

from the action of a yet to be identified enzyme remains to be established. On the other hand, the continued ability of fragmented LPs to interact with HA probably reflects the lack of proteolytic modification within the C-terminal disulfide-bonded loops.

Very little is known about the half-life and turnover of LP in the cartilage matrix. In canine experimental OA, the synovial fluid levels of LP and the rate of loss of this glycoprotein from cultured cartilage explants increases several-fold within 3 months after disease induction [66, 111]. In contrast, the synovial fluid levels of LP are markedly decreased in disused joints [111]. These findings are in close agreement with the progressive disappearance of the link-rich, more saturated aggregates from the cartilage matrix in experimental OA and with the maintenance of these fast-sedimenting aggregates in disuse atrophy [18, 112]. Although articular cartilage from both canine OA and disused joints exhibit enhanced levels of matrix degrading enzymes, these cartilages differ in their HA content: it is markedly reduced in OA and unchanged in disuse. The same holds true for human OA cartilage. Since, in contrast to the disuse process, the OA process is apparently irreversible, one might argue that the loss of both HA and link-rich aggregates prognosticates articular cartilage destruction.

Half of the HA molecules synthesized by cultured explants of normal articular cartilage diffuse rapidly into the culture medium [113]. The newly synthesized HA molecules remaining within the matrix are quite large, but with time they are gradually depolymerized to give a molecular size distribution similar to that observed for the endogenous HA [113, 114]. As no hyaluronidase has been identified thus far in the cartilage matrix, it has been suggested that this depolymerization may result from the action of oxygen-derived free radicals [115]. On the other hand, chondrocytes do have the capacity to internalize and degrade HA to small oligosaccharides within a low pH lysosomal compartment, with the endocytosis being mediated via cell surface CD44/HA receptors [116]. Factors that upregulate chondrocyte catabolism, such as interleukin-1 and the 29 kDa fibronectin fragment, also cause an increased expression of CD44 at the cell surface [117].

As cartilage is bathed by synovial fluid, many investigators have studied the effects of exogenous HA upon matrix metabolism. The addition of HA of relatively high molecular mass ($M_r = 2 \times 10^5$) to the culture medium of cartilage explants inhibits the synthesis of both HA and aggrecan molecules in a concentration-dependent manner [115]. This effect, which is reversible upon removal of the HA from the culture medium, may be mediated via the induction of nitric oxide synthase through activation of the transcriptional regulator factor kB [118]. Conversely, the addition of HA tetrasaccharides or hexasaccharides to the culture medium of cartilage explants does not change the rate of synthesis of either HA or aggrecan but reduces the rate of loss of HA from the tissue [115]. It is possible that these small oligosaccharides compete with endogenous HA molecules for the CD44 and/or other receptors involved in the internalization and breakdown of HA.

VI. PRODUCTS OF THE METABOLISM OF OTHER MATRIX COMPONENTS

The metabolism of other cartilage matrix components has received much less attention, and, as a consequence, very little is known about the mechanisms regulating their degradation during normal turnover or in disease. The small non-aggregating PGs might display longer half-lives than aggrecan molecules [119]. The content of biglycan declines after maturity; further, the proportion of degraded forms free of GAG may reach up to 15% in old age [120]. Decorin is found as a GAG-substituted form at all ages; a nonglycanated form can, however, be detected in limited amounts in adult cartilage. The degree of substitution of KS-containing fibromodulin and lumican also decreases with aging [121].

Upon stimulation with IL-1, both native and fragmented forms of decorin are lost from the cartilage matrix, but the nature of the enzyme(s) involved in this catabolic event remains to be established. This cytokine also markedly reduces the rate of synthesis of biglycan and decorin in explants of normal cartilage [122]. In OA cartilage, the concentrations of biglycan and decorin have been reported to be either enhanced [123] or unchanged [124]. This discrepancy may be explained by the fact that these two studies used antibodies recognizing different epitopes. In the first study, the epitopes were located near the C termini of the two small PGs and thus were able to recognize both intact and degraded forms of the molecules. In the second study, the antibodies were directed against epitopes located near the N termini of the molecules and thus probably recognized only the intact forms of decorin and biglycan.

Degradation products from noncollagenous proteins could also provide useful information about the pathologic changes taking place in cartilage. An elevation in the synovial fluid levels of cartilage oligomeric matrix protein (COMP) does not seem specific for a particular form of joint disease [125]. These levels also do not correlate with the rate of joint destruction in RA patients [126]. In contrast, longitudinal studies of patients with joint disease have indicated that a high serum level of COMP tends to prognosticate rapid articular cartilage destruction [25]. Little is known about the metabolism of COMP in cartilage and it is therefore difficult to put these findings in perspective. Further, recent studies have shown that COMP is found in significant amounts in synovium and several other connective tissues and have suggested that it can no longer be considered a cartilage-specific protein [127]. However, COMP, and especially its disease-specific degradation fragments [128], appear to hold great promise as markers of metabolic processes in articular cartilage and other joint tissues.

VII. OTHER PRODUCTS OF CHONDROCYTE METABOLISM

When stimulated by bacterial lipopolysaccharide and proinflammatory cytokines such as IL-1, chondrocytes synthesize an inducible isoform of nitric oxide (NO) synthase (iNOS) [22, 129], an induction that can be markedly inhibited by anti-inflammatory cytokines such as interleukin-4 and interleukin-10 [130], as well as by nonsteroidal anti-inflammatory drugs [131]. Once induced, this iNOS generates large amounts of NO and L-citrulline for a sustained period of time through the oxidation of the guanidino nitrogen of L-arginine. It has been estimated that chondrocyte-derived NO contributes significantly to the total NO produced in the joint cavity in inflammatory arthritides [132].

Several experimental studies implicate NO in the pathophysiology of the arthritic joint, as this highly reactive radical not only inhibits the synthesis of both PGs and type II collagen [132, 133] by chondrocytes but also may induce apoptosis [134]. Further, NO may interact with superoxides to produce tissue-damaging peroxynitrites and hydroxyl radicals [135]. Adding strength to this hypothesis are the results of *ex vivo* analyses of human arthritic cartilage that showed that NO

synthase is expressed by the chondrocytes of diseased, but not normal tissue [136]. However, there is also evidence that NO may have a protective role during the inflammatory response [130]. These two effects may manifest themselves at different concentrations of NO. This seems plausible since the induction of low levels of NO in chondrocytes stimulates prostaglandin production, whereas maximal stimulation of NO results in inhibition of prostaglandin synthesis [129].

As chondrocytes are capable of producing hydrogen peroxide [137], this potential mechanism of matrix degradation cannot be discounted. Even at low concentrations, oxygen-derived free radicals (ODFR) inhibit glycolysis and induce a rapid depletion in ATP. The depletion in ATP is further compounded by a direct nonenzymatic hydrolysis of ATP leading to a rapid increase in inorganic pyrophosphate (PPi) levels [138]. This effect of ODFR on ATP depletion is reversible as long as the exposure of chondrocytes to ODFR does not last more than 1 to 2 hours. Long-term exposure to ODFR leads to peroxidation of membrane lipids and cell death. ODFR also promote the degradation or denaturation of various cartilaginous matrix components. Thus, ODFR depolymerize HA and can degrade collagen, LP, and PG either directly or indirectly by activating latent proteinases and/or inactivating inhibitors of proteinases.

By being degraded by several inorganic pyrophosphatases, including alkaline phosphatase, PPi is a critical source of phosphate for the deposition of basic calcium phosphate crystals [139]. PPi itself is the byproduct of many synthetic reactions in the cell [139] and the direct product of nucleoside triphosphate pyrophosphohydrolases (NTPPPH) [140].

In idiopathic chondrocalcinosis, the deposition of calcium pyrophosphate dihydrate (CPPD) crystals in articular cartilage is strongly linked to substantial increases in NTPPPH activity and PPi concentrations [141]. CPPD crystal deposition commonly complicates cartilage injury and OA, a condition in which its appearance prognosticates joint destruction [142]. The crystals have the capacity to promote cartilage degeneration as well as acute and chronic synovitis [141]. TGF-β is unique in its capacity to markedly upregulate extracellular elaboration of PPi by the chondrocytes [143], a response that is further increased by epidermal growth factor [144] but suppressed by IL-1 [145].

Several components of the complement system, including C1q, have been reported to be secreted by normal and OA chondrocytes, but their potential roles in matrix homeostasis and chondrocyte metabolism are largely hypothetical [146]. Likewise, nothing is known about the possible functions of a protein termed YLK-40 that appears to be secreted by both chondrocytes and synoviocytes and whose serum and synovial levels are enhanced in various arthritides [147]. Chondrocytes also secrete fibronectin: in both OA and RA, the cartilage matrix exhibits a 10- to 20-fold increase in content of this ubiquitous protein [148]. Although TGF-β markedly increases fibronectin synthesis by normal chondrocytes, this growth factor alone is not sufficient to explain such an accumulation in diseased cartilage; therefore, either intact or degraded fibronectin molecules are likely to originate from the synovial fluid. In contrast to intact molecules, fibronectin fragments markedly affect the metabolism of chondrocytes. Indeed, at the high concentrations found in synovial fluids from diseased joints, these fragments stimulate the liberation of IL-1 and upregulate cartilage catabolism both *in vivo* and *in vitro* [149]. It is interesting that at lower concentrations, the same fragments have an anabolic effect, thought to be mediated by IGF-1, upon matrix metabolism [150].

VIII. CONCLUDING STATEMENT

The cartilage matrix contains several molecules that are found in much higher concentrations than in other tissues. The attention that aggrecan and collagen type II are receiving as potential markers of specific metabolic alterations in cartilage disease will likely extend to less abundant molecules found to play key roles in the maintenance of matrix homeostasis. As our understanding of the function and metabolism of these molecules improves, so will their potential as markers of the irreversible destabilization of the collagenous meshwork or of other specific alterations in cartilage matrix organization.

Acknowledgments

The preparation of this manuscript was supported in part by Grant 3.4597.98 from the Funds for Medical Scientific Research (Belgium), by the FDS of the UCL, Grants AR39239 and AG4736 from the National Institutes of Health, the Greater Chicago Area Chapter of the Arthritis Foundation, and the Arthritis and Orthopedics Institute at Rush-Presbyterian-St. Luke's Medical Center.

References

1. Atencia, L. J., McDevitt, C. A., Nile, W. B., and Sokoloff, L. (1989). Cartilage content of an immature dog. *Connect. Tissue Res.* **18**, 235–242.
2. Hascall, V. C. (1988). Proteoglycans: The chondroitin sulfate/keratan sulfate proteoglycan of cartilage. *ISI Atlas Sci. Biochem.*, pp. 189–198.
3. Hardingham, T. E., Fosang, A., and Dudhia, J. (1992). Aggrecan, the chondroitin sulfate/keratan sulfate proteoglycan from cartilage. *In* "Articular Cartilage and Osteoarthritis" (K. E. Kuettner, R. Schleyerbach, J. G. Peyron, and V. C. Hascall, eds.), pp. 5–20. Raven Press, New York.
4. Mow, V. C., Holmes, M. H., and Lai, W. M. (1984). Fluid transport and mechanical properties of articular cartilage: A review. *J. Biomech.* **17**, 377–394.
5. Maroudas, A., Miizrahi, J., Katz, E. P., Watchel, E. J., and Soudry, M. (1986). Physicochemical properties and functional behavior of normal and osteoarthritic human cartilage. *In* "Articular Cartilage Biochemistry" (K. E. Kuettner, R. Schleyerbach, and V. C. Hascall, eds.), pp. 311–329. Raven Press, New York.
6. Mow, V. C., Fithran, D. C., and Kelly, M. A. (1990). Fundamentals of articular cartilage and meniscus biomechanics. *In* "Articular Cartilage and Knee Joint Function. Basic Science and Arthroscopy" (J. W. Ewing, ed.), pp. 1–18. Raven Press, New York.
7. Poole, C. A. (1992). The chondron and its pericellular environment. *In* "Articular Cartilage and Osteoarthritis" (K. E. Kuettner, R. Schleyerbach, J. G. Peyron, and V. C. Hascall, eds.), pp. 201–220. Raven Press, New York.
8. Heinegard, D., Lorenzo, P., and Sommarin, Y. (1995). Articular cartilage matrix proteins. *In* "Osteoarthritic Disorders" (K. E. Kuettner and V. M. Goldberg, eds.), pp. 229–237. American Academy of Orthopedic Surgeons, Rosemont, MD.
9. Brighton, C. T., and Heppenstall, R. B. (1971). Oxygen tension in zones of the epiphyseal plate, the metaphysis and diaphysis. *J. Bone Jt. Surg., Am. Vol.* **53A**, 719–728.
10. Clark, C. C., Tolin, B. S., and Brighton, C. T. (1991). The effect of oxygen tension on proteoglycan synthesis and aggregation in mammalian growth plate chondrocytes *J. Orthop. Res.* **9**, 477–484.
11. Marcus, R. E., and Srivastava, V. M. L. (1973). Effect of low oxygen tensions on glucose metabolizing enzymes in cultured articular chondrocytes. *Proc. Soc. Exp. Biol. Med.* **143**, 488–491.
12. Spencer, C. A., Palmer, T. N., and Mason, R. M. (1990). Intermediary metabolism in the Swarm rat chondrosarcoma chondrocyte. *Biochem. J.* **265**, 911–914.
13. Mason, R. M., and Sweeney, C. (1994). The relationship between proteoglycan synthesis in Swarm chondrocytes and pathways of cellular energy and UDP-sugar metabolism. *Carbohydr. Res.* **255**, 255–270.
14. Urban, J. P. G., Hall, A. C., and Ghel, K. A. (1993). Regulation of matrix synthesis rates by the ionic and osmotic environment of articular chondrocytes. *J. Cell. Physiol.* **154**, 262–270.
15. Palmoski, M. J., and Brandt, K. D. (1984). Effect of static and cyclic compressive loading on articular cartilage plugs in vitro. *Arthritis Rheum.* **27**, 675–681.
16. Parkkinen, J. J., Mammi, M. J., Helminen, H. J., and Tammi, M. (1992). Local stimulation of proteoglycan synthesis in articular cartilage explants by dynamic compression in vitro. *J. Orthop. Res.* **10**, 610–620.
17. Kim, Y.-J., Sah, R. L.-Y., Grodzinski, A. L., Plaas, A. H. K., and Sandy, J. D. (1994). Mechanical regulation of cartilage biosynthetic behavior: Physical stimuli. *Arch. Biochem. Biophys.* **311**, 1–12.
18. Palmoski, M. J., Perricone, E., and Brandt, K. D. (1979). Development and reversal of proteoglycan aggregation defect in normal canine knee cartilage after immobilization. *Arthritis Rheum.* **22**, 508–517.
19. Pita, J. C., Muller, F. J., Manicourt, D. H., Buckwalter, J. A., and Ratcliffe, A. (1992). Early matrix changes in experimental osteoarthritis and joint disuse atrophy. *In* "Articular Cartilage and Osteoarthritis" (K. E. Kuettner, R. Schleyerbach, J. G. Peyron, and V. C. Hascall, eds.), pp. 455–469. Raven Press, New York.
20. Salter, R. B. (1989). The biologic concept of continuous passive motion of synovial joints. *Clin. Orthop.* **242**, 12–25.
21. Aydelotte, M. B., and Kuettner, K. E. (1993). Heterogeneity of articular chondrocytes and cartilage matrix. *In* "Joint Cartilage Degradation. Basic and Clinical Aspects" (J. F. Woessner, Jr. and D. S. Howell, eds.), pp. 37–65. Dekker, New York.
22. Hayashi, T., Abe, E., Yamate, T., Taguchi, Y., and Jasin, H. (1997). Nitric oxide production by superficial and deep articular chondrocytes. *Arthritis Rheum.* **40**, 261–269.
23. Hauselmann, H. J., Flechtenmacher, J., Mollenhauer, J., Kuettner, K. E., and Aydelotte, M. B. (1994). Differences in responsiveness and in receptor numbers for interleukin-1 between adult human chondrocytes from superficial and deep zones of articular cartilage. *Trans. Orthop. Res. Soc.* **19**, 363.
24. Hinek, A., and Poole, A. R. (1988). The influence of vitamin D metabolites on the calcification of cartilage matrix and the C-propeptide of type II collagen (chondrocalcin). *J. Bone Miner. Res.* **3**, 421–429.
25. Mansson, B., Carey, D., Alini, M., Ionescu, M., Rosenberg, L. C.,

Poole, A. R., Heinegard, D., and Saxne, T. (1995). Cartilage and bone metabolism in rheumatoid arthritis. Differences between rapid and slow progression of disease identified by serum markers of cartilage metabolism. *J. Clin. Invest.* **95**, 1071–1077.

26. Shinmei, M., Ito, K., Matsuyama, S., Yoshihara, Y., and Matsuzawa, K. (1993). Joint fluid carboxy-terminal type II procollagen peptide as a marker of cartilage collagen biosynthesis. *Osteoarthritis Cartilage* **1**, 121–128.

27. Eyre, D. R., Wu, J. J., and Woods, P. E. (1992). Cartilage-specific collagens: Structural studies. *In* "Articular Cartilage and Osteoarthritis" (K. E. Kuettner, R. Schleyerbach, J. G. Peyron, and V. C. Hascall, eds.), pp. 119–131. Raven Press, New York.

28. Monnier, V. M., and Cerami, A. (1981). Non-enzymatic browning in vivo. Possible process for aging of long-lived proteins. *Science,* **211**, 491–493.

29. Poole, A. R. (1992). Immunology of cartilage. *In* Osteoarthritis: Diagnosis and Medical/Surgical Management" (R. Moskowitz, D. S. Howell, V. M. Goldberg, and H. J. Mankin, eds.), pp. 155–189. Saunders, Philadelphia.

30. Dodge, G. R., and Poole, A. R. (1989). Immunohistochemical detection and immunochemical analysis of type II collagen degradation in human normal, rheumatoid and osteoarthritic articular cartilages and in explants of bovine articular cartilage cultured with interleukin-1. *J. Clin. Invest.* **83**, 647–661.

31. Barrett, A. J. (1978). The possible role of neutrophil proteinases in damage to articular cartilage. *Agents Actions* **8**, 15–18.

32. Wu, J.-J., Lark, M. W., Chun, L. E., and Eyre, D. R. (1991). Sites of stromelysin cleavage in collagen II, IX, X and XI. *J. Biol. Chem.* **266**, 5625–5628.

33. Kozaci, L. D., Buttle, D. J., and Hollander, A. P. (1997). Degradation of type II collagen, but not proteoglycan correlates with matrix metalloproteinase activity in cartilage explant cultures. *Arthritis Rheum.* **40**, 164–174.

34. Murphy, G., Cockett, M. I., Stephens, P. E., Smith, B. J., and Doherty, A. J. P. (1987). Stromelysin is an activator of pro-collagenase. A study with natural and recombinant enzymes. *Biochem. J.* **248**, 265–268.

35. Knauper, V., Lopez-Otin, C., Smith, B., Knight, G., and Murphy, G. (1996). Biochemical characterization of human collagenase-3. *J. Biol. Chem.* **271**, 1544–1550.

36. Nagase, H. (1997). Activation mechanisms of matrix metalloproteinases. *Biol. Chem.* **378**, 151–160.

37. Miller, E. J., Harris, E. D., Jr., Chung, E., Finch, J. E., Jr., McCroskery, P. A., and Butler, W. T. (1976). Cleavage of type II and III collagen with mammalian collagenase: Site of cleavage and primary structure at the NH$_2$-terminal portion of the smaller fragment released from both collagens. *Biochemistry* **15**, 787–792.

38. Hasty, K. A., Pourmotabbed, T. F., Golberg, G. I., Thompsonn, J. P., Spinella, D. G., Stevens, R. M., and Mainardi, C. L. (1990). Human neutrophil collagenase: A distinct gene product with homology to other matrix metalloproteinases. *J. Biol. Chem.* **265**, 11421–11424.

39. Mitchell, P. G., Magna, H. A., Reeves, L. M., Lopresti-Morrow, L. L., Yocum, S. A., Rosner, P. J., Geghegan, K. F., and Hambor, J. E. (1996). Cloning, expression and type II collagenolytic activity of matrix metalloproteinase-13 from human osteoarthritic cartilage. *J. Biol. Chem.* **97**, 761–768.

40. Dodge, G. R., Pidoux, I., and Poole, A. R. (1991). The degradation of type II collagen in rheumatoid arthritis: An immunoelectron microscopic study. *Matrix* 11, 330–338.

41. Hollander, A. P., Pidoux, I., Reiner, A., Rorabeck, C., Bourne, R., and Poole, A. R. (1995). Damage to type II collagen in aging and osteoarthritis starts at the articular surface and then extends into the cartilage with progressive degeneration. *J. Clin. Invest.* **96**, 2859–2869.

42. Billinghurst, R. C., Dahlberg, L., Ionescu, M., Reiner, A., Bourne, R., Rorabeck, C., Mitchell, P., Hambor, J., Diekmann, O., Tschesche, H., Chen, J., Van Wart, H., and Poole, A. R. (1997). Enhanced cleavage

of type II collagen by collagenases in osteoarthritic articular cartilage. *J. Clin. Invest.* **99**, 1534–1545.

43. Murphy, G., and Reynolds, J. J. (1993). Extracellular matrix degradation. *In* "Connective Tissue and Its Heritable Disorders. Molecular Genetic and Medical Aspects" (P. M. Royce and B. Steinmann, eds.), pp. 287–316. Wiley-Liss, New York.

44. Sinigaglia, L., Varenna, M., Binelli, L., Bartucci, F., Arrigoni, M., Ferrara, R., and Abbiati, G. (1995). Urinary and synovial pyridinium crosslink concentrations in patients with rheumatoid arthritis and osteoarthritis. *Ann. Rheum. Dis.* **54**, 144–147.

45. Black, D., Marabani, M., Sturrock, R. D., and Robins, S. P. (1989). Urinary excretion of hydroxypyridinium crosslinks of collagen in patients with rheumatoid arthritis. *Ann. Rheum. Dis.* **48**, 641–644.

46. Seibel, M. J., Duncan, A., and Robins, S. P. (1989). Urinary hydroxypyridinium crosslinks provide indices of cartilage and bone involvement in arthritic diseases. *J. Rheumatol.* **16**, 964–970.

47. Robins, S. P., Seibel, M. J., and McLaren, A. L. (1990). Collagen markers in urine in human arthritis. *In* "Methods in Cartilage Research" (A. Maroudas and K. Kuettner, eds.), pp. 348–352. Academic Press, London.

48. Astbury, C., Bird, H. A., McLaren, A. M., and Robins, S. P. (1994). Urinary excretion of pyridinium crosslinks of collagen correlated with joint damage in arthritis. *Br. J. Rheumatol.* **33**, 11–15.

49. Thompson, P. W., Spector, T. D., James, I. T., Henderson, E., and Hart, D. J. (1992). Urinary collagen crosslinks reflect radiographic severity in knee osteoarthritis. *Br. J. Rheumatol.* **31**, 759–761.

50. MacDonald, A. G., McHenry, P., Robins, S. P., and Reid, D. M. (1994). Relationship of urinary pyridinium crosslinks to disease extent and activity in osteoarthritis. *Br. J. Rheumatol.* **33**, 16–19.

51. Eyre, D. R., Dickson, I. R., and Van Ness, K. P. (1988). Collagen crosslinking in human bone and articular cartilage. Age-related changes in the content of mature hydroxypyridinium residues. *Biochem. J.* **252**, 495–500.

52. Gough, A. K. S., Peel, N. F. A., Eastell, R., Holder, R. L., Lilley, J., and Emery, P. (1994). Excretion of pyridinium crosslinks correlates with disease activity and appendicular bone loss in early rheumatoid arthritis. *Ann. Rheum. Dis.* **53**, 14–17.

53. Garnero, P., and Delmas, P. D. (1996). Measurements of biochemical markers: Methods and limitations. *In* "Principles of Bone Biology" (J. P. Bilezikian, L. G. Raisż, and G. A. Rodan, eds.), pp. 1277–1291. Academic Press, San Diego, CA.

54. Sah, R. L.-Y., Grodzinski, A. L., Plaas, A. H. K., and Sandy, J. D. (1992). Effects of static and dynamic compression on matrix metabolism in cartilage explants. *In* "Articular Cartilage and Osteoarthritis" (K. E. Kuettner, R. Schleyerbach, J. G. Peyron, and V. C. Hascall, eds.), pp. 373–392. Raven Press, New York.

55. Sandy, J. D. (1992). Extracellular metabolism of aggrecan. *In* "Articular Cartilage and Osteoarthritis" (K. Kuettner, R. Schleyerbach, J. Peyron, and V. C. Hascall, eds.), pp. 21–33. Raven Press, New York.

56. Mok, S. S., Masuda, K., Hauselmann, H. J., Aydelotte, M. B., and Thonar, E. J.-M. A. (1994). Aggrecan synthesized by mature bovine chondrocytes suspended in alginate. Identification of two distinct metabolic matrix pools. *J. Biol. Chem.* **269**, 33021–33027.

57. Maroudas, A., Palla, G., and Gilav, E. (1992). Racemization of aspartic acid in human articular cartilage. *Connect. Tissue Res.* **27**, 1–8.

58. Maroudas, A., Uchitel, N., Bayliss, M. T., and Gilav, E. (1994). Racemization of aspartic acid in proteoglycans from human articular cartilage. *Trans. Orthop. Res.* **19**, 3 (abstr.).

59. Lohmander, S. (1977). Turnover of proteoglycans in guinea pig costal cartilage. *Arch. Biochem. Biophys.* **180**, 93–101.

60. van Kampen, G. P., van de Stadt, R. J., van de Laar, M. A. F. J., and van der Korst, J. K. (1992). Two distinct metabolic pools of proteoglycans in articular cartilage. *In* "Articular Cartilage and Osteoarthritis" (K. E. Kuettner, R. Schleyerbach, J. G. Peyron, and V. C. Hascall, eds.), pp. 281–289. Raven Press, New York.

61. Hardingham, T. E. (1988). Biosynthesis, assembly and turnover of cartilage proteoglycans. *In* "Control of Tissue Damage" (A. Glauert, ed.), pp. 41–54. Elsevier, Amsterdam.

62. Kuettner, K. E., Thonar, E. J.-M. A., and Aydelotte, M. B. (1990). *In* "Cartilage Changes in Osteoarthritis" (K. D. Brandt, ed.), pp. 3–11. Indiana University School of Medicine, Indianapolis.

63. Bayliss, M. T. (1992). Metabolism of animal and human osteoarthritic cartilage. *In* "Articular cartilage and Osteoarthritis" (K. E. Kuettner, R. Schleyerbach, J. G. Peyron, and V. C. Hascall, eds.), pp. 487–500. Raven Press, New York.

64. Häuselmann, H. J., Masuda, K., Hunziker, E. B., Neidhart, M., Mok, S. S., Michel, B. A., and Thonar, E. J.-M. A. (1996). Adult human chondrocytes cultured in alginate form a matrix similar to native human articular cartilage. *Am. J. Physiol.* **40**, C742–C752.

65. Caroll, G. (1989). Measurement of sulfated glycosaminoglycans and proteoglycan fragments in arthritic synovial fluid. *Ann. Rheum. Dis.* **48**, 17–24.

66. Ratcliffe, A. M., Doherty, M., Maini, R. N., and Hardingham, T. E. (1988). Increased levels of proteoglycan components in the synovial fluids of patients with acute joint disease. *Ann. Rheum. Dis.* **47**, 826–832.

67. Witter, J., Roughley, P. J., Webber, C., Roberts, N., Keystone, E., and Poole, A. R. (1987). The immunologic detection and characterization of cartilage proteoglycan degradation products in synovial fluids of patients with arthritis. *Arthritis Rheum.* **30**, 519–529.

68. Saxne, T. D., and Heinegard, D. (1992). Synovial fluid analysis of two groups of proteoglycan epitopes distinguishes early and late cartilage lesions. *Arthritis Rheum.* **35**, 385–390.

69. Thonar, E. J.-M. A., Manicourt, D. H., Williams, J. M., Fukuda, K., Campion, G. V., Sweet, B. M. E., Lenz, M. E., Schnitzer, T. J., and Kuettner, K. E. (1992). Serum keratan sulfate: A measure of cartilage proteoglycan metabolism. *In* "Articular Cartilage and Osteoarthritis" (K. E. Kuettner, R. Schleyerbach, J. G. Peyron, and V. C. Hascall, eds.), pp. 429–445. Raven Press, New York.

70. Poole, A. R., Ionescu, M., Swan, A., and Dieppe, P. A. (1994). Changes in cartilage metabolism in arthritis are reflected by altered serum and synovial fluid levels of the cartilage proteoglycan aggrecan. *J. Clin. Invest.* **94**, 25–33.

71. Sandy, J. D., Neame, P. J., Boynton, R. E., and Flannery, C. R. (1991). Catabolism of aggrecan in cartilage explants. Identification of a major cleavage site within the interglobular domain. *J. Biol. Chem.* **266**, 8683–8685.

72. Sandy, J. D., Flannery, C. R., Neame, P. J., and Lohmander, L. S. (1992). The structure of aggrecan fragments in human synovial fluid. Evidence for the involvement in osteoarthritis of a novel proteinase which cleaves the Glu^{373}-Ala^{374} bond of the interglobular domain. *J. Clin. Invest.* **89**, 1512–1516.

73. Lohmander, L. S., Neame, P. J., and Sandy, J. D. (1993). The structure of aggrecan fragments in human synovial fluid. Evidence that aggrecanase mediates cartilage degradation in inflammatory joint disease, joint injury and osteoarthritis. *Arthritis Rheum.* **36**, 1214–1222.

74. Hughes, C. E., Caterson, B., Fosang, A. J., Roughley, P. J., and Mort, J. S. (1995). Monoclonal antibodies that specifically recognize neoepitope sequences generated by aggrecanase and matrix metalloproteinase cleavage of aggrecan: Application to catabolism in situ and in vitro. *Biochem. J.* **305**, 799–804.

75. Lark, M. W., Williams, H., Hoerrner, L. A. Weidner, J., Ayala, J. M., Harper, C. F., Christen, A., Olszewski, J., Konteatis, Z., Webber, R., *et al.* (1995). Quantification of a matrix metalloproteinase-generated aggrecan G1 fragment using monospecific anti-peptide serum. *Biochem. J.* **307**, 245–252.

76. Lark, M. W., Gordy, J. T., Weidner, J. R., Ayala, J., Kimura, J. H., Williams, H. R., Mumford, R. A., Flannery, C. R., Carlson, S. S., Iwata, M., and Sandy, J. D. (1995). Cell-mediated catabolism of aggrecan.

Evidence that cleavage of the aggrecanase site (Glu^{373}-Ala^{374}) is a primary event in proteolysis of the interglobular domain. *J. Biol. Chem.* **270**, 2550–2556.

77. Fosang, A. J., Last, K., Gardiner, P., Jackson, D. C., and Brown, L. (1995). Development of a cleavage-site-specific monoclonal antibody for detecting metalloproteinase-derived aggrecan fragments: Detection of fragments in human synovial fluid. *Biochem. J.* **310**, 337–343.

78. Singer, I. I., Kawka, D. W., Bayne, E. K., Donatelli, S. A., Weidner, J. R., Williams, H. A., Ayala, J. M., Mumford, R. A., Lark, M. W., Glant, T. T., *et al.* (1995). A metalloproteinase-generated neoepitope is induced and immunolocalizes in articular cartilage during inflammatory arthritis. *J. Clin. Invest.* **95**, 2178–2186.

79. Fosang, A. J., Last, K., and Maciewicz, R. A. (1996). Aggrecan is degraded by matrix metalloproteinases in human arthritis. Evidence that matrix metalloproteinases and aggrecanase activities can be independent. *J. Clin. Invest.* **98**, 2292–2299.

80. Lark, M. W., Bayne, E. K., Flanagan, J., Harper, C. F., Hoerrner, L. A., Hutchinson, N. I., Singer, I. I., Donatelli, S. A., Weidner, J. R., Williams, H. R., Mumford, R. A., and Lohmander, L. S. (1997). Aggrecan degradation in human cartilage. Evidence for both metalloproteinase and aggrecanase activity in normal, osteoarthritic and rheumatoid joints. *J. Clin. Invest.* **100**, 93–106.

81. Roberts, C. R., Roughley, P. J., and Mort, J. S. (1989). Degradation of human proteoglycan aggregate induced by hydrogen peroxide. Protein fragmentation, amino acid modification and hyaluronic acid cleavage. *Biochem. J.* **259**, 805–811.

82. Ilic, M. Z., Handley, C. H., Robinson, H. C., and Mok, M. T. (1992). Mechanism of catabolism of aggrecan by articular cartilage. *Arch. Biochem. Biophys.* **294**, 115–122.

83. Louakis, P., Schrikande, A., Davis, G., and Maniglia, C. A. (1992). N-terminal sequencing of proteoglycan fragments isolated from medium of interleukin-1 treated articular cartilage cultures. *Biochem. J.* **284**, 589–593.

84. Rosenberg, L., Wolfenstein-Todel, C., Margolis, R., Pal, S., and Strider, W. (1976). Proteoglycans from bovine proximal humeral articular cartilage. Structural basis for the polydispersity of proteoglycan subunits. *J. Biol. Chem.* **251**, 6439–6444.

85. Heinegard, D. (1977). Polydispersity of cartilage proteoglycans. Structural variation with size and buoyant density of the molecules. *J. Biol. Chem.* **252**, 1980–1989.

86. Bayliss, M. T., and Ali, S. Y. (1978). Age-related differences in the composition and structure of human articular cartilage proteoglycans. *Biochem. J.* **176**, 683–693.

87. Morgelin, M., Paulsson, M., Hardingham, T. E., Heinegard, D., and Engel, J. (1988). Cartilage proteoglycans. Assembly with hyaluronate and link protein as studied by electron microscopy. *Biochem. J.* **253**, 175–185.

88. Flannery, C. R., Lark, M. V., and Sandy, J. D. (1992). Identification of a stromelysin cleavage site within the interglobular domain of human aggrecan: Evidence for proteolysis at this site in vivo in human articular cartilage. *J. Biol. Chem.* **267**, 1008–1014.

89. Fosang, A. J., Neame, P. J., Last, K., Hardingham, T. E., Murphy, G., and Hamilton, J. A. (1992). The interglobular domain of cartilage aggrecan is cleaved by Pump, gelatinases and cathepsin B. *J. Biol. Chem.* **267**, 19470–19474.

90. Arner, E. C. (1994). Effect of animal age and chronicity of interleukin-1 exposure on cartilage proteoglycan depletion in vivo. *J. Orthop. Res.* **12**, 321–330.

91. Lewthwaite, J., Blake, S. M., Hardingham, T. E., Warden, P. J., and Henderson, B. (1994). The effect of recombinant human interleukin-1 receptor antagonist on the induction phase of antigen induced arthritis in the rabbit. *J. Rheumatol.* **21**, 467–472.

92. Cawston, T. (1993). Blocking cartilage destruction with metalloproteinase inhibitors: A valid therapeutic target. *Ann. Rheum. Dis.* **52**, 769–770.

93. Mort, J. S., Pidoux, I., and Poole, A. R. (1993). Direct evidence for metalloproteinases mediating matrix degradation in interleukin-1 stimulated human articular cartilage. *Matrix* **13**, 95–102.

94. Andrews, H. J., Plumpton, T. A., Harper, G. P., and Cawston, T. E. (1992). A synthetic peptide metalloproteinase inhibitor, but not TIMP, prevents the breakdown of proteoglycan within articular cartilage in vitro. *Agents Actions* **37**, 147–154.

95. Buttle, D. J., Handley, C. J., Ilic, M. Z., Saklatvala, J., Murata, M., and Barrett, A. J. (1993). Inhibition of cartilage proteoglycan release by a specific inactivator of cathepsin B and an inhibitor of matrix metalloproteinases: Evidence for two converging pathways of chondrocyte-mediated proteoglycan degradation. *Arthritis Rheum.* **36**, 1709–1717.

96. Seed, M. P., Ismaiel, S., Cheung, C. Y., Thompson, T. A., Gardner, C. R., Atkins, R. M., and Elson, C. J. (1993). Inhibition of interleukin-1 beta induced rat and human cartilage degradation in vitro by the metalloproteinase inhibitor U27391 *Ann. Rheum. Dis.* **52**, 37–43.

97. Roughley, P. J., White, R. J., and Poole, A. R. (1985). Identification of a hyaluronic acid-binding protein that interferes with the preparation of high-buoyant density proteoglycan aggregates from adult human cartilage. *Biochem. J.* **231**, 129–138.

98. Fosang, A. J., Last, K., Knauper, V., Murphy, G., and Neame, P. J. (1996). Degradation of cartilage aggrecan by collagenase-3 (MMP-13). *FEBS Lett.* **380**, 17–20.

99. Bayne, E. K., MacNaul, K. L., Donatelli, S. A., Christen, A., Griffin, P. R., Hoernerr, L. A., Calaycay, J. R., Ayala, J. M., Chapman, K., and Hagmann, W. (1995). The use of an antibody against the matrix metalloproteinase-generated aggrecan neoepitope FVDIPEN-CCOH to assess the effects of stromelysin-1 in a rabbit model of cartilage degradation. *Arthritis Rheum.* **38**, 1400–1409.

100. Morales, T. I., and Hascall, V. C. (1988). Correlated metabolism of proteoglycans and hyaluronic acid in bovine cartilage organ cultures. *J. Biol. Chem.* **263**, 3632–3638.

101. Morales, T. I., and Hascall, V. C. (1989). Effects of interleukins and lipopolysaccharides on protein and carbohydrate metabolism in bovine articular cartilage organ cultures. *Connect. Tissue Res.* **19**, 255–275.

102. Webber, C., Glant, T. T., Roughley, P. J., and Poole, A. R. (1987). The identification and characterization of two populations of aggregating proteoglycans of high buoyant density isolated from post-natal human articular cartilages of different ages. *Biochem. J.* **248**, 735–740.

103. Scott, J. E. (1992). Oxygen and the connective tissues. *Trends Biochem. Sci.* **17**, 340–343.

104. Bayliss, M. T., Venn, M., Maroudas, A., and Ali, S. Y. (1983). Structure of proteoglycans from different layers of human articular cartilage. *Biochem. J.* **209**, 387–400.

105. Manicourt, D.-H., Pita, J. C., Thonar, E. J.-M. A., and Howell, D. S. (1991). Proteoglycans non-dissociatively extracted from different zones of canine normal articular cartilage: Variations in the sedimentation profile of aggrecan with degree of physiological stress. *Connect. Tissue Res.* **26**, 231–246.

106. Caterson, B., Highes, C. E., Johnstone, B., and Mort, J. S. (1992). Immunological markers of cartilage proteoglycan metabolism in animal and human osteoarthritis. *In* "Articular Cartilage and Osteoarthritis" (K. E. Kuettner, R. Schleyerbach, J. G. Peyron, and V. C. Hascall, eds.), pp. 415–427. Raven Press, New York.

107. Ishiguro, N., Uebelhart, D., Thonar, E. J.-M. A., *et al.* (1992). Immunolocalization of atypical chondroitin sulfate chains reacting with the 3-B-3 monoclonal antibody following chymopapain-induced injury in the rabbit. *Orthop. Res. Soc. Trans.* **17**, 278.

108. Prehm, P. (1986). Mechanism, localization and inhibition of hyaluronate synthesis. *In* "Articular Cartilage Biochemistry" (K. E. Kuettner, R. Schleyerbach, and V. C. Hascall, eds.), pp. 81–91. Raven Press, New York.

109. Weigel, P. H., and Hascall, V. C. (1997). Hyaluronan synthases *J. Biol. Chem.* **272**, 13997–14000.

110. Roughley, P. J., Nguyen, Q., and Mort, J. S. (1992). The role of proteinases and oxygen radicals in the degradation of human articular cartilage. *In* "Articular Cartilage and Osteoarthritis" (K. E. Kuettner, R. Schleyerbach, J. G. Peyron, and V. C. Hascall, eds.), pp. 305–317. Raven Press, New York.

111. Ratcliffe, A., Beauvais, P. J., and Saed-Nejad, F. (1994). Differential levels of synovial fluid aggrecan aggregate components in experimental osteoarthritis and joint disuse. *J. Othop. Res.* **12**, 464–473.

112. Manicourt, D.-H., Thonar, E. J.-M. A., Pita, J. C., and Howell, D. S. (1989). Changes in the sedimentation profile of proteoglycan aggregates in the early stages of experimental canine osteoarthritis. *Connect. Tissue Res.* **23**, 33–50.

113. Ng, C. K., Handley, C. J., Mason, R. M., and Robinson, H. C. (1989). Synthesis of hyaluronate in cultured bovine articular cartilage. *Biochem. J.* **263**, 761–767.

114. Holmes, M. W. A., Bayliss, M. T., and Muir, H. (1988). Hyaluronic acid in human articular cartilage. Age-related changes in content and size. *Biochem. J.* **250**, 435–441.

115. Ng, C. K., Handley, C. J., Preston, B. N., Robinson, H. C., Bolis, S., and Parker, G. (1995). Effect of exogenous hyaluronan and hyaluronan oligosaccharides on hyaluronan and aggrecan synthesis and catabolism in adult articular cartilage explants. *Arch. Biochem. Biophys.* **316**, 596–606.

116. Hua, Q., Knudson, C. B., and Knudson, W. (1993). Internalization of hyaluronan by chondrocytes occur via receptor-mediated endocytosis. *J. Cell Sci.* **106**, 365–375.

117. Chow, G., Knudson, C. B., Homandberg, G., and Knudson, W. (1995). Increased expression of CD44 in bovine articular chondrocytes by catabolic cellular mediators *J. Biol. Chem.* **270**, 27734–27741.

118. McGee, C. M., Lowenstein, C. J., Horton, M. R., Wu, J., Bao, C., Chin, B. Y., Choi, A. M. K., and Noble, P. W. (1997). Hyaluronan fragments induce nitric-oxide synthase in murine macrophages through a nuclear factor kB-dependent mechanism *J. Biol. Chem.* **272**, 8013–8018.

119. Campbell, M. A., and Handley, C. J. (1987). The effect of retinoic acid on proteoglycan turnover in bovine articular cartilage cultures. *Arch. Biochem. Biophys.* **258**, 143–155.

120. Witsch-Prhem, P., Miehlke, R., and Kresse, H. (1992). Presence of small proteoglycan fragments in normal and arthritic human cartilage. *Arthritis Rheum.* **35**, 1042–1052.

121. Plaas, A. H. K., Barry, F. P., and Wong-Palms, S. (1992). Keratan sulfate substitution on cartilage matrix molecules. *In* "Articular Cartilage and Osteoarthritis" (K. E. Kuettner, R. Schleyerbach, J. G. Peyron, and V. C. Hascall, eds.), pp. 69–79. Raven Press, New York.

122. von den Hoff, H., de Koning, M., van Kampen, J., and van der Rost, J. (1995). Interleukin-1 reversibly inhibits the synthesis of biglycan and decorin in intact articular cartilage in culture. *J. Rheumatol.* **22**, 1520–1526.

123. Cs-Szabo, G., Melching, L. E., Roughley, P. J., and Glant, T. T. (1997). Changes in messenger RNA and protein levels of proteoglycans and link protein in human osteoarthritic cartilage samples. *Arthritis Rheum.* **40**, 1037–1045.

124. Poole, A. R., Rosenberg, L. C., Reiner, A., Ionescu, M., Bogoch, E., and Roughley, P. J. (1996). The contents and distributions of the proteoglycans decorin and biglycan in normal and osteoarthritic human articular cartilages. *J. Orthop. Res.* **14**, 681–689.

125. Saxne, T., and Heinegard, D. (1992). Cartilage oligomeric matrix protein: A novel marker of cartilage turnover detectable in synovial fluid and blood. *J. Rheumatol.* **31**, 583–591.

126. Mansson, B., Geborek, P., and Saxne, T. (1997). Cartilage and bone macromolecules in knee joint synovial fluid in rheumatoid arthritis: Relation to development of knee or hip joint destruction. *Ann. Rheum. Dis.* **56**, 91–96.

127. DiCesare, P. E., Carlson, C. S., Stollerman, E. S., Chen, F. S., Leslie, M., and Perris, R. (1997). Expression of cartilage oligomeric matrix protein by human synovium. *FEBS Lett.* **412**, 249–252.

128. Vilim, V., Lenz, M. E., Vytasek, R., Masuda, K., Pavelka, K., Kuettner, K. E., and Thonar, E. J.-M. A. (1997). Characterization of monoclonal antibodies recognizing different fragments of cartilage oligomeric matrix protein in human body fluids. *Arch. Biochem. Biophys.* **341**, 8–16.

129. Stadler, J., Stefanovic-Racic, M., Billiar, T. R., Curran, R. D., McIntyre, L. A., Georgescu, H. I., Simmons, R. L., and Evans, C. H. (1991). Articular chondrocytes synthesize nitric oxide in response to cytokines and lipopolysaccharide. *J. Immunol.* **147**, 3915–3920.

130. Lyons, C. R. (1995). The role of nitric oxide in inflammation. *Adv. Immunol.* **60**, 323–371.

131. Aeberhard, E. E., Henderson, S. A., Arabolos, N. S., Griscavage, J. M., Castro, F. E., Barrett, C. T., and Ig Naro, L. J. (1995). Nonsteroidal anti-inflammatory drugs inhibit expression of the inducible nitric oxide synthase gene. *Biochem. Biophys. Res. Commun.* **208**, 1053–1059.

132. Stefanovic-Racic, M., Stadler, J., and Evans, C. H. (1993). Nitric oxide and arthritis. *Arthritis Rheum.* **36**, 1036–1044.

133. Cao, M., Westerhausen-Larson, A., Niyibizi, C., Kavalkovich, K., Georgescu, I., Rizzo, C. F., Hebda, P. A., Stefanovic-Racic, M., and Evans, C. H. (1997). Nitric oxide inhibits the synthesis of type II collagen without altering Col2A1 mRNA abundance: Prolyl hydroxylase as a possible target. *Biochem. J.* **324**, 305–310.

134. Blanco, F. J., Ochs, R. L., Schwarz, H., and Lotz, M. (1995). Chondrocyte apoptosis induced by nitric oxide. *Am. J. Pathol.* **146**, 75–85.

135. Hogg, N., Darley-Usmar, V. M., Wilson, M. T., and Moncada, S. (1992). Production of hydroxyl radicals from the simultaneous generation of superoxide and nitric oxide. *Biochem. J.* **281**, 419–424.

136. Amin, A. R., Di Cesare, P. E., Vyas, P., Attur, M., Tzeng, E., Billiar, T., Stucnin, S., and Abramson, S. B. (1995). The expression and regulation of nitric oxide synthase in human osteoarthritis affected chondrocytes. *J. Exp. Med.* **182**, 2097–2102.

137. Tiku, M. L., Liesch, J. B., and Robertson, F. M. (1990). Production of hydrogen peroxide by rabbit articular chondrocytes. Enhancement by cytokines. *J. Immunol.* **145**, 690–696.

138. Kwam, B. J., Fragonas, E., Degrassi, A., Kwam, C., Matulova, M., Pollesello, P., Zanetti, F., and Vittur, F. (1995). Oxygen-derived free radical (ODFR) action on hyaluronan (HA), on two HA ester derivatives, and on the metabolism of articular chondrocytes. *Exp. Cell Res.* **218**, 79–86.

139. Oyajobi, B. O., Russell, R. G., and Caswell, A. M. (1994). Modulation of ectonucleoside triphosphate pyrophosphatase activity of human osteoblast-like bone cells by 1 alpha, 25 dihydroxyvitamin D3, 24R,25 dihydroxyvitamin D3, parathyroid hormone and dexamethasone. *J. Bone Miner. Res.* **9**, 1259–1266.

140. Howell, D. S., Martel-Pelletier, J., Pelletier, J.-P., Morales, S., and Muniz, O. (1984). NTP pyrophosphohydrolase in human chondrocalcinotic and osteoarthritic cartilage II. Further studies on histologic and subcellular distribution. *Arthritis Rheum.* **27**, 193–199.

141. Ryan, L. M., and McCarty, D. J. (1997). Calcium pyrophosphate crystal deposition disease, pseudogout and articular chondrocalcinosis. *In* "Arthritis and Allied Conditions" (W. J. Koopman, ed.), pp. 2103–2126. Williams & Wilkins, Baltimore, MD.

142. Dieppe, P., Cushnaghan, J., and McAlindon, T. (1992). Epidemiology, clinical course and outcome of knee osteoarthritis. *In* "Articular Cartilage and Osteoarthritis" (K. E. Kuettner, R. Schleyerbach, J. G. Peyron, and V. C. Hascall, eds.), pp. 617–627. Raven Press, New York.

143. Rosenthal, A. K., Cheung, H. S., and Ryan, L. M. (1991). Transforming growth factor b 1 stimulates inorganic pyrophosphate elaboration by porcine cartilage. *Arthritis Rheum.* **34**, 904–911.

144. Rosenthal, A. K., and Ryan, L. M. (1994). Aging increases growth factor induced inorganic pyrophosphate elaboration by articular cartilage. *Mech. Ageing Dev.* **75**, 35–44.

145. Lotz, M., Rosen, F., McCabe, G., Quach, J., Blanco, F., Dudler, J., Solan, J., Goding, J., Seegmiller, J. E., and Terkeltaub, R. (1995). Interleukin-1 β suppresses transforming growth factor-induced inorganic pyrophosphate (PPi) production and expression of the PPi-generating enzyme PC-1 in human chondrocytes. *Proc. Natl. Acad. Sci. U.S.A.* **92**, 10364–10368.

146. Bradley, K., North, J., Saunders, D., Schwaeble, W., Jeziorska, M., and Woolley, D. E. (1996). Synthesis of classical pathway complement components by chondrocytes. *Immunology* **88**, 648–656.

147. Johansen, J. S., Jensen, H. S., and Price, P. A. (1993). A new biochemical marker for joint injury. Analysis of YKL-40 in serum and synovial fluid. *Br. J. Rheum.* **32**, 949–955.

148. Lust, G., and Burton-Wurster, N. (1992). Fibronectin in osteoarthritis: Comparison of animal and human diseases. *In* "Articular Cartilage and Osteoarthritis" (K. E. Kuettner, R. Schleyerbach, J. G. Peyron, and V. C. Hascall, eds.), pp. 447–500. Raven Press, New York.

149. Xie, D. L., Hui, F., Meyers, R., and Homandberg, G. A. (1994). Cartilage chondrolysis by fibronectin fragments is associated with release of several proteinases: Stromelysin plays a major role in chondrolysis. *Arch. Biochem. Biophys.* **311**, 205–212.

150. Homandberg, G. A., and Hui, F. (1994). High concentrations of fibronectin fragments cause short-term catabolic effects in cartilage tissue while lower concentrations cause continuous anabolic effects. *Arch. Biochem. Biophys.* **311**, 213–218.

CHAPTER 22

Fluid Dynamics of the Joint Space and Trafficking of Matrix Products

PETER A. SIMKIN   University of Washington, Seattle, Washington 98195

I. INTRODUCTION

A large and growing body of literature attests to the broad current interest in cartilage-derived molecules as "markers" of damage and repair across a wide variety of joint diseases [1–3]. Specific markers and the rationale for their use are examined in detail elsewhere in this volume. This chapter will aim to put such data in the context of normal and pathologic joint physiology. In so doing, important caveats in the interpretation of marker data will be introduced and potential strategies for dealing with them will be discussed.

II. INTERPRETATION OF MARKER DATA AND STRATEGIES FOR DEALING WITH THEM

The underlying assumptions are straightforward. Both in normal and in abnormal joints, articular cartilage is thought to be backed by an impermeable barrier of subchondral bone. Although this assumption clearly deserves more intensive study, particularly in the setting of inflammatory joint disease, it will be accepted for the purpose of this chapter. It means that any product of cartilaginous injury or degradation must leave that tissue by passing into the overlying synovial fluid. Sampling of that fluid and measurements of its marker content may therefore provide insights in to the extent of the lesion. Further, such data may help evaluate the potential healing response to injury and the effectiveness of therapeutic interventions. Because markers are subsequently cleared from the synovial fluid into plasma, it has also been thought that simple measurements in blood may have similar value.

Measurements of marker concentration comprise virtually all of the published marker data. How useful are such static findings in this book about dynamics of bone and cartilage metabolism? All synovial fluid solutes are molecules in transit. Some move mainly from plasma into the joint (i.e., glucose and oxygen), others move mainly from the joint back into plasma (i.e., lactate, carbon dioxide, and cartilaginous "markers"), and most simply move back and forth in the ongoing equilibrium which characterizes any specific compartment of the body's extracellular space. When we aspirate an aliquot of synovial fluid, we arrest this process. Measurements in such aspirates characterize a moment in the joint just as a still frame characterizes but a moment in a moving picture. To extend the analogy, a single photograph of a busy avenue would reveal measurable numbers of pedestrians and automobiles. No matter how carefully one counted, however, such a snapshot could tell little or nothing about how fast each individual moved, how great was the overall traffic flow, or where everyone was going. If one's interest was narrower, as in police cars or men in overcoats, the photo would reveal even less. To begin to understand what is really going on, one must incorporate time in the measurements and evaluate the differing rates that characterize each participant in the scene. This limitation poses a fundamental problem for those interested in specific synovial fluid solutes and underscores the importance of interpreting the findings of aspirates within a dynamic context.

In considering the dynamics of large synovial solutes, the most relevant data have come not from cartilaginous markers but from studies of serum albumin. Such data are useful primarily for the perspective they provide on synovial lymphatic outflow. Small molecules (roughly those having molecular masses less than 10,000) are able to diffuse directly into plasma across the fenestrae of synovial blood vessels and are therefore cleared more rapidly from the joint. For larger molecules, however, the sole route of egress is thought to be convective transport through lymphatics. These valved vessels lie within the synovial interstitium; there they take up interstitial fluid, including all of its dissolved solutes, and send it on its way back to the bloodstream. That path has classically been thought to end at the thoracic duct, but evidence suggests that earlier vascular access may sometimes occur, presumably through blood vessels perfusing regional lymph nodes [4].

Albumin kinetics have been studied in joints primarily through studies using radiolabeled molecules [5–7]. Briefly, serum albumin is tagged *in vitro* with radioiodide and a precisely quantified dose is injected into the joint space. Serial gamma counts are then obtained over the joint for a period of hours and their log values are plotted against time. Such studies usually yield a highly linear declining function whose slope can be readily expressed either as a simple rate constant (in min^{-1}) or as a half-life (in min) (Fig. 1). At the conclusion of the experiment, the joint space is aspirated and the residual labeled albumin is quantified in a measured volume of synovial fluid. It is then a simple matter to take the initial counts injected, correct that number for the fraction known to have left the joint and the physical decay of the isotope, and calculate the distribution volume of the remainder by mass balance. The product of that volume (in ml) and the removal rate constant (in min^{-1}) provide a clearance rate for albumin (in ml/min) that is considered the best available measure of articular lymphatic flow [6, 8].

Proteins up to the size of IgM macroglobulin have been found to leave human knees at the same rate as albumin [9–

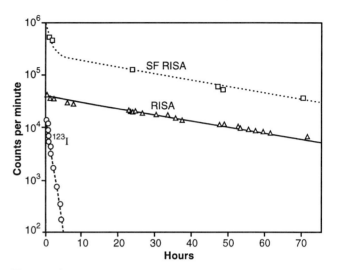

FIGURE 1   Kinetics of albumin removal from a human knee. Radiolabeled albumin (RISA) was injected at time 0 and followed serially by external counting (△) and in synovial fluid aspirates (□). After a brief equilibration period, both curves decline at the same constant rate, which may be expressed as a half-life or in min^{-1}. The latter rate constant may be multiplied by the volume of distribution to provide a clearance value in ml/min. The more rapid curve labeled ^{123}I illustrates removal of free iodide which was followed concurrently [5]. Reproduced from Wallis *et al.* [5], with permission.

11]. This means that one may multiply the concentration of such a protein (in, for instance, mg/ml) by the albumin clearance (in ml/min) to calculate a flux rate for the protein of interest (mg/min). Since most joints would presumably be studied under steady-state conditions, the flux out should equal the flux in. This influx rate is of great potential interest in converting marker studies from a static to a dynamic basis. The influx into the joint of a solely cartilage-derived molecule should provide a true indicator of "release" and thus of the rate of cartilage catabolism.

Similarly, of course, the product of the distribution volume of albumin and the concentration of a comparable protein should provide an appropriate estimate of the intra-articular mass of that protein. Previous investigators interested in marker mass have based their calculations on the synovial fluid volume, either that recovered by aspiration, that measured by indicator dilution, or a combination of the two [12, 13]. It seems most unlikely, however, that any marker found in the synovial fluid would not also be distributed through the synovial interstitial tissue. Studies with radiolabeled albumin invariably show a distribution volume that is larger than that of synovial fluid. Pilot studies also found that this larger volume did not change between 24 and 72 hours (see Fig. 1). These findings are consistent with the concept of a synovial interstitial volume that is limited by a functionally impermeable capsule and that remains in passive equilibrium with a smaller volume of included synovial fluid. It is the larger, interstitial volume that should be considered in estimating the mass and/or the dynamics of an intra-articular solute (Fig. 2).

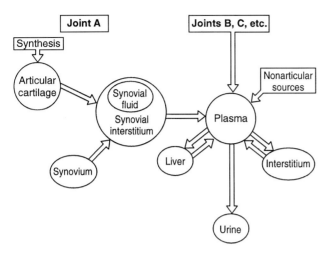

FIGURE 2 In a hypothetical knee (joint A), cartilage matrix turnover reflects the balance between ongoing synthesis and loss. "Lost" molecules enter the synovial fluid and equilibrate throughout the synovial interstitium. Degradation, which can potentially occur at many sites, produces putative "marker" molecules that are cleared from the joint into plasma by the lymphatics. In plasma, the markers mix with like molecules from other joints as well as from nonarticular sources. From plasma, markers may redistribute into other interstitial spaces, may be further processed (primarily in the liver), or may be excreted into the urine. The marker literature consists mainly of concentration measurements in synovial fluid and plasma [3]. Reproduced from Simkin and Bassett [3], with permission.

Figure 2 also illustrates some of the inherent problems when concentrations are measured not in synovial fluid but in the far more accessible plasma. If a given arthritic joint is indeed in the steady state, the rate of cartilage products released into the joint will be equalled by the rate at which those same products are passed on to the plasma pool. There, however, these products will be admixed with and diluted by the same products from all other joints in the body. This major problem limits the hope that plasma values will be useful in interpreting the degree of involvement in any single joint. The plasma pooling could be seen as an advantage in the use of markers to assess therapeutic response in a polyarticular process such as rheumatoid arthritis. Two additional concerns must be addressed, however, in any such attempt. First, most hyaline cartilage is nonarticular and many "cartilaginous" molecules are also found in tissues other than cartilage, such as the synovial matrix. Input from these sources will obviously dilute the interpretation of plasma findings as indicators of well-being in articular cartilage. The second and most important concern is that concentrations in plasma, like those in synovial fluid, are just as dependent on removal as they are on input. Most of this removal is thought to be hepatic, but some of it may be renal, some may be redistribution into other tissue compartments, and we know very little about how these rates vary among individuals. This concern is potentially adressable, but plasma concentrations will remain of limited value until we can place them in a meaningful kinetic context.

These concerns can be illustrated by some of the findings on hyaluronan. This polymeric disaccharide enters the plasma from many different tissues, with indirect evidence indicating that the peritoneum may be quantitatively the most important source. Local kinetics vary greatly among tissues, with the posterior chamber of the eye having perhaps the slowest turnover ($t_{1/2} \cong 70$ hr), the anterior chamber the fastest ($t_{1/2} \cong 1$ hr), and other tissues, including the synovium, falling somewhere in between. Entry into plasma from joints is accelerated by local inflammation and is also related clearly to the timing and extent of physical activity. Hyaluronan degradation may occur locally in tissues or subsequently in the liver. In the liver, the rate of removal from the blood is size dependent, with larger polymers being taken up more rapidly than shorter ones. The complexity of these factors illustrates some of the formidable difficulties inherent in any attempt to use plasma measurements of hyaluronan to provide meaningful information about what is happening in any specific joint. Unfortunately, the same concern applies to most plasma measurements of markers derived from cartilage.

In practice, the articular methodology shows clearly that the clearance of radiolabeled albumin is significantly faster from the knees of patients with rheumatoid arthritis (RA) than it is from patients with osteoarthritis (OA). This was true both in the initial series from Seattle and in a large study from London that focused on corticosteroid effects on hyaluronan levels [5, 6, 14]. Mean values were the same in both studies: 0.07 ml/min in RA (and in ankylosing spondylitis) and 0.04 ml/min in OA. In the British study, intra-articular corticosteroids were administered to all subjects and the study was repeated after 2 weeks and again after 2 months. Albumin clearance fell to mean rates of 0.03 and 0.04 ml/min at these intervals in RA but remained steady at 0.04 ml/min in the OA patients. Patients with ankylosing spondylitis were also studied and their albumin clearance also fell markedly after corticosteroid injections. Thus, the available evidence in humans indicates that albumin clearance (which can be considered as a measure of lymphatic drainage) is accelerated in inflammatory disease and is markedly diminished when the inflammation is effectively treated (Table I).

Comparable findings have been shown in experimental animals. Using both intra-articular pyrophosphate crystals and anterior cruciate ligament resection, Myers et al. [15, 16] have found that inflammation markedly accelerates the clearance of albumin from canine knees. Clearance increased (estimated by comparison with studies of the unmanipulated, contralateral knee) by approximately 20-fold in the intense inflammation induced by large amounts of crystals. It was also highly significant, however, when the inflammatory response was low grade, as it was with small amounts of crystals and in a common surgically-induced model of osteoarthritis (Table II). In unpublished work, Simkin et al. have used IL-1 α to induce synovitis in caprine carpal and tarsal joints and in each case, the clearance of albumin from inflamed joints was

TABLE I. Clearance of Labeled Albumin from Arthritic Knees of Human Patients

Conditions	N	C_{RISA}	C_{RISA} 2 weeks poststeroid	C_{RISA} 2 months poststeroid	Reference
OA	11	0.039 ± 0.010	n.d.	n.d.	[5]
RA	9	0.071 ± 0.008	n.d.	n.d.	[5]
OA	8	0.04 ± 0.01	0.04 ± 0.01	0.04 ± 0.01	[14]
RA	8	0.07 ± 0.01	0.03 ± 0.01	0.04 ± 0.01	[14]
AS	6	0.07 ± 0.02	0.04 ± 0.01	0.03 ± 0.01	[14]

Note. C_{RISA}, clearance of radioiodinated serum albumin in ml/min; OA, RA, and AS are osteoarthritis, rheumatoid arthritis, and ankylosing spondylitis. Values are mean $\pm$ S.E.M.

substantially greater than when the same joints were studied under control conditions both before and after the acute experimental inflammation [P. A. Simkin and J. E. Bassett, unpublished observations]. Thus in animal studies as well as in the studies of people with arthritis, the articular inflammatory response includes a significant acceleration of protein clearance.

These rates of protein clearance are essential determinants of the concentration of every synovial solute. In fact, the rate of removal from the joint is every bit as critical to the intrasynovial concentration as is the rate of entry. This simple fact has obvious applications for the interpretation of marker studies. A number of these investigators have, for instance, compared synovial fluid concentrations found in rubjects with rheumatoid arthritis with those found in subjects with osteoarthritis. Since the clearance from RA knees is approximately twice that found in OA, a finding of comparable synovial fluid concentrations would not mean that the release rate into the RA knee was also the same; instead it would be twice as great. Similarly, an RA marker concentration after a corticosteroid injection that was unchanged from the preinjection value would mean that the release of that marker had been cut in half. This is true because the articular clearance after injec-

tions is also halved. These simple illustrations show that it is, and will always be, extremely dangerous to use marker concentrations to draw conclusions about differences between diseases, responses to therapy, or any other comparison between joints unless the clearance kinetics have also been assessed.

Note that the critical determinants are the clearance rates (in ml/min). The flux rate (mg/min) is not critical because the flux in will always equal the flux out in the steady state. The intrasynovial volume is also not critical in determining concentration. A constant input of a marker molecule will rapidly lead to a steady concentration when the synovial fluid volume is small and will take considerably longer when the volume is large. The endpoint steady-state concentration will be the same, however, regardless of the effusion volume (Fig. 3).

One of the most disappointing aspects of marker studies has been the wide range of synovial fluid concentrations observed for virtually every cartilaginous marker in aspirates from virtually every diagnostic category. Values spanning two or more orders of magnitude are more the rule than the exception and this broad range has greatly limited the practical application of the method. Much of this variation, of course, reflects lack of homogeneity in any patient group. Among

TABLE II. Albumin Clearance and Volume Determinations in Canine Knees with and without Experimental Joint Disease

Condition	N	C_{RISA} (ml/min)	Va (ml)	Vd (ml)	Reference
500 μg CPPD	3	33.7	2.2 ± 0.6	36.6 ± 11.0	[15]
0.5 μg CPPD	3	6.7	1.4 ± 1.1	6.4 ± 2.1	[15]
0.05 μg CPPD	6	2.7	0.8 ± 0.6	3.8 ± 1.1	[15]
contra	13	1.5	0.2 ± 0.2	2.7 ± 0.1	[15]
cruciate	6	3.8	1.1 ± 0.9	9.2 ± 3.6	[16]
contra	6	1.4	0.1 ± 0.1	3.7 ± 0.9	[16]

Note. C_{RISA}, the clearance of radioiodinated serum albumin; CPPD, the mass of calcium phyrophosphate dihydrate crystals injected; cruciate indicates surgical transection of the anterior cruciate ligament; contra, the contralateral knee in each series of animals; Va, the aspirated volume of synovial fluid; Vd, the distribution volume of labeled albumin. Values are mean $\pm$ S.D.

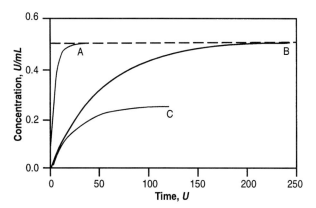

FIGURE 3 Effect of volume (mL) and clearance rate (mL per unit of time) on the solute concentration (U/mL) in a well-mixed knee receiving solute at a constant rate of 1 U per unit of time. The knee of patient A has a volume of 10 mL, whereas the knee of patient B has a volume of 100 mL. When both knees are cleared at a constant rate of 2 mL per unit of time, they both attain the same solute concentration of 0.5 U/mL, although the larger volume requires much more time to reach equilibrium. The knee of patient C also has a volume of 100 mL and receives material at the same rate. However, it is cleared at twice the rate of patient B (4 mL per unit of time) and therefore goes to an equilibrium solute concentration half as great. This figure illustrates that steady-state concentrations of any solute reflect the balance of input and output and are independent of volume [3]. Reproduced from Simkin and Bassett [3], with permission.

rheumatoid subjects, for instance, both sexes are likely to be represented and there will always be a significant range of patient age, disease duration, effusion duration, therapeutic measures in use, and intensity of the inflammatory response. Each of these factors may play a role in the intrasynovial input or clearance of specific marker molecules. Some of the observed variation must reflect real differences in marker release that carry important information about the condition and the prognosis of the studied joint. One may hope that quantification of lymphatic outflow, by allowing conversion of static synovial fluid concentrations to dynamic marker release rates, will help to sort out the logical mechanisms that underlie the current diversity of findings.

The foregoing discussion has focused on proteins "comparable" to albumin. Many of the intrasynovial molecules of greater current interest do not fit this description. Solutes with molecular masses of 10,000 or less will be cleared not only by lymphatics but will also pass through microvascular fenestrae and be cleared directly into the venous circulation. Because the rate of synovial plasma flow greatly exceeds the rate of lymphatic drainage, venous clearance could easily accelerate the clearance of IL-1 or TNF α, for instance, by an order of magnitude compared to that of albumin. There are no available data that allow estimation of the passive transport rates for such solutes. Obviously, the specific cellular uptake of such cytokine molecules adds huge additional complications to any consideration of their articular dynamics.

At the other end of the size spectrum, markers released from cartilage may not resemble the compact, globular struc-

ture of albumin but may instead be much larger and more linear strands of aggrecan (or its catabolites), type II collagen, or other cartilage constituents. It is now clear that such macromolecules do not leave the joint as readily as does albumin. This issue was addressed by Page-Thomas *et al.*, who found the mean clearance half-life for large proteoglycan molecules ($M_r = 2.5 \times 10^6$) leaving the rabbit knee to be 12.5 hr in contrast to 3.9 hr for albumin in the same joints [17]. A more striking difference was reported by Coleman *et al.*, who also used rabbit knees but studied hyaluronan kinetics with a different experimental approach. Their mean half-lives were 26.3 hr for hyaluronan and 1.23 hr for albumin [18]. These findings lead to an inescapable conclusion: marker molecules, which are large in mass and/or configuration, are partially reflected back into the joint space as fluid flows into terminal lymphatides through the interstitial matrix of the synovium. More work remains to be done in defining just what are the critical molecular dimensions, in evaluating the effects of local inflammation on this sieving function of the synovium, and in distinguishing between the fractions that are cleared into lymphatics, reflected back into the joint, or locally degraded. That work will be facilitated by Levick's simple approach comparing half-lives of markers to that of albumin in order to quantify the extent of reflection [19].

III. CONCLUSIONS

Studies of cartilaginous markers have been limited primarily to measurements of concentration in synovial fluid and in plasma. When such data are used to compare different conditions or to follow the same condition serially, the work necessarily assumes that the clearance does not vary between conditions, between individuals, or within the same individual over time. Unfortunately, those assumptions are demonstrably false. To fulfill the marker promise of information regarding "release" from cartilage, the kinetics of these molecules must be examined together with their concentration. Fortunately, relatively simple techniques, largely based on concurrent studies of serum albumin as a reference solute, may go a long way to remedy this situation.

References

1. Lohmander, L. S. (1994). Articular cartilage and osteoarthritis: The role of molecular markers to monitor breakdown, repair and disease. *J. Anat.* **184**, 477–492.
2. Poole, A. R., and Dieppe, P. (1994). Biological markers in rheumatoid arthritis. *Semin. Arthritis Rheum.* **23** (Suppl. 2), 17–31.
3. Simkin, P. A., and Bassett, J. E. (1995). Cartilage matrix molecules in serum and synovial fluid. *Curr. Opin. Rheumatol.* **7**, 346–351.
4. Rayan, I., Thonar, E. J.-M. A., Chen, L. M., Lenz, M. E., and Williams, J. M. (1998). Regional differences in the rise in blood levels of antigenic keratan sulfate and hyaluronan after chymopapain induced knee joint injury. *J. Rheumatol.* **25**, 521–526.

5. Wallis, W. J., Simkin, P. A., Nelp, W. B., and Foster, D. M. (1985). Intraarticular volume and clearance in human synovial effusions. *Arthritis Rheum.* **28**, 441–449.

6. Wallis, W. J., Simkin, P. A., and Nelp, W. B. (1987). Protein traffic in human synovial effusions. *Arthritis Rheum.* **30**, 57–63.

7. Simkin, P. A., and Benedict, R. S. (1990). Iodide and albumin kinetics in normal canine wrists and knees. *Arthritis Rheum.* **33**, 73–79.

8. Levick, J. R. (1995). Fluid movement across synovium in healthy joints: Role of synovial fluid macromolecules. *Ann. Rheum. Dis.* **54**, 417–423.

9. Rodnan, G. P., and MacLachlan, M. J. (1960). The absorption of serum albumin and gammaglobulin from the knee joint of man and rabbit. *Arthritis Rheum.* **3**, 152–157.

10. Sliwinski, A. F., and Zvaifler, N. J. (1969). The removal of aggregated and nonaggregated autologous gamma globulin from rheumatoid joints. *Arthritis Rheum.* **12**, 504–514.

11. Weinberger, A., and Simkin, P. A. (1989). Plasma proteins in synovial fluids of normal human joints. *Semin. Arthritis Rheum.* **19**, 66–76.

12. Geborek, P., Saxne, T., Heinegard, D., and Wollheim, F. A. (1988). Measurement of synovial fluid volume using albumin dilution upon intraarticular saline injection. *J. Rheumatol.* **15**, 91–94.

13. Delecrin, J., Oka, M., Kumar, P., Takahashi, S., Kotoura, Y., Yamamuro, T., and Daculsi, G. (1992). Measurement of synovial fluid volume: A new dilution method adapted to fluid permeation from the synovial cavity. *J. Rheumatol.* **19**, 1746–1752.

14. Pitsillides, A. A., Will, R. K., Bayliss, M. T., and Edwards, J. C. W. (1994). Circulating and synovial fluid hyaluronan levels: Effects of intraarticular corticosteroid on the concentration and the rate of turnover. *Arthritis Rheum.* **37**, 1030–1038.

15. Myers, S. L., Brandt, K. D., and Eilam, O. (1995). Even low-grade synovitis significantly accelerates the clearance of protein from the canine knee. Implications for measurement of synovial fluid "markers" of osteoarthritis. *Arthritis Rheum.* **38**, 1085–1091.

16. Myers, S. L., O'Connor, B. L., and Brandt, K. D. (1996). Accelerated clearance of albumin from the osteoarthritic knee: Implications for interpretation of concentrations of "cartilage markers" in synovial fluid. *J. Rheumatol.* **23**, 1744–1748.

17. Page-Thomas, D. P., Bard, D., King, B., and Dingle, J. T. (1987). Clearance of proteoglycan from joint cavities. *Ann. Rheum. Dis.* **46**, 934–937.

18. Coleman, P. J., Scott, D., Ray, J., Mason, R. M., and Levick, J. R. (1997). Hyaluronan secretion into the synovial cavity of rabbit knees and comparison with albumin turnover. *J. Physiol.* **503**, 645–656.

19. Levick, J. R. (1998). A method for estimating macromolecular reflection by human synovium, using measurements of intra-articular half lives. *Ann. Rheum. Dis.* **57**, 339–344.

CHAPTER 23

In Vitro Models of Cartilage Metabolism

H. J. HÄUSELMANN AND E. HEDBOM

Department of Rheumatology and Physical Medicine, Section of Matrix Biology, Center of Experimental Rheumatology, University Hospital Zürich, Zürich, Switzerland

I. ABSTRACT

There is a hierarchy of culture systems that can be employed as models in studies of cartilage metabolism. From the biological point of view, the best system is the (organ) culture of explanted cartilage slices. Cell proliferation, which may complicate the interpretation of metabolism data, can be avoided in these cultures. The bovine species is preferable, showing negligible cell proliferation under normal culture conditions. Human adult articular cartilage is a potentially good alternative, but major disadvantages include limited supply of material and heterogeneity of samples due to difficulties in controlling for age and subclinical degenerative processes. The organ culture system, with the anabolic and catabolic pathways balanced to maintain homeostasis, is very useful for studying synthesis, turnover, and drug responses with respect to the metabolism of matrix macromolecules. However, for some types of studies, e.g., those concerning assembly of matrix macromolecules or evaluation of cell surface receptors, this culture system is less suitable. In addition, the presence of a large matrix containing polyanionic macromolecules generally makes extraction and analysis of mRNA or proteins more difficult. Therefore, systems with isolated chondrocytes are widely used. The monolayer culture, although offering technical advantages, is in many cases the least desirable system. Phenotypic changes occur more rapidly even at high density conditions and anchorage-dependent growth is likely to cause other unwanted, more subtle changes. Suspension cultures of chondrocytes in agarose, alginate, or other gel forming systems exhibit several interesting features. The gels minimize inappropriate cell–cell interactions and stabilize or reestablish the differentiated chondrocyte phenotype. Cells isolated from different cartilage layers and different joints can be compared when cultured under initially controlled conditions. The three-dimensional gel suspension cultures can readily be used to study the metabolism of proteoglycans and other glycoproteins newly synthesized and laid down in the pericellular matrix. Studies of this kind are likely to provide new insights in chondrocyte biology and repair of cartilage lesions.

II. OVERVIEW OF *IN VITRO* MODELS OF CARTILAGE METABOLISM

In adult articular cartilage, living chondrocytes comprise only 2–5% of the tissue volume, the remainder being occupied by the extracellular matrix, which has a decisive influence on the biomechanical properties of the tissue [1]. The chondrocytes are responsible not only for the generation of extracellular matrix during growth and development, but also for its maintenance by finely tuned synthesis and degradation of matrix macromolecules. The importance of the chondrocytes in adult cartilage is illustrated by the pathological changes in osteoarthritis. Here, a disturbed metabolism under the influence of altered biomechanical loading conditions results in a loss of equilibrium in the turnover of matrix constituents and, as a consequence, in a disintegration of the matrix.

The macromolecules known to be present in cartilage extracellular matrices are extensively described in other sections of this book. Studies of these molecules have dramatically increased our knowledge regarding their structures and genetic relationships, whereas information about their supramolecular organization and spatial distribution within the cartilage matrix still is relatively limited. Moreover, many aspects of the regulation of the biosynthesis, processing, and control over deposition and degradation of matrix constituents are poorly understood. It is obvious that the appropriate function of cartilage requires a coordinated expression of several genes coding for both major and minor components of the tissue. However, many of the necessary regulatory mechanisms and proteins involved therein remain to be identified.

The mature articular chondrocyte embedded in its extracellular matrix is a resting cell with no measurable mitotic activity and a very low rate of matrix production and degradation. However, the fact that chondrocytes, even from old individuals, after enzymatic release from articular cartilage and transfer to cell culture can become reactivated and start to divide and produce extracellular matrix indicates that the metabolic state of these cells is strictly controlled by their microenvironment. Likewise, chondrocytes *in vivo* may respond to structural changes in the extracellular matrix. For example, the partial degradation and loss of proteoglycans observed in initial stages of osteoarthritis [2, 3] lead to chondrocyte proliferation and increased collagen and proteoglycan (PG) biosynthesis [4, 5].

Mature articular cartilage is in many respects heterogeneous. There are differences between species and between different joints. Even within a single joint, there is variation in cartilage properties. It is important to consider that many features of articular cartilage vary with the depth in the tissue. The cell density is highest near the articular surface where the chondrocytes appear flattened and are oriented parallel to the surface. Cells of the deeper cartilage layers are more spherical and those of the deepest zone are usually slightly extended in the direction perpendicular to the surface. By a number of criteria, the cells of different layers, but particularly the surface layer versus the deep layers, exhibit differences in their properties, including rate of synthesis of various components and different ratios of specific molecules produced [6, 7]. Some of these differences have been shown to persist in primary cell cultures [6, 8].

Another important matter is the cell/matrix relationship in terms of relative proportions and the quality of the interaction. Stockwell observed that the thickness of cartilage within a given joint of a quadruped animal was related to the body weight of the animal [9]. However, cellularity was not related to the thickness of cartilage present, but instead was related to the joint surface area. This means that larger and heavier animals have more matrix per cell. Human knee joint cartilage, which has to cope with unusually high loads because of the bipedal nature of man, is particularly thick and enriched in extracellular matrix. Accordingly, the cell/matrix ratio of this special articular cartilage is extremely low [9, 10].

The issues introduced above are all related to cartilage cell biology and biochemistry. They can be addressed in experimental studies. In this context, *in vivo* cartilage models are often too complicated and impractical to use and, hence, *in vitro* models are preferable in many cases. Among the different possible testing systems, a hierarchy can be recognized that includes: (1) the intact joint, together with all the biomechanical forces that are placed on it; (2) the cells and their matrix in tissue culture; and (3) culture of isolated cells after release from the extracellular matrix. Cultures of cartilage slices or isolated chondrocytes have proven to be very useful tools in studies of the metabolic activity and regulation of cartilage cells and their surrounding matrix, for example with respect to the formation of PG, the assembly of the latter into PG aggregates, and their turnover [11, 12]. In addition, systems with bare chondrocytes in culture are extremely valuable as models, offering possibilities to isolate single parameters, to determine specific cell-matrix interactions, and to dissect intrinsic cellular properties (e.g., cell shape) from extrinsic matrix-induced properties.

Numerous studies have focused on the behavior of chondrocytes in different culture systems (Fig. 1, Table I). Investigators have tried to relate the properties of cells maintained in culture to those within articular cartilage tissue [8, 13, 14] to define the unique properties of chondrocytes as opposed to those of other cells (particularly fibroblasts [15]), and to develop culture conditions that accurately maintain the cartilage phenotype [16–20]. With few exceptions, only culture conditions that allow the cells to maintain a spherical cell shape and prevent spreading and outgrowth of cell processes can preserve the chondrogenic phenotype [20–25]. A culture condition that certainly supports this phenotype is organ culture [12]. Cultures in agarose [16, 18, 26, 27], in alginate [28–30], possibly in collagen gel [20, 31, 32], in high density monolayer cultures [33–36], and in suspension cultures in spinner flasks [8, 37, 38] or roller bottles [35, 38] produce, at least for a certain period of time, phenotypically stable chondrocytes from several different species. With the

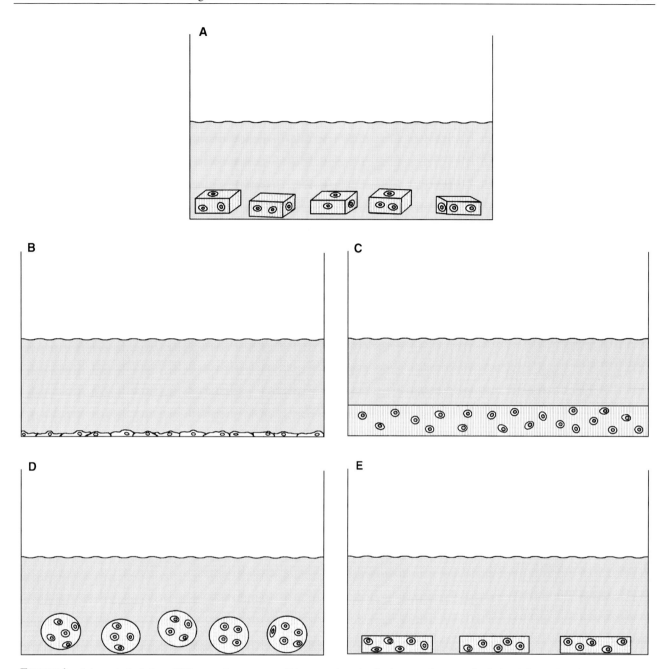

FIGURE 1   Schematic depiction of different culture systems. (A) organ culture (explant) system demonstrating isolated pieces of cartilage immersed in culture medium; (B) monolayer system demonstrating chondrocytes adherent to a plastic surface; (C–E) three-dimensional gel systems showing suspended chondrocytes at the bottom of the culture dish with medium on top, in the case of the agarose system (C), suspended chondrocytes in alginate beads (D), or alginate diskettes (E).

exception of primary cultures of bovine and human articular chondrocytes in alginate beads [19] and of a clonal population of a mature human chondrosarcoma cell line [25], there is no information available regarding the long-term stability (i.e., over several months) of the phenotype in such cultures.

The common feature of the chondrogenic culture conditions is that the chondrocytes are allowed to encapsulate themselves in a pericellular matrix consisting of collagen II and large aggregating PG together with a number of other collagenous and noncollagenous matrix proteins. The cell-associated matrix that is formed is, at least in three-dimensional culture systems like agarose and alginate, apparently very similar to native cartilage matrix in its composition [14, 19, 26, 39, 40].

TABLE I.   Comparison of Different Chondrocyte Culture Systems

	Explant	Gel suspension	Monolayer
Biological aspects			
Preservation of the chondrocyte phenotype	Excellent	Very good in agarose or alginate gel	Depends on seeding density; poor if cells are seeded at low density
Persistence of differences between chondrocyte subpopulations	Yes	Yes, at least to some extent	Has not been shown
Persistence of matrix-dependent control of chondrocyte behavior	Yes	Disrupted initially but becomes gradually reestablished	No
Metabolic activity with respect to matrix constituents	Similar as *in vivo*: steady state, with slow turnover of matrix macromolecules	Enhanced anabolic activity, turnover rate similar as *in vivo*	Strongly stimulated anabolism; studies of metabolism difficult
Cell proliferation	No	Yes, but slow	Yes, rapid growth to reach confluent state; possible to prepare large amounts of cells from small samples
Technical aspects			
Handling	Difficult	Less difficult	Easy
Homogeneity among replicate samples	Not very good	Good	Good
Detection of gene expression	Difficult to isolate mRNA; low signal strength	Easy to isolate mRNA, particularly in the case of alginate cultures	Easy to isolate mRNA; high signal strength
Quantification of specific gene products, isolation of macromolecules	Relatively difficult, the presence of a compact extracellular matrix hampers extraction	Less difficult	Easy
Studies of supramolecular organization of matrix constituents	Possible but difficult	Possible	Limited possibilities, not very useful
Nutrition of cultured cells	May be poor; varies with the shape and quality of the specimen	Good and constant in most cases	Good and constant

Note: See text for references.

A. Organ (Explant) Culture System and Isolated Chondrons

The extracellular matrix of cartilage tissue is substantially different from the sparser, less-organized matrix that is laid down initially by cultured chondrocytes following their isolation (Fig. 2). For some applications, it is preferable to use an experimental model in which chondrocytes are kept within the matrix structure that is assembled *in vivo*. This type of *in vitro* system preserves the immediate environment of the chondrocyte with its macromolecules, including cell-binding proteins, as well as the collagen "basket" or "chondron" organization of the fibrillar network in the territorial matrix surrounding the chondrocyte; thus, it permits a more realistic evaluation of signals transmitted from and to the chondrocytes through the complex architecture of the tissue. Furthermore, articular organ cultures maintain the proper cellular and matrix topography of the tissue. This level of organization is considered to be essential for the normal physiology of the tissue.

The pioneering work of Fell [41] showed that it was possible to maintain cartilage in organ culture. Since then, articular

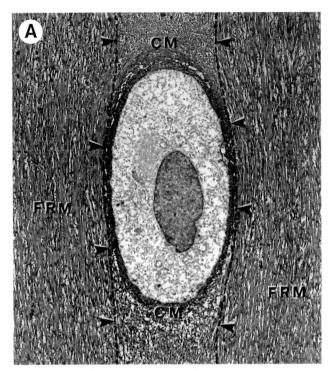

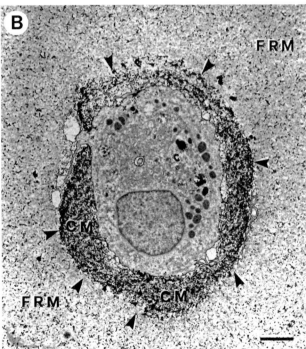

FIGURE 2   Electron micrographs of adult human articular chondrocytes cultured in articular cartilage tissue (A) and alginate gel (B). (A) Chondrocyte in normal adult human knee joint cartilage. (B) Chondrocyte isolated from adult human knee joint cartilage and cultured in alginate gel for 30 days. The alginate bead and tissue were fixed, stained, embedded, and sectioned according to the protocol described in van Osch *et al.* [75]. Delineation of the border between cell-associated matrix (pericellular and territorial matrix, CM) and further removed matrix compartments (interterritorial matrix, FRM) is indicated by arrowheads and a dotted line in (A) and by arrowheads in (B). Bar, 2.5 mm.

cartilage from various species and from differently aged animals has been successfully maintained in explant culture [42]. In more thorough studies of cartilage metabolism, bovine cultures have been used most frequently. Initial work by Hascall *et al.* demonstrated a spontaneous resorption of matrix PG in either calf or steer cartilage when cultured in the presence of medium alone (basal cultures) [43]. This was different from the metabolic state of normal cartilage, where the amount of PG within the extracellular matrix is kept at a remarkably constant level. However, cultures of calf articular cartilage in the presence of 20% fetal calf serum (FCS) revealed a precise balance between anabolic and catabolic pathways, keeping the PG mass at steady state. The half-life of total PG initially present in the calf tissue culture was approximately 21 days [44]. These findings could be confirmed and extended in additional experiments in which ^{35}S-sulfate precursors were used to specifically label the PG. Newly synthesized molecules were retained in the matrix and continuously released into the culture medium at a constant rate corresponding to a half life of 21 days [44]. Measurements of the biosynthesis of PG by a short pulse in the presence of ^{35}S-sulfate showed constant rates of PG synthesis over the entire experimental period, adequately compensating for losses of PG through catabolic pathways.

The advantages of cartilage explant cultures with chondrocytes that are able to keep matrix homeostasis similar to homeostasis *in vivo* have inspired a number of researchers to choose this model system to investigate different aspects of PG metabolism in further detail. Studies have been performed specifically concerning the regulation of PG synthesis [43], PG turnover [45–47], and the response of cartilage to damage by proteinases [48], lipopolysaccharides [47], and interleukin-1 [12, 45, 49, 50]. In addition, it should be noted that the organ cultures also maintain constant levels of collagen type II for several weeks [47, 51]. The initial work of Hascall *et al.* [43] showed synthesis of cartilage-specific type II collagen and suggested a balanced metabolism for this component. Furthermore, electron microscopy studies have shown that after 50 days of culture in the presence of FCS, the collagen fibers keep their morphological integrity and characteristic banding pattern [51].

The cartilage organ culture model is ideal for investigating the effects of various agents on cartilage metabolism. It is of particular interest to assess the ability of therapeutic agents to protect cartilage from damage and to enhance repair processes. In such studies, it is often relevant to use culture medium not supplemented with large quantities of FCS, since maintenance of cartilage homeostasis may represent the aim and not the starting point. For example, several independent research groups have presented evidence that growth factors like transforming growth factor-β1 (TGF-β1) and insulin-like growth factor-1 (IGF-1) are able to maintain or restore PG homeostasis in explant cultures of bovine articular cartilage [44, 52, 53].

A limiting factor of the organ culture system is that the PG cannot be extracted in significant amounts with solvents that do not dissociate the PG-aggregates into their component parts [54, 55]. This has been circumvented by cutting very thin sections [7] and treating these with purified collagenase prior to extraction with an associative solvent. However, due to its technical difficulty and time consuming behavior, this procedure is not used routinely.

An alternative for studying chondrocyte metabolism is to isolate and culture chondrons. Chondrons are structural units in cartilage consisting of one or more chondrocytes, the cell-associated and territorial matrix with the enclosing capsule. While chondron structure and molecular anatomy have been fairly well described [56], studies of chondron metabolism have received limited attention because of the limited yield and viability after mechanical isolation of chondrons. One reported method of enzymatic chondron isolation appears to be relatively simple, gives a better yield of viable chondrons, and therefore provides an attractive *in vitro* model system to study chondrocyte metabolism within the confines of its natural three-dimensional pericellular microenvironment [57].

B. High Density Monolayer Cultures

Growth and expression of the differentiated phenotype of chondrocytes from different origins and species are known to be highly dependent on cell density or cell–cell contact [27, 33, 58]. Chondrocytes placed in low density monolayers spread along the culture surface and, over time, come to resemble fibroblasts [59, 60]. This morphologic transformation has been noted to have the functional correlate that the dedifferentiating chondrocytes downregulate their synthesis of cartilage-specific macromolecules (e.g., the most abundant collagen II and the large aggregating keratan sulfate-containing chondroitin sulfate-PG aggrecan) and upregulate the synthesis of collagen I [23, 61, 62]. Some investigators have therefore utilized primary, short-term, high cell density monolayer cultures [35, 36], which synthesize molecules *in vitro* that are indistinguishable from those made *in vivo*, at least with respect to PG [63]. The phenotypic expression as monitored by PG and collagen II synthesis is maintained during the first 10–15 cell doublings but, at least in the cases of chick or bovine chondrocytes, slow phenotypic transition leads to a marked decrease of collagen II expression and a significant expression of collagen I after approximately 7–14 days [40, 64, 65].

As stated above, the expression of collagen I polypeptides by cartilage cells cultured in monolayers often is considered a marker for the loss of the chondrocyte phenotype. However, Kolettas *et al.* [66] demonstrated, using sensitive detection with reverse transcriptase/polymerase chain reaction, that chondrocytes in normal fresh intact human ar-

ticular cartilage expressed collagen $\alpha1(I)$ mRNA. Whether this indicates protein secretion is not yet clear. The same authors also showed that despite the morphological differences between chondrocytes cultured as monolayers (fibroblastoid appearance) and chondrocytes cultured over agarose (spherical), under both culture conditions the cells expressed markers at mRNA and protein levels characteristic of cartilage. Thus, the cells in both systems expressed collagens II and IX as well as the major constituents of the large PG aggregates, aggrecan and link protein, but not the cell surface PG syndecan. On the basis of these data, Kolettas *et al.* [66] proposed that the loss of the chondrocyte phenotype is associated with loss of one or more cartilage-specific molecules rather than with the appearance of noncartilage-specific molecules.

An interesting alternative to the use of chondrocytes from normal cartilage for propagation in monolayer cultures has been explored by Block *et al.* [25], who developed cell lines from adult human chondrosarcoma for this purpose. The availability of a stable clonal chondrocytic cell population synthesizing normal cartilage PG in long-term culture provided opportunities to examine the influence of cell shape and physical state on the biosynthesis of chondrocyte-specific macromolecules. The confounding issues of inherent dedifferentiation and chondrocyte heterogeneity could be excluded from these studies. Although the chondrocytes exhibited abnormal regulation of growth, which may be associated with abnormalities in the control of gene expression, the stability of the phenotype with respect to PG production in this particular low density monolayer culture system demonstrated that dedifferentiation does not always occur whenever chondrocytes show a flattened morphology and a high proliferation rate. Therefore, the control of aggrecan biosynthesis may be distinct from influences related to cell shape.

Apart from the influence of direct physical contacts of cells with their surroundings and the specific properties of differently established cell lines, phenotypic expression and stability may critically depend on the presence of soluble factors (e.g., cytokines). Indeed, monolayer cultures have been employed in several studies concerning the effects of such factors on chondrocyte activities. This may be because the technical procedures are simple and convenient and many variables are relatively well controlled, which should give a good accuracy in the experiments. The disadvantage that the studied cells may be phenotypically different from normal chondrocytes is sometimes less considered. Interestingly, some of the reported results indicate that exogenously added factors may preserve the chondrocyte phenotype and prevent dedifferentiation. For example, Sailor *et al.* showed that human recombinant bone morphogenetic protein-2, a member of the TGF-β superfamily, promoted the phenotype of articular chondrocytes from 14-day-old calves in cell culture. In addition, the cytokine did not induce differentiation to a hypertrophic phenotype, suggesting a potential for future use of human recombinant bone morphogenetic protein-2 and other related proteins in treatment of osteoarthritis and repair of articular cartilage [64].

Monolayer cultures with a high cell density may be quite useful for studying the intracellular events involved in PG biosynthesis [63] and, in some cases, the process of PG aggregation [67]. Only very little cell-associated matrix is accumulated in these cultures, and the chondrocytes secrete newly synthesized macromolecules more or less directly into the medium. As a consequence, PG and other matrix components synthesized in the presence of radiolabeled precursors can be recovered from the medium in relatively large amounts with a high specific radioactivity [68]. For the same reason, cultures of this type are not useful for examining PG turnover or for studies of mechanisms and molecules involved in matrix assembly.

C. Suspension Culture Systems

Cells grown in suspension or in three-dimensional gels like agarose [16, 18, 26, 27] or alginate [28–30] keep their spherical shape, divide, and reestablish an abundant cell-associated matrix (Figs. 3 and 4). Once integrated within

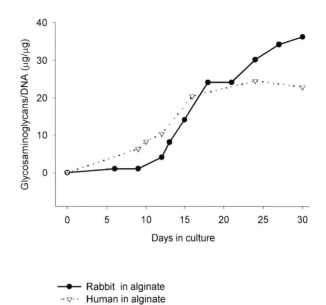

Rabbit in alginate
Human in alginate

FIGURE 4   Accumulation of glycosaminoglycans in relation to cell number in rabbit and human chondrocytes cultured in alginate. Chondrocytes were isolated from normal rabbit and human articular cartilage and cultured in alginate for 30 days in the presence of 10% fetal calf serum. The increase in glycosaminoglycans was determined using a slightly modified protocol of the alcian blue precipitation method [82]. DNA was measured using the Hoechst dye 33258 [68a].

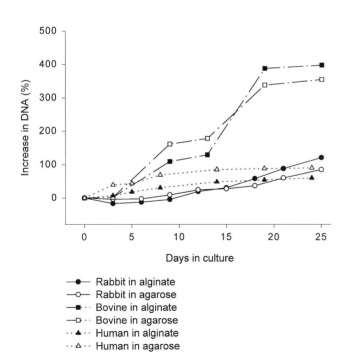

—●— Rabbit in alginate
—○— Rabbit in agarose
—■·· Bovine in alginate
—□·· Bovine in agarose
··▲·· Human in alginate
··△·· Human in agarose

FIGURE 3   Proliferation of human, bovine, and rabbit chondrocytes cultured in three-dimensional culture systems. Chondrocytes were isolated from normal human, bovine, and rabbit articular cartilage and cultured in either agarose or alginate for approximately 20 days in the presence of 10% fetal calf serum. The increase in cell number over time was determined by quantifying DNA of the seeded cells at various time points using the fluorescent dye 33258 from Hoechst [68a]. The numbers are expressed as percent increase from baseline (day 0).

the matrix, PGs appear to undergo limited degradation by factors released by the cells. The chondrocytes retain phenotypic stability for several months [19]. In particular, agarose and alginate, which represent the two most widely employed gel systems, have been used extensively to examine the effect of different agents on synthesis and turnover of PG by articular chondrocytes of several species [18, 26, 29, 55, 69, 70]. These *in vitro* models are also useful in comparing the properties of specific cell populations from different regions of articular cartilage or from different joints [71]. For example, some cells in preparations from the whole thickness of articular cartilage do not surround themselves with an abundant extracellular matrix [55, 72]. These chondrocytes are derived from the most superficial layer and they show a specific metabolic behavior that is very different from that of cells derived from deeper layers of articular cartilage. Likewise, chondrocytes from different joints (e.g., ankle versus knee joint) demonstrate differences in their metabolic behavior with respect to PG synthesis and degradation under the influence interleukin-1 [71].

One attractive attempt to explain the ineffective healing response of cartilage lesions was to postulate the absence of an appropriate stimulatory regulator [73]. This hypothesis has led to a large number of studies exploring the effect of exogenous growth factors on articular chondrocytes *in vitro*. The rate of cell divisions, the state of cell differentiation, and the types of matrix components synthesized in different matrix compartments can be altered by the addition of exogenous cytokines to chondrocyte cultures [74, 75]. A further level of complexity has been introduced by the suggestion that components of the extracellular matrix may act locally to modulate the activity of cytokines. To examine this question further, a suspension culture system (alginate) may be suitable because it allows matrix proteins such as fibrillar collagens to become incorporated in an assembled matrix surrounding the chondrocytes [76].

In addition, gel suspension cultures can be used as a source of matrix-embedded chondrocytes to be tested in biomechanical experiments. Gels containing suspended chondrocytes with their newly formed and laid down matrix can be loaded after various culture times in order to determine stress-strain relationships [26]. Interestingly, the results can be correlated to different stages of matrix assembly modified by different cytokines and growth factors.

1. Specific Advantages of the Alginate Gel System

a. Solubilization of the Gel and Release of the Chondrocytes after a Certain Time in Culture   A disadvantage of most gel suspension culture systems is the lack of methods for depolymerization of the gel-forming component under mild conditions. As a consequence, there is no possibility to release the cells after a certain time in culture. For the same reason, PG of the newly synthesized and laid down matrix cannot be extracted in significant amounts unless denaturing solvents are used which dissociate the PG-aggregates into their component parts [54, 55] (Fig. 5). Under these circumstances the cells can not be used in the form of isolated chondrocytes for further examinations, e.g., for the characterization of intracellular regulatory molecules using molecular biology and/or immunohistochemical techniques. The specific property of alginate to depolymerize in the presence of substances that form soluble complexes with calcium ions offers an elegant possibility to circumvent these obstacles.

b. Characterization of Macromolecules in Different Matrix Compartments   In adult articular cartilage, matrix compartmentalization was originally characterized according to histological criteria. Hunziker [77] has proposed that the definition of the different compartments should be based on the organization of the collagen network. The cell-associated matrix is made up of two compartments, the pericellular compartment around the plasmalemma (rich in PG) and, adjacent to this, the territorial (or capsular) matrix with a fine network of collagen fibrils extending around individual or nests of chondrocytes. The outermost interterritorial matrix constitutes the largest domain in adult articular cartilage. The agarose system is able to keep cultured chondrocytes phenotypically stable and permits formation of a new, dense pericellular matrix consisting of aggregating PG and collagen fibers, the latter forming a basket-like structure [6].

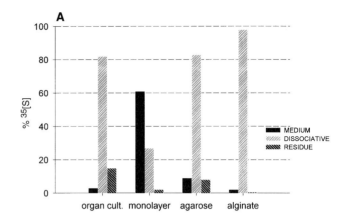

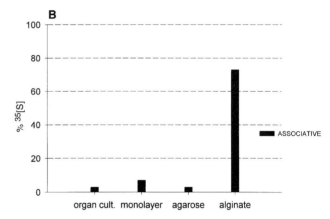

FIGURE 5   Comparison of extractibility of ^{35}S-sulfate-proteoglycans synthesized by human chondrocytes in different *in vitro* models of cartilage metabolism. The results are depicted as percent of total ^{35}S-proteoglycans synthesized during a 4-h incubation in the presence of ^{35}S-sulfate. (A) At the end of this incubation, the medium used for radiolabeling was removed and the gel was extracted with 4 M GuHCl (dissociative extraction). The residue reflects radiolabeled proteoglycans that were recovered in a pellet after centrifugation of the 4 M GuHCl extract. (B) In parallel cultures, the labeling medium was removed at the end of the incubation and the gel was extracted with 0.2 M GuHCl (associative extraction). In the case of the alginate, the gel was first solubilized (see Section III, Techniques, in this chapter).

This newly synthesized and assembled matrix resembles the combined pericellular and territorial matrix seen in cartilage *in vivo*. In contrast to the matrix assembled and laid down in cartilage *in vivo*, no further-removed interterritorial matrix is formed in the agarose system.

Interestingly, the extracellular matrix of chondrocytes cultured in alginate gel is composed of two compartments: the cell-associated matrix, believed to correspond to the pericellular and territorial matrix compartments, and the further-removed matrix, a compartment that is thought to correspond to the interterritorial areas of the articular cartilage matrix [14, 78]. Due to the unique advantage of the alginate system to offer quick solubilization of the gel and release of the cells after a certain time in culture, most of the aggrecan molecules in each compartment are readily extractable. Therefore, it is possible to study these molecules in their native aggregated state [29] (Fig. 5). Using this approach, most newly synthesized ^{35}S-aggrecan molecules capable of binding to HA become incorporated into the cell-associated matrix [14, 78]. Aggrecan molecules that reached the further-removed matrix during the first 24 h following synthesis were found to lack a functional HA-binding region upon entering this compartment. This suggested that molecules released extracellularly with an immature, as yet nonfunctional HA-binding region, have a much greater chance of reaching the further-removed interterritorial areas of the matrix than those whose HA-binding domain is already functional.

c. Examination of PG Metabolism in the Two Different Matrix Compartments It is generally agreed that PG, including aggrecan, the most abundant PG in cartilage, turns over more rapidly than collagens. In cultured adult bovine articular cartilage explants maintaining steady-state conditions, the half-life of aggrecan is fairly short (7–41 days) [79]. However, measurement of racemization of aspartic acid in aggrecan isolated from adult human articular cartilage led Maroudas [80] to suggest that the average half-life of this aggregating PG in human adult articular cartilage is actually closer to two years. The discrepancy between the long average half-life of aggrecan molecules in human articular cartilage and the shorter half-life of aggrecan synthesized *in vitro* remains to be clarified. An interesting possibility is that the majority of aggrecan molecules in human articular cartilage is present in a matrix compartment that escapes the more rapid turnover typical of newly synthesized ^{35}S-aggrecan molecules *in vitro*. Lohmander was the first to propose that the cartilage matrix contains at least two compartments of PG turning over at different rates, a hypothesis supported by his study of guinea pig costal cartilage [81]. Evidence in support of this contention was also obtained from another study that compared the rate of turnover of aggrecan molecules present in the cell-associated and further-removed compartments of the matrix formed by mature bovine articular chondrocytes in alginate beads. The results showed that aggrecan molecules incorporated in the cell-associated matrix turn over more rapidly ($t_{1/2}$ = 15 days) than those deposited in the further removed matrix ($t_{1/2}$ = >95 days) [78].

Since normal human adult articular cartilage is difficult to obtain, very few attempts have been made to study the metabolism of aggrecan in this tissue. It is not clear to what extent the information about the metabolism of nonhuman articular chondrocytes can be applied in trying to understand the changes these cells and their synthesized products undergo with aging and in disease (i.e., osteoarthritis). Studies have shown that the matrix formed by adult human chondrocytes in alginate beads is composed of two compartments: a thin rim of cell-associated matrix which corresponds to the pericellular and territorial matrix of articular cartilage and a more abundant further-removed matrix, the possible equiv-

alent of the interterritorial matrix in the tissue [14]. On day 30 of culture, the relative and absolute volumes occupied by the cells and each of the two matrix compartments in the beads were nearly identical to those in native articular cartilage, although the number of collagen fibers laid down in the alginate system was clearly less than in *in vivo* cartilage (Fig. 2). Further, the concentration of aggrecan in the cell-associated matrix was similar to that in adult human articular cartilage and was approximately 40 times higher than in the further-removed matrix compartment. Fluorescence-activated cell sorting revealed that the cell-associated matrix was built upon the cell membrane in part via interactions between hyaluronan and CD44-like receptors. Approximately 25% of the aggrecan molecules synthesized by the chondrocytes during a 4 h pulse in the presence of ^{35}S-sulfate on day 9 of culture were retained in the cell-associated matrix where they turned over with a half-life of 29 days. Most ^{35}S-aggrecan molecules reached the further-removed matrix compartment where they turned over much more slowly ($t_{1/2}$ >100 days). These results add support to the contention that, comparable to the bovine species, aggrecan molecules of the pericellular and territorial areas in adult human articular cartilage matrix are more susceptible to degradation by proteolytic enzymes than those which belong to the interterritorial areas further removed from the cells. Despite these encouraging findings, the morphometric and biochemical characterization of the different matrix compartments of chondrocytes cultured in alginate needs to be established further; and it has yet to be shown that these two compartments can be reliably separated at various time points in culture.

III. TECHNIQUES

A. Cell Culture Systems

1. HARVESTING OF CARTILAGE

Intact, not opened metacarpophalangeal or shoulder joints (10 months old calves or 18–24 months old steers) are obtained from a local slaughterhouse. Human knee or ankle joints are obtained from organ donors from regional organ banks or medical examiner offices after institutional approval. Cartilage tissue should be prepared within 24 h after death. In all cases, articular cartilage in the joints should appear normal and free of osteoarthritic lesions or other visible abnormalities. Articular cartilage slices are aseptically dissected from the joints, immediately placed in Ham's F12 medium supplemented with 5% FBS and 50 μg/ml gentamicin, and then minced with a scalpel into small pieces (3 × 3 × 1–2 mm).

2. ISOLATION OF CHONDROCYTES

For all cell culture systems, chondrocytes are isolated using sequential digestion of the articular cartilage matrix with pronase E (0.4%) and bacterial collagenase P (0.025%) at

37°C [29]. After extensive rinsing and filtering through a series of screens, the cells are ready for plating as monolayers in plastic dishes or for encapsulation within the various gels.

3. Encapsulation of Cells in Agarose or Alginate Gel

The cells are seeded in 1% low temperature gelling Sea Plaque agarose (F.M.C. Corp.) at a density of 4×10^5 cells/well corresponding to 4×10^6 cells/ml of gel (slight modifications of the methods described for the culture of rabbit [16] and bovine [55] chondrocytes in agarose gel) or encapsulated in alginate beads at a density of either 4×10^6 or 8×10^6 cells/ml of alginate gel. The lower cell density is chosen for metabolic studies, whereas the higher density is suitable for comparative morphometric and biochemical studies. The procedure for the preparation of chondrocyte cultures in alginate beads has been described by Häuselmann et al. [29]. Briefly, the cells are suspended in sterile filtered 1.2% low viscosity alginate gel (Keltone LV, Kelco Corp.) and slowly extruded through a 22 gauge needle in a dropwise fashion into a 102 mM CaCl$_2$ solution. After instantaneous gelation, the beads are allowed to polymerize further for a period of 10 min in CaCl$_2$ solution. Following four washes in 10 volumes of 0.15 M NaCl and one wash in Ham's F12 medium, the beads are finally placed in complete culture medium (Ham's F12/DMEM medium, containing 10% FBS, 50 μg/ml gentamicin, and 25 μg/ml ascorbic acid). Agarose and alginate cultures are maintained in 24-well plates at 37°C in a humidified atmosphere of 5% CO$_2$ in air. The medium (1ml medium per 10^6 cells) is changed daily.

4. Synthesis of Proteoglycans

Between day 7 and 9 in culture, chondrocytes in alginate beads or agarose are fed with fresh complete medium containing ^{35}S-sulfate (20 μCi/ml). After different periods of time, the medium is harvested and analyzed. Following solubilization of the alginate beads in sodium citrate/EDTA, the two matrix compartments are separated by centrifugation, to separate the cell-associated compartment in the pellet (CM) from the further removed compartment in the supernatant (FRM). PGs in the CM and FRM are solubilized using 4 M guanidine HCl buffered at pH 5.8. Agarose cultures are extracted directly with 4 M guanidine HCl. In addition, agarose gels are treated with 0.5 M NaOH to complete the solubilization (residue). Radioactivity (cpm) in ^{35}S-PG in the dissociative extracts and labeling media is determined by subjecting an aliquot of each solution to chromatography on Sephadex G-25 (PD 10 columns), followed by liquid scintillation counting of the material eluting in the void volume (V$_o$) of the column.

5. Accumulation of Newly Synthesized Proteoglycans in Different Extracellular Matrix Compartments

In order to measure total PG accumulation in the beads with time in culture, and to compare the CM with the FRM, isolated human chondrocytes are cultured in alginate for up to 50 days. The content of PG in the 4 M guanidine HCl extracts of the CM and FRM compartments is measured by alcian blue precipitation [82].

6. Degradation of Newly Synthesized Proteoglycans with Respect to Different Matrix Compartments

Between day 7 and 9 of culture, beads containing articular chondrocytes are removed from the batch culture. The culture medium is replaced with fresh complete medium containing ^{35}S-sulfate at 20 μCi/ml, followed by incubation of alginate or agarose cultures at 37°C. After 4 h, the cultured beads and agarose layers are washed four times for a total of 4 h with fresh culture medium at 4°C, using gentle rocking to promote removal of unincorporated ^{35}S-sulfate. The beads are distributed into 24-well culture plates (five beads/well) and cultured for an additional period of time with daily changes of complete medium. The same procedure is used for agarose cultures. The medium is collected daily from each culture. For each time point studied, the beads or agarose cultures are collected, the beads solubilized, and the ^{35}S-PG in each of the two matrix compartments isolated and stored frozen at −80°C. At the completion of the experiment, all samples, including those from cultures not subjected to a period of chase, are analyzed at the same time to obviate the need to correct for decay in ^{35}S-sulfate activity.

7. Study of the Movement of Newly Synthesized ^{35}S-Proteoglycans (Only in Alginate Beads)

Between day 7 and 9 of culture, beads are removed from the batch culture and incubated at 37°C in fresh complete medium. The culture medium is replaced with fresh complete medium containing ^{35}S-sulfate at a final concentration of 50 μCi/ml. After 30 min, the medium is harvested and the beads are washed extensively (2 × 30 min) at 4°C with cold medium supplemented with MgSO$_4$ to a final concentration of 1.5 mM, then washed again (1 × 30 min) at 4°C with cold complete culture medium to remove excess unincorporated label. After the washing procedure, the beads are placed in 24-well culture plates (five beads/well) and fed with 0.4 ml of complete medium. At various time points of chase (up to 24 h), the medium is removed, the beads solubilized, and the resulting suspension centrifuged to separate the CM compartment from the FRM compartment. For each time point, ^{35}S-PGs of the medium and 4 M guanidine HCl extracts of the pellet and supernatant are measured.

B. Organ Culture System

For organ culture systems, small pieces of bovine cartilage (1–$2 \times 3 \times 3$ mm) are distributed ($\sim$100 mg wet weight of cartilage slices/vial corresponding to roughly 4×10^6 cells) in sterile plastic vials which contain 4 ml of culture medium (Dulbecco's modified Eagle's medium, containing 1g/l glucose and supplemented with organic buffers and nonessential amino acids) [43] and are incubated at 37°C in humidified atmosphere with 5% CO_2 in air for approximately five days without changing the medium. At this time metabolic studies can be performed.

1. SYNTHESIS OF PROTEOGLYCANS

Before labeling, each culture is preincubated in fresh medium for 1 h, and this medium is then replaced with 2 ml of labeling medium containing 40 μCi of ^{35}S-sulfate. Labeling can be performed at 37°C for times between 20 min and overnight, depending on the experiment [43, 83]. The tissue is washed three times with medium and then distributed in vials (100 mg tissue/vial) containing medium appropriate for each experiment.

2. DEGRADATION OF NEWLY SYNTHESIZED PROTEOGLYCANS WITH RESPECT TO DIFFERENT MATRIX COMPARTMENTS

When studying the turnover of ^{35}S-labeled PG in cartilage explants, tissue from a single steer is maintained in 30 ml medium containing 20% FCS for six days, then labeled for 6 h with 300 μCi of ^{35}S-sulfate in 10 ml of medium containing 20% FCS [45]. The tissue is then washed three times with medium before being distributed into vials (100 mg tissue/vial) containing medium appropriate for each experiment.

IV. A WORD OF CAUTION

In adult human cartilage, the half-lives of PG and collagen are on the order of 1 year. In contrast, the reported half-lives of newly synthesized PG of chondrocytes cultured as monolayers, as suspension in spinner cultures or agarose gels, or even as organ cultures are on the order of days to weeks. This is true for chondrocytes from young or old animals as well as from cells from human adult articular cartilage. Surprisingly, half-lives of newly synthesized PG in chondrocytes cultured in alginate beads have repeatedly been shown to be on the order of 30–100 days. These large differences between the latter turnover rates and the *in vivo* rates, with the exception of the alginate culture system, require some consideration. Several problems seem to be involved, such as type of PG that has been synthesized, how these newly synthesized PGs are assembled and held in the tissue, and also by what mech-

anism these PGs are turned over. All this has to be kept in mind if one uses *in vitro* models that are relevant to processes of aging and degeneration [80]. It is obvious that isolated and cultured chondrocytes behave differently than chondrocytes residing in a nearly normal extracellular matrix, as in an explant. In the latter we can attempt to understand how a chondrocyte maintains and regulates the extracellular matrix. This is different from a chondrocyte in cell culture, which is given the task of reconstructing a matrix. Therefore, it is of crucial importance to use the *in vitro* model appropriate to the research question which one would like to answer.

V. FUTURE PROSPECTS

It is generally agreed that superficial cartilage lesions do not heal. Hence, erosions or traumatic injuries limited to the cartilage do not induce any processes leading to repair of the tissue. In contrast, in the case of a full thickness defect that penetrates to the subchondral bone, cells presumably derived from the bone marrow are capable of filling the defect and producing a repair tissue that may develop into hyaline-like cartilage. This is true particularly if young rabbits are used as the experimental model. However, after some months this hyaline-like cartilage is transformed into fibrocartilage rich in collagen type I. This fibrocartilage is inferior to normal hyaline cartilage with respect to biomechanical properties. The biological basis for this "imperfect repair" is not understood and the phenotypic properties of the chondrocytes derived from the subchondral bone marrow are not known.

A report by Brittberg *et al.*, describing the first results of a study of chondrocyte transplantation in patients with cartilage defects [84], has revived the concept of cell isolation, subsequent culture, and transplantation into (osteo)chondral lesions. The concept is based on biological experiments initiated in the 1960s, that demonstrated that cells transplanted into chondral defects have the capacity to proliferate and transform into mature chondrocytes capable of synthesizing a cartilaginous matrix to fill out the defect. Although these first results have attracted the attention of a number of scientists and physicians, two major problems can be identified.

1. The harvest of sufficient amounts of cells in older patients is very difficult. The solution to this problem has been to let the isolated chondrocytes adhere on plastic and then culture them in monolayers for 2–3 weeks under conditions of enhanced cell proliferation.

2. Two months after transplantation, in which the multiplied cells are injected as a cell suspension, the dominant part of the repair tissue develops into fibrous cartilage not possessing the same superior biomechanical properties as hyaline cartilage. This phenomenon could be related to

the fact that isolated chondrocytes cultured on plastic or other surfaces dedifferentiate into fibroblast-like cells, with a decreased synthesis of cartilage-specific molecules like aggrecan and collagen II as a consequence.

For these reasons, new interest in the application of gel suspension culture systems during and/or after the period of proliferation of chondrocytes *in vitro* has arisen. The potential advantages of such cultures are not restricted to the fact that the cell environment is physically stabilized and that the cells are kept well in place (osteochondral lesions) after transplantation. These three-dimensional cultures, as outlined in the sections above, offer possibilities to obtain controlled cell multiplication in a phenotypically stable fashion. It is noteworthy that growth factors have been shown to stimulate the proliferation of chondrocytes, induce the differentiation of mesenchymal cells into chondrocytes, and stimulate the synthesis of cartilage-specific macromolecules. Improved protocols for the culture of adult human chondrocytes in gel suspension systems are likely to offer novel opportunities in the treatment of articular cartilage lesions.

Acknowledgments

The authors thank Drs. Klaus Kuettner, Margaret Aydelotte, and Eugene Thonar, Rush Medical College, Department of Biochemistry, Rush-Presbyterian-St. Luke's Medical Center, Chicago, for their competent help in establishing the alginate culture system during a post-doctoral fellowship.

Figure 2 was kindly provided by Prof. E. B. Hunziker, M. E. Müller Institute for Biomechanics, University of Bern, Switzerland.

References

1. Stockwell, R. A. (1979). Biology of cartilage cells. *In* "Biological Structure and Function" (R. Harrison and R. McMinn, eds.), Vol. 7. Cambridge University Press, Cambridge, UK.

2. Eyre, D. R., McDevitt, C. A., Billingham, M. E., and Muir, H. (1980). Biosynthesis of collagen and other matrix proteins by articular cartilage in experimental osteoarthrosis. *Biochem. J.* **188**, 823–837.

3. McDevitt, C. A., Gilbertson, E. M. M., and Muir, H. (1977). An experimental model of osteoarthritis; early morphological and biochemical changes. *J. Bone Jt. Surg.* **59**, 25–29.

4. Mankin, H. J., and Lipiello, L. (1971). The glycosaminoglycans of normal and arthritic cartilage. *J. Clin. Invest.* **50**, 1712–1719.

5. Nimni, M., and Deshmukh, K. (1973). Differences in collagen metabolism between normal and osteoarthritic human articular cartilage. *Science* **181**, 751–752.

6. Aydelotte, M. B., and Kuettner, K. E. (1988). Differences between subpopulations of cultured bovine articular chondrocytes. I. Morphology and cartilage matrix production. *Connect. Tissue Res.* **18**, 205–222.

7. Bayliss, M. T., Venn, M., Maroudas, A., and Ali, S. F. (1983). Structure of proteoglycans from different layers of human articular cartilage. *Biochem. J.* **209**, 387–400.

8. Scheinberg, R. D., Ehrlich, M. G., Lipiello, L., and Mankin, H. J. (1982). Degradative enzyme activity in isolated chondrocyte populations. *Clin. Orthop. Relat. Res.* **164**, 279–286.

9. Stockwell, R. A., and Meachim, G. (1979). The chondrocytes. *In* "Adult Articular Cartilage" (M. A. R. Freeman, ed.), 2nd ed., pp. 69–144. Pitman Medical, Turnbridge Wells.

10. Vignon, E., Arlot, M., Patricot, L. M., and Vignon, G. (1976). The cell density of human femoral head cartilage. *Clin. Orthop.* **121**, 303–308.

11. Lohmander, L. S., and Kimura, H. J. (1986). Biosynthesis of cartilage proteoglycan. *In* "Articular Cartilage Biochemistry" (K. E. Kuettner, R. Schleyerbach, and V. C. Hascall, eds.), pp. 93–111. Raven Press, New York.

12. Handley, C. J., McQuillan, D. J., Campbell, M. A., and Bolis, S. (1986). Steady-state metabolism in cartilage explants. *In* "Articular Cartilage Biochemistry" (K. E. Kuettner, R. Schleyerbach, and V. C. Hascall, eds.), pp. 163–179. Raven Press, New York.

13. Zanetti, M., Ratcliffe, A., and Watt, F. M. (1985). Two subpopulations of differentiated chondrocytes identified with a monoclonal antibody to keratan sulfate. *J. Cell Biol.* **101**, 53–59.

14. Häuselmann, H. J., Masuda, K., Hunziker, E. B., Neidhart, M., Mok, S. S., Michel, B. A., and Thonar, E. J.-M. A. (1996). Adult human articular chondrocytes cultured in alginate gel form a matrix similar to native human articular cartilage. *Am. J. Physiol. (Cell Physiol.)* **271**, 742–752.

15. Lust, G., Nuki, G., and Seegmiller, J. E. (1976). Inorganic pyrophosphate and proteoglycan metabolism in cultured human articular chondrocytes and fibroblasts. *Arthritis Rheum.* **19**, 479–487.

16. Benya, P. D., and Shaffer, J. D. (1982). Dedifferentiated chondrocytes reexpress the differentiated collagen phenotype when cultured in agarose gels. *Cell* **30**, 215–224.

17. Adolphe, M., and Benya, P. (1992). Different types of cultured chondrocytes—the *in vitro* approach to the study of biological regulation. *In* "Biological Regulations of the Chondrocytes" (M. Adolphe, ed.), pp. 105–139. CRC Press, Boca Raton, FL.

18. Aydelotte, B. A., Schleyerbach, R., Zeck, B. J., and Kuettner, K. E. (1986). Articular chondrocytes cultured in agarose gel for study of chondrocytic chondrolysis. *In* "Articular Cartilage Biochemistry," (K. E. Kuettner, R. Schleyerbach, and V. Hascall, eds.), pp. 235–254. Raven Press, New York.

19. Häuselmann, H. J., Fernandes, R. J., Mok, S. S., Schmid, T. M., Block, J. A., and Aydelotte, M. B. (1994). Phenotypic stability of bovine articular chondrocytes after long-term culture in alginate beads. *J. Cell Sci.* **107**, 17–27.

20. Solursh, M., Jensen, K. L., Reiter, R. S., Schmid, T. M., and Linsenmayer, T. F. (1986). Environmental regulation of type X collagen production by cultures of limb mesenchyme, mesectoderm, and sternal chondrocytes. *Dev. Biol.* **117**, 90–101.

21. Glowacki, J., Trepman, E., and Folkman, J. (1983). Cell shape and phenotypic expression in chondrocytes. *Proc. Soc. Exp. Biol. Med.* **172**, 93–98.

22. Newman, P., and Watt, F. M. (1988). Influence of cytochalasin D-induced changes in cell shape on proteoglycan synthesis by cultured articular chondrocytes. *Exp. Cell Res.* **178**, 199–210.

23. von der Mark, K. (1986). Differentiation, modulation and dedifferentiation of chondrocytes. *Rheumatology* **10**, 272–315.

24. Watt, F. M. (1986). The extracellular matrix and cell shape. *Trends Biochem. Sci.* **11**, 482–485.

25. Block, J. A., Inerot, S. E., Gitelis, S., and Kimura, J. H. (1991). The effects of long term monolayer culture on the proteoglycan phenotype of a clonal population of mature human malignant chondrocytes. *Connect. Tissue Res.* **26**, 295–313.

26. Buschmann, M. D., Gluzband, Y. A., Grodzinsky, A. J., Kimura, J. H., and Hunziker, E. B. (1992). Chondrocytes in agarose culture synthesize a mechanically functional extracellular matrix. *J. Orthop. Res.* **10**, 745–758.

27. Bruckner, P., Hörler, I., Mendler, M., Houze, Y., Winterhalter, K. H., Eich-Bender, S. G., and Spycher, M. (1989). Induction and prevention

of chondrocyte hypertrophy in culture. *J. Cell Biol.* **109**, 2537–2545.

28. Guo, J., Jourdian, G. W., and MacCallum, D. K. (1989). Culture and growth characteristics of chondrocytes encapsulated in alginate beads. *Connect. Tissue Res.* **19**, 277–297.

29. Häuselmann, H. J., Aydelotte, M. B., Schumacher, B. L., Kuettner, K. E., Gitelis, S. H., and Thonar, E. J.-M. A. (1992). Synthesis and turnover of proteoglycans by human and bovine articular chondrocytes cultured in alginate beads. *Matrix* **12**, 116–129.

30. Bonaventure, J., Kadhom, N., Cohen-Solal, L., Ng, K. H., Bourguignon, J., Lasselin, C., and Freisinger, P. (1994). Reexpression of cartilage-specific genes by dedifferentiated human articular chondrocytes cultured in alginate beads. *Exp. Cell Res.* **212**, 97–104.

31. Kimura, T., Yasui, N., Ohsawa, S., and Ono, K. (1984). Chondrocytes embedded in collagen gels maintain cartilage phenotype during long-term cultures. *Clin. Orthop. Relat. Res.* **186**, 231–239.

32. Maor, G., von der Mark, K., Reddi, H., Heinegard, D., Franzen, A., and Silbermann, M. (1987). Acceleration of cartilage and bone differentiation on collagenous substrata. *Collagen Relat. Res.* **7**, 351–370.

33. Solursh, M., and Meier, S. (1974). Effects of cell density on the expression of differentiation by chick embryo chondrocytes. *J. Exp. Zool.* **187**, 311–322.

34. Meats, J. E., Elford, P. R., Bunning, R. A. D., and Russell, R. G. G. (1985). Retinoids and synovial factor(s) stimulate the production of plasminogen activator by cultured human chondrocytes. A possible role for plasminogen activator in the resorption of cartilage in vitro. *Biochim. Biophys. Acta* **838**, 161–169.

35. Kuettner, K. E., Pauli, B. U., Gall, G., Memoli, V. A., and Schenk, R. K. (1982). Synthesis of cartilage matrix by mammalian chondrocytes *in vitro. J. Cell Biol.* **93**, 743–750.

36. Watt, F. M. (1988). Effect of seeding density on stability of the differentiated phenotype of pig articular chondrocytes in culture. *J. Cell Sci.* **89**, 373–378.

37. Deshmukh, K., Kline, W., and Sawyer, B. (1976). Role of calcium in the phenotypic expression of rabbit articular chondrocytes in culture. *FEBS Lett.* **67**, 48–51.

38. Norby, D. P., Malemud, C. J., and Sokoloff, L. (1977). Differences in the collagen types synthesized by lapine articular chondrocytes in spinner and monolayer cultures. *Arthritis Rheum.* **20**, 709–716.

39. Dessau, W., Sasse, J., Timpl, R., Jilek, F., and von der Mark, K. (1978). Synthesis and extracellular deposition of fibronectin in chondrocyte cultures. Response to the removal of extracellular cartilage matrix. *J. Biol. Chem.* **79**, 342–355.

40. von der Mark, K., Gauss, V., von der Mark, H., and Müller, P. K. (1977). Relationship between cell shape and type of collagen synthesized as chondrocytes lose their cartilage phenotype in culture. *Nature* **267**, 531–532.

41. Poole, A. R. (1989). Honor Bridget Fell, Ph.D. D.Sc., F.R.S., D.B.E., 1900–1986, The scientist and her contributions. *In Vitro Cell Biol.* **25**, 450–453.

42. Sokoloff, L. (1980). *In* "The Joints and Synovial Fluid" (L. Sokoloff, ed.), Vol. 2, pp. 1–26. Academic Press, New York.

43. Hascall, V. C., Handley, C. J., McQuillan, D. J., Hascall, G. K., Robinson, H. C., and Lowther, D. A. (1983). The effect of serum on biosynthesis of proteoglycans by bovine articular cartilage in culture. *Arch. Biochem. Biophys.* **224**, 206–223.

44. Morales, T. I. (1993). Articular organ cultures: In vitro models of matrix homeostasis, resorption or repair. *In* "Joint Cartilage Degradation; Basic and Clinical Aspects" (J. F. Woessner, Jr. and D. S. Howell, eds.), Vol. 12, pp. 261–280. Dekker, New York.

45. Campbell, M. A., Handley, C. J., Hascall, V. C., Campbell, R. A., and Lowther, D. A. (1984). Turnover of proteoglycans in cultures of bovine articular cartilage. *Arch. Biochem. Biophys.* **234**, 275–289.

46. Hascall, V. C., Morales, T. I., Hascall, G. K., Handley, C. J., and McQuillan, D. (1983). Biosynthesis and turnover of proteoglycans in organ culture of bovine articular cartilage. *J. Rheumatol., Suppl.* **10**, 45–52.

47. Morales, T., Wahl, L. M., and Hascall, V. C. (1984). The effect of bacterial lipopolysaccharides on the biosynthesis and release of proteoglycans from calf articular cartilage cultures. *J. Biol. Chem.* **259**, 6720–6729.

48. Bartholomew, J. S., Handley, C. J., and Lowther, D. A. (1985). The effects of trypsin treatment on proteoglycan biosynthesis by bovine articular cartilage. *Biochem. J.* **227**, 429–437.

49. Tyler, J. A. (1985). Chondrocyte-mediated depletion of articular cartilage proteoglycans in vitro. *Biochem. J.* **225**, 493–507.

50. Sandy, J. D., Neame, P. J., Boynton, R. E., and Flannery, C. R. (1991). Catabolism of aggrecan in cartilage explants. *J. Biol. Chem.* **266**, 8683–8685.

51. Tian, X., Chen, S., Morales, T. I., and Hascall, V. C. (1989). Biochemical and morphological studies of steady state and lipopolysaccharide treated bovine articular cartilage explant cultures. *Connect. Tissue Res.* **19**, 195–218.

52. Luyten, F. P., Hascall, V. C., Nissely, S. P., Morales, T. I., and Reddi, A. H. (1988). Insulin-like growth factors maintain steady state metabolism of proteoglycans in bovine articular explants. *Arch. Biochem. Biophys.* **267**, 416–425.

53. Morales, T. I. (1994). Transforming growth factor β and insulin-like growth factor-1 restore proteoglycan metabolism of bovine articular cartilage after depletion by retinoic acid. *Arch. Biochem. Biophys.* **315**, 190–198.

54. Barone-Varelas, J., Schnitzer, T. J., Meng, Q., Otten, L., and Thonar, E. J.-M. A. (1991). Age-related differences in the metabolism of proteoglycans in bovine articular cartilage explants maintained in the presence of insulin-like growth factor-1. *Connect. Tissue Res.* **26**, 101–120.

55. Aydelotte, M. B., Greenhill, R. R., and Kuettner, K. E. (1988). Differences between sub-populations of cultured bovine articular chondrocytes II. Proteoglycan metabolism. *Connect. Tissue Res.* **18**, 223–234.

56. Poole, C., Flint, M., and Beaumont, B. (1987). Chondrons in cartilage: ultrastructural analysis of the pericellular microenvironment in adult human articular cartilage. *J. Orthop. Res.* **5**, 509–522.

57. Lee, G. M., Poole, C. A., Kelley, S. S., Chang, J., and Caterson, B. (1997). Isolated chondrons: a viable alternative for studies of chondrocyte metabolism *in vitro. Osteoarthritis Cartilage* **5**, 261–274.

58. Kosher, R. A. (1983). The chondroblast and the chondrocyte. *In* "Cartilage" (B. K. Hall, ed.), Vol. 1, pp. 59–85. Academic Press, New York.

59. Holtzer, H., Abbott, J., Lash, J., and Holtzer, S. (1960). The loss of phenotypic traits by differentiated cells *in vitro. Proc. Natl. Acad. Sci. U.S.A.* **46**, 1533–1542.

60. Sokoloff, L., Malemud, C. J., Srivastava, V. M. L., and Morgan, W. D. (1973). In vitro culture of articular chondrocytes. *Fed. Proc.* **32**, 1499–1502.

61. Abbott, J., and Holtzer, H. (1966). The loss of phenotype traits by differentiated cells III. The reversible behaviour of chondrocytes in primary cultures. *J. Cell Biol.* **28**, 473–487.

62. Aulthouse, A. L., Beck, M., Griffey, E., Sanford, J., Arden, K., Machado, M. A., and Horton, W. A. (1989). Expression of the human chondrocyte phenotype *in vitro. In Vitro Cell Dev. Biol.* **25**, 659–668.

63. Thonar, E. J.-M. A., Buckwalter, J. A., and Kuettner, K. E. (1986). Maturation-related differences in the structure and composition of proteoglycan synthesized by chondrocytes from bovine articular cartilage. *J. Biol. Chem.* **261**, 2467–2474.

64. Sailor, L. Z., Hewick, R. M., and Morris, E. A. (1996). Recombinant human bone morphogenetic Protein-2 maintains the articular chondrocyte phenotype in long-term culture. *J. Orthop. Res.* **14**, 937–945.

65. Hering, T. M., Kollar, J., Huynh, T. D., Varelas, J. B., and Sandell, L. J. (1994). Modulation of extracellular matrix gene expression in bovine high-density chondrocyte cultures by ascorbic acid and enzymatic resuspension. *Arch. Biochem. Biophys.* **314**, 90–98.

66. Kolettas, E., Buluwela, L., Bayliss, M. T., and Muir, H. I. (1995). Expression of cartilage-specific molecules is retained on long-term culture of human articular chondrocytes. *J. Cell Sci.* **108**, 1991–1999.

67. Kimura, J. H., Hardingham, T. E., and Hascall, V. C. (1980). Assembly of newly synthesized proteoglycan and link protein into aggregates in cultures of chondrosarcoma chondrocytes. *J. Biol. Chem.* **255**, 7134–7143.

68. Lohmander, L. S. (1990). Biosynthesis of cartilage proteoglycan: An analysis of posttranslational events by different *in vitro* labeling protocols. *In* "Methods in Cartilage Research" (A. Maroudas and K. E. Kuettner eds.), pp. 148–152. Academic Press, San Diego, CA.

68a. Kim, Y. J., Sah, R. L., Doong, J. Y., and Grodzinsky, A. J. (1988). Fluorometric assay of DNA in cartilage explants using Hoechst 33258. *Anal. Biochem.* **174**, 168–176.

69. Häuselmann, H. J., Oppliger, L., Michel, B. A., Stefanovic-Racic, M., and Evans, C. H. (1994). Nitric oxide and proteoglycan biosynthesis by human articular chondrocytes in alginate culture. *FEBS Lett.* **352**, 361–364.

70. Häuselmann, H. J., Stefanovich-Racic, M., Michel, B. A., and Evans, C. H. (1998). Differences in nitric oxide production by superficial and deep human articular chondrocytes: Implication for proteoglycan turnover in inflammatory joint diseases. *J. Immunol.* **160**, 1444–1448.

71. Chubinskaya, S., Huch, K., Mikecz, K., Cs-Szabo, G., Hasty, K. A., Kuettner, K. E., and Cole, A. (1996). Chondrocyte MMP-8: Upregulation of neutrophil collagenase by interleukin-1ß in human cartilage from knee and ankle joints. *Lab. Invest.* **74**, 232–240.

72. Häuselmann, H. J., Flechtenmacher, J., Michal, L., Shinmei, M., Kuettner, K. E., and Aydelotte, M. B. (1996). The superficial layer of human articular cartilage is more susceptible to Interleukin-1-induced damage than the deeper layers. *Arthritis Rheum.* **39**, 478–488.

73. Mankin, H. J. (1962). Localization of tritiated thymidine in articular cartilage of rabbits. *J. Bone Jt. Surg., Am. Vol.* **44**, 688–698.

74. Sporn, M. B., and Robberts, A. B. (1990). TGF-beta: Problems and prospects. *Cell Regul.* **1**, 875–882.

75. van Osch, G. J., van den Berg, W. B., Hunziker, E. B., and Häuselmann, H. J. (1998). Differential effects of IGF-1 and TGF-β2 on the assembly of proteoglycans in pericellular and territorial matrix by cultured bovine articular chondrocytes. *Osteoarthritis Cartilage* **6**, 187–195.

76. Qi, W.-N., and Scully, S. P. (1997). Extracellular collagen modulates the regulation of chondrocytes by transforming growth factor-β1. *J. Orthop. Res.* **15**, 483–490.

77. Hunziker, E. B. (1992). Articular structure in humans and experimental animals. *In* "Articular Cartilage and Osteoarthritis" (K. E. Kuettner, R. Schleyerbach, J. G. Peyron, and V. C. Hascall, eds.), pp. 183–199. Raven Press, New York.

78. Mok, S. S., Masuda, K., Häuselmann, H. J., Aydelotte, M. B., and Thonar, E. J.-M. A. (1994). Aggrecan synthesized by mature bovine chondrocytes suspended in alginate: Identification of two distinct metabolic matrix pools. *J. Biol. Chem.* **269**, 33021–33027.

79. van Kampen, G. P. J., van de Stadt, R. J., van de Laar, M. A. F. J., and van der Korst, J. K. (1992). Two distinct metabolic pools of proteoglycans in articular cartilage. *In* "Articular Cartilage and Osteoarthritis" (K. E. Kuettner, R. Schleyerbach, J. G. Peyron, and V. C. Hascall, eds.), pp. 281–289. Raven Press, New York.

80. Maroudas, A., Bayliss, M. T., Uchitel-Kaushansky, N., Schneiderman, R., and Gilav, E. (1998). Aggrecan turnover in human articular cartilage: Use of aspartic acid racemization as a marker of molecular age. *Arch. Biochem. Biophys.* **350**, 61–71.

81. Lohmander, S. (1977). Turnover of proteoglycans in guinea pig costal cartilage. *Arch. Biochem. Biophys.* **180**, 93–101.

82. Björnsson, S. (1993). Simultaneous preparation and quantitation of proteoglycans by precipitation with alcian blue. *Anal. Biochem.* **210**, 282–291.

83. McQuillan, D. J., Handley, C. J., Robinson, H. C., Ng, K., Tzaicos, C., Brooks, P. R., and Lowther, D. A. (1984). The relation of protein synthesis to chondroitin sulphate biosynthesis in cultured bovine cartilage. *Biochem. J.* **224**, 977–988.

84. Brittberg, M., Lindahl, A., Nilsson, A., Ohlsson, C., Isaksson, O., and Peterson, L. (1994). Treatment of deep cartilage defects in the knee with autologous chondrocyte transplantation. *N. Engl. J. Med.* **331**, 879–895.

CHAPTER 24

Animal Models of Cartilage Breakdown

CARLOS J. LOZADA   Division of Rheumatology and Immunology, University of Miami School of Medicine, Miami, Florida 33136; Jackson Memorial Hospital, Miami, Florida 33136

ROY D. ALTMAN   Division of Rheumatology and Immunology, University of Miami School of Medicine, Miami, Florida 33136; Miami Veterans Affairs Medical Center, Miami, Florida 33136

I. INTRODUCTION

Osteoarthritis (OA) is the most common rheumatic disease, affecting as much as 12% of the U.S. population between the ages of 25 and 74 [1]. Although variable in its presentation, OA often carries significant morbidity. In addition, the cost of OA to society is significant. This cost is related to the high prevalence of OA, reduced avocational and vocational activities of patients with OA, the occasional loss of the patient's ability at self care, and the related drain on health resources [2]. With significant improvement in our understanding of the etiopathogenesis of OA, there have been changes in the conceptual approach to management which provide new emphasis on potential preventive measures and a more comprehensive approach to treatment [3]. Guidelines for the management of OA at specific sites are being developed and reported [4, 5].

Therapeutic considerations must appreciate that OA is no longer considered "degenerative" or "wear and tear" arthritis, but rather it involves dynamic biomechanical and biochemical processes [6]. Much of the joint damage that occurs in OA is through active remodeling, involving all the joint structures [7]. Although articular cartilage continues to be at the center of change, OA is increasingly viewed as a disease of all the joint tissues, and, therefore, as the failure of the joint as an organ system. The desired goal of osteoarthritis (OA) researchers is "chondroprotection," or the ability to preserve not only cartilage but the entire joint from the arthritic process. Many have attempted to attach this label to OA drugs but they have been unable to show the "disease modifying" effect [8].

In a 1996 workshop of the Osteoarthritis Research Society (OARS) [9], it was recommended that the term "structure modifying drugs" be used to describe medications that would

339

have been classified before as "chondroprotective." The term "chondroprotective" was branded as "misleading," because OA is a disease not only of the cartilage but of the entire joint. These structure-modifying drugs would be intended to prevent, retard, stabilize, or reverse the development of OA. Because of the natural history of OA, any benefits from these would only be apparent after several years of observation, making clinical trials a very challenging undertaking. Animal models of OA should increasingly play an important role, as they are more expedient ways of assessing structure modification potential in a new therapeutic intervention. Measures used to identify structure modification would include radiographic assessments of joint space, such as fluoroscopically positioned anteroposterior radiographs of the knee, or MRI. However, none of these is particularly useful in the study of preclinical OA and, therefore, animal models are the best way of studying disease modification at that stage.

Because in all likelihood OA involves different pathogenetic pathways, it is unlikely that one animal model could be optimal for all of its presentations. The study of OA's natural history or of therapeutic interventions using human subjects has been hindered by the fact that OA commonly presents at a late stage of disease and, thus, evaluating early disease is difficult. Obtaining tissue samples is also a problem in most cases. Other difficulties include determining disease duration, standardization difficulties, and difficulties grading pathological change [10].

Animal models have evolved that are being used to evaluate both symptomatic and the new disease-modifying therapies. They provide readily available study specimens (synovial fluid, cartilage, etc.) of superior quality as well as easily available controls. These models provide a bridge between tissue culture findings and human OA.

II. FACTORS IN SELECTING AN ANIMAL MODEL OF OSTEOARTHRITIS (OA)

The choice of animal model at a particular site or for a particular study involves several factors. Abnormalities to be studied should be compared to those seen in the model. Mechanism of disease induction in the model may also be important. Most models involve surgical destabilization of the joint, but the injection of irritants or enzymes into the joints and spontaneous models have been used as well. All of these models reproduce certain aspects of OA but none is capable of mimicking all aspects of human disease [11].

Factors that determine the actual model selected include similarity to human OA (or to the aspect of OA to be studied), anatomic similarity to a human joint, reproducibility of lesions, availability of the animal, and cost of the animal (including housing). Rate and degree of progression of the

OA also is important. In previous reviews, animal models of OA have been classified by mechanism of disease induction or by the animal used [12]. Some of the more useful models include the Pond-Nuki model of anterior cruciate ligament transection in dogs [13, 14], the Hulth-Telhag model that involves meniscectomy and anterior cruciate ligament transection in rabbits, the Moskowitz model of partial meniscectomy in rabbits [15–17], congenital hip dysplasia in dogs [18], and gluteal myectomy and tendonotomy in guinea pigs. Other models include spontaneous osteoarthritis in horses [19], Rhesus monkeys [20], guinea pigs, mice [21], and domestic animals [22]. In this chapter, models will be classified based on the animal being used for study. Models induced through surgical destabilization of the joint will be emphasized.

III. CANINE MODELS OF OA

Canine models have multiple advantages over other animal models. First of all, the amount of cartilage available is clearly more than adequate for study, including biochemical evaluation. This obviates the need for pooling specimens that can introduce error. Dogs are relatively easy to care for when compared to other animals. They do have the disadvantages of requiring more space and being more costly than other models such as the lapine and murine models. The OA also tends to develop more slowly in dogs than in other animals.

A. The Pond-Nuki (Anterior Cruciate Ligament Transection) Model

This model was reported on by Pond and Nuki in 1973. Transecting the anterior cruciate ligament (ACL) of the stifle joint (hind limb knee) produces the OA lesions (Figs. 1–4). Transection of the ACL is generally done by blind stab incision. Greyhounds and beagles have been used for study [23]. Several therapies for OA such as hyaluronic acid injections [24, 25], glycosaminoglycan polysulfuric esters (Figs. 3, 4) [26], and pentosan polysulfate [27], have been tested using this model. Early lesions include focal softening, fibrillation, and erosions of cartilage (Fig. 1a). These occur more prominently in the medial aspect of the medial tibial plateau, with less severe changes noted at the lateral tibial plateau and the femoral condyles. Histological examination shows fibrillation, deep cartilage clefts, and eventual erosions [28]. Metachromatic staining confirms loss of cartilage (Fig. 2).

The density of cartilage cells increases with time and clones of cells are common. There is also synovial vascular proliferation with villous folds and, occasionally, adhesions. Meniscal pathology is observed as well. About 20–40% of the dogs develop medial meniscal fibrillation or tears. These are often seen in the posterior horn of the meniscus.

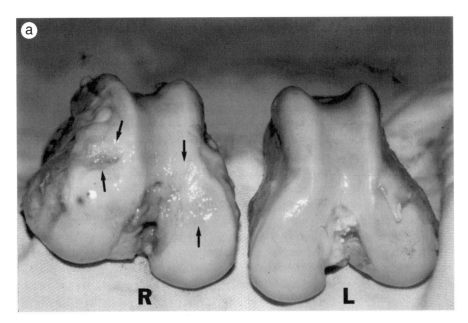

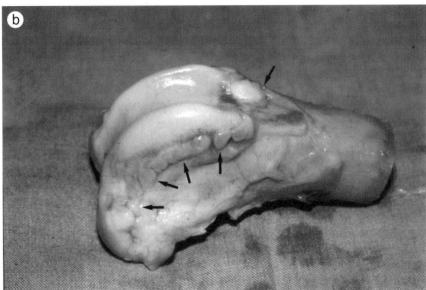

FIGURE 1 Gross anatomy of the canine model of osteoarthritis. Osteoarthritis develops following transection of the anterior cruciate ligament of the right hind limb stifle (knee) of the dog. (A) The unoperated left stifle has a normal appearance of the surface, whereas the operated stifle develops ulcers on the medial inferior and lateral anterior surfaces (arrows). (B) Large osteophytes develop along the margins of the joint and high in the intercondylar groove (arrows).

As in human disease, osteophytes are part of the clinical picture. Formation of these osteophytes is noted around the proximal limit of the femoral trochlea (Fig. 1b). These changes can be seen beginning at 2 weeks. They progress over time (in both size and number) and eventually can involve the tibial femoral and patellar borders. Increased vascularity has been seen in these areas using dye injection techniques.

Synovial fluid is present in variable amounts, usually ranging from 2 to 20 ml in the first 4 weeks and around 1 ml at 24 weeks or later. Except for immediately after surgery (when there can be over 5000 red cells/ml), the fluid is largely non-bloody and noninflammatory, with white blood cell counts of less than 1000 WBC/ml (80% mononuclear) at 4 weeks. The fluid is loose with a poor mucin clot (Ropes test).

Cartilage changes are extensive and occur throughout the entire cartilage; they are not limited to weight-bearing areas. Cartilage water content is increased and it swells more when immersed in saline [29]. Transmission electron microscopy reveals that the collagen fibers and perilacunar network are

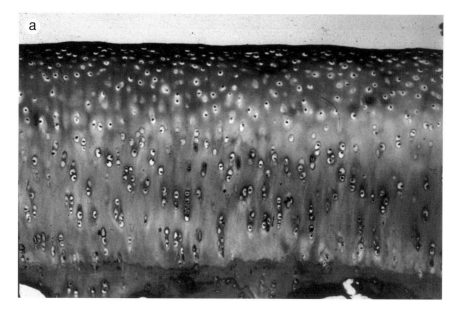

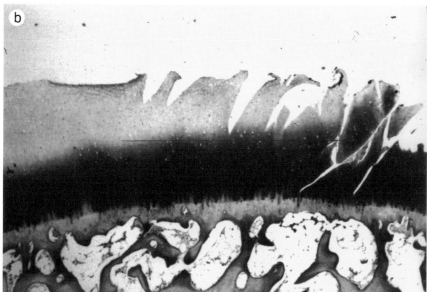

FIGURE 2   Histology of the canine model of osteoarthritis. Osteoarthritis develops following transection of the anterior cruciate ligament of the right hind limb stifle (knee) of the dog. (A) The surface is
intact, proteoglycan staining is evenly distributed through the tissue, the chondrocytes appear normal in
number and distribution, the tidemark is intact, and there is no invasion of the zone of calcified cartilage
(safranin O, 400X). (B) The surface is markedly disrupted with fissures deep into the radial zone of
cartilage, there is loss of proteoglycan staining, and chondrocyte proliferation is seen in some of the
fragments at higher power (safranin O, 40X).

abnormally separated. Collagen synthesis is increased ten
fold [30], type II collagen is less glycosylated, and type I
Collagen is not found. Chondrocytes have been observed to
have prominent Golgi membranes and vacuolar changes, indicating increased synthetic activity. Proteoglycans are more
easily extracted and have high galactosamine:glucosamine
molar ratios. This constitutes evidence for formation of
smaller aggregates of proteoglycans.

The Pond-Nuki model of OA has several advantages and
similarities to human disease. However, in addition to the
disadvantages of dog models in general, it also produces disease and cartilage changes that only progress to a certain
extent. Therefore, it is unlike certain subsets of human OA
in this respect. Nevertheless, overall it is a very practical and
useful model that appears to be valid for the study of potential
structure/disease modifying drugs in OA [31, 32].

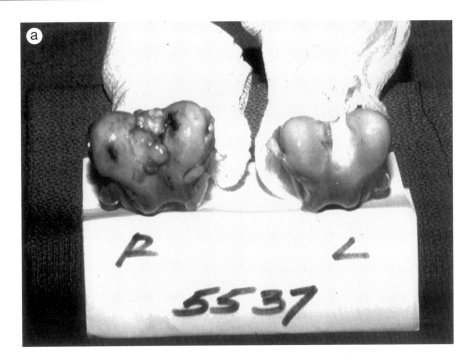

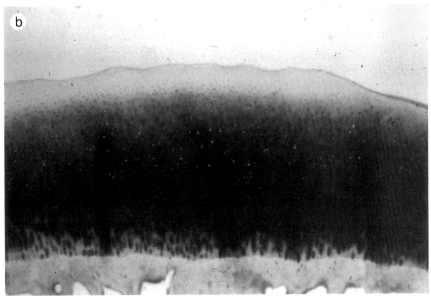

FIGURE 3 Canine model of osteoarthritis treated with pentosan polysulfate. (A) Gross anatomy shows no change in surface of the untreated left stifle, contrasted with relatively minor surface disruptions of the right stifle accentuated by the presence of carbon black. (B) Histologic findings include near normal anatomic changes except for minor surface disruption (safranin O; 40X).

B. Other ACL Transection Models

Other ACL transection models also have been used. They differ mainly in the way that the transection is done and the type of dog used. Some models employ an arthroscopic technique [33]. It has the advantage of direct visualization of tissues and avoidance of cartilage or vascular damage while performing the transection. Medial arthrotomy has also been used to transect the ACL [34].

Dorsal root ganglionectomy has been used by Brandt and others to accelerate OA changes in ACL transection models. The general concept is that deafferentiation of the extremity will deprive the central nervous system of afferent input from nociceptive or proprioceptive nerve fibers. This leads to recurrent joint trauma and progression of OA. However, dorsal root ganglionectomy alone has not induced OA up to 16 months after the procedure [35, 36]. Perhaps articular cartilage injury, as would be expected to occur after

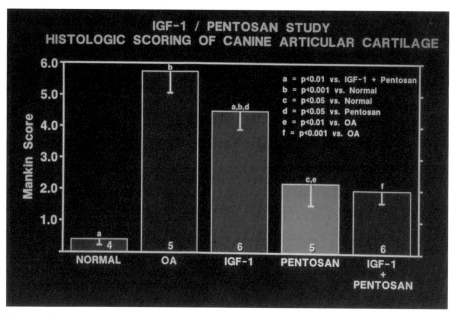

FIGURE 4 Canine model of osteoarthritis treated with pentosan polysulfate. Summary of histologic findings by the Mankin scoring system [ref]. Insulin-like growth factor-1 (IGF-1) was not as effective as pentosan polysulfate alone or in combination with pentosan in surpressing the development of the histologic lesions of osteoarthritis (adapted from Rogachefsky *et al.* [27]).

ACL transection, is necessary for the development of the Charcot-like arthropathy in this model. When the dorsal root ganglionectomy is followed 2 weeks later by ACL transection [37], articular cartilage breaks down within 3 weeks, in contrast to other ACL models in which cartilage can remain hypertrophic for up to 3 years [38].

C. Biochemical Studies Using ACL Models

Serum markers of OA have been studied using ACL transection models. Serum levels of markers of aggrecan degradation and synovial metabolism have been studied. Levels of both antigenic keratan sulfate (a marker for aggrecan degradation) and hyaluronan (a marker of synovial metabolism and proliferation) have been shown to increase by 1–2 weeks after transection of ACL and to remain elevated for at least 13 weeks [39]. These changes precede the development of OA lesions in these models.

In other studies, cartilage from cruciate-deficient dogs has been shown to release more proteoglycan into synovial fluid and also *in vitro* into culture media than cartilage from control animals. The amounts of chondroitin sulfate, keratan sulfate, and link protein released into the synovial fluid were significantly elevated over those in control dogs [40].

Cartilage proteoglycans have been studied in further detail using both ACL transection models and disuse atrophy models. In normal dogs, proteoglycan aggregate size differs by cartilage layer. Slow sedimenting aggregates were found mainly in the superficial zone, with twice as much hyaluronic acid in this zone as compared to deeper layers. These aggregates were not link protein stabilized. *In vitro*, the size of hyaluronic acid, the size of the proteoglycan monomers, and the ability to form proteoglycan-hyaluronic acid aggregates were the same in the two layers. In the ACL-deficient dogs and also in the disuse atrophy model, changes were observed that included decreases in the amount of fast sedimenting proteoglycans at 14 weeks [41].

Monoclonal antibodies that recognize abnormal epitopes in chondroitin sulfate chains have been used in ACL transection models. Strong immunohistochemical staining of cartilage, denoting atypical chondroitin chain structure, has been noted in the superficial zones and around chondrocyte clusters [42].

D. Meniscectomy Models

In meniscectomy models, the amount of damage to cartilage and joint appears to be related to the amount of meniscus removed. Medial compartments were usually affected whereas lateral compartments had little damage regardless of whether a partial or complete meniscectomy had been performed.

E. Immobilization Models

In contrast to contact areas of cartilage, where cartilage damage can occur through mechanical compression and by prevention of diffusion of synovial fluid, absence of weight bearing in contact-free areas can have notable consequences, but for different reasons. There can be diminished synovial fluid production by atrophic synovial membrane and a lack of cartilage nutrition secondary to reduced synovial fluid diffusion related to joint limitation. Dog right hind knee joints were immobilized with a cast at 90 degree flexion of the hip and the knee for varying periods of time from 6 days to 8 weeks in one study [43]. The dogs were permitted to ambulate on three legs. Defects in sulfate incorporation into the matrix were described; proteoglycan synthesis was affected from day 6. After 3 weeks of immobilization, new proteoglycans were no longer forming hyaluronate aggregates. There was progressive loss of metachromatic staining and cartilage thickness. Interestingly, the problem was almost completely reversed with remobilization, although other studies have not shown such a degree of reversibility.

F. Spontaneous Models

Joint laxity and degeneration at the hip have been studied in spontaneous canine models. Several breeds of dogs, but especially Labrador retrievers and German shepherds, can be used for study because of the incidence of hip dysplasia. It is unknown whether the cartilage and ligament abnormalities or the joint laxity are primary [44]. Nevertheless, pathologic and biochemical changes are eventually seen that have similarities to human OA.

Cartilage abnormalities can be seen on gross examination as early as 3 months. There is dulling and softening of the cartilage with flaking, erosions, and fibrillation. There is a loss of proteoglycans with decreased metachromatic stain and an increase in fibronectin [45].

Disadvantages to using spontaneous models of disease include disease reproducibility, time lapse between birth and development of disease, and cost. In other animals, such as mice and guinea pigs, these concerns can be somewhat ameliorated.

IV. LAPINE (RABBIT) MODELS OF OA

Rabbit models of OA have several advantages. Small size and low cost are the most obvious of these. Lapine OA also progresses at a faster rate than the canine OA. Almost complete denudation of cartilage can be seen as early as 20 to 25 weeks in rabbits. Therefore, these models lend themselves to shorter studies and to studying severe disease. On the other hand, only small amounts of cartilage are available for biochemical study. This leads to specimen pooling. Given the small joints, a degree of surgical skill is required for obtaining acceptable specimens.

A. The Moskowitz (Medial Meniscectomy) Model

In 1973, Moskowitz described this model that attempts to mimic a meniscal tear causing human OA. It has been used to study therapeutic agents such as chloroquine and glycosaminoglycan products [46–48]. OA is achieved by surgically freeing the medial meniscus of the rabbit from the anterior pole to the midmedial collateral ligament. Partial excision (one-third to one-fourth) of the anterior aspect of the meniscus is done as well. It is thought that this meniscus then acts as a partially attached loose body that can alter the biomechanical forces across the joint and/or destabilize the knee.

Cartilage changes usually begin to occur within 4 to 8 weeks. There is cartilage pitting, ulceration, and fissuring. These gross changes can be seen using carbon black mapping [49]. Osteophyte formation occurs on the medial femoral condyle and the inner aspect of the medial tibial plateau. These osteophytes occur as early as 1 week after the surgery and occur in more than 75% of rabbits after 4 weeks. Cyst formation has been seen as well. Cartilage changes (pitting and erosions) occur principally on the medial femoral condyles. They also occur on the medial tibial plateaus [50]. Osteochondrocytes are present in 95% of tibias and are seen on the medial femoral condyle and the inner aspect of the medial tibial plateau.

In terms of histology, there is a disruption of the cartilage surface, chondrocyte proliferation, and chondrocyte cloning (Fig. 5). This proliferation of clones represents an effort at repair. There is also decreased Safranin-o staining. Synovitis is absent or mild. Changes continue to evolve between months 1 and 6. Initially there is increased cell replication not only in cartilage but also in subchondral bone, raising the possibility that early OA changes in humans may also involve subchondral bone. These changes have been shown through increased incorporation of tritiated thymidine, radiolabeled sulfate, and tritiated glycine, which indicate increased DNA, proteoglycan, and protein synthesis, respectively. Cell replication and protein synthesis eventually decrease because there is OA progression [51]. This particular sequence of glycosaminoglycan synthesis and cell replication is similar to that found in human disease [52].

Work using the partial-meniscectomized New Zealand white rabbit has been used to study the activity of matrix metalloproteinases (see Chapter 10), in particular matrix metalloproteinase-3 (MMP-3) [53]. Lesions at 4 weeks postmeniscectomy showed prominent inflammation of the synovium and an increase in MMP-3 activity in synovial cultures. There was a normalization of levels by week 8, but a second increase was observed at week 12 in synovial cultures. In chondrocyte cultures, there was an increase in MMP-3 activity at week 8 but none at week 4 or week 12 (when compared to control rabbits). Inhibition of the MMP-3 activity

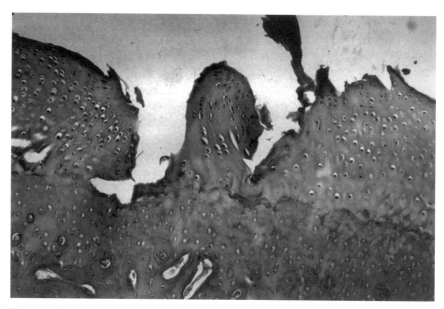

FIGURE 5   In the lapine model of osteoarthritis, osteoarthritis develops following partial medial meniscectomy of the right hind limb stifle (knee) of the rabbit, producing a massive disruption of cartilage by 12 weeks. There are large fissures, cloning of chondrocytes, loss of proteoglycan staining, dusruption of the tidemark, and many empty lacunae reflecting advanced osteoarthritis.

could be achieved by adding recombinant tissue inhibitor of metalloproteinase-1 (TIMP-1) to the cultures. This sequence of activation of MMP activity, synovial production followed by chondrocyte production, may provide insights into the early pathogenic sequences in OA.

B. Lateral Meniscectomy Model

In this model, OA is induced by partially resecting the lateral meniscus of the rabbit knee. Small portions of the fibular collateral and sesamoid ligaments also are resected [54–56]. This produces ulceration and gross degeneration of the medial and lateral tibial condyles. There is exposure of subchondral bone and osteophyte formation as well. Histologically, there is loss of proteoglycans as identified through decreased metachromatic staining. Cartilage fissuring, ulceration, and chondrocyte clones also were seen.

C. ACL Transection in the Rabbit

Unilateral transection of the ACL has been used for the induction of rabbit knee joint OA. In one study, 9 weeks after the surgery femora and tibiae from 11 study and contralateral control knees were obtained. Cartilage damage occurred predominantly on the posteromedial aspects of the joint and, to a lesser extent, on the anterolateral aspects [57].

New Zealand White (NZW) rabbits with closed epiphyses have been used in this model, and hyaluronic acid also has been studied with this model [58]. The NZW rabbits typically undergo unilateral ACL resection with contralateral arthrotomy (sham) and can then be used as their own controls. At 4 weeks after ACL transection, no full-thickness ulceration usually is observed. By 8 weeks, four of ten animals in one study had developed full-thickness ulceration of the medial femoral condyles. At 12 weeks, six of ten had developed such lesions. Using a computerized video analysis system, cartilage thickness and area showed decreases over time in all regions of the joint [59].

D. Rabbit Immobilization Model

The metabolism of hyaluronan in rabbits has been studied with an immobilization model (using a splint). It has been demonstrated that plasma levels of hyaluronan did not increase during immobilization but did increase in the 24 hours following remobilization [60]. This suggests that hyaluronan accumulates in the joint during immobilization. This accumulation could potentially lead to increased levels of IL-1, which in turn could increase prostromelysin and procollagenase mRNA transcription and lead to joint damage [61].

E. Rabbit Chymopapain Model

This model of chemical induction of disease has been used to study keratan sulfate as a marker for OA activity. In the cartilage injury seen in this model, serum keratan sulfate levels rise rapidly and return to baseline. As matrix proteoglycans are depleted, bone markers, such as bone-specific collagen cross-links appear in serum. This sequence of events illustrates the linkage of cartilage metabolism to bone metabolism [62].

V. GUINEA PIG MODELS OF OA

Models using guinea pigs include spontaneous OA and partial medial meniscectomy. A papain-induced model of knee OA also has been used.

A. Spontaneous OA

Guinea pigs develop spontaneous OA of the knee and other joints. Because cartilage destruction occurs mostly in the medial tibial plateau, the lateral side often is used as an internal control [63]. In Dunkin Hartley guinea pigs, the changes can be seen as early as 3 months of age and are age related. In one particular study, biochemical indices of OA were compared between 2-month- and 22-month-old guinea pigs. Collagen concentrations decreased over time as proteoglycan content increased in tibial cartilage [64]. Radiographic changes at 22 months included marginal osteophytes of the tibia and femur, sclerosis of the subchondral bone of the tibial plateau, femoral condyle cysts, and calcification of the collateral ligaments.

The relation of OA of the knee to weight has been explored in Hartley albino guinea pigs. Two groups of 20 male guinea pigs each were maintained on the same diet, but the guinea pigs in one of the groups were allowed to eat as much as they desired. Ten animals from each group were sacrificed at 9 months. The animals in the group limited to 30–35 g of feed per day weighed 28% less and the severity of their OA lesions was reduced by 40%. The other half of the animals were killed at 18 months and the animals in the restricted diet group were 29% lighter and had a 56% reduction in the severity of their OA [65].

This model also has been effectively used to investigate the expression of chondroitin sulfate epitopes. At 3 months, the time of the very earliest evidence of cartilage fibrillation, atypical chondroitin 6-sulfate chains can be identified in medial tibial plateau proteoglycans but not in the lateral compartment of the knee or in the hip [66]. They were seen principally in the superficial zone of cartilage.

B. Meniscectomy Model

Partial medial meniscectomy in the guinea pig knee has been used as a model of OA. In one study, the changes in the knee joint were evaluated at 1, 2, 3, 6, and 12 weeks postsurgery. Changes were observed as early as 1 week postsurgery. There were foci of moderate to severe cartilage degeneration in the medial tibial plateau and the femoral condyle. At 2 weeks, the degeneration was more extensive, with evidence of early osteophyte formation on the medial side of the femur and/or tibia in some of the animals. Severity of the changes increased progressively at weeks 3, 6, and 12 [67].

VI. OVINE MODELS OF OA

As in the case of canine models, ovine models offer the advantage of a larger animal with the opportunity of doing topographical studies of the cartilage and easy sampling with ample supply of cartilage and synovial fluid.

A. Meniscectomy Model

Some investigators have used a model in which the OA is induced by meniscectomy, particularly using purebred Merino sheep [68]. Lateral meniscectomy is performed in the stifle joint. Increased synthesis of dermatan sulfate proteoglycans 1 and 2 has been described in lateral tibial and femoral cartilage. There also was increased catabolism of aggrecan. Experiments in this model have shown that there is a topographical variation in proteoglycan synthesis by articular cartilage related to mechanical stress. These data suggest that an altered chondrocyte phenotypic expression of proteoglycans because of abnormal mechanical loading may be an early event in human OA [69]. Intra-articular hyaluronic acid (HA) injections have been evaluated using this model.

VII. SIMIAN MODELS OF OA

Spontaneous models of OA, particularly in Rhesus monkeys, have been studied. Two principal forms of arthritis have been identified in these monkeys: osteoarthritis and calcium pyrophosphate dihydrate crystal deposition disease. Spondyloarthropathy has also been described. Studies of these primates have been done at the Caribbean Primate Research Center in Cayo Santiago, Puerto Rico [70]. The primates were allowed to range free and their disease resembles spontaneous human OA with respect to age, sex, joint histology, and cartilage composition. Evidence of OA has been found in 20% of females and 4% of males in the center [71].

Free-ranging monkeys have had a significantly higher prevalence of "degenerative joint diseases" (osteoarthritis and/or pseudogout) based on radiographic findings and passive knee joint extension than caged animals of the same age [72]. The spontaneous OA incidence increased with age and, in females, with increased parity. As in humans, the disease was characterized by persistence of the chondrocyte density typical of the cartilage of young animals [73].

VIII. MURINE MODELS

Mice are easy to keep and develop and reproduce rapidly when compared to larger animals. They, however, do not provide large quantities of cartilage or synovial fluid for study. The topography of the cartilage itself is also not adequately studied. These models have been used extensively, however, particularly for the study of cytokines, growth factors, nitric oxide pathways, and cyclooxygenase expression in OA. Interesting work has been done in murine models trying to explain the mechanism of action of tetracyclines in the arthritides [74].

In one particular model, OA was induced by injection of highly purified bacterial collagenase into mouse knee joints. This produced cartilage loss on the lateral tibial plateau and osteophytes on the margin of the lateral tibial plateau. There was good correlation between the size of the osteophytes and the degree of cartilage loss for both the lateral and medial aspects of the joints [75].

Spontaneous models also exist, such as the STR/ort mice. Eighty five percent of male mice develop OA of the medial tibial cartilage by 35 weeks of age. It has been postulated that these changes involve abnormal catecholamine metabolism with changed activity and distribution of monoamine oxidase [76]. Low-grade histological lesions appeared within 10–20 weeks of age. In one study, the level of aggrecan was 2-fold greater in the tibial cartilage of 16–19 week STR/ort mice when compared to the control CBA mice with normal cartilage.

In another study, at 20 weeks of age, STR/ort and CBA tibial cartilage was analyzed for aggrecan gene transcription using a quantitative reverse transcription-polymerase chain reaction (RT-PCR). The samples of cartilage from the STR/ort medial and lateral tibial plateaus had 2.8- and 4.6-fold greater amounts of aggrecan cDNA per milligram of wet cartilage than those from the CBA tibial plateau. There were no differences in the cellularity of tibial cartilage between the species of mice [77].

The expression of cytokines such as IL-1 α, IL-1 β, and IL-6, as well as of growth factors such as insulin-like growth factor 1 (IGF-1) and transforming growth factor β (TGF β) have been studied in STR/ort mice. This was done using a nonradioactive in situ hybridization method using digoxigenin-labeled oligonucleotide probes to study expression of the cytokines and growth factors. At 20 weeks of age, STR/ort mice with no OA lesions showed positive expression for all of the cytokines and growth factors. At 35 weeks of age, areas with OA lesions coexisted with apparently normal cartilage, but signals for both cytokines and growth factors were increased when compared to control CBA mice. At 50 weeks of age, the expression of the factors was still elevated.

Interestingly, those STR/otr mice that had not developed OA by age 50 weeks had much reduced expression of both the growth factors and the cytokines when compared with those mice that developed OA [78].

IX. ANIMAL MODELS OF RHEUMATOID ARTHRITIS (RA)

Several animal models have been used in the investigation of pathogenetic mechanisms and therapeutics of rheumatoid arthritis (RA). Among the most commonly used models are adjuvant arthritis and collagen-induced arthritis. Other models include severe combined immunodeficient (SCID) mice implanted with human synovial tissues and human HLA-DR4-CD4 transgenic mice [79].

A. Adjuvant Arthritis

Experimental arthritis has been induced by injection of agents with the capacity to elicit an indirect immune response (adjuvants). Adjuvant arthritis (AA) is the classic example. The arthritis is produced through the injection of mineral oil and complete Freund's adjuvant (contains mycobacterial antigens) into rats [80]. Traditionally, the complete Freund's adjuvant has been thought to be the critical component. However, it has been shown that incomplete Freund's adjuvant (without mycobacterial antigens) along with pristane (a mineral oil) can induce arthritis in mice and rats [81, 82]. It is thought that regardless of whether the main immune stimulus is the mycobacterial antigen or the mineral oil, the targets of the autoimmune response are heat shock proteins [HSP] (highly conserved from species to species) [83]. Passive transfer of a T-cell clone responding to mycobacterial HSP 60 has been shown to produce disease in naive recipient animals. Immunization with HSP60, however, did not induce disease in the same study and actually afforded protection to the immunized animals [84].

Onset of disease in AA typically occurs within 19 days and presents as an acute inflammatory reaction with extensive bone loss. Macrophage-derived cytokines are prominent and include IL-1, TNF, and IL-6. There is also polyclonal activation of T cells and B cells with resulting production of multiple autoantibodies against heat shock proteins and cartilage. The presence of cytokines also leads to eventual synovial hypertrophy, expression of adhesion molecules, and abnormal expression of MHC type II molecules.

B. Collagen-Induced Arthritis

Type II collagen induces an erosive polyarthritis in certain strains of rats, mice, and higher primates. The role of cytokines and lymphocyte responses in inflammatory arthritis are being gradually elucidated with the help of this model. The collagen is usually injected intraperitoneally. The propensity for developing this collagen induced arthritis (CIA) is linked to the expression of certain MHC type II molecules and is characterized by synovitis, the production of pathogenic autoreactive antibodies that can fix and activate complement, much like in human RA [85]. Human RA cartilage and synovium contain antibodies to type II collagen at a prevalence greater than that in serum. Collagen-induced arthritis has been particularly useful in the study of the role of cytokines and other inflammatory mediators in RA. Multiple fragments and preparations of type II collagen (CII) can result in induction of arthritis. In one study, cynomolgus monkeys were immunized with chicken, human, or monkey CII or cyanogen bromide (CB)-generated peptide fragments of chicken CII emulsified in Freund's complete adjuvant. Clinical arthritis developed in all groups immunized with intact CII or with all major cyanogen bromide fragments except CB8 [68].

Type II orally administered collagen has been successful in preventing collagen-induced arthritis when fed to animals prior to the intraperitoneal injection of antigen. It also has been used to successfully treat the arthritis once induced. Attempts to develop immune tolerance by treating human RA with oral type II collagen have been relatively unsuccessful [87]. The presence of B cells appears to be crucial to the development of CIA because B cell-deficient mice do not develop the disease [88].

Various markers of cartilage breakdown have been investigated using this model. Studies in genetically susceptible Rhesus monkeys have revealed that during periods of active CIA, plasma c-reactive protein (CRP) is increased. There also are increased urinary excretion rates of the collagen cross-links hydroxylysylpyridinoline (HP) and lysylpyridinoline (LP) [89]. In one particular study in Rhesus monkeys with CIA, HP (the predominant cross-link in cartilage) was increased 9- to 15-fold as compared to a 4- to 6-fold increase in LP (the predominant cross-link in bone). This suggested a predominant destruction of cartilage in this particular model. Anti-CD 4 therapy has been tested in this model and has been effective [90].

In a study using murine CIA, the role of aggrecanase and matrix metalloproteinases (MMPs) in cartilage destruction was assessed [91]. The generation of the neoepitopes NITEGE373 (for aggrecanase) and VDIPEN341 (for MMP) were studied using immunoperoxidase microscopy with specific antipeptide antibodies in normal and stromelysin-1 deficient knockout mice with CIA. High levels of both epitopes were detected in areas with depletion of glycosaminoglycans but before significant cartilage erosion occurred. Chondrocyte periarticular matrix showed particularly high levels of both epitopes, suggesting that stimulated chondrocytes can synthesize and/or activate both enzymes.

Suppressors or inhibitors of TNF-α also have been tested using CIA. In one study, a type IV phosphodiesterase inhibitor (rolipram) was tested in murine CIA [92]. Upon treatment with this compound, bone marrow-derived macrophage production of TNF-α and IL-12 was suppressed. Reduced interferon gamma production and increased IL-10 production were also noted. These results appeared to indicate that this compound may favor a T helper type 2 response (Th2) while suppressing T helper type 1 response (Th1). Synergistic effects were seen when this compound was used in combination therapy for CIA with anti-CD4 monoclonal antibodies.

The administration of IL-4 has also been shown to suppress disease activity in CIA, raising the possibility that it also might do so in human disease [93]. Furthermore, daily intraperitoneal administration of a monoclonal antibody against IL-4 (starting on the day of immunization with CII) for 10 days has been shown to increase both the incidence and severity of CIA [94].

The importance of IL-6 in the development of CIA has also been demonstrated. Mice with null mutations for IL-6 introduced into their genome were protected from CIA. They also had a reduced antibody response to CII and a lack of inflammatory cells and tissue damage in their knee joints [95].

X. ANIMAL MODEL OF SERONEGATIVE SPONDYLARTHROPATHY-B27 TRANSGENIC RAT

Rats and mice transgenic for the human HLA-B27 gene have been used as experimental models for the human spondylarthropathies [96]. In a particular rat strain (HLA-B27 transgenic), spontaneous inflammation develops. It can involve peripheral and vertebral joints, the gastrointestinal lining, male genital tract, skin, nails, and even the heart. If these rats are kept in a sterile environment, the inflammation tends not to occur. The level of expression of HLA-B27 seems to correlate with the degree of inflammation. The disease can be transferred to nontransgenic rats through bone marrow cell transfer.

XI. CONCLUSIONS

These animal models continue to serve as bridges to understanding human disease. The fact that so many models continue to be used underscores the complexity of OA/RA and their etiopathogeneses. Different models are better at mimicking different aspects of human disease. No perfect model exists. It would be impossible to argue, however, that these models have not immensely increased our knowledge of the pathology, pathogenesis, and biochemistry of OA.

Models that involve cruciate ligament section, total or partial meniscectomies, or combined ligament/meniscal resection models are thought to most closely resemble human OA. This is certainly true for posttraumatic human OA. These models have been criticized as only representing this subset of disease but, nevertheless, are the most often used animal models of OA. To date, the models of RA are even less representative of the human disease. Transgenic technology has provided a model very similar to the typical human spondylarthropathy, ankylosing spondylitis. Practical concerns, such as experience with a model, cost, animal size, and ease of care continue to be powerful forces in deciding which model to use at a particular institution.

References

1. Lawrence, R. C., Hochberg, M. C., Kelsey, J. L. *et al.* (1989). Estimates of the prevalence of selected arthritic and musculoskeletal diseases in the United States. *J. Rheumatol.* **16**, 427–441.

2. Levy, E., Ferme, A., Perocheau, D., and Bono, I. (1993). Socioeconomic costs of osteoarthritis in France. *Rev. Rhum. Mal. Osteo-Articulaires* **60**, 63S–67S.

3. Lozada, C. J., and Altman, R. D. (1997). Management of osteoarthritis *In* "Arthritis and Allied Conditions" (W. J. Koopman, ed.), 13th ed., pp. 2013–2025. Williams & Wilkins, Baltimore, MD.

4. Hochberg, M. C., Altman, R. D., Brandt, K. D., Clark, B. M., Dieppe, P. A., Griffin, M. R. *et al.* (1995). Guidelines for the medical management of osteoarthritis: Part II. Osteoarthritis of the knee. *Arthritis Rheum.* **38**, 1541–1546.

5. Hochberg, M. C., Altman, R. D., Brandt, R. D., Clark, B. M., Dieppe, P. A., Griffin, M. R. *et al.* (1995). Guidelines for the medical management of osteoarthritis: Part I. Osteoarthritis of the hip. *Arthritis Rheum.* **38**, 1535–1540.

6. Hutton, C. W. (1989). Osteoarthritis: The cause not result of joint failure? *Ann. Rheum. Dis.* **48**, 958–961.

7. Liang, M. H., and Fortin, P. (1991). Management of osteoarthritis of the hip and knee. *N. Engl. J. Med.* **325** (2), 125–127.

8. Lozada, C. J., and Altman, R. D. (1997). Chondroprotection in osteoarthritis. *Bull. Rheum. Dis.* **46**, 5–7.

9. Altman, R., Brandt, K., Hochberg, M., Moskowitz, R. *et al.* (1996). Design and conduct of clinical trials in patients with osteoarthritis: Recommendations from a task force of the Osteoarthritis Research Society. *Osteoarthritis Cartilage* **4**, 217–243.

10. Altman, R. D., and Dean, D. D. (1990). Osteoarthritis research: Animal models. *Semin. Arthritis Rheum.* **19** (Suppl. 1), 21–25.

11. Carney, S. L. (1991). Cartilage research, biochemical, histologic and immunohistochemical markers in cartilage, and animal models of osteoarthritis. *Curr. Opin. Rheumatol.* **3**, 669–675.

12. Moskowitz, R. W. (1984). Experimental models of osteoarthritis. *In* "Osteoarthitis: Diagnosis and Management" (R. W. Moskowitz, D. S. Howell, Goldberg, V. M. *et al.*, eds.), pp. 109–129. Saunders, Philadelphia.

13. Pelletier, J. P., Martel-Pelletier, J., Altman, R. D. *et al.* (1983). Collagenolytic activity and collagen matrix breakdown of the articular cartilage in the Pond-Nuki dog model of osteoarthritis. *Arthritis Rheum.* **26**, 866–874.

14. Pond, M. J., and Nuki, G. (1973). Experimentally-induced osteoarthritis in the dog. *Ann. Rheum. Dis.* **32**, 387–388.

15. Moskowitz, R. W., Davis, W., Sammarco, J. *et al.* (1973). Experimentally induced degenerative joint lesions following partial meniscectomy in the rabbit. *Arthritis Rheum.* **16**, 397–405.

16. Moskowitz, R. W. (1977). Osteoarthritis-studies with experimental models. *Arthritis Rheum.* **20**, S104–S108.

17. Moskowitz, R. W., Howell, D. S., Goldberg, V. M. *et al.* (1979). Cartilage proteoglycan alterations in an experimentally induced model of rabbit osteoarthritis. *Arthritis Rheum.* **22**, 155–163.

18. Schnell, G. B. (1959). Canine hip dysplasia. *Lab. Invest.* **8**, 1178–1189.

19. Alwan, W. H., Carter, S. D., Bennett, D., May, S. A. *et al.* (1990). Cartilage breakdown in equine osteoarthritis: Measurement of keratan sulfate by an ELISA system. *Res. Vet. Sci.* **49**, 56–60.

20. Chateauvert, J. M., Grynpas, M. D., Kessler, M. J., and Pritzker, K. P. (1990). Spontaneous osteoarthritis in Rhesus macaques. II. Characterization of disease and morphometric studies. *J. Rheumatol.* **17**, 73–83.

21. Silberberg, R. (1977). Epiphyseal growth and osteoarthrosis in blotchy mice. *Exp. Cell Biol.* **45**, 1–8.

22. Skoloff, L. (1969). "The Biology of Degenerative Joint Disease," pp. 18–21. University of Chicago Press, Chicago.

23. Howell, D. S., Pita, J. C., Muller, F. J., Manicourt, D. H., and Altman, R. D. (1991). Treatment of osteoarthritis with tiaprofenic acid: Biochemical and histological protection against cartilage breakdown in the Pond-Nuki canine model. *J. Rheumatol.* **18** (Suppl. 27), 138–142.

24. Abatangelo, G., Botti, P., Del Bue, M., Gei, G. *et al.* (1989). Intraarticular sodium hyaluronate injections in the Pond-Nuki experimental model of osteoarthritis in dogs. I. Biochemical results. *Clin. Orthop.* **241**, 278–285.

25. Schiavinato, A., Lini, E., Guidolin, D., Pezzoli, G. *et al.* (1989). Intraarticular sodium hyaluronate injections in the Pond-Nuki experimental model of osteoarthritis in dogs. II. Morphological findings. *Clin. Orthop.* **241**, 286–299.

26. Altman, R. D., Dean, D. D., Muniz, O. E., and Howell, D. S. (1989). Therapeutic treatment of canine osteoarthritis with glycosaminoglycan polysulfuric acid ester. *Arthritis Rheum.* **32**, 1300–1307.

27. Rogachefsky, R. A., Dean, D. D., Howell, D. S., and Altman, R. D. (1993). Treatment of canine osteoarthritis with insulin-like growth factor-1 (IGF-1) and sodium pentosan polysulfate. *Osteoarthritis Cartilage* **2**, 105–114.

28. Johnson, R. G. (1986). Transection of the canine anterior cruciate ligament: A concise review of experience with this model of degenerative joint disease. *Exp. Pathol.* **30**, 209–213.

29. Altman, R. D., Tennenbaum, J., Latta, L. *et al.* (1984). Biomechanical and biochemical properties of dog cartilage in experimentally induced osteoarthritis. *Ann. Rheum. Dis.* **43**, 83–90.

30. Eyre, D. R., McDevitt, C. A., Billingham, M. E. J. *et al.* (1980). Biosynthesis of collagen and other matrix proteins in articular cartilage in experimental osteoarthrosis. *Biochem. J.* **188**, 823–837.

31. Altman, R. D., Dean, D. D., Muniz, O. E. *et al.* (1989). Therapeutic treatment with glycosaminoglycan polysulfuric acid ester(GAGPS) suppresses neutral metalloproteinases and cartilage swelling in the Pond–Nuki dog model of osteoarthritis. *Arthritis Rheum.* **32**, 759–766.

32. Altman, R. D., Dean, D. D., Muniz, O. E. *et al.* (1989). Prophylactic treatment of canine osteoarthritis with glycosaminoglycan polysulfuric acid ester (GAGPS). *Arthritis Rheum.* **16**, 759–766.

33. Marshall, K. W., and Chan, A. D. (1996). Arthroscopic anterior cruciate ligament transection induces canine osteoarthritis. *J. Rheumatol.* **23**, 338–343.

34. Visco, D. M., Hill, M. A., Widmer, W. R., Johnstone, B., and Myers, S. L. (1996). Experimental osteoarthritis in dogs: A comparison of the Pond–Nuki and medial arthrotomy methods. *Osteoarthritis Cartilage* **4**, 9–22.

35. O'Connor, B., Palmoski, M., and Brandt, K. (1985). Neurogenic acceleration of degenerative joint lesions. *J. Bone. Jt. Surg., Am. Vol.* **67A**, 562–572.

36. O'Connor, B. L., Visco, D. M., and Brandt, K. D. (1989). The development of experimental osteoarthritis (OA) in dogs with extensively deafferented knee joints. *Arthritis Rheum.* **32** (Suppl. 4), S106.

37. Yu, L. P., Jr., Smith, G. N., Jr., Brandt, K. D., Myers, S. L., O'Connor, B. L., and Brandt, D. A. (1992). Reduction of the severity of canine osteoarthritis by prophylactic treatment with oral doxycycline. *Arthritis Rheum.* **35**, 1150–1159

38. Brandt, K. D. (1991). Transection of the anterior cruciate ligament in the dog: A model of osteoarthritis. *Semin. Arthritis Rheum.* **21** (Suppl. 2), 22–32.

39. Thonar, E. J., Mausda, K., Lenz, M. E., Hauselmann, H. J. *et al.* (1995). Serum markers of systemic disease processes in osteoarthritis. *J. Rheumatol.* **22** (Suppl. 43), 68–70.

40. Ratcliffe, A., Billingham, M. E. J., Saed-Nejad, F., Muir, H. *et al.* (1992). Increased release of matrix components from articular cartilage in experimental canine osteoarthritis. *J. Orthop. Res.* **10**, 350–358.

41. Howell, D. S., Muller, F., and Manicourt, D. H. (1992). A mini review: Proteoglycan aggregate profiles in the Pond-Nuki model of osteoarthritis and in canine disuse atrophy. *Br. J. Rheumatol.* **31** (Suppl. 1), 7–11.

42. Caterson, B., Highes, C. E., Johnstone, J. B., and Mort, J. S. (1992). Immunological markers of cartilage proteoglycan metabolism in animal and human osteoarthritis. *In* "Articular Cartilage and Osteoarthritis" (K. E. Kuettner, R. Schleyerbach, J. G. Peyron, and V. C. Hascall, eds.), pp. 415–427. Raven Press, New York.

43. Palmoski, M., Perricone, E., and Brandt, K. D. (1997). Development and reversal of a proteoglycan aggregate defect in normal canine knee cartilage after immobilization. *Arthritis Rheum.* **22**, 508–517.

44. Lust, G., Beilman, W. T., Dueland, D. J. *et al.* (1980). Intraarticular volume and hip joint instability in dogs with hip dysplasia. *J. Bone Jt. Surg., Am. Vol.* **62A**, 576–582.

45. Wurster, N. B., and Lust, G. (1982). Fibronectin in osteoarthritic canine articular cartilage. *Biochem. Biophpys. Res. Commun.* **109**, 1094–1101

46. Moskowitz, R. W., Goldberg, V. M., Rosner, I. A. *et al.* (1981). Specific drug therapy of experimental osteoarthritis. *Semin. Arthritis Rheum.* **11** (Suppl. 1), 127–129.

47. Howell, D. S., Munoz, O. E., and Carreno, M. R. (1986). The effect of glycosaminoglycan polysulfate ester (GAGPE) on proteoglycan degrading enzyme activity in an animal model of osteoarthritis (OA). *Adv. Inflammation Res.* **11**, 197–205.

48. Carreno, M. R., Muniz, O. E., and Howell, D. S. (1986). The effect of glycosaminoglycan polysulfate ester on articular cartilage in experimental osteoarthritis: Effects on morphological variables of disease severity. *J. Rheumatol.* **13**, 490–497.

49. Meachim, G. (1972). Light microscopy of India ink preparations of fibrillated cartilage. *Ann. Rheum. Dis.* **31**, 457–464.

50. Malemud, C. J., Goldberg, V. M., and Moskowitz, R. W. (1986). Pathological, biochemical and experimental therapeutic studies in meniscectomy models of osteoarthritis in the rabbit—its relationship to human joint pathology. *Br. J. Clin. Pract.* **43**, 21–31.

51. Radin, E. L. (1984). Biomechanical considerations. *In* "Osteoarthritis, Diagnosis and Management" (R. W. Moskowitz, D. S. Howell, V. M. Goldberg *et al.*, eds.), pp. 93–108. Saunders, Philadelphia.

52. Mayor, M. B., and Moskowitz, R. W. (1974). Metabolic studies in experimentally-induced degenerative joint disease in the rabbit. *J. Rheumatol.* **1**, 17–23.

53. Mehraban, F., Lark, M. W., Ahmed, F. N., Xu, F., and Moskowitz, R. W. (1998). Increased secretion and activity of matrix metalloproteinase-3 in synovial tissues and chondrocytes from experimental osteoarthritis. *Osteoarthritis Cartilage* **6**, 286–294.

54. Colombo, C., Butler, M., O'Byrne, E. *et al.* (1983). I. Development of knee joint pathology following lateral meniscectomy and section of the fibular collateral and sesamoid ligaments. *Arthritis Rheum.* **26**, 875–886.

55. Colombo, C., Butler, M., Hickman, L. *et al.* (1983). A new model of osteoarthritis in rabbits. II. Evaluation of anti-osteoarthritic effects of selected antirheumatic drugs administered systemically. *Arthritis Rheum.* **26**, 1132–1139.

56. Butler, M., Colombo, C., Hickman, L. *et al.* (1983). A new model of osteoarthritis in rabbits. III. Evaluation of anti-osteoarthritic effects of selected drugs administered intraarticularly. *Arthritis Rheum.* **26**, 1380–1386.

57. Chang, D. G., Iverson, E. P., Schinagl, R. M., Sonoda, M. *et al.* (1997). Quantitation and localization of cartilage degeneration following the induction of osteoarthritis in the rabbit knee. *Osteoarthritis Cartilage* **5**, 357–372.

58. Yoshioka, M., Shimizu, C., Harwood, F. L., Coutts, R. D., and Amiel, D. (1997). The effects of hyaluronan during the development of osteoarthritis. *Osteoarthritis Cartilage* **4**, 251–260.

59. Yoshioka, M., Coutts, R. D., Amiel, D., and Hacker, S. A. (1996). Characterization of a model of osteoarthritis in the rabbit knee. *Osteoarthritis Cartilage* **4**, 87–98.

60. Konttinen, Y. T., Michelsson, J. E., Gronblad, M., Jaakola, L., and Honkanen, V. (1991). Plasma hyaluronan levels in rabbit immobilization osteoarthritis: Effect of remobilization. *Scand. J. Rheumatol.* **20**, 392–396.

61. Malemud, C. J. (1992). Markers of osteoarthritis and cartilage research in animal models. *Curr. Opin. Rheumatol.* **5**, 494–502.

62. Williams, J. M., Uebelhart, J. D., Onghi, D., Kuettner, K. E., and Thonar, E. J. (1992). Animal models of cartilage repair. *In* "Articular Cartilage and Osteoarthritis" (K. E. Kuettner, R. Schleyerbach, J. G. Peyron, and V. C. Hascall, eds.), pp. 511–526. Raven Press, New York.

63. De Bri, E., Jonsson, K., Reinholt, F. P., and Svensson, O. (1996). Focal destruction and remodeling in guinea pig arthrosis. *Acta Orthop. Scand.* **67**(5), 498–504.

64. Jimenez, P. A., Glasson, S. S., Trubetskoy, O. V., and Haimes, H. B. (1997). Spontaneous osteoarthritis in Dunkin Hartley guinea pigs: Histologic, radiologic, and biochemical changes. *Lab. Anim. Sci.* **47**(6), 598–601.

65. Bendele, A. M., and Hulman, J. F. (1991). Effects of body weight restriction on the development and progression of spontaneous osteoarthritis in guinea pigs. *Arthritis Rheum.* **34**, 1180–1184.

66. Caterson, B., Hughes, C. E., Johnstone, B., and Mort, J. S. (1992). Immunological markers of cartilage proteoglycan metabolism in animal and human osteoarthritis. *In* "Articular Cartilage and Osteoarthritis" (K. E. Kuettner, R. Schleyerbach, J. G. Peyron, and V. C. Hascall, eds.), pp. 415–427. Raven Press, New York.

67. Bendele, A. M. (1987). Progressive chronic osteoarthritis in femorotibial joints of partial medial meniscectomized guinea pigs. *Vet. Pathol.* **24**, 444–448.

68. Smith, M. M., Little, C. B., Rodgers, K., and Ghosh, P. (1997). Animal models used for the evaluation of anti-osteoarthritis drugs. *Pathol. Biol.* **45**, 313–320.

69. Little, C. B., Ghosh, P., and Bellenger, C. R. (1996). Topographic variation in biglycan and decorin synthesis by articular cartilage in the early stages of osteoarthritis: An experimental study in sheep. *J. Orthop. Res.* **14**, 433–444.

70. Pritzker, K. P., Chateauvert, J., Grynpas, M. D., Renlund, R. C., Turnquist, J. *et al.* (1989). Rhesus macaques as an experimental model for degenerative arthritis. *P. R. Health Sci. J.* **8**, 99–102.

71. Rothschild, B. M., Hong, N., and Turnquist, J. E. (1997). Naturally occurring inflammatory arthritis of the spondyloarthropathy variety in Cayo Santiago rhesus macaques (*Macaca mulatta*). *Clin. Exp. Rheumatol.* **15**, 45–51.

72. Kessler, M. J., Turnquist, J. E., Pritzker, K. P., and London, W. T. Reduction of passive extension and radiographic evidence of degenerative knee joint diseases in cage-raised and free-ranging aged rhesus monkeys (*Macaca mulatta*). *J. Med. Primatol.* **15**, 1–9.

73. Chateauvert, J. M., Grynpas, M. D., Kessler, M. J., and Pritzker, K. P. (1990). Spontaneous osteoarthritis in rhesus macaques. II. Characterization of disease and morphometric studies. *J. Rheumatol.* **17**, 73–83.

74. Amin, A. R., Attur, M. G., Thakker, G. D., Patel, P. D. *et al.* (1996). A novel mechanism of action of tetracyclines: Effects on nitric oxide synthases. *Proc. Natl. Acad. Sci. U.S.A.* **26**, 14014–14019.

75. van Osch, G. J., van der Kraan, P. M., van Valburg, A. A., and van den Berg, W. B. (1996). The relation between cartilage damage and osteophyte size in a murine model for osteoarthritis in the knee. *Rheumatol. Int.* **16**, 115–119.

76. Chayen, J., Bitensky, L., and Chambers, M. G. (1996). Modulation of murine osteoarthritis. *Cell Biochem. Funct.* **14**, 57–61.

77. Gaffen, J. D., Bayliss, M. T., and Mason, R. M. (1997). Elevated aggrecan mRNA in early murine osteoarthritis. *Osteoarthritis Cartilage* **5**, 227–233.

78. Chambers, M. G., Bayliss, M. T., and Mason, R. M. (1997). Chondrocyte cytokine and growth factor expression in murine osteoarthritis. *Osteoarthritis Cartilage* **5**, 301–308.

79. Houri, J. M., and O'Sullivan, F. X. (1995). Animal models in rheumatoid arthritis. *Curr. Opin. Rheumatol.* **7**, 201–205.

80. Billingham, M. E. J. (1995). Adjuvant arthritis: The first model. *In* "Mechanisms and Models in Rheumatoid Arthritis" (B. Henderson, J. C. W. Edwards, and E. R. Pettipher, eds.), pp. 389–410. Academic Press, London.

81. Wooley, P. H., Seibold, J. R., Whalen, J. D., and Chapdelaine, J. M. (1989). Pristane-induced arthritis. The immunological and genetic features of an experimental murine model of autoimmune disease. *Arthritis Rheum.* **32**, 1022–1030

82. Kleinau, S., Erlandsson, H., Holmdahl, R., and Klareskog, L. (1991). Adjuvant oils induce arthritis in the DA rat. I. Characterization of the disease and evidence for an immunological involvement. *J. Autoimmunol.* **4**, 871–880.

83. van Eden, W., Hogervorst, E. J., Hensen, E. J. *et al.* (1989). A cartilage-mimicking T-cell epitope on a 65K mycobacterial heat-shock protein: Adjuvant arthritis as a model for human rheumatoid arthritis. *Curr. Topi. Microbiol. Immunol.* **145**, 27–43.

84. van der Zee, R., Anderton, S. M., Prakken, A. B., Liesbeth Paul, A. G., and van Eden, W. (1998). T cell responses to conserved bacterial heat-shock-protein epitopes induce resistance in experimental autoimmunity. *Semin. Immunol.* **10**, 35–41.

85. Myers, L. K., Rosioniec, E. F., Cremer, M. A., and Kang, A. H. (1997). Collagen-induced arthritis, an animal model of autoimmunity. *Life Sci.* **61**, 1861–1878.

86. Shimozure, Y., Yamane, S., Fujimoto, K., Terao, K. *et al.* (1998). Collagen-induced arthritis in nonhuman primates: Multiple epitopes of type II collagen can induce autoimmune-mediated arthritis in outbred cynomolgus monkeys. *Arthritis Rheum.* **41**, 507–514.

87. Cremer, M. A., Rosloniec, E. F., and Kang, A. H. (1998). The cartilage collagens: A review of their structure, organization, and role in the pathogenesis of experimental arthritis in animals and in human rheumatic disease. *J. Mol. Med.* **76**, 275–278.

88. Svensson, L., Jirholt, J., Holmdahl, R., and Jansson, L. (1998). B cell-deficient mice do not develop type II collagen-induced arthritis (CIA). *Clin. Exp. Immunol.* **111**, 521–526.

89. 't Hart, B. A., Bank, R. A., De Roos, J. A., Brok, H. *et al.* (1988). Collagen-induced arthritis in rhesus monkeys: Evaluation of markers for inflammation and joint degradation. *Br. J. Rheumatol.* **37**, 314–323.

90. Ranges, N. A., Fortin, S., Barger, M. T., Sriram, S. *et al.* (1988). In vivo modulation of murine collagen induced arthritis. *Int. Rev. Immunol.* **4**, 83–90.

91. Singer, II., Scott, S., Kawka, D. W., Bayne, E. K. *et al.* (1997). Aggrecanase and metalloproteinase-specific aggrecan neo-epitopes are induced in the articular cartilage of mice with collagen II-induced arthritis. *Osteoarthritis Cartilage* **5**, 407–418.

92. Ross, S. F., Williams, R. O., Mason, L. J., Mauri, C. *et al.* (1997). Suppression of TNF-alpha expression, inhibition of Th1 activity, and amelioration of collagen- induced arthritis by rolipram. *J. Immunol.* **159**, 6253–6259.

93. Horsfall, A. C., Butler, D. M., Marinova, L., Warden, P. J. *et al.* (1997). Suppression of collagen-induced arthritis by continuous administration of IL-4. *J. Immunol.* **159**, 5687–5696.

94. Yoshino, S. (1998). Effect of a monoclonal antibody against interleukin-4 on collagen-induced arthritis in mice. *Br. J. Pharmacol.* **123**, 237–242.

95. Alonzi, T., Fattori, E., Lazzaro, D., Costa, P. *et al.* (1998). Interleukin 6 is required for the development of collagen-induced arthritis. *J. Exp. Med.* **187**, 461–468.

96. Hammer, R. E., Maika, S. D., Richardson, J. A., Tang, J. P. *et al.* (1990). Spontaneous inflammatory disease in transgenic rats expressing HLA-B27 and human beta 2m: An animal model of HLA B27-associated human disorders. *Cell* **63**, 1099–1112.

PART III

Markers of Bone and Cartilage Metabolism

A. Quantification: Technical Aspects
(Chapters 25–31)

B. Clinical Applications
(Chapters 32–46)

CHAPTER 25

Genetic Approaches to Metabolic Bone Diseases

ANDRÉ G. UITTERLINDEN, JOHANNES P. T. M. VAN LEEUWEN, HUIBERT A. P. POLS

Department of Internal Medicine III, Erasmus University Medical School, 3000 Rotterdam, The Netherlands

I. ABSTRACT

The molecular genetic dissection of the complex trait osteoporosis into its composite genetic factors has been initiated, but not without generating considerable controversy. Osteoporosis candidate genes have appeared and disappeared as true susceptibility genes and have also been proposed as candidate genes in the context of other diseases. In this chapter we will address several of the mainly methodological issues underlying such controversy. Advantages and disadvantages of the approaches undertaken to identify the true osteoporosis genes are described and complicating factors are discussed and illustrated. However, in spite of the many difficulties that still must be overcome, the molecular genetic approach to analyzing osteoporosis holds great promise to delineate the pathophysiological mechanisms underlying this disease. Furthermore, genetic insights will also be valuable for diagnostic strategies and, most importantly, will help in designing therapeutic intervention strategies based on an understanding of the molecular mode of action of the proteins involved.

II. INTRODUCTION

A. Genetic Diseases

The concept of "genetic" diseases has substantially evolved, due not only to new insights into the genetic nature of disease but also because of the availability of methods to identify and characterize genetic factors predisposing a person to disease. The importance of acquiring knowledge on such genetic risk factors lies in the possibility of [1] determining a "risk profile" at a very early stage, through molecular genetic techniques, even before the disease is presented clinically, and (2) designing therapeutic intervention strategies on the basis of knowledge of the molecular action of the proteins involved.

Initially, genetic diseases were defined as single Mendelian traits, usually with an early onset of the disease and relatively fast progression, that showed clear Mendelian inheritance patterns in families. Since it was recognized in 1980 that the genetic inheritance patterns of these monogenic diseases could be followed using naturally occurring DNA sequence variations [1], molecular genetic technology soon allowed the isolation of the genes responsible for diseases such as Duchenne muscular dystrophy, cystic fibrosis, Huntington's disease, and several others. By 1998, the chromosomal position of more than 500 disease genes of the estimated 3000 monogenic diseases had been determined, and close to one hundred have been cloned and characterized.

In the area of bone metabolism, the accumulation of knowledge about the molecular genetic nature of disease had led to important discoveries. Among the cloned disease genes responsible for Mendelian bone disorders are the genes encoding collagen type Iα1 (located on chromosome 17q22) and collagen type Iα2 (located on chromosome 7q22.1); these are responsible for most forms of what is the best known and characterized genetic bone disease, osteogenesis imperfecta (OI). This inherited brittle-bone disorder predisposes a patient to easy fracturing of bones, even with little trauma, and to skeletal deformity. The condition involves either qualitative or quantitative alterations in type I collagen protein that are the result of a variety of possible small point mutations or small deletions/duplications within one of the genes that encodes the chains of the collagen type I protein. While bone fragility is common to all forms of OI, the clinical phenotypic presentation is remarkably variable, ranging from lethal perinatal forms to only a mild increase in fracture frequency. Underlying this range of variation is the so-called locus and allelic heterogeneity (i.e. the disease phenotype varies according to which gene is mutated and according to the type and location of the mutation).

B. Complex Traits

The characterization of the molecular genetic basis of osteogenesis imperfecta and other, by current standards, relatively simple genetic disorders is still changing our concept of disease. Analysis of such diseases not only illustrates the vast and devastating effects simple mutations can have, but also generates novel technological tools accelerating the process of gene discovery and mutation detection. Together, this provides the basis to tackle the more challenging problems of the common multifactorial diseases such as osteoporosis. Many of the most important medical conditions in the western world are usually not characterized by simple Mendelian inheritance patterns, early onset, and straightforward diagnostic criteria, and, most importantly, occur much more frequently in the population. Whereas cystic fibrosis, for example, has an estimated population incidence of 1 in 3000, and the combined incidence of all forms of OI is about 1 in 10,000, common diseases such as diabetes, hypertension, asthma, manic depression, and osteoporosis occur in 5–50% of the elderly population. In view of the increase in the maximum life expectancy of men and women in our society, these common disease will even further increase in frequency and the search

for the responsible genes has become a priority in medical research. Unlike the relatively straightforward genetics of the monogenic disorders, common diseases have a multifactorial nature (genetic and environmental conditions interact), are multigenic (multiple genes are involved), and usually have a late onset with variable clinical manifestations. It is therefore not surprising that these diseases are referred to as complex traits. However, due to the successful application of molecular genetic techniques to monogenic diseases, unravelling of the etiology of complex traits by genetic means now has become a feasable mission [2]. In the field of bone metabolism, the main target disease is, of course, osteoporosis.

The genetic dissection of the complex traits follows similar analytical strategies for many of the common diseases, including osteoporosis. First, evidence from twin studies is sought to demonstrate and estimate the heritability of the trait (or one or more of its composite features) and the influence of environmental factors. Epidemiological studies are needed to quantify the variability of a trait and to identify potentially modifying environmental factors. Genetic epidemiological studies applying molecular genetic tools can then identify chromosomal regions harboring putative candidate genes. Finally, candidate gene studies will establish the contribution of particular gene variants in explaining the variation of the trait and their relationship to gene-environment interactions, and, last but not least, will investigate the underlying molecular mechanisms.

C. Osteoporosis

In the field of metabolic bone diseases, genetic studies are focused on osteoporosis, and therefore osteoporosis is the main subject of this chapter. In particular, studies have been initiated to identify gene variants underlying the genetic control of bone mineral density (BMD), one of the main risk factors of osteoporosis. Evidence from twin and family studies suggests that genetic factors play a major role in determining BMD. Twin studies of peak BMD and postmenopausal BMD have shown high concordance rates for monozygotic twin pairs in comparison to dizygotic twin pairs, with estimates of the heritability ranging from 50–80% [3, 4]. In addition, first-degree relatives of osteoporotic patients and daughters of mothers with osteoporosis were shown to have reduced BMD [5–8]. Finally, segregation analysis in families has shown that bone mineral density is under polygenic control [9, 10]. Bone density can be considered to be a result of the balance between bone formation and bone resorption. Therefore, it can be expected that aspects of the proces of bone turnover are under genetic control. Indeed, several twin studies have shown that biochemical markers of bone formation (such as osteocalcin and bone-specific alkaline phosphatase) and markers of bone resorption (such as ICTP, the pyridinoline cross-linked carboxy-terminal telopeptide of the

TABLE I. Brief Glossary of Genetic Terms

Allele	One of several alternative forms of a DNA sequence at a specific chromosomal location (locus). At each autosomal chromosomal locus in a cell, two alleles are present, one inherited from the mother, the other from the father
Haplotype	A series of alleles found at linked loci on a single chromosome (phase)
Kbp	Kilobasepairs (1.10^3 bp)
Linkage	The tendency of DNA sequences to be inherited together as a consequence of their close proximity on a chromosome
Linkage disequilibrium	Nonrandom association of alleles at linked loci
Locus	A unique chromosomal location defining the position of a particular DNA sequence
Mbp	Megabasepairs (1.10^6 bp)
Microsatellite	A locus consisting of tandemly repetitive sequence units the size of which is (arbitrarily) defined as 1–5 bp
Minisatellite	A locus consisting of tandemly repetitive sequence units the size of which is (arbitrarily) defined as 6 bp or more
Mutation	An alteration in the DNA sequence
Polymorphism	The existence of two or more alleles at a frequency of at least 1% in the population
QTL	Quantitative trait locus; a gene that influences quantitative variation in a trait
RFLP	Restriction fragment length polymorphism
VNTR	Variable number of tandem repeats; a polymorphic micro- or minisatellite

type I collagen) have strong genetic components contributing to their variation in the population [11–13]. In the genetic analyses of bone turnover and BMD, the strongest genetic effects were observed for premenopausal peak BMD, and the effects became less with age. Taken together, this indicates that several parameters of osteoporosis are genetically determined but that gene-environment interactions also seem to play an important role, especially at older ages.

As the Human Genome Project progresses, a plethora of knowledge is becoming available about the function of genes and the genetic variants of these genes that exist in the population. Although this has led to many molecular genetic studies of osteoporosis, it has also created controversy and misunderstanding. In this chapter, several mainly methodological factors that can influence the outcome and interpretation of such studies will be discussed and illustrated with examples. Table I lists brief explanations of some of the genetic terms frequently used throughout the text.

III. ANALYTICAL CONSIDERATIONS

There are several steps in the analytical process of the identification of DNA sequence changes that are responsible for variations in the several composite phenotypic characteristics underlying osteoporosis. These involve, for example, the definition of the phenotype of osteoporosis (diagnostic criteria), the choice of study designs, and the types of DNA markers and method of genotyping used in the analyses. Table II lists some of the possible pitfalls in genetic association studies by category. Here we will discuss several steps in the analytical

process with some emphasis on the molecular genetic aspects and the possible complicating factors encountered.

A. Diagnostic Considerations

The aim of osteoporosis gene hunts is to ultimately produce a map of osteoporosis genes, variants of which contribute to one or more of the composite features of the osteoporotic phenotype. In this respect, the diagnostic criteria used to define osteoporosis form an important lead in the genetic analysis of the disease. In other words, the genetic variation can be correlated with a variety of biological endpoints, all of which are relevant for osteoporosis but to a different extent. According to the generally accepted definition, osteoporosis is characterized by reduced bone mineral density and microarchitectural deterioration of bone tissue leading to an increased fracture risk [14]. Of these, fractures and BMD can be measured and used in genetic analyses, but the deterioration of the bone architecture is less easy to quantify.

At first sight, fractures may seem the diagnostic criterion of choice because they are a discrete and clinically relevant endpoint of the disease. However, there are several drawbacks to their use in genetic analyses. Fractures usually occur at a more advanced age (mean age is about 70 years), severely complicating the study of relatives (brothers and sisters) of patients. Patients and/or relatives might not live in the same neighborhood, they might have already died, and they might also suffer from other diseases. In addition, the definition of what constitutes an osteoporotic fracture can vary. For example, different types of fracture can be discerned, such as

TABLE II.   Pitfalls in Genetic Association Studies

Epidemiological
1. Sample size is too small, leading to chance findings

2. Population is biased due to selection, admixture, inbreeding, etc.

3. Environmental factors differ between populations

Genetic
1. Allelic heterogeneity; different alleles are associated in different populations

2. Locus heterogeneity; gene effects differ between populations due to genetic drift and the founder effect

3. Linkage disequilibrium; one or more adjacent genes are the true susceptibility loci instead of the locus being tested

Molecular genetic
1. Low genetic resolution; unjustified grouping of alleles due to insufficient methodological discriminatory power

2. Anonymous polymorphisms; there is no known functional effect of the polymorphism to provide a direct biological explanation of the association

vertebral vs nonvertebral fractures and hip fracture vs wrist fracture, each of which may have a different set of risk factors and concomitantly might have a different set of risk genes.

Bone mineral density as a diagnostic criterion is only one of the major risk factors, but it also is one that is relatively easy to measure. However, it has to be taken into account that bone density changes with age under normal conditions. In the first decades of life BMD increases gradually to reach the peak bone mass in the third decade, whereas BMD in elderly individuals, and especially in postmenopausal women, bone mass is also influenced by the rate of bone loss. Each of these conditions has separate sets of risk factors and also environmental factors influencing the outcome. Nevertheless, several early studies showed that BMD is under strong genetic control, and therefore it is not surprising that most molecular genetic analyses have focused on BMD as the main outcome variable. BMD values follow a normal distribution in the population and can therefore be considered as a quantitative trait. Although this can complicate the analysis (i.e. what is a "low" BMD?), this feature can also be exploited to improve the efficiency of genetic strategies to localize BMD genes (see section III.C.1).

B. Molecular Genetic Considerations

1. CANDIDATE GENES

Many protein products and their corresponding genes are already known to play important roles in bone metabolism (see Fig. 1). Furthermore, with the advent of molecular genetics it has become relatively easy to determine genetic variation in these genes. Consequently, many molecular genetic studies on osteoporosis have chosen one or more of these already known genes to investigate their role in explaining some of the genetic variance in the different phenotypic endpoints of osteoporosis. This approach is thus also known as the candidate gene approach. Candidate genes can be selected on the basis of their involvement in a particular biochemical pathway in bone metabolism. An example of this is the vitamin D receptor gene which was the very first gene suggested to be involved in the genetic regulation of BMD by the pioneering studies of Drs. Eisman and Morrison [15]. In addition, genes involved in the estrogen endocrine system, such as the estrogen receptor gene, are important candidates in view of the importance of estrogen for bone metabolism, which is illustrated, for example, by effects of menopause on BMD. By using anonymous polymorphisms, variants of the estrogen receptor gene were found to be associated with BMD [16], but other researchers could not replicate this finding [17]. Further examples of candidate genes selected on the basis of bone biology are polymorphisms described in the genes for interleukin-6 and transforming growth factor ß. Variants of these genes have also been found to be associated with differences in bone density [18, 19] but these observations have not yet been confirmed by other investigators.

One can also experimentally identify such genes by methods developed to identify genes being expressed specifically in a certain tissue, for example bone tissue. One such a method is representational difference analysis, or RDA [20]. This method is based on generating a "fingerprint" of a representative set of hundreds of cDNA fragments derived from two or more sources of mRNA, such as normal vs tumour cells, bone tissue vs liver tissue, etc. The fingerprints consist of PCR products that are generated using degenerate or specific primers and can be produced, e.g., by electrophoretic separation or by DNA chip technology. By comparing such fingerprints, cDNA fragments that are expressed specifically or more abundantly in a particular source of mRNA can be identified.

Alternatively, candidate genes can be identified by methods highlighting the importance of particular genes in the development of bone tissue, such as in transgenic and knockout mice. Examples of this include the interleukin-4 transgenic mouse, that results in an osteoporotic mouse [21], and the

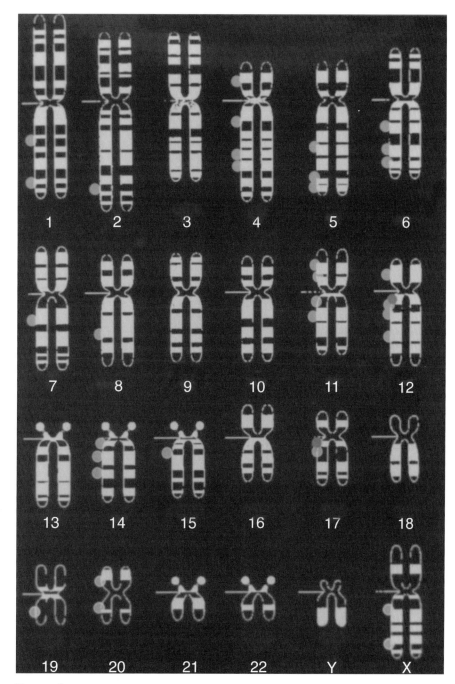

FIGURE 1   The human karyotype highlighting some of the locations of possible candidate genes for osteoporosis. The VDR-COL2A1 locus on chromosome 12 and the COLIA1 locus on chromosome 17 are indicated with darker shading, both of which are discussed in more detail in the text.

cfos-proto-oncogene knockout mouse [22] and the NF-κB1 and NF-κB2 double knockout mouse [23], both of which result in an osteopetrotic mouse. Occasionally, human "knock-out experiments of nature" are described as case reports that identify such genes. For example, a 28-year-old man with a loss-of-function mutation of the estrogen receptor α gene had osteoporosis [24].

Another important method for identifying candidate genes is based on genetic studies involving the study of transmission of a mutation in pedigrees suffering from monogenetic disorders that lead to distorted bone metabolism. In such cases, a gene will be identified for which severe mutations have a dramatic effect on bones or bone metabolism. For example, loss-of-function mutations in the gene for the vitamin D receptor are responsible for the bone disease that characterizes hypocalcemic 1α,25-dihydroxyvitamin D-resistant rickets [25, 26]. This gene will be discussed in more detail below. Similarly, several girls with loss-of-function mutations in the aromatase P450 gene, who cannot synthesize estrogen, develop osteoporosis [27], but no population-based studies of this gene have been published. In other pedigree studies, a locus for "high peak bone density" and the locus for osteoporosis pseudoglioma syndrome, a recessive disorder characterized by juvenile-onset blindness and osteoporosis, were mapped to the same region on chromosome 11 by positional cloning studies [28, 29], suggesting the presence of a gene effecting bone density. All of these disorders involve severe phenotypes caused by particular mutations, e.g., in the coding sequence of the disease gene. However, mutations elsewhere in the gene, for example in regulatory areas responsible for control of expression of the gene, could have more subtle effects. Albeit small, such effects could be relevant with respect to osteoporosis, especially through an accumulative effect during life.

Although the candidate gene approach has been shown to be fruitful, there are several drawbacks. First, detailed molecular genetic knowledge on the gene must exist before it can be studied. This means that the gene must have been cloned and linked to some extent with bone metabolism. This severely compromises the comprehensiveness of this approach because only about 5% of the total number of human genes has been cloned and characterized and only a few of these are genes that are actually involved in bone metabolism. Therefore, major genes related to bone metabolism might still be unknown. Another disadvantage of the candidate gene approach is the fact that it may provide a biased view. Using this approach, the genome is not randomly searched for genes that contribute to osteoporosis but rather a selected gene is studied. If a weak association is found with bone density, for example, it will be hard to dismiss it in view of the amount of work that went into the study and the pressure to publish or patent. These potential drawbacks become even more pertinent when anonymous sequence variants in or outside the gene are studied, i.e., those sequence changes that by themselves do not code for a different protein or result in differences in regulation of the expression of the gene.

2. GENOME SEARCHES

A more objective approach is to not make any presumption about a possible role of a particular gene but rather to randomly search the complete genome to identify only those regions in the genome that contain putative candidate genes which contribute to osteoporosis. Genome search approaches involve genetic studies to find evidence of cotransmission of DNA marker alleles and the phenotype of interest [1]. Because the chromosomal location of such markers is known or can be easily determined, this principle is also known as positional cloning. Positional cloning strategies were first applied to identify genes responsible for monogenic diseases, such as Duchenne muscular dystrophy and cystic fibrosis, but later it was realized that the same principle could be used to dissect more complex genetic traits by identifying the composite genetic factors. Initially, the diseases under study included psychological and behavorial traits, such as bipolar disorder and schizophrenia. Many difficulties were encountered in the study design, especially in designing guidelines for what to declare a positive linkage, but eventually these were properly addressed [30]. The many lessons learned led first to the successful analysis of type I diabetes that resulted in the identification of several genomic loci with positive linkage [31, 32]. Currently it is hard to think of a common trait that is not the subject of one or more genome searches.

Chromosomal areas shared between individuals are "identical by state" (IBS), but not necessarily "identical by descent" (IBD). The latter requires individuals to share a common ancestor who has transmitted the chromosomal area (over several generations) to them. Most genome search approaches rely on the identification of chromosomal areas that are identical by descent in unrelated individuals who have the same disease phenotype, e.g., low BMD and/or more than one fracture. Supposedly, such individuals share one or more chromosomal regions containing a sequence variant of one or more osteoporosis genes derived from a common ancestor. To ensure that such areas are identical by descent and not identical by state, sibs (i.e., brothers and sisters) who share a phenotype are analyzed. Sharing one allele of a given locus among sibs with similar phenotypes and sharing the same locus (but possibly with different alleles) between different sib pairs indicate the involvement of a certain locus (chromosomal area) in the phenotype of interest. The chromosomal regions are analyzed using anonymous polymorphic markers (usually CA/GT-microsatellites) scattered over the genome with a spacing of 10–20 centiMorgan (cM) (see Section III.B.3). Genome searches rely on the availability of hundreds of well-documented family samples and on an infrastructure to scan hundreds of polymorphic markers in these samples. With improved genotyping technology this approach has become feasible, but it still is laborious and costly. When performed in humans, genome searches have the drawback that samples from hundreds of well-characterized patients and their relatives have to be collected. Alternatively, it is possible to perform such genome searches in crosses of inbred mice which have, for example, very low and very high BMD. Although helpful for identifying BMD genes, the usefulness of this approach for the identification of human osteoporosis genes is somewhat hampered by the evolutionary distance between mice and men.

In general, a drawback of the genome search approach is the fact that, as a result of genome scans with current technology, only the approximate position of several chromosomal regions containing putative candidate genes will be identified. The precision of this position usually depends on the number of families analyzed and the number of markers used in the study. On average this will result in a region of 5–10 cM, corresponding roughly with 5–10 million basepairs (Mbp), to be searched further for candidate genes. Because 1 Mbp can contain up to one hundred genes it still is a formidable task to identify the candidate gene itself. One is looking for one or a few functional DNA polymorphisms (point mutations, small deletions, or insertions, etc.) amidst the several hundred present in such an area. Therefore, the most likely and efficient approach to construct an osteoporosis gene map will be a combination of genome searches and candidate gene analyses. Genome searches will identify and rank the most important regions in the genome while the available knowledge on bone metabolism genes and candidate gene studies will aid in identifying the true osteoporosis genes within those regions.

3. DNA SEQUENCE VARIATION

Crucial to any genetic association analysis is the detection of variations in the basepair sequence of the genomic or mitochondrial DNA between different individuals and the ability to relate this to variation in the phenotypic characteristic of interest. By definition, DNA sequence variations are termed polymorphic if they occur at a population frequency of one percent or more, as opposed to mutations responsible for a genetic disease that occur at frequencies of less than one percent.

Monogenic diseases are usually caused by mutations having severe effects, such as those in the coding regions of disease genes leading to crucial amino acid changes or in regulatory regions with considerable effects on expression of the gene. In contrast, polymorphisms are thought to underlie the more subtle variations in genes thought to be responsible for the normal distribution of most phenotypic characteristics of complex traits. Disease mutations arise through relatively recent DNA sequence changes in a given founder individual and usually do not tend to be very old in evolutionary terms. Polymorphisms are usually much older and, because selection has little influence on their spreading in the population, polymorphisms are much more frequent. It has been estimated that about one in every 200–300 bp of the total estimated 3 billion basepairs in the human genome is polymorphic in the population [33]. Although this implies that it will not be very difficult to find polymorphisms, it also poses the considerable problem of identifying which of these are in fact responsible for explaining variation of the phenotype of interest.

a. Types of DNA Sequence Variation DNA sequence polymorphisms come in many shapes [34], the most simple one being a single nucleotide polymorphism, or SNP, of which the human genome contains several million, both in coding and in noncoding regions of the genome. The human genome is estimated to contain roughly 80,000 genes, with

about 200,000 SNPs estimated to be situated in the coding regions of these genes [35, 36]. Another frequent type of DNA sequence variation involves the tandem repetition of short sequence motifs. Depending on the length of these motifs, they are arbitrarily referred to as microsatellites or short tandem repeats (with a motif length of up to 6 bp), or minisatellites (motif length >6 bp). Due to the sometimes highly polymorphic variation in number of repeat units, these sequences are termed variable number of tandem repeats, or VNTRs. Microsatellites with short motifs, such as the GT (or CA) repeats, are present in an estimated 100,000 copies per haploid genome and are spread throughout the chromosomes. These characteristics make them highly suitable as genetic markers for use in genome scans. Minisatellites occur less frequently but still can be informative markers in association analyses when located in the neighborhood of genes of interest. One example of this, the VNTR 1 kb 3′ of the collagen type IIα1 (COL2A1) gene, will be discussed in Section b4.

b. Genotyping Methods for Detecting DNA Sequence Variation The methodology used to determine polymorphism at a particular locus of interest is of considerable importance in the association analysis, especially when anonymous polymorphisms are used. The applicability of anonymous DNA markers in genetic association analysis is based on the assumption that one or more alleles of this marker is supposedly in linkage with a true susceptibility polymorphism (caused by a functional sequence variation) elsewhere in the gene. To increase the chance of detecting such a linkage, it is therefore of crucial importance to identify as many alleles as possible. Two examples can illustrate this: the direct molecular haplotyping protocol that was developed for genotyping three adjacent RFLPs at the VDR locus and the heteroduplexing protocol that was developed for genotyping a VNTR at the COL2A1 locus.

b.1 Single Nucleotide Polymorphisms (SNPs): There are many methods of detecting single nucleotide polymorphisms [34, 37] but few are suited for application on a large scale, as is required in genetic association analyses when hundreds of samples have to be analyzed. The most robust and most widely applied method is the detection of the single nucleotide polymorphisms (SNPs) as a restriction fragment length polymorphism (RFLP) within a PCR fragment generated from the locus and detected by electrophoretic separation. Examples include the BsmI, ApaI, and TaqI polymorphisms within the VDR gene. In RFLP typing, the presence or absence of a particular nucleotide change leads to presence or absence of a recognition site for a particular restriction enzyme. A prerequisite for this method is, of course, knowing the location of the nucleotide change within the palindromic (4–6 bp) recognition site of any one of the few hundred existing restriction enzymes. Although this limits the RFLP method to certain classes of SNPs, there are molecular genetic ways of creating an artificial recognition site conditional on the presence or absence of a certain sequence variation through mutagenic PCR. An example, the COLIA1 Sp1 G to T polymorphism, will be discussed in Section III.D.1.b.

DNA chip technology [38] has made it possible to screen several hundreds of SNPs in a semiautomated fashion. In this technique, a hundred to several thousand different oligonucleotides corresponding to the gene or sequence of interest are attached in an ordered fashion to a microarray of about 1 cm^2. Subsequently, fluorescently labelled PCR products are generated from the sample to be analyzed and hybridized to the array. The pattern of hybridization is analyzed by confocal microscopic scanning and a positive signal indicates existence of homology between oligos and the sample. Thus, depending on the oligonucleotides on the array and the sample, one can genotype by testing for a certain number of possible point mutations in a gene or analyse expression patterns by testing for the presence or absence of a particular gene product (as mRNA). Sofar, the technology for genotyping has been applied to find sequence variation in hypervariable HIV proteins [39] and in detecting mutations in the cystic fibrosis transmembrane regulator gene gene [40] and the BRCA-1 breast cancer gene [41]. It is expected that it will surely lead to considerable increases in the throughput of screening SNPs in the analysis of candidate genes and in other applications in the analysis of complex traits including osteoporosis.

A special case is presented when several polymorphisms of interest are located close to each other, e.g., in adjacent genes or in the 5′ and 3′ regulatory region of a certain gene. Although each can be analyzed separately, the informativeness (i.e. the number of alleles that can be discriminated at a certain locus) of the analyses can be increased by analyzing them in relation to each other. This can be accomplished by determining which of the alleles of each of the polymorphic sites are on the same chromosome; in other words, determine the phase (or linkage) of the alleles. The phase of a set of such alleles is called a haplotype. The linkage of polymorphisms can be disturbed by chromosomal recombination events. This is rarely observed for polymorphisms separated by relatively short distances and/or in linkage disequilibrium (see also Section III.B.3.c) but is seen more frequently for polymorphisms further apart.

The construction of haplotypes can be based on two polymorphisms at, for example, 100 bp distance or several polymorphisms at a distance of up to several Mbp. Haplotypes can be determined in essentially two ways: by genetic analysis and by molecular analysis. In genetic analysis, the cotransmission of such alleles is determined in some form of pedigree analysis such as in multigenerational pedigrees or in sib pairs. The pattern of combination of cotransmitted alleles observed in a given pedigree then indicates which alleles are in phase. The more accurate molecular analysis for haplotyping can be straightforward for polymorphisms at a relatively short distance of about 500 bp (e.g., by allele-specific sequencing). However, for longer distances of up to several kb, more sophisticated technology has to be applied, such as long-range PCR combined, e.g., with double or triple restriction enzyme digestion. An example of this, direct molecular haplotyping at the VDR locus, will be discussed in the next section. For still longer distances of up to several Mbp, no molecular methods are available and one has to rely on genetic analyses. Because collecting family samples requires large efforts in terms of time, money, and manpower, the genetic analyses are laborious and cumbersome. In contrast, molecular analyses do not require additonal samples and can be done directly in DNA from only the individual of interest.

b.2 Direct Molecular Haplotyping at the VDR Locus: For association analysis using the VDR locus, initially three adjacent RFLPs were described within intron 8 (an anonymous BsmI and ApaI RFLP) and exon 9 (a TaqI RFLP leading to a silent amino acid codon change, see Fig. 2). Two alleles at each RFLP can be discerned: one with and one without the recognition site of the restriction enzyme, indicated by lower and upper case letters, respectively (such as B and b for the BsmI RFLP). Because these RFLPs are anonymous and are not the true susceptibility sequence changes, they merely serve as markers for a functional sequence change(s) elsewhere in the VDR gene or in a nearby gene. By simply analyzing coincidence of alleles at each of the RFLP loci in the same individuals, it was discovered that the BsmI and TaqI RFLPs were in strong linkage disequilibrium; i.e., the "B" allele almost always occurred together with the "t" allele of the TaqI RFLP and vice versa [15]. However, the ApaI RFLP in between them showed no linkage with these RFLPs, indicating that Bsm (or Taq) is not a good marker for alleles detected by the ApaI RFLP. This suggested that more alleles in this region of the VDR locus exist which could be detected if the ApaI RFLP could be analyzed in relation to the BsmI and TaqI RFLP. Determining the phase of linkage between the three RFLPs (haplotyping) could detect this and thereby considerably increase the informativeness. Figure 2 shows that it is possible to produce such "direct molecular haplotypes" by generating a large PCR product spanning the three RFLP sites and subsequently digesting this PCR product with all three restriction enzymes [42]. Application of this genotyping protocol in a large population-based study revealed the existence of five different haplotype alleles combining to form 12 different genotypes. In particular, the existence of haplotype alleles baT (48%), bAT (11%), and bAt (1%) indicates that the same BsmI allele (b) is, in fact, a group of alleles. Thus, when using for example only the Bsm I RFLP, unjustified grouping will obscure possible linkage of one of these haplotype alleles with a true susceptibility allele. Indeed, when the single RFLPs and the direct molecular haplotyping protocol were applied in a large population-based association analysis of the VDR locus with BMD, an association with BMD was demonstrated only when the haplotype

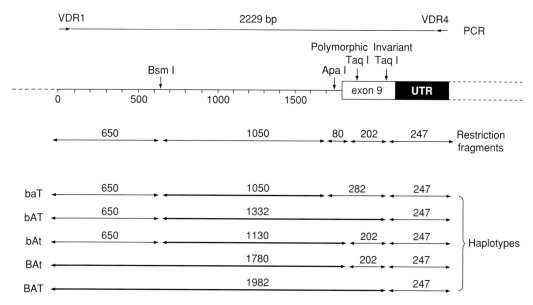

FIGURE 2 Direct molecular haplotyping of three adjacent RFLPs at the VDR gene locus. A 2229 bp long PCR product is generated spanning three RFLP sites at the 3′ end of the VDR gene. Subsequent simultaneous digestion with the three restriction enzymes results in the generation of particular restriction fragments, indicated in bold. These are indicative of the combined presence or absence of the three recognition sites on a single chromosome and thereby establish phase or a molecular haplotype of the three polymorphic sites. In a Dutch population of more than 2000 subjects, five different haplotypes could be distinguished. Lower case letters indicate presence of the recognition site, upper case letters indicate absence. UTR, untranslated region.

alleles were analyzed and not when any of the single RFLPs were tested [42].

b.3 Variable Number of Tandem Repeats: Variable Number of Tandem Repeat (VNTR) polymorphisms are ususally analyzed simply by generating a PCR fragment including the VNTR sequence and separating the resulting allelic fragments, which differ by size, by gel electrophoresis. For long VNTRs (>500 bp and repeat units of >30 bp) this is done in agarose gels, whereas for shorter fragments (such as the GT repeats) this is done in polyacrylamide gels using radioactivity to detect the allelic fragments. To ease the operation and increase the throughput of genotyping, especially for the GT-microsatellites, the detection step and electrophoresis step have been semiautomated by introducing fluorescent labels and detection by laser technology and, by separating fragments by capillary electrophoresis. VNTRs can display substantial polymorphism on the basis of difference in the number of tandem repeat units with up to several hundred alleles. This informativity can be even further increased by detecting sequence heterogeneity among the repeat units. An example of this is heteroduplex analysis of the VNTR 1 kb 3′ of the collagen type IIα1 (COL2A1) gene.

b.4 VNTR heteroduplexing at the COL2A1 locus: Heteroduplex analysis is based on the different electrophoretic mobility of heteroduplex molecules vs homoduplex molecules. Heteroduplex molecules are formed in solution by first denaturing the double stranded PCR fragment and subsequently allowing the strands to basepair again by renaturation. In case a small sequence difference between otherwise identical alleles is present (for example a 3-bp deletion), after renaturation, the homoduplex alleles are formed again but heteroduplex molecules are also formed consisting of the plus-strand of one allele basepaired to the minus strand of the other allele and vice versa. Due to the presence of the sequence difference in the two strands constituting such heteroduplex molecules, a small area is present where there is no perfect basepairing and which, as a result, has a different spatial structure. This leads to anomalous electrophoretic behavior, although the length of both the homoduplex and the heteroduplex molecules is the same. Heteroduplexing is therefore suitable to distinguish alleles of identical size but with small sequence changes.

Because the COL2A1 gene product is abundantly present in cartilage, an important target tissue in osteoarthritis, sequence variation in this gene has been analyzed in relation to radiographic osteoarthritis [43]. The COL2A1 gene is a very complex gene of more than 30 kb containing 54 exons, making routine sequence comparison of the gene a difficult task. Therefore, association analyses have been performed with polymorphic markers instead, in particular using a polymorphic AT-rich minisatellite VNTR 1 kb 3′ of the gene. Using different populations and different genotyping systems to analyze the VNTR, association studies have not been able to show a consistent relationship of VNTR alleles with osteoarthritis. Most genotyping systems of this VNTR are based on separating the VNTR alleles simply by size [44, 45].

By using a newly developed heteroduplexing assay to genotype this VNTR, Wilkin *et al.* [46] and Uitterlinden, *et al.* [47] have revealed substantial sequence heterogeneity within the VNTR. In a population of 963 individuals, a total of 29 different COL2A1 VNTR heteroduplex alleles could be discriminated, of which several, in particular alleles 4A (with a population frequency of 25%) and 4B (15%), could not be discriminated by other systems [47]. Uitterlinden *et al.* [47] were able to demonstrate an association of specifically these two alleles with joint space narrowing at the knee, a characteristic of osteoarthritis thought to be due to degeneration of joint cartilage. When the analyses was repeated at lower genetic resolution (e.g., by combining the 29 heteroduplex alleles into six homoduplex alleles based on size), no associations could be observed [Uitterlinden *et al.*, unpublished data]. This again highlights the importance of the genotyping system for distinguishing allelic variants and of the need for optimal genetic informativeness in association analyses.

c. Multiple Adjacent Polymorphisms—Linkage Disequilibrium The use of functional polymorphisms as genetic markers makes the interpretation of association analyses rather straightforward. However, the functionality of polymorphisms can usually only be established through laborious molecular biological and cell biological experiments. Therefore, the application of "nonfunctional" polymorphisms makes the testing of a particular locus in association analyses much more feasible because these are very abundant in the human genome and they do not require scrutiny to establish functionality. When an anonymous polymorphism is used, an asociation between the characteristic of interest and one of the marker alleles presumes that one of the marker alleles is in linkage (is on the same chromosome) more often than expected, with a truly causative susceptibility allele of a polymorphism elsewhere in the gene. This means the marker polymorphism and the susceptibility locus are in linkage disequilibrium (LD).

The distance over which linkage disequilibrium extends can vary and depends on the population structure and the markers used [48, 49]. For normal noninbred populations, the LD usually is up to a few hundred kilobasepairs. Because such an area can harbor tens of genes, associations found with anonymous polymorphisms should therefore be interpreted cautiously. This is especially important in view of the fact that functionally related genes tend to be located in close proximity of each other and often also show coordinated expression patterns. Well known examples include the 80 Major Histocompatibility Complex genes within 4 Mbp on chromosome 6p21.3, the immunoglobulin heavy chain gene cluster on chromosome 14q32.3 and the immunoglobulin light chain gene clusters on chromosomes 2p12 and 22q11, the α-globin gene cluster on chromosome 16p13.3, and the four HOX genes clusters on chromosomes 2p, 7, 12, and 17.

In the case of the VDR gene, association studies with the currently available polymorphisms can not exclude a nearby gene as the true susceptibility gene, or that the association might involve concerted effects of one or more adjacent genes. A good candidate in this respect might be the 25-hydroxyvitamin D 1-α-hydroxylase gene, which has been shown to be responsible for the pseudovitamin D deficiency rickets (PDDR) disease phenotype [50] and which is mapped on chromosome 12q13.3, in close proximity of the VDR gene locus [50, 51]. Mapping studies to determine the exact location of the PDDR gene and its distance from the VDR gene locus and polymorphism studies of this disease locus are necessary to clarify this issue.

Functional polymorphisms also can be in linkage disequilibrium with other functional polymorphisms, whereby either one or more sequence changes in the same gene or in nearby genes can contribute to the phenotype of interest. An example of this is the protective effect of the V64I allele of the CCR2 chemokine receptor gene on HIV-1 disease progression and complete linkage disequilibrium between this allele and the CCR5-Δ32 allele, a point mutation in the regulatory region of the CCR5 gene, located nearby on chromosome 3 [52].

c.1 Short Range Linkage Disequilibrium: An example of a candidate gene in osteoporosis in which linkage disequilibrium plays a role is the presence of three adjacent polymorphisms in the VDR gene over a distance of 2 kb. Each of these has been used in the several dozens of association analyses of VDR polymorphisms with bone density, but usually the RFLPs have not been analyzed in relation to each other. A direct molecular haplotyping method to genotype the three loci simultaneously revealed five different haplotypes underlying the distribution of alleles at these loci (see Fig. 2). Several additional polymorphisms at the VDR locus also have been identified, none of which has a clear functional effect on VDR expression characteristics. These include a FokI RFLP at the translation initiation site, a multiallelic polyA stretch in the 3' untranslated region (UTR), and several SNPs in the 3' UTR. LD between these polymorphisms has been shown to differ between the different polymorphic sites and also among different populations [53]. Therefore, the interpretation of association results using these different polymorphisms is complicated, especially in the absence of knowledge on any functional sequence change in linkage with any of the polymorphisms.

c.2 Long Range Linkage Disequilibrium: Another example of the importance of linkage disequilibrium is illustrated by the association between the VDR locus and osteoarthritis [54, 55]. Because the collagen type IIα1 gene, an important candidate gene in osteoarthritis, is located close to the VDR gene (see Fig. 3), the results found with the

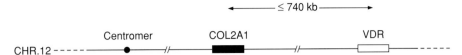

FIGURE 3   Adjacent location of the VDR and the COL2A1 gene loci near the centromeric area on the long arm of chromosome 12 at 12q12–13.

VDR locus could be explained by linkage disequilibrium of a VDR allele with a true susceptibility allele at the COL2A1 locus. However, unlike the situation for the three RFLPs at the VDR locus, the molecular phase of alleles at loci which are so far apart can not be determined directly. This can only be done by analysing cotransmission of alleles in pedigrees or by likelihood methods estimating the haplotype frequencies at the population level [56]. Although evidence has been obtained by the latter method for the existence of linkage disequilibrium between alleles at the VDR and COL2A1 loci [Uitterlinden *et al.*, unpublished data] this could not explain the association between the VDR locus and osteoarthritis. The LD was weak and no LD could be identified between the VDR and COL2A1 risk alleles. Furthermore, associations were found of the VDR risk alleles and the COL2A1 risk alleles, each with a different characteristic of osteoarthritis [54; Uitterlinden *et al.*, unpublished data]: VDR with osteophytes and COL2A1 with joint space narrowing.

c.3 Linkage Disequilibrium in Genome Searches: In genome searches, LD between alleles of anonymous markers and true susceptibility alleles in genes is exploited to identify candidate gene regions. Using sib-pair designs and a minimum number of markers to cover the genome (usually 200–400), areas of 5–20 million basepairs are identified in which the candidate gene containing a susceptibility polymorphism is situated. In normal populations LD extends over relatively short distances (typically less than 1 Mbp), but in isolated populations (such as the Fins, or island inhabitants, etc.) LD can extend over much larger distances (10–20 Mbp), thereby reducing the number of markers needed to identify such candidate gene areas [49]. Although such populations are useful in genome searches, a potential drawback of this approach is the fact that the genetic makeup of such populations can be peculiar due to their isolated nature (founder effect), and this can lead to the identification of only a subset of the total number of candidate genes for a complex trait.

Many genome searches for complex traits, such as those using sib pairs, rely on the identification of areas that are identical-by-descent (IBD) because they were inherited from the same ancestor or a limited number of ancestors. The average size of IBD segments (or the extent of LD) is determined by the number of ancestors and the number of generations that separates given individuals from such a common ancestor. If this is a recent ancestor, the number of markers needed to scan the genome is limited to a few hundred, whereas detection of more distant ancestral IBD segments requires thousands of markers. Extensive LD due to a founder effect can also be exploited to limit the number of affected individuals necessary for a genome search. This has been demonstrated for the monogenic disorder benign recurrent intrahepatic cholestasis, in which case only three patients were sufficient to localize the disease gene [57]. Similarly, it might be used to map composite genetic factors of more complex traits in isolated inbred populations.

Genotyping technology has developed rapidly but it still relies on sequentially typing single locus markers one at a time and subsequent massive genome comparison to identify the IBD regions among the many regions that are not. Alternative methods (such as the genome mismatch scanning method or GMS) have therefore been developed to identify only those regions that are IBD. GMS is based on the selective amplification, out of total genomic DNA, of perfect homoduplexes such as can be expected in chromosomal areas that are IBD. In combination with DNA chip technology, this method even allows genome searches to be performed without the necessity of genotyping microsatellites by gel electrophoresis [58], thereby substantially reducing the effort and costs. Although promising, this approach still requires rigourous testing to establish its robustness and ease of use to make it a reasonable alternative for microsatellite genotyping.

C. Genetic Epidemiological Considerations

1. STUDY DESIGNS

An important prerequisite for measuring genetic effects in association studies is the size of the sample used in the study. Although power calculations can be made, they heavily rely on what is expected, e.g., with respect to the size of effects. Intuitively it is clear that small sample sizes can only measure large effects and small effects can only be measured in large samples. Genome searches in a few hundred sib pairs will identify only those chromosomal areas that contain genes that have relatively large effects (explaining, e.g., approximately 1–2 standard deviation [SD] in variation of the BMD). Consequently, negative results from association studies on candidate genes in a sample of, say, a few hundred subjects can not exclude the genes under study as having relatively small effects. Nevertheless, such genes can be of considerable importance, e.g., in contributing to epistatic effects (see Section III.C.2.b).

The study design for candidate gene analyses differs from that for genome searches. The evaluation of candidate gene polymorphisms is most frequently done in case-control or population-based studies. In association studies, usually a case-control design is used to evaluate risk factors for discrete outcome variables such as osteoporotic fracture. Allele frequencies of susceptibility gene variants are then compared as a measure of association. Over- or underrepresentation of a particular susceptibility allele and Hardy-Weinberg disequilibrium in the cases compared to controls then indicates association with the trait of interest. When continuous variables such as BMD are analyzed in this way, much information is lost when arbitrary cutoff values to define low and/or high BMD are rigorously applied. Therefore, such variables are usually analyzed in population-based studies to determine if, for example, the mean BMD values display genotype-dependent differences.

In genome searches, the most common and robust approach is the sib-pair design. In this method, the difference in trait values (e.g., BMD) for a pair of sibs is squared and examined as a function of the number of alleles that the pair have derived from a common parent IBD at a certain marker locus. A negative regression of the squared difference on the number of shared alleles indicates linkage between the marker and the quantitative trait locus (QTL). Although usually sibs are selected at random, choosing sib pairs that are concordant for either high or low trait values or are extremely discordant can substantially increase the power of QTL mapping studies [59].

A special case of sib-pair analysis of complex traits is presented by twin studies [60]. In this respect, dizygotic (DZ) twins can be regarded as same-age sibs, a feature that can be a considerable advantage in genetic studies in view of the fact that most traits show age-related variation in expression. Furthermore, paternity is usually less of a dispute than in normal sib-pair studies and, not unimportantly, most twins tend to be cooperative research subjects. Initially, twin studies were used to estimate the "heritability" of a particular trait. This is done by comparing the similarity of a particular phenotypic characteristic in the members of monozygous versus dizygous twin pairs. Because monozygous twins (MZ) share 100% of their genetic constitution, whereas dizygous share only 50%, traits with a high heritability are expected to be more similar between members of monozygous twin pairs than between members of dizygous twins. This approach can be applied to provide heritability estimates of traits as such, but it can also be used in association studies of candidate gene variants. This has the advantage that ethnically matched controls are automatically analyzed, but also that estimates are obtained of genetic variance as well as how much of the variance is not accounted for by the polymorphism. Although the twin model has gained increasing popularity in studying the relative contribution of genetic and environmental factors to traits, it is not without problems. The major one is

that the excess similarity of MZ twins can be due not only to genetic identity, but also to more similar postnatal environments compared to DZ twins.

2. INTERACTIONS

Despite the presence of a genetic variant, phenotypic expression of such a variation might not always be observed. Such "reduced penetrance" usually involves interaction of the protein product with other factors that are endogenous (i.e., other proteins), exogenous (i.e., other biomolecules such as necessary cofactors), or a combination of both. Several different epidemiological models can be constructed to investigate interactions between genetic susceptibility and other risk factors [61] but here we will focus on two examples: gene-environment interaction and epistatic phenomena.

a. Gene-Environment Studies The action of particular proteins depends heavily on the bioavailability of particular ligands that are necessary to induce their action in a target cell. An example in the field of bone research is the vitamin D endocrine system in which the ligand—1,25α-dihydroxyvitamin D$_3$—is necessary for the vitamin D receptor to exert its effect as a transcription factor and start the cascade of cellular events by switching on other genes. In relation to the reported association of VDR polymorphisms with BMD, only a small number of studies have analyzed the influence of vitamin D as a possible modulating factor of this association. In a short-term intervention study, serum calcium and osteocalcin response to vitamin D treatment appeared to be VDR-genotype dependent [62]. In addition, in more long-term intervention studies, a VDR genotype-dependent effect on BMD in response to vitamin D treatment also has been observed [63, 64]. In relation to other disease phenotypes related to pleiotropic effects of VDR polymorphisms, the influence of vitamin D can be of relevance. For example, in the Framingham study it was demonstrated that serum vitamin D levels modulate the risk for knee osteoarthritis [65]. In view of the association found between VDR polymorphisms and risk for knee osteoarthritis, this observation suggests that the VDR-vitamin D gene-environment interaction might contribute to risk modification for knee osteoarthritis.

In a study by Krall *et al.* [66], the association between VDR genotype and bone loss was most evident in individuals with the BB VDR genotype and low calcium intake (i.e., less than 650 mg/day). Other studies in subjects with relatively high calcium intake of more than 800 mg/day, such as the Ofely study and the Rotterdam study, did not observe strong associations between VDR polymorphisms and BMD. Also, in subjects from the Framingham study, calcium intake modulated VDR genotype-dependent differences in BMD such that subjects with the bb genotype and with a calcium intake >800 mg/day had 7–12% higher BMD [67]. The influence of dietary calcium intake on VDR genotype-related differences is most likely mediated through the vitamin D endocrine system as a major regulator of intestinal calcium absorption. Indeed, several small studies have presented evidence to suggest such an effect [68–70]. Taken together, these results suggest that the relationship between VDR genotype and bone density, but also other pleiotropic effects, might be modulated by dietary calcium intake, possibly through influencing intestinal calcium absorption.

b. Epistasis In a cell, gene products do not act by themselves but are always acting in a rich environment of other gene products. Consequently, genetic variants of a protein will interact with other protein variants, resulting in a kaleidoscope of possible interactions reflecting the underlying genetic diversity. This can involve more general protein interactions such as the basic transcription and translation machinery but can also be very specific for a particular metabolic pathway. In bone metabolism, for example, the production of bone-specific matrix proteins is under the control of bone-specific transcription factors, such as the VDR-regulated expression of osteocalcin. Therefore, such interactions imply that polymorphisms of one gene can influence the effect of gene variants of the other interacting gene. Interaction between genes can simply be additive or subtractive but also can be hierarchical in that the effect of one gene can be dominant over the other. This can be the case, for example, for upstream genes over downstream genes in a metabolic pathway. Thus, epistasis (interaction deviation, synergism) occurs when the combined effect of two or more genes on a phenotype can not be predicted as the sum of their separate effects. An example of an epistatic phenomenon in osteoporosis would be two gene variants, A and B, each of which is associated with, for example, 0.05 g/cm^2 reduced BMD, while their combined presence leads to a BMD which is reduced by 0.2 g/cm^2.

With the expected progress in the construction of an osteoporosis gene map in the coming years, epistatic phenomena are expected to be of considerable importance in explaining some of the genetic variance. The study of epistasis in human populations requires considerable sample sizes, especially when the expected effects are modest, and is therefore currently possible only for genes with major effects on a phenotype of interest. This situation can be somewhat improved by analysis of populations with reduced genetic diversity, such as the so-called isolated populations now frequently exploited in linkage disequilibrium mapping (see Section III.B.3.c). Animal studies, however, currently provide better possibilities for unraveling epistatic phenomena. An example is the description of epistasis in mapping experiments of colon and lung tumor susceptibility genes in Recombinant Congenic (RC) inbred mice [71, 72]. These studies revealed a number of interacting loci with epistatic effects on cancer susceptibility. Such congenic strains are made by inbreeding of second generation backcrosses from parental strains with different phenotypes. As a result RC strains share 87.5% of the genetic background of one parent while 12.5% is derived from the other parent and spread through the genome as unlinked segments. Thus, the genetic complexity of "the study population" is reduced, greatly facilitating the identification of chromosomal areas contributing to the phenotype of interest and allowing the study of their interaction.

D. Biological Considerations

1. FUNCTIONAL RELEVANCE OF POLYMORPHISMS

The interpretation of association analyses is critically dependent on the type of sequence variation used as a genetic marker. Anonymous polymorphisms are used as genetic markers to indicate whether a certain chromosomal area is associated with the characteristic of interest. In other words, the position of a putative candidate gene is indicated. However, in such cases, IBS is established rather than IBD and therefore the association results can be influenced by factors such as the population structure, LD, allelic heterogeneity, and locus heterogeneity. This is the case for the associations of VDR genotype and BMD using, e.g., the anonymous RFLP polymorphisms at the 3' end of the gene. The situation is considerably improved, however, when a polymorphism has been shown to have functional consequences such as allele-specific expression levels or conformations. In this case, a particular allele is expected to show similar associations in different populations. An example of a functional sequence variation in a candidate gene in relation to osteoporosis is the G to T substitution in an Sp1 binding site in the first intron of the collagen type Iα1 gene.

a. Vitamin D Receptor Polymorphisms The vitamin D receptor gene as part of the vitamin D endocrine system was recognized early on as an important candidate gene for osteoporosis given its role as a major transcription factor in bone metabolism. The pioneering work of Morrison and Eisman on VDR polymorphisms in relation to serum osteocalcin levels and BMD used three anonymous RFLPs as genetic markers in twin studies and in a cohort of 311 postmenopausal women. Initially, in a study of female twins, associations of the BsmI RFLP were reported with the serum concentration of the noncollageneous bone matrix protein osteocalcin, a marker of bone formation [73]. Subsequently, several studies analyzed the association of VDR polymorphisms with BMD but reported varying results. A meta-analysis from data of 16 of these studies concluded that there was a weak association with a small overall effect, with VDR genotype accounting for about 2% of the variation in bone density [74].

However, the use of anonymous RFLPs precluded a functional explanation of the underlying mechanism of the association. In the initial study of Morrison *et al.* [15], it was suggested that sequence variation in the 3' untranslated region of the VDR gene could be related to differences in expression of the gene. Some studies have suggested differential expression of VDR alleles whereby the "BAt" allele was expressed at a 30% lower level than the "baT" allele [75]. Another VDR polymorphism was described that created a second ATG translation initiation site in the coding region preceeding the original one by three amino acids. A functional significance of this polymorphism was suggested in view of its association with differential transactivation of a vitamin D response element [76]. However, another study indicated no genotype-related differences in VDR gene expression [77]. This leaves the use of anonymous RFLPs in the study of VDR polymorphisms and disease still complicating the interpretation of the association results. However, together with the gene-environment studies discussed in Section III.C.2.a, there is a convincing body of evidence to suggest allelic variation of some kind at this locus, either in the VDR gene and/or in a nearby gene involved in vitamin D metabolism, underlies the genotype-related differences observed in the association studies.

b. The Collagen Type Iα1 Sp1 Polymorphism   The group of Ralston (Aberdeen, UK) detected a common guanine (G) to thymidine (T) polymorphism at the first base of a binding site for the transcription factor Sp1 in the first intron of the COLIA1 gene (see Fig. 4). They found the T allele (with a population frequency of about 18%) to be associated with low bone density and increased prevalence of osteoporotic

vertebral fracture [78]. Importantly, these observations have been extended in a large population-based cohort study of 1778 postmenopausal women in the Netherlands [79]. In this study, the same T allele was associated with low bone density at the spine and hip. The differences increased with age to become 10–20% between extreme genotypes in the oldest age group of women of 75–80 years, suggesting the COLIA1 polymorphism to be a marker for accelerated bone loss in older women. In addition, women with the GT and TT genotype were found to have a 1.4–2.8-fold increased risk for osteoporotic nonvertebral fracture which was found to be largely independent of BMD.

The exact mechanisms by which the different COLIA1 alleles relate to bone density and fracture risk is not known but they might relate to differences in bone quality as well as quantity. Preliminary studies have shown that oligonucleotides corresponding to the T allele bind the Sp1 protein with greater affinity than those corresponding to the G allele, and subjects who are heterozygous for the polymorphism have a three-fold greater abundance of transcripts derived from the T allele than the G allele (Hobson, Grant, and Ralston, unpublished data). This indicates that the T allele may be associated with a disturbance in the relative abundance of COLIA1 and COLIA2 mRNAs, which would translate to a similar disturbance for the proteins. Normally, the proteins are expressed in a ratio of 2:1 for the COLIA1: COLIA2, the same ratio as in the final collagen type Iα1 protein which consists of three helices. This disturbance of the ratio would be analogous to the situation in osteogenesis

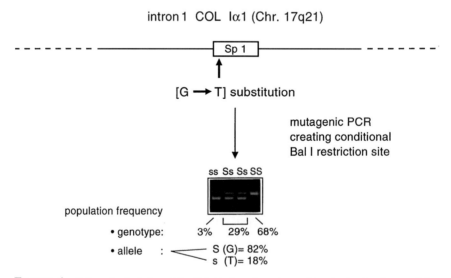

FIGURE 4   Schematic depiction of the Sp1 binding site polymorphism in the first intron of the collagen type Iα1 gene, its detection by mutagenic PCR, and distribution of alleles and genotypes in a Dutch population (n = 1778). The PCR test is based on using a primer that is partially mismatched immediately adjacent to the site of the mutation. During PCR the primer will introduce a BalI recognition site only in alleles carrying the T-substitution in the Sp1 site. Little "s" indicates presence of the BalI recognition site in the Sp1 site and, thus, presence of the T-substitution; big "S" indicates absence of the BalI site and thus presence of the wild type G nucleotide at that position.

imperfecta for the so-called null mutations (in which one of the alleles is not expressed or is very poorly expressed [80]).

2. PLEIOTROPIC EFFECTS OF GENE VARIANTS

Another important issue to address in relation to the biological implications of genetic association studies are the so-called pleiotropic effects of gene variants. Pleiotropy (or polypheny) means that a particular gene (or variants thereof) plays a role in more than one biological process and therefore can have more effects than just the one being analyzed when testing a certain hypothesis. When such biological processes are to a large extent independent, pleiotropy will not substantially influence the outcome and interpretation of association studies. However, when processses are, in one way or the other, related to each other, pleiotropy is crucial to explaining the underlying mechanisms of associations observed with a certain gene variant. Alternatively, certain relations of disease phenotypes can be exploited to suggest that pleiotropic effects of a certain gene may play a role and thereby provide clues to the identification of candidate genes. An example of this includes the relationship of menopause with BMD and the effects of the estrogen endocrine system on menopause, but also on bone density and cardiovascular disease. From this it can be expected that genes and variants thereof involved in explaining the (demonstrated) genetic contribution to age of first and last menstruation might also have an effect on BMD and cardiovascular disease.

Although in fact almost all gene products can be expected to display pleiotropic effects to some extent, certain genes will be more evident candidates than others. An example of these are transcription factors, such as the family of steroid hormone receptors, that are involved in regulating the expression of a number of downstream genes in a given metabolic pathway. A well-established example of a gene displaying pleiotropic effects in the field of metabolic bone disease is the vitamin D receptor gene and its association with BMD as well as with several other diseases. Initally, the VDR gene was analyzed in relation to BMD, but soon other disease phenotypes that were related to osteoporosis were analyzed in relation to VDR gene variants. The example of VDR and osteoarthritis also illustrates several of the analytical considerations discussed previously.

a. The Vitamin D Endocrine System and Osteoarthritis
Osteoporosis and osteoarthritis are common age-related diseases involving the skeleton and the joints, respectively. Low bone density is an essential feature of osteoporosis whereas several epidemiological studies have shown bone density to be increased in subjects with osteoarthritis. Radiographic osteoarthritis (ROA) is commonly defined using the Kellgren score. This score is a composite score largely based on the assessment of two different characteristics: osteophytes and narrowing of the joint space. Osteophytes are osseous and cartiliginous neoplastic protrusions forming mostly at the margin of osteoarthritic joints, while joint space narrowing is thought to be due to degeneration of cartilage. These relationships and characteristics suggest the VDR gene as a candidate gene for osteoarthritis; the suggestion becomes even more pertinent when it's chromosomal location is taken into consideration. The VDR gene is located close to the collagen type IIA1 (COL2A1) gene that encodes the most abundant protein in cartilage and is also a major candidate gene in osteoarthritis. Although some studies have implicated the COL2A1 gene in the etiology of osteoarthritis, controversy still exists because other studies could not. Nevertheless, because of possible linkage disequilibrium between both loci (see section III.A), associations found with one gene (the "marker" gene) could be explained by linkage of the marker allele with sequence variation in the other gene. Therefore, both genes have to be analyzed in relation to (separate features of) osteoarthritis.

In a group of 846 men and women from the Rotterdam study, Uitterlinden *et al.* [54] have indeed identified the "baT" VDR haplotype allele to be associated with a 2.3-fold increased risk for osteoarthritis as diagnosed using the Kellgren score. Importantly, this relationship was independent of bone density thereby making this parameter less likely to mediate the relationship. Similarly, in a different study, the "T" VDR allele (as in the "baT" allele) was also found to be associated with an increased risk for osteoarthritis by the group of Spector [54]. However, because anonymous RFLPs in the VDR gene were analyzed, these observations still could not exclude the COL2A1 gene from being involved as the true susceptibility locus in the association with osteoarthritis.

In an effort to further explore and disentangle these relationships, we analyzed the composite features of ROA (osteophytes and joint space narrowing at the knee) in relation to VDR genotype and to COL2A1 genotype, separately and independently of the presence of ROA as diagnosed by the Kellgren score. Surprisingly, the same VDR allele was associated with the presence of osteophytes (as assessed independently of the presence of ROA) whereas no association of VDR alleles could be observed for the joint space narrowing. Subsequently, when individual features of ROA were analyzed in the same individuals by COL2A1 genotype as determined by the heteroduplexing genotyping method (see Section III.B.3.b.4), a COL2A1 VNTR allele was found to be associated with a two-fold increased risk for joint space narrowing but not for osteophytes [Uitterlinden *et al.*, unpublished data]. Neither did we find an association of COL2A1 genotype with osteoarthritis as assessed using the Kellgren score. This latter observation indicates that the COL2A1 gene locus does not seem to have a strong effect on the overall Kellgren score but might play a role in the process of cartilage degeneration. Importantly, these results imply that the results found with the VDR allele can not be explained by linkage disequilibrium of alleles at this locus with the COL2A1 gene locus, but rather suggest that the VDR gene itself is involved in the etiology of osteoarthritis. This notion is further supported by observations of serum vitamin D levels in relation to osteoarthritis in subjects from the Framingham study [65]. In this longitudinal study, low serum vitamin D levels were found to be associated with increased risk of osteoarthritis and with increased risk of progression of osteoarthritis. This suggests the possible existence of gene-environment interactions influencing the genetic association of VDR gene variants with osteoarthritis.

b. Vitamin D Receptor Polymorphisms in Other Diseases
The vitamin D endocrine system is also a known regulator of, for example, parathyroid hormone synthesis and secretion. Primary hyperparathyroidism (HPT) involves reduced calcium-mediated suppression of the secretion of parathyroid hormone. In some, but not all, association analyses VDR polymorphisms were found to be associated with primary HPT [81]. Vitamin D is also known to have immunomodulatory properties by influencing, e.g., T-cell growth and is also known to influence pancreatic insulin secretion. Allelic variation in the VDR was found to influence susceptibility to insulin-dependent diabetes mellitus [82]. Another example involves prostate cancer risk, which is increased at low sunlight exposure and low 1,25-D serum levels and which was shown to be associated with VDR polymorphisms [83].

In view of the cell growth and differentiation regulatory characteristics of the vitamin D endocrine system in a wide variety of cell types, it is tempting to hypothesize that at least a part of the risk for all of the disease phenotypes discussed above is caused by a loss of control by the vitamin D endocrine system with age. This notion is further supported by the increase in frequency of all of the disease phenotypes with age, and the fact that in the elderly, low vitamin D levels have been previously observed to be common [84].

IV. PERSPECTIVES

A. The "Osteoporosis Gene Map"

Studies on the genetic basis of osteoporosis are important in identifying new genes that act as regulators of bone density, bone quality, and fractures. Genome searches have been initiated that will result in identification of chromosmal areas containing candidate genes and also provide a first order hierarchy of genes with large effects and genes with smaller effects. Overlap of this candidate chromosomal area map with the (still growing) map of existing osteoporosis candidate genes will ultimately identify the really important genes. Furthermore, the identification of pleiotropic effects of candidate genes in other disease phenotypes, such as obesity, menopause, osteoarthritis, etc., might also lead to identification of osteoporosis risk genes.

With the current state of the Human Genome Project, with relatively few genes characterized and the catalogue of hu-

man sequence variation still in its infancy, functional polymorphisms in candidate genes are still scarce. This makes them only suitable for use in candidate gene association studies. However, when more of the human genetic variation is catalogued, it will be possible to perform genome wide analyses of sequence variants in, e.g., all osteoporosis genes and measure their contribution to the osteoporotic phenotype in different populations. This will open the way to accurately quantifying interactions between the genome and environments rather than to analyzing one particular gene-environment interaction. In view of the expected enormous increase in gene variants, the analysis of these gene variants and their interaction with each other and with the environment will also require subtantial developments in the methodology of DNA analysis. One such molecular genetic development, the DNA chip technology, is expected to be of considerable importance in streamlining the analysis of the plethora of DNA sequence variation.

B. Diagnostic Developments

Genetic markers for osteoporosis can be useful clinically in identifying individuals at risk of osteoporosis and in targeting preventive treatment. For example, the association between COLIA1 genotypes and osteoporotic fracture in postmenopausal women, coupled with the divergence of bone density values with increasing age in different genotype groups, raises the possibility that genotyping at the polymorphic COLIA1 Sp1 site may give information on susceptibility to osteoporotic fracture that could complement that which can be gained by bone density measurements alone.

Although very promising in terms of their early predictive power, the specificity and sensitivity of genetic markers must also be considered in relation to existing risk factors, such as BMD and age. The absence of knowledge on the mechanisms whereby several genetic variants of certain genes exert their effect effectively limits their use in clinical practice. In addition, the psychological burden of knowing one is a carrier and the cost-effectiveness of screening programs need serious consideration. However, genetic approaches are very useful ways to obtain insights into the pathophysiological mechanisms of osteoporosis and, in general, into diseases of bone metabolism. Finally, they will be very helpful in the design of new therapeutic intervention strategies for osteoporosis by selection of drugs based on understanding the molecular mode of action.

References

1. Botstein, D, White, D. L., Skolnick, M., and Davis, R. W. (1980). Construction of a genetic linkage map in man using restriction fragment length polymorphisms. *Am. J. Hum. Genet.* **32**, 314–331.
2. Lander, E. S., and Schork, N. J. (1994). Genetic dissection of complex traits. *Science* **265**, 2037–2048.

3. Smith, D. M., Nance, W. E., Kang, K. W., Christian, J. C., and Johnston, C. C. (1973). Genetic factors in determining bone mass. *J. Clin. Invest.* **52**, 2800–2808.

4. Pocock, N. A., Eisman, J. A., Hopper, J. L., Yeates, M. G., Sambrook, P. N., and Ebert, S. (1987). Genetic determinants of bone mass in adults: A twin study. *J. Clin. Invest.* **80**, 706–710.

5. Evans, R. A., Marel, G. M., Lancaster, E. K., Kos, S., Evans, M., and Wond, S. Y. P. (1988). Bone mass is low in relatives of osteoporotic patients. *Ann. Intern. Med.* **109**, 870–873.

6. Seeman, E., Hopper, J. L., Bach, L. A., Cooper, M. E., Parkinson, E., McKay, J., and Jerums, G. (1989). Reduced bone mass in daughters of women with osteoporosis. *N. Engl. J. Med.* **320**, 554–558.

7. Krall, E. A., and Dawson-Hughes, B. (1993). Heritable and life-style determinants of bone mineral density. *J. Bone Miner. Res.* **8**, 1–9.

8. Jouanny, P., Guillemin, F., Kuntz, C., Jeandel, C., and Pourel, J. (1995). Environmental and genetic factors affecting bone mass. *Arthritis. Rheum.* **38**, 61–67.

9. Livshits, G., Pavlovsky, O., and Kobyliansky, E. (1996). Population biology of human aging: segregation analysis of bone age characteristics. *Hum. Biol.* **68**, 539–554.

10. Gueguen, R., Jouanny, P., Guillemni, F., Kuntz, C., Pourel, J., and Siest, G. (1995). Segregation analysis and variance components analysis of bone mineral density in healthy families. *J. Bone Miner. Res.* **10**, 2017–2022.

11. Kelly, P. J., Hopper, J. L., Macaskill, G. T., Pocock, N. A., Sambrook, P. N., and Eisman, J. A. (1991). Genetic factors in bone turnover. *J. Clin. Endocrinol. Metab.* **72**, 808–813.

12. Tokita, A., Kelly, P. J., Nguyen, T. V., Qi, J.-C., Morrison, N. A., Risteli, L., Risteli, J., Sambrook, P. N., and Eisman, J. A. (1994). Genetic influences on type I collagen synthesis and degradation: Further evidence for genetic regulation of bone turnover. *J. Clin. Endocrinol. Metab.* **78**, 1461–1466.

13. Garnero, P., Arden, N. K., Griffiths, G., Delmas, P. D., and Spector, T. D. (1996). Genetic influence on bone turnover in postmenopausal twins. *J. Clin. Endocrinol. Metab.* **81**, 140–146.

14. Kanis, J. A., Melton, L. J., Christiansen, C., Johnston, C. C., and Khaltaev, N. (1994). The diagnosis of osteoporosis. *J. Bone Miner. Res.* **9**, 1137–1141.

15. Morrison, N. A., Qi, J. C., Tokita, A., Kelly, P. J., Crofts, L., Nguyen, T. V., Sambrook, P. N., and Eisman, J. A. (1994). Prediction of bone density from vitamin D receptor alleles. *Nature* **367**, 284–287.

16. Kobayashi, S., Inoue, S., Hosoi, T., Ouchi, Y., Shiraki, M., and Orimo, H. (1996). Association of bone mineral density with polymorphism of the estrogen receptor gene. *J. Bone Miner. Res.* **11**, 306–311.

17. Han, K. O., Moon, I. G., Kang, Y. S., Chung, H. G., Min, H. K., and Han, I. K. (1997). Nonassociation of estrogen receptor genotypes with bone mineral density and estrogen responsiveness to hormonal replacement therapy in Korean postmenopausal women. *J. Clin. Endocrinol. Metab.* **82**, 991–995.

18. Murray, R. E., McGuigan, F., Grant, S. F. A., Reid, D. M., and Ralston, S. H. (1997). Polymorphisms of the interleukin-6 gene are associated with bone mineral density. *Bone* **21**, 89–92.

19. Langdahl, B. L., Knudsen, J. Y., Jensen, H. K., Gregersen, N., and Eriksen, E. F. (1997). A sequence variation:713-8delC in the transforming growth factor-beta 1 gene has higher prevalence in osteoporotic women than in normal women and is associated with very low bone mass in osteoporotic women and increased bone turnover in both osteoporotic and normal women. *Bone* **3**, 289–294.

20. Liang, P., and Pardee, A. B. (1992). Differential display of eukaryotic messenger RNA by means of the polymerase chain reaction. *Science* **257**, 967–971.

21. Lewis, D. B., Liggitt, H. D., Effmann, E. L., Motley, T., Teitelbaum, S. L., Jepsen, K. J., Goldstein, S. A., Bonadio, J., Carpenter, J., and Perlmutter, R. M. (1993). Osteoporosis induced in mice by overproduction of interleukin 4. *Proc. Natl. Acad. Sci. U.S.A.* **90**, 11618–11622.

22. Grigoriadis, A. E., Wang, Z. Q., Cecchini, M. G., Hofstetter, W., Felix, R., Fleisch, H., and Wagner, E. F. (1994). c-Fos: A key regulator of osteoclast-macrophage lineage determination and bone remodelling. *Science* **266**, 443–448.

23. Iotsova, V., Caamano, J., Loy, J., Lewin, A., and Bravo, R. (1997). Osteopetrosis in mice lacking NF-κB1 and NFκB2. *Nat. Med.* **3**, 1285–1289.

24. Smith, E. P., Boyd, J., Frank, G. R., Takahashi, H., Cohen, R. M., Specker, B., Williams, T. C., Lubahn, D. B., and Korach, K. S. (1994). Estrogen resistance caused by a mutation in the estrogen-receptor gene in a man. *N. Engl. J. Med.* **331**, 1056–1061.

25. Hughes, M. R., Malloy, P. J., Kieback, D. G., Kesterson, R. A., Pike, J. W., Feldman, D., and O'Malley, B. W. (1988). Point mutations in the human vitamin D receptor gene associated with hypocalcemic rickets. *Science* **242**, 1702–1705.

26. Malloy, P. J., Weisman, J., and Feldman, D. (1994). Hereditary 1α, 25-dihydroxyvitamin D-resistant rickets resulting from a mutation in the vitamin D receptor deoxyribonucleic acid-binding domain. *J. Clin. Endocrinol. Metab.* **78**, 313–316.

27. Morishima, A., Grumbach, M. M., Simpson, E. R., Fisher, C., and Qin, K. (1995). Aromatase deficiency in male and female siblings caused by a novel mutation and the physiological role of estrogens. *J. Clin. Endocrinol. Metab.* **80**, 3689–3698.

28. Gong, Y., Vikkula, M., Boon, L., Liu, J., Beighton, P., Ramesar, R., Peltonen, L., Somer, H., Hirose, T., Dallapiccola, B., de Paepe, A., Swoboda, W., Zabel, B., Superti-Furga, A., Steimann, B., Brunner, Han, G., Jans, A., Boles, R. G., Adkins, W., van den Boogaard, M.-J., Olsen, B. R., and Warman, M. L. (1996). Osteoporosis-pseudoglioma syndrome, a disorder affecting skeletal strength and vision, is assigned to chromosome region 11q12–13. *Am. J. Hum. Genet.* **59**, 146–151.

29. Johnson, M. L., Gong, G., Kimberling, W., Recker, S. M., Kimmel, D. B., and Recker, R. R.. (1997). Linkage of a gene causing high bone mass to human chromosome 11 (11q12–13). *Am. J. Hum. Genet.* **60**, 1326–1332.

30. Lander, E., and Kruglyak, L. (1995). Genetic dissection of complex traits: Guidelines for interpreting and reporting linkage results. *Nat. Genet.* **11**, 241–247.

31. Davies, J. L., Kawaguchi, Y., Bennett, S. T., Copeman, J. B., Cordell, H. J., Pritchard, L. E., Reed, P. W., Gough, S. C. L., Jenkins, S. C., Palmer, S. M., Balfour, K. M., Rowe, B., Farall, M., Barnett, A. H., Bain, S. C., and Todd, J. A. (1994). A genome-wide search for human type I diabetes susceptibility genes. *Nature* **371**, 130–136.

32. Hashimoto, L., Habita, C., Beressi, J., Delepine, M., Besse, C., Cambon-Thomsen, A., Deschamps, I., Rotter, J., Djoulah, S., James, M., Froguel, P., Weissenbach, J., Lathrop, G., and Julier, C. (1994). Genetic mapping of a susceptibility locus for insulin-dependent diabetes mellitus on chromosome 11q. *Nature* **371**, 161–164.

33. Cooper, D. N., and Krawczak, M. (1993). "Human Gene Mutation." BIOS Scientific Publishers, Oxford, UK.

34. Uitterlinden, A. G., and Vijg, J. (1994). "Two-Dimensional DNA Typing: A Parallel Approach to Genome Analysis." Ellis Horwood, Chichester, UK.

35. Collins, F. C., Guyer, M. S., and Chakravarti, A. (1997). Variations on a theme: Cataloging human DNA sequence variation. *Science* **278**, 1580–1581.

36. Marshall, E. (1997). 'Playing chicken' over gene markers. *Science* **278**, 2046–2048.

37. Uitterlinden, A. G. (1995). Gene- and genome-scanning by two-dimensional DNA typing. *Electrophoresis* **16**, 186–196.

38. Fodor, S. P. A., Read, J. L., Pirrung, M. C., Stryer, L., Lu, A. T., and Solas, D. (1991). Light-directed, spatially addressable parallel chemical synthesis. *Science* **251**, 767–773.

39. Kozal, M. J., Shah, N., Shen, N., Yang, R., Fucini, R., Merigan, T. C., Richman, D. D., Morris, D., Hubell, E., Chee, M., and Gingeras, T. R. (1996). Extensive polymorphisms observed in HIV-1 clade B protease gene using high-density oligonucleotide arrays. *Nat. Med.* **2**, 753–759.

40. Cronin, M. T., Fucini, R. V., Kim, S. M., Masino, R. S., Wespi, R. M., and Miyada, C. G. (1996). Cystic fibrosis mutation detection by hybridization to light-generated DNA probe arrays. *Hum. Mutat.* **7**, 244–255.

41. Hacia, J. G., Brody, L. C., Chee, M. S., Fodor, S. P. A., and Collins, F. S. (1996). Detection of heterozygous mutations in BRCA1 using high density oligonucleotide arrays and two-colour fluorescence analysis. *Nat. Genet.* **14**, 441–447.

42. Uitterlinden, A. G., Pols, H. A. P., Burger, H., Huang, Q., van Daele, P. L. A., van Duijn, C. M., Hofman, A., Birkenhäger, J. C., and van Leeuwen, J. P. T. M. (1996). A large scale population based study of the association of vitamin D receptor gene polymorphisms with bone mineral density. *J. Bone Miner. Res.* **11**, 1242–1248.

43. Knowlton, R. G., Katzenstein, P. L., Moskowitz, R. W., Weaver, C. J., Malemud, M. N., Parthria, S. A., Jimenez, S. A., and Prockop, D. J. (1990). Genetic linkage of a polymorphism in the type II procollagen gene (COL2A1) to primary osteoarthritis associated with mild chondrodysplasia. *N. Engl. J. Med.* **322**, 526–530.

44. Stoker, N. G., Cheah, K. S. E., Griffin, J. R., Pope, F. M., and Solomon, E. (1985). A highly polymorphic region 3′ to the human type II collagen gene. *Nucleic Acids Res.* **13**, 4613–4622.

45. Berg, E. S., and Olaisen, B. (1993). Characterization of the COL2A1 VNTR polymorphism. *Genomics* **16**, 350–354.

46. Wilkin, D., Koprinikar, K. E., and Cohn, D. H. (1993). Heteroduplex analysis can increase the informativeness of PCR-amplified VNTR markers: Application using a marker tightly linked to the COL2A1 gene. *Genomics* **15**, 372–375.

47. Uitterlinden, A. G., Huang, Q., Pols, H. A. P., and van Leeuwen, J. P. T. M. (1998). Population analysis of the collagen type IIα1 3′ variable number of tandem repeat polymorphism by heteroduplex genotyping. *Electrophoresis* **19**, 661–666.

48. Peterson, A. C., Rienzo, A. D., Lehesjoki, A.-E., de la Chapelle, A., Slatkin, M., and Freimer, N. (1995). The distribution of linkage disequilibrium over anonymous genome regions. *Hum. Mol. Genet.* **4**, 887–894.

49. Laan, M., and Pääbo, S. (1997). Demographic history and linkage disequilibrium in human populations. *Nat. Genet.* **17**, 435–438.

50. Kitanaka, S., Takeyama, K.-I., Murayama, A., Sato, T., Okumura, K., Nogami, M., Hasegawa, Y., Niimi, H., Yanagisawa, J., Tanaka, T., and Kato, S. (1998). Inactivating mutations in the 25-hydroxyvitamin D₃ 1α-hydroxylase gene in patients with pseudovitamin D-deficiency rickets. *N. Engl. J. Med.* **338**, 653–661.

51. St.-Arnaud, R., Messerlian, S., Moir, J. M., Omdahl, J. L., and Glorieux, F. H. (1997). The 25-hydroxyvitamin D 1-alpha-hydroxylase gene maps to the pseudovitamin D deficiency rickets (PDDR) disease locus. *J. Bone Miner. Res.* **12**, 1552–1559.

52. Kostrikis, L. G., Huang, Y., Moore, J. P., Wolinsky, S. M., Zhang, L., Guo, Y., Deutsch, L., Phair, J., Neumann, A. U., and Ho, D. D. (1998). A chemokine receptor CCR2 allele delays HIV-1 disease progression and is associated with a CCR5 promotor mutation. *Nat. Med.* **4**, 350–353.

53. Ingles, S. A., Haile, R. W., Henderson, B. E., Kolonel, L. N., Nakaichi, G., Shi, C.-Y., Yu, M. C., Ross, R. K., and Coetzee, G. A. (1997). Strength of linkage disequilibrium between two vitamin D receptor markers in five ethnic groups: Implications for association studies. *Cancer Epidemiol. Biomarkers Prev.* **6**, 93–98.

54. Uitterlinden, A. G., Burger, H., Huang, Q., Odding, E., van Duijn, C. M., Hofman, A., Birkenhäger, J. C., van Leeuwen, J. P. T. M., and Pols, H. A. P. (1997). Vitamin D receptor genotype is associated with radiographic osteoarthritis at the knee. *J. Clin. Invest.* **100**, 259–263.

55. Keen, R. W., Hart, D. J., Lanchbury, J. S., and Spector, T. D. (1997). Association of early osteoarthritis at the knee with a TaqI polymorphism of the vitamin D receptor gene. *Arthrtis Rheum.* **40**, 1444–1449.

56. Terwilliger, J. D., and Ott, J. (1994). "Handbook of Human Linkage." Johns Hopkins University Press, Baltimore MD.

57. Houwen, R. H. J., Baharloo, S., Blankenship, K., Raeymakers, P., Juyn, J., Sandkuijl, L. A., and Freimer, N. (1994). Genome screening by searching for shared segments: Mapping a gene for benign recurrent intrahepatic cholestasis. *Nat. Genet.* **8**, 380–386.

58. Cheung, V. G., Gregg, J. P., Gogolin-Ewens, K. J., Bandong, J., Stanley, C. A., Baker, L., Higgins, M. J., Nowak, N. J., Shows, T. B., Ewens, W. J., Nelson, S. F., and Spielman, R. S. (1998). Linkage-disequilibrium mapping without genotyping. *Nat. Genet.* **18**, 225–230.

59. Risch, N., and Zhang, H. (1995). Extreme discordant sib-pairs for mapping quantitative trait loci in humans. *Science* **268**, 1584–1589.

60. Martin, N., Boomsma, D., and Machin, G. (1997). A twin-pronged attack on complex traits. *Nat. Genet.* **17**, 387–392.

61. Ottman, R. (1990). An epidemiologic approach to gene-environment interaction. *Genet. Epidemiol.* **7**, 177–185.

62. Howard, G., Nguyen, T., Morrison, N., Watanabe, T., Sambrook, P., Eisman, J, and Kelly, P. (1995). Genetic influences on bone density: Physiological corellates of vitamin D receptor gene alleles in premenopausal women. *J. Clin. Endocrinol. Metab.* **80**, 2800–2805.

63. Matsuyama, T., Ishii, S., Tokita, A., Yabuta, K., Yamamori, S., Morrison, N. A., and Eisman, J. A. (1995). VDR gene polymorphisms and vitamin D analog treatment in Japanese. *Lancet* **345**, 1238–1239.

64. Graafmans, W. C., Lips, P., Ooms, M. E., van Leeuwen, J. P. T. M., Pols, H. A. P., and Uitterlinden, A. G. (1997). The effect of vitamin D supplementation on the bone mineral density of the femoral neck is associated with vitamin D receptor genotype. *J. Bone Miner. Res.* **12**, 1241–1245.

65. McAlindon, T. E., Felson, D. T., Zhang, Y., Hannan, M. T., Aliabadi, P., Weissman, B., Rush, D., Wilson, P. W. F., and Jacques, P. (1996). Relation of dietary intake and serum levels of vitamin D to progression of osteoarthritis of the knee among participants in the Framingham study. *Ann. Intern. Med.* **125**, 353–359.

66. Krall, E. A., Parry, P., Lichter, J. B., and Dawson-Hughes, B. (1995). Vitamin D receptor alleles and rates of bone loss: Influence of years since menopause and calcium intake. *J. Bone Miner. Res.* **10**, 978–984.

67. Kiel, D. P., Myers, R. H., Cupples, L. A., Kong, X. F., Zhu, X. H., Ordovas, J., Schaefer, E. J., Felson, D. T., Rush, D., Wilson, P. W., Eisman, J. A., and Holick, M. F. (1997). The BsmI vitamin D receptor restriction fragment length polymorphism (bb) influences the effect of calcium intake on bone mineral density. *J. Bone Miner. Res.* **12**, 1049–1057.

68. Wishart, J. M., Horowitz, M., Need, A. G., Scopacasa, F., Morris, H. A., Clifton, P. M., and Nordin, B. E. (1997). Relations between calcium intake, calcitriol, polymorphisms of the vitamin D receptor gene, and calcium absorption in premenopausal women. *Am. J. Clin. Nutr.* **65**, 798–802.

69. Ongphiphadhanakul, B., Rajatanavin, R., Chanprasertyothin, S., Chailurkit, L., Piaseu, N., Teerarungsikul, K., Sirisriro, R., Komindr, S., and Puavilai, G. (1997). Vitamin D receptor gene polymorphism is associated with urinary calcium excretion but not with bone mineral density in postmenopausal women. *J. Endocrinol. Invest.* **20**, 592–596.

70. Gennari, L., Becherini, L., Gonelli, M. L., Cepollaro, C., Martini, S., Mansani, R., and Brandi, M. L. (1997). Vitamin D receptor genotypes and intestinal calcium absorption in postmenopausal women. *Calcif. Tissue Int.* **61**, 460–463.

71. Fijneman, R. J. A., de Vries, S. S., Jansen, R. C., and Demant, P. (1996). Complex interactions of new quantitative trait loci, *Sluc1, Sluc2, Sluc3,* and *Sluc4,* that influence the susceptibility to lung cancer in the mouse. *Nat. Genet.* **14**, 465–467.

72. Van Wezel, T., Stassen, A. P. M., Moen, C. J. A., Hart, A. A. M., van der Valk, M. A., and Demant, P. (1996). Gene interactions and single gene effects in colon tumour susceptibility in mice. *Nat. Genet.* **14**, 468–470.

73. Morrison, N. A., Yeoman, R., Kelly, P. J., and Eisman, J. A. (1992). Contribution of trans-acting factor alleles to normal physiological

variability: Vitamin D receptor gene polymorphisms and circulating osteocalcin. *Proc. Natl. Acad. Sci. U.S.A.* **89**, 6665–6669.

74. Cooper, G. S., and Umbach, D. M. (1996). Are vitamin D receptor polymorphisms associated with bone mineral density? A meta-analysis. *J. Bone Miner. Res.* **11**, 1841–1849.

75. Verbeek, W., Gombart, A. F., Shiohara, M., Campbell, M., and Koeffler, H. P. (1997). Vitamin D receptor: No evidence for allele-specific mRNA stability in cells which are heterozygous for the TaqI restriction enzyme polymorphism. *Biochem. Biophys. Res. Commun.* **238**, 77–80.

76. Arai, H., Miyamaoto, K.-I., Taketani, Y., Yamamoto, H., Iemori, Y., Morita, K., Tonai, T., Nishisho, T., Mori, S., and Takeda, E. (1997). A vitamin D receptor gene polymorphism in the translation initiation codon: Effect on protein activity and relation to bone mineral density in Japanese women. *J. Bone Miner. Res.* **12**, 915–921.

77. Mocharla, H., Butch, A. W., Pappas, A. A., Flick, J. T., Weinstein, R. S., de Togni, P., Jilka, R. L., Roiberson, P. K., Parfitt, A. M., and Manolagas, S. C. (1997). Quantification of vitamin D receptor mRNA by competitive polymerase chain reaction in PBMC: lack of correspondence with common allelic variants. *J. Bone Miner. Res.* **12**, 726–733.

78. Grant, S. F. A., Reid, D. M., Blake, G., Herd, R., Fogelman, I., and Ralston, S. H. (1996). Reduced bone density and osteoporotic vertebral fracture associated with a polymorphic Sp1 binding site in the collagen type Iα1 gene. *Nat. Genet.* **14**, 203–205.

79. Uitterlinden, A. G., Burger, H., Huang, Q., Yue, F., McGuigan, F. E. A., Grant, S. F. A., Hofman, A., van Leeuwen, J. P. T. M., Pols, H. A. P., and Ralston, S. H. (1998). Relation of alleles at the collagen type Iα1 gene to bone density and risk of osteoporotic fractures in postmenopausal women. *N. Engl. J. Med.* **338**, 1016–1021.

80. Willing, M. C., Deschenes, S. P., Scott, D. A., Byers, P. H., Slayton, R. L., Pitts, S. H., Arikat, H., and Roberts, E. J. (1994). Osteogenesis imperfecta type I: Molecular heterogeneity for COLIA1 null alleles of type I collagen. *Am. J. Hum. Genet.* **55**, 638–647.

81. Carling, T., Kindmark, A., Helleman, P., Lundgren, E., Ljunghall, S., Rastad, J., Akerstrom, G., and Melhus, H. (1995). Vitamin D receptor genotypes in primary hyperparathyroidism. *Nat. Med.* **1**, 1309–1311.

82. McDermott, M. F., Ramachandran, A., Ogunkolade, B. W., Aganna, E., Curtis, D., Boucher, B. J., Snehalatha, C., and Hitman, G. A. (1997). Allelic variation in the vitamin D receptor influences susceptibility to IDDM in Indian Asians. *Diabetologia* **40**, 971–975.

83. Taylor, J. A., Hirvonen, A., Watson, M., Pittman, G., Mohler, J. L., and Bell, D. A. (1996). Association of prostate cancer with vitamin D receptor gene polymorphism. *Cancer. Res.* **56**, 4108–4110.

84. Van der Wielen, R. P. J., Lowik, M. R. H., van den Berg, H., de Groot, L. C. P. G. M., Haller, J., Moreiras, O., and van Staveren, W. (1995). Serum vitamin D concentrations among elderly people in Europe. *Lancet* **346**, 207–210.

CHAPTER 26

Measurement of Calcium, Phosphate, Parathyroid Hormone, and Vitamin D

HEINRICH SCHMIDT-GAYK Department of Endocrinology, Laboratory Group,
D-69126 Heidelberg, Germany

I. CALCIUM AND PHOSPHORUS

A. Calcium in Serum

Calcium in serum (or plasma) is found in three fractions, namely the ionized fraction (Ca^{2+}), the complexed fraction, and the protein-bound fraction. The sum of the three fractions is the total serum (or plasma) calcium, which is fairly constant in a healthy person. In a healthy person, approximately 50% is ionized and 5–10% is bound to low molecular weight ligands (i.e., bicarbonate, lactate, phosphate, and citrate). Sometimes the calcium bound to low molecular weight ligands is described as "complexed" calcium. 40–45% is protein-bound (mainly to albumin, less to globulins). For routine purposes it is sufficient to determine the concentration of total calcium together with the concentration of total protein and/or albumin. The concentration of total protein or albumin might be necessary for the calculation of corrected serum calcium. The normal ranges are shown in Table I [1].

1. CURRENT ASSAY TECHNOLOGY

a. Atomic Absorption Spectrometry (AAS) Atomic absorption spectrometry is the reference method for the determination of total calcium [2, 3]. Calcium in serum and urine is diluted sufficiently with lanthanum chloride solution, which binds interfering substances such as proteins and phosphates. When introduced into a flame, the dissociated free calcium atom absorbs light from the characteristic wavelengths (e.g., 422.7 nm) produced by a hollow cathode lamp with a calcium filament. The imprecision within the series is <1% and between series is <2%.

b. Flame Atomic Emission Spectroscopy (FAES) For routine purposes, flame atomic emission spectroscopy and photometry (see next section) are used in most clinical chemistry laboratories. Serum or plasma is diluted with distilled water (which may contain lithium), sprayed into a flame of acetylene/air (2300°C), and vaporized. Some interference of sodium is corrected by a sodium containing solution (140 mmol/l) for calibration.

TABLE I.   Reference Ranges for Calcium in
Serum (or Plasma, Ammonium Heparinate)

Total calcium		
Age	mg/dl	mmol/l
<28 days	7.1–10.8	1.75–2.70
1–12 months	8.2–10.8	2.05–2.70
1–20 years	8.6–10.6	2.14–2.65
Adults	8.8–10.4	2.2–2.6
Ionized calcium		
Adults	4.6–5.4	1.15–1.35

The fraction of ionized calcium/total calcium is
47–57%. From Schmidt-Gayk [1].

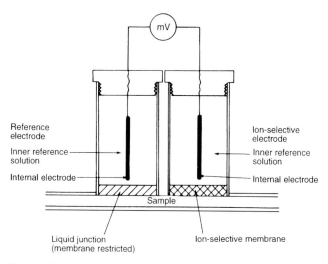

FIGURE 1   Schematic diagram of a typical flow-through ISE-reference electrode measuring cell.

Simultaneously, the emission of sodium, potassium, lithium, and calcium may be measured. Lithium is used as an internal standard to correct for variations in flame intensity. FAES is used for high throughput automated multichannel clinical chemistry analyzers (e.g. Olympus Co., Japan) or high throughput stand alone electrolyte analyzers (sodium, potassium, calcium; e.g. Eppendorf, Hamburg, Germany). Because of technical improvements, highly precise measurements are possible, with coefficients of variation within series below 0.5% and from series to series below 0.8%. In addition to serum calcium determination, FAES can be used successfully for the determination of calcium in feces.

c. Photometry   Calcium complexes with ortho-cresolphthalein-complexone [4] or Arsenazo III [5]. At pH 10–12, calcium yields a red complex with ortho-cresolphthalein-complexone, which is measured at 570–575 nm. The complex is stabilized by KCN, thereby eliminating interference from heavy metals. By adding 8-hydroxychinoline, interference of magnesium is eliminated [6]. Photometry is used in many high throughput automated multichannel clinical chemistry analyzers (e.g., Hitachi, Japan). Within assay coefficients of variation of 1% and between assay coefficients of variation of <2% are obtained. An enzymatic method for assaying calcium in serum and urine with porcine pancreatic α-amylase also has been published [7]. In this assay, calcium activates α-amylase yielding a product which is monitored at 405 nm.

d. Ion Selective Electrodes (ISE) for Ionized Calcium   A typical Ca^{2+} ion selective electrode (Fig. 1) [8] consists of an assembly in which a Ca^{2+} selective membrane encloses an inner reference solution of $CaCl_2$ held within a stem of plastic or glass. An internal reference electrode, usually Ag/AgCl, is immersed in the inner reference solution. In its simplest form this consists of a standard aqueous solution of $CaCl_2$, usually saturated with AgCl to prevent dissolution of the AgCl from the internal reference electrode, and containing NaCl and KCl in physiological concentrations.

Calcium ISEs in routine use in clinical chemistry are based on so-called liquid membranes in which an ion-selective electroactive substance, or "ionophore," is dissolved in an organic liquid phase which is trapped within a polymeric matrix, usually polyvinyl chloride (PVC). The cell is completed by an external reference electrode in junction with the analyte solution. The affinity of the ion exchanger for the free ionized calcium imparts the selective permeability to the membrane, though with a very high resistance to mass transport. According to the Nernst equation, the cell will develop a potential for a given free ionized calcium activity in the analyte solution. The commercialized equipment with thermostat-controlled flow-through electrodes, automated calibration, and pH correction have made the determination of ionized calcium as easy as modern blood gas analysis [9]. Within assay coefficients of variation of 1% and between assay coefficients of variation of <2% are obtained [10].

e. Fluorometric Titration   Fluorometric titration with ethylene glycol tetraacetic acid (EGTA) is used in the Corning 940 calcium analyzer (Corning). This method has a wide linear range, and good precision (coefficients of variation of 1–3% within series) and recovery [11]. However, this method is susceptible to interferences by copper, iron, zinc, and certain drugs such as sulfadiazine, heparin, and acetylsalicylic acid [12]. This method has been very successfully used for the determination of serum and urinary calcium, especially in the smaller laboratory and in pediatric laboratories.

f. Conclusions   Is there a preferred method for the determination of serum calcium? Electrolyte-balanced heparin used in syringes may produce a bias in the measurement of ionized calcium concentration in specimens with abnormally low protein concentration [13]. However, in patients with multiple myeloma or hyperlipidemia, ionized serum calcium is superior to FAES or photometry, because in the latter methods the volume of serum proteins or serum lipids decreases the volume of serum water so that FAES or photometry yield falsely low values for electrolytes. In patients receiving large amounts of citrate (multiple transfusions, cardiopulmonary bypass surgery, hepatic transplantation), the monitoring of ionized calcium is of great importance [14, 15].

In patients with hypercalcemia, if ionized calcium is compared with total calcium without correction for total protein or albumin, ionized calcium appears to be a slightly better indicator of elevated calcium states than total calcium [16].

Using photometry, the Arsenazo III method increased calibration stability (from 12 hours using ortho-cresolphthalein-complexone to 48 hours with Arsenazo III [5]). However, citrate interfered in the Arsenazo III method, whereas there was no interference in the ortho-cresolphthalein-complexone method [17]. In addition, falsely elevated serum calcium levels were reported in two patients with IgM paraproteinemia when the Arsenazo III dye binding method was used, whereas normal results were obtained in these patients when measuring ionized calcium and total calcium (by atomic absorption spectrophotometry and by the ortho-cresolphthalein-complexone method) [18].

For routine laboratory services, hospitals, or practicing physicians, FAES or photometry is clearly adequate. However, there are also some routine hospital laboratories that have switched to ionized calcium. For intensive care units with patients receiving multiple transfusions or large amounts of citrate, the determination of ionized calcium is necessary.

2. PREANALYTICAL CONSIDERATIONS

Preanalytical variability is mainly caused by posture and prolonged venous occlusion if blood samples are taken using a tourniquet. The effect of venous occlusion on serum calcium, protein, phosphorus, and magnesium concentrations is shown in Table II [19–21].

There are various formulas that can be used for the correction of serum calcium:

(a) according to the concentration of albumin [22]:

corrected Ca (mg/dl)
= measured Ca (mg/dl) − albumin (g/dl) + 4.0

or, recalculated for the SI-system of units:

corrected Ca (mmol/l)
= measured Ca (mmol/l) − 0.025 × albumin (g/l) + 1.0

(b) according to the concentration of total protein [20]:

corrected Ca (mg/dl)
= measured Ca (mg/dl)/(0.6 + TP/19.4)

TABLE II. Effect of Venous Occlusion on Serum Calcium, Protein, Phosphorus, and Magnesium Concentrations

Constituent	Baseline	3-min tourniquet	p
Total calcium (mg/dl)	9.64	9.87	<0.01
(mmol/l)	2.41	2.47	
Total protein (g/dl)	6.9	7.3	<0.001
Corrected calcium (mg/dl)	10.11	10.09	n.s.
(mmol/l)	2.528	2.523	
Phosphorus (mg/dl)	3.22	3.19	n.s.
Magnesium (mg/dl)	2.09	2.13	n.s.
Ionized calcium (mg/dl)	4.62	4.62	n.s.
(mmol/)	1.155	1.155	

The correction of calcium was performed according to Husdan [20], which is a slight modification of a formula obtained by Parfitt [21]. From Husdan [19].

where TP is the serum total protein concentration (g/dl), or, recalculated using the SI system of units:

corrected Ca (mmol/l)
= measured Ca (mmol/l)/(0.6 + TP/194)

where TP is the serum total protein concentration (g/l).

At a total protein concentration of 77.6 g/l divided by 194, a value of 0.4 is obtained. This means that at a protein concentration of 77.6 g/l, the corrected calcium is the same as the measured value. The formula of Husdan [20] was compared with the formula of Payne [22] by applying them to 100 patients with primary hyperparathyroidism and 100 healthy controls; a better separation of these groups was made using the formula of Husdan. It is assumed that the method of albumin determination influences the albumin correction method.

In addition to effects of venous occlusion, physiological protein fluctuations in a standing or a recumbent position are mainly responsible for intraindividual serum calcium variability [23]. Furthermore, some false low normal ranges have been published in healthy blood donors. This occurs because the connection to the blood bag is cut after the donation and an extra tube of blood is then collected for the determination of calcium [24]. After blood donation, however, the serum protein concentration is significantly lower than before the donation.

3. BIOLOGICAL VARIABILITY: DIURNAL RHYTHMS AND SEASONAL VARIATIONS

The semidiurnal variations (8 AM–6 PM) of total and ionized calcium and of intact parathyroid hormone (PTH) are shown in Figure 2. By applying the formula of Husdan [20], almost no circadian variation of serum calcium was observed from 9 AM to 5 PM [25]. Seasonal variations were not observed

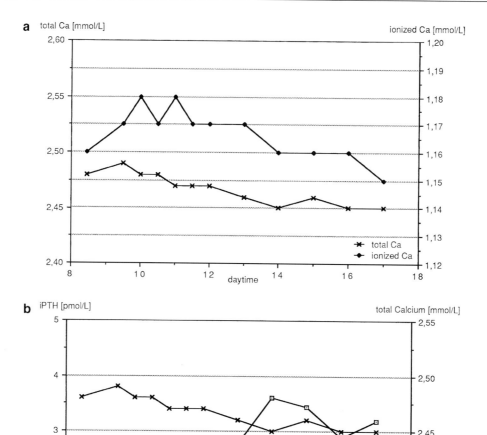

FIGURE 2 Semidiurnal variation of serum calcium and parathyroid hormone in healthy adults. (A) total and ionized calcium; (B) total calcium and intact parathyroid hormone; (C) total calcium corrected for total protein (according to Husdan [14]) and intact parathyroid hormone; and (D) ionized calcium and intact parathyroid hormone.

for serum calcium in a health examination survey in more than 2000 men [26].

B. Calcium in Urine

1. Preanalytical and Analytical Considerations

There are various recommendations regarding the collection and treatment of urine samples for the determination of calcium (Table III) [27].

Weber [28] found in freshly collected urine samples a mean calcium concentration of 2.39 mmol/l with and without acidification by HCl. Because acidification would decrease the concentration of uric acid and excludes pH determination in the collected sample, the following recommendation can be made: If electrolytes (sodium, potassium, calcium, magnesium, chloride), glucose, uric acid, urea, creatinine, albumin, protein, α-amylase, or β-NAG are to be determined in urine samples with modern automated equipment (e.g., Roche Diagnostics/Hitachi, Roche/Cobas, Olympus AU series, Beckman CX series, Kone Analyzer, Instrumentation Laboratory/Monarch), flame photometers or atomic absorption spectroscopy, the urine should be collected without additives and analyzed within hours after collection, according to this literature survey.

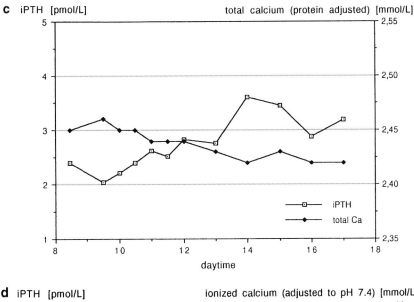

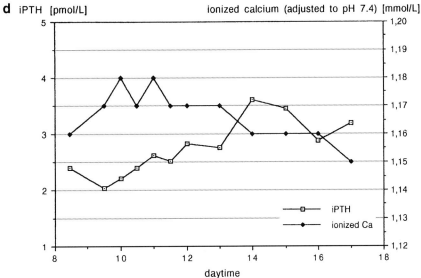

FIGURE 2 *(continued)*

2. BIOLOGICAL VARIATION

a. Diurnal and Seasonal Variation of Urinary Calcium Excretion   In normal individuals, a diurnal variation of urinary calcium excretion has been found [29]. The maximum urinary calcium excretion is observed between 10 AM and 2 PM according to Min *et al.* [29], and between 10 AM and 6 PM according to Wisser *et al.* [30]. The diurnal variation of urinary calcium in fasting individuals is remarkably similar to that of sodium [29]. For the detection of hypercalciuria, an overnight urine collection may be used for screening purposes.

We did not observe a seasonal variation of urinary calcium in patients with calcium-containing kidney stones. In contrast, Robertson *et al.* [31] found increased urinary calcium in the summer months compared to the winter months. The results of Robertson might be explained by a lesser vitamin D supply in the winter months in Leeds (England) than in Heidelberg (Germany).

b. Other Factors Influencing the Urinary Excretion of Calcium   Normal 24 hour urinary calcium excretion rates are 120–320 mg (3–8 mmol) in men, 100–280 mg (2.5–7 mmol) in women, or 2–4 mg/kg body weight in either sex. Higher urinary calcium levels are observed in many patients with increased intestinal calcium absorption and/or increased bone resorption with or without hypercalcemia. However, because parathyroid hormone increases the tubular reabsorption of calcium, some patients with primary

Table III.   Collection and Storage of Urine for Determination of Calcium Content

Author	Year	Recommendation
Documenta Geigy	1968	Ca-urate is precipitated in acidified urine
Doerner	1992	add 5 ml concentrated HCl after collection
Frings	1975	no addition of HCl
Gowans	1986	add HCl after collection until pH 5–6 is obtained
Greiling	1995	add 5 ml HCl, 6 mol/l, to the container before collection is started, after collection acidify with HCl to pH 1
Guder	1986	add thymol to the container before collection is started
Gunn	1992	acidify after collection
Hauptmann	1992	no addition for pediatric purposes
Jahnen	1989	no difference between acidified and untreated divided samples
Keller	1991	no addition, analyze as soon as possible after collection
Manz	1984	no addition for pediatric purposes
Misselwitz	1981	no addition for pediatric purposes
Ng	1984	no difference between acidified and untreated samples if assayed within six hours
Nordin	1976	add antibacterial substance (e.g., thymol) before collection is started, after collection fill 25 ml into a separate container and add two drops of concentrated HCl
Paunier	1970	add 10 ml of concentrated HCl/l urine after collection (pediatrics)
Richterich	1971	add thymol to the container before collection is started, after collection add 10 ml of concentrated HCl/l urine
Thomas	1998	add 10 ml of concentrated HCl after collection and raise the temperature of the sample
Tietz	1987	add 5 ml HCl, 6 mol/l, to the container before collection is started, after collection acidify with HCl to pH 3–4, do not use more than 10 ml of HCl, 6 mol/l
Weber	1989	immediately after collection, no difference was noted between samples collected with and without acidification by HCl.

From Schmidt-Gayk [27].

hyperparathyroidism present with normal urinary calcium excretion.

Urinary calcium is often increased in recurrent stone formers and is significantly related to urinary sodium excretion (dietary sodium consumption). In one review, Massey and Whiting [32] stated that for every 100 mmol of sodium (6 g NaCl) excreted, there is approximately a 1 mmol loss of urinary calcium in normocalciuric healthy populations. In addition, urinary calcium is related to urinary urea excretion (dietary protein consumption). Hess and coworkers [33] observed that there is a relationship between protein overconsumption and upregulation of calcitriol (1,25-dihydroxyvitamin D_3) synthesis.

Whereas a high dietary calcium intake decreases the risk of kidney stones, probably by inhibiting intestinal oxalate absorption, additional pharmaceutical calcium intake in large doses (1000 mg or more) may increase the risk of kidney stone formation by hypercalciuria, which is detectable for some hours following large oral doses. Therefore, it is recommended that additional pharmaceutical calcium intake should be divided into two doses of 500 mg each (taken in the morning and evening) or even into three doses. In healthy persons,

for every 1000 mg (25 mmol) of additional oral calcium intake, urinary calcium increases by about 60 mg (1.5 mmol). The metabolic evaluation of patients with recurrent idiopathic calcium nephrolithiasis [34] yielded the following results: the most frequent risk factor was hypercalciuria (39%), followed by hyperoxaluria (32%) and low volume (32%), hypocitraturia (29%), hyperuricosuria (23%), and hypomagnesiuria (19%). After immobilization (e.g., after tetraplegia) urinary calcium increases to amounts of about 600 mg per 24 h caused by excessive bone resorption.

Low urinary calcium excretion is observed in renal insufficiency, vitamin D deficiency, and other hypocalcemic states. In hypercalcemic states, relatively low urinary calcium is observed in patients on thiazide medication and in patients with Addison's disease (cortisol and mineralocorticoid deficiency) and familial hypocalciuric hypercalcemia (FHH).

C. Phosphorus in Serum

Phosphorus is present in blood chiefly as inorganic and organic phosphates; nearly all of the latter resides in the erythrocytes. Determination is often referred to as inorganic phosphorus rather than inorganic phosphate, since the phosphate determined is usually reported in terms of phosphorus [12].

1. CURRENT ASSAY TECHNOLOGY

a. Molybdate Method for the Determination of Inorganic Phosphate Most methods depend on the reaction of phosphate ions with molybdate to form a colorless phosphomolybdate complex such as $(NH_4)_3[(PO_4(MoO_3)_{12}]$, which can be measured directly by UV absorption at 340 nm or after reduction to a complex heteropolymer, molybdenum blue, at 600–700 nm [35]. The former method is the most commonly used by discrete analyzers because of its speed, good precision, accuracy, and reagent stability. To prevent protein precipitation, a solubilizing agent such as Tween 80 is necessary in the reagents. In the application of Roche Diagnostics for the Hitachi automated analyzers (e.g., Hitachi 717), the final concentrations of the reagents in the assay are: ammonium-molybdate 1.0 mmol/l; sulfuric acid 0.35 mol/l; sodium chloride 44 mmol/l; and a detergent. Measurement is performed at 340 nm, with an additional reading at 660 nm to correct for interference. In another adaptation, a blank absorbance is measured at 340 nm and at 376 nm [36].

The intra-assay coefficient of variation (imprecision) is usually less than 2% for the phosphomolybdate method, and the interassay coefficient of variation is usually below 3% with automated analyzers. Recovery is in the range of 98–103%. Turbidity may interfere in the phosphomolybdate method, yielding falsely high values. In addition, high hemoglobin and bilirubin concentrations interfere. High citrate concentrations yield falsely low results because citrate competes with phosphate for binding at the molybdate ion. In addition, mannit from infusion therapy and phenothiazines form complexes with phosphomolybdate, yielding falsely low values [6].

Pseudohyperphosphatemia has previously been reported in patients with paraproteins [37]. Some studies have shown that interference is due to turbidity caused by precipitation of the paraprotein by the acid reagent used in both visible and ultra-violet spectrophotometric methods [38]. Other investigators have identified the presence of a phosphate-binding immunoglobulin. Savory and Pearce [36] evaluated an improved methodology of Roche Diagnostics (Roche UK Ltd., Sussex, UK) containing a detergent-modified reagent, which was compared with the standard kit supplied by the same manufacturer. Using the original reagent, pseudohyperphosphatemia was found in 27% (12 of 45) of the samples. The modified reagent was free from interference, with no significant difference between results from serum and protein-free supernatants.

b. Enzymatic Method for the Determination of Inorganic Phosphate An enzymatic method for the determination of phosphate in serum and urine has been described [39], and applications have been published for the Hitachi 717 and Bayer/Technicon RA-XT analyzers (Bayer Diagnostics, Munich, Germany). In this method, phosphate ions react with inosine in the presence of purine nucleoside phosphorylase to form hypoxanthine; this is oxidized by xanthin oxidase to uric acid with production of hydrogen peroxide. The latter is measured with the aid of a chromogen system, the colored product being measured at 555 nm. Enzymatic phosphate determination on the Hitachi 717 and Bayer/Technicon RA-XT analyzers gave within-run coefficients of variation of 2.2% and interassay coefficients of variation of 3%. The adapted method was linear up to 3.2 mmol/l phosphate. No interference was found for bilirubin up to 270 μmol/l and for hemoglobin up to 114 μmol/l. The correlation ($r = 0.99$) to the automated molybdenum blue method was very good. The values of control sera were on average 4.1% lower than the declared values for the molybdenum blue methods [39].

2. REFERENCE RANGES

In normal healthy subjects, the total phosphate concentration in plasma is 3.9 mmol/l, of which only 0.8–1.4 mmol/l is inorganic phosphate, the remainder being phospholipids and other organic compounds (for review on plasma phosphate, see Crook and Swaminathan [35]). Approximately 10% of plasma inorganic phosphate is nonfiltrable or protein-bound, and 6% is complexed with calcium or magnesium; 84% of plasma phosphate is free and present as HPO_4^{2-} and $H_2PO_4^{-}$, the relative proportion depending on the pH.

The reference ranges for fasting plasma or serum phosphate vary greatly with age. During the first six months of life, phosphate concentrations are 1.6–2.5 mmol/l (5.0–7.8 mg/dl). Thereafter the values decrease significantly. At 4–8 years of age, the phosphate concentration range is 1.2–1.8 mmol/l (3.7–5.4 mg/dl) and at 10 years of age it is, 1.1–1.7 mmol/l (3.5–5.3 mg/dl). No sex difference is observed in childhood, but during puberty the phosphate concentration decreases abruptly to the range observed in young adults: 0.8–1.45 mmol/l (2.5–4.5 mg/dl) in males and 0.9–1.4 mmol/l (2.8–4.7 mg/dl) in females [40]. The levels decline slightly in adults of both sexes until middle age; thereafter they increase in elderly females and decrease slightly in elderly males. Increased bone resorption occurring in a substantial proportion of women after menopause may be responsible for some of the increase in serum phosphate seen in older women.

3. PREANALYTICAL CONSIDERATIONS

Specimens for phosphate measurements should be obtained from a fasting patient in the morning, e.g., from 7 AM to 9 AM. Hyperglycemia and hyperinsulinemia, as occurring during standard oral glucose tolerance tests or after a regular meal, may lead to hypophosphatemia due to a shift of phosphate from the extracellular to the intracellular space [41].

Serum or plasma should be separated from cells within one hour after collection of the specimen. Hemolysis must be avoided because phosphate may be split off from labile esters in the erythrocytes. Plasma or serum may be stored at 4°C for several days, or in the frozen state for several months. The concentration of phosphate in serum is 0.06–0.10 mmol/l higher than that in plasma because intracellular phosphate is released from platelets and erythrocytes during clotting. This is especially marked in patients with thrombocytosis. Citrate, oxalate, and EDTA should not be used as anticoagulants because they interfere with the formation of the phosphomolybdate complex.

4. BIOLOGICAL VARIATION

A mean level of about 1.0 mmol/l is observed in healthy volunteers in the morning (7 AM–10 AM), rising to 1.2 mmol/l from 3 AM–5 PM and 1.3 mmol/l at midnight [42]. The semidiurnal variation of serum phosphate and intact PTH in nonfasting healthy subjects is shown in Figure 3. The diurnal rhythm of phosphate in plasma is abolished in fasting subjects [43]. A similar rhythm as in healthy persons, with higher levels in the evening and during the night, was observed in patients on hemodialysis, but phosphate levels were generally higher than those of healthy persons [44].

D. Phosphate in Urine

In healthy subjects, the net intestinal absorption of phosphate is linearly related to dietary intake; about 50–75% of ingested phosphate is absorbed and excreted into the urine. The bulk of the absorbed amount occurs by diffusion; only a small percentage is mediated by vitamin D metabolites (mainly by calcitriol). Therefore, urinary phosphate is a valuable indicator of nutrition (meat, dairy products) and is often above the normal range of 25–35 mmol/24 h in overnutrition. There exists a circadian rhythm for phosphate excretion, with higher levels in the afternoon and during sleep (about 6 mmol/4 hr) than in the morning (about 4 mmol/4 hr) [45]. In fasting individuals, the circadian variation of urinary phosphate excretion vanishes [29].

The tubular maximum of phosphate reabsorption related to the glomerular filtration rate (TmP/GFR) is the best method to calculate renal tubular reabsorption of phosphate. TmP/GFR can be easily determined using the fasting urinary and plasma concentrations of phosphate and creatinine and a nomogram of Walton and Bijvoet [46]. Increased parathyroid hormone, volume expansion (e.g., increased sodium intake), or a phosphaturic factor in oncogenic osteomalacia decrease tubular phosphate reabsorption (lower TmP/GFR). TmP/GFR displays a similar circadian rhythm as described above for the serum phosphate levels: TmP/GFR starts at about 0.85 mmol/l in the morning and approaches 1.0 mmol/l in the evening and 1.2 mmol/l at 3 AM during sleep [45].

II. PARATHYROID HORMONE AND PARATHYROID HORMONE-RELATED PROTEIN (PTHRP)

A. Parathyroid Hormone

The concentration of calcium ions in blood, along with calcitriol and calcitonin, is mainly regulated by parathyroid

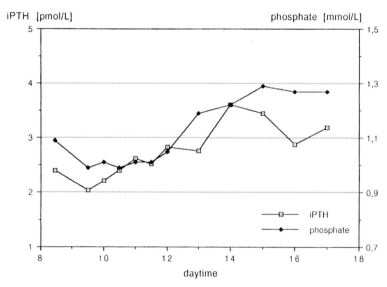

FIGURE 3   Semidiurnal variation of serum phosphate and intact PTH in nonfasting healthy subjects.

hormone (PTH; parathyrin) (see also Chapter 13). In patients with disorders of calcium metabolism, measurement of serum PTH plays an important role, specifically to differentiate hypercalcemia due to primary hyperparathyroidism from other hypercalcemic disorders in which a high serum calcium level tends to suppress the secretion of PTH. In the differential diagnosis of hypocalcemia, serum PTH measurement is useful to distinguish hypoparathyroidism from other causes of elevated PTH levels. In patients with renal failure, PTH measurements are most often performed to estimate the degree of secondary hyperparathyroidism.

PTH is an 84 amino acid peptide, the extreme aminoterminal sequence of which is required for its calcemic bioactivity. Measurement of serum PTH concentrations was complicated for a long time by the fact that several fragments of the hormone circulate in blood as a result of the metabolism of PTH both peripherally and within the parathyroid gland [47]. Intact PTH is cleaved, mainly by the liver, between the amino acid residues 34–38, into fragments. Nevertheless, intact PTH does not accumulate in patients with severe liver disease [48].

The N-terminal fragments are cleared quickly from the circulation and are detectable only in low concentrations [49]. Only in some patients with renal failure have significant concentrations of N-terminal fragments been determined [50]. The N-terminal fragment has been isolated and sequenced as PTH1–37 [51]. In contrast to the normally low concentrations of the N-terminal fragment, midregion and C-terminal fragments disappear less rapidly from the circulation and thus are present in higher concentrations. It is not entirely clear if the midregional and C-terminal fragments are biologically totally inactive. These fragments are, however, inactive in stimulating the renal adenylate cyclase. Measurement of intact PTH in serum was further complicated by the fairly low amounts of the intact hormone (1–6 pmol/l) due to its short half-life of 2–4 min [52] compared with >ten-fold longer half-lives of some noncalcemic fragments.

1. IMMUNOASSAYS FOR PTH

The immunoheterogeneity of PTH in serum has led to the development of several different PTH radioimmunoassays (RIAs), many of which detected a specific part of the hormone ("fragment assays"). The most widely used PTH RIAs were directed against the midregion or C-terminal part of the hormone. Although these assays detected mainly biologically inactive fragments of PTH, many of them could discriminate patients with primary hyperparathyroidism from normal subjects [53]. In some circumstances, especially in renal dysfunction, the elevated results obtained by these assays had to be interpreted with caution, because midregion and C-terminal fragments are removed from the circulation mainly by glomerular filtration [47]. In the differential diagnosis of hypercalcemia, these assays were not as useful as

assays for intact PTH. Furthermore, many PTH RIAs were not sensitive enough to distinguish normal from subnormal PTH values [54].

The best way to study the secretory activity of the parathyroid glands is to measure the biologically active intact PTH(1–84) molecule. This became possible in 1987 by application of the two-site immunoradiometric assay (IRMA) technique to the measurement of PTH [55–57]. This method overcame the limitations of older assays [54, 58] because it is both sensitive enough to detect the low amounts of intact hormone in normal subjects and specific enough to prevent nonspecific serum effects and cross-reaction with inactive fragments. Hence, in clinical practice there is no need for "fragment-specific" PTH assays anymore. The subsequent part of this chapter therefore only discusses the clinical application of two-site immunometric assays employing two different antibodies to detect exclusively the intact hormone.

2. NORMAL RANGE OF SERUM INTACT PTH

The results obtained by different two-site assays of intact PTH are remarkably similar. This is because detection is restricted to a relatively homogeneous group of circulating peptides (the intact or mainly intact hormone) and the use of identical standards (synthetic hPTH (1–84)) [49, 55–57, 59, 60]. Most assays have a normal range in adults of ~1–6 pmol/l, roughly equivalent to 10–60 ng/l. Intact PTH levels increase slightly with age but are similar in men and women and are only slightly influenced by some lifestyle factors [61]. Intact PTH values are slightly lower in children aged 2–15 [62].

3. PREANALYTICAL AND ANALYTICAL CONSIDERATIONS

Intact PTH is somewhat unstable in serum when stored for more than six hours at room temperature [63]; the presumed degradation is less severe in EDTA-plasma. The decrease in intact PTH detected by several investigators was 15–30% in the first 24 hours [59, 60, 63], whereas no significant decrease was seen within the first six hours in serum or unseparated blood [60], or even for 24 hours if the serum was stored at 4°C [59]. Intact PTH levels were stable in EDTA-treated plasma even for 48 hours at room temperature. Therefore, EDTA-treated plasma is the preferred sample material when samples have to be shipped and stored at room temperature for more than a few hours. Incomplete filling of EDTA-treated tubes may sometimes result in falsely low measurements of intact PTH, possibly due to high concentrations of EDTA (shift of pH). However, serum is required for some of the commercially available assays.

The secretion of PTH is pulsatile [64] and shows diurnal variations with minor increases during the day and a peak at night. Serum PTH levels are also influenced by oral calcium and phosphate intake. During the day, serum PTH levels parallel the serum phosphate levels, as shown in Figure 3. The pulsatility of intact PTH secretion is shown in Figures 4

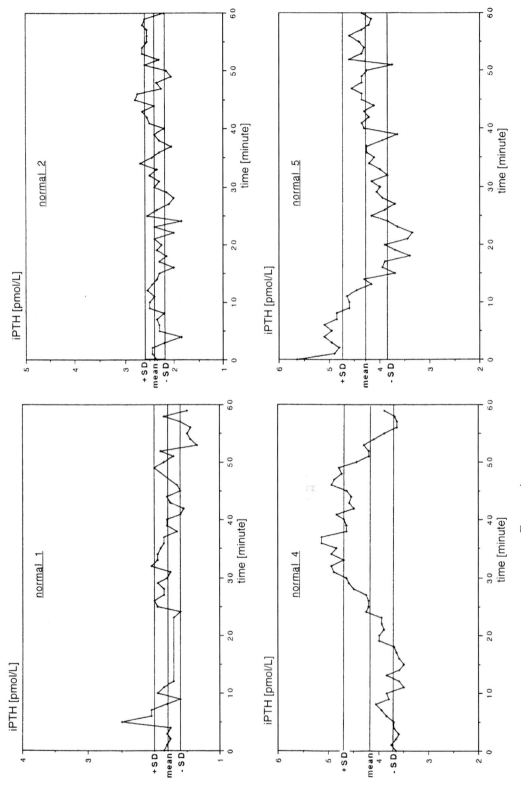

FIGURE 4   Pulsatility of intact PTH secretion in healthy persons.

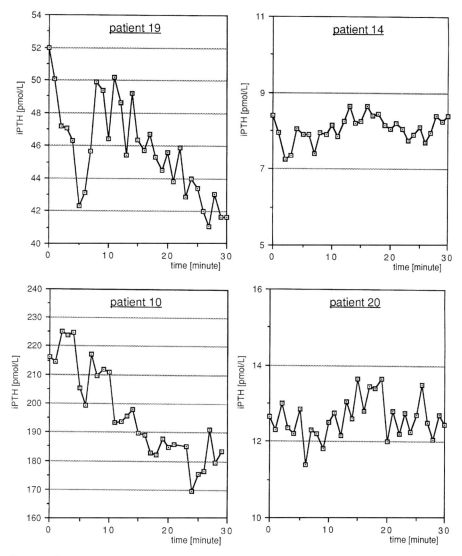

FIGURE 5   Pulsatility of intact PTH secretion in patients with primary hyperparathyroidism.

(healthy subjects) and 5 (patients with primary hyperparathyroidism).

Results with intact PTH assays are relatively independent of renal function and are not influenced by excessive amounts of accumulated hormone fragments [65], unlike results with some RIAs for midregion or C-terminal PTH fragments. However, Lepage *et al.* [66] have shown that when serum from healthy individuals and uremic patients was fractionated by HPLC, two immunoreactive peaks could be detected by the Nichols two-site intact PTH assay. One peak was shown to comigrate with synthetic PTH(1–84), and a second, more hydrophilic peak, was shown to accumulate in renal failure and accounted for 40–60% of the total immunoreactivity in these patients, compared with 10–20% in healthy individuals. This large interfering fragment might be PTH(7–84).

B. Parathyroid Hormone-Related Protein (PTHrP)

Hypercalcemia is a frequent complication of many types of malignancies. The humoral form of the syndrome (HHM, humoral hypercalcemia of malignancy) shares several biochemical features with primary hyperparathyroidism (pHPT). This led to the successful isolation and purification of PTHrP from various human tumors and the cloning of cDNA from a lung tumor cell line. The aminoterminal end of PTHrP shows a sequence homology to the aminoterminal biologically active end of PTH, with eight of 13 amino acid residues being identical. *In vitro*, the amino-terminal fragment of PTHrP (residues 1–34) and PTH(1–34), the sequence which is responsible for most known biological effects of PTH, have a very similar biological activity on bone and kidney. PTHrP

TABLE IV. Current Methodology for the Measurement of PTHrP

Author et al.	Year	Ref.	Method	Antibodies against	Sensit. pmol/l	Elevated (%)	Elevated (n/n)
Budayr	1989	67	RIA	(1–34)	1.7	55	36/65
						71	30/42 ST
Kao	1990	67	RIA	(1–34)	1–2	47	17/36
						53	10/19 ST
Henderson	1990	67	RIA	(1–34)	8	50	19/38
						52	15/29 ST
Burtis	1990	67	RIA	(109–138)	2	100	30/30
			IRMA	(1–36)/(37–74)	1	83	25/30
Grill	1991	67	RIA	(1–40)	2	100	27/27 ST
						64	11/17 BM
Ratcliffe	1991	67	RIA	(1–34)	12	3	1/30
			RIA	(37–67)	57	7	2/31
			IRMA	(1–34)/(37–67)	0.23	100	31/31
Ratcliffe	1991	67	IRMA	(1–34)/(37–67)	0.23	95	35/37
Bucht	1992	68	RIA	(63–77)	8.4	58	11/19
Pandian	1992	69	IRMA*	(1–36)/(37–74)	0.1	91	42/46 ST
Blind	1993	70	RIA	(53–84)	5	69	11/16 ST
			IRMA*	(1–40)/(60–72)	0.3	44	7/16 ST
Fraser	1993	71	IRMA*	(1–40)/(60–72)	0.7	46	44/95
Ikeda	1994	72	IRMA	(1–34)/(50–83)	0.5	100	46/46 ST
Dominguez	1996	73	IRMA*	(1–40)/(60–72)	0.3	100	6/6 ST
Gao	1997	74	ILMA	(1–34)/(53–84)	0.2	89	40/45 ST
INCSTAR**	1998		IRMA	(1–40)/(57–80)	0.2		

ST, solid tumors; BM, bone metastases; *, Test produced by Nichols Institute, San Juan Capistrano, CA; **, Test produced by INCSTAR Corporation, Stillwater, MN; data from the package insert. For references up to 1991, see [67].

mRNA isolated from several tissues encoded PTHrP proteins of different length between 139 and 173 amino acids with an identical common sequence. It is now believed that PTHrP plays a major pathogenetic role in more than 75% of cases of HHM (see also Chapter 14).

1. IMMUNOASSAYS FOR PTHrP

The introduction of PTH assays specific for the intact hormone has facilitated the differential diagnosis of hypercalcemia. Immunoassays of PTHrP, however, further improve this differentiation. In addition, increased interest in measurements of PTHrP in the circulation arose from the possible role of PTHrP as a tumor marker in normocalcemic malignancy and its possible hormonal function in physiology. Because the known biological activity of PTHrP is restricted to its amino-terminal part, most immunoassays were directed against PTHrP(1–34), (1–37), or (1–40), or larger fragments that contain PTHrP(1–34). Direct radioimmunoassays for amino-terminal PTHrP were, however, often not sensitive enough to detect the very low concentrations occurring in healthy persons and some of the patients with HHM. This situation resembles the difficulties with assays

for amino-terminal PTH. Initially, radioimmunoassays were developed for the sequences PTHrP(1–34), (1–37), (1–40), (37–67), (53–84), and (109–138). Later, immunoradiometric assays (IRMA), immunoluminometric assays (ILMA), and other two-site sandwich assays with better sensitivity and specificity were developed. The different approaches used to measure PTHrP are summarized in Table IV [67–74] (for references up to 1991, see [67]).

a. Radioimmunoassays for PTHrP Ratcliffe et al. [67] produced several monoclonal antibodies to PTHrP(1–34) using PTHrP coupled to bovine thyroglobulin as antigen. For use as a tracer, [Tyr⁰]-PTHrP(1–34) was radioiodinated with ¹²⁵I. None of the antibodies cross-reacted with PTH(1–34), and inhibition studies with peptide subfragments of PTHrP (1–34) indicated that all recognize a central region extending from residues 9–18 to between residues 23 and 34. In addition, the lack of cross-reaction of the monoclonal antisera with PTH(1–34) suggested that the binding sites were not at the extreme N-terminus where homology with PTH is greatest. All antibodies tested cross-reacted with native PTHrP in cell culture fluids from human keratinocytes and squamous cancer cell lines. Very high concentrations of PTHrP (80 μg/l) were detected in human and bovine milk. This result suggests that human and bovine PTHrP are similar. A polyclonal antiserum raised to the same conjugate exhibited even higher avidity than the monoclonal antisera. The avidity of the monoclonal antibodies was not sufficiently high to allow direct measurement of PTHrP in serum. However, they were used to extract PTHrP from 5 to 10 ml of serum prior to measurement by radioimmunoassay.

Ratcliffe *et al.* [67] reported in 1991 that direct radioimmunoassays for PTHrP(1–34) and for PTHrP(37–67) were not able to discriminate between patients with HHM, pHPT, and control subjects. In contrast, after affinity extraction of 5 ml of plasma, the radioimmunoassay for PTHrP(1–34) separated patients with HHM (high) from healthy controls (low) and patients with pHPT (low). Bucht *et al.* [68] developed a radioimmunoassay for PTHrP(63–77) which took five days of incubation to achieve a sensitivity of 8.4 pmol/l. Normal persons were undetectable, and 14 of 19 patients with HHM had measurable levels ranging from 8.4 to 145 pmol/l. The levels of PTHrP(63–77) were increased in renal failure.

b. Two-Site Immunometric Assays for PTHrP. A two-site IRMA [67] showed undetectable (<0.23 pmol/l) levels of PTHrP in control subjects and in patients with pHPT and significantly increased concentrations in patients with HHM (mean 6.1 pmol/l, range 0.46–26.5 pmol/l). This two-site IRMA used a mouse monoclonal antibody to PTHrP(1–34) coupled to cellulose particles for immunoextraction of N-terminal immunoreactivity and a rabbit antiserum to PTHrP(37–67) that is indirectly labeled with ^{125}I-PTHrP(37–67) for quantifying the bound analyte. For the purpose of comparison, this assay is designated in this paper as PTHrP(1–67). As a standard, PTHrP(1–86) was used. In chronic renal failure and normocalcemic malignancy, plasma concentrations of PTHrP(1–67) were below or close to the detection limit of the assay.

The high values obtained by direct radioimmunoassays, intermediate values with the extracted radioimmunoassays, and relatively low values with the IRMA suggest that the radioimmunoassays cross-react with circulating immunoreactive species, whereas the IRMA has highly restricted cross-reactivity.

Burtis *et al.* [67] developed an IRMA directed toward PTHrP(1–74) and a radioimmunoassay directed toward PTHrP(109–138). Sixty normal subjects had low or undetectable plasma PTHrP(1–74) concentrations (mean, 1.9 pmol/l) and undetectable PTHrP(109–138) concentrations (<2.0 pmol/l). Patients with HHM had elevated levels of both PTHrP(1–74) (mean 20.9 pmol/l) and PTHrP(109–138) (mean 23.9 pmol/l). The plasma concentrations of both PTHrP assays correlated with the levels of urinary cyclic AMP excreted. In some patients, the concentrations decreased after the tumors were resected. Patients with chronic renal failure had plasma PTHrP(1–74) concentrations similar to those of the normal subjects, but their plasma PTHrP(109–138) concentrations were elevated (mean 29.6 pmol/l). The levels of both peptides were normal in patients with pHPT and in those with hypercalcemia due to various other causes. An anti-PTHrP(1–36) immunoaffinity column failed to extract PTHrP(109–138) immunoactivity from plasma, suggesting that the C-terminal region circulates as a separate peptide.

Blind *et al.* [70] developed a radioimmunoassay for PTHrP (53–84), which cross-reacts with PTHrP(1–86) but not with the shorter synthetic peptides PTHrP(38–64) and PTHrP(67–86). Synthetic human PTHrP(1–86) was used as a standard and for tracer preparation. The assay has a detection limit of 5 pmol/l with a normal range of less than 5–21 pmol/l. Radioimmunoassays for PTHrP(1–34), (1–37), (1–40), (53–84), (63–77), and (109–138) are often not sensitive enough to detect PTHrP in healthy persons, often exhibiting higher normal levels than two-site IRMAs and increased peptide concentrations in renal failure. Therefore, for clinical use in patients with HHM and for the differentiation of hypercalcemia, only IRMAs or other two-site assays should be used. These are more sensitive, more specific, and are not influenced by kidney function.

2. PREANALYTICAL CONSIDERATIONS

A careful investigation on the stability of endogenous PTHrP in blood, serum, or plasma using a immunoradiometric assay has shown that correct sample handling is extremely important [75]. When blood was separated within 15 min of collection, PTHrP levels in serum and heparinized plasma were significantly lower than in EDTA plasma. PTHrP was unstable in blood kept at 20°C for four hours, and inclusion of protease inhibitors reduced, but failed to abolish, this instability. In blood collected in the presence of EDTA, inclusion of leupeptin either alone or in combination with pepstatin and aprotinin increased the mean half-time of disappearance from 3.9 to 10.1 and 11.2 hours, respectively. In contrast, when blood containing EDTA was separated within 15 min, PTHrP was stable in plasma at 20°C for at least four hours. As a result of the instability of PTHrP immunoreactivity in whole blood at ambient temperatures, blood collected in EDTA should be separated within 15 min and the plasma frozen until assay. Gao *et al.* [74] obtained similar results for the stability of PTHrP in EDTA plasma. As a general rule, peptides (like PTH, ACTH, PTHrP) are more stable in EDTA plasma than in serum.

3. NORMAL RANGE

Most normal persons have undetectable concentrations of PTHrP even with the two-site assays. Ratcliffe *et al.* [67] found a normal range below 0.24 pmol/l, Pandian *et al.* [69] below 1.5 pmol/l, Fraser *et al.* [71] below 2.6 pmol/l, and Gao *et al.* [74] below 1.0 pmol/l. Because levels in most normal persons are not measurable, nothing is known about circadian, seasonal, or menstrual variation. Increased levels are observed during pregnancy and lactation [76].

III. VITAMIN D AND VITAMIN D METABOLITES

A. Measurement of Vitamin D$_2$ (Ergocalciferol) and Vitamin D$_3$ (Cholecalciferol)

Determination of the serum concentrations of the native vitamins D$_2$ and D$_3$ only provides information about recent exposure to either nutritional vitamin D or to UV radiation. Within hours, vitamin D is removed from the circulation and reappears again a few hours later as 25(OH)D (calcidiol, see next section). Measurements of the native forms of vitamin D are therefore not useful for assessing the human vitamin D status. They have, however, application in evaluating the vitamin content of natural or vitamin D-enriched foods or pharmaceutical products.

B. Measurement of 25-hydroxyvitamin D

For several reasons, 25-hydroxyvitamin D (25(OH)D) is the ideal parameter to indicate the access of the organism to vitamin D: vitamin D is rapidly transformed into 25(OH)D, the product is mainly confined to the extracellular compartment and is tightly bound to vitamin D-binding protein (DBP), and it has a very long half-life in blood. Indeed, many data in animals and humans have shown that plasma levels of 25(OH)D are the best markers of imminent or existing vitamin D deficiency. Moreover, 25(OH)D, being the vitamin D metabolite with the highest serum concentration, is relatively easy to measure. In most countries, 25(OH)D$_2$ constitutes less than 10% and 25(OH)D$_3$ more than 90% of the total 25(OH)D concentration. This is because vitamin D is mostly produced by UV radiation, which yields vitamin D$_3$, and vitamin D$_2$ containing drugs are less used than vitamin D$_3$ preparations (see also Chapter 15).

1. CURRENT ASSAY TECHNOLOGY

Many techniques are available for the measurement of 25(OH)D. These techniques include the original competitive protein-binding assay (using DBP as binding protein and ^{3}H-25(OH)D as tracer), radioimmunoassays using tritiated 25(OH)D or iodinated analogs of vitamin D as tracers, high-performance liquid chromatography (HPLC), and mass spectrometry after extensive purification (Table V) [77–84]. The techniques for the determination of 25(OH)D all agree fairly well with each other and, in fact, confirm the earlier estimates of the total "vitamin D" content of serum using a

bioassay in which serum extracts were given to D-deficient animals and growth plate characteristics were measured as end points. Some assays for 25(OH)D, however, do not use proper extraction techniques prior to the assay and some "matrix" components of serum (probably lipids) may then interfere with the assay results, giving rise to spuriously elevated values. Falsely elevated values have been reported for assays with ethanol extraction [77, 79].

In addition, when DBP is used as a binding protein, several vitamin D metabolites will compete for the same single binding site so that other metabolites besides 25(OH)D will be measured. This especially applies to 24,25(OH)$_2$D and 25,26(OH)$_2$D, which normally circulate in blood in a relatively fixed ratio (roughly 10% and 2%, respectively) with 25(OH)D, so that without purification prior to the assay, a mild overestimation of the total 25(OH)D content will be obtained. This small overestimation (20%) is, however, of little clinical importance in view of the wide biological range of normal 25(OH)D levels and therefore hampers in no way the clinical benefit of such nonchromatographic assays, when at least nonspecific interference by serum matrix components has been excluded.

We compared different detergents for use in the radioimmunoassay for 25(OH)D and confirmed the results of Kobayashi [81]: polyvinylalcohol (PVA) increased the binding and solubility of 25(OH)D better than the detergents Tween, Triton, or Brij. Therefore, *we* use PVA in the radioimmunoassay for 25(OH)D. However, in our scintillation proximity assay (SPA) system (radioimmunoassay without separation), the differences are less pronounced compared to the DASP separation system of Kobayashi [81]. *We* use antibodies against 1,25-dihydroxyvitamin D highly cross-reacting for 25(OH)D and the Amersham SPA system. The SPA system consists of a second antibody tagged with a fluorophore which only emits light if tritium decays nearby (that is ^{3}H-25(OH)D decaying at the first antibody). Table V shows that there has been a trend to use acetonitrile for extraction. In addition, there is a trend to use gelatin as a stabilizing agent according to Toss [77]. Furthermore, combining gelatin and PVA in the assay buffer is recommended. Dextrane-coated charcoal separation is often replaced by second antibody separation or the Amersham SPA system, a method which omits the separation step.

Table VI [85–90] gives an overview of chromatographic methods for determination of 25(OH)D.

In addition to the automated HPLC method of Schöneshöfer (Table VI), Quesada [91] published a continuous cleanup/preconcentration procedure of hydroxyvitamin D$_3$ metabolites in plasma [91] that may be coupled on-line with an HPLC with a UV detector. Therefore, it is now possible to set up a totally automated HPLC system. By the introduction of fluorescence or electrochemical detection, the amount of serum necessary for the measurement of 25(OH)D has decreased from

TABLE V. Overview of Competitive Protein-Binding Assays (Using Vitamin D-Binding Protein as Binding Protein and ^{3}H-25(OH)D as Tracer), Radioimmunoassays Using Tritiated 25(OH)D, or Iodinated Analogs of Vitamin D as Tracers

Author	Year	Extraction	Chroma-tography	Binding protein	Incubation time	°C	Vol. ml	Recovery %	Solubilizing agents	Separation/ Detection
Belsey	1971	C/MeOH	SA	D(−)RS	days		0.8	75–85	LP (human)	LP Precip.
Haddad	1971	Ether	SA	KC	1 h	RT	1.1	64.1	7% EtOH	DCC
Bayard	1972	C/MeOH	TLC	D(−)HS	14 + 4 h	4°C	1.0	20–25	2% EtOH	Florisil
Edelstein	1974	C/MeOH	LH 20	D(−)RS	30 min	RT	1.1	80	7% EtOH	DCC
Preece	1974	C/MeOH	SA	D(−)RS	16 h	4°C	0.5	90	2% EtOH	DCC
Belsey	1974	EtOH	–	D(−)RS	2 h		1.0	95–100	1% EtOH	DCC
Offermann	1974	EtOH	–	KC	1 h	4°C	1.0	97–100	1% EtOH	DCC
Bouillon	1976	D/MeOH	LH 20	D(−)RS	1 h	0°C	1.0	82	8% EtOH, LP	DCC
Shimotsuji	1976	C/MeOH	LH 20	D(−)RS	30 min		1.0	91.6	6.5% EtOH	DCC
Justova	1976	N/MeOH/T	–	D(−)HS	2 h	4°C	1.5	95–110	1.3% EtOH	DCC
Pettifor	1976	EtOH	–	D(−)RS	3 h	4°C	1.0	96–102	1% EtOH	DCC
Garcia-P	1976	EtOH	–	D(−)RS	2 h	4°C	1.0	91	9% EtOH	DCC
Morris	1976	EtOH	–	D(−)HS	2 h	4°C	1.0	83	10% EtOH	DCC
Ellis	1977	EtOH	SA	HS	1.5 + 1 h		1.0	n.d.	10% EtOH Triton X-405	DCC
Mason	1977	EtOH	SA	KC	2 h	4°C	2.46	95.3	6.1% EtOH	DCC
Schmidt-Gayk	1977	EtOH	–	D(−)RS	1 h	0°C	1.07	90	6.5% EtOH	DCC
Aksnes	1978	C/MeOH	SA	D(−)HS	3 h	0°C	1.1	80	10% EtOH 2% PVA	DCC
Delvin	1980	Ether	SA	BAG	1 h	4°C	1.07	90.1	7% EtOH	DCC
Keck	1981	D/MeOH	HPLC	D(−)KC	2 h	RT	1.1	50	4.5% EtOH	DCC
Toss	1981	D/MeOH	LH 20	D(−)RS	1 h	4°C	1.28	n.d.	6.2% EtOH 1.7% Gelatin	DCC
Lambert	1981	MeOH/ MeCl$_2$	Lipidex + HPLC	RS	2 h	0−5°C		no data 86.3	0.1% bovine serum albumin	DCC
Wood	1983	EtOH	–	rabbitS	2 h	4°C	0.57	n.d.	12.3% EtOH	DCC
Hummer	1984	Acetonitrile	Sep-Pak	Ab	20 h	4°C	0.55	94–115	4.5% EtOH	DCC
Bothe	1984	Acetonitrile	–	rabbitS	1 h	4°C	0.435	92	8% Acetonitrile 0.2% Gelatin	DCC
Bouillon	1984	EtOH	–	D(−)RS	1 h	4°C	0.55	101–103	9.1% EtOH 0.01% Ovalb.	DCC : false high!*
		CYH/EA	–	D(−)RS	1 h	4°C	0.55	105 ± 1	,,	DCC
		CYH/EA	–	Ab	1 h	4°C	0.55	105 ± 1	,,	DCC
Prószynska	1985	Extrelut	–	D(−)RS	2−20 h	4°C	0.57	99–108	12.3% EtOH	DCC
Hollis	1985	Acetonitrile	–	Ab	2 h	4°C	0.55	108	9.1% EtOH 0.04% Gelatin	DAB
Shephard [78]	1987	Acetonitrile	SP C18	D(−)RS	days		0.8	83.5	LP (human)	LP Precip.
Dean [79]	1988	C/MeOH	SP C18	D(−)RS	2 h	4°C	1.0	102	1% EtOH	DCC**
Fuchs [80]	1991	Acetonitrile	–	D(−)HS	1 + 1 h	4°C	0.46	92	0.005% T20 0.2% Gelatin	DAB
Kobayashi [81]	1992			Ab	4.5 h	4°C	0.25	85	1% PVA 0.1% Gelatin	DASP
Kobayashi [82]	1993	C/MeOH	IAC	Ab	4 h	4°C	0.225	81.2	1% PVA 0.1% Gelatin	EIA
Hollis [83]	1993	Acetonitrile	–	Ab	90 min	RT	1.075	85–115	≅5% EtOH 0.04% Gelatin	DAB

continued

| Author | Year | Extraction | Chroma-tography | Binding protein | Incubation | | | Recovery % | Solubilizing agents | Separation/Detection |
					time	°C	Vol. ml			
INCSTAR [84]	1993	Acetonitrile		Ab	90 min	RT	1.075	85–115	,,	DAB
Schmidt-Gayk this paper	1998	Acetonitrile	–	Ab	12 h	RT	0.32	92	0.01% PVA 0.1% Gelatin	SPA

Abbreviations: Ab, antibody; BAG, bovine α_1-globulin fraction; CYH/EA, cyclohexane/ethylacetate; C, chloroform (CHCl$_3$); D, dichloromethane (CH$_2$Cl$_2$); D(−), vitamin D deficient serum; DAB, double antibody separation; DASP, double antibody solid phase; DCC, dextran-coated charcoal; EIA, enzyme immunoassay; EtOH, ethanol; HPLC, high-performance liquid chromatography; HS, human serum; KC, kidney cytosol, rat kidney cytosol***; LH 20, Sephadex LH 20 column chromatography; LP, lipoprotein; MeOH, methanol; MeCl$_2$, methylene chloride; N, ammoniumsulfate (NH$_4$)$_2$SO$_4$; Ovalb, ovalbumin; PVA, polyvinyl alcohol, MW 2000; rabbitS, rabbit serum; RS, rat serum; RT, room temperature; SA, silicic acid; SPA, scintillation proximity assay; SP C18, Sep-Pak C$_{18}$; TLC, thin layer chromatography; T20, Tween 20. *, Falsely high results after ethanol precipitation (extraction) if no chromatography is included. **, Falsely high results after ethanol precipitation (extraction) if no chromatography is included. Rat kidney cytosol (KC) was used in some assays as binding protein. However, this contains more or less serum with vitamin D-binding protein (DBP), and this might be the effective protein. (For references before 1987, see [77].)

about 500 μl with UV absorption methods to 200 μl with fluorescence detection to 20 μl with electrochemical detection [88]. Further information on assays for vitamin D metabolites can be obtained from the reviews by Bouillon [92], Porteous [93], Ohyama [94] and Schmidt-Gayk [77, 95, 96].

2. STANDARDIZATION OF ASSAYS

1 mol/l of vitamin D metabolites yields an absorption of 16,500 at 254 nm and of 18,300 at 265 nm wavelength. For pure standard solutions in ethanol it is recommended to prepare a concentration of 100 μmol/l and to check absorbance in a quartz glass cuvette in a spectrophotometer (it should be 1.83 at 265 nm). Alternatively, a concentration of 25 μmol/l is prepared, the absorbance of which should be 0.458 at 265 nm. These stock solutions are then further diluted to the desired concentrations of standard solutions.

3. NORMAL RANGE OF 25-HYDROXYVITAMIN D IN SERUM OR PLASMA

As far as normal 25(OH)D ranges are concerned, marked seasonal variation, geographical influences, and methodological issues have to be taken into account (Table VII) [97]. For example, using nonchromatographic competitive protein-binding assays, we adopted as a normal range for the southwest of Germany (Heidelberg) 50–250 nmol/l for the summer and 25–125 nmol/l for the winter.

With the introduction of 25(OH)D assays, it became evident that low levels of this metabolite are quite frequent in many populations when vitamin D supplementation of food is not the rule and sun exposure is relatively low for climatic or cultural reasons. To define subclinical vitamin D deficiency, Bouillon *et al.* [98] have proposed the use of a vitamin D challenge test. This test is considered positive if, in the absence of histological or biochemical signs of vitamin D deficiency, a rapid increase in serum 1,25(OH)$_2$D$_3$ is observed after supplementation with physiological amounts of vitamin

D or 25(OH)D. In addition, in studies of ultraviolet light irradiation, Mawer and co-workers [100] found 1,25(OH)$_2$D$_3$ increases of more than 5 ng/l if the starting level of 25(OH)D was below 20 ng/ml (50 nmol/l).

Serum or plasma levels of 25(OH)D below 5 ng/ml are usually considered severe vitamin D deficiency. Values between 6 and 10 ng/ml should be diagnosed as mild vitamin D deficiency, and between 11 and 20 ng/ml as a suboptimal supply by which bone and mineral homeostasis can be reasonably maintained through adaptive mechanisms (i.e., increased renal 1-alpha-hydroxylation, mild secondary hyperparathyroidism). The amounts of 20–100 ng/ml (50–250 nmol/l) of 25(OH)D are regarded as optimal levels.

4. SEASONAL VARIATION

A study of the vitamin D supply of 2889 apparently healthy, independently living German women aged 35 to 75 years showed that more than 25% of the participants had suboptimal vitamin D supply (<20 ng/ml = <50 nmol/l) during the winter months (October to May). About 5% had vitamin D deficiency (levels below 10 ng/ml [25 nmol/l]), as shown in Figure 6A.

Guillemant and co-workers [101] noted that in healthy young men in France, low levels of 25(OH)D in March were accompanied by elevations in the level of intact PTH. Higher levels of 25(OH)D in September yielded lower levels of intact PTH compared to March. In contrast to the seasonal variation of 25(OH)D and intact PTH, there was no seasonal variation of 1,25(OH)$_2$D$_3$ (mean concentration 37.7 ng/l in September and 38.2 ng/l in March) [101]. These data suggest that low levels of 25(OH)D in the winter months result in decreased intestinal calcium absorption with mild secondary hyperparathyroidism [103], which in turn stimulates the renal 1-alpha-hydroxylase to keep 1,25(OH)$_2$D$_3$ in the normal range.

It has been observed that even in the United States, with the availability of vitamin D fortified milk (400 IU/l),

TABLE VI. Overview of Chromatographic Methods for the Determination of 25(OH)D

Author	Ref.	Year	Method	Extraction	Column	Solvents	Gradient	Recovery %	Detection
Lambert	[77]	1977	LH20 HPLC	MeOH/MeCl$_2$	C18	MeOH/water	–	88	UV
Eisman	[77]	1977	HPLC	MeOH/chloroform	SA	hexane/ isopropanol	–	72.2	UV
Gilbertson	[77]	1977	HPLC	Chloroform/MeOH	SA	EtOH/hexane	–	95	UV
Schaefer	[77]	1978	LH20 HPLC	MeOH/MeCl$_2$	SA	isopropanol/ MeCl$_2$	–	no data	UV
Jones	[77]	1978	HPLC	MeOH/chloroform	(1) SA (2) C18	iso/hexane MeOH/H$_2$O	–	89.1	UV
Shepard	[77]	1979	LH20 L5000 HPLC	MeOH/MeCl$_2$	SA	hexane/ isopropanol	–	74.4	UV
Dabek	[77]	1981	HPLC	SP C18	SA	hexane/ isopropanol	–	93	UV
Parviainen	[77]	1981	2x LH20 HPLC	MeOH/chloroform	SA	hexane/ isopropanol	–	68.8	UV
Trafford	[77]	1981	L5000 2 HPLC runs	EtOH	SA	hexane/ isopropanol	–	91.2–104.5	UV
Turnbull	[77]	1982	HPLC	Acetonitrile SP C18	SA	hexane/ isopropanol	–	54.9	UV
Norris	[77]	1986	HPLC	SP C18	(1) SA (2) C18	hexane/iso MeOH/H$_2$O	–	50	UV
Mawer	[77]	1987	HPLC	Acetonitrile	SA	hexane/ isopropanol	–	70.1	UV
Lindbäck	[77]	1987	HPLC	Acetonitrile	C18	MeOH/water	–	no data	MS
Iwata	[77]	1990	HPLC	C18	C8	Acetonitrile/ NaCl 0.2 M	(1) 80:20 (2) 85:15	76.9	Fluorescence
Mayer	[85]	1990	LH20 HPLC	MeOH/MeCl$_2$	SA	hexane/ isopropanol	–	77	UV
Aksnes	[86]	1992	HPLC	MeOH/iso/hexane	C18	MeOH/water	–	−85.3	UV
Shimizu	[87]	1992	SP Sil HPLC	MeOH/MeCl$_2$	SA	MeOH/MeCl$_2$	–	57.4	Fluorescence
Masuda	[88]	1997	HPLC	MeOH/MeCl$_2$	SA	hexane/ isopropanol	–	no data	EC
Takeuchi	[89]	1997	BEC18OH BEC18 HPLC		SA		–		UV
Schöneshöfer	[90]	1998	HPLC, automated	MeOH	RP	Acetonitrile/ pH 2 buffer	–	−95	UV

Abbreviations: as in Table I, additionally BEC18OH, Bond Elut C18OH; BEC18, Bond Elut C18; EC electrochemical detection; iso, isopropanol; LH20, Sephadex LH 20 chromatography; L5000, Lipidex 5000 chromatography; MeCl$_2$, methylene chloride, dichloromethane; MS, mass spectrometry; RP, reverse phase; SP Sil, Sep Pak silica cartridge; UV, ultraviolet absorption. (For references before 1990, see [77].)

hypovitaminosis D is common in March and in September in general medical inpatients, including those with vitamin D intakes exceeding the recommended daily amount and those without apparent risk factors for vitamin D deficiency [104]. Of 290 consecutive patients on a general medical ward, 164 patients (57%) were considered to be vitamin D-deficient (25(OH)D below 15 ng/ml [37.5 nmol/l]), of whom 65 (22%) were considered severely vitamin D-deficient (25(OH)D below 8 ng/ml [20 nmol/l]). A total of 63% of the patients studied in March and 49% of those studied in September had serum 25(OH)D concentrations of 15 ng/ml or less.

5. INCREASED LEVELS OF 25-HYDROXYVITAMIN D

Vitamin D intoxication with vitamin D$_3$ or D$_2$ yields high levels of 25(OH)D, whereas intoxication with dihydrotachysterol or 5,6-trans-25-hydroxyvitamin D is not detected by the assays for 25(OH)D. Assays employing vitamin D binding protein (DBP) as the binding protein normally recognize 25(OH)D$_3$ and 25(OH)D$_2$ equally well. Most cases of vitamin D intoxication occur as a consequence of large intakes of pharmaceutical preparations of vitamin D. In the past, standard high dose vitamin D prophylaxis was in some

TABLE VII.   Normal Range of 25-Hydroxyvitamin D (25(OH)D) in Serum

Author	Year	n	Country	Range (nmol/l)	Mean (±SD)	Remarks
Bayard	1972	18	France	25–60	38	
Belsey	1974	15	USA	50–250	88	
Bouillon	1976	51	Belgium		33 ± 10	May
Bothe	1990	37	Germany	15–270	109	Sep.
		46		<8–120	30	Dec.–Jan.
Dabek	1981	10	Finland	20–120	30	Nov.–May
		16		33–120	64	May–Oct., HPLC
Edelstein	1974	18	England		38 ± 14	Chromatography
Garcia-Pasqual	1976	18	Switzerland	62–153	100 ± 24	
Gilbertson	1977	24	USA	14–60	38 ± 13	Feb., HPLC
Haddad	1971	40	USA	28–138	68 ± 27	May and Jun.
Hollis	1985	50	USA		65 ± 28	HPLC
Jones	1978	25	Canada	23–60	40 ± 10	Dec., HPLC
Justova	1976	30	Czechoslovakia	50–105	72 ± 13	May–Sep.
Keck	1981	17	Germany		30 ± 15	Oct., HPLC + CPBA
					8.2 ± 2.3	Apr.
Lambert	1977	10	USA, MN		63 ± 5	Sep., HPLC
Mason	1977	?	Australia	33–110	72 ± 20	Fall season
Morris	1976	35	England	13–181	67	Nov.–Dec., 20–40 y
		15		0–104	27	May–Jun., 65–75 y
Nayer	1977	11	Belgium	40–93	58 ± 17	
Offermann	1974	50	Germany		90 ± 42	
Parviainen	1981	16	Finland		55 ± 12	Oct.–Nov., HPLC
Pettifor	1976	286	South Africa		77 ± 25	Children 1–18 y
Preece	1974	38	England	10–55	30 ± 14	Adults, early winter
		14		10–50	28 ± 12	Children, early winter
Stryd	1979	10	USA, MI	20–60	33 ± 15	Jan., HPLC
		10		52–117	78 ± 25	Jun., HPLC
Trafford	1981	11	England		60 ± 28	Aug., HPLC
Turnbull	1982	24	England		50 ± 19	Apr.–Jul., HPLC

Note: For references see Bothe and Schmidt-Gayk [97].

countries used in infants (e.g., four oral doses of 15 mg = 600,000 IU), which may lead to hypercalcemia, hypercalciuria, and nephrocalcinosis in susceptible infants.

C. Measurement of 1,25-Dihydroxyvitamin D (1,25(OH)₂D, Calcitriol)

The conversion of 25(OH)D to $1,25(OH)_2D$ was initially thought to be exclusively limited to the kidney (distal tubular cells of the nephron), and this origin remains the main source of circulating $1,25(OH)_2D$ even now that other cells seem to be able to produce the same metabolite [73]. Other cells or tissues have been shown to produce $1,25(OH)_2D$ *in vitro*, such as bone cells, intestine, and white blood cells. It is doubtful that these tissues actually contribute to the circulating $1,25(OH)_2D$ level because in acute situations after bilateral nephrectomy, no radioactive $1,25(OH)_2D_3$ can be detected after injection of its labeled precursor. Low levels, however, can be found in anephric subjects loaded chronically with sufficient precursor vitamin D.

Plasma levels of $1,25(OH)_2D$ (calcitriol) depend mainly on renal function, the levels of intact PTH, and the supply to the organism of calcium and phosphate. Among the other hormones, only growth hormone and IGF I have well-documented stimulatory effects, whereas the effects of other hormonal and humoral factors are disputed or limited to some lower species. As for other vitamin D metabolites, $1,25(OH)_2D$ is tightly bound to the serum vitamin D-binding protein and probably only the free hormone is available for cellular entry, receptor occupation, and therefore biological activity. This hypothesis, like that concerning other free

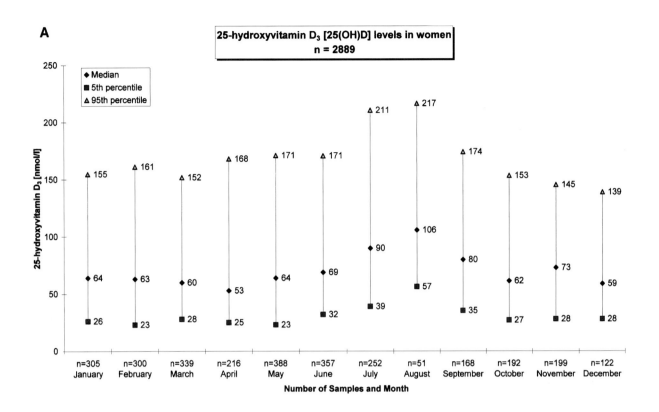

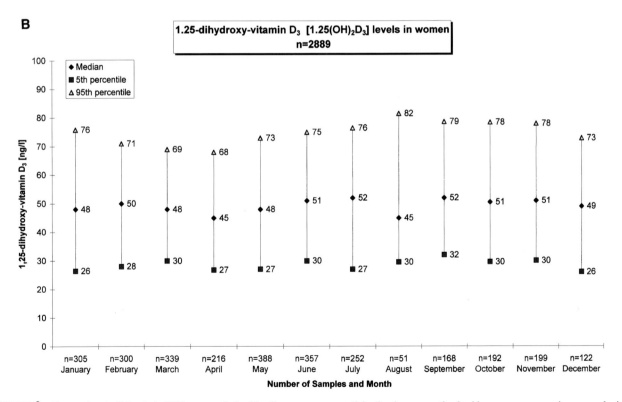

FIGURE 6   Serum vitamin D levels in 2889 apparently healthy German women participating in a preventive health program or a routine gynecological investigation. (A) 25(OH)D levels, and (B) 1,25(OH)$_2$HD$_3$ levels.

Table VIII.   Overview of the Published Techniques for the Measurement of Calcitriol

Author	Year	Ref.	Extraction	Purification	Serum, ml	Assay	x ± SD range ng/l	Sens. ng/l or pg/vial	Separation
Brumbaugh	1974	95	MeOH/C	SA, LH20, Celite	20	D(−)CIMRRA	39 ± 8		Filter
Eisman	1976	95	$MeCl_2$	LH20, HPLC	5	D(−)CIMRRA	29	10	PEG
Clemens	1978	95	$MeCl_2$	LH20, HPLC	10–20	RIA	35	20 pg	DCC
Björkhem	1979	95	C/MeOH	LH20, HPLC, RP-HPLC	20	ID-MF	55 ± 10	5	
Clemens	1979	95	$MeCl_2$	LH20, HPLC	10	RIA	41	10	DCC
O'Riordan	1979	95	$MeCl_2$	LH20, HPLC	5–10	RIA	41 ± 2.5	10	DCC
Taylor	1979	95	$MeCl_2$	LH20, HPLC	5	D(−)CIMRRA	33 ± 14	2.6 pg	DCC
Bouillon	1980	95	CYH/EA	LH20, HPLC	5	RIA	38	3–4	DCC
Peacock	1980	95	Acetone/$MeCl_2$	LH20, HPLC	5	RIA D(−)CIMRRA	44.2	7.2 2.6	DCC DCC
Mallon	1980	95	$MeCl_2$/MeOH	LH20	2–5	D(−)CIMRRA	31.3	1.5	PEG
Stern	1980	95	isopropylether	HPLC	1	Bioassay, ^{45}Ca release	33 ± 6	2	–
Gray	1981	95	MeOH/C	LH20, HPLC	2	RIA	57	10	DCC
Dokoh	1981	95	Clin Elut (DE)	HPLC	0.5	D(−)CIMRRA	55 ± 13	1	DCC
Jongen	1981	95	n-hexane/iso/ n-butanol	HPLC	5	NCIMRRA	52 ± 11	1–2 pg	DCC
Dabek	1981	95	MeOH/C	LH20	5	D(−)CIMRRA	42 ± 14	4–5 pg	PEG
Parviainen	1981	95	hexane/iso	RP-HPLC	2–3	D(−)CIMRRA	children	1 pg	DCC
Imawari	1982	95	MeOH/ ethylacetate	LH20, HPLC	2	CIMRRA	37 ± 11 26–62	2	DCC
Manolagas	1982	95	Clin Elut (DE)	–	1–2	cytoreceptor (intact cells)	34 ± 11	2	–
Duncan	1983	95	diethylether	SA, HPLC	2–3	normal rabbit IMRRA	35 ± 11	1 pg	DCC
Rhodes (extraction)	1983	95	acetonitrile	SPC_{18}, HPLC	2	not assayed			
Fraher	1983	95	acetonitrile	SPC_{18}, HPLC	2	RIA	42 20–65	2	DCC
Gray	1983	95	ethyl acetate/ cyclohexane	HPLC	3	RIA	38 m 31 f	5	DCC
Scharla	1984	95	Extrelut-1	HPLC	1	RIA 25 yr elderly 77 yr	55 ± 12 32 ± 12	3	DCC
Reinhardt	1984	95	acetonitrile	SPC_{18}, SPSA	0.2–1	CTCRRA	37	1.5 pg	DCC
Kao	1984	95	HCl/MeOH	BEC_{18}, $BENH_2$	3	D(−)CIMRRA	25 ± 7	<5	PEG
Nicholson	1985	95	Clin Elut (DE)	SA column		cytoreceptor (intact cells)	39 ± 10	1 pg	–
De Leenheer	1985	95	benzene	HPLC	1.5	RIA	52 ± 15	5	DCC
De Leenheer	1985	95	benzene	HPLC	1.5	NCIMRRA	54 ± 31	5	DCC
Hummer	1985	95	$MeCl_2$/MeOH	LH20, HPLC	3–5	RIA RRA	62 ± 16 35 ± 4	1.6 pg 2.6 pg	DCC DCC
Blayau	1986	95	MeOH/$MeCl_3$	SPC_{18}, HPLC	2	BMGRRA	50 39–69	5.8	DCC
Hollis	1986	95	acetonitrile	(a) BEC_{18}, or (b) $BEC_{18}OH$	0.5–1	CTCRRA,NE	28 ± 11	0.7 pg	DCC
Hartwell	1988	95	$MeCl_2$/MeOH	LH20, HPLC	3–5	CTCRRA D(−)CIMRRA	38 38	1.5 pg 6.7 pg	DCC

continues

continued

Author	Year	Ref.	Extraction	Purification	Serum, ml	Assay	$x \pm SD$ range ng/l	Sens. ng/l or pg/vial	Separation
Jongen	1988	95	acetonitrile	SPC_{18}, HPLC	4	NCIMRRA	52 ± 11	1–2 pg	DCC
Oftebro	1988	95	diethylether	SPC_{18}, SPSA	2	CTCRRA	42 ± 10	4	DCC
					20	GC-MS-SIM	45 ± 7	2.5	–
Armbruster	1990	95	Extrelut-1	HPLC	1	RIA, 20–34 yr	63	3.75	DAB
Mawer	1990	106	acetonitrile	SPC_{18}, HPLC	1–3	RIA	35	1.25 pg	DCC
Koyama	1992	107	$MeCl_2$	SPSA	0.5	PIMRRA,NE	37 ± 11	0.45 pg	ABSP
Wildermuth	1993	108	Extrelut-1	SPSA	0.5	RIA	32–80	2.7	SPA
Watanabe	1994	109	acetonitrile	$BEC_{18}OH$	1	BMGRRA	–	0.5 pg	DCC
Wei	1994	110	acetonitrile	$BEC_{18}OH$	0.5–1	BMGRRA	30–70	0.5 pg	DCC
Withold "Gamma-B"	1995	111	immunoextraction, kit	–	0.3–0.5	RIA, ^{125}I-tracer	39 19–74	3	DASP
Hollis	1996	112	acetonitrile	$BEC_{18}OH$, silica cartridge	0.5	RIA, ^{125}I-tracer	16–56	2.4	DAB
Kobayashi	1997	113	Chem Elut column	immunosorbent	0.5	RRA	36 ± 10		DCC
Takeuchi	1997	114	acetonitrile	$BEC_{18}OH$	0.5	CTCRRA		1.25 pg	DCC

Abbreviations: ABSP, antibody solid phase; $BEC_{18}OH$, Bond Elut $C_{18}OH$ cartridge; BMGRRA, bovine mammary gland, RRA; C, chloroform ($CHCl_3$); CIMRRA, chicken intestinal mucosa RRA; CTCRRA, calf thymus cytosol RRA; D(−), vitamin D deficient; DAB, double antibody separation; DASP, double antibody solid phase; DCC, dextran-coated charcoal; HPLC, high-performance liquid chromatography; ID-MF, isotope dilution-mass fragmentography; LH 20, Sephadex LH 20 column chromatography; MeOH, methanol; $MeCl_2$, methylene chloride, dichloromethane; NCIMRRA, normal chicken intestinal mucosa RRA; PEG, polyethyleneglycol; PIMRRA, pig intestinal mucosa RRA; RIA, radioimmunoassay; RRA, radioreceptorassay; SA, silicic acid; SPA, scintillation proximity assay; SPC_{18}, Sep-Pak C_{18} cartridge; SPSA, Sep Pak silicic acid cartridge. For references before 1990 see Schmidt-Gayk *et al.* [95].

steroid and thyroid hormones, is based both on clinical and on experimental observations (see also Chapter 15).

1. CURRENT ASSAY TECHNOLOGY

Many different calcitriol measurements have been published. Some of them are rather imprecise, as an international laboratory comparison study has shown [78]. Reference levels also varied greatly due to differences in extraction, purification, quantitation, and separation, but also to the use of different solvents and detergents. Table VIII [106–114] gives an overview of the published calcitriol measurement techniques.

As shown in Table VIII, there is a trend towards the use of acetonitrile or solid phases for extraction, and immunoextraction is employed in a commercial kit and by scientific groups. In addition, there is a trend to use bovine mammary gland for the receptor, which can be prepared in large amounts (more than 100,000 assays from one mammary gland) and which is very specific and sensitive. In radioimmunoassays, there is a trend to use antisera against $1,25(OH)_2D_3$ conjugated via the side chain (carbon 25, O'Riordan) or carbon 11 (Kobayashi). In the assay buffer, gelatin often is used as a stabilizing agent, as in the assay of 25(OH)D according to Toss (cited in Bothe and Schmidt-Gayk [97]). Furthermore, it is recommended to combine gelatin and a detergent in very low concentrations (Triton X-100, 0.0001% [v/v]) in the assay buffer to improve

the solubility of calcitriol. In addition, kits with ^{125}I-labeled tracer are available. With the Amersham scintillation proximity assay system, a separation step is no longer necessary.

2. BIOLOGICAL VARIATION

While seasonal variations in serum 25(OH)D are rather obvious, such changes are often absent in $1,25(OH)_2D$ levels [69, 75]. Results from our own studies, including 2889 apparently healthy German women aged 35–75 years, are shown in Figure 6B.

Minor alterations of $1,25(OH)_2D$ are observed across the menstrual cycle. Thus, serum levels of $1,25(OH)_2D$ are slightly higher during the luteal phase compared with the early follicular phase [116]. Hormone replacement therapy (HRT) increases $1,25(OH)_2D$ slightly within the normal range from about 130 to 150 pmol/l (52 to 60 ng/l, mean values) [117]. Alterations caused by HRT may be caused by alterations in the concentrations of DBP.

Acknowledgments

The support of Dr. Eberhard Blind, Würzburg, Germany; Prof. Roger Bouillon, Leuven, Belgium; Dr. Klaus Herfarth, Heidelberg, Germany; and Hans-Jürgen Roth, Heidelberg, Germany, is gratefully acknowledged.

References

1. Schmidt-Gayk, H., and Thomas, L. (1992). Mineralhaushalt und Neben-schilddrüse, Harnsteine. *In* "Labor und Diagnose" (L. Thomas, ed.), pp. 341–386. Die Medizinische Verlagsgesellschaft, Marburg.

2. Cali, J. P., Bowers, G. N., Jr., and Young, D. S. (1973). A referee method for the determination of total calcium in serum. *Clin. Chem.* **19**, 1208–1213.

3. Welch, M. W., Hamar, D. W., and Fettman, M. J. (1990). Method comparison for calcium determination by flame atomic absorption spectrophotometry in the presence of phosphate. *Clin. Chem.* **36**, 351–354.

4. Corns, C. M., and Ludman, C. J. (1987). Some observations on the nature of the calciumcresolphthalein complexone reaction and its relevance to the clinical laboratory. *Ann. Clin. Biochem.* **24**, 345–351.

5. Janssen, J. W., and Helbing, A. R. (1991). Arsenazo III: An improvement of the routine calcium determination in serum. *Eur. J. Clin. Chem. Clin. Biochem.* **34**, 197–201.

6. Walmsley, T. A., and Fowler, R. T. (1981). Optimum use of 8-hydroxyquinoline in plasma calcium determinations. *Clin. Chem.* **27**, 1782.

7. Kayamori, Y., and Katayama, Y. (1994). Enzymatic method for assaying calcium in serum and urine with porcine pancreatic (-amylase. *Clin. Chem.* **40**, 781–784.

8. Buckley, B. M., and Russell, L. J. (1988). The measurement of ionised calcium in blood plasma. *Ann. Clin. Biochem.* **25**, 447–465.

9. Vanstapel, F. J., and Lissens, W. D. (1984). Free ionised calcium—a critical survey. *Ann. Clin. Biochem.* **21**, 339–351.

10. Bowers, G. N., Jr., Brassard, C., and Sena, S. F. (1986). Measurement of ionized calcium in serum with ion-selective electrodes: A mature technology that can meet the daily service needs. *Clin. Chem.* **32**, 1437–1447.

11. Gowans, E. M. S., and Fraser, C. G. (1986). Five methods for determining urinary calcium compared. *Clin. Chem.* **32**, 1560–1562.

12. Henry, J. B. (1996). Analytical techniques. *In* "Clinical Diagnosis and Management by Laboratory Methods" (J. B. Henry, ed.), 19th ed. Saunders, Philadelphia.

13. Lyon, M. E., Guajardo, M., Laha, T., Malik, S., Henderson, P. J., and Kenny, M. A. (1995). Electrolyte balanced heparin may produce a bias in the measurement of ionized calcium concentration in specimens with abnormally low protein concentration. *Clin. Chim. Acta* **233**, 105–113.

14. Mann, S. W., Buckley, B. M., Roberts, K. D., and Green, A. (1988). Changes in plasma ionised calcium concentration during pediatric cardiopulmonary bypass surgery. *Ann. Clin. Biochem.* **25**, 226–227.

15. Kost, G. J., Jammal, M. A., Ward, R. E., and Safwat, A. M. (1986). Monitoring of ionized calcium during human hepatic transplantation. *Am. J. Clin. Pathol.* **86**, 61–70.

16. Ladenson, J. H., Lewis, J. W., McDonald, J. M., Slatopolsky E., and Boyd, J. C. (1978). Relationship of free and total calcium in hypercalcemic conditions. *J. Clin. Endocrinol. Metab.* **48**, 393–397.

17. Gawosky, J. M., and Walsh, D. (1989). Citrate interference in assays of total calcium in serum. *Clin. Chem.* **35**, 2140–2141.

18. John, R., Oleesky, D., Issa, B., Scanlon, M. F., Williams, C. P., Harrison, C. B., and Child, D. F. (1997). Pseudohypercalcemia in two patients with IgM paraproteinaemia. *Ann. Clin. Biochem.* **34**, 694–696.

19. Husdan, H., Rapoport, A., Locke, S., and Oreopoulos, D. (1974). Effect of venous occlusion of the arm on the concentration of calcium in serum, and methods for its compensation. *Clin. Chem.* **20**, 529–532.

20. Husdan, H., Rapoport, A., and Locke, S. (1973). Influence of posture on the serum concentration of calcium. *Metab. Clin. Exp.* **22**, 788–797.

21. Parfitt, A. M. (1969). Chlorothiazide-induced hypercalcemia in juvenile osteoporosis and hyperparathyroidism. *N. Engl. J. Med.* **281**, 55–59.

22. Payne, R. B., Little, A. J., Williams, R. B., and Milner, J. R. (1973). Interpretation of serum calcium in patients with abnormal serum proteins. *Br. Med. J.* **4**, 643–646.

23. Pedersen, K. O. (1972). On the cause and degree of intraindividual serum calcium variability. *Scand. J. Clin. Lab. Invest.* **30**, 191–199.

24. Kaiser, C., Müller, H. A. G., Schmitt, Y., Geisen, H. P., and Schott, F. J. (1994). Should reference values for calcium be revised? *Klin. Lab.* **40**, 599–602.

25. Herfarth, K., Drechsler, S., Imhoff, W., Schlander, M., Engelbach, M., Maier, A., and Schmidt-Gayk, H. (1992). Calcium regulating hormones after oral and intravenous calcium administration. *Eur. J. Clin. Chem. Clin. Biochem.* **30**, 815–822.

26. Ljunghall, S., Hedstrand, H., Hellsing, K., and Wibell, L. (1977). Calcium, phosphate and albumin in serum. *Acta Med. Scand.* **201**, 23–30.

27. Schmidt-Gayk, H. (1992). Urinary calcium. *Klin. Lab.* **38**, 614–615.

28. Coe, F. L., Parks, J. H., and Moore, E. S. (1979). Familial idiopathic hypercalciuria. *N. Engl. J. Med.* **300**, 337–340.

29. Min, H. K., Jones, J. E., and Flink, E. B. (1966). Circadian variations in renal excretion of magnesium, calcium, phosphorus, sodium, and potassium during frequent feeding and fasting. *Fed. Proc.* **25**, 917–921.

30. Wisser, H., Doerr, P., Stamm, D., Fatranska, M., Giedke, H., and Wever, R. (1973). Circadian rhythm of electrolytes, catecholamines and 17-hydroxycorticosteroids in urine. *Klin. Wochenschr.* **51**, 242–246.

31. Robertson, W. G., Gallagher, J. C., Marshall, D. H., Peacock, M., and Nordin, B. E. C. (1974). Seasonal variations in urinary excretion of calcium. *Br. Med. J.* **4**, 436–437.

32. Massey, L. K., and Whiting, S. J. (1996). Dietary salt, urinary calcium, and bone loss. *J. Bone Miner. Res.* **11**, 731–736.

33. Hess, B., Ackermann, D., Essig, M., Takkinen, R., and Jaeger, P. (1995). Renal mass and serum calcitriol in male idiopathic calcium renal stone formers: Role of protein intake. *J. Clin. Endocrinol. Metab.* **80**, 1916–1921.

34. Hess, B., Hasler-Strub, U., Ackermann, D., and Jaeger, P. (1997). Metabolic evaluation of patients with recurrent idiopathic calcium nephrolithiasis. *Nephrol. Dial. Transplant.* **12**, 1362–1368.

35. Crook, M., and Swaminathan, R. (1996). Disorders of plasma phosphate and indications for its measurement. *Ann. Clin. Biochem.* **33**, 376–396.

36. Savory, D. J., and Pearce, C. J. (1995). Paraprotein interference causing pseudohyperphosphataemia: Evaluation of an improved methodology. *Ann. Clin. Biochem.* **32**, 498–501.

37. Cohen, A. M., Magazanik, A., van-der Lijn, E., Shaked, P., and Levinsky, H. (1994). Pseudohyperphosphataemia incidence in an automatic analyzer. *Eur. J. Clin. Chem. Clin. Biochem.* **32**, 559–561.

38. Bowles, S. A., Tait, R. C., Jefferson, S. G., Gilleece, M. H., and Haeney, M. R. (1994). Characteristics of monoclonal immunoglobulins that interfere with serum inorganic phosphate measurement. *Ann. Clin. Biochem.* **31**, 249–254.

39. Zimmermann, K., Jenckel-Loss, G., Fiedler, H., and Weber, R. (1993). Evaluation of enzymatic phosphate determination in comparison with the molybdenum blue method. *Klin. Lab.* **39**, 777–780.

40. Cherian, A. G., and Hill, J. G. (1978). Percentile estimates of reference values for fourteen chemical constituents in sera of children and adolescents. *Am. J. Clin. Pathol.* **69**, 24–31.

41. Kemp, G. J., Blumsohn, A., and Morris, B. W. (1992). Cellular phosphate shifts during oral glucose loading. *Clin. Chem.* **38**, 2338–2339.

42. Markowitz, M., Rotkin, L., and Rosen, J. F. (1981). Circadian rhythms of blood minerals in humans. *Science* **213**, 672–674.

43. Fraser, W. D., Logue, F. C., Christie, J. P., Cameron, D. A., O'Reilly, D. St. J., and Beastell, G. H. (1994). Alteration of the circadian rhythm of intact parathyroid hormone following a 96-hour fast. *Clin. Endocrinol.* **40**, 523–528.

44. Ring, T., Sanden, A. K., Hansen, H. H. T., Halkier, P., Nielsen, C., and Fog, L. (1995). Ultradian variation in serum phosphate concentration in patients on haemodialysis. *Nephrol. Dial. Transplant.* **10**, 59–63.

45. Kemp, G. J., Blumsohn, A., and Morris, B. W. (1992). Circadian changes

in plasma phosphate concentration, urinary phosphate excretion, and cellular phosphate shifts. *Clin. Chem.* **38**, 400–402.

46. Walton, R. J., and Bijvoet, O. L. M. (1975). Nomogram for derivation of renal threshold phosphate concentration. *Lancet* **2**, 309–310.

47. Martin, K. J., Hruska, K. A., Freitag, J. J., Klahr, S., and Slatopolsky, E. (1979). The peripheral metabolism of parathyroid hormone. *N. Engl. J. Med.* **301**, 1092–1098.

48. Klein, G. L., Enures, D. B., Colonna, J. D., Berquist, W. E., Goldstein, L. I., Busuttil, R. W., and Deftos, L. J. (1989). Absence of hyperparathyroidism in severe liver disease. *Calcif. Tissue Int.* **44**, 330–334.

49. Klee, G. G., Preissner, C. M., Schryver, P. G., Taylor, R. L., and Kao, P. C. (1992). Multisite immunochemiluminometric assay for simultaneously measuring whole-molecule and amino-terminal fragments of human parathyrin. *Clin. Chem.* **38**, 628–635.

50. Gao, P., Schmidt-Gayk, H., Dittrich, K., Nolting, B., Maier, A., Roth, H. J., Seemann, O., Reichel, H., Ritz, E., and Schilling T. (1996). Immunochemiluminometric assay with two monoclonal antibodies against the N-terminal sequence of human parathyroid hormone. *Clin. Chim. Acta* **245**, 39–59.

51. Hock, D., Mägerlein, M., Heine, G., Ochlich, P. P., and Forssmann, W.-G. (1997). Isolation and characterization of the bioactive circulating human parathyroid hormone, hPTH-1-37. *FEBS Lett.* **400**, 221–225.

52. Brasier, A. R., Wang, C. A., and Nussbaum, S. R. (1988). Recovery of parathyroid hormone secretion after parathyroid adenomectomy. *J. Clin. Endocrinol. Metab.* **66**, 495–500.

53. Schmidt-Gayk, H., Schmitt-Fiebig, M., Hitzler, W., Armbruster, F. P., and Mayer, E. (1986). Two homologous radioimmunoassays for parathyrin compared and applied to disorders of calcium metabolism. *Clin. Chem.* **32**, 57–62.

54. Armitage, E. K. (1986). Parathyrin (parathyroid hormone): Metabolism and methods for assay. *Clin. Chem.* **32**, 418–424.

55. Blind, E., Schmidt-Gayk, H., Armbruster, F. P., and Stadler, A. (1987). Measurement of intact human parathyrin by an extracting two-site immunoradiometric assay. *Clin. Chem.* **33**, 1376–1381.

56. Brown, R. C., Aston, J. R., Weeks, I., and Woodhead, J. S. (1987). Circulating intact parathyroid hormone measured by a two-site immunochemiluminometric assay. *J. Clin. Endocrinol. Metab.* **65**, 407–414.

57. Nussbaum, S. R., Zahradnik, R. J., Lavigne, J. R., Brennan, G. L., Nozawa-Ung, K., Kim, L. Y., Keutmann, H. T., Wang, C. A., Potts, J. T., Jr., and Segré, G. V. (1987). Highly sensitive two-site immunoradiometric assay of parathyrin, and its clinical utility in evaluating patients with hypercalcemia. *Clin. Chem.* **33**, 1364–1367.

58. Blind, E., Schmidt-Gayk, H., Scharla, S., Flentje, D., Fischer, S., Göhring, U., and Hitzler, W. (1988). Two-site assay of intact parathyroid hormone in the investigation of primary hyperparathyroidism and other disorders of calcium metabolism compared with a midregion assay. *J. Clin. Endocrinol. Metab.* **67**, 353–360.

59. Bouillon, R., Coopmans, W., De Groote, D. E., Radoux, D., and Eliard, P. H. (1990). Immunoradiometric assay of parathyrin with polyclonal and monoclonal region-specific antibodies. *Clin. Chem.* **36**, 271–276.

60. Ratcliffe, W. A., Heath, D. A., Ryan, M., and Jones, S. R. (1989). Performance and diagnostic application of a two-site immunoradiometric assay for parathyrin in serum. *Clin. Chem.* **35**, 1957–1961.

61. Landin-Wilhelmsen, K., Wilhelmsen, L., Lappas, G., Rosen, T., Lindstedt, G., Lundberg, P. A., Wilske, J., and Bengtsson, B. A. (1995). Serum intact parathyroid hormone in a random population sample of men and women: Relationship to anthropometry, life-style factors, blood pressure, and vitamin D. *Calcif. Tissue Int.* **56**, 104–108.

62. Shaw, N. J., Wheeldon, J., and Brocklebank, J. T. (1990). Indices of intact serum parathyroid hormone and renal excretion of calcium, phosphate, and magnesium. *Arch. Dis. Child.* **65**, 1208–1211.

63. Levin, G. E., and Nisbet, J. A. (1994). Stability of parathyroid hormone-related protein and parathyroid hormone at room temperature. *Ann. Clin. Biochem.* **31**, 497–500.

64. Prank, K., Nowlan, S. J., Harms, H. M., Kloppstech, M., Brabant, G., Hesch, R. D., and Sejnowski, T. J. (1995). Time series prediction of plasma hormone concentration. Evidence for differences in predictability of parathyroid hormone secretion between osteoporotic patients and normal controls. *J. Clin. Invest.* **95**, 2910–2919.

65. Blind, E., Raue, F., Reichel, H., and Schmidt-Gayk, H. (1992). Validity of intact plasma parathyrin measurements in chronic renal failure as determined by two-site immunoradiometric assays with N- or C-terminal capture antibodies. *Clin. Chem.* **38**, 2345–2347.

66. Lepage, R., Roy, L., Brossard, J.-H., Rousseau, L., Dorais, C., Lazure, C., and D'Amour, P. (1998). A non-(1–84) circulating parathyroid hormone (PTH) fragment interferes significantly with intact PTH commercial assay measurements in uremic samples. *Clin. Chem.* **44**, 805–809.

67. Ratcliffe, W. A., Norbury, S., Stott, R. A., Heath, D. A., and Ratcliffe, J. G. (1991). Immunoreactivity of plasma parathyrin-related peptide: Three region-specific radioimmunoassays and a two-site immunoradiometric assay compared. *Clin. Chem.* **37**, 1781–1787.

68. Bucht, E., Eklund, A., Toss, G., Lewensohn, R., Granberg, B., Sjöstedt, U., Eddeland R., and Torring, O. (1992). Parathyroid hormone-related peptide, measured by a midmolecule radioimmunoassay, in various hypercalcemic and normocalcemic conditions. *Acta Endocrinol.* **127**, 294–300.

69. Pandian, M. R., Morgan, C. H., Carlton, E., and Segré, G. V. (1992). Modified immunoradiometric assay of parathyroid hormone-related protein: Clinical application in the differential diagnosis of hypercalcemia. *Clin. Chem.* **38**, 282–288.

70. Blind, E., Raue, F., Meinel, T., Bucher, M., Manegold, C., Ebert, W., Vogt-Moykopf, I., and Ziegler, R. (1993). Levels of parathyroid hormone-related protein in hypercalcemia of malignancy: Comparison of midregional radioimmunoassay and two-site immunoradiometric assay. *Clin. Invest.* **71**, 31–36.

71. Fraser, W. D., Robinson, J., Lawton, R., Durham, B., Gallacher, S. J., Boyle, I. T., Beastall, G. H., and Logue, F. C. (1993). Clinical and laboratory studies of a new immunoradiometric assay of parathyroid hormone-related protein. *Clin. Chem.* **39**, 414–419.

72. Ikeda, K., Ohno, H., Hane, M., Yokoi, H., Okada, M., Honma, T., Yamada, A., Tatsumi, Y., Tanaka, T., Saito, T., Hirose, S., Mori, S., Takeuchi, Y., Fukumoto, S., Terukina, S., Iguchi, H., Kiriyama, T., Ogata, E., and Matsumoto, T. (1994). Development of a sensitive two-site immunoradiometric assay for parathyroid hormone-related peptide: Evidence for elevated levels in plasma from patients with adult T-cell leukemia/lymphoma and B-cell lymphoma. *J. Clin. Endocrinol. Metab.* **79**, 1322–1327.

73. Dominguez, A. S., Olivie, M. A. A., Sousa, T. R., Alvarez, M. L. T., Perez, D. R., Novoa, R. A., and Garcia-Mayor, R. V. G. (1996). Plasma parathyroid hormone-related protein levels in patients with cancer, normocalcemic and hypercalcemic. *Clin. Chim. Acta* **244**, 163–172.

74. Gao, P., Eberle, A. M., and Schmidt-Gayk, H. (1997). One-step two-site immunochemiluminometric assay for parathyroid hormone-related protein. *In* "Calcium Regulating Hormones and Markers of Bone Metabolism: Measurement and Interpretation" (H. Schmidt-Gayk, E. Blind, and H.-J. Roth, eds.), 2nd ed., pp. 79–83. Clin. Lab. Publications, Heidelberg.

75. Hutchesson, A. C. J., Hughes, S. V., Bowden, S. J., and Ratcliffe, W. A. (1994). In vitro stability of endogenous parathyroid hormone-related protein in blood and plasma. *Ann. Clin. Biochem.* **31**, 35–39.

76. Lippuner, K., Zehnder, H.-J., Casez, J.-P., Takkinen, R., and Jaeger, P. (1996). PTH-related protein is released into the mother's bloodstream during lactation: Evidence for beneficial effects on maternal calcium-phosphate metabolism. *J. Bone Miner. Res.* **11**, 1394–1399.

77. Schmidt-Gayk, H., Armbruster, F. P., and Bouillon, R., eds. (1990). "Calcium Regulating Hormones, Vitamin D Metabolites, and Cyclic AMP. Assays and their Clinical Application." Springer-Verlag, Berlin.

78. Shephard, G. S., Carlini, S. M., Hanekom, C., and Labadarios, D. (1987). Analysis of 25-hydroxyvitamin D in plasma using solid phase extraction. *Clin. Chim. Acta* **167**, 231–236.

79. Dean, B., Kolavcic, M. S., Wark, J. D., and Harrison, L. C. (1988). Chromatography of serum on Sep-pak C18 corrects falsely elevated vitamin D metabolite levels measured by protein binding assay. *Clin. Chim. Acta* **176**, 169–178.

80. Fuchs, D., Zahn, I., Roth, H.-J., and Schmidt-Gayk, H. (1991). Improved competitive protein binding assay (CPBA) with second antibody separation for the diagnosis of hyper- and hypovitaminosis D. *9th Workshop on Vitam. D*, Paris, Abstr., p. 240.

81. Kobayashi, N., Ueda, K., and Shimada, K. (1992). Evaluation of solubilizing agents for 25-hydroxyvitamin D_3 immunoassays. *Clin. Chim. Acta* **209**, 83–88.

82. Kobayashi, N., Ueda, K.,Tsutsumi, M., Tabata, Y., and Shimada, K. (1993). Enzyme immunoassay for plasma 25-hydroxyvitamin D_3 employing immunoaffinity chromatography as a pretreatment method. *J. Steroid Biochem. Mol. Biol.* **44**, 93–100.

83. Hollis, B. W., Kamerud, J. Q., Selvaag, S. R., Lorenz, J. D., and Napoli, J. L. (1993). Determination of vitamin D status by radioimmunoassay with an ^{125}I-labeled tracer. *Clin. Chem.* **39**, 529–533.

84. INCSTAR (1993). Package insert given by the manufacturer.

85. Mayer, E., and Schmidt-Gayk, H. (1990). Simultaneous determination of 25-hydroxyvitamin D_2 and 25-hydroxyvitamin D_3 by high-performance liquid chromatography. *In* "Calcium Regulating Hormones, Vitamin D Metabolites, and Cylic AMP. Assays and their Clinical Application" (H. Schmidt-Gayk, F. P. Armbruster, and R. Bouillon, eds.), pp. 247–257. Springer-Verlag, Berlin.

86. Aksnes, L. (1992). A simplified high-performance liquid chromatographic method for determination of vitamin D_3, 25-hydroxyvitamin D_2 and 25-hydroxyvitamin D_3 in human serum. *Scand. J. Clin. Lab. Invest.* **52**, 177–182.

87. Shimizu, M., Gao, Y., Aso, T., Nakatsu, K., and Yamada, S. (1992). Fluorometric assay of 25-hydroxyvitamin D_3 and 24R,25-dihydroxyvitamin D_3 in plasma. *Anal. Biochem.* **204**, 258–264.

88. Masuda, S., Okano, T., Kamao, M., Kanedai, Y., and Kobayashi, T. (1997). A novel high-performance liquid chromatographic assay for vitamin D metabolites using a coulometric electrochemical detector. *J. Pharm. Biomed. Anal.* **15**, 1497–1502.

89. Takeuchi, A., Ishida, Y., Sekimoto, H., Masuda, S., Okano, T., Nishiyama, S., Matsuda, I., and Kobayashi, T. (1997). Simplified method for the determination of 25-hydroxy and 1,25-dihydroxy metabolites of vitamins D_2 and and D_3 in human plasma. Application to nutritional studies. *J. Chromatogr. B* **691**, 313–319.

90. Schöneshöfer, M., Zolchow, S., and Seipelt, P. (1997). Routine method for the specific determination of serum 25-hydroxycholecalciferol (calcidiol) levels using the liquid-chromatographic ALCATM-system. *Clin. Lab.* **43**, 985–991.

91. Quesada, J. M., Ortiz-Boyer, F., Fernández-Romero, J. M., and Luque de Castro, M. D. (1997). Continuous cleanup/preconcentration procedure of hydroxyvitamin D_3 metabolites in plasma. *In* "Vitamin D, Chemistry, Biology and Clinical Applications of the Steroid Hormone" (A. W. Norman, R. Bouillon, and M. Thomasset, eds.), pp. 739–740. Printing and Reprographics, University of California, Riverside.

92. Bouillon, R. (1983). Radiochemical assays for vitamin D metabolites: Technical possibilities and clinical applications. *J. Steroid Biochem.* **19**, 921–927.

93. Porteous, C. E., Coldwell, R. D., Trafford, D. J. H., and Makin, H. L. J. (1987). Recent developments in the measurement of vitamin D and its metabolites in human body fluids. *J. Steroid Biochem.* **28**, 785–801.

94. Ohyama, Y., Hayashi, S., Usui, E., Noshiro, M., and Okuda, K. (1997). Assay of vitamin D derivatives and purification of vitamin D hydroxylases. *In* "Methods in Enzymol 021" (D. B. McCormick, J. W. Suttle, and C. Wagner, eds.), Vol. 282, pp. 186–199. Academic Press, San Diego, CA.

95. Schmidt-Gayk, H., Blind, E., and Roth, H. J., eds. (1997). "Measurement and Interpretation of Calcium Regulating Hormones and Markers of Bone Metabolism," 2nd ed. Clin. Lab. Publications, Heidelberg.

96. Schmidt-Gayk, H., Bouillon, R., and Roth, H. J., (1997). "Measurement of vitamin D and its metabolites (calcidiol and calcitriol) and their clinical significance. *Scand. J. Clin. Lab. Invest.* **57** (Suppl. 227), 35–45.

97. Bothe, V., and Schmidt-Gayk, H. (1990). Competitive protein-binding assay for the diagnosis of hyper- and hypovitaminosis D. *In* "Calcium Regulating Hormones, Vitamin D Metabolites, and Cyclic AMP: Assays and their Clinical Application" (H. Schmidt-Gayk, F. P. Armbruster, and R. Bouillon, eds.), pp. 258–279. Springer-Verlag, Berlin.

98. Bouillon, R. A., Auwerx, J. H., Lissens, W. D., and Pelemans, W. K. (1987). Vitamin D status in the elderly: Seasonal substrate deficiency causes 1,25-dihydroxycholecalciferol deficiency. *Am. J. Clin. Nutr.* **45**, 755–763.

99. Peacock, M., Selby, P. L., Francis, R. M., Brown, W. B., and Hordon, L. (1985). Vitamin D deficiency, insufficiency, sufficiency and intoxication. What do they mean? *In* "Vitamin D. A Chemical, Biochemical and Clinical Update," pp. 569–570. de Gruyter, Berlin and New York.

100. Mawer, E. B., Berry, J. L., Sommer-Tsilenis, E., Beykirch, W., Kuhlwein, A., and Rohde, B. T. (1984). Ultraviolet irradiation increases serum 1,25-dihydroxyvitamin D in vitamin-D-replete adults. *Mine. Electrolyte Metab.* **10**, 117–121.

101. Guillemant, J., Cabrol, S., Allemandou, A., Peres, G., and Guillemant, S. (1995). Vitamin D-dependent seasonal variation of PTH in growing male adolescents. *Bone* **17**, 513–516.

102. Clements, M. R., Johnson, L., and Fraser, D. R. (1987). A new mechanism for induced vitamin D deficiency in calcium deprivation. *Nature* **325**, 62–65.

103. Chapuy, M. C., Schott, A. M., Garnero, P., Hans, D., Delmas, P. D., and Meunier, P. J., and EPIDOS Study Group. (1996). Healthy elderly French women living at home have secondary hyperparathyroidism and high bone turnover in winter. *J. Clin. Endocrinol. Metab.* **81**, 1129–1133.

104. Thomas, M. K., Lloyd-Jones, D. M., Thadhani, R. I., Shaw, A. C., Deraska, D. J., Kitch, B. T., Vamvakas, E. C., Dick, I. M., Prince, R. L., and Finkelstein, J. S. (1998). Hypovitaminosis D in medical inpatients. *N. Engl. J. Med.* **338**, 777–783.

105. Jongen, M. J. M., van der Vijgh, W. J. F., van Beresteyn, E. C. H., van den Berg, H., Bosch, R., Hoogenboezem, T., Visser, T. J., and Netelenbos, J. C. (1982). Interlaboratory variation of vitamin D metabolite measurements. *J. Clin. Chem. Clin. Biochem.* **20**, 753–756.

106. Mawer, E. B., Berry, J. L., Cundall, J. P., Still, P. E., and White, A. (1990). A sensitive radioimmunoassay using a monoclonal antibody that is equipotent for ercalcitriol and calcitriol (1,25-dihydroxy vitamin D_2 and D_3). *Clin. Chim. Acta* **190**, 199–210.

107. Koyama, H., Prahl, J. M., Uhland, A., Nanjo, M., Inaba, M., Nishizawa, Y., Morii, H., Nishii, Y., and DeLuca, H. F. (1992). A new, highly sensitive assay for 1,25-dihydroxyvitamin D not requiring high-performance liquid chromatography: Application of monoclonal antibody against vitamin D receptor to radioreceptor assay. *Anal. Biochem.* **205**, 213–219.

108. Wildermuth, S., Dittrich, K., Schmidt-Gayk, H., Zahn, I., and O'Riordan, J. L. H. (1993). Scintillation proximity assay for calcitriol in serum without high pressure liquid chromatography. *Clin. Chim. Acta* **220**, 61–70.

109. Watanabe, Y., Kubota, T., Suzumura, E., Suzuki, T., Yonezawa, M., Ishigama, T., Ichikawa, M., and Seino, Y. (1994). 1,25-dihydroxyvitamin D radioreceptor assay using bovine mammary gland receptor and non-high performance liquid chromatographic purification. *Clin. Chim. Acta* **225**, 187–194.

110. Wei, S., Tanaka, H., Kubo, T., Ichikawa, M., and Seino, Y. (1994). A multiple assay for vitamin D metabolites without high-performance liquid chromatography. *Anal. Biochem.* **222**, 359–365.

111. Withold, W., Wolff, T., Degenhardt, S., and Reinauer, H. (1995). Evaluation of a radioimmunoassay for determination of calcitriol in human sera employing a ^{125}I-labelled tracer. *Eur. J. Clin. Chem. Clin. Biochem.* **33**, 959–963.

112. Hollis, B. W., Kamerud, J. Q., Kurkowski, A., Beaulieu, J., and Napoli, J. L. (1996). Quantification of circulating 1,25-dihydroxyvitamin D by radioimmunoassay with an ^{125}I-labeled tracer. *Clin. Chem.* **42**, 586–592.

113. Kobayashi, N., Imazu, T., Kitahori, J., Mano, H., and Shimada, K. (1997). A selective immunoaffinity chromatography for determination of plasma 1α,25-dihydroxyvitamin D_3: application of specific antibodies raised against a 1,25-dihydroxyvitamin D_3-bovine serum albumin conjugate linked through the 11α-position. *Anal. Biochem.* **244**, 374–383.

114. Takeuchi, A., Ishida, Y., Sekimoto, H., Masuda, S., Okano, T., Nishiyama, S., Matsuda, I., Kobayashi, T. (1997). Simplified method for the determination of 25-hydroxy and 1α,25-dihydroxy metabolites of vitamins D_2 and D_3 in human plasma. Application to nutritional studies. *J. Chromatogr. B* **691**, 313–319.

115. Hine, T. J., and Roberts, N. B. (1994). Seasonal variation in serum 25-hydroxy vitamin HD_3 does not affect 1,25-dihydroxy vitamin D. *Ann. Clin. Biochem.* **31**, 31–34.

116. Thys-Jacobs, S., and Alvir, M. A. J. (1995). Calcium-regulating hormones across the menstrual cycle: Evidence of a secondary hyperparathyroidism in women with PMS. *J. Clin. Endocrinol. Metab.* **80**, 2227–2232.

117. van Hoof, H. J. C., van der Mooren, M. J., Swinkels, L. M. J. W., Rolland, R., and Benraad, Th. J. (1994). Hormone replacement therapy increases serum 1,25-dihydroxyvitamin D: A 2-year prospective study. *Calcif. Tissue Int.* **55**, 417–419.

CHAPTER 27

Measurement of Biochemical Markers of Bone Formation

KIM E. NAYLOR AND RICHARD EASTELL

Bone Metabolism Group, Section of Medicine, Division of Clinical Sciences, Northern General Hospital,
The University of Sheffield, S5 7AU Sheffield, United Kingdom

I. ABSTRACT

Biochemical markers of bone formation are measured in serum and each reflects a different stage of osteoblast differentiation. Many assays, both in house and commercial, are available for their measurement. New assays are being developed to improve sensitivity and specificity to bone. It is important to understand the requirements for sample collection and handling for each assay when planning research protocols. It is also beneficial to understand which markers are best suited to provide the information required. This chapter aims to review the current assays available for the measurement of biochemical markers of bone formation and to describe possible sources of variability in those measurements. This includes preanalytical variability, such as that caused by sample collection and storage and the effects of repeat freeze–thaw cycles, and analytical variability, such as that caused by cross-reactivity. There have been reports of discordant results between assays measuring the same analyte; possible reasons for these discrepancies are discussed in this chapter. Also, biological variables, such as age and gender effects, menstrual, circadian, and seasonal variations are considered. The effects of fracture, exercise, and nonbone diseases on biochemical markers of bone formation are also discussed.

II. INTRODUCTION

Biochemical markers of bone formation are measured in serum and reflect osteoblast activity. The biochemical markers of bone formation each reflect a different stage of osteoblast differentiation. During bone formation, the matrix is produced before mineralization occurs; hence the propeptides of type I procollagen are early markers of bone formation, as they are released prior to the synthesis of type I collagen which forms around 90% of bone matrix. Bone alkaline phosphatase is also an early osteoblast marker because it is a cell membrane enzyme present in preosteoblasts and osteoblasts. Osteocalcin is a later marker of osteoblast differentiation; although its exact function is unknown, it has a strong affinity for hydroxyapatite crystals of mineralized bone.

Traditional methods for the assessment of bone turnover have several drawbacks. Imaging techniques such as isotope bone scans require specialized equipment and can not be repeated frequently. Bone biopsies are invasive and only reflect bone turnover in a local area of the skeleton. However, histomorphometry does provide information about cellular activity. Whole body calcium kinetic studies are time consuming and require precise execution. However, these methods do provide a "gold standard" to which new biochemical markers of bone turnover can be compared to validate their utility for clinical use.

A good biochemical marker of bone formation should be specific for bone tissue and reflect only formation and not resorption. It should also correlate to a gold standard method of bone formation measurement. If assays are intended to be used routinely, then it would be preferable if the method was not cumbersome or time consuming and also was relatively inexpensive with readily available reagents.

III. ALKALINE PHOSPHATASE

A. Total Alkaline Phosphatase

Alkaline phosphatase is a membrane-bound enzyme of uncertain function that hydrolyzes phosphate esters (with maximum activity at pH 9). (See also Chapter 9.) Serum total alkaline phosphatase (TAP) is an established marker of bone formation that has been shown to correlate with bone mineralization as measured by calcium kinetic methods [1]. It is generally measured by an automated colorimetric method using paranitrophenyl phosphate. The method is readily available and relatively inexpensive and has good reproducibility. However, TAP is not specific to bone; it is produced by most body tissues, liver being the main nonskeletal source. As a bone formation marker, TAP is useful in detecting dramatic changes in bone turnover, for example in Paget's disease of bone, but is less reliable in identifying subtle changes in bone turnover that occur in osteoporosis [2].

The most common causes of elevated TAP are bone disease (with increased osteoblast activity) or cholestatic liver disease. Total alkaline phosphatase is elevated in severe bone disease, such as Paget's disease of bone, osteomalacia, and metastatic bone disease, but it is not usually elevated in osteoporosis. Because of the occurrence of alkaline phosphatase in nonskeletal tissues, it can be elevated due to various reasons. For example, during the last trimester of pregnancy, alkaline phosphatase activity is elevated due to the placental isoenzyme. Liver disease, such as intra- or extrahepatic cholestasis, can also cause elevated TAP. Elevated TAP can

also be due to malignancy, with bone or liver involvement or direct production by the tumor. A placental-like isoenzyme, Regan, has been identified in patients with malignant disease, particularly in carcinoma of the bronchus. Alkaline phosphatase is decreased in the bone disease hypophosphatasia and in other diseases such as hypothyroidism and coeliac disease, and in patients treated with glucocorticoid therapy. There is seasonal variability in TAP, with lower levels reported in the summer compared to the winter [3].

B. Bone-Specific Alkaline Phosphatase

Due to the contribution of alkaline phosphatase from nonskeletal sources, TAP lacks sensitivity and specificity for measuring bone formation. Circulating TAP consists of several isoenzymes of alkaline phosphatase. Four genes have been identified that code for alkaline phosphatase. The genes that code for germ cell, placental, and intestinal isoforms are on chromosome 2. The tissue nonspecific alkaline phosphatase gene codes for liver, kidney, and bone alkaline phosphatase and is located on chromosome 1 [4]. These isoforms differ by their posttranslational modification which provides a basis for their analytical separation.

There are several techniques that have been adopted to quantify the liver- and bone-specific isoenzymes, including heat inactivation, chemical inhibition, electrophoresis, wheat germ lectin precipitation, and immunoassays [5]. Commercially available assays are listed in Table I. The heat inactivation method utilizes the half-inactivation time of alkaline phosphatase isoenzymes at 56°C [6]. This method of heat inactivation is also used to determine the activity of placental or 'Regan' isoenzymes, because these are more stable at 65°C than bone or liver alkaline phosphatases. Because cross-reactivity can occur with intestinal alkaline phosphatase, it is better to use fasting blood samples for this analysis. Electrophoresis is a suitable separation method because the liver isoform is more negatively charged than the bone isoform. Several methods are available using separation by electrophoresis. However, this technique is generally tedious and quantification is sometimes difficult due to the overlap

TABLE I.   Commercial Assays Available for Measurement of Bone Alkaline Phosphatase

Assay	Manufacturer	Method
Tandem-R Ostase	Hybritech Inc., San Diego, CA	IRMA
Alkphase-B	Metra Biosystems Inc., Mountain View, CA	ELISA
Iso-ALP	Roche Diagnostics, Germany	Wheat germ lectin ppt with colorimetric method

of isoforms. The correlation between some of these methods is not good, possibly due to poor specificity. Electrophoresis allows the accurate quantitation of the various isoforms of alkaline phosphatase with selective inhibition (e.g., with neuraminadase or wheat germ lectin) improving separation [7].

Wheat germ lectin precipitation of the bone isoenzyme is a quick and inexpensive assay for bone alkaline phosphatase (BAP) [8]. Wheat germ lectin preferentially binds to the N-acetylglucosamine residues on the bone isoenzyme. Total enzyme activity is measured in the untreated sample and in the supernatant remaining after wheat germ lectin precipitation, which contains the liver isoenzyme. Hence BAP activity can be calculated by subtraction. A problem with this technique is the variation in affinity of wheat germ lectin for the bone isoenzyme. There can be variation in lectin reactivity even within the same batch. Therefore, it is important to prepare the correct lectin concentration. Cord blood is an ideal standard for the assay because it contains BAP only. The wheat germ lectin precipitation method is not suitable for patients with obstructive liver disease because biliary alkaline phosphatase can precipitate with the bone fraction. Biliary alkaline phosphatase can be converted to the liver isoform by pretreatment of the sample with a detergent such as Triton-X. Wheat germ lectin precipitation can also be incorporated as a pretreatment to electrophoresis to improve resolution [9].

Immunoassays have been developed that utilize monoclonal antibodies. These have been directed at both the liver [10] and the bone isoform [11–14]. These methods provide a rapid and convenient alternative to other measurement methods. Garnero et al. [11] reported that BAP, measured by immunoradiometric assay, was more sensitive than TAP for clinical investigation of patients with metabolic bone disease. A study in patients with metastatic bone disease [15] reported a slight advantage in the measurement of bone over total alkaline phosphatase for monitoring the treatment of patients. Enzyme immunoassays have also been developed that find BAP more sensitive than TAP [12, 13]. These assays showed good correlation with other methods of measuring BAP. Price et al. [16] compared BAP measured by immunometric assay and enzyme immunocapture assay. From studies in children, it was found that the two types of assay appeared to recognize different isoforms. Although the measurement of BAP may be more sensitive than that of TAP, Woitge et al. [17] have raised the issue that TAP provides sufficient diagnostic information for most clinical situations. However, BAP may be more useful if the patient has liver disease or only a small increase in bone turnover (e.g., mild Paget's disease, osteoporosis).

There is no specific patient preparation required for the measurement of BAP. However, if TAP is measured in the procedure, blood samples should be collected after an overnight fast to avoid increased intestinal alkaline phosphatase. Price [18] reported that less than 10% total activity was lost in samples stored at 4°C for 3 days or 3 months at −20°C.

For long term storage, −70°C is recommended. It is also advisable to centrifuge turbid samples or those containing particles prior to assay. The immunoassay kits specify the use of serum. Samples should not be subjected to more than three freeze–thaw cycles. In patients with liver disease, the lipid containing biliary fraction of alkaline phosphatase can be affected by repeat freeze–thaw cycles, which can distort the electrophoretic pattern [18]. If very high levels are found for BAP it is preferable to measure the sample by a second method to rule out liver contribution, or measure other bone formation markers to confirm bone involvement [7].

C. Biological Variability

Alkaline phosphatase is cleared from the blood slowly as it has a half-life of around 40 hours [19]. This results in low day-to-day variability in this biochemical marker. There is a circadian rhythm for the bone isoform which results in diurnal variation of the marker, but this is small and parallels the reduction in serum albumin at night. A seasonal rhythm has been observed for BAP [20]. Serum BAP was significantly higher during the winter months compared to the summer in both men and women. According to Woitge and coworkers [20], seasonal effects explained 12% of the variability of BAP.

Age, sex, and hormonal status all affect alkaline phosphatase levels [7]. In children, BAP correlates with height velocity and weight gain until puberty, when there is a dramatic increase [9]. Studies of the effect of gender in adults have produced conflicting results. Bone alkaline phosphatase is reported to increase after the sixth decade of life in both sexes [21]. There are hormonal effects on BAP as well; it is elevated during the luteal phase of the menstrual cycle [22]. Bone-specific alkaline phosphatase has also been shown to increase during pregnancy, with a peak during the third trimester [23], in comparison to nonpregnant nonlactating controls, and this reflects an increase in bone remodeling. An increase in TAP during pregnancy can also be attributed to the placental isoform.

There is an increase in alkaline phosphatase in high bone-turnover states due to disease or menopausal status. The established methods for BAP measurement, such as electrophoresis, chemical inhibition, and heat inactivation, show only small increases due to osteoporosis, whereas newer methods show increases of a much greater magnitude with respect to age and menopausal status [9].

Fractures are another confounding factor to be considered when measuring biochemical markers of bone turnover. There is a significant increase in TAP of about 30% 2 weeks after tibial shaft fractures [24]. Serum BAP showed an initial decrease during the first 8 weeks following fracture, then a 40% increase by week 10, which was significantly higher than the first day following fracture. Both total and bone alkaline

TABLE II.   Commercial Assays Available for Measurement of Osteocalcin

Assay	Manufacturer	Analyte	Method
Bovine osteocalcin	Biomedical Technologies Inc., Stoughton, MA	intact bovine osteocalcin	RIA
Intact osteocalcin	Biomedical Technologies Inc., Stoughton, MA	intact human osteocalcin	ELISA
Midtact osteocalcin	Biomedical Technologies Inc., Stoughton, MA, USA	intact and N-terminal fragment human osteocalcin	ELISA
LUMItest osteocalcin	BRAHMS, Berlin, Germany	intact human osteocalcin	LIA
OSCAtest osteocalcin	BRAHMS, Berlin, Germany	intact human osteocalcin	RIA
OSTK-PR	CIS Bio International, Gif-sur-Yvette, France	intact bovine osteocalcin	RIA
ELSA-OST-NAT	CIS Bio International, Gif-sur-Yvette, France	intact human osteocalcin	IRMA
ELSA-OSTEO	CIS Bio International, Gif-sur-Yvette, France	intact and N-terminal fragment human osteocalcin	IRMA
Osteocalcin	DAKO, Glostrup, Denmark	intact osteocalcin	ELISA
Osteocalcin	Diagnostic Systems Laboratories, Webster, TX, USA	intact human osteocalcin	RIA
Osteocalcin	Incstar Corp., Stillwater, MN, USA	intact bovine osteocalcin	RIA
N-tact Osteo SP	Incstar Corp., Stillwater, MN, USA	intact osteocalcin	IRMA
Novocalcin	Metra Biosystems, Mountain View, CA, USA	intact bovine osteocalcin	ELISA
Mitsubishi, Yuka BGP IRMA	Yuka Medias Co. Ltd., Tokyo, Japan	intact human osteocalcin	IRMA
Human osteocalcin	Nichols Inst., San Juan Capistrano, CA, USA	intact and fragment human osteocalcin	IRMA
N-MID osteocalcin	Osteometer A/S, Herlev, Denmark	intact and N-terminal fragment human osteocalcin	IRMA
Osteocalcin	Takara Shuzo Co., Otsu, Shiga Japan	undercarboxylated osteocalcin	ELISA

Note: Abbreviations: RIA, radioimmunoassay; ELISA, enzyme linked immunosorbent assay; LIA, luminescence immunoassay.

phosphatase continued to increase during the 20 week study period.

Exercise can also affect bone formation markers. Serum BAP has been reported to increase by about 40% during the first month of resistance exercise training, although this increase was not significant on resting days when compared to baseline values [25]. A study of endurance trained athletes found no difference in BAP in the athletes compared to population-based age- and sex-matched controls [26].

IV. OSTEOCALCIN

A. Assays for Osteocalcin

Osteocalcin is an established, extensively used biochemical marker of bone formation. It is commonly measured by both in house methods and commercial kits with various assay formats [27]. These include high performance liquid chromatography (HPLC), radioimmunoassay (RIA), immunoradiometric assay (IRMA), enzyme linked immunosorbent assay (ELISA), and luminescence immunoassay (LIA). Commercially available assays are listed in Table II. Because bovine osteocalcin exhibits homology with the C-terminal region of human osteocalcin, many assays use antibodies directed against the C-terminal region of the bovine osteocalcin molecule. However, other assays have been developed which utilize antisera directed against human osteocalcin [28–31]. Garnero *et al.* [28] found a human-specific IRMA to be more sensitive than a bovine RIA for the clinical investigation of metabolic bone disease. There have been several reports of discordant results obtained with osteocalcin measured by different laboratories using similar methods [32] and also different assay formats [33, 34]. This has resulted in conflicting

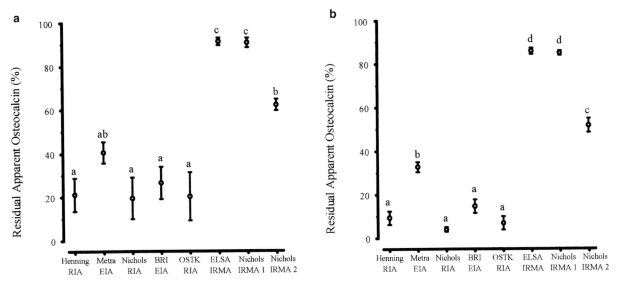

FIGURE 1   Effect of sample storage at (a) 4°C for 2 weeks and (b) at 4°C for 4 weeks on the concentration of osteocalcin measured by eight different assays. Results (mean ± SEM) are expressed relative to control samples stored at −75°C. Overall significance of the differences between methods by analysis of variance was $P < 0.0001$ for both storage conditions. Symbols without a common letter are significantly different ($P < 0.05$, Scheffé test). From Blumsohn *et al.* [33], with permission.

reports of the changes in osteocalcin due to different factors such as ethnicity, age, sex, and disease [27]. Although there is good correlation between assays in healthy control patients and osteoporotic patients, differences are particularly marked in patients with impaired renal function or renal failure [30, 31].

Because there is poor agreement with the manufacturers' reference ranges, it is important to establish reference ranges for healthy controls and patients with metabolic bone disease. In order to standardize results, Delmas and coworkers [32] recommended that results should be expressed as a percentage of serum osteocalcin in a normal population. A study carried out with commercial assays found discordant results even when the results were normalized to healthy controls [33]. Analytical variability is a possible source of discordant results. Discrepancies could be attributed to sample collection and handling, epitope specificity, quantitation of the assay standards, and immunoreactivity with the multiple forms of the osteocalcin molecule found in serum [34].

The effects of sample collection and handling are somewhat dependent on the osteocalcin assay that is intended for use, but the following are general guidelines. The intact osteocalcin molecule is very unstable in serum samples [35], hence sample collection and storage must be rapid if the intact osteocalcin molecule is to be measured. It is preferable to keep the blood at 2–8°C immediately after collection and during sample handling. The sample should be stored in the freezer within 1 hour of sample collection. Furthermore, it is important to keep the sample at 2–8°C during assay preparation, particularly for the measurement of intact osteocalcin. It is preferable to use a fresh sample for analysis and to avoid repeat freeze–thaw cycles. Reduced concentrations have been

reported after two or three freeze–thaw cycles [34, 36]. For short-term sample storage, −20°C is adequate, but −70°C is required for long-term storage [27] (Fig. 1). There is a drastic effect of hemolysis, which results in up to 90% lower values for osteocalcin concentration, hence it is advisable to reject hemolysed samples for analysis [34]. Lipemia also affects results because osteocalcin bound to lipid has reduced immunoreactivity. The type of sample collected should also be taken into consideration, as different anticoagulants can affect osteocalcin concentrations in plasma. In the study by Power *et al.* [36], serum concentrations were found to be up to three-fold higher than those in matched plasma samples. Structural stability of osteocalcin depends on calcium. Some osteocalcin assays are sensitive to calcium [34, 37], as they may have antisera directed against conformational epitopes, hence chelating agents should not be used in blood collection tubes. Improved stability has been observed for assays that measure both the intact and the large N-terminal midfragment of osteocalcin.

One of the most likely causes of the discordant results found for different assays is the ability of the assay to detect the different osteocalcin peptides. Circulating osteocalcin is heterogeneous; in addition to the intact molecule there are several osteocalcin fragment molecules [38, 39] (see also Chapter 3). These fragments are the result of proteolyic hydrolysis of peptide bonds involving arginine residues. Garnero *et al.* [35] characterized various immunoreactive forms of human osteocalcin using monoclonal antibodies. In healthy subjects, the intact molecule (1–49) was found to account for around 36% of total osteocalcin, the large N-terminal midfragment (1–43) accounted for around 30%, and the remainder consisted of smaller N-terminal, mid, and C-terminal

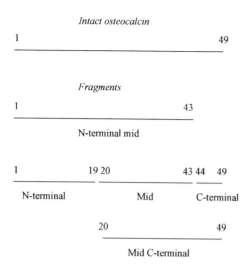

Intact osteocalcin

1   49

Fragments

1   43

N-terminal mid

1   19 20   43 44   49

N-terminal   Mid   C-terminal

20   49

Mid C-terminal

FIGURE 2   Proposed immunoreactive forms of osteocalcin in normal adult serum. Adapted from Garnero *et al.* [35], *J. Bone Miner. Res.* 1995; **9**, 255–264 with permission of the American Society for Bone and Mineral Research.

fragments (Fig. 2). There has been some speculation that the fragment may be produced by bone resorption; however, levels of the large N-terminal midfragment were not altered by bisphosphonate therapy in patients with Paget's disease of bone. Proteolytic degradation of the intact molecule occurs both *in vivo* and *in vitro*. If an assay detects the intact osteocalcin exclusively, then samples must be handled with great care by maintaining low temperature conditions to minimize degradation. This is not so critical for an assay that measures both the intact and N-terminal midfragment molecule, which has improved sample stability [40]. The generation of osteocalcin fragment molecules is not fully understood. It is possible that the fragments of osteocalcin could be derived from osteoblast synthesis, catabolism of the intact molecule in bone, or proteolysis in blood or other tissues [7]. It is also not known if fragment generation is altered by metabolic bone diseases. These questions need to be addressed to improve the clinical utility of osteocalcin assays (see also Chapter 3).

Assays have been developed that measure undercarboxylated osteocalcin by either hydroxyapatite precipitation or specific antibodies that recognize undercarboxylated osteocalcin [41, 42]. Undercarboxylated osteocalcin in the serum appears to increase with age [27, 43]. This is attributed to the decrease in vitamin K with respect to age. Most available assays do not distinguish between the degree of carboxylation of osteocalcin and therefore may overestimate bone formation because undercarboxylated osteocalcin is less likely to be incorporated into the bone matrix. A study by Vergnaud *et al.* [42] reported an increase in the undercarboxylated osteocalcin but not in total osteocalcin to be predictive of hip fracture risk in elderly women. It may be of benefit to specifically measure undercarboxylated osteocalcin in elderly populations. As the carboxylation of osteocalcin is vitamin K-

dependent then any drugs that affect vitamin K status, such as anticoagulants, will potentially affect the proportion of undercarboxylated osteocalcin in the circulation (see also Chapters 3 and 32).

B. Biological Variability

Osteocalcin has a half-life in the circulation of around 5 minutes, resulting in high circadian variability. It is rapidly metabolized by the kidney, hence osteocalcin levels are affected by renal function; if the renal function is impaired, osteocalcin levels will be elevated. Osteocalcin has a circadian rhythm with a nocturnal peak and an afternoon nadir [44]. Nielsen *et al.* [45] proposed that endogenous serum cortisol controls the circadian rhythm of circulating osteocalcin. Greenspan *et al.* [46] examined diurnal variation of biochemical markers of bone turnover in an elderly population. The diurnal variation in osteocalcin and bone alkaline phosphatase was found to be present with no gender-related differences. A seasonal rhythm for osteocalcin in young adults was reported by Thomsen *et al.* [47] who found the annual amplitude to be 23%. The highest levels were found to be in February, with a nadir in July. A similar trend was found by Douglas *et al.* [48], who reported higher levels of osteocalcin in the spring compared to autumn. The level of carboxylation of the osteocalcin was not different at the two time points. Woitge *et al.* reported osteocalcin to be around 15% higher in the winter compared to summer levels in both men and women. The seasonal rhythm for osteocalcin appears to mirror that seen for BAP, although it is less pronounced and accounts for 2% of the variability in serum osteocalcin [20].

Osteocalcin levels are higher in children compared to adults. In children, osteocalcin correlates with growth velocity rather than with age and the level of osteocalcin peaks during puberty. Vanderschueren *et al.* [49] found serum osteocalcin to be higher in men than in women and they observed an age-related decline. There was a temporary increase in osteocalcin concentration in women in the sixth decade, suggesting bone turnover is stimulated by menopause [49]. There is a significant increase in osteocalcin levels during the luteal phase of the menstrual cycle [22]. It has been reported that although other bone formation markers are elevated during pregnancy, osteocalcin is not and this is possibly due to placental degradation of osteocalcin [50].

Osteocalcin is elevated in high bone-turnover states; however, alkaline phosphatase appears to be superior in the determination of disease severity in Paget's disease of bone, although there are conflicting reports on levels in osteoporotic patients. Serum osteocalcin levels have been reported to fall rapidly with glucocorticoid administration in healthy young men [51]. The effect was found to be dose dependent and was attributed to the reduced biosynthesis of osteocalcin by osteoblasts.

Serum osteocalcin is increased following fracture. Obrant *et al.* [52] found osteocalcin to positively correlate with time elapsed after fracture, with an average two-fold increase after 60 days. Levels remained elevated for the 3 months of the study [52]. Osteocalcin has also been reported to increase for the first 4 days post fracture, then decrease until 5 weeks, after which there is an increase of around 35% by 20 weeks, in comparison to day 1 of the fracture [24]. Joerring *et al.* [53] found that following Colles' fracture, osteocalcin increased by 44% ($P < 0.001$) within 1 week compared to baseline (fracture sustained less than 24 hours earlier) and had returned to baseline at 9 months.

Osteocalcin concentration is significantly increased by around 20% in response to resistance exercise during the first month of training, both on exercise and training days [25]. Changes in plasma volume should be taken into account when interpreting the changes in biochemical markers during exercise [54].

V. PROPEPTIDES OF TYPE I PROCOLLAGEN

A. Assays for Propeptides of Type I Procollagen

Because type I collagen is such an abundant protein in the bone matrix, it is reasonable to consider the propeptides of type I procollagen as potential markers of bone formation. The carboxy-terminal propeptide of type I procollagen (PICP) correlates with histomorphometric measurement of bone formation in osteoporotic patients [55]. Assays for PICP are available in both RIA [56] and ELISA [57] format (Table III).

There have been several reported assays for the amino-terminal propeptide of type I procollagen (PINP) [58]. Ebeling *et al.* [59] developed an ELISA for PINP based on synthetic peptides (residues 7–24 from human proα1 (I) chain). The results were disappointing, with poor relationships to other markers of bone formation. Others have shown close correlation between PINP and other bone formation

markers [60, 61]. PINP can occur as both an intact and a fragment molecule. It has been suggested that measurement of the intact molecule is preferable, as it is too large to undergo glomerular filtration [62].

There are no special patient preparation requirements. The propeptides of type I procollagen are relatively robust and serum samples may be stored for up to 5 days at 2–8°C. A minimum of −20°C is recommended for long term storage [56]. Repeat freeze–thaw cycles, although not recommended, do not appear to affect concentrations.

The metabolism of human propeptides of type I procollagen is not fully understood. From rat studies it was found that both propeptides of type I procollagen are cleared by liver endothelial cells (PICP by the mannose receptors [63] and PINP by scavenger receptors [64]). It may not be suitable to measure these markers in patients with liver disease. PICP appears to be less sensitive and specific than other biochemical markers of bone formation [65, 66]. This may be due to the contribution of PICP from tissues other than bone that contain type I procollagen. Although there is little published data on PINP as a biochemical marker of bone formation, preliminary reports have shown PINP to be a more dynamic marker than PICP and other bone formation markers [67–69], particularly for monitoring the response to antiresorptive therapy. The differences may be due to the different clearance mechanisms of the two propeptides. PICP clearance is sensitive to hormonal changes (e.g., IGF-I, thyroid hormone) which are particularly relevant in studies during puberty, pregnancy, and menopause. Measurement of these markers of bone collagen formation may be useful in diseases of impaired collagen formation such as osteogenesis imperfecta [57].

B. Biological Variation

The propeptides of type I procollagen have a relatively short half-life in the rat (for PICP, 6 to 9 minutes, and for PINP 1 minute). PICP has a circadian rhythm with a nocturnal peak and an afternoon nadir. Unlike osteocalcin, the circadian rhythm does not appear to depend on endogenous serum cortisol levels [70]. There does not appear to be a seasonal variation in levels of PICP. Woitge *et al.* [20] reported that, like other biochemical markers of bone formation, PICP was higher in women in the winter compared to summer; however, this difference was not statistically significant.

There may be a significant contribution to serum PICP from nonbone type I procollagen sources [55]. Type I collagen is the most abundant type of collagen in the body and it is therefore possible that some of the procollagen propeptides present in serum could be from nonbone sources. Because bone is a metabolically active tissue with higher turnover than soft tissues, type I procollagen peptides should theoretically mainly reflect type I bone collagen formation.

TABLE III. Commercial Assays Available for Measurement of Propeptides of Type I Procollagen

Assay	Manufacturer	Analyte	Method
Procollagen PICP	Orion Diagnostica, Turku, Finland	PICP	RIA
Procollagen intact PINP	Orion Diagnostica, Turku, Finland	PINP	RIA
Prolagen-C	Metra Biosystems Inc., Palo Alto, CA	PICP	ELISA
OSCAtest PICP	BRAHMS Diagnostica GmbH, Berlin, Germany	PICP	RIA

TABLE IV. Biochemical Markers of Bone Formation in Mid-Puberty (Tanner Stages II and III) Relative to the Mean Levels in Adults

	Mid-pubertal level, mean ± SEM[a]	Relative level[b]
OC (μg/l)	42.9 ± 2.3	9.3
TAP (μkat/l)	5.2 ± 0.2	5.2
iBAP (μg/l)	86.5 ± 4.0	9.0
wBAP (μkat/l)	4.4 ± 0.2	10.4
PICP (μg/l)	290 ± 14	3.3

[a]Mean level in Tanner stages II and III.

[b]Mean mid-pubertal level expressed as a ratio to the mean level in adults.

Abbreviations: OC, osteocalcin; TAP, total alkaline phosphatase; iBAP, immunoreactive bone alkaline phosphatase; wBAP, wheat germ lectin bone alkaline phosphatase; PICP, C-terminal propeptide of type I procollagen. From Blumsohn et al. [66].

PICP is higher in children compared to adults, but not by as much as other biochemical markers of bone formation (Table IV). However, PINP appears to be elevated by a similar magnitude as other bone formation markers [67]. PICP decreases with age in men, but no change was found with age in women up to the sixth decade of life [56]. There does not appear to be a significant increase in PICP due to menopause, but PICP increases in older women [71]. PINP shows a more dynamic response to estrogen therapy in menopausal women than does PICP [72]. During pregnancy, PICP is elevated, with a peak during the third trimester [23].

The procollagen propeptides are cleared by the liver and therefore are elevated in patients with liver disease. They are not filtered by the kidney and therefore renal function has no effect on their serum levels, making them useful markers in patients with impaired renal function. The effect of fracture on type I procollagen C-terminal propeptide was studied in Colles' fracture patients [53]. PICP was elevated at 2 weeks post fracture (21%, $P < 0.05$) and was still elevated at week 5 of the study. At 9 months, the levels were not significantly different than baseline (samples taken within 24 hours of fracture). Exercise does not appear to have an effect on PICP, with no significant changes reported with resistance training exercise [25]. In endurance trained athletes, PICP was reported to be lower in runners than in controls [26].

VI. SUMMARY

New assays are being developed to improve sensitivity and specificity to bone of the biochemical markers of bone formation. Because many are intended for commercial use, they are designed to be less cumbersome and time consuming. It is important to understand which analyte the assay is measuring, particularly with osteocalcin assays. This will have an impact on sample handling and interpretation of results. It is also beneficial to know which markers are best suited to provide the information required. For example, the procollagen propeptides are useful in osteogenesis imperfecta patients. In diseases with very high bone turnover changes, such as Paget's disease, total alkaline phosphatase is adequate to assess bone turnover. In diseases with more subtle changes in bone turnover, such as osteoporosis, bone-specific markers are more suitable. It is important to consider confounding factors that may affect the bone formation markers. Variability can be reduced by establishing a sample collection protocol with samples taken at a specific time of day within specified time limits after an overnight fast. Confounding factors should be considered such as age, gender, physical activity, renal function, and recent fractures. In addition, other factors such as medication should also be taken into account when interpreting results. It is advisable for each laboratory to establish reference ranges from a local population for each marker, if possible for both males and females over several age ranges (i.e., pre-pubertal and pubertal children, premenopausal and postmenopausal women). As more assays become available and more centers measure biochemical markers of bone turnover, it may be beneficial to initiate an interlaboratory quality assurance scheme.

References

1. Charles, P., Poser, J. W., Mosekilde, L., and Jensen, F. T. (1985). Estimation of bone turnover evaluated by ^{47}Ca-kinetics. Efficiency of serum bone gamma-carboxyglutamic acid-containing protein, serum alkaline phosphatase, and urinary hydroxyproline excretion. J. Clin. Invest. 76, 2254–2258.

2. Delmas, P. D. (1988). Biochemical markers of bone turnover in osteoporosis. In "Osteoporosis" (B. L. Riggs and L. J. Melton, III, eds.), pp. 297–316. Raven Press, New York.

3. Devgun, M. S., Paterson, C. R., and Martin, B. T. (1981). Seasonal changes in the activity of serum alkaline phosphatase. Enzyme 26, 301–305.

4. Fishman, W. H. (1990). Alkaline phosphatase isoenzymes: Recent progress. Clin. Biochem. 23, 99–104.

5. Van Hoof, V. O., and De Broe, M. E. (1994). Interpretation and clinical significance of alkaline phosphatase isoenzyme patterns. Crit. Rev. Clin. Lab. Sci. 31, 197–293.

6. Moss, D. W., and Whitby, L. G. (1975). A simplified heat-inactivation method for investigating alkaline phosphatase isoenzyme in serum. Clin. Chim. Acta 61, 63–71.

7. Calvo, M. S., Eyre, D. R., and Gundberg, C. M. (1996). Molecular basis and clinical application of biological markers of bone turnover. Endocr. Rev. 17, 333–368.

8. Rosalki, S. B., and Foo, A. Y. (1984). Two new methods for separating and quantifying bone and liver alkaline phosphatase isoenzymes in plasma. Clin. Chem. 30, 1182–1186.

9. Crofton, P. M. (1992). Wheat-germ lectin affinity electrophoresis for alkaline phosphatase isoforms in children: Age-dependent reference ranges and changes in liver and bone disease. Clin. Chem. 38, 663–670.

10. Lawson, G. M., Katzman, J. A., Kimlinger, T. K., and O'Brien, J. F. (1985). Isolation and preliminary characterization of a monoclonal antibody that interacts preferentially with the liver isoenzyme of human alkaline phosphatase. *Clin. Chem.* **31**, 381–385.

11. Garnero, P., and Delmas, P. D. (1993). Assessment of the serum levels of bone alkaline phosphatase with a new immunoradiometric assay in patients with metabolic bone disease. *J. Clin. Endocrinol. Metab.* **77**, 1046–1053.

12. Gomez, B., Jr., Ardakani, S., Ju, J., Jenkins, D., Cerelli, M. J., Daniloff, G. Y., and Kung, V. T. (1995). Monoclonal antibody assay for measuring bone-specific alkaline phosphatase activity in serum. *Clin. Chem.* **41**, 1560–1566.

13. Hata, K., Tokuhiro, H., Nakatsuka, K., Miki, T., Nishizawa, Y., Morii, H., and Miura, M. (1996). Measurement of bone-specific alkaline phosphatase by an immunoselective enzyme assay method. *Ann. Clin. Biochem.* **33**, 127–131.

14. Hill, C. S., and Wolfert, R. L. (1989). The preparation of monoclonal antibodies which react preferentially with human bone alkaline phosphatase and not liver alkaline phosphatase. *Clin. Chim. Acta* **186**, 315–320.

15. Piovesan, A., Berruti, A., Torta, M., Cannone, R., Sperone, P., Panero, A., Gorzegno, G., Termine, A., Dogliotti, L., and Angeli, A. (1997). Comparison of assay of total and bone-specific alkaline phosphatase in the assessment of osteoblast activity in patients with metastatic bone disease. *Calcif. Tissue Int.* **61**, 362–369.

16. Price, C. P., Milligan, T. P., and Darte, C. (1997). Direct comparison of performance characteristics of two immunoassays for bone isoform of alkaline phosphatase in serum. *Clin. Chem.* **43**, 2052–2057.

17. Woitge, H. W., Seibel, M. J., and Ziegler, R. (1996). Comparison of total and bone specific alkaline phosphatase in patients with nonskeletal disorders or metabolic bone disease. *Clin. Chem.* **42**, 1796–1804.

18. Price, C. P. (1993). Multiple forms of human serum alkaline phosphatase: Detection and quantitation. *Ann. Clin. Biochem.* **30**, 355–372.

19. Crofton, P. M. (1982). Biochemistry of the alkaline phosphatase isoenzymes. *Crit. Rev. Clin. Lab. Sci.* **16**, 161–194.

20. Woitge, H. W., Scheidt-Nave, C., Kissling, C., Leidig-Bruckner, G., Meyer, K., Grauer, A., Scharla, S. H., Ziegler, R., and Seibel, M. J. (1998). Seasonal variation of biochemical indexes of bone turnover: Results of a population-based study. *J. Clin. Endocrinol. Metab.* **83**, 68–75.

21. Duda, R. J., O'Brein, J. F., Katzmann, J. A., Peterson, J. M., Mann, K. G., and Riggs, B. L. (1988). Concurrent assays of circulating bone gla-protein and bone alkaline phosphatase: Effects of sex, age and metabolic bone disease. *J. Clin. Endocrinol. Metab.* **66**, 951–957.

22. Nielsen, H. K., Brixen, K., Bouillon, R., and Mosekilde, L. (1990). Changes in biochemical markers of osteoblastic activity during the menstrual cycle. *J. Clin. Endocrinol. Metab.* **70**, 1431–1437.

23. Cross, N. A., Hillman, L. S., Allen, S. H., Krause, G. F., and Vieira, N. E. (1995). Calcium homeostasis and bone metabolism during pregnancy, lactation and postweaning: A longitudinal study. *Am. J. Clin. Nutr.* **61**, 514–523.

24. Bowles, S. A., Kurdy, N., Davis, A. M., France, M. W., and Marsh, D. R. (1996). Serum osteocalcin, total and bone specific alkaline phosphatase following isolated tibial shaft fracture. *Ann. Clin. Biochem.* **33**, 196–200.

25. Fujimura, R., Ashizawa, N., Watanabe, M., Mukai, N., Amagai, H., Fukubayashi, T., Hayashi, K., Tokuyama, K., and Suzuki, M. (1997). Effect of resistance exercise training on bone formation and resorption in young male subjects assessed by biomarkers of bone metabolism. *J. Bone Miner. Res.* **12**, 656–662.

26. Brahm, H., Strom, H., Piehl-Aulin, K., Mallmin, H., and Ljunghall, S. (1997). Bone metabolism in endurance trained athletes: A comparison to population-based controls based on DXA, SXA, quantitative ultrasound, and biochemical markers. *Calcif. Tissue Int.* **61**, 448–454.

27. Power, M. J., and Fottrell, P. F. (1991). Osteocalcin: Diagnostic methods and clinical applications. *Crit. Rev. Clin. Lab. Sci.* **28**, 287–335.

28. Garnero, P., Grimaux, M., Demiaux, B., Preaudat, C., Seguin, P., and Delmas, P. D. (1992). Measurement of serum osteocalcin with a human-specific two-site immunoradiometric assay. *J. Bone Miner. Res.* **7**, 1389–1398.

29. Taylor, A. K., Linkhart, S. G., Mohan, S., and Baylink, D. J. (1988). Development of a new radioimmunoassay for human osteocalcin: Evidence for a mid molecule epitope. *Metab., Clin. Exp.* **37**, 872–877.

30. Masters, P. W., Jones, R. G., Purves, D. A., Cooper, E. H., and Cooney, J. M. (1994). Commercial assays for serum osteocalcin give clinically discordant results. *Clin. Chem.* **40**, 358–363.

31. Diego, E. M. D., Guerrero, R., and de la Piedra, C. (1994). Six osteocalcin assays compared. *Clin. Chem.* **40**, 2071–2077.

32. Delmas, P. D., Price, P. A., and Mann, K. G. (1990). Validation of the bone gla protein (osteocalcin) assay. *J. Bone Miner. Res.* **5**, 3–11.

33. Blumsohn, A., Hannon, R. A., and Eastell, R. (1995). Apparent instability of osteocalcin in serum as measured with different commercially available immunoassays. *Clin. Chem.* **41**, 318–319.

34. Tracy, R. P., Andrianorivo, A., Riggs, B. L., and Mann, K. G. (1990). Comparison of monoclonal and polyclonal antibody-based immunoassays for osteocalcin: A study of sources of variation in assay results. *J. Bone Miner. Res.* **5**, 451–461.

35. Garnero, P., Grimaux, M., Seguin, P., and Delmas, P. D. (1994). Characterization of immunoreactive forms of human osteocalcin generated in vivo and in vitro. *J. Bone Miner. Res.* **9**, 255–264.

36. Power, M. J., O'Dwyer, B., Breen, E., and Fottrell, P. F. (1991). Osteocalcin concentrations in plasma prepared with different anticoagulants. *Clin. Chem.* **37**, 281–284.

37. Bouillon, R., Vanderschueren, D., Van Herck, E., Nielsen, H. K., Bex, M., Heyns, W., and Van Baelen, H. (1992). Homologous radioimmunoassay of human osteocalcin. *Clin. Chem.* **38**, 2055–2060.

38. Taylor, A. K., Linkhart, S., Mohan, S., Christenson, R. A., Singer, F. R., and Baylink, D. (1990). Multiple osteocalcin fragments in human urine and serum as detected by a midmolecule osteocalcin radioimmunoassay. *J. Clin. Endocrinol. Metab.* **70**, 467–472.

39. Gundberg, C., and Weinstein, R. S. (1986). Multiple immunoreactive forms in uremic serum. *J. Clin. Invest.* **77**, 1762–1767.

40. Rosenquist, C., Qvist, P., Bjarnason, N., and Christiansen, C. (1995). Measurement of a more stable region of osteocalcin in serum by ELISA with two monoclonal antibodies. *Clin. Chem.* **41**, 1439–1445.

41. Merle, B., and Delmas, P. D. (1990). Normal carboxylation of circulating osteocalcin (bone Gla protein) in Paget's disease of bone. *Bone Miner.* **11**, 237–245.

42. Vergnaud, P., Garnero, P., Meunier, P. J., Breart, G., Kamihagi, K., and Delmas, P. D. (1997). Undercarboxylated osteocalcin measured with a specific immunoassay predicts hip fracture in elderly women: The EPIDOS study. *J. Clin. Endocrinol. Metab.* **82**, 719–724.

43. Szulc, P., Arlot, M., Chapuy, M., Duboeuf, F., Meunier, P. J., and Delmas, P. D. (1994). Serum undercarboxylated osteocalcin correlates with hip bone mineral density in elderly women. *J. Bone Miner. Res.* **9**, 1591–1595.

44. Eastell, R., Calvo, M. S., Burritt, M. F., Offord, K. P., Russell, R. G. G., and Riggs, B. L. (1992). Abnormalities in circadian patterns of bone resorption and renal calcium conservation in type I osteoporosis. *J. Clin. Endocrinol. Metab.* **74**, 487–494.

45. Nielsen, H. K., Brixen, K., Kassem, M., Charles, P., and Mosekilde, L. (1992). Inhibition of the morning cortisol peak abolishes the expected morning decrease in serum osteocalcin in normal males: Evidence of a controlling effect of serum cortisol on the circadian rhythm in serum osteocalcin. *J. Clin. Endocrinol. Metab.* **74**, 1410–1414.

46. Greenspan, S. L., Dresner-Pollak, R., Parker, R. A., London, D., and Ferguson, L. (1997). Diurnal variation of bone mineral turnover in elderly men and women. *Calcif. Tissue Int.* **60**, 419–423.

47. Thomsen, K., Eriksen, E. F., Jorgensen, J. C. R., Charles, P., and Mosekilde, L. (1989). Seasonal variation of bone-Gla protein. *Scand. J. Clin. Lab. Invest.* **49**, 605–611.

48. Douglas, A. S., Miller, M. H., Reid, D. M., Hutchison, J. D., Porter, R. W., and Robins, S. P. (1996). Seasonal differences in biochemical parameters of bone remodelling. *J. Clin. Pathol.* **49**, 284–289.

49. Vanderschueren, D., Gevers, G., Raymaekers, G., Devos, P., and Dequeker, J. (1990). Sex and age-related changes in bone and serum osteocalcin. *Calcif. Tissue Int.* **46**, 179–182.

50. Rodin, A., Duncan, A., Quartero, H. W. P., Pistofidis, G., Mashiter, G., Whitaker, K., Crook, D., Stevenson, J. C., Chapman, M. G., and Fogelman, I. (1989). Serum concentrations of alkaline phosphatase isoenzymes and osteocalcin in normal pregnancy. *J. Clin. Endocrinol. Metab.* **68**, 1123–1127.

51. Godschalk, M. F., and Downs, R. W. (1988). Effect of short-term glucocorticoids on serum osteocalcin in healthy young men. *J. Bone Miner. Res.* **3**, 113–115.

52. Obrant, K. J., Merle, B., Bejui, J., and Delmas, P. D. (1990). Serum bone-gla protein after fracture. *Clin. Orthop.* **258**, 300–303.

53. Joerring, S., Jensen, L. T., Anderson, G. R., and Johansen, J. S. (1992). Types I and III procollagen extension peptides in serum respond to fracture in humans. *Arch. Orthop. Trauma Surg.* **111**, 265–267.

54. Brahm, H., Piehl-Aulin, K., and Ljunghall, S. (1997). Bone metabolism during exercise and recovery: The influence of plasma volume and physical fitness. *Calcif. Tissue Int.* **61**, 192–198.

55. Parfitt, A. M., Simon, L. S., Villanueva, A. R., and Krane, S. M. (1987). Procollagen type I carboxy-terminal extension peptide in serum as a marker of collagen biosynthesis in bone. Correlation with bone formation rates and comparison with total alkaline phosphatase. *J. Bone Miner. Res.* **2**, 427–436.

56. Melkko, J., Niemi, S., Risteli, L., and Risteli, J. (1990). Radioimmunoassay for the carboxyterminal propeptide of human type I procollagen (PICP). *Clin. Chem.* **36**, 1328–1332.

57. Winterbottom, N., Vernon, S., Freeman, K., Daniloff, G., and Seyedin, S. (1993). A serum immunoassay for the C-terminal propeptide of type I collagen. *J. Bone Miner. Res.* **8**, S341 (abstr.).

58. Risteli, J., Niemi, S., Kauppila, S., Melkko, J., and Risteli, L. (1995). Collagen propeptides as indicators of collagen assembly. *Acta Orthop. Scand.* **66**, 183–188.

59. Ebeling, P. R., Peterson, J. M., and Riggs, B. L. (1992). Utility of type I procollagen propeptide assays for assessing abnormalities in metabolic bone disease. *J. Bone Miner. Res.* **7**, 1243–1250.

60. Linkhart, S. G., Linkhart, T. A., Taylor, A. K., Wergedal, J. E., Bettica, P., and Baylink, D. J. (1993). Synthetic peptide-based immunoassay for amino-terminal propeptide of type I procollagen: application for evaluation of bone formation. *Clin. Chem.* **39**, 2254–2258.

61. Orum, O., Hansen, M., Jensen, C. H., Sorensen, H. A., Jensen, L. B., Horslev-Petersen, K., and Teisner, B. (1996). Procollagen type I N-terminal propeptide (PINP) as an indicator of type I collagen metabolism: ELISA development, reference interval, and hypovitaminosis D induced hyperparathyroidism. *Bone* **19**, 157–163.

62. Melkko, J., Kauppila, S., Niemi, S., Risteli, L., Haukipuro, K., Jukkola, A., and Risteli, J. (1996). Immunoassay for intact amino-terminal propeptide of human type I procollagen. *Clin. Chem.* **42**, 947–954.

63. Smedsrod, B., Melkko, J., Risteli, L., and Risteli, J. (1990). Circulating C-terminal propeptide of type I procollagen is cleared mainly via the mannose receptor in liver endothelial cells. *Biochem. J.* **271**, 345–350.

64. Melkko, J., Hellevik, T., Risteli, L., Risteli, J., and Smedsrod, B. (1994). Clearance of NH_2-terminal propeptides of types I and III procollagen is a physiological function of the scavenger receptor in liver endothelial cells. *J. Exp. Med.* **179**, 405–412.

65. Hassager, C., Fabbri-Mabelli, G., and Christiansen, C. (1993). The effect of the menopause and hormone replacement therapy on serum carboxyterminal propeptides of type I collagen. *Osteoporosis Int.* **3**, 50–52.

66. Blumsohn, A., Hannon, R. A., Wrate, R., Barton, J., Al-Dehaimi, A. W., Colwell, A., and Eastell, R. (1994). Biochemical markers of bone turnover in girls during puberty. *Clin. Endocrinol.* **40**, 663–670.

67. Naylor, K. E., Blumsohn, A., Hannon, R. A., Peel, N. F. A., and Eastell, R. (1996). Different responses of carboxy and amino terminal propeptides of type I procollagen in three clinical models of high bone turnover. *J. Bone Miner. Res.* **11**, S194 (abstr.).

68. Garnero, P., Vergnaud, P., and Delmas, P. D. (1997). Amino terminal propeptide of type I collagen (PINP) is a more sensitive marker of bone turnover than C-terminal propeptide in osteoporosis. *J. Bone Miner. Res.* **12**, S497 (abstr.).

69. Tahtela, R., Turpeinen, M., Sorva, R., and Karonen, S. L. (1997). The aminoterminal propeptide of type I procollagen: Evaluation of a commercial radioimmunoassay kit and values in healthy subjects. *Clin. Biochem.* **30**, 35–40.

70. Schlemmer, A., Hassager, C., Alexanderson, P., Fledelius, C., Pedersen, B. J., Kristensen, L. O., and Christiansen, C. (1997). Circadian variation in bone resorption is not related to serum cortisol. *Bone* **21**, 83–88.

71. Eastell, R., Peel, N. F. A., Hannon, R. A., Blumsohn, A., Price, A., Colwell, A., and Russell, R. G. G. (1992). Effect of age on bone collagen in older women. *Bone* **13**, 275

72. Suvanto-Luukkonen, E., Risteli, L., Sundstrom, H., Penttinen, J., Kauppila, A., and Risteli, J. (1997). Comparison of three serum assays for bone collagen formation during postmenopausal estrogen-progestin therapy. *Clin. Chim. Acta* **266**, 105–116.

CHAPTER 28

Measurement of Biochemical Markers of Bone Resorption

MARIUS E. KRAENZLIN Endocrine Clinic, Basel, Switzerland

MARKUS J. SEIBEL Department of Medicine, Division of Endocrinology and Metabolism, University of Heidelberg Medical School, Heidelberg, Germany

I. ABSTRACT

In the past, a major difficulty in the diagnosis and management of metabolic bone diseases has been the lack of convenient and accurate means by which the metabolic state of the bone could be monitored. There has been significant progress in the development of bone resorption markers with regard to specificity and sensitivity. The longest established marker of bone resorption was hydroxyproline, but hydroxyproline is not specific to bone collagen. There is, therefore, much interest in collagen products that are more specific for bone, including galactosylhydroxylysine, the collagen cross-links (pyridinoline and deoxypyridinoline) and their related telopeptides, and bone sialoprotein. The pyridinolines and the related collagen fragments (telopeptides) are the most extensively studied markers of bone resorption. This chapter reviews progress in this area, particularly the analytical aspects and the factors contributing to the variability of the various bone resorption assays.

II. INTRODUCTION

Considerable progress has been made in the development of assays of biochemical markers for the assessment of bone formation and bone resorption. Currently available bone resorption markers are summarized in Table I. Changes in bone resorption can be assessed by measurement of urinary hydroxyproline, galactosyl-hydroxylysine, pyridinoline cross-links, fragments of collagen type I (telopeptides), tartrate-resistant acid phosphatase, and bone sialoprotein. Efforts have also been made to demonstrate the clinical utility of biochemical markers of bone turnover in the identification and definition of osteoporotic risk, early diagnosis of metabolic

Hydroxyproline

Hydroxylysine glycosides

Pyridinium cross-links and related collagen fragments (telopeptides)

Tartrate-resistant acid phosphatase

Bone sialoprotein

bone disease, determination of effective therapy for those with established disease, and monitoring therapeutic effects.

The bone matrix is composed of approximately 70% mineral and 30% organic matter. The latter consists of collagen, noncollagenous proteins, and proteoglycans. The main structural protein of bone is type I collagen, which constitutes approximately 90% of the organic matrix (see Chapters 1 and 11). During the process of bone resorption, collagen and the other constituents of the organic matrix are degraded by the action of various proteases. The resulting breakdown products, as well as the the enzymes produced by active osteoclasts and the other components involved in osteoclast regulation and function, are consecutively released into the circulation and partly eliminated by the kidney. Most assays for bone resorption measure collagen degradation products, such as hydroxyproline, hydroxlysine glycosides, the 3-hydroxy-pyridinium cross-links (pyridinoline and deoxypyridinoline), and their higher molecular weight derivates originating from the nonhelical region of the collagen molecule (amino- and carboxy-terminal telopeptides). Other noncollageneous markers are tartrate-resistant acid phosphatase (an osteoclast enzyme) and bone sialoprotein (an adhesion protein in bone) (see also Chapters 4 and 9).

The value of a biochemical marker of bone turnover depends on several criteria. The ideal marker should be specific to the tissue being monitored. In the case of bone, this applies to osteocalcin, but not, for example, to hydroxyproline or its peptides. Furthermore, the marker should be easily measurable in serum or urine by specific and sensitive techniques. Other criteria that determine the value of biochemical markers include knowledge of the factors that control synthesis and metabolism as well as the biological variability. With most markers, there is still only limited information available about their metabolism and the factors that influence their production and degradation.

This chapter will review the progress in improving diagnostic markers for bone resorption, particularly the analytical aspects and the various factors contributing to the variability of these assays. The clinical application of the bone resorption assays will be reviewed in Chapters 32–46.

III. HYDROXYPROLINE

The best established and most widely used marker of bone resorption traditionally was urinary hydroxyproline (OHPr).

Hydroxyproline occurs mainly in fibrillar collagens, where it accounts for 13–14% of the total amino acid content. Hydroxyproline is produced as a result of the posttranslational modifications of proline by prolyl hydroxylase during collagen synthesis (see Chapter 1). The amino acid occurs almost exclusively in collagen and therefore its urinary levels are considered to reflect collagen turnover in bone and other tissues [1].

There are, however, several problems with using hydroxyproline as a marker for bone resorption. First, the amino acid is not specific for bone. It is found in all collagens, not just type I [1]. Second, the use of hydroxyproline as a quantitative measure of collagen breakdown is hampered by the fact that the free amino acid is reabsorbed by the kidneys and eventually degraded in the liver into products that can not be detected by the hydroxyproline assay. Furthermore, it has been suggested that about 10% of the total urinary hydroxyproline pool is released during the proteolytic processing of newly synthesized procollagen and therefore is indicative of collagen formation [2]. Thus, urinary hydroxyproline is derived from breakdown of all types of collagen in the body and, at least in part, also from collagen-containing foods in the diet.

Measurement of urinary hydroxyproline involves acid hydrolysis of the OHPr-containing peptides by adding an equal volume of 12 N HCl to the urine and heating at 100–105°C for 10–18 hours. This hydrolysis step is required to measure total amounts of OHPr, as more than 90% of urinary OHPr is peptide-bound. The acid hydrolysis is followed by oxidation of free hydroxyproline to pyrrole with chloramine T, and the colorimetric reaction of the pyrrole with p-dimethyl-aminobenzaldehyde (Ehrlich reagent) is measured. The urinary OHPr concentrations are read from a standard curve based on aqueous OHPr solutions that are run simultaneously with the samples [3–7]. The intra- and interassay variation reported for the colorimetric assay ranges from 2–10% and 8–15%, respectively. The recovery ranges from 70–90% and the sensitivity is on the order of 5 μmol/l [4, 5, 8]. Injection of iodinated contrast medium is known to interfere with hydroxyproline determination [9]. The iothalamic acid contained in contrast medium reduces the optical extinction by 12–84%, depending on the amount of iodinated contrast medium. The iodide ions are probably released during thermal hydrolysis and reduced to iodine by chloramine T, and at the same time the chloramine T is inactivated and thus is not available to oxidize OHPr [9].

In addition to the colorimetric assay, several high-performance liquid chromatography (HPLC) methods for measuring urinary hydroxyproline have been published. Hydroxyproline, like most imino and amino acids, absorbs only weekly in the ultraviolet-visible region and possesses no native fluorescence. Therefore, a hydroxyproline derivative is needed to allow photometric or fluorimetric detection. Dimethylaminoazobenzene-4-sulfonyl chloride, phenylisothio-cyanate, o-phthaladehyde, and 4-chlor-7-nitrobenzo-2-oxa-

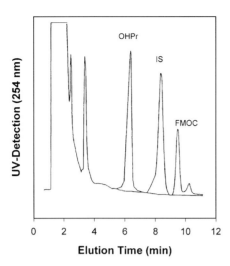

FIGURE 1   Separation of urinary hydroxyproline (OHPr) by high performance liquid chromatography. IS, internal standard; FMOC, 9-fluorenylmethyl-chlorformate.

1,3-diazole have been used as derivatization agents [10–12]. The separation is then performed on a reverse-phase column followed by UV-detection. Quantitation of OHPr is done by using an internal or external standard (Fig. 1). The intra- and interassay variation, as well as recovery and sensitivity described for the HPLC, are considerably better than for the colorimetric method; the interassay variation is 4–5% and analytical recovery ranges from 95–110%.

OHPr measurements are usually performed in a fasting urine sample collected over two hours in the morning and expressed as OHPr/creatinine ratio. In adults, a higher 24 hour OHPr excretion has been reported for men than for women, reflecting the difference in total body collagen mass. This difference disappears when corrections are made for urinary creatinine [7].

IV. GLYCOSYLATED HYDROXYLYSINE

Hydroxylysine is another amino acid unique to collagen and collagen-like peptides. Similar to OHPr, hydroxylysine is produced by a posttranslational modification of lysine during collagen synthesis. Unlike OHPr, these amino acids can then undergo further modification by glycosylation, giving rise to galactosyl hydroxylysine (GH) and glucosylgalactosyl hydroxylysine (GGH) [13, 14]. This subsequent glycosylation of hydroxylysine differs in collagens from different tissues. The monoglycosylated galactosyl-hydroxylysine is enriched in bone compared with the disaccharide form, glucosyl-galactosyl-hydroxylysine, which is the major form in skin. Although hydroxylysine is found in all collagens, GH is five- to seven-fold more concentrated in type I collagen of bone than in type I collagen of skin. Measurements of GH are therefore thought to reflect mainly resorption of bone col-

lagen [13, 14]. In addition, hydroxylysine glycosides, unlike hydroxyproline, are apparently not significantly metabolized prior to urinary excretion and are not affected by diet. Because of this, it has been estimated that urinary hydroxylysine glycosides can account for 50–100% of collagen breakdown and not the 10–25% estimated for OHPr [13]. Under normal conditions, hydroxylysine glycosides represent 80% of the total urinary hydroxylysine. 10% of the hydroxylysine is present in the free form and the remainder is peptide-bound, suggesting that free hydroxylysine is largely metabolized and not excreted [15]. This ratio of free to peptide-bound forms varies with age; the free and peptide-bound hydroxylysine are most prominent in children [15].

The major difficulty with measuring urinary hydroxylysine glycosides has been the methods involved in their determination. The procedure generally consists of separation by ion-exchange chromatography followed by amino acid analysis [16, 17]. A new method for measuring these glycosides has been introduced, comprising the conversion of the amino groups into fluorescent derivatives prior to their separation by reverse-phase (HPLC) [18]. GH is derivatized by adding dansyl chloride to the urine samples. A hydrolytic pretreatment is not required. The separation is carried out by reverse-phase HPLC involving a gradient elution system. Quantitation of the measured analyte is performed using an external standard extracted from urine or with commercially available purified lysine [19]. Intra- and interassay variations are in the order of 5–8% and 6–7%, respectively [20, 21]. The sensitivity appears to be on the order of picomoles [18]. Although the introduction of the HPLC method for measurement of the glycosylated hydroxylysine is an improvement, the method still remains technically demanding and slow.

There have been some reports on the value of GH in the evaluation of metabolic and metastatic bone disease. However, more testing needs to be done to determine the usefulness of this procedure in clinical practice [18, 20, 22, 23].

V. COLLAGEN CROSS-LINKS

A. 3-Hydroxy-Pyridinium Cross-Links of Collagen

The pyridinium cross-links, pyridinoline or hydroxylysylpyridinoline (PYD) and deoxypyridinoline or lysylpyridinoline (DPD), are receiving considerable attention as the most promising markers of bone resorption (Fig. 2). PYD and DPD are derived from hydroxylysine and lysine residues within the collagen molecule and are found in mature, but not immature or newly synthesized, type I, II, and III collagens [24, 25]. The cross-links covalently link collagen molecules between two telopeptides and a triple-helical sequence at two intermolecular sites and therefore stabilize collagen fibrils (Fig. 3). Of the two forms, PYD and DPD, PYD is the major

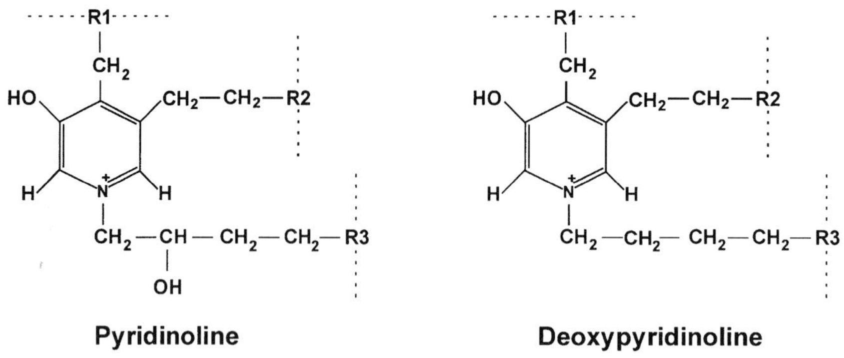

Pyridinoline   **Deoxypyridinoline**

FIGURE 2   Molecular structure of pyridinoline cross-links. R1 and R2 are telopeptide sequences and R3 represents a helical sequence; for the free cross-links, R1, R2, and R3 = $-CH(COOH)NH_2$.

cross-link in all connective tissues, whereas DPD is found in high amounts in mineralized tissue. In human bone, for example, the DPD:PYD ratio is 1:3.5, as compared to a ratio of 1:10 in human cartilage. Significant amounts of DPD are found in bone and dentin only, with very small amounts in the aorta and ligaments. DPD is therefore considered to be specific for bone collagen degradation. PYD and DPD, in contrast to OHPr, are completely absent from the collagen of normal skin (see also Chapter 2).

During collagen breakdown, the pyridinoline cross-links are released and cleared by the kidneys. In urine, PYD and DPD are present as both free amino acid derivatives (about 40%) and as oligopeptide-bound fractions (about 60%) [26]. The free form can be measured directly, whereas the conjugated form has to be hydrolyzed before assay, in which case the total amount of PYD and DPD is determined [27]. The relatively normal values for DPD excretion in patients with renal dysfunction support the notion that cross-link excretion

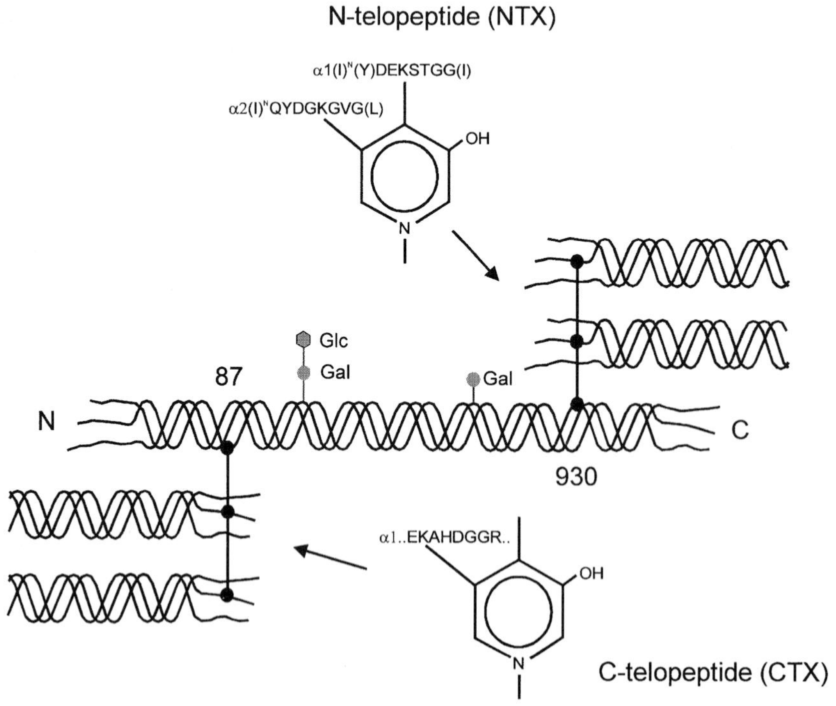

FIGURE 3   Schematic representation of the intermolecular cross-linking in type I collagen and the locations of the peptide sequence selected for the N-terminal (NTX) and C-terminal (CTX) immunoassays (modified and adapted from references [25, 55, 62]).

is generally unaffected by changes in renal function [28]. They are apparently not metabolized within the body and their levels are, in contrast to OHPr, not influenced by diet. However, there is evidence that some free PYD and DPD excreted into the urine is produced by the kidney [29].

There are two principal methods for measuring urinary levels of pyridinoline cross-links. The first technique involves extensive hydrolysis of the urine followed by ion exchange chromatography and HPLC analysis. Detection is based on the intrinsic fluorescence of these compounds. Although these assays have been and will remain the reference methods, they are cumbersome and labor intensive. The second method employs antibodies against the free amino acids or the peptides containing the cross-link component. Several immunoassays for the free pyridinolines or small peptides and for the (cross-linked) N- and C-terminal telopeptide in urine or serum have been described.

1. HPLC METHOD FOR COLLAGEN CROSS-LINKS

Urine samples are usually hydrolyzed with 6 N HCl at 107°C for 16 hours in order to convert all cross-link components into the peptide-free form. By omitting the hydrolysis step, only the peptide-free fraction of PYD and DPD is measured. Following a partition chromatography step (CF1 cellulose), the pyridinoline cross-link components are separated by reverse-phase ion-paired HPLC. Eluting fluorescence peaks are quantified using an external PYD and/or DPD standard extracted from bone or urine (Fig. 4) [30, 31].

A problem in the interpretation of results obtained by HPLC was the lack of a functional internal standard. Although recovery for PYD and DPD from hydrolysis to identification is usually between 80 and 90% or higher, the addition of an internal standard is required in order to improve

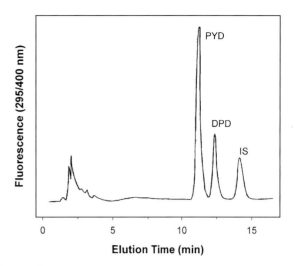

FIGURE 5 Separation of urinary pyridinoline cross-links (pyridinoline [PYD] and deoxypyridinoline [DPD]) by reverse-phase high performance liquid chromatography, with the addition of an internal standard (IS), acetyl-pyridinoline (reproduced from Robins [33a], with permission).

the precision of the overall method. This internal standard is particularly necessary to correct for between-sample variation in recovery [27]. A number of reports have described the succesful use of either isodesmosine, derived from elastin, or acetyl-pyridinoline, a semi-synthetic derivative, as internal standards [27, 32, 33] (Fig. 5) [332]. Mean recoveries of PYD and DPD, monitored using the internal standard isodesmosine, were 97% and 93%, respectively, and interassay variation was lowered from 15.1 to 5.3% for PYD and from 20.8 to 4.6% for DPD [27, 32]. Although the use of an internal standard has considerably improved analytical precision, the HPLC procedure is not yet standardized, and results from different laboratories are not necessarily comparable. Laboratories using the same standard usually provide values with a correlation coefficient of $r > 0.95$, but values may differ in absolute terms. Therefore, an accepted international reference material is urgently needed to enable comparison among different laboratories and centers [34, 35].

The coefficient of variation for the determination of PYD varies between 4 and 8%, and for DPD between 6 and 10%, with a detection limit of 1 pmol. Calculated as a coefficient of variation, the overall reproducibility of the complete analysis, including CF1 column fractionation, was found to be 12–16% [30, 36, 37]. The pyridinoline measurements are usually performed on a fasting urine sample collected over two hours in the morning and are expressed as a cross-link/creatinine ratio. The values in fasting morning urine samples correlate well with the 24 hour output of PYD and DPD [27, 28].

Sulfasalazine (salicyloazosulfapyridine), a compound used in treating rheumatoid arthritis or chronic inflammatory bowel disease, has been reported to interfere with the determination of pyridinoline in treated individuals [38]. Sulfasalazine is metabolized into sulfapyridine and 5-aminosalicylic

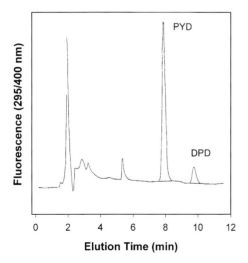

FIGURE 4 Separation of urinary pyridinoline cross-links (pyridinoline [PYD] and deoxypyridinoline [DPD]) by reverse-phase high performance liquid chromatography.

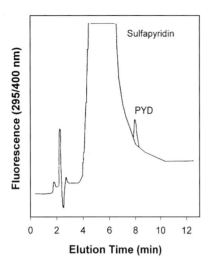

FIGURE 6   High performance liquid chromatogram of pyridinoline cross-links illustrating the interference by sulfapyridine.

acid by intestinal bacteria. These metabolites are absorbed and then excreted in the urine. Sulfapyridine and 5-aminosalicylic acid peaks elute at a retention time similar to that of the peaks for PYD and DPD (Fig. 6). The retention time of sulfapyridine or its derivative can be delayed, and thereby separated from the pyridinoline peaks, by increasing the solvent heptabutyric acid (HFBA) [38].

2. IMMUNOASSAYS FOR COLLAGEN CROSS-LINKS

Since 1995, considerable progress has been made in developing immunoassays against the free amino-acids or against peptides containing the cross-links. All of these newer assays offer considerable advantages in the ease and speed of analysis, but usually at the expense of precision and reproducibilty.

An ELISA for the direct measurements of free cross-link components in urine was developed initially using polyclonal, and later monoclonal, antibodies [39, 40]. This assay did not, however, distinguish between PYD and DPD, as both cross-links showed similar reactivity with the antibodies. An intra-assay variation of approximately 7% and interassay variation of 11%, as well as a sensitivity of 25 nmol/l, have been reported [39]. An ELISA based on a monoclonal antibody has been described that shows 100% reactivity with free DPD and exhibits less than 2% cross-reactivity with PYD [41]. The intra- and interassay variations were 4–8% and 4–13.7%, respectively, with a sensitivity of 2 nM DPD. Another immunoassay developed by the same group measures both free PYD and free DPD in urine, with the monoclonal antibody employed showing similar affinity for each cross-link [40]. Peptides larger than approximately 1000 Da exhibited minimal cross-reactivity in this assay. In early 1998, the immunoassay for free DPD in urine was for the first time established on an automated system, making this assay now also feasible for large scale routine analyses [42]. The results obtained with the two immunoassays for free cross-links (in-

cluding the automated version) correlated well with values for total DPD measured by HPLC.

An important consideration when using the immunoassays for pyridinium cross-links in urine is the knowledge of the normal physiological variations that occur in the excretion of the free cross-link fraction. It has been shown that the proportion of free pyridinolines is smaller in elderly subjects than in adolescents and in healthy adults. In particular, elderly subjects with vitamin D deficiency seem to excrete a lower amount of free cross-link components than healthy subjects. In the elderly, a change in the molecular distribution of pyridinoline cross-links is observed; elderly people have an increased proportion of the largest peptide-bound forms (particularly >10,000 Da) and a decreased proportion of free pyridinolines and the smallest peptide-bound forms [43]. Consequently, the increase in urinary cross-links often seen in subjects over the age of 70 years is mainly due to a increase in the peptide-bound (i.e. high molecular weight) fraction [44]. This seems to indicate that changes in cross-link metabolism are at least partly responsible for the age-related increase in urinary cross-link concentration. Furthermore, in patients treated with bisphosphonates or hormone replacement therapy, it has been suggested that changes in the free fraction of immunoreactive cross-links do not reflect the changes in the excretion of total pyridinolin cross-links. In a short-term study on intravenous pamidronate treatment of Paget's disease, no reduction of the excretion of free DPD, but a markedly decreased excretion of the peptide-bound fraction was observed [45, 46]. This finding, however, has not been confirmed by others [47]. To circumvent the problem of the variable excretion of free pyridinolines, prior to immunoassay, a hydrolysis-step may be performed such that the total DPD concentration (i.e., the sum of free and peptide-bound fractions) can be measured [47].

B. Immunoassays for Collagen Telopeptides

The main molecular sites involved in collagen cross-linking are the short nonhelical peptides at both ends of the collagen molecule, termed amino- (N-) and carboxy- (C-) terminal telopeptides. In normal collagen, these telopeptides are each linked via pyridinium or pyrrole compounds to the helical portion of neighboring collagen molecules (Fig. 3) [25, 48–51]. During collagen breakdown, N- and C-terminal telopeptide fragments of various sizes, still attached to the helical portions of a nearby molecule by a pyridinium cross-link, are released into the circulation. The majority of these fragments are relatively small and readily cleared by the kidneys.

It has been demonstrated that type I collagen molecules can undergo β-isomerization of the aspartic acid residue within its C-telopeptides [52, 53]. This process of spontaneous posttranslational modification has been attributed to protein aging [52]. As a consequence of this isomerization, type I collagen molecules may be present in bone matrix as either linear (α) or β-isomerized C-telopeptides. Changes in the level of β-isomerization were found to reflect the metabolic status of pagetic bone [53, 54]. In Paget's disease, a much larger increase in the urinary excretion of the linear, nonisomerized form than the β-isomerized C-telopeptides has been observed.

In the early 1990s, a competitive inhibition ELISA was developed for the measurement of N-terminal cross-linked telopeptide (NTX) fragments in the urine [55]. This assay is based on a monoclonal antibody that specifically recognizes an epitope embedded in the α–2 chain of the N-telopeptide fragment (Fig. 3). The compound still contains the pyridinium cross-link, but this antibody does not recognize the pyridinoline or deoxypyridinoline cross-link per se. Thus, the antibody appears to react only with a conformational epitope which is specific for the cross-linking site of bone collagen [55]. Collagen must be broken down to small cross-linked peptides that contain the exact sequence before antibody binding occurs with the NTX antigen. Furthermore, the antibody also recognizes such peptides in culture medium conditioned by osteoclasts that are resorbing human bone particles *in vitro* [56, 57]. These data suggest that the NTX-peptide is a direct product of osteoclastic proteolysis and appears not to be metabolized further [55]. There is some contention about this specificity, however. Although the antibody recognizes a cross-link-containing sequence from the α–2 chain N-telopeptide, the cross-link is not involved in the epitope, and cross-reaction with skin-derived peptides has been reported [48, 58].

The NTX assay is calibrated using standard amounts of human bone collagen digested with bacterial collagenases. The intra- and interassay variability, expressed as a coefficient of variation, is on average 8% and 10% respectively, or higher at low concentration, and the sensitivity is 20–25 nM [59–61]. It has also been reported that the assay exhibits nonlinear recovery for sample dilutions prepared in assay buffer. This nonlinear recovery, however, could be corrected for by sample dilutions made in urine at low analyte concentrations [61]. This assay requires no hydrolysis or pretreatment of the urine.

Generally the measurement is performed in a second morning spot urine. Results are reported as bone collagen equivalents (BCE), in nM, corrected for creatinine excretion to compensate for differences in urine dilution.

In 1994, an ELISA for the measurement of the cross-linked part of the C-terminal telopeptide region of type I collagen in urine has been introduced [62]. For this assay, a synthetic octapeptide sequence (EKAHD-β-GGR) specific for the beta-isomerized form of the C-telopeptide α-1 chain was used to generate polyclonal and later monoclonal antibodies (β-CTX assay) (Fig. 3) [63]. This particular sequence of amino acids was chosen as the antigen because it contains the lysine of the C-telopeptide domain which participates in intermolecular cross-linking. Due to the compact structure of this peptide, protection from further degradation when excreted in the urine was anticipated [55, 62]. The intra- and interassay coefficients of variation are 6–8% and 8%, respectively [59, 61, 62]. At low concentrations, however, the assay exhibits poor precision [61]. The detection limit is 0.2–0.5 μg/ml.

A radioimmunoassay based on monoclonal antibodies recognizing the linear nonisomerized peptide form (αCTX) of the same amino acid sequence has also been developed [64]. This assay shows less than 2% cross-reactivity with the β-isomerized form (βCTX). Intra- and interassay variations for this assay are 3–5% and 4–6.5%, respectively [64].

More recently, a new assay for the measurement of CTX in serum has been developed. This sandwich ELISA utilizes monoclonal antibodies that recognize only the double-stranded beta-isomerized octapeptide sequence EKAHD-β-GGR [65]. The intra- and interassay coefficients for this assay are 6–7% and 9%, respectively, and the detection limit is 10 ng/ml [65].

In the meanwhile, a serum assay has been developed for the N-terminal telopeptide of type I collagen ("serum NTX"). The monoclonal antibody used is identical to the urinary assay. Clinical studies have shown that results obtained by the two new serum assays correlate well with their respective urinary analytes. In metabolic and malignant bone disease, however, the serum NTX assay appears to be slightly more sensitive than the serum CTX assay [65a].

Another immunoassay for the C-telopeptide cross-link domain applicable to serum was described earlier [66]. This radioimmunoassay is based on a polyclonal antibody against purified cross-linked peptides (ICTP), prepared by digesting human bone collagen with bacterial collagenase, or with trypsin, and purified by reverse-phase separations on HPLC [66]. The same material is also used for the calibration of the assay. The intra- and interassay coefficients of variation are 5–8% and 6–9%, respectively [67, 68]. A nonspecific binding of approximately 10% has been reported [67, 68]. The detection limit is on the order of 0.34 μg/L [66]. The main mechanism of its removal from blood is via the kidney because of the small size of the ICTP antigen. Glomerular filtration rates of $\leq$50 ml/min lead to a significant retention of this peptide [66]. Lipemic serum also appears to interfere with the assay. Although this was the first assay available for the assessment of bone resorption from serum samples, the results from clinical applications are somewhat disappointing and suggest that it lacks specificity.

VI. TARTRATE-RESISTANT ACID PHOSPHASTASE

The acid phosphatases are a heterogenous group of enzymes that hydrolyze phosphomonoesters at low pH with the release of phosphoric acid (see Chapter 9). There are five isoenzymes of acid phosphatase in serum, the major sources of which are bone, prostate, platelets, erythrocytes, and the spleen [69–72]. These isoenzymes differ inmolecular size, sensitivity towards various inhibitors, and electrophoretic mobility in acidic native polyacrylamic gels [69–71]. According to their relative electrophoretic mobility, serum acid phosphatase isoenzymes have been classified as type 0, 1, 2, 3a, 4, 5a, and 5b isoenzymes [71, 72]. Based on their sensitivity to inhibition by L(+)-tartrate, serum acid phosphatase isoenzymes are also divided into two classes, namely tartrate-sensitive (TSAP) and tartrate-resistant acid phosphatase (TRAP). However, one should bear in mind that the suscebility to L(+)-tartrate is not completely tissue specific [69–72]. The only TRAP isoenzymes present in serum are type 5a and 5b.

The skeleton is rich in acid phosphatase activity [73–75]. While osteoclasts show the greatest abundance in type 5b TRAP, some activity has also been shown in osteoblasts and osteocytes [76–78]. Generally, TRAP is used as cytochemical marker to distinguish osteoclasts from other bone cells [79–81].

In serum, TRAP can be measured either by spectrophotometric techniques or by immunoassay. A variety of spectrophotometric and kinetic assays for serum TRAP have been developed [70, 71, 82–91]. These assays differ in many aspects, including the type and concentrations of substrate, assay buffer, and pH of the reaction. The most widely used kinetic assay measures the hydrolysis of p-nitrophenol phosphate in the presence of sodium tartrate [82]. This assay takes into account several possible interferences. To minimize the interferences of noncompetitive inhibitors, the serum samples are diluted five-fold and the substrate concentration is increased. The diluted serum samples are then preincubated at 37°C for one hour before assay to inactivate erythrocytic TRAP activity released by hemolysis. To minimize the effect of platelet-derived TRAP activity, which may be released during clotting, the clotting time should be kept to a minimum, (i.e. 1–2 hours at room temperature) [82]. The reported intra- and interassay variation are 5% and 10%, respectively, and the recovery of exogenous added purified TRAP activity to human serum is $110 \pm 10\%$ [82].

The major drawback of the kinetic assays is the fact that these methods do not distinguish between TRAP activity derived from osteoclasts or from other sources. Consequently, they lack specificity and sensitivity for the osteoclastic isoenzyme. To improve the specificity and sensitivity of serum TRAP measurements, several immunoassays have been developed. Again, however, most of these immunoassay were not developed using osteoclastic TRAP as antigen. The first reported immunoassays used a immunoprecipitation approach based on a polyclonal antibody directed against a partially purified osteoclastic-like 5b TRAP recovered from the spleen of a patient with hairy-cell leukemia; alternatively, antibodies against porcine uteroferrin, which resembles osteoclastic TRAP, were used [92–94]. TRAP activity of the immune complex was then determined using a kinetic assay. However, the specificity of the antisera employed in these immunoprecipitation assays has not been evaluated, and it seems of further disadvantage that serum TRAP "levels" are still determined on the basis of the enzyme activity.

Immunoassays measuring protein concentration rather than enzyme activity have been developed [95–98]. An ELISA for serum type 5b osteoclastic TRAP using polyclonal antibodies against partially purified hairy cell leukemia spleen type 5b TRAP has been described [95]. The antibody reacted with the lysosomal type 5b TRAP in osteoclasts but showed no cross-reactivity with partially purified acid phosphatases from normal human spleen, prostatic acid phosphatase, or acid phosphatase extracted from osteoblasts [95]. Intra- and interassay variations are both less than 10% for this assay. Another ELISA is based on polyclonal antibodies against human cord plasma TRAP [96]. The antibody used in this assay cross-reacted with extracts of bone, but not with extracts obtained from spleen, erythrocytes, platelets, prostate or osteoblasts. Intra- and interassay variations are reported to be less than 12.5% and, analytical recovery varied from 94–106%. Since 1996, the first assays based on poly- and monoclonal antibodies against TRAP purified from human bone were described [98, 99]. The polyclonal antisera were employed in a competitive fluorescence immunoassay and were shown to immunohistochemically recognize osteoclasts from human bone and alveolar macrophages from human lung tissue, but not cells from human spleen tissue [99]. The two monoclonal antibodies raised against human osteoclastic type 5b TRAP were found to recognize different epitopes and therefore allowed the development of a two-site fluorescence immunoassay [98]. In this latter assay, the intra- and interassay coefficients of variation are both less than 5%, analytical recovery is $98.9 \pm 3.3\%$, and a sensitivity of less than 0.1 μg/l has been demonstrated. Although available evidence indicates that immunoassays for measurement of osteoclastic type 5b TRAP are promising, only limited data on clinical application of these assays are available.

VII. BONE SIALOPROTEIN

Bone sialoprotein (BSP) is a glycosylated protein with an apparent Mw of 70–80 kDa (core protein: 34 kDa) that accounts for approximately 5–10% of the noncollageneous proteins of the bone extracellular matrix [100, 101]. High amounts of BSP are expressed in active osteoblasts and, to a lesser degree, in osteoclast-like cell lines [102–104]. Compared to other noncollageneous proteins, the tissue distribution of BSP is relatively restricted; the protein or its mRNA is detected mainly in mineralized tissues such as bone and dentin and at the interface of calcifying cartilage and bone. However, BSP related immunoreactivity has also been demonstrated in placental trophoblasts and platelets [105,

106]. BSP contains an Arg-Gly-Asp (RGD) integrin recognition sequence, improves the attachment of osteoblasts and osteoclasts to surfaces, binds preferentially to the alpha2-chain of collagen type I, nucleates hydroxyapatite crystal formation *in vitro*, and appears to enhance osteoclast-mediated bone resorption [107–109]. The protein is therefore considered to play an important role in cell-matrix-adhesion processes and in the supramolecular organization of the extracellular matrix of mineralized tissues.

Several immunoassays for the determination of bone sialoprotein in serum have been developed [110–112]. All of these assays are based on polyclonal antisera against BSP. In terms of normal ranges, biological and pathological variability, and response to osteotropic treatment, most experience has been collected using a homologous radioimmunoassay [112, 113]. This assay uses bone sialoprotein isolated from human bone by standard extraction procedures and final purification by wide pore reverse-phase HPLC. The anti-BSP-antibodies against human BSP were raised in chicken. In this particular assay, the coefficients of variation were 6.1–7.0% for intraassay variability, and 9.2–9.4% for interassay variability. The lower detection limit is 0.7 ng/mL, and recovery after spiking of human samples with purified BSP ranged between 92 and 108%. Importantly, no cross-reactivity was observed with a number of noncollagenous proteins, such as osteocalcin, osteopontin, and osteonectin, or with bone alkaline phosphatase [112] (Fig. 7).

Employing the aforementioned radioimmunoassay, normal values for serum BSP ranged between 4.0 and 23.5 ng/mL (mean 11.8 ± 4.6 ng/mL). In healthy adults, serum BSP values were generally found to be unrelated to body measures, liver or kidney function, or lumbar bone density. However, serum BSP levels were significantly lower in premenopausal women than in males or postmenopausal females. Interestingly, in postmenopausal females, serum BSP levels were

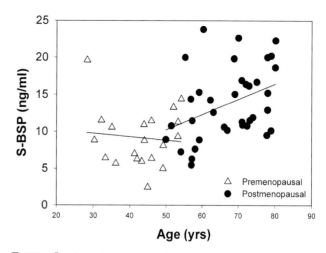

FIGURE 8 Serum bone sialoprotein (BSP) levels in healthy female subjects according to menopausal status. Reproduced from Seibel *et al.* [113], *J. Clin. Endocrinol. Metab.* **81**, 3289–3294, 1996; © The Endocrine Society.

correlated with chronological age ($r = 0.41$, $p < 0.001$) (Fig. 8) but not with age at menopause or with the duration of menopause. In contrast, no relation with age was seen in males and premenopausal females [113].

Results indicate that serum BSP reflects processes associated with osteoclast activity and bone resorption rather than osteoblast activity. Serum BSP is greatly elevated in patients with multiple myeloma (depending on the disease stage), and treatment with intravenous bisphosphonates results in a rapid fall of serum BSP values, paralelling the changes seen in urinary cross-link concentrations [112, 114]. Thus, serum BSP is presently considered as marker of bone resorption.

As seen with many other biomarkers of bone metabolism, serum BSP shows typical changes related to biological influences, such as diurnal, day-to-day, and menstrual variability, as well as changes with somatic growth and season [114, 115].

VIII. VARIABILITY

The appropriate interpretation of biochemical marker results should consider all sources of variability, which include not only the analytical performance characteristics of the method but also the biological variability of the markers, as well as the influence of preanalytical conditions. The total variability is the sum of the biological and analytical variations ($SD_{TOT}^2 = SD_B^2 + SD_A^2$) [116]. Ideally, the biochemical marker, and the assays used to measure it, should possess minimal and predictable biological variability and should be influenced as little as possible by preanalytical conditions. However, this often is not the case. The factors that confound measurements of biochemical markers to a variable degree are circadian rhythm, diet, age, sex, menstrual cycle, liver function, kidney clearance, as well as thermal stability, storage, and repeated freeze-thaw cycles (Table II).

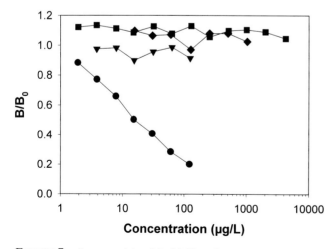

FIGURE 7 Cross-reactivity of Anti-BSP-antibody with noncollagenous proteins (● bone sialoprotein (BSP), ▼ bone alkaline phosphatase, ■ osteocalcin, ♦ osteonectin) (reproduced from Karmatschek *et al.* [112]).

TABLE II.   Sources of Variability

Analytical performance of the assay
Diurnal variation
Day-to-day variability
Variability due to menstrual cycle
Seasonal variability
Variation with growth and age
Kidney function
Analyte stability
Specimen collection
Storage of the samples

A. Analytical Performance

The analytical performances of the various bone resorption assays have been described above and are summarized in Table III.

B. Diurnal Variation

Most biochemical markers show significant diurnal variations, with highest values in the early morning hours and lowest values during the afternoon and at night. In 1970, it was demonstrated that the excretion of OHPr follows a circadian rhythm and this circadian rhythm is fairly constant from day to day [8]. Diurnal variation in pre- and postmenopausal women, as well as in men, has now been reported by many investigators for all biochemical markers of bone turnover, including the pyridinium cross-links, the telopeptide markers, tartrate-resistant acid phosphatase and bone sialoprotein [28, 61, 67, 115, 117–123].

Although some authors reported diurnal changes as high as ±100% of the daily mean, most studies found amplitudes between ±15–30%. Diurnal variation appears not to be affected by age, menopause, bed rest, or physical activity [120]. Although in postmenopausal women bone turnover is higher than in premenopausal women, the circadian variation is similar for both pre- and postmenopausal women and, thus, is not influenced by sex hormones [120, 122]. In osteoporotic women, it has been suggested that the increase in bone resorption at night may persist longer into the morning and that this may account in part for the greater bone loss in osteoporotic women [117]. However, this could not be confirmed for elderly women with osteopenia [120]. The circadian rhythm is also not influenced by season [124]. The etiology of these diurnal variations is unknown. Several hormones also showing circadian variation, such as parathyroid hormone, growth hormone, and cortisol, may be implicated

TABLE III.   Markers of Bone Resorption

Marker	Analyte	Tissue of origin	Assay method	Sensitivity	Intra-assay CV (%)	Interassay CV (%)	Commercially available assay
Hydroxyproline (OHPr)	Hydroxproline	Bone, cartilage, soft tissue, skin, blood	Colorimetric HPLC	5 μM/L 1 pM/L	2–10 2–4	8–15 5–8	Hypronosticon, Organon Teknika, Netherlands Hydroxyproline, BioRad Laboratories, Germany
Hydroxylysine glykosides	Galactosyl-hydroxylysine (GHYL)	Bone, soft tissue, skin, complement	HPLC	1 pM/L	5–8	6–7	
Pyridinoline (PYD)	Total PYD	Bone, cartilage, tendon, blood vessels	HPLC	1 pM/L	4–8	7–15	Crosslinks, BioRad Laboratories, Germany
	Free PYD (and free DPD)		ELISA	7.5 mM	7	11	Pyrilinks, Metra Biosystems, Inc., USA
Deoxypyridinoline (DPD)	Total DPD	Bone, dentin	HPLC	1 pM/L	6–10	8–12	Crosslinks, BioRad Laboratories, Germany
	Free DPD	Bone, dentin	ELISA	2 nM	4–8	4–14	Pyrilinks-D, Metra Biosystems, Inc., USA
Cross-linked telopeptides	N-telopeptide (NTX)	Bone	ELISA	20–25 nM/L	8	10	Osteomark, Ostex International, Inc., USA
	C-telopeptide (CTX)	Bone	ELISA RIA	0.2–0.5 μg/ml	6–8 3–5	8 4–6.5	CrossLaps, Osteometer Biotech, Denmark
	C-telopeptide (ICTP)	Bone	RIA	0.5 μg/L	5–8	6–9	ICTP, Orion Diagnostica, Finland
Tartrate-resistant acid phosphatase	TRAP	Bone, blood	Colorimetric RIA	<0.1μg/L	5 <5	10 <5	
Bone sialoprotein (BSP)	Sialoprotein	Bone, dentin, cartilage, platelets	RIA ELISA	0.7 ng/ml	6–7	9	

in affecting bone metabolism, [125–128]. Most markers of bone turnover do reflect the circadian rhythm of bone remodeling. Thus, controlling the time point of sampling is crucial to provide clinically relevant information.

C. Day-to-Day Variability

Biochemical markers of bone turnover not only vary within a single day (diurnal variation) but also exhibit a considerable variation between consecutive days [27, 61, 116]. This intraindividual day-to-day variability is apparently largely due to genuine variations in marker levels and not to analytical imprecision. Expressed as a coefficient of variation, the day-to-day variation in cross-link excretion measured by HPLC was 16–26% [27, 28]. A similar variability has been reported for free pyridinoline immunoassays (7–25%), for the N-terminal telopeptide (NTX, 13–35%), and for the C-terminal telopeptide assay (CTX, 12–35%), as well as for the tartrate-resistant acid phosphatase (TRAP, 10–12%) [61, 129–131]. In general, serum markers for bone formation show less day-to-day variability than urine markers for bone resorption. This may be related mostly to the difficulties associated with collecting accurately timed urine samples. The day-to-day variability adds a considerable variation to the measurements of biochemical markers, and this, in contrast to the diurnal variation, can not be controlled.

D. Variability Due to the Menstrual Cycle

Bone turnover varies with the menstrual cycle with an overall amplitude of 10–20% [115, 132–134]. Although not all available data show the same significance, there is substantial evidence that bone formation is higher during the luteal than the follicular phase [132], whereas the bone resorption markers are higher during the mid-follicular, late-follicular, and early luteal phase [134]. Cyclical changes in bone turnover have also been reported in postmenopausal women treated with sequential estrogen/progestagen regimens, showing decreases during estrogen treatment and increases during progestagen treatment [135, 136]. In general, the variability due to menstrual cycle is not so important in clinical practice, because most women evaluated for osteoporosis are postmenopausal. However, in premenopausal women with metabolic bone disease, the menstrual variability should be taken into account and the timing for sampling is probably best during the first 3–7 days of the menstrual cycle.

E. Seasonal Variability

A seasonal rhythm for measures of calcium homeostasis has been shown by a number of investigators. Serum levels of 25-OH vitamin D and urinary calcium excretion are elevated in late summer and decreased in winter, whereas parathyroid hormone levels tend to decrease during winter [137–143]. Only few data are available as to whether season influences bone turnover [138, 144–147]. It has been shown that bone turnover is increased during winter, with more pronounced changes in females than in males [144]. Furthermore, the seasonal increase in turnover tends to coincide with a significant reduction in serum 25-OH vitamin D, suggesting that the increase in bone turnover during the winter period may be due, at least in part, to subclinical vitamin D deficiency [144].

F. Variation with Growth and Age

During childhood, and particularly during puberty, biochemical markers of bone turnover levels are much higher than during adulthood because of the contribution of growth and modeling as well as remodeling of bone [7, 84, 148, 149]. In girls, estradiol seems to be the major determinant of the increase in bone turnover, with a peak during the rapid growth phase of Tanner stages II and III. After the age of 50, there is a more or less linear increase in levels of bone turnover markers both in men and in women. In women, the age-dependence of the marker levels is more pronounced and mainly due to menopause. Bone resorption increases by about 50% within 6–12 months after menopause [113, 150–153].

G. Kidney Function

Mild to moderate renal impairment was shown to have no significant influence on the total excretion of pyridinoline cross-links, and urinary values usually do not change until a creatinine clearance of <25 ml/min is reached [28, 44, 154]. In contrast, the serum levels of the C-terminal telopeptide ICTP are strongly affected by renal function and tend to increase with a glomerular filtration rate of ≤50 ml/min [66]. In patients with renal failure, serum BSP levels tend to increase, and in this group, highest values are seen in patients with renal insufficiency and secondary hyperparathyroidism [113].

H. Analyte Stability, Specimen Collection, and Storage

Both the free and conjugated forms of PYD and DPD have been shown to be stable in urine samples kept at room temperature for several weeks [27, 155]. Several reports show that pyridinium cross-links can be stored at -20°C for years [27, 155–157]. Repeated freezing and thawing of urine samples up to ten times had no effect on the concentrations of the pyridinolines [155]. Similar stability has been reported in part for the N-terminal (NTX) and C-terminal (CTX) telopeptides, except for the serum C-terminal telopeptide (ICTP) which lost up to 12% when stored at room temperature for five days [61, 62, 66]. The stability properties of glycosylated hydroxylysine have not been fully characterized, but it may be necessary to add boric acid to preserve the urine samples [158]. TRAP activity declines rapidly at room temperature and during frozen storage at -20°C but retains its activity when stored at -70°C [82]. Multiple freezing–thawing (for up to three cycles) did not appear to have a significant effect on TRAP serum activity [123].

Pyridinium cross-links are unstable when subjected to intensive UV irradiation. After exposure to natural light for three hours, no changes in PYD and DPD could be demonstrated, whereas pyridinolines in the aqueous standard were rapidly degraded [159–161]. The increased pyridinoline photolysis in the aqueous standards compared with urinary pyridinolines may be attributed to the fact that the intensity of incident UV light is higher in aqueous solutions. Photolysis of the pyridinoline standard solution is prevented by storage in amber vials [160]. The rate of pyridinoline photolysis is also pH dependent (i.e., the rate increases with increasing pH) [159]. It has also been shown that the sensitivity to UV light is greater for free pyridinoline than for total pyridinoline [161]. The telopeptides NTX and CTX are not affected by UV light exposure [161]. Serum BSP levels are rather stable, both at room temperature and -20°C, and have been shown to not change significantly during repeated freeze–thaw cycles. The evidence shows, therefore, that random urine samples can be used for measurement of urinary pyridinolines, however, placing the urine samples in the dark within two hours of collection is recommended [159].

Measurement of bone resorption markers is usually performed in fasting urine samples over two hours or in a fasting spot sample in the morning which is corrected for urinary creatinine. Alternatively, timed 24-hour urine collection can be performed and the excretion rate of the marker determined. Both approaches are subject to some difficulties. Creatinine output has been reported to be fairly constant with time (variations within 10%) and to correlate with lean body mass [162], but there are also reports suggesting that the correction for creatinine in a urine spot sample could be misleading. On the other hand, timed 24-hour urine collections are subject to inevitable inaccuracies due to collection errors. In general, similar results are obtained from either 24-hour, 2-hour, or spot urine collections. It should be kept in mind, however, that the slope of diurnal changes is steepest during the morning hours (see diurnal variation), which is usually the time at which urine samples are collected. Therefore, if spot urine is used for measurement of bone resorption markers, the time of collection should be controlled as closely as possible.

In conclusion, there are a number of sources of variability that need to be taken into account. To overcome some of these limitations due to preanalytic and biological variability, standardized sampling, storage, and transport to the laboratory are mandatory for appropriate interpretation of the results.

References

1. Prockop, D. J., and Kivirikko, K. I. (1984). Heritable diseases of collagen. *N. Engl. J. Med.* **311**, 376–386.
2. Smith, R. (1980). Collagen and disorders of bone. *Clin. Sci.* **59**, 215–221.
3. Woessner, J. F. (1961). The determination of hydroxyproline in tissue and protein samples containing small proportions of this imino acid. *Arch. Biochem. Biophys.* **93**, 440–447.
4. Kivirikko, K. I., Laitinen, O., and Prockop, D. J. (1967). Modifications of a specific assay for hydroxyproline in urine. *Ana. Biochem.* **19**, 249–255.
5. Podenphant, J., Larsen, N. E. and Christiansen, C. (1984). An easy and reliable method for determination of urinary hydroxyproline. *Clin. Chim. Acta* **142**, 145–148.
6. Sela, B. A., and Doolman, R. (1991). Refinement of a specific assay for hydroxyproline in urine. *Clin. Chim. Acta* **203**, 91–94.
7. Hodgkinson, A., and Thompson, T. (1982). Measurement of the fasting urinary hydroxyproline:creatinine ratio in normal adults and its variation with age and sex. *J. Clin. Pathol.* **35**, 807–811.
8. Mautalen, C. A. (1970). Circadian rhythm of urinary total and free hydroxyproline excretion and its relation to creatinine excretion. *J. Lab. Clin. Med.* **75**, 11–18.
9. Scalella, P. (1982). Interference by iodinated contrast media in total urinary hydroxyproline measurement. *Lancet* **1**, 907.
10. Reed, P., Holbrook, I. B., Gardner, M. L. G., and McMurray, J. R. (1991). Simple, optimized liquid-chromatographic method for measuring total hydroxyproline in urine evaluated. *Clin. Chem.* **37**, 285–290.
11. Casari, E., Ferrero, C. A., Grazioli, V., and Murone, M. (1992). Performance of a modified HPLC method to determine total hydroxyprolinuria in 2-h urine samples. *Clin. Chem.* **38**, 2337–2338.
12. Dawson, C. D., Jewett, S., and Driskoll, W. J. (1988). Liquid-chormatographic determination of total hydroxyproline in urine. *Clin. Chem.* **34**, 1572–1574.
13. Cunningham, L. W., Ford, J. D. and Segrest, J. P. (1967). The isolation of identical hydroxylysyl glycosides from hydrolysates of soluble collagen and from human urine. *J. Biol. Chem.* **242**, 2570–2571.
14. Krane, S. M., Kantrowitz, F. G., Byrns, M., Pinnell, S. R., and Singer, F. R. (1977). Urinary excretion of hydroxylysine and its glycosides as an index of collagen degradation. *J. Clin. Invest.* **39**, 819–827.
15. Askenasi, R. (1975). Urinary excretion of freee hydroxylysine, peptide-bound hydroxylysine and hydroxylysyl glycosides in physiological conditions. *Clin. Chim. Acta* **59**, 87–92.
16. Segrest, J. P., and Cunningham, L. W. (1970). Variations in human urinary O-hydroxylysyl glycoside levels and their relationship to collagen metabolism. *J. Clin. Invest.* **49**, 1497–1509.
17. Krane, S. M., Kantrowittz, F. G., Byrne, M., Pinnell, S. R. and Singer, F. R. (1977). Urinary excretion of hydroxylysine and its glycosides as an index of collagen degradation. *J. Clin. Invest.* **59**, 819–827.
18. Moro, L., Modricky, C., Stagni, N., Vittur, F., and Bernard, B. (1984). High-performance liquid chromatographic analysis of urinary hydroxylysyl glycosides as indicator of collagen turnover. *Analyst* **109**, 1621–1622.
19. Moro, L., Battista, C., Modricky, C., Rovis, L., and de Bernard, B. (1989). High-Performance liquid chromatographic preparation of galactosyl-hydroxylysine, a specific bone collagen marker. *J. Chromatogr.* **490**, 285–292.
20. Moro, L., Modricky, C., Rovis, L., and de Bernard, B. (1988). Determination of galactosyl hydroxylysine in urine as a means for the identification of osteoporotic women. *Bone Miner.* **3**, 271–276.
21. Moro, L., Gazzarrini, C., Modricky, C., Rovis, L., de Bernard, B., Galligioni, E., Crivellari, D., Morassut, S., and Monfardini, S. (1990). High predictivity of galactosyl-hydroxylysine in urine as an indicator of bone metastases from breast cancer. *Clin. Chem.* **36**, 772–774.

22. Bettica, P., Moro, L., Robins, S. P., Taylor, A. K., Talbot, J., Singer, F. R., and Baylink, D. J. (1992). Bone-resorption markers galactosyl hydroxylysine, pyridinium crosslinks, and hydroxyproline compared. *Clin. Chem.* **38**, 2313–2318.

23. Moro, L., Mucelli, R. S., Gazzarrini, C., Modricky, C., Marotti, F., and de Bernard, B. (1988). Urinary beta-1-galactosyl-0-hydroxylysine (GH) as a marker of collagen turnover of bone. *Calcif. Tissue Int.* **42**, 87–90.

24. Robins, S. P. (1983). Cross-linking of collagen. Isolation, structural characterization and glycosylation of pyridinoline. *Biochem. J.* **215**, 167–173.

25. Eyre, D. R., Paz, M. A. and Gallop, P. M. (1984). Cross-linking in collagen and elastin. *Annu. Rev. Biochem.* **53**, 717–748.

26. Delmas, P. D., Gineyts, E., Bertholin, A., Garnero, P., and Marchand, F. (1993). Immunoassay of pyridinoline crosslink excretion in normal adults and in Paget's disease. *J. Bone Miner. Res.* **8**, 643–648.

27. Colwell, A., Russell, R. G. G., and Estell, R. (1993). Factors affecting the assay of urinary 3-hydroxy pyridinium crosslinks of collagen as markers of bone resorption. *Eur. J. Clin. Invest.* **23**, 341–349.

28. McLaren, A. M., Isdale, A. H., Whitings, P. H., Bird, H. A., and Robins, S. P. (1993). Physiological variations in the urinary excretion of pyridinium crosslinks of collagen. *Br. J. Rheumatol.* **32**, 307–312.

29. Colwell, A., and Eastell, R. (1996). The renal clearance of free and conjugated pyridinium cross-links of collagen. *J. Bone Miner. Res.* **11**, 1976–1980.

30. Black, D., Duncan, A., and Robins, S. P. (1988). Quantitative analysis of the pyrdinium crosslinks of collagen in urine using ion-paired reversed-phase high- performance liquid chromatography. *Anal. Biochem.* **169**, 197–203.

31. Uebelhart, D., Gineyts, E., Chapuy, M.-C. and Delmas, P. D. (1990). Urinary excretion of pyridinium crosslinks: A new marker of bone resorption in metabolic bone disease. *Bone Miner.* **8**, 87–96.

32. Pratt, D. A., Daniloff, Y. N., Duncan, A., and Robins, S. P. (1992). Automated analysis of the pyridinium crosslinks of collagen in tissue and urine using solid-phase extraction and reversed-phase high-performance liquid chromatography. *Anal. Biochem.* **207**, 168–175.

33. Robins, S. P., Stead, D. A. and Duncan, A. (1994). Precautions in using internal standard to measure pyridinoline and deoxypyrinoline in urine. *Clin. Chem.* **40**, 2322–2323.

33a. Robins, S. P. (1997). Measurement of pyridinium crosslinks by HPLC and immunoassay. *In* "Calcium Regulating Hormones and Markers of Bone Metabolism: Measurement and Interpretation" (H. Schmidt-Gayk, *et al.* eds.), pp. 135–140. Clin. Lab. Publications, Heidelberg.

34. Calabresi, E., Lasagni, L., Franceschelli, F., Bartolini, L., Serio, M., and Brandi, M. L. (1994). Use of an internal standard to measure pyridinoline and deoxypyridinoline in urine. *Clin. Chem.* **40**, 336–337.

35. Robins, S. P., Duncan, A., Wilson, N., and Evans, B. J. (1996). Standardization of pyridinium crosslinks, pyridinoline and deoxypyridinoline, for use as biochemical markers of collagen degradation. *Clin. Chem.* **42**, 1621–1626.

36. Seibel, M. J., Duncan, A. and Robins, S. P. (1989). Urinary hydroxypyridinium crosslinks provide indices of cartilage and bone involvement in arthritic disease. *J. Rheumatol.* **16**, 964–970.

37. Seibel, M. J., Baylink, D. J., Farley, J. R., Epstein, S., Yamauchi, M., Eastell, R., Pols, H. A., Raisz, L. G., and Gundberg, C. M. (1997). Basic science and clinical utility of biochemical markers of bone turnover—a Congress report. *Exp. Clin Endocrinol Diabetes* **105**, 125–133.

38. Peel, N. F. A., al-Dehaimi, A. W., Colwell, A., Russell, R. G. G. and Eastell, R. (1994). Sulfasalazine may interfere with HPLC assay of urinary pyridinium crosslinks. *Clin. Chem.* **40**, 167–168.

39. Seyedin, S. M., Kung, V. T., Daniloff, Y. N., Hesley, R. P., Gomez, B., Nielsen, L. A., Rosen, H. N., and Zuk, R. F. (1993). Immunoassay for urinary pyridinoline: The new marker of bone resorption. *J. Bone Miner. Res.* **8**, 635–641.

40. Gomez, B., Ardakani, S., Evans, B. J., Merrel, L. D., Jenkins, D. K., and Kung, V. T. (1996). Monoclonal antibody assay for free urinary pyridinium cross-links. *Clin. Chem.* **42**, 1168–1175.

41. Robins, S. P., Woitge, H., Hesley, R., Ju, J., Seyedin, S., and Seibel, M. J. (1994). Direct enzyme-linked immunoassay for urinary deoxypyridinoline as a specific marker for measuring bone resorption. *J. Bone Miner. Res.* **9**, 1643–1649.

42. Seibel, M. J., Woitge, H., Auler, B., Kissling, C., and Ziegler, R. (1998). Urinary free deoxypyridinoline: Comparison of a new automated chemiluminescence immunoassay with HPLC and ELISA techniques. *Clin. Lab.* **44**, 129–135.

43. Kamel, S., Brazier, J., Neri, V., Picard, C., Samson, L., Desmet, G., and Sebert, J. L. (1995). Multiple molecular form of pyridinoline crosslinks excreted in human urine evaluated by chromatographic and immunoassay methods. *J. Bone Miner. Res.* **10**, 1385–1392.

44. Seibel, M. J. (1997). Clinical use of pyridinium crosslinks. *In* Calcium Regulating Hormones and Markers of Bone Metabolism: Measurement and Interpretation (H. Schmidt-Gayk *et al.*, eds.), pp. 157–169. Clin. Lab. Publications, Heidelberg.

45. Garnero, P., Shih. W. J., Gineyts, E., Karpf, D. B. and Delmas, P. D. (1994). Comparison of new biochemical markers of bone turnover in late postmenopausal osteoporotic women in response to alendronate treatment. *J. Clin. Endocrinol. Metab.* **79**, 1693–1700.

46. Randall, A. G., Kent, G. N., Garcia-Webb, P., Bhagat, C. I., Pearce, D. J., Gutteridge, D. H., Prince, R. L., Stewart, G., Stuckey, B., Will, R. K., Retallack, R. W., Price, R. I., and Ward, L. (1996). Comparison of biochemical markers of bone turnover in paget disease treated with pamidronate and a proposed model for the relationships between measurements of different forms of pyridinoline cross-links. *J. Bone Miner. Res.* **11**, 1176–1184.

47. Blumsohn, A., Naylor, K. E., Assiri, A. M., and Eastell, R. (1995). Different responses of biochemical markers of bone resorption to bisphosphonate therapy in paget disease. *Clin. Chem.* **41**, 1592–1598.

48. Knott, L., and Bailey, A. J. (1998). Collagen cross-links in mineralizing tissues: A review of their chemistry, function and clinical relevance. *Bone* **22**, 181–187.

49. Hanson, D., and Eyre, D. R. (1996). Molecular site specificity of pyridinoline and pyrrole crosslinks in type I collagen of human bone. *J. Biol. Chem.* **247**, 26508–26516.

50. Knott, L., Tarlton, J. F., and Bailey, A. J. (1997). Chemistry of collagen cross-linking: Biochemical changes in collagen during the partial mineralization of turkey leg tendon. *Biochem. J.* **322**, 535–542.

51. Kuypers, R., Tyler, M., Kurth, L. B., Jenkins, I. D., and Horgan, D. J. (1992). Identification of the loci of the collagen-associated Ehrlich chromagen in type I collagen confirms its role as a trivalent crosslink. *Biochem. J.* **283**, 129–136.

52. Fledelius, C., Johnsen, A. H., Cloos, P. C., Bonde, M. and Qvist, P. (1997). Characterization of urinary degradation products derived from type I collagen. Identification of a beta-isomerized Asp-Gly sequence within the C-terminal telopeptide (alpha1) region. *J. Biol. Chem.* **272**, 9755–9763.

53. Garnero, P., Fledelius, C., Gineyts, E., Serre, C. M., Vignot, E., and Delmas, P. D. (1997). Decreased beta-isomerization of the C-terminal telopeptide of type I collagen alpha 1 chain in Paget's disease of bone. *J. Bone Miner. Res.* **12**, 1407–1415.

54. Garnero, P., Gineyts, E., Schaffer, A. V., Seaman, J., and Delmas, P. D. (1998). Measurement of urinary excretion of nonisomerized and beta-isomerized forms of type I collagen breakdown products to monitor the effects of the bisphosphonate zoledronate in Paget's disease. *Arthritis Rheum.* **41**, 354–360.

55. Hanson, D. A., Weis, M. A., Bollen, A. M., Maslan, S. L., Singer, F. R., and Eyre, D. R. (1992). A specific immunoassay for monitoring human bone resorption: Quantitation of type I collagen cross-linked N-telopeptides in urine. *J. Bone Miner. Res.* **7**, 1251–1258.

56. Eyre, D. R. (1995). The specificity of collagen crosslinks as markers of bone and connective tissue degradation. *Acta. Orthop. Scand.* **66**, 166–170.

57. Apone, S., Fevold, K., Lee, M., and Eyre, D. R. (1998). A rapid method for quantifying osteoclast activity in vitro. *J. Bone Miner. Res.* **9**, S178 (abstr.).

58. Robins, S. P. (1995). Collagen cross-links in metabolic bone disease. *Acta Orhop. Scand.* **66**.

59. Garnero, P., Gineyts, E., Arbault, P., Christiansen, C., and Delmas, P. D. (1995). Different effects of bisphosphonate and estrogen therapy on free and peptide-bound cross-links excretion. *J. Bone Miner. Res.* **10**, 641–649.

60. Gertz, B. J., Hanson, D. A., Quan, H., Harris, S. T., Genant, H. K., Chesnut, CH. H., III, and Eyre, D. R. (1994). Monitoring bone resorption in early postmenopausal women by an immunoassay for crosslinked collagen peptides in urine. *J. Bone Miner. Res.* **9**, 135–142.

61. Ju, H.-S. J., Leung, S., Brown, B., Stringer, M. A., Leigh, S., Scherrer, C., Shepard, K., Jenkins, D., Knudsen, J., and Cannon, R. (1997). Comparison of analytical performance and biological variability of three bone resorption assays. *Clin. Chem.* **43**, 1570–1576.

62. Bonde, M., Qvist, P., Fledelius, C., Riis, B. J., and Christiansen, C. (1994). Immunoassay for quantifying type I collagen degradation products in urine evaluated. *Clin. Chem.* **40**, 2022–2025.

63. Fledelius, C., Kolding, I., Bonde, M., Cloos, P., and Christgau, S. (1996). Specificity of the Crosslaps ELISA and the MabA7 ELISA. *Osteoporosis Int.* **6**(Suppl.1), PMO440.

64. Bonde, M., Fledelius, C., Qvist, P., and Christiansen, C. (1996). Coated tube radioimmunoassay for c-telopeptides of type I collagen to assess bone resorption. *Clin. Chem.* **42**, 1639–1644.

65. Bonde, M., Garnero, P., Fledelius, C., Qvist, P., Delmas, P. D., and Christiansen, C. (1997). Measurement of bone degradation products in serum using antibodies reactive with an isomerized form of an 8 amino acid sequence of the c-telopeptide of type I collagen. *J. Bone Miner. Res.* **12**, 1028–1034.

65a. Woitge, H. W., Oberwittler, H., Farahmand, I., Lang, M., Ziegler, R., and Seibel, M. J. (1999). Novel serum assays for bone resorption. *J. Bone Miner. Res.* **14** (in press).

66. Risteli, J., Elomaa, I., Niemi, S., Novamo, A., and Risteli, L. (1993). Radioimmunoassay for the pyridinoline cross-linked carboxy-terminal telopeptide of type I collagen: A new serum marker of bone collagen degradation. *Clin. Chem.* **39**, 635–640.

67. Hassager, C., Risteli, J., Risteli, L., Jensen, S. B., and Christiansen, C. (1992). The diurnal variation in serum markers of type I collagen synthesis and degradation in healthy premenopausal women. *J. Bone Miner. Res.* **7**, 1307–1311.

68. Eriksen, E. F., Charles, P., Melsen, F., Mosekilde, L., Risteli, L., and Risteli, J. (1993). Serum markers of type I collagen formation and degradation in metabolic bone disease: Correlation with bone histomorphometry. *J. Bone Miner. Res.* **8**, 127–132.

69. Romas, N. A., Rose, N. R., and Tannenbaum, M. (1979). Acid phosphatase: New developments. *Hum. Pathol.* **10**, 501–512.

70. Yam, L. T. (1974). Clinical significance of human acid phosphatases. *Am. J. Med.* **56**, 604–616.

71. Li, C. Y., Chuda, R. A., Lam, K.-W., and Yam, L. T. (1973). Acid phosphatases in human plasma. *J. Lab. Clin. Med.* **82**, 446–460.

72. Lam, K. W., Lai, L., and Yam, L. T. (1978). Tartrate-resistant acid phosphatase activity measured by electrophoresis *and acrylamide gel*. *Clin. Chem.* **24**, 309–312.

73. Vaes, G., and Jacques, P. (1965). The assay of acid hydrolases and other enzymes in bone tissue. *Biochem. J.* **97**, 380–388.

74. Wergedal, J. E. (1970). Characterization of bone acid phosphatase activity. *Proc. Soc. Exp. Biol. Med.* **134**, 244–247.

75. Hammarstrom, L. E., Hanker, J. S., and Toverud, S. U. (1971). Cellular differences in acid phosphatase isoenzymes in bone and teeth. *Clin. Orthop.* **78**, 151–155.

76. Lau, K.-H. W., Stepan, J. J., Yoo, A., Mohan, S., and Baylink, D. J. (1991). Evidence that tartrate-resistant acid phosphatases from osteoclastomas and hairy cell leukemia spleen are members of a multigene family. *Int. J. Biochem.* **23**, 1237–1244.

77. Wergedal, J., Lau, K.-H. W., and Baylink, D. J. (1988). Fluoride and bovine bone extract influence cell proliferation and phosphatase activities in human bone cell cultures. *Clin. Orthop. Relat. Res.* **233**, 274–282.

78. Bianco, P., Ballanti, P., and Bonucci, E. (1988). Tartrate resistent acid phosphatase activity in rat osteoblasts and osteocytes. *Calcif. Tissue Int.* **73**, 167–171

79. Minkin, C. (1982). Bone acid phosphatase: Tartrate-resistant acid phosphatase as a marker of osteoclast function. *Calcif. Tissue Int.* **34**, 285–290.

80. Wergedal, J. E., and Baylink, D. J. (1984). Characterization of cells isolated and cultured from human bone. *Proc. Soc. Exp. Biol. Med.* **176**, 27–31.

81. Lam, K. W., Lee, P., Li, C. Y. and Yam, L. T. (1980). Immunological and biochemical evidence for identity of tartrate-resistant isoenzymes of acid phosphatases from human spleen and tissues. *Clin. Chem.* **26**, 420–422.

82. Lau, K. H. W., Onishi, T., Wergedal, J. E., Singer, F. R., and Baylink, D. J. (1987). Characterization and assay of tartrate-resistant acid phosphatase activity in serum: Potential use to assess bone resorption. *Clin. Chem.* **33**, 458–462.

83. Stepan, J. J., Pospichal, J., Presl, J. and Pacovsky, V. (1987). Bone loss and biochemical indices of bone remodelling in surgically induced postmenopausal women. *Bone* **8**, 279–284.

84. Stepan, J. J., Tesarova, A., Havranek, T., Jodl, J., Normankova, J., and Pacovsky, V. (1985). Age and sex dependency of the biochemical indices of bone remodelling. *Clin. Chim. Acta* **151**, 273–283.

85. Stepan, J. J., Silinkova-Malkova, E., Havranek, T., Formankova, J., Zichova, M., Lachmanova, J., Strakova, M., Broulik, P., and Pacovsky, V. (1983). Relationship of plasma tartrate resistant acid phosphatase to the bone isoenzyme of serum alkaline phosphatase in hyperparathyroidism. *Clin. Chim. Acta* **133**, 189–200.

86. Cooper, J. D. H., Turnell, D. C., and Price, C. P. (1982). The estimation of serum acid phosphatase using alpha-naphthyl phosphate as substrate: Observation on the use of fast red TR salt in the assay. *Clin. Chem.* **126**, 297–306.

87. Bais, R., and Edwards, J. B. (1976). An optimized continuous-monotoring procedure for semiautomated determination of serum acid phosphatase activity. *Clin. Chem.* **22**, 2025–2028.

88. Lam, K. W., Burke, D. S., Siemens, M., Cipperly, V., Li, C. Y., and Yam, L. T. (1982). Characterization of serum acid phosphatase associated with dengue hemorrhagic fever. *Clin. Chem.* **28**, 2296–2299.

89. Warren, R. J., and Moss, D. W. (1977). An automated continuous-monitoring procedure for the determination of acid phosphatase activity in serum. *Clin. Chim. Acta* **77**, 179–188.

90. Omene, J. A., Glew, R. H., Baig, H. A., Robinson, D. B., Brock, W., and Chamber, J. P. (1981). Determination of serum acid and alkaline phosphatase using 4-methylumbelliferyl phosphate. *Afr. J. Med. Sci.* **10**, 9–18.

91. Nakanishi, M., Yoh, K., Uchida, K., Maruo, S., and Matsuoka, A. (1998). Improved method for measuring tartrate-resistant acid phosphatase activity in serum. *Clin. Chem.* **44**, 221–225.

92. Lam, K. W., Siemens, M., Sun, T., Li, C.Y., and Yam, L. T. (1982). Enzyme-immunoassay for tartrate-resistant acid phosphatase. *Clin. Chem.* **28**, 467–470.

93. Echetebu, Z. O., Cox, T. M., and Moss, D. W. (1987). Antibodies to

porcine uteroferrin used in measurement of human tartrate-resistant acid phosphatase. *Clin. Chem.* **33**, 1832–1836.

94. Whitaker, K. B., Cox, T. M., and Moss, D. W. (1989). An immunoassay of human band-5 ("tartrate-resistent") acid phosphatase that involves the use of anti-porcine uteroferrin antibodies. *Clin. Chem.* **35**, 86–89.

95. Kraenzlin, M. E., Lau, K.-H. W., Liang, L., Freeman, T. K., Singer, F. R., Stepan, J., and Baylink, D. J. (1990). Development of an immunoassay for human serum osteoclastic tartrate-resistant acid phosphatase. *J. Clin. Endocrinol. Metab.* **71**, 442–451.

96. Cheung, C. K., Panesar, N. S., Haines, C., Masarei, J., and Swaminathan, R. (1995). Immunoassay of a tartrate-resistant acid phosphatase in serum. *Clin Chem.* **41**, 679–686.

97. Ott, S. M. (1993). Clinical effects of bisphosphonates in involutional osteoporosis. *J. Bone Miner. Res.* **8** (Suppl. 2), S597–S606.

98. Halleen, J., Hentunen, T. A., Karp, M., Käkönen, S. M., Petterson, K., and Väänänen, H. K. (1998). Characterization of serum tartrate-resistant acid phosphatase and development of a direct two-site immunoassay. *J. Bone Miner. Res.* **13**, 683–687.

99. Halleen, J., Hentunen, T. A., Hellman, J., and Vaananen, H. K. (1996). Tartrate-resistant acid phosphatase from human bone: Purification and development of an immunoassay. *J. Bone Miner. Res.* **11**, 1444–1452.

100. Fisher, L. W., McBride, O. W., Termine, J. D., and Young, M. F. (1990). Human bone sialoprotein: Deduced protein sequence and chromosomal localization. *J. Biol. Chem.* **265**, 2347–2351.

101. Oldberg, A., Franzen, A., and Heinegard, D. (1985). Isolation and characterization of two sialoproteins present only in bone. *Biochem. J.* **232**, 715–724.

102. Chen, J., Shapiro, H. S., and Wrana, J. L. (1991). Localization of bone sialoprotein (BSP) expression to sites of mineral tissue formation in fetal rat tissue by in-situ hybridization. *Matrix* **11**, 133–143.

103. Shapiro, H. S., Chen, J., Wrana, J. L., Zhang, Q., Blum, M., and Sodek, J. (1993). Characterization of porcine bone sialoprotein: Primary structure and cellular expression. *Matrix* **13**, 431–440.

104. Fujisawa, R., Butler, W. T., Brunn, J. C., Zhou, H. Y., and Kuboki, Y. (1993). Differences in composition of cell-attachment sialoproteins between dentin and bone. *J. Dent. Res.* **72**, 1222–1226.

105. Young, M. F., Kerr, J. M., Ibaraki, K., Heegaard, A. M., and Robey, P. G. (1992). Structure, expression, and regulation of the major non-collagenous matrix proteins of bone. *Clin. Orthop.* **281**, 275–294.

106. Chenu, C., and Delmas, P. D. (1992). Platelets contribute to circulating levels of bone sialoprotein in human. *J. Bone Miner. Res.* **7**, 47–54.

107. Ross, F. P., Chappel, J., Alvarez, J. I., Sander, D., Butler, W. T., Farach-Carson, M. C., Mintz, K. A., Robey, P. G., Teitelbaum, S. L., and Cheresh, D. A. (1993). Interactions between the bone matrix proteins osteopontin and bone sialoprotein and the osteoclast integrin alpha v beta 3 potentiate bone resorption. *J. Biol. Chem.* **268**, 9901–9907.

108. Fujisawa, R., Nodasaka, Y., and Kuboki, Y. (1995). Further characterization of interaction between bone sialoprotein (BSP) and collagen. *Calcif. Tissue Int.* **56**, 140–144.

109. Hunter, G. K., Kyle, C. L., and Goldberg, H. A. (1994). Modulation of crystal formation by bone phosphoproteins: Structural specificity of the osteopontin-mediated inhibition of hydroxyapatite formation. *Biochem. J.* **300**, 723–728.

110. Saxne, T., Zunino, L., and Heineg (1995). Increased release of bone sialoprotein into synovial fluid reflects tissue destruction in rheumatoid arthritis. *Arthritis Rheum.* **38**, 82–90.

111. Ohno, U., Matsuyama, T., Ishii, S., Hata, H., and Kuboki, Y. (1995). Measurement of human immunoreactive bone sialoprotein (BSP) in normal adults and in pregnant women. *J Bone Miner. Res.* **10** (Suppl.1), S476 (abstr.).

112. Karmatschek, M., Maier, I., Seibel, M. J., Woitge, H. W., Ziegler, R., and Armbruster, F. P. (1997). Improved purification of human bone sialoprotein and development of a homologous radioimmunoassay. *Clin. Chem.* **43**, 2076–2082.

113. Seibel, M. J., Woitge, H. W., Pecherstorfer, M., Karmatschek, M., Horn, E., Ludwig, H., Armbruster, F. P., and Ziegler, R. (1996). Serum immunoreactive bone sialoprotein as a new marker of bone turnover in metabolic and malignant bone disease. *J. Clin. Endocrinol. Metab.* **81**, 3289–3294.

114. Woitge, H. W., Knothe, A., Ziegler, R., and Seibel, M. J. (1998). Seasonal changes in bone turnover: Results of a prospective longitudinal study. *In preparation.*

115. Li, Y., Woitge, W., Kissling, C., Lang, M., Oberwittler, H., Karmatschek, M., Armbruster, F. P., von Schickfus, A. R., Ziegler, R., and Seibel, M. J. (1998). Biological variability of serum immunoreactive bone sialoprotein. *Clin. Lab.* **44**, 553–555.

116. Jensen, J. B., Kollerup, G., Sorensen, A., and Sorensen, O. H. (1997). Intraindividual variability of bone markers in the urine. *Scand. J. Clin. Lab. Invest.* **57**, 29–34.

117. Eastell, R., Calvo, M. S., Burritt, M. F., Offord, K. P., Russell, R. G. G., and Riggs, B. L. (1992). Abnormalities in circadian patterns of bone resorption and renal calcium conservation in type I osteoporosis. *J. Clin. Endocrinol. Metab.* **74**, 487–494.

118. Schlemmer, A., Hassager, C., Jensen, S. B., and Christiansen, C. (1992). Marked diurnal variation in urinary excretion of pyridinium cross-links in premenopausal women. *J. Clin. Endocrinol. Metab.* **74**, 476–480.

119. Pagani, F., and Panteghini, M. (1994). Diurnal rhythm in urinary excretion of pyridinium crosslinks. *Clin. Chem.* **40**, 952–953.

120. Schlemmer, A., Hassager, C., Pedersen, B., and Christiansen, C. (1994). Posture, age, menopause, and osteopenia do not influence the circadian variation in the urinary excretion of pyridinium crosslinks. *J. Bone Miner. Res.* **9**, 1883–1888.

121. Bollen, A. M., Martin, M. D., Leroux, B. G., and Eyre, D. R. (1995). Circadian variation in urinary excretion on bone collagen cross-links. *J. Bone Miner.Res.* **10**, 1885–1890.

122. Eastell, R., Simmons, P. S., Assiri, A. M., Burritt, M. F., Russell, R. G. G., and Riggs, B. L. (1992). Nyctohemeral changes in bone turnover assessed by serum bone gla-protein concentration and urinary deoxypyridinoline excretion: Effect of growth and aging. *Clin. Sci.* **83**, 375–382.

123. Schmeller, N. T., and Bauer, H. W. (1983). Circadian variation of different fractions of serum acid phosphatase. *Prostate* **4**, 391–395.

124. Nielsen, H. K., Brixen, K., and Mosekilde, L. (1990). Diurnal rhythm and 24-hour integrated concentrations of serum osteocalcin in normals: Influence of age, sex, season, and smoking habits. *Calcif. Tissue Int.* **47**, 284–290.

125. Markowitz, M. E., Arnaud, S., Rosen, J. F., Thorpy, M., and Laximinarayan, S. (1988). Temporal interrelationships between the circadian rhythms of serum parathyroid hormone and calcium concentrations. *J. Clin. Endocrinol. Metab.* **67**, 1068–1073.

126. Calvo, M. S., Eastell, R., Offord, K. P., Bergstralh, E. J., and Burritt, M. F. (1991). Circadian variation in ionized calcium and intact parathyroid hormone: Evidence for sex differences in calcium homeostasis. *J. Clin. Endocrinol. Metab.* **72**, 69–76.

127. Nielsen, H. K., Laurberg, P., Brixen, K., and Mosekilde, L. (1991). Relations between diurnal variations in serum osteocalcin, cortisol, parathyroid hormone, and ionized calcium in normal individuals. *Acta Endocrinol.* **124**, 391–398.

128. Ebeling, P. R., Butler, P. C., Eastell, R., Rizza, R. A., and Riggs, B. L. (1991). The nocturnal increase in growth hormone is not the cause of the nocturnal increase in serum osteocalcin. *J. Clin. Endocrinol. Metab.* **73**, 368–372.

129. Popp-Snijders, C., Lips, P., and Netelenbos, J. C. (1996). Intra-individual variation in bone resorption markers in urine. *Ann. Clin. Biochem.* **33**, 347–348.

130. Blumsohn, A., Hannon, R. A., al-Dehaimi, A. W., and Eastell, R. (1994). Short-term intraindividual variability of markers of bone turnover in healthy adults. *J. Bone Miner. Res.* **9** (Suppl.1), S153.

131. Panteghini, M., and Pagani, F. (1995). Biological variation in bone-derived biochemical markers in serum. *Scand. J. Clin. Lab. Invest.* **55**, 609–616.

132. Nielsen, H. K., Brixen, K., Bouillon, R., and Mosekilde, L. (1990). Changes in biochemical markers of osteoblastic activity during the menstrual cycle. *J. Clin. Endocrinol. Metab.* **70**, 1431–1437.

133. Schlemmer, A., Hassager, C., Risteli, J., Risteli, L., Jensen, S. B., and Christiansen, C. (1993). Possible variation in bone resorption during the normal menstrual cycle. *Acta Endocrinol.* **129**, 388–392.

134. Gorai, I., Chaki, O., Nakayama, M., and Minaguchi, H. (1995). Urinary biochemical markers for bone resorption during the menstrual cycle. *Calcif. Tissue Int.* **57**, 100–104.

135. Johansen, J. S., Jensen, S. B., Riis, B. J., and Christiansen, C. (1990). Time-dependent variations in bone turnover parameters during 2 months cyclic treatment with different doses of combined estrogen and progestagen in postmenopausal osteoporosis. *Metab. Clin. Exp.* **39**, 1122–1126.

136. Christiansen, C., Riis, B. J., Nilas, L., Rodbro, P., and Deftos, L. (1985). Uncoupling of bone formation and resorption by combined oestrogen and progestagen therapy in postmenopausal osteoporosis. *Lancet*, 800–801.

137. Juttman, J. R., Visser, T. J., Buurman, C., De Kam, E., and Birkenhäger, J. C. (1981). Seasonal fluctuations in serum concentrations of vitamin D metabolites in normal subjects. *Br. Med. J.* **282**, 1349–1352.

138. Overgaard, K., Nilas, L., Sidenius Johansen, J., and Christiansen, C. (1988). Lack of seasonal variation in bone mass and biochemical estimates of bone turnover. *Bone* **9**, 285–288.

139. Scharla, S., Scheidt-Nave, C., Leidig, G., Seibel, M. J., and Ziegler, R. (1996). Lower serum 25-hydroxyvitamin D is associated with increased bone resorption markers and lower bone density at the proximal femur in normal females: A population-based study. *Exp. Clin. Endocrinol. Diabetes* **104**, 289–292.

140. Morgan, D. B., Rivlin, R. S., and Davis, R. (1972). Seasonal changes in the urinary excretion of calcium. *Am. J. Clin. Nutr.* **25**, 652–654.

141. Lips, P., Hakeng, H. L., Jongen, M. J. M., and van Ginkel, F. C. (1983). Seasonal variation in serum concentrations of parathyroid hormone in elderly people. *J. Clin. Endocrinol. Metab.* **57**, 204–206.

142. Krall, E. A., Sahyoun, N., Tannenbaum, S., Dallal, G. E., and Dawson-Hughes, B. (1989). Effect of vitamin D intake on seasonal variations in parathyroid hormone secretion in postmenopausal women. *N. Engl. J. Med.* **321**, 1777–1783.

143. Chapuy, M.-C., Schott, A. M., Garnero, P., Delmas, P. D., and Meunier, P. J. (1996). Healthy elderly French women living at home have secondary hyperparathyroidism and high bone turnover in winter. *J. Clin. Endocrinol. Metab.* **81**, 1129–1133.

144. Woitge, H., Scheidt-Nave, C., Kissling, C., Leidig, G., Meyer, K., Grauer, A., Scharla, S., Ziegler, R., and Seibel, M. J. (1998). Seasonal variation of biochemical indices of bone turnover: Results of a population based study. *J. Clin. Endocrinol. Metab.* **83**, 68–75.

145. Hyldstrup, L., McNair, P., Jensen, G. F., and Transbol, I. (1986). Seasonal variations in indices of bone formation precede appropriate bone mineral changes in normal men. *Bone* **7**, 167–170.

146. Vanderschueren, D., Gevers, G., Dequeker, J., Geusens, P., Nijs, J., Devos, P., De Roo, M., and Bouillon, R. (1991). Seasonal variation in bone metabolism in young healthy subjects. *Calcif. Tissue Int.* **49**, 84–89.

147. Thomsen, K., Eriksen, E. F., Jorgensen, J., Charles, P., and Mosekilde, L. (1989). Seasonal variation in serum bone gla protein. *Calcif. Tissue Int.* **49**, 84–89.

148. Krabbe, S., Hummer, L., and Christiansen, C. K. (1984). Longitudinal study of calcium metabolism in male puberty. Bone mineral content; and serum levels of alkaline phosphatase; phosphate and calcium. *Acta Paediatr. Scand.* **73**, 750–755.

149. Hyldstrup, L., McNair, P., Jensen, G. F., Nielsen, H. R., and Transbol, I. (1984). Bone mass as referent for urinary hydroxyprolin excretion: Age and sex-related changes in 125 normals and in primary hyperparathyroidism. *Calcif. Tissue Int.* **36**, 639–644.

150. Eastell, R., Delmas, P. D., Hodgson, S. F., Eriksen, E. F., Mann, K. G., and Riggs, B. L. (1988). Bone formation rate in older normal women: Concurrent assessment with bone histomorphometry, calcium kinetics, and biochemical markers. *J. Clin. Endocrinol. Metab.* **67**, 741–748.

151. Kelly, P. J., Pocock, N. A., Sambrook, P. N., and Eisman, J. A. (1989). Age and menopause-related changes in indices of bone turnover. *J. Clin. Endocrinol. Metab.* **69**, 1160–1165.

152. Hassager, C., Colwell, A., Assiri, A. M., and Christiansen, C. (1992). Effect of menopause and hormone replacement therapy on urinary excretion of pyridinium crosslinks: A longitudinal and cross-sectional study. *Clin. Endocrinol.* **37**, 45–50.

153. Seibel, M. J., Woitge, H. W., Scheidt-Nave, C., Kissling, C., Leidig, G., Grauer, A., Scharla, S., and Ziegler, R. (1994). Urinary hydroxypyridinium crosslinks of collagen in population-based screening for overt vertebral osteoporosis: Results of a pilot study. *J. Bone Miner. Res.* **9**, 1433–1440.

154. Robins, S. P. (1990). Collagen markers in urine in human arthritis. *In* "Methods in Cartilage Research" (A. Maroudas, and K. E. Kuettner, eds.), pp. 348–352. Academic Press, London.

155. Gerrits, M. I., Thijssen, J. H., and van Rijn, H. (1995). Determination of pyridinoline and deoxypyridinoline in urine, with special attention to retaining their stability. *Clin. Chem.* **41**, 571–574.

156. Beardsworth, L. J., Eyre, D. R., and Dickson, I. R. (1990). Changes with age in the urinary excretion of lysyl- and hydroxylysylpyridinoline, two new markers of bone collagen turnover. *J. Bone Miner. Res.* **5**, 671–676.

157. Seibel, M. J., Gartenberg, F., Silverberg, S. J., Ratcliffe, A., Robins, S. P., and Bilezikian, J. P. (1992). Urinary hydroxypyridinium cross-links of collagen in primary hyperparathyroidism. *J. Clin. Endocrinol. Metab.* **74**, 481–486.

158. Blumsohn, A., Hannon, R. A., and Eastell, R. (1995). Biochemical assessment of skeletal activity. *Phys. Med. Rehab. Clin. North Am.* **6**, 483–505.

159. Colwell, A., Hamer, A., Blumsohn, A., and Eastell, R. (1996). To determine the effects of ultraviolet light, natural light and ionizing radiation on pyridinium cross-links in bone and urine using high-performance liquid chromatography. *Eur. J. Clin. Invest.* **26**, 1107–1114.

160. Walne, A. J., James, I. T., and Perret, D. (1995). The stability of pyridinium crosslinks in urine and serum. *Clin. Chim. Acta* **240**, 95–97.

161. Blumsohn, A., Colwell, A., Naylor, K. E., and Eastell, R. (1995). Effect of light and gamma-irradiation on pyridinolines and telopeptides of type I collagen in urine. *Clin. Chem.* **41**, 1195–1197.

162. Heymsfield, S. B., Artega, C., McManus, B. S., Smith, J., and Moffitt, S. (1983). Measurements of muscle mass in humans: Validity of the 24 hour urinary creatinine method. *Am. J. Clin. Nutr.* **37**, 478–494.

CHAPTER 29

Validation of Local and Systemic Markers of Bone Turnover

KIM BRIXEN AND ERIK FINK ERIKSEN

Aarhus Bone and Mineral Research Group, Aarhus Amtssygehus, Denmark

I. INTRODUCTION

Assessment of bone turnover (i.e., the amount of bone renewed during the bone remodelling process) remains essential in understanding bone physiology, pathophysiology, and response to treatment. Unfortunately, direct measurement of bone turnover in the whole skeleton is only possible by combined calcium-kinetics and balance or histomorphometric analysis of bone biopsies, and both methods are impractical in clinical use. A long and growing list of biochemical markers that can be measured in the blood or urine have been used or proposed to provide easy, albeit indirect, means of assessing bone turnover. Moreover, bone tissue concentrations of growth factors produced by bone cells have been proposed to reflect bone turnover.

In addition to technical demands on precision, accuracy, and specificity, biochemical markers should be validated by comparison with independent measurement of bone formation and resorption in terms of amount of work or rate of work and not merely by clinical experience. The combined calcium

kinetics and balance studies are considered the golden standard because they measure bone turnover at the organ level (i.e., the whole skeleton). Strontium can replace calcium in the kinetic studies. These methods, however, have some inherent limitations. They are very cumbersome and require admission of patients to a metabolic ward for weeks. Furthermore, bone formation and resorption rates are not mathematically independent and the measurement error of the resorption rate is rather larg [1]. Histomorphometric analysis of bone biopsies provides another possibility for validation; however, this method has another set of limitations. First, histomorphometry only reflects turnover in the bone tissue actually sampled (usually the iliac crest). Turnover is also much greater in cancellous compared with cortical bone, which comprises approximately 80% of the skeleton. Second, the invasive nature of the procedure precludes more than two to three repeated measurements in each patient. Third, bone resorption is often measured as static parameters (e.g., osteoclast covered surfaces) which do not necessarily reflect the true resorption rate. Thus, whether one uses calcium kinetics or bone histomorphometry for the validation of biochemical bone markers, the results may be biased by the tight biological coupling between bone formation and resorption in almost all clinical situations.

Another significant confounder when validating bone markers in serum and urine is the significant day-to-day variation for all markers studied so far [2]. This variability amounts to 15–30%, which of course affects the ability to demonstrate significant correlations [3]. Some of the variation can be overcome by repeated sampling, but this has only been performed in very few of the studies reviewed here.

II. VALIDATION OF BIOCHEMICAL MARKERS BY CALCIUM KINETICS

A. Biochemical Markers of Bone Formation

The ideal marker of bone formation should be a structural protein released into the blood in a rate proportional to its incorporation into bone, and the fraction released should be unchanged by disease. It should have a well-characterized function and should not be released unaltered during bone resorption. Furthermore, its metabolic pathway and serum half-life should be known. Osteoblasts produce collagen, a number of noncollagenous matrix proteins, enzymes, and growth factors, all of which participate in the regulation of bone mineralization. Although none of these meet all the ideal demands, several can be measured in serum as fairly reliable indicators of osteoblastic activity.

1. OSTEOCALCIN

In one study, serum levels of osteocalcin were compared with bone formation rates as measured by calcium kinetics in normal healthy volunteers [4] (Table I, Fig. 1). Another study was unable to demonstrate a significant correlation in 19 normal volunteers [5], probably due to the relatively small number of subjects and a small range of turnover in this group. A study comprising twelve young and eleven older

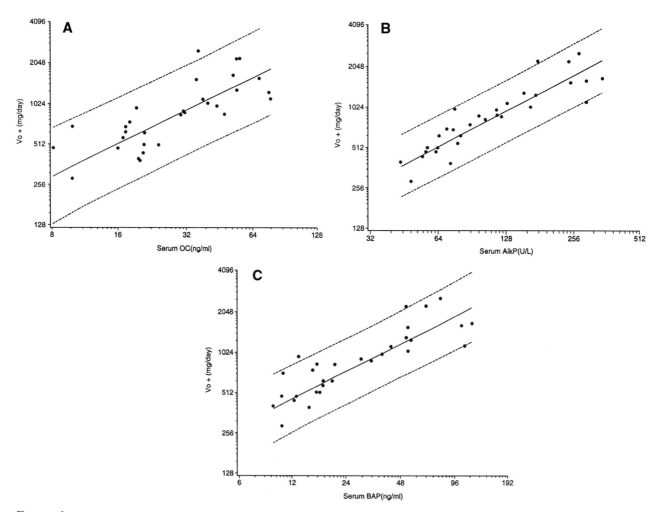

FIGURE 1   Relationship between calcium kinetic bone formation rates (Vo+) and biochemical markers of bone formation (serum-osteocalcin [OC], serum total alkaline phosphatase [TAP], and serum bone specific alkaline phosphatase [BAP] in young healthy females. From Weaver *et al.*, *J. Bone Miner. Res.* 1997; **12**, 1714–1720 [4], with permission of the American Society for Bone and Mineral Research.

TABLE I. Pearson Correlation Coefficients between Calcium Kinetic Mineralization Rates (m) and Resorption Rates (r) and Various Biochemical Markers of Bone Formation and Resorption in Serum and Urine from Young Healthy Females

	S-OC	S-TAP	S-BAP	S-TRAP	U-OHP/Cr	U-NTX/Cr
m	0.82	0.92	0.90	0.77	0.94	0.88
r	0.66	0.81	0.72	0.71	0.79	0.70

S-OC, serum osteocalcin; S-TAP, serum total alkaline phosphatase; S-BAP, serum bone-specific alkaline phosphatase; S-TRAP, serum tartrate resistant acid phosphatase; U-OHP/Cr, urinary hydroxyproline/creatinine ratio; U-NTX/Cr, urinary N-telopeptide of type I collagen/creatinine ratio.

From Weaver *et al.*, *J. Bone Miner. Res.* 1997; **12**, 1714–1720 [4], with permission of the American Society for Bone and Mineral Research.

women did not find any significant correlation between serum osteocalcin and mineralization rate when both groups were pooled. The correlation was significant, however, when the two groups were analyzed separately [6].

In patients with high- and low-turnover bone diseases (myxedema, thyrotoxicosis, and primary hyperparathyroidism) as well as osteoporosis, significant correlations between mineralization rate and serum osteocalcin have been demonstrated [5, 7].

2. ALKALINE PHOSPHATASE

A number of studies have demonstrated significant correlations between serum alkaline phosphatase and bone formation rate as assessed by calcium kinetics in normal patients [4] (Table I, Fig. 1) and in patients with high- and low-turnover states [8], renal failure complicated with adynamic bone, aluminium-related osteomalacia, secondary hyperparathyroidism [9], and renal failure treated with CAPD [10, 11]. Serum bone-specific alkaline phosphatase (BAP) is a sensitive marker of adynamic bone disease in renal failure as evaluated by histomorphometry [12]. In 19 normal individuals, no correlation between serum BAP and bone formation rate could be found [5]. Some [8], but not all [4], studies have found that BAP correlates more closely with mineralization rate than does total alkaline phosphatase (Table I).

3. CARBOXY-TERMINAL PROPEPTIDE OF TYPE I PROCOLLAGEN

Carboxy-terminal propeptide of type I procollagen (PICP) has been validated as a marker of bone formation by studies demonstrating significant correlations of PICP with mineralization rate as measured by calcium-kinetics in normal volunteers [5, 13] and in patients with osteoporosis [5, 13] and high- and low-turnover bone diseases [5]. PICP did not, however, show a correlation with mineralization rate in patients

with untreated renal failure [14] or in patients undergoing treatment with peritoneal dialysis [15]. PICP correlated with mineralization rate in patients with high- and low turnover states [16] and rheumatoid arthritis [17].

4. ASSESSMENT OF OSTEOBLASTIC SECRETION RATES FOR MARKERS OF BONE FORMATION

The serum levels of a given bone marker depend on several factors: (1) the osteoblastic secretion rate, (2) the number of osteoblasts currently involved in bone formation (i.e. bone turnover), and (3) the metabolic clearance rate of the marker (in most cases, this depends on filtration and tubular treatment in the kidneys). In order to isolate the effects of a single osteoblastic secretion of formative markers, Charles *et al.* [5] investigated the effects of correction for bone turnover on marker levels in serum in normal individuals, in patients with a variety of metabolic bone diseases characterized by increased or reduced levels of calciotropic hormones (thyrotoxicosis, myxedema, primary hyperparathyroidism, osteomalacia), and in patients with osteoporosis. They corrected for bone turnover by dividing S-OC, S-PICP, and S-TAP by the calcium kinetic mineralization rate (m). This correction revealed significant differences in "apparent" osteoblastic secretion rate of all three markers (Fig. 2). Single osteoblastic secretion of PICP was significantly reduced in primary hyperparathyroidism, thyrotoxicosis, and osteomalacia but was similar to that of normals in myxedema and osteoporosis. Secretion of OC remained similar to that of normals in all diseases except osteomalacia, highlighting the crucial role of vitamin D in the regulation of osteocalcin secretion. Secretion of alkaline phosphatase was similar to that of normals in primary hyperparathyroidism and thyrotoxicosis but significant increases were seen in myxedema, osteoporosis, and osteomalacia. This analysis depends on the assumption that the metabolic clearance rates for the markers were similar for all diseases. Furthermore, it is assumed that the incorporation of ^{45}Ca into bone matrix is the same for all diseases. Nevertheless, the study indicates that that marker levels depend not only on turnover, but also on ambient concentrations of calciotropic hormones and disease-specific alterations in osteoblastic function and clearance of the marker. Apart from osteomalacia, osteocalcin revealed the least pertubations over the disease spectrum studied.

B. Growth Factors

Osteoblasts produce a number of local growth factors such as insulin-like growth factors (IGFs), transforming growth factor-beta (TGF-β), and interleukins, as well as a number of specific binding proteins such as IGF-binding proteins 1–6. None of these are unique for bone cells and data suggest that they may act in autocrine, paracrine, and endocrine fashions (see also Chapters 6 and 7).

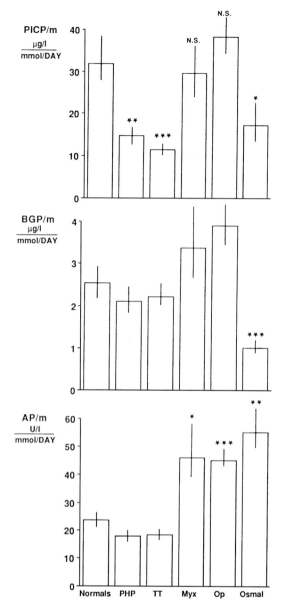

FIGURE 2   "Apparent" osteoblastic secretion of PICP, osteocalcin (OC) and total alkaline phosphatase (TAP) in various metabolic bone diseases (primary hyperparathyroidism [PHP], thyrotoxicosis [TT], myxedema [Myx], osteoporosis [Op], osteomalacia [Osmal] and normal controls. From Charles *et al.*, *Calcif. Tissue Int.* 1992; **51**, 406–411 [5], with permission.

IGFs and TGF-β, however, are stored in large amounts in the bone matrix. Pheilschifter *et al.* [18] demonstrated that the concentration of TGF-β extracted from the bone matrix obtained from Jamshidi biopsies from the iliac crest correlated with osteoblast- ($r = 0.28$, $n = 247$, $p < 0.0001$) and osteoclast- ($r = 0.34$, $n = 66$, $p = 0.005$) covered surfaces measured in bone biopsies from breast cancer patients. Also, bone matrix TGF-β in the femoral head correlated with osteoblast- ($r = 0.49$, $n = 62$, $p > 0.0001$) and osteoclast- ($r = 0.25$, $n = 62$, $p = 0.046$) covered surfaces in the cancellous bone of the femoral head in patients undergoing hip

replacement. In the same population of breast cancer patients, bone matrix IGF-I also correlated with osteoblast- ($r = 0.16$, $p = 0.01$) and osteoclast- ($r = 0.16$, $p = 0.001$) covered surfaces whereas bone matrix IGF-II only correlated with osteoblast-covered surfaces ($r = 0.19$, $p < 0.001$) [19]. These data suggest that measurement of biochemical substances in the bone matrix itself may be used as markers of bone turnover.

The concentration of growth factors in the bone matrix, however, only explained 4–6% of the variation in the histomorphometric indices of bone turnover. Furthermore, osteoblast- and osteoclast-covered surfaces do not necessarily reflect bone turnover. Direct assessment of bone turnover necessitates dynamic histomorphometry using intra-vital tetracycline labelling. Finally, histomorphometry is usually performed on transiliac biopsies with a diameter of 6–9 mm, and the use of Jamshidi biopsies with a diameter of only 2 mm may decrease precision. Despite these cautionary notes, the measurement of growth factors such as IGFs, TGF-β, and interleukin-6, or binding proteins, and in particular IGFBP-5, may hold a great potential as bone markers in a broader sense (e.g., as markers reflecting proliferative potential of osteoblasts).

C. Biochemical Markers of Bone Resorption

The ideal marker of bone resorption should be a degradation product of a matrix component not found in any other tissue. Its serum level should not be under separate endocrine control and it should not be reutilized in new bone formation. During the degradation of collagen, several metabolites are released into circulation and excreted in the urine, some of which are specific for bone or predominantly originate from bone (see Chapters 19 and 28). Furthermore, osteoclasts produce several enzymes among which tartrate-resistant acid phosphatase, with some reservations, may be used as a marker of bone resorption (see Chapters 9 and 28). The close metabolic control of calcium absorption, excretion, and nonresorptive release from bone, as well as reutilization during bone formation, however, precludes the use of serum levels of calcium or urinary calcium excretion as a measure of bone resorption.

1. HYDROXYPROLINE

The urinary hydroxyproline/creatinine ratio correlates with bone resorption in normal healthy volunteers, and in patients with osteoporosis [20] and high- and low-turnover state metabolic diseases [21], as assessed by calcium kinetics [4] (Fig. 3, Table I).

2. COLLAGEN CROSS-LINKS

The urinary excretion of the amino-terminal telopeptide of type I collagen (NTX)-creatinine ratio correlates with bone resorption in normal healthy volunteers [4] (Fig. 3, Table I), as assessed by calcium kinetics. Similarly, urinary total deoxypyridinoline (DPD) correlates with the bone resorption rate in

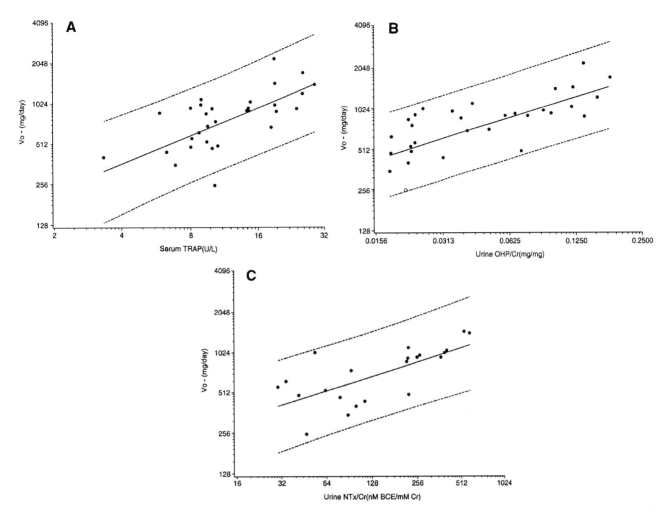

FIGURE 3   Relationship between calcium kinetic bone resorption rates (Vo−) and biochemical markers of bone resorption (serum tartrate-resistant acid phosphatase [TRAP], urinary hydroxyproline/creatinine ratio [OHP/Cr], urinary telopeptide of type I collagen/creatinine ratio [NTX/Cr]. From Weaver *et al., J. Bone Miner. Res.* 1997; **12**, 1714–1720 [4], with permission of the American Society for Bone and Mineral Research.

patients with osteoporosis [20]. Another telopeptide, carboxy-terminal cross-linked telopeptide of type I collagen (ICTP), can be measured in serum. ICTP has also been shown to correlate to the bone resorption rate as assessed by calcium kinetics in patients with high- and low-turnover bone disease and osteoporosis, but not in normals [13].

3. TARTRATE-RESISTANT ACID PHOSPHATASE

Serum tartrate-resistant acid phosphatase correlates with bone resorption in normal healthy volunteers as assessed by calcium kinetics [4] (Fig. 3, Table I).

III. VALIDATION OF BIOCHEMICAL MARKERS BY BONE HISTOMORPHOMETRY

Bone histomorphometry offers the most detailed analysis of bone remodeling, but the interpretation of histomorphome-

tric findings in relation to biochemical markers is hampered by the fact that the biopsy core only reflects bone remodeling in a small area of the total skeleton. Moreover, the relative contribution of cortical, endocortical, and cancellous envelopes to total remodeling activity and subsequent production rates of individual markers is not known in detail. Finally, the bone biopsy will tell very little about factors that may affect the degradation of a given bone marker. The analysis will, therefore, only compare indices pertaining to the production rate of a given marker and marker levels. Thus, many confounding factors affect correlation analyses between biochemical markers and bone histomorphometry. Despite these limitations, such analyses are important for the validation of individual bone markers. It is the only way to assess the degree to which bone turnover, single cell activity, and possible mineralization defects affect bone markers levels.

The production rates of most bone markers mainly depend on the number of resorptive or formative cells currently active. This number depends on two factors: (1) activation frequency (i.e., initiation rate of new remodeling cycles) and

TABLE II.   Calculation of Volume Referent Indices of Resorption and Formation in Cortical and Cancellous Bone

Index	Abbreviation	Formula
Bone resorption rate volume referent	BRS.R/BV	aES × RsR/BS × S/V
Bone formation rate volume referent	BFR/BV	MAR × MS/BS × S/V
Bone balance volume referent	dBV/BV	BFR/BV − BRs.R/BV

aES, active erosion surface (osteoclastic and mononuclear surface); RsR/BS, linear erosion rate; MAR, mineral appositional rate; MS/BS, mineralizing surface; S/V, surface-to-volume ratio.

(2) single cell activity at individual remodeling sites. Bone histomorphometry is the only technique that is able to separate these two variables.

Most studies comparing histomorphometry and biochemical markers have mainly used surface estimates as indices reflecting osteoblastic and osteoclastic activity. Osteoblastic, osteoid, mineralization, or resorption surfaces do not separate between single cell activity and activation rate. Very low turnover with low cellular activity and prolongation of all phases (and consequently low production rates) can theoretically lead to increases in surface extension similar to those seen in a high turnover state with increased cellular activity (and elevated production rates) [22]. It is, therefore, preferable to compare volume referent histomorphometric indices (e.g., combining tetracycline-derived indices and surface estimates) to avoid these confounders. Standard formulae permit the calculation of volume referent indices of cancellous and cortical indices of bone resorption and formation based on the use of the surface to volume ratio (Table II) [22].

A. Assessment of Bone Turnover in Normal Individuals

Eastell et al. [6] assessed bone formation rates using multiple methods in 12 younger (age, 30–41 years) and 11 older (age, 55–73 years) healthy individuals. Bone formation was higher in the older women than in the younger women based on measurements of osteocalcin (1.67 ± 0.07 [SE] versus 1.14 ± 0.10 nmol/L; $p < 0.01$), serum bone-specific alkaline phosphatase activity (388 ± 42 versus 223 ± 22 nkatal/L, $p < 0.01$), and bone formation rate by histomorphometry of iliac biopsy ($31.1 \pm 4.9\%$ versus $15.1 \pm 2.7\%$/year; $p < 0.01$). However, bone formation was similar in the two groups when accretion rates were assessed by calcium kinetics (5.9 ± 1.0 versus 7.5 ± 1.2; $p = NS$). This latter discrepancy was ascribed to several age-related factors: reduced mineralization of completed osteons and lack of correction for the decrease in total skeletal calcium in the older group.

Younger women exhibited significant correlations between osteocalcin and volume referent formation rates and calcium kinetic accretion rates. No such correlation was demonstrable for bone-specific alkaline phosphatase (Table III) [6]. In this younger group, osteocalcin also correlated significantly to bone-specific alkaline phosphatase and bone formation rate correlated to calcium accretion. In older women, neither osteocalcin nor bone-specific alkaline phosphatase correlated to histomorphometric formation rates. However, osteocalcin correlated significantly to calcium kinetic accretion rate. Serum osteocalcin also correlates with bone formation rate as measured by histomorphometry in healthy men [23].

B. Assessment of Bone Turnover in Patients with Various Metabolic Bone Diseases

1. RENAL OSTEODYSTROPHY

Coutteneye et al. [12] investigated the correlation between bone-specific alkaline phosphatase and adynamic bone disease in 103 hemodialysis patients. They performed a bone biopsy after double tetracycline labeling and correlated the histomorphometric indices of bone turnover to serum levels of intact PTH, osteocalcin, and the bone-specific isoenzyme of alkaline phosphatase (BAP). In 38 (37%) of the patients the diagnosis of adynamic bone disease was established by bone histomorphometry. The authors established a cut off

TABLE III.   Correlation Matrices Describing the Relations between Different Biochemical Markers

	Young women			Old women			All women		
	S-BAP	BFR/BV	Accr. rate	S-BAP	BFR/BV	Accr. rate	S-BAP	BFR/BV	Accr. rate
S-Oc	0.58*	0.76*	0.71*	0.55	0.07	0.83	0.70*	0.63*	0.37*
S-BAP		0.40	0.47		0.00	0.23		0.46*	0.10
BFR/BV			0.88*			0.27			0.32

S-Oc, S-osteocalcin; S-BAP, S-bone-specific alkaline phosphatase; BFR/BV, volume referent histomorphometric bone formation rate; Accr. rate, calcium accretion by ^{45}Ca kinetics. Reprinted with permission from Eastell et al. Bone formation rate in older normal women: Concurrent agreement with bone histomorphometry, calcium kinetics, and biochemical markers. J. Clin. Endocrinol. Metab. 1988; 67, 741–748 [6]. © The Endocrine Society.

value of ≤27 U/L for the bone isoenzyme of alkaline phosphatase, ≤14 μg/L for osteocalcin, and ≤150 pg/ml for intact PTH. Analysis of receiver–operator curves revealed that bone-specific alkaline phosphatase and intact PTH were the best indices for the detection of adynamic bone disease, as indicated by a sensitivity of 78.1% and 80.6% and a specificity of 86.4% and 76.2%, respectively. Furthermore, it was calculated that the positive predictive value for the proposed cutoff values was 75% for bone-specific alkaline phosphatase, 65% for intact PTH, and 55% for osteocalcin. The authors, therefore, concluded that bone-specific alkaline phosphatase (BAP) was the best serum marker to evaluate adynamic bone disease in patients with renal failure.

Urena *et al.* [24] investigated 42 hemodialysis patients with bone histomorphometry and assessment of bone specific alkaline phosphatase (BAP), total alkaline phosphatase (TAP), and PTH. They found that patients with a high-turnover bone disease exhibited significantly higher plasma BAP levels than patients with normal or low bone turnover (66.9 ± 63.5 ng/mL versus 10.8 ± 4.2 ng/mL). BAP levels were positively correlated with osteoclast surface (r = 0.39, p < 0.0001), osteoclast number/mm^2 (r = 0.36, p < 0.001), osteoblast surface (r = 0.50, p < 0.005), and bone formation rate (r = 0.91, p < 0.0001). The bone formation rate revealed a better correlation with plasma BAP levels than with levels of TAP or PTH. Plasma BAP levels >20 ng/mL showed the highest sensitivity and specificity for the diagnosis of high-turnover bone disease and formally excluded patients with low-turnover bone disease or who were normal. The authors concluded that both serum PTH and BAP were useful in the separation of high- and low-turnover renal osteodystrophy.

Joffe *et al.* [25] tried to assess whether bone histology could be predicted by clinical assessment and noninvasive techniques in patients on peritoneal dialysis. No correlations were found between clinical symptoms, biochemical markers, radiographic bone surveys, BMC measurements, and bone histology. The authors concluded that bone histology cannot be comprehensively predicted by bone markers.

Charhon *et al.* [26] correlated serum osteocalcin (S-OC), serum total alkaline phosphatase (S-TAP), and serum immunoreactive PTH (S-iPTH) to dynamic histomorphometry in 42 patients undergoing chronic hemodialysis. Serum osteocalcin was markedly increased (64.0 ± 74.8 [± SD] versus 6.2 ± 2.2 ng/ml) in normal subjects. Furthermore, osteocalcin significantly correlated with S-TAP (r = 0.53) and S-iPTH (r = 0.55) levels. S-OC was significantly higher in the 14 patients with high-turnover renal osteodystrophy (138.5 ± 90.8 ng/ml) than in the 28 patients with the low-turnover disease (26.8 ± 14.8 ng/ml). S-OC was significantly correlated with the cellular parameters of bone resorption and formation (r = 0.57–0.69) and with the dynamic parameters of bone formation (r = 0.62–0.82). The extent of stainable bone aluminum was significantly negatively correlated with S-OC

(r = −0.51) and S-iPTH (r = −0.33), but not with S-TAP. These authors concluded that measurement of S-OC allowed better discrimination between low- and high-turnover renal osteodystrophy than S-TAP. In patients with low-turnover disease, however, S-OC did not permit discrimination between patients with or without osteomalacia.

Mazzafero *et al.* [14] investigated whether markers of bone collagen formation (S-PICP) and degradation (S-ICTP) could provide indirect estimates of the rate of bone turnover. They also measured serum intact and C-terminal PTH, osteocalcin, and total alkaline phosphatase (TAP). A transiliac bone biopsy for histomorphometry was also performed. As shown in other studies, S-PTH, S-OC, and S-TAP were correlated to static histomorphometric parameters of resorption and formation. Serum-PICP showed a slightly positive correlation with S-OC (0.365, p < 0.01), but not with PTH, TAP, or histomorphometric indices of bone resorption and formation. In another study, however, Coen *et al.* [27] reported a highly significant correlation between S-PICP and dynamic (tetracycline-based) histomorphometric indices of bone turnover. Urinary excretion of total pyridinoline (U-PYD) correlates with parameters of bone resorption in patients undergoing hemodialysis [28] (see Chapter 39).

2. OTHER METABOLIC BONE DISEASES

Lauffenburger *et al.* [29] investigated two groups of patients: (1) those with low-turnover bone disease (osteoporosis) before and after fluoride treatment, and (2) those with high-turnover bone disease (Paget's disease) before and after bisphosphonate treatment with etidronate. The authors assessed the following histomorphometric indices: osteoblast surface (ObS/BS), osteoid surface (OS/BS), osteoclast number (N.ocl/BS), and erosion surface (ES/BS). The histomorphometric parameters were correlated to serum total alkaline phosphatase (TAP), urinary hydroxyproline (HyPro), calcium kinetic accretion rate (m), and calcium kinetic resorption rate (r). In both patient groups, bone formation indices were significantly correlated (ObS/BS/m, r = 0.85; OS/BS/m, r = 0.83; and AP/m, r = 0.97). Bone resorption indices correlated less well than bone formation indices (Oc.N/BS/r, r = 0.68 and ES/BS/r, r = 0.63). Hydroxyproline correlated significantly with the sum of r + m (r = 0.97).

Eriksen *et al.* [16] measured serum levels of the pyridinoline cross-linked telopeptide domain of type I collagen (ICTP) as a marker of bone resorption and serum carboxyterminal propeptide of type I procollagen (PICP) as a marker of bone formation [16]. Serum levels of the two antigens were correlated to histomorphometric indices of bone resorption and bone formation calculated from iliac crest bone biopsies in a group of 18 individuals with high- and low-turnover bone disease (myxedema, primary hyperparathyroidism, and thyrotoxicosis).

Mean S-ICTP and S-PICP values differed widely among the three groups. Mean S-PICP values in patients with thyrotoxicosis and primary hyperparathyroidism were three and two times higher, respectively, than in patients with myxedema. S-ICTP values revealed even more pronounced differences among the three groups. Matrix degradation assessed from S-ICTP was three times greater than the degradation rate seen in primary hyperparathyroidism and four times greater than that seen in myxedema. The differences in bone formation rates as assessed by bone histomorphometry (BFR/BV) revealed relative differences similar to those seen for PICP. This was not the case, however, for S-ICTP. Patients with myxedema revealed the lowest values for volume referent resorption rate (BRs.R/BV), but cancellous bone resorption rates in patients with thyrotoxicosis were lower than those seen in patients with primary hyperparathyroidism, despite the pronounced differences in ICTP between the two groups.

Linear regression of S-ICTP on BRs.R/BV was significant ($r = 0.51$, $p < 0.03$). S-ICTP also correlated significantly to cancellous bone balance ($r = 0.45$, $p < 0.03$). No significant regressions on other histomorphometric resorption indices were demonstrable (Table IV). S-PICP was significantly correlated with the mineral appositional rate ($r = 0.53$, $p < 0.05$) and volume-referent bone formation rate ($r = 0.61$, $p < 0.01$). The correlation with bone turnover (expressed as the activation frequency) was also highly significant ($r = 0.61$, $p < 0.01$) (Table V). No significant correlations with wall thickness or bone balance were demonstrable. The relative contribution of PICP and ICTP to cancellous bone balance was assessed by bone histomorphometry and revealed that the variation in ICTP was the only significant determinant.

3. HYPERCALCEMIC STATES

The use of serum osteocalcin (S-OC) to discriminate between hypercalcemia due to malignant disease and primary hyperparathyroidism was studied in 25 patients with primary hyperparathyroidism and in 24 patients with bone metastases with or without hypercalcemia [30]. Despite similar levels of hypercalcemia, S-OC was increased in patients with primary hyperparathyroidism (14.2 ± 9.6 ng/ml, $p < 0.001$), while it was decreased in patients with malignant hyper-

TABLE IV. Regression of S-ICTP on Histomorphometric Indices of Cancellous Bone Resorption and Turnover

Variable	r	p
Erosion depth, μm	0.48	<0.05
Linear resorption rate (BMU), μm/day	0.27	NS
Volume referent resorption rate, %/year	0.61	<0.01
BMU balance, μm	−0.58	<0.05
Volume referent bone balance, %/year	−0.4	<0.05
Activation frequency, year^{-1}	0.46	NS

From Eriksen *et al. J. Bone Miner. Res.* 1993; **8**, 127–132 [16], with permission of the American Society for Bone and Mineral Research.

TABLE V. Regression of S-PICP on Histomorphometric Indices of Cancellous Bone Formation and Turnover

Variable	r	p
Wall thickness, μm	−0.01	NS
Mineral appositional rate, μm/day	0.53	<0.05
Bone formation rate, %/year	0.61	<0.01
BMU balance, μm	−0.49	NS
Volume referent cancellous bone balance, %/year	−0.15	NS
Activation frequency, year^{-1}	0.61	<0.01

From Eriksen *et al. J. Bone Miner. Res.* 1993; **8**, 127–132 [16], with permission of the American Society for Bone and Mineral Research.

calcemia (3.1 ± 2.8 ng/ml, $p < 0.001$) and normal in patients with bone metastases without hypercalcemia (6.6 ± 2.7 ng/ml). In primary hyperparathyroidism, S-OC was correlated with serum immunoreactive parathyroid hormone ($r = 0.90$), calcium ($r = 0.73$), and adenoma weight ($r = 0.79$). After parathyroidectomy, S-OC slowly returned to normal values within two to six months, suggesting that S-OC reflects increased bone turnover rather than a direct effect of PTH on osteocalcin synthesis (see Chapter 40). Iliac crest biopsies were performed in 11 patients with primary hyperparathyroidism and in nonaffected areas in nine cancer patients. Serum-OC was significantly correlated with all parameters reflecting bone formation but not with parameters for bone resorption. Patients with bone metastases were analyzed according to the presence or the absence of hypercalcemia. In contrast to normocalcemic patients who had normal S-OC levels, hypercalcemic patients exhibited reduced osteocalcin levels and lower bone formation at the cellular level ($p < 0.05$).

4. OSTEOPOROSIS

The urinary excretion of the pyridinoline cross-links PYD and DPD, specific markers of bone and cartilage collagen degradation, was evaluated along with serum osteocalcin (S-OC) and urinary hydroxyproline (U-OHP) in 36 elderly women with vertebral osteoporosis [31]. The same women also had an iliac crest biopsy performed. The authors found that urinary pyridinoline cross-links, but not hydroxyproline, correlated significantly with histologic resorption, assessed by osteoclast surface ($r = 0.35$, $p < 0.05$ for Pyr; $r = 0.46$, $p < 0.01$ for DPD). In addition, PYD and DPD were correlated with the bone formation rate as well as the serum osteocalcin level ($r = 0.69–0.80$, $p < 0.0001$). These data indicate that PYD and DPD are sensitive markers of bone turnover in elderly women with vertebral osteoporosis. The authors concluded that the poor correlation between markers of bone resorption and histological assessment of bone resorption indicated the low sensitivity of iliac crest histomorphometry in the measurement of resorption rate of the skeleton. A surface estimate is a poor index for comparison with volume-dependent variables such as biochemical markers of bone remodeling because it depends on both activation frequency and cellular activity at individual resorption foci. The conclusion drawn seems therefore somewhat premature.

Brown *et al.* [32] investigated the correlation between serum osteocalcin (S-OC) levels and bone remodeling in osteoporosis. Mean ($\pm$ SD) S-OC was normal (7.0 ± 3.3 ng/ml) in 26 patients with untreated postmenopausal osteoporosis. Nine patients, however, exhibited osteocalcin values either above (n = 4) or below (n = 5) the normal values obtained in 35 age-matched control women (6.9 ± 1.3 ng/ml). Serum osteocalcin correlated positively with osteoid volume, osteoid surfaces, mineralizing surfaces, and bone formation rate, but not with erosion surfaces. Based on normal values for osteoid volume, the authors classified patients as having either high (HF, n = 9), normal (NF, n = 12), or low osteoid formation (LF, n = 5). Serum osteocalcin (mean $\pm$ SEM) was significantly lower in the LF group (2.7 ± 0.9 ng/ml) and significantly higher in the HF group (9.7 ± 0.8 ng/ml) than in the NF group (7.0 ± 0.6 ng/ml). Somewhat surprisingly, serum total alkaline phosphatase (S-TAP) and urinary hydroxyproline (U-OHP) did not discriminate between these three groups and did not correlate significantly with any of the histomorphometric indices. The authors concluded that S-OC could predict the histological profile in postmenopausal osteoporosis and suggested that the marker might be useful both in the diagnosis and in the control of treatment effects in osteoporotic patients. The use of osteocalcin in this area is, however, hampered by its sensitivity to ambient vitamin D levels and the degree of hyperparathyroidism in individual patients.

IV. CONCLUSIONS

Serum and urine markers of bone resorption and formation are valuable tools for the investigation of metabolic bone diseases and the evaluation of treatment effects in clinical trials. Numerous histomorphometric and calcium kinetic studies have demonstrated that marker levels, despite the inherent profound variability, reflect the activity of resorptive and formative cell populations quite well in groups of individuals. The studies have, however, also revealed that the serum or urine concentration of a given bone marker has to be evaluated in the context of numerous other factors influencing the formation rate and clearance rate of that marker.

References

1. Eriksen, E. F., Hodgson, S. F., Eastell, R., Cedel, S. L., O'Fallon, W. M., and Riggs, B. L. (1990). Cancellous bone remodeling in type 1 (postmenopausal) osteoporosis: Quantitative assessment of rates of formation, resorption, and bone loss at tissue and cellular levels. *J. Bone Miner. Res.* **5**, 311–319.

2. Blumsohn, A., and Eastell, R. (1992). Prediction of bone loss in postmenopausal women. *Eur. J. Clin. Invest.* **22**, 764–766.

3. Peel, N., and Eastell, R. (1993). Measurement of bone mass and turnover. *Baillières Clin. Rheumatol.* **7**, 479–498.

4. Weaver, C. M., Peacock, M., Martin, B. R., McCabe, G. P., Zhao, J., Smith, D. L., and Wastney, M. E. (1997). Quantification of biochemical markers of bone turnover by kinetic measures of bone formation and resorption in young healthy females. *J. Bone Miner. Res.* **12**, 1714–1720.

5. Charles, P., Hasling, C., Risteli, L., Risteli, J., Mosekilde, L., and Eriksen, E. F. (1992). Assessment of bone formation by biochemical markers in metabolic bone disease: Separation between osteoblastic activity at the cell and tissue level. *Calcif. Tissue Int.* **51**, 406–411.

6. Eastell, R., Delmas, P. D., Hodgson, S. F., Eriksen, E. F., Mann, K. G., and Riggs, B. L. (1988). Bone formation rate in older normal women: Concurrent assessment with bone histomorphometry, calcium kinetics, and biochemical markers. *J. Clin. Endocrinol. Metab.* **67**, 741–748.

7. Wand, J. S., Green, J. R., Hesp, R., Bradbeer, J. N., Sambrook, P. N., Smith, T., Hampton, L., Zanelli, J. M., and Reeve, J. (1992). Bone remodelling does not decline after menopause in vertebral fracture osteoporosis. *Bone Miner.* **17**, 361–375.

8. Brixen, K., Nielsen, H. K., Eriksen, E. F., Charles, P., and Mosekilde, L. (1989). Efficacy of wheat germ lectin-precipitated alkaline phosphatase in serum as an estimator of bone mineralization rate: Comparison to serum total alkaline phosphatase and serum bone Gla-protein. *Calcif. Tissue Int.* **44**, 93–98.

9. Cochran, M., Neville, A., and Marshall, E. A. (1994). Comparison of bone formation rates measured by radiocalcium kinetics and double-tetracycline labeling in maintenance dialysis patients. *Calcif. Tissue Int.* **54**, 392–398.

10. Joffe, P., Hyldstrup, L., Heaf, J. G., Podenphant, J., and Henriksen, J. H. (1992). Bisphosphonate kinetics in patients undergoing continuous ambulatory peritoneal dialysis: Relations to dynamic bone histomorphometry, osteocalcin and parathyroid hormone. *Am. J. Nephrol.* **12**, 419–424.

11. Jarava, C., Armas, J. R., Salgueira, M., and Palma, A. (1996). Bone alkaline phosphatase isoenzyme in renal osteodystrophy. *Nephrol. Dial. Transplant.* **11** (Suppl. 3), 43–46.

12. Couttenye, M. M., D'Haese, P. C., Van, H. V., Lemoniatou, E., Goodman, W., Verpooten, G. A., and De, B. M. (1996). Low serum levels of alkaline phosphatase of bone origin: A good marker of adynamic bone disease in haemodialysis patients. *Nephrol. Dial. Transplant.* **11**, 1065–1072.

13. Charles, P., Mosekilde, L., Risteli, L., Risteli, J., and Eriksen, E. F. (1994). Assessment of bone remodeling using biochemical indicators of type I collagen synthesis and degradation: Relation to calcium kinetics. *Bone Miner.* **24**, 81–94.

14. Mazzaferro, S., Pasquali, M., Ballanti, P., Bonucci, E., Costantini, S., Chicca, S., De, M. S., Perruzza, I., Sardella, D., and Taggi, F. (1995). Diagnostic value of serum peptides of collagen synthesis and degradation in dialysis renal osteodystrophy. *Nephrol. Dial. Transplant.* **10**, 52–58.

15. Joffe, P., Heaf, J. G., and Jensen, L. T. (1995). Type I procollagen propeptide in patients on CAPD: Its relationships with bone histology, osteocalcin, and parathyroid hormone. *Nephrol. Dial. Transplant.* **10**, 1912–1917.

16. Eriksen, E. F., Charles, P., Melsen, F., Mosekilde, L., Risteli, L., and Risteli, J. (1993). Serum markers of type I collagen formation and degradation in metabolic bone disease: Correlation with bone histomorphometry. *J. Bone Miner. Res.* **8**, 127–132.

17. Kroger, H., Risteli, J., Risteli, L., Penttila, I., and Alhava, E. (1993). Serum osteocalcin and carboxyterminal propeptide of type I procollagen in rheumatoid arthritis. *Ann. Rheum. Dis.* **52**, 338–342.

18. Pfeilschifter, J., Diel, I., Scheppach, B., Bretz, A., Krempien, R., Erdmann, J., Schmid, G., Reske, N., Bismar, H., Seck, T., Krempien, B., and Ziegler, R. (1998). Concentration of transforming growth

factor beta in human bone tissue: Relationship to age, menopause, bone turnover and bone volume. *J. Bone Miner. Res.* **13**, 716–730.

19. Seck, T., Scheppach, B., Scharla, S., Diel, I., Blum, W. F., Bismar, H., Schmid, G., Krempien, B., Ziegler, R., and Pfeilschifter, J. (1998). Concentration of insulin-like Growth factor (IGF)-I and -II in iliac crest bone matrix from pre- and postmenopausal women: Relationship to age, menopause, bone turnover, bone volume, and circulating IGF's. *J. Clin. Endocrinol. Metab.* **83**, 2331–2337.

20. Eastell, R., Colwell, A., Hampton, L., and Reeve, J. (1997). Biochemical markers of bone resorption compared with estimates of bone resorption from radiotracer kinetic studies in osteoporosis. *J. Bone Miner. Res.* **12**, 59–65.

21. Charles, P., Poser, J. W., Mosekilde, L., and Jensen, F. T. (1985). Estimation of bone turnover evaluated by 47Ca-kinetics. Efficiency of serum bone gamma-carboxyglutamic acid-containing protein, serum alkaline phosphatase, and urinary hydroxyproline excretion. *J. Clin. Invest.* **76**, 2254–2258.

22. Eriksen, E. F. (1986). Normal and pathological remodeling of human trabecular bone: Three dimensional reconstruction of the remodeling sequence in normals and in metabolic bone disease. *Endocr. Rev.* **7**, 379–408.

23. Clarke, B. L., Ebeling, P. R., Jones, J. D., Wahner, H. W., O'Fallon, W. M., Riggs, B. L., and Fitzpatrick, L. A. (1996). Changes in quantitative bone histomorphometry in aging healthy men. *J. Clin. Endocrinol. Metab.* **81**, 2264–2270.

24. Urena, P., Hruby, M., Ferreira, A., Ang, K. S., and De, V. M. (1996). Plasma total versus bone alkaline phosphatase as markers of bone turnover in hemodialysis patients. *J. Am. Soc. Nephrol.* **7**, 506–512.

25. Joffe, P., Heaf, J. G., and Jensen, C. (1996). Can bone histomorphometry be predicted by clinical assessment and noninvasive techniques in peritoneal dialysis? *Miner. Electrolyte Metab.* **22**, 224–233.

26. Charhon, S. A., Delmas, P. D., Malaval, L., Chavassieux, P. M., Arlot, M., Chapuy, M. C., and Meunier, P. J. (1986). Serum bone Gla-protein in renal osteodystrophy: Comparison with bone histomorphometry. *J. Clin. Endocrinol. Metab.* **63**, 892–897.

27. Coen, G., Mazzaferro, S., Ballanti, P., Bonucci, E., Bondatti, F., Manni, M., Pasquali, M., Perruzza, I., Sardella, D., and Spurio, A. (1992). Procollagen type I C-terminal extension peptide in predialysis chronic renal failure. *Am. J. Nephrol.* **12**, 246–251.

28. Urena, P., Ferreira, A., Kung, V. T., Morieux, C., Simon, P., Ang, K. S., Souberbielle, J. C., Segré, G. V., Drueke, T. B., and De Vernejoul, M. C. (1995). Serum pyridinoline as a specific marker of collagen breakdown and bone metabolism in hemodialysis patients. *J. Bone Miner. Res.* **10**, 932–939.

29. Lauffenburger, T., Olah, A. J., Dambacher, M. A., Guncaga, J., Lentner, C., and Haas, H. G. (1977). Bone remodeling and calcium metabolism: A correlated histomorphometric, calcium kinetic, and biochemical study in patients with osteoporosis and Paget's disease. *Metab. Clin. Exp.* **26**, 589–606.

30. Delmas, P. D., Demiaux, B., Malaval, L., Chapuy, M. C., Edouard, C., and Meunier, P. J. (1986). Serum bone gamma carboxyglutamic acid-containing protein in primary hyperparathyroidism and in malignant hypercalcemia. Comparison with bone histomorphometry. *J. Clin. Invest.* **77**, 985–991.

31. Delmas, P. D., Schlemmer, A., Gineyts, E., Riis, B., and Christiansen, C. (1991). Urinary excretion of pyridinoline crosslinks correlates with bone turnover measured on iliac crest biopsy in patients with vertebral osteoporosis. *J. Bone Miner. Res.* **6**, 639–644.

32. Brown, J. P., Delmas, P. D., Malaval, L., Edouard, C., Chapuy, M. C., and Meunier, P. J. (1984). Serum bone Gla-protein: A specific marker for bone formation in postmenopausal osteoporosis. *Lancet* **1**, 1091–1093.

CHAPTER 30

Genetic Markers of Joint Disease

MICHEL NEIDHART, RENATE E. GAY, AND STEFFEN GAY

Center for Experimental Rheumatology, Department of Rheumatology, University Hospital, Zürich, Switzerland

I. ABSTRACT

Association between specific class I and II HLA (human leukocyte antigen) alleles with various autoimmune diseases has been established. The association of the HLA-B2702 allele with ankylosing spondylitis and the association of defined HLA-DRB1 alleles, which share a common epitope, with rheumatoid arthritis (RA) are particularly strong. For the most part, however, these associations have been defined in Caucasian and Asian populations and caution is required in extrapolating these findings to other racial or ethnic groups. The occurrence and dosage of these HLA-DRB1 alleles affect the course and outcome of RA. The mechanisms underlying the association of particular HLA alleles with autoimmune disease may involve "molecular mimicry" between foreign antigens and HLA molecules and/or other self-antigens, altered antigen presentation, and bias during thymocyte development. Non-HLA genes and environmental factors also are involved in the pathogenesis of RA and may influence the effects of HLA alleles. Of particular interest are the genes located within or near the HLA region on chromosome 6p21, for example, the tumor-necrosis factor (TNF) and prolactin (Prl) genes. In addition, new molecular techniques are resulting in the rapid identification of other candidate genes, among them genes in the T-cell receptor β-chain locus and the genes that encode adhesion molecules, cytokines and their receptors, neuroendocrine factors, tumor suppressor molecules, proteolytic enzymes, and various structural proteins.

II. GENETIC MARKERS AND ENVIRONMENTAL FACTORS

Both genetic and environmental factors are involved in the etiology of rheumatoid arthritis (RA). The relationship of these with each other and with joint disease is complex, as both genes and environment may act in a protective manner or render individuals susceptible to disease. Family studies have confirmed that "autoimmunity" is a dominant Mendelian trait [1]. First-degree relatives are at an increased risk for developing RA. Mothers more often confer susceptibility to RA on their offspring than do fathers [2]. In monozygotic twins, the concordance for RA is 10–21%, whereas the rate is significantly lower in dizygotic twins [3–7]. These data must be interpreted cautiously, however, as twins can differ in terms of crucial aspects of the immune response such as in the somatic rearrangement of immunoglobulin and T-cell receptor (TCR) genes. When considering the genetic component of susceptibility, it is important to bear in mind that nongenetically determined factors may account for greater than 50% of disease susceptibility [8]. Environmental factors that may particularly influence autoimmune disease include infectious agents and reproductive behaviors [9]. Nevertheless, the majority of autoimmune diseases are known to be associated, at least partly, with processes that are dependent on the products of the human major histocompatibility complex (MHC) genes, including human leukocyte antigen (HLA) genes, which, in turn, may account for some of the genetic susceptibility [10].

III. GENETIC MARKERS ASSOCIATED WITH THE HUMAN MAJOR HISTOCOMPATIBILITY COMPLEX

Molecules within the human MHC complex were originally recognized through their ability to provoke rejection of grafts exchanged between different individuals. The clusters of class I, II, and III genes in the MHC complex on chromo-some 6p21 are illustrated in Figure 1. Clearly, mediation of graft rejection is not the physiological role of the HLA system. It subsequently has been established that HLA molecules play a major role in regulating the immune system by influencing the differentiation of thymocytes and by permitting the deletion of autoreactive T cells and the positive selection of particular T-cell subpopulations. In addition, mature T lymphocytes only recognize and respond correctly to antigens when they are presented in association with HLA molecules.

Class I HLA genes encode the 45-kDa transmembrane α-chain glycoprotein, which is associated with β_2-microglobulin on the cell surface. Class I HLA molecules are expressed on most cell types. They play an important role in the elimination of virally infected cells; the viral antigens on the surface of infected cells are presented in the context of class I HLA molecules to CD8+ cytotoxic T lymphocytes permitting lysis of the infected cells prior to viral replication.

Class II HLA genes encode glycoproteins that form transmembrane heterodimers composed of 32-kDa α-chains bound noncovalently to 28-kDa β-chains. Class II HLA molecules are expressed predominantly on B lymphocytes, macrophages, and dendritic cells. Their expression also can be induced by a variety of cytokines, for example γ-interferon. They are primarily involved in the presentation of foreign antigens by macrophages, for example to CD4+ T lymphocytes during the initiation and propagation of the immune response. These antigens are presented as antigenic peptide

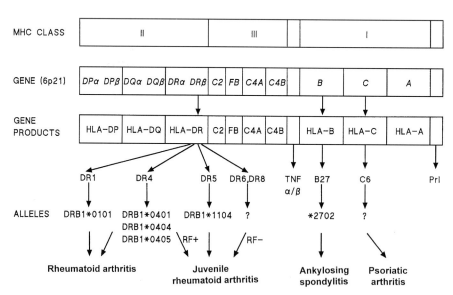

MHC COMPLEX

FIGURE 1   Map of the human major histocompatibility complex (MHC). The HLA class I, II, and III molecules are encoded in distinct regions on chromosome 6p. The HLA class II region contains three subregions: DP, DQ, and DR. Each of these contains a variable number of α- and β-chains. Class I HLA-B27 and -C6, as well as class II HLA-"DR1," -"DR4," -"DR5" and -"DR6," are associated with joint diseases. For example, the DRB1*0101 ("DR1"), *0401, *0404, and *0405 ("DR4") alleles are associated with rheumatoid arthritis. The tumor necrosis factor (TNF α/β) and prolactin (Prl) genes are in close proximity to the HLA regions.

fragments, which are derived from internalized proteins by lysosomal degradation.

The HLA antigens initially were detected using lymphocytoxicity tests. In this procedure, which was developed in the mid-1970s, various HLA-antisera are allowed to react with specific antigens on the cell surface of lymphocytes from a given individual. In the case of a positive reaction, the addition of complement induces cell lysis. The process is stopped with formalin and the "damaged" lymphocytes are stained with eosin. Several problems are associated with this method, in particular the usually low titers and cross-reactivity of the antisera (e.g., anti-HLA-"B27" can cross-react with HLA-"B7" and HLA-"B22"). Therefore, each antiserum must be carefully tested using a defined panel of cells. The development of flow cytometric and ELISA techniques has provided valid alternatives. Flow cytometry is now employed routinely for the identification of class I HLA-"B27"-positive individuals, using commercially available FITC-conjugated murine anti-HLA-B27 monoclonal antibodies to stain the patient's leukocytes. Unfortunately, double-labeling with PE-conjugated anti-HLA-B7 monoclonal antibody is rarely performed. Although flow cytometry is rapid and reliable, it is expensive; however, recent data show that flow cytometry is preferable to the lymphocytotoxicity technique [11]. A sandwich ELISA for detection of serum HLA-"B27" has been developed in which the plate is coated with an anti-HLA-"B27" monoclonal antibody; after incubation with serum, bound HLA-"B27" is revealed using a HRP-conjugated anti-β_2-microglobulin monoclonal antibody. The advantages of this approach are the low costs and the use of patient serum rather than cells; however, cross-reactivity with HLA-"B7" remains a limitation and requires careful analysis of results.

A hallmark of the HLA gene products is their polymorphism, that is, the enormous degree of interindividual structural variability. The delineation of the HLA polymorphism has led to an effort to relate these genetic differences to the propensity of an individual to develop autoimmunity. The introduction of DNA typing greatly facilitated the detection of HLA polymorphisms. Initially, the technique of so-called restriction fragment length polymorphism (RFLP) analysis was employed. With the further development of molecular biological techniques, in particular the polymerase chain reaction (PCR), the serological identification of HLA markers in joint disease is becoming obsolete [12], at least in experimental laboratories. The first commercially available test was based on the reverse dot plot hybridization principle [13]. Other PCR tests include multiple primer pairs and control templates, and the use of automated DNA sequencers also is being evaluated. However, PCR techniques may fail to reveal differences in HLA sequences if they lie outside the area being probed.

In contrast to the early serological nomenclature, the current names of the HLA alleles include the specific DNA sequence and are, therefore, definitive. The domains of the class II HLA molecules that lie extracellulary form the peptide groove and act as the contact point for interaction of the antigens with the TCR. It is in these domains that most of the polymorphisms are found, lying in three "hypervariable" regions. Most of the polymorphisms of HLA-DR reside in the DRB1 locus, where the β-chain component of most classic DR specificities is encoded. Alleles at this locus are designated by the locus indicator, followed by an asterisk and then the allelic designation. For example, HLA-"DR1" and HLA-"DR4," which are associated with RA [14–16], are now designated HLA-DRB1 *0101 to *0104 and *0401 to *0419, respectively. That is, four alleles are detected by HLA-"DR1" alloantisera and 19 by HLA-"DR4" alloantisera. Clearly, use of the terms "DR1" and "DR4" is imprecise and the data generated in the past using alloantisera-based techniques reflect this imprecision. Consequently, such terms have been placed in quotation marks throughout this chapter.

The associations of specific HLA molecules with particular joint diseases are indicated in Figure. 1. The HLA-linked diseases (e.g., diseases linked to HLA-"B8", HLA-"B27", and HLA-"DR4") are intimately bound up with autoimmune processes, as indicated in Table I. The genetic association is usually described in terms of conferring susceptibility to, or risk for, the particular disease. The degree of risk conferred by a given HLA allele can be calculated as the estimated relative risk (rr). A relative risk of >1 suggests that the HLA allele may be positively associated with the disease.

A. Association of Class I HLA Molecules with Autoimmune Disease

Class I HLA gene products are divided into type A, B, and C molecules (Fig. 1). A very strong association with class I HLA-"B27" is found for ankylosing spondylitis (rr = 85–91 in Caucasians, but is ten-fold less in African blacks) [17, 18]. The consistency of this finding lends support to the concept that the HLA-"B27" alleles are involved directly in the pathogenesis of ankylosing spondylitis. Among the nine distinct HLA-"B27" alleles, HLA-B *2702 is the more frequent in this disease, whereas HLA-B *2705 is the wild type and HLA-B *2703 does not appear to be associated with an increased risk [12]. These alleles produce single substitutions in the amino acid sequence of the HLA-"B27" molecule and, thus, may be associated with functional differences with respect to peptide binding, T-cell recognition, or both. Interestingly, transgenic human-HLA-"B27" rats experience an illness strikingly similar to human ankylosing spondylitis [19, 20]. A germ-free environment markedly reduces the incidence of disease in these rats, implicating a role for microorganisms.

The incidence of HLA-"B27" is also high in other autoimmune diseases, particularly in Reiter's syndrome (rr = 37) and the reactive arthritides (rr between 14 and 29) [17, 21]. A possible mechanism for the pathogenesis of

TABLE I.   Association of Class I HLA-"B8" and -"B27" and Class II HLA-"DR4"
Polymorphisms with Auto-Immune Diseases

Diseases	Class I HLA		Class II HLA	
	Serology	Alleles	Serology	Alleles
HLA-"B8"-associated				
Myasthenia gravis	A2, B8, B13	—	DP	DPB1*0402
Dermatitis herpetiformis	B8	—	DR3, DQ2	—
Graves' disease	B8, B35	—	DP	DPB1*0402
			DR3, DR17	—
Chronic viral hepatitis	A1, B8	—	DR3, DR4	—
Celiac disease	A1, B8	—	DR3, DR7	—
			DQ2	DQB1*0201
Myositis	B7, B8	—	DR3, DR8	—
Type I diabetes	B8, B15, B35	—	DR3	—
			DR4	DRB1*0401, 2, 5, 8, 10, 14
			DQ2	DQB1*0201
			DQ7	DQB1*0304
			DQ8	DQB1*0302
HLA-"B27"-associated				
Ankylosing spondylitis	B27	*2702	DR4	DRB1*0401
HLA-"DR4"-associated				
Subacute thyroiditis	B35, B67	—	DR4	—
Rheumatoid arthritis	—	—	DR1	DRB1*0101
			DR4	DRB1*0401, 4, 5
			DR10	DRB1*1001
			DR14	DRB1*1402
			DQ8	DQB1*0301
Juvenile rheumatoid arthritis	—	—	DR4	—
			DR6	—
			DR8	—
			DR5	DRB1*1104

HLA-"B27"-associated diseases is that peptides from arthritogenic bacteria with homology to endogenous self-peptides elicit an autoimmune T-cell response upon infection [22]. Alternatively, class II HLA molecules could present class I HLA peptides, leading to HLA-"B27"-associated arthritis, for example. Patients with ankylosing spondylitis do have autoantibodies to HLA-"B27" [23]. Cross-reaction of HLA-"B27" sequences with microbial products of *Klebsiella pneumoniae* or other microorganisms (e.g., *Salmonella, Shighella, Yersinia* spp.) have been described [24]. Certain subtypes of HLA-B27 (*2701, 2704, 2705, and 2706) could present peptides from arthritogenic bacteria and peptides derived from HLA-"B27" itself [22].

Other class I HLA associations include the inflammatory myopathies [25], chronic viral hepatitis [26], myasthenia gravis [27, 28], Graves' thyrotoxic disease [28, 29], subacute thyroiditis [30, 31], acute anterior uveitis, autoimmune type I (insulin-dependent) diabetes, and psoriasis vulgaris [24] (rr between 3 and 18). As illustrated in Table I, associations with class I and class II HLA molecules are not exclusive. The relative risk of a combination of class I HLA-"B8" with class II HLA-DPB1*0402 is additive, reaching 10 to 11 for myasthenia gravis and 6 for Graves' disease [28]. Most autoimmune

diseases related to HLA-"B8" also are associated with class II HLA-"DR3" and/or HLA-"DR4".

B. Association of Class II HLA Molecules and Autoimmune Disease

Class II gene products are divided into products encoded in the DP, DQ, and DR regions. Each of these regions encodes a variable number of both α- and β-chains. The HLA-DR region contains a single α-chain gene, designated DRα, that does not exhibit significant allelic variation. In contrast, the genes encoding the HLA-DR β-chains are highly polymorphic and vary in number among different individuals in the population. Many of these DRβ genes are nonfunctional pseudogenes (ψDRB), although all "haplotypes" contain at least one functional DRB1 gene and many haplotypes contain a second functional DRB gene (e.g., DRB3, DRB4, or DRB5). A haplotype is a set of genes, usually linked, which are passed together from generation to generation. The presence of haplotypes is usually established by conducting family studies, wherein the inheritance pattern and linkage can be determined.

Some HLA-DRB1 gene products, the "DR3" (alleles *0301 to 0304) molecules, are associated with organ-specific diseases such as dermatitis herpetiformis (rr = 17), chronic viral hepatitis (rr = 14), Addison's adrenal disease, celiac disease, type I diabetes, Sjögren's syndrome, and Graves' disease (rr between 4 and 11) [24, 26, 32]. Juvenile Sjögren's syndrome is associated with both HLA-"DR3" and "DR52" [33]. In addition to HLA-"DR3" and some class I HLA gene products (e.g., HLA-"B8"), Graves' disease also could be associated with HLA-"DR17" [29].

Furthermore, some "DR4" products of the HLA-DRB1 gene (alleles *0401 to 0419) have been associated with autoimmune type I diabetes and RA (rr = 6 for both) [24]. The analysis of association of type I diabetes and HLA began with the discovery of weak relations to class I HLA-"B8" or HLA-"B15" and has progressed to the discovery of close associations with class II antigens. The combination of "DR3" and "DR4" alleles is an especially high risk factor for type I diabetes (rr = 14) [34]. The associated HLA-DRB1 alleles are multiple: *0401, *0402, *0405, *0408, *0410, and *0414 [24, 35, 36]. In addition, heterozygozity of an HLA-"DR1" allele is associated with an increased risk of the development of retinopathy [37]. In RA, the HLA antigen association remains with specific alleles of HLA-"DR1" and HLA-"DR4" [14–16, 38, 39]. In monozygotic twins, a five-fold risk for RA concordance is seen in twins who are HLA-"DR4" positive [40].

The HLA-DRB1 gene products, "DR5" (alleles *1101–1113 and *1201–1203), are associated with Hashimoto's autoimmune thyroid disease, primary myxedema, and seronegative juvenile RA (rr between 2 and 3) [21, 41]. In patients with juvenile RA, the HLA-"DR5" split DRB1 *1104 is associated with a risk of chronic iridocyclitis (rr = 8) [42]. Other HLA-DRB1 gene products associated with juvenile RA are HLA-"DR6" and HLA-"DR8" in seronegative patients and HLA-"DR4" in seropositive patients [41].

Patients with chronic viral hepatitis commonly have immunologic manifestations, including autoantibodies and concurrent autoimmune diseases. Disease susceptibility is associated with class I HLA-"A1" and HLA-"B8," the presence of antinuclear autoantibodies is associated with class II HLA-"DR3," while concurrent immunologic diseases (e.g., thyroiditis and Sjögren's syndrome) are associated with HLA-"DR4" gene products [26]. In Caucasians with systemic lupus erythematosus (SLE) or Sjögren's syndrome, the HLA associations (e.g., HLA-"DR2," HLA-"DR3," or HLA-"DQ") are related more directly to the presence of particular autoantibodies (e.g., Ro/SS-A, La/SS-B, or antiribosomal P) than to the disease process [43–46]. In the "normal" population and patients with SLE, complement component C2 deficiency is associated with the HLA-"A25," "B18," and "DR2" haplotype [47].

The association of HLA with autoimmune diseases also includes "DQ" molecules, particularly "DQ2," "DQ6," "DQ7,"

and "DQ8." Dermatitis herpetiformis and celiac disease are associated with HLA-"DQ2" [32, 48, 49]. Type I diabetes is related to HLA-"DQ2," "DQ7," and "DQ8," or more precisely to the presence of Arg at position 52 of the DQ α-chain and the absence of Asp at position 57 of the DQ β-chain [50]. Multiple sclerosis is associated with HLA-DQB1 *0602 ("DQ6") [51, 52]. Autoimmune thyroid diseases could be associated with HLA-"DQ7" [53, 54]. The findings in Hashimoto's thyroid disease are controversial [55, 56].

Some HLA-"DR2" products derived from the DRB1 *1501 to 1504 or *1601 to *1606 alleles are risk factors for Goodpasture's syndrome (rr between 13 and 16), multiple sclerosis, and SLE (rr between 3 and 4) [24, 45, 51]. In contrast, the HLA-"DR2" alleles are underrepresented in type I diabetes, autoimmune chronic hepatitis, and RA [57]; HLA-"DR2"-positive patients (e.g., DRB1*1601) have less severe diseases, implying that "DR2" is a "poor-responder" or a protective gene. In type I diabetes, HLA-DRB1 *0403, *0404, and *0406 [36], and in SLE, HLA-"DQ1" also could represent protective alleles [58].

There are, however, important ethnic differences in the associations. First, in a given population, an association with class I HLA alleles can be potentiated through an increased incidence of specific class II alleles. For example, in Scotland, ankylosing spondylitis is associated with both HLA-"B27" and DRB1 *0401 [59]. Secondly, different alleles are associated with the same autoimmune diseases in different regions of the world. For example, in Caucasians, class I HLA-"B8" and class II HLA-"DR3" are associated with inflammatory myositis, whereas in the Japanese, these diseases are associated with HLA-"B7" and HLA-"DR8" [25]. In the eastern Baltic region, in addition to class I HLA-"B35" and class II HLA-DRB1 *0408, type I diabetes is associated with HLA-DQB1 *0304 ("DQ7") [35], whereas in Spain and Chile, it is associated with HLA-DQB1 *0201 ("DQ2") or *0302 ("DQ8") [9, 60]. The ethnic differences that have been reported for the association of RA with class II HLA alleles are discussed below.

IV. HLA-DRB1 ALLELES AND RHEUMATOID ARTHRITIS

The clinical heterogeneity of RA is well known; some cases are very mild and self-limiting, whereas others progress to a profoundly debilitating erosive disease and may include extraarticular manifestations. In this disease, the destructive potential of the synovial membrane is a characteristic feature. It is possible that an exogenous antigen, likely an infectious organism, targets the synovium. The observation that HLA molecules function by specifically binding antigenic peptides and presenting them to T lymphocytes has supported the concept of an antigen-driven response. However, major progress in our understanding of the pathologic events leading to RA can be expected only if single mechanism models are abandoned. Such models are oversimplistic and underestimate the complexity of the disease. In particular, full recognition of the importance of nonimmune tissues and mechanisms in pathogenesis of RA will open new avenues of research and innovative conceptual approaches [61]. Nevertheless, in RA, the current opinion is that at least one of the multiple genetic risk determinants, which may not be pathologic if occurring alone, is linked to the HLA region [10, 38, 62, 63].

Thus, seropositive RA (in the sense of high levels of IgM rheumatoid factors) has been associated with HLA-"DR4" [14] and to specific alleles, namely HLA-DRB1 *0401 or *0404 in Caucasians and *0405 in Asians [15, 16, 39, 64]. In some other ethnic groups, however, RA has been associated with HLA-"DR1" [65, 66] (HLA-DRB1*1001 ("DR10") in Spanish [67] and Israeli populations [68] or HLA-DRB1 *1402 ("DR14") in Yakima Indians [69]). In an attempt to explain these ethnic differences, the "shared epitope" hypothesis was proposed [70]. Almost all racial-ethnic groups share the association of RA with the DRβ-encoded amino acid sequence motif QKRAA, QRRAA, or RRRAA from residues 70 to 74 of the DR β-chain [63, 71, 72]. The shared epitopes are a set of conserved amino acid residues in the third hypervariable region of the HLA-DR β-chain. The "DR4" allele, DRB1 *0401, is characterized by the QKRAA motif (arginine versus lysine substitution at position 71), the "DR1" allele and other "DR4" alleles by the QRRAA motif, whereas the "DR10" allele DRB1 *1001 is characterized by the RRRAA motif (arginine versus glycine substitution at position 70). It has been claimed that the QKRAA sequence in particular, which characterizes the HLA-DRB1 *0401 allele, might contribute to RA [72, 73]. The significance of these motifs in disease risk remains controversial, however. For example, in African-Americans, a specific association with the shared epitope is not observed [74]. Furthermore, in some reports, the degree of risk for RA is weaker for "DR1"- than for "DR4"-associated alleles [75, 76]. These observations suggest that the shared epitope may not be entirely functionally equivalent when it occurs in the context of different HLA-DR molecules or in the setting of different genetic backgrounds; thus, these motifs may not offer a complete explanation for the HLA association with RA [77].

In contrast to autoimmunity, which is a dominant familial phenotype [1], inheritance of the HLA-"DR1" and "DR4" alleles is a recessive trait [16]. The presence of particular alleles increases disease susceptibility and severity as their penetration increases. Thus, in seropositive juvenile RA, heterozygosity for HLA-DRB1 *0401/*0404 shows the strongest association with disease [78]. In adult RA, patients who are homozygous or heterozygous for DRB1 *0401 and *0404 show more severe and erosive disease [64, 79]. In patients who are homozygous for DRB1 *0401 or *0404, as well as in heterozygous patients showing both DRB1 *0101 and *0401, extra-articular manifestations such as nodules, vasculitis, or

Felty's syndrome are frequently observed [62, 64, 73, 79]. These observations suggest that these HLA-DRB1 alleles are subject to a "dose-response" effect.

A. Extra-articular Manifestations

IgM rheumatoid factors are one of the most characteristic laboratory parameters in RA, and the specificity of their association with disease is increased when their titer is high. They are defined as reacting with the Fc portion of IgG. Interestingly, half of human polyclonal IgM rheumatoid factors also show positive ELISA reactions with affinity-isolated HLA class I molecules ("A2" and "B7") [80]. This may reflect antigenic overlap between products of several members of the immunoglobulin gene superfamily. The pathological significance of these findings remains unknown, however.

In RA, patients who are HLA-"DR1" or HLA-"DR4" show high levels of IgM rheumatoid factors, erythrocyte sedimentation rates (ESR), platelet counts, and C-reactive protein (CRP), often with depressed hemoglobin levels [66]. Thus, it has been claimed that seronegative (prognostically good) and seropositive patients (prognostically worse)—in the sense of high levels of IgM rheumatoid factors—can be distinguished by the presence of HLA-DRB1 *0101 or *0401 alleles [38, 63, 73]. HLA typing is usually considered to be a costly and unnecessary procedure for the diagnosis of inflammatory rheumatoid diseases. However, these genetic markers alone [81], or combined with either IgM rheumatoid factors [82] or ESR and CRP [73], could indicate the outcome in early RA.

The T lymphocyte control of production of rheumatoid factors may explain the observation that IgM rheumatoid factor positivity is an HLA-dependent phenomenon. According to this concept, the levels of memory T lymphocytes (CD45RA−, CD45RO+) in the peripheral blood correlate with the serum levels of IgM rheumatoid factors [83]. The higher risk of IgM rheumatoid factors positivity is observed in patients who carry the HLA-DRB1 *0401 allele with the HLA-"DQ8" DQB1 *0301 allele (rr = 5) [73]. The role of HLA-"DQ8" molecules in RA has been suggested by experiments using transgenic mice [84]. Interestingly, DQA1-incompatibility and DQB1-incompatibility between mother and fetus often results in a favorable course of RA in the mother [85]. The influence of DQ-incompatibility is more prominent than DRB1-incompatibility.

A number of studies have reported a higher frequency of HLA-"DR4" in patients with extra-articular disease, such as Felty's syndrome and vasculitis [86, 87]. The presence of both HLA-DRB1 *0101 and *0401 alleles in heterozygous patients has been associated with vasculitis (rr = 3) [73].

Clear differences in RA susceptibility exist between males and females and these may be attributable to hormonal status. Gender-related factors influence the disease penetrance associated with HLA-DRB1 alleles. Thus, the effect of HLA-DRB1 risk alleles on prognosis and pathogenesis should be considered separately for men and women [88]. Males have a higher threshold requirement for developing RA and this may explain why RA in males has a closer association with HLA risk alleles [7]. The decreased testosterone concentration observed in male patients with RA, which is associated with HLA-"B15," could restore the susceptibility to that observed in women [89].

Furthermore, in RA, the diurnal rhythm of prolactin (Prl)—an immunostimulatory hormone—shows a peak at about 2 AM, possibly contributing to the nocturnal worsening of symptoms. The Prl gene is in close proximity (telomeric) to the HLA region on the short arm of chromosome 6. The effects of breast feeding and nulliparity are modified by the HLA-"DR4" status, suggesting an interaction between genetic and reproductive risk factors in the etiology of RA [90]. The Prl response to thyrotropin-releasing hormone is increased in women with RA, particularly in HLA-"DR4"-positive cases. The associations between HLA-"DR4" (and corresponding DRB1 alleles) and reproductive risk factors could be due to linkage disequilibrium between the HLA complex, abnormal regulation of the expression of the Prl gene, or polymorphism of the Prl protein, which could influence the pathological processes [91]. Linkage disequilibrium refers to alleles of two linked genes that tend to be passed together from generation to generation and thus occur paired more frequently that would be expected from the frequencies of the individual genes.

B. Degradation of Cartilage and Bone

In RA, an early study reported a higher frequency of HLA-"DR4" in patients with erosions revealed by radiological changes [92]. More recently, severe articular damage has been associated with HLA-DRB1 *0401 and/or *0404 in Caucasians [64, 66, 79, 82]. A five-year prospective study supports the view that DRB1 *0101 is associated with early inflammatory arthritis, whereas the HLA-"DR4" alleles (*0401 and *0404) are more specifically associated with progression to "aggressive" RA [93]. One study [94] examined 169 patients enrolled in a multicenter trial of minocycline therapy for RA and found that the rate of progression of radiographic erosions was correlated with the presence and dosage of HLA-DRB1 alleles encoding some of the shared epitopes (*0401 and/or *0404).

In addition to high levels of rheumatoid factors, IgG anti-type II collagen autoantibodies are characteristic of RA. Proliferative T-cell responses to type II collagen occur in some healthy individuals, suggesting that thymic tolerance for this antigen may be incomplete [95]. Moreover, most patients with RA show no evidence of a T-cell response to type II collagen, which may indicate that peripheral tolerance to this antigen develops in response to cartilage breakdown. However, in a minority of patients, T- and B-cell responses to type II collagen persist and may contribute to joint damage. Thus, although the antigen(s) that initiates RA remains elusive, it has been shown that many patients have autoimmunity directed to type II collagen.

The argument against this concept is that, in RA, the association—if any—between anti-type II collagen autoantibodies and HLA-"DR4" is very weak [96]. Similarly, there is no significant correlation between the serum levels of IgM rheumatoid factors and IgG anti-type II collagen autoantibodies [83]. On the other hand, experiments with transgenic mice have shown that HLA-"DR1" is capable of presenting peptides derived from human type II collagen, suggesting that this class II HLA molecule is capable of mediating an autoimmune response [39]. It is unlikely, however, that the susceptibility to RA is a simple immune response gene phenomenon that is specific for type II collagen.

Markers for joint diseases, such as cartilage oligomeric matrix protein (COMP) that is produced by chondrocytes and synovial fibroblasts, may provide additional information. Low molecular weight COMP fragments and autoantibodies to COMP can be detected in synovial fluids from patients with RA but not osteoarthritis. HLA-"B27"-positive patients with inflammatory arthritides other than RA exhibited patterns of greater degradation of COMP in synovial fluid than HLA-"B27"-negative patients [97]. Furthermore, in RA, a preliminary study showed that patients with RA-associated HLA-DRB1 alleles (e.g., *0101, *0401 and/or *0404) had increased serum levels of COMP, compared with other RA patients [98], suggesting an association with more severe joint disease.

A working hypothesis can be synthesized in which HLA-"DR1" and HLA-"DR4" gene products have distinct influences on inflammation, extra-articular manifestations, and cartilage degradation (Fig. 2). According to this hypothesis, HLA-"DR1" patients have a more inflammatory disease, whereas HLA-"DR4" patients have a more aggressive disease in the sense of progressive joint destruction. These two processes may occur independently [61].

V. MOLECULAR MECHANISMS

It appears likely that particular HLA alleles are involved directly in the pathogenesis of joint disease. One mechanism by which HLA alleles may predispose an individual to autoimmune disease relates to the role of HLA molecules in guiding the process of T-cell development in the thymus [99]. The end result is a fine balance of discrimination between self and nonself. In view of the complexity of this process, it is not surprising that, to a certain extent, autoantibodies to various antigens can occur in all individuals. The mouse model of type II collagen-induced arthritis provides evidence that

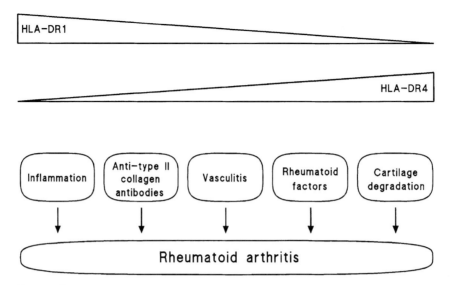

FIGURE 2   Class II HLA-"DR1" and -"DR4" in rheumatoid arthritis (RA): distinct associations with inflammatory processes, IgG anti-type II collagen antibodies, vasculitis, IgM rheumatoid factors, and cartilage degradation.

thymic selection events can influence susceptibility to this disease [100]. Experiments with human transgenic mouse lines have provided new information concerning the potential mechanisms by which HLA alleles may confer disease susceptibility [19, 20, 39, 84, 101]. For example, HLA-"DQ8" transgenic mice showed increased susceptibility to collagen-induced arthritis, whereas HLA-"DQ6" transgenic mice displayed reduced susceptibility, and HLA-"DR2" transgenic mice did not develop the disease [84]. Interestingly, in HLA-"DR8" transgenic mice, injection of the HLA-DRB1 *0402 peptide (which does not confer genetic predisposition to RA) resulted in a reduced incidence of collagen-induced arthritis. This was accompanied by decreased production of interferon-γ, interleukin-12, and IgG2a anti-type II collagen autoantibody, whereas the release of interleukin-4 was increased. Possibly, the DRB1 *0402 peptide presented by HLA-"DQ8" favors the negative selection of autoreactive thymocytes and induces a protective Th2 response. Because HLA-DR alleles are not distributed randomly among patients with RA, it can be anticipated that the T-cell repertoire also will be biased.

A second potential mechanism relates to the concept of "molecular mimicry." As illustrated in Figure 3, T lymphocyte recognition of antigen is normally restricted to the individual's own HLA molecules. Allelic differences in HLA structure may result in subtle differences between individuals in the presentation of antigen to T lymphocytes. One study shows that specific TCR recognition is influenced by HLA polymorphism [102]. The reason for the HLA-"B27" association with ankylosing spondylitis may relate to the specific peptides that are bound and presented to CD8+ T lymphocytes by these molecules [12]. In addition, the same antigen can be presented differently by the HLA-"B27" molecules

associated with either low or high risk of disease, resulting in T-cell responses to different epitopes [103].

Because HLA-DR alleles are not randomly distributed among patients with RA, it can be anticipated that the T-cell repertoire also will be biased. The RA-associated DRB1 *0401 and *0404 alleles encode HLA molecules that preferentially bind negatively charged amino acids of the antigenic sequence (Asp, Glu), in contrast to other HLA-"DR4" molecules that preferentially bind positively charged amino acids (Arg, Lys) [104]. In addition, residue 71, which in the DRB1 *0401 sequence presents an arginine versus lysine substitution, plays a critical role in T-lymphocyte stimulation, either through direct contact with the TCR or by changing the orientation or conformation of the HLA/peptide complex [105]. Interestingly, the shared epitope of HLA-"DR1" and HLA-"DR4" that is associated with RA binds the 70-kDa human and bacterial heatshock proteins [72, 106] and shows homology with a segment of the gp 110 protein of the Epstein-Barr virus [24]. Thus, specific HLA molecules may be biased in their ability to present particular autoantigens, or cross-reactive foreign antigens, to T lymphocytes [73, 107]. In this biased context, antigenic peptides from particular infectious agents with homology to endogenous self peptides could be presented and, subsequently, elicit an autoimmune response [22].

In addition, the HLA molecule itself can be an autoantigen. In some cases, peptides derived from specific HLA molecules can be recognized by T lymphocytes [108]. In such a case, molecular mimicry may occur between foreign antigens and portions of disease-associated HLA molecules [109]. Consequently, autoantibodies against specific HLA molecules (e.g., anti-HLA-"B27") can be detected [23]. The T lymphocytes

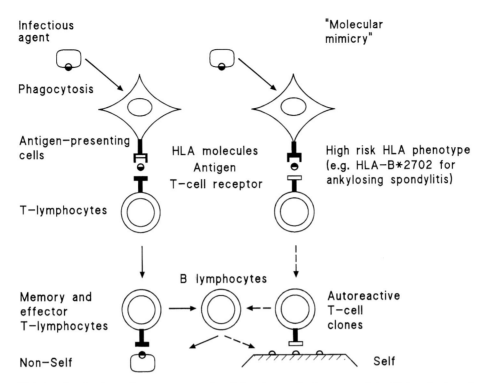

FIGURE 3   Foreign antigens are presented to T lymphocytes in the context of the HLA molecule and T-cell receptor for antigen. "Normal" cellular and humoral immune responses (right) lead to the clearance of an infectious agent. However, specific HLA molecules can present differently (left), producing potential autoreactive T lymphocytes; if they encounter a structure in the body similar to the presented epitope (molecular mimicry), they begin an auto-immune reaction, including the triggering of autoantibody production by B lymphocytes.

may be involved in both the initiation and maintenance of the disease process. The HLA-"DR1" amino acid sequence that is associated with RA (QKRAAA) lies adjacent to the antigen-binding cleft of the molecule and can be presented to CD4+ T lymphocytes. The corresponding HLA-DRB1 allele (*0101) has been associated with the inflammatory phase of RA [93], including the T-cell response to type II collagen [73]. Similar HLA-DRB1 QKRAA sequences are also expressed by numerous infectious agents, e.g., *Brucella ovis*, *Escherichia coli*, *Lactobacillus lactis*, and Epstein-Barr virus [110]. Thus, this amino acid sequence could represent an antigenic epitope common to several different infectious agents and could be involved in molecular mimicry. This concept illustrates the complex interplay of hereditary and shared environmental factor in the pathogenesis of joint diseases. Again, many factors other than specific HLA haplotypes must be involved because many normal individuals carry the shared epitope motif and do not develop arthritis.

RA probably arises as a consequence of the activation of only a few cells within the joints. The development of molecular biology techniques (*in situ* hybridization and *in situ* PCR) has permitted the analysis of the synovial membrane at the cellular level and has opened a fascinating new horizon to exploration. These studies have indicated a third possible

mechanism, in which the immune responses of T and B lymphocytes are accompanied (or even preceded) by viral activation of synovial fibroblasts and/or macrophages (Fig. 4). Specific HLA molecules might affect the susceptibility of these cells to viral attachment or infection. A persistent intra-articular viral infection might play an important role in the pathogenesis of certain forms of chronic arthritis (e.g., Parvovirus B19, Epstein-Barr virus, human T-cell leukemia virus-I, hepatitis C, mumps, and rubella viruses, as well as retroviruses) [111, 112]. In the early stages of RA, proliferation and activation of synovial fibroblasts precedes the influx of leukocytes [113]. The aggressive transformed-like fibroblasts attach to bone and cartilage and destroy the joint through local production of proteolytic enzymes, such as cathepsins (B and L) and matrix metalloproteinases (MMP-1, -9, -13, and -14). During this process, chemoattractants (e.g., osteopontin and interleukin-16) could be responsible for the infiltration of leukocytes. In this context, specific HLA-"DR" molecules associated with RA severity may favor the autoimmune and inflammatory responses. Thereafter, soluble factors (e.g., interleukin-1, tumor necrosis factor-alpha [TNF-α], and osteopontin) stimulate the release of proteolytic enzymes by chondrocytes and fibroblasts, which in turn lead to exacerbation of joint destruction [114, 115].

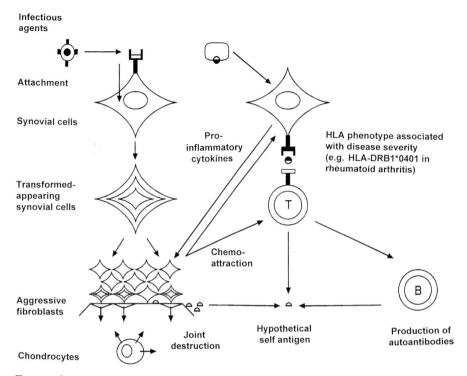

FIGURE 4   HLA-"DR" molecules as bystanders in rheumatoid arthritis. Infectious agents activate synovial fibroblasts and macrophages. Specific HLA molecules favor the viral attachment or infection. The synovial fibroblasts proliferate, destroy the joint via proteolytic enzymes, and attract mononuclear cells. Subsequently, specific HLA molecules favor a severe inflammation and, through the action of pro-inflammatory cytokines, could exacerbate joint destruction by chondrocytes and synovial fibroblasts.

The search for additional, non-HLA genes involved in autoimmunity has focused primarily on candidate gene families such as TCR, immunoglobulin, and cytokine genes. Until recently, the results for RA have been inconclusive. However, it seems that TCR-α chain SSCP—an amino acid allelic variant—could be highly associated with RA [116]. Another study showed that the presence of TCR-β polymorphisms enhanced the risk of RA in HLA-"DR4"-positive individuals [117]. The most intriguing evidence relates to TNF-α production in chronic inflammatory diseases. This cytokine is thought to be involved in the pathogenesis of RA; it is increased in synovial fluid, mediates bone erosion and synovial fibroblast proliferation, and its gene (TNF-α/β) is located within the class I and class III HLA loci on chromosome 6p in humans.

VI. MICROSATELLITE ALLELES

A large number of informative genetic markers, designated "microsatellites," have been identified throughout the human genome. Microsatellite markers consist of unique genetic regions that contain repeated elements, most often dinucleotide repeats. The number of these repeats commonly varies greatly between individuals. Several thousand microsatellites have been identified and assigned to specific chromosomal regions [7, 118]. For example, microsatellite-based methods enabled the demonstration of an association between the fibrillin-1 gene (FBN1 haplotype) on chromosome 15q with systemic sclerosis [119]; previously, a defect in this gene showing autosomal dominance had been described in Marfan syndrome.

Within the TNF locus, five microsatellites have been recognized, two for TNF-α and three for TNF-β. RA could be associated with TNF-α microsatellite polymorphisms, as has been shown for some other autoimmune diseases (e.g., multiple sclerosis, dermatitis herpetiformis, celiac disease, and SLE) [49, 120–124]. Differences were seen between men and women and according to age at onset [123]. Whether the association of specific TNF-α microsatellite alleles with RA is independent of the HLA-DRB1 shared epitope remains controversial, however [121, 122, 125–127].

Candidate genes that predispose an individual to RA have been identified using fluorescence-based microsatellite marker analysis and affected sib-pair linkage studies [128]. Common gene loci for disease susceptibility found in Japan and Europe [129, 130] are chromosome loci D1s214, D8s556, and the region of chromosome X between DXs1047 and

DXs1227. These regions contain candidate genes that may be important in the pathogenesis of RA, such as the TNF receptor II gene near D1s214 and the CD154 (CD40 ligand) gene near DXs1047–DXs1227. Other candidate genes identified by the microsatellite method and linkage analysis in affected siblings are those for interleukin-2, interleukin-5 receptor, interferon-γ [130], CD80 (B7.1), and CD86 (B7.2) [130]. CD80 and CD86, as well as CD28 ligands, act as important costimulatory molecules during antigen presentation. These studies confirmed that non-HLA loci account for more than 50% of genetic susceptibility to RA.

VII. CONCLUSIONS

Considerable effort has been expended in establishing that HLA-DR alleles are involved in the predisposition and outcome of joint diseases. It has been established that some HLA-DRB1 alleles play a role in RA, at least in Caucasian and Asian patients. Routine HLA-DRB1 typing early in the course of disease could help the decision of treatment strategy; however, such decisions still must be guided primarily by clinical parameters. Little is known about the molecular mechanisms by which the HLA-"DR" polymorphism contribute to the pathogenesis of RA. The shared epitope concept represents the first of several hypotheses. The results of other studies defining additional influences of genes on chromosome 6 have been less consistent, with the possible exception of the TNF and prolactin genes. In spite of the association of TNF-α microsatellite polymorphisms with long-term RA outcome, their contribution to the pathogenesis is not yet clear. In HLA-DRB1 *0401-positive individuals, an association has been found between RA and alleles of two highly polymorphic microsatellite markers lying close to the prolactin gene locus. The most exciting findings have been generated through the examination of non-HLA genes. It is anticipated that some of the genes identified by microsatellite analyses of immunorelevant loci (e.g., TCR β-chain locus, adhesion molecules, cytokines and their receptors) will concur with the current concepts of the inflammatory and immune processes that are pathologically important in RA. In view of the current understanding of the pathogenesis of RA, it is not clear that whether these polymorphisms will play a decisive role or merely be contributory factors. Rather, the discovery of other gene polymorphisms (e.g., in the genes that encode neuroendocrine factors, tumor suppressor genes, proteolytic enzymes, and structural proteins), identification of anti-apoptotic molecules in synovial fibroblasts (e.g., sentrin), as well as clarification of the roles of exogenous and endogenous retroviral sequences, is more likely to represent the decisive breakthroughs that permit a clear understanding of the genetic basis of RA.

References

1. Sels, F., Westhovens, R., Edmonds, M. P., Vandermeulen, E., and Dequeker, J. (1997). HLA typing in a large family with multiple cases of different autoimmune diseases. *J. Rheumatol.* **24**, 859–869.
2. Koumantaki, Y., Giziaki, E., Linos, A., Kontomerkos, A., Kaklamanis, P., Vaiopoulos, G., Mandas, J., and Kaklamani, E. (1997). Family history as a risk factor for rheumatoid arthritis: A case control study. *J. Rheumatol.* **24**, 1522–1526.
3. Bellamy, N., Duffy, D., Martin, N., and Matthews, J. (1992). Rheumatoid arthritis in twins: A study of aetiopathogenesis based on the Australian Twin Registry. *Ann. Rheum. Dis.* **51**, 588–593.
4. Silman, A. J., MacGregor, A. J., Thompson, W., Holligan, S., Cathy, D., Farhan, A., and Ollier, W. E. (1993). Twin concordance rates for rheumatoid arthritis: Results from a nationwide study. *Br. J. Rheumatol.* **32**, 903–907.
5. Jarvinen, P., and Aho, K. (1995). Twin studies in rheumatic diseases. *Semin. Arthritis Rheum.* **24**, 19–28.
6. MacGregor, A. J., Bamber, S., and Silman, A. J. (1994). A comparison of the performance of different methods of disease classification for rheumatoid arthritis. Results of analysis from a nationwide twin study. *J. Rheumatol.* **21**, 1420–426.
7. Ollier, W. E., and MacGregor, A. (1995). Genetic epidemiology of rheumatoid disease. *Br. Med. Bull.* **51**, 267–285.
8. Leslie, R. D., and Hawa, M. (1994). Twin studies in auto-immune disease. *Acta Genet. Med. Gemellol.* **43**, 71–81.
9. Perez, F., Calvillan, M., Santos, J. L., and Carrasco, E. (1996). Incidence of type I (insulin dependent) diabetes mellitus in Santiago, Chile: The role of immunogenetic and environmental factors. *Rev. Med. Chile* **124**, 1177–1186.
10. Weyand, C. M., and Goronzy, J. J. (1997). Pathogenesis of rheumatoid arthritis. *Med. Clin. North Am.* **81**, 29–55.
11. Munoz, E., Gonzales, R., Acasuso, M., Cisnal, A., Solana, R., Pérez, V., and Collantes, E. (1997). Flow cytometric HLA-B27 typing versus cytotoxicity using gene typing as a reference technique. *Arthritis Rheum.* **40** (Suppl.), S212.
12. Frankenberger, B., Breitkopf, S., Albert, E., Scholz, S., Keller, E., Schattenkirchner, M., Weiss, E. H., and Kellner, H. (1997). Routine molecular genotyping of HLA-B27 in spondyloarthropathies overcomes the obstacles of serological typing and reveals an increased B *2702 frequency in ankylosing spondylitis. *J. Rheumatol.* **24**, 899–903.
13. Buyse, I., Decorte, R., Cuppens, H., Semana, G., Edmonds, M. P., Marynen, P., and Cassiman J. J. (1993). Rapid DNA typing of class II HLA antigens using the polymerase chain reaction and reverse dot plot hybridization. *Tissue Antigens* **41**, 1–14.
14. Stastny, P. (1978). Association of the B-cell alloantigen DRw4 with rheumatoid arthritis. *N. Engl. J. Med.* **398**, 869–874.
15. Stastny, P., Fernandez-Vina, M., Cerna, M., Havelka, S., Ivaskova, E., and Vavrincova, P. (1993). Sequences of HLA alleles associated with arthritis in adults and children. *J. Rheumatol.* **37** (Suppl.), 5–8.
16. Hasstedt, S. J., Clegg, D. O., Ingles, L., and Howard, R. H. (1994). HLA-linked rheumatoid arthritis. *Am. J. Hum. Genet.* **55**, 738–746.
17. Bender, K. (1992). Das HLA-system. 5th ed., *Biotest, Suppl.*, pp. 1–66.
18. Adebajo, A., and Davis, P. (1994). Rheumatic diseases in African blacks. *Semin. Arthritis Rheum.* **24**, 139–153.
19. Hammer, R. E., Maika, S. D., Richardson, J. A., Tang, J. P., and Taurog, J. D. (1990). Spontaneous inflammatory disease in transgenic rats expressing HLA-B27 and human β2m: An animal model of HLA-B27 associated human disorders. *Cell* **63**, 1099–1112.
20. Taurog, J. D., Richardson J. A., Croft, J. T., Simmons, W. A., Zhiou, M., Fernandez-Sueiro, J. L., Balish, E., and Hammer, R. E. (1994). The germfree state prevents development of gout and joint inflammatory disease in HLA-B27 transgenic rats. *J. Exp. Med.* **180**, 2359–2364.

21. Arnett, F. C. (1994). Histocompatibility typing in the rheumatic diseases. Diagnostic and prognostic implications. *Rheum. Dis. Clin. North Am.* **20**, 371–390.

22. Garcia, F., Marina, A., Albar, J. P., and Lopez-de-Castro, J. A. (1997). HLA-B27 presents a peptide from a polymorphic region of its own molecule with homology to proteins from arthritogenic bacteria. *Tissue Antigens* **49**, 23–28.

23. Tani, Y., Tiwana, H., Hukuda, S., Nishioka, J., Fielder, M., Wilson, C., Bansal, S., and Ebringer, A. (1997). Antibodies to Klebsiella, Proteus, and HLA-B27 peptides in Japanese patients with ankylosing spondylitis and rheumatoid arthritis. *J. Rheumatol.* **24**, 109–114.

24. Braun W. E. (1992). HLA molecules in autoimmune diseases. *Clin. Biochem.* **25**, 187–191.

25. Furuya, T., Hakoda, M., Higami, K., Ueda, H., and Kashiwazaki, S. (1997). Association of HLA class I and class II alleles with Japanese myositis patients. *Arthritis Rheum.* **40** (Suppl.), S148.

26. Czaja, A. J. (1997). Extrahepatic immunologic features of chronic viral hepatitis. *Dig. Dis.* **15**, 125–144.

27. Barnton, E. N., Smikle, M., and Morgan, O. S. (1992). Myasthenia gravis and HLA phenotypes in Jamaicans. *South Med. J.* **85**, 904–906.

28. Ratanachaiyavong, S., Fleming, D., Janer, M., Demaine, A. G., Wilcox, N., Newsom-Davis, J., and McGregor, A. M. (1994). HLA-DPB1 polymorphisms in patients with hyperthyroid Graves' disease and early onset myasthenia gravis. *Autoimmunity* **17**, 99–104.

29. Inoue, D., Sato, K., Sugawa, H., Akamizu, T., Maeda, M., Inoko, H., Tsuji, K., and Mori, T. (1993). Apparent genetic difference between hypothyroid patients with blocking-type thyrotropin receptor antibody and those without, as shown by restriction fragment length polymorphism analyses of HLA-DP loci. *J. Clin. Endocrinol. Metab.* **77**, 606–610.

30. Rubin, R. A., and Guay, A. T. (1991). Susceptibility to subacute thyroiditis is genetically influenced: Familial occurence in identical twins. *Thyroid* **1**, 157–161

31. Ohsako, N., Tamai, H., Sudo, T., Mukuta, T., Tanaka, H., Kuma, K., Kimura, A., and Sasazuki, T. (1995). Clinical characteristics of subacute thyroiditis classified according to human leucocyte antigen typing. *J. Clin. Endocrinol. Metab.* **80**, 3653–3656.

32. Setterfield, J., Bhogal, B., Black, M. M., and McGibbon, D. H. (1997). Dermatitis herpetiformis and bullous pemphigoid: A developing association confirmed by immuno-electronmicroscopy. *Br. J. Dermatol.* **136**, 253–256.

33. Ostuni, P. A., Ianniello, A., Sfriso, P., Mazzola, G., Andretta, M., and Gambari, P. F. (1996). Juvenile onset of primary Sjögren's s syndrome: Report of 10 cases. *Clin. Exp. Rheumatol.* **14**, 689–693.

34. Thomson, G. (1995). HLA disease associations: Models for the study of complex human genetic disorders. *Crit. Rev. Clin. Lab. Sci.* **32**, 183–219.

35. Ilonen, J., Koskinen, S., Nejentsev, S., Sjoroos, M., Knip, M., Schwartz, E. I., Adojaan, B., Kovalchuk, L., and Sochnevs, A. (1997). HLA DQB1 *0304 DRB1 *0408 haplotype associated with insulin dependent diabetes mellitus in populations in the eastern Baltic region. *Tissue Antigens* **49**, 532–534.

36. Undlien, D. E., Friede, T., Rammensee, H. G., Joner, G., Dahljorgensen, K., Sovik, O., Akselsen, H. E., Knutsen, I., Ronningen, K. S., and Thorsby, E. (1997). HLA encoded genetic predisposition in IDDM: DR4 subtypes may be associated with different degrees of protection. *Diabetes* **46**, 143–149.

37. Falk, A. A. K., Knip, J. M., Ilonen, J. S., and Laatikainen, L. T. (1997). Genetic markers in early diabetic retinopathy of adolescent with type I diabetes. *J. Diabetes Comp.* **11**, 203–207.

38. Weyand, C. M., and Goronzy, J. J. (1990). Disease-associated human histocompatibility leucocyte antigen determinants in patients with seropositive rheumatoid arthritis. Functional role in antigen-specific and allogeneic T cell recognition. *J. Clin. Invest.* **85**, 1051–1057.

39. Rosloniec, E. F., Brand, D. D., Myers, L. K., Whittington, K. B., Gumanovskaya, M., Zaller, D. M., Woods, A., Altmann, D. M., Stuart, J. M., and Kang, A. H. (1997). An HLA DR1 transgene confers susceptibility to collagen induced arthritis elicited with human type II collagen. *J. Exp. Med.* **185**, 1113–1122.

40. Jawaheer, D., Thompson, W., MacGregor, A. J., Carthy, D., Davidson, J., Dyer, P. A., Silman, A. J., and Ollier, W. E. (1994). "Homozygosity" for the HLA-DR shared epitope contributes the highest risk for rheumatoid arthritis concordance in identical twins. *Arthritis Rheum.* **37**, 681–686.

41. Nepom B. S. (1991). The immunogenetics of juvenile rheumatoid arthritis. *Rheum. Dis. Clin. North Am.* **17**, 825–842.

42. Melin-Aldana, H., Giannini, E. H., Taylor, J., Lovell, D. J., Levinson, J. E., Passo, M. H., Ginsberg, J., Burke, M. J., and Glass, D. N. (1992). Human leukocyte antigen-DRB1*1104 in the chronic iridocyclitis of pauciarticular juvenile rheumatoid arthritis. *J. Pediatr.* **121**, 56–60.

43. Harley, J. B., Alexander, E. L., Bias, W. B., Fox, O. F., Provost, T. T., Reichlin, M., Yamagata, H., and Arnett, F. C. (1986). Anti-Ro/SS-A and anti-La/SS-B in patients with Sjögren's syndrome. *Arthritis Rheum.* **29**, 196–206.

44. Hamilton, R. G., Harley, J. B., Bias, W. B., Roebber, M., Reichlin, M., Hochberg, M. C., and Arnett, F. C. (1988). Two RO (SS-A) autoantibody responses in systemic lupus erythematosus: Correlation of HLA-DR/DQ specificities with quantitative expression of Ro (SS-A) autoantibody. *Arthritis Rheum.* **31**, 496–505.

45. Arnett, F. C., and Reveille, J. D. (1992). Genetic of systemic lupus erythematosus. *Rheum. Dis. Clin. North Am.* **18**, 865–870.

46. Arnett, F. C., Reveille, J. D., Moutsopoulos, H. M., Georgescu, L., and Elkon, K. B. (1996). Ribosomal P autoantibodies in systemic lupus erythematosus. Frequencies in different ethnic groups and clinical and immunogenetic associations. *Arthritis Rheum.* **39**, 1833–1839.

47. Aurajo, M. N. T., Silva, N. P., Andrade, L. E. C., Sato, E. I., Gerbasedelima, M., and Leser, P. G. (1997). C2 deficiency in blood donors and lupus patients: Prevalence, clinical characteristics and HLA associations in the Brazilian population. *Lupus* **6**, 462–466.

48. Hall, M. A., Lanchbury, J. S., Lee, J. S., Welsh, K. I., and Ciclitara, P. J. (1993). HLA-DQ2 second-domain polymorphism may explain increased trans-associated risk in celiac disease and dermatitis herpetiformis. *Hum. Immunol.* **12**, 284–292.

49. Manus, R. M., Wilson, A. G., Mansfield, J., Weir, D. G., Duff, G. W., and Kelleher, D. (1996). TNF2, a polymorphism of the tumor necrosis-alpha gene promoter, is a component of the celiac disease major histocompatibility complex haplotype. *Eur. J. Immunol.* **26**, 2113–2118.

50. McDermott, M. F., Schmidt-Wolf, G., Sinha, A. A., Koo, M., Porter, M. A., Briant, L., Cambon-Thomsen, A., MacLaren, N. K., Fiske, D., Bertera, S., Truscco, M., Amos, C. I., McDevitt, H. O., and Kastner, D. L. (1996). No linkage or association of telomeric and centromeric T-cell receptor beta-chain markers with susceptibility to type 1 insulin-dependent diabetes in HLA-DR4 multiplex families. *Eur. J. Immunogenet.* **23**, 361–370.

51. Spurkland, A., Celius, E. G., Knutsen, I., Beiske, A., Thorsby, E., and Vartdal, F. (1997). The HLA DQ (alpha 1 *0102, beta 1 *0602) heterodimer may confer susceptibility to multiple sclerosis in the absence of the HLA DR (alpha 1 *01, beta 1 *1501) heterodimer. *Tissue Antigens* **50**, 15–22.

52. Stewart, G. J., Teutsch, S. M., Castle, M., Heard, R. N. S., and Benetts, B. H. (1997). HLA DR, DQA1 and DQB1 associations in Australian multiple sclerosis patients. *Eur. J. Immunogenet.* **24**, 81–92.

53. Badenhoop, K., Schwarz, G., Walfish, P. G., Drummond, V., Usadel, K. H., and Bottazzo, G. F. (1990). Susceptibility to thyroid autoimmune disease: Molecular analysis of HLA-D region genes identifies new markers for goitrous Hashimoto's thyroiditis. *J. Clin. Endocrinol. Metab.* **71**, 1131–1137.

54. Tandon, N., Zhiang, L., and Weetman, A. P. (1991). HLA association with Hashimoto's thyroiditis. *Clin. Endocrinol.* **34**, 383–386.

55. Jenkins, D., Penny, M. A., Fletcher, J. A., Jacobs, K. H., Mijovic, C. H., Franklyn, J. A., and Sheppard, M. C. (1992). HLA class II gene polymorphism contributes little to Hashimoto's thyroiditis. *Clin. Endocrinol.* **37**, 141–145.

56. Roman, S. H., Greenberg, D., Rubinstein, P., Wallenstein, S., and Davies, T. F. (1992). Genetics of autoimmune thyroid disease: Lack of evidence for linkage to HLA within families. *J. Clin. Endocrinol. Metab.* **74**, 496–503.

57. Congia, M., Clemente, M. G., Dessi, C., Cucca, F., Mazzoleni, A. P., Frau, F., Lampis, R., Cao, A., Lai, M. E., and DeVirgillis, S. (1996). HLA class II genes in chronic hepatitis C virus-infection and associated immunological disorders. *Hepatology* **24**, 1338–1341.

58. Fouad, F., Johny, K., Kaaba, S., Alkarmi, T. O., Shama, P., and al Harbi, S. (1994). MHC in systemic lupus erythematosus: A study on a Kuwaiti population. *Eur. J. Immunogenet.* **21**, 11–14.

59. McGarry, F., Field, M., Chaudhuri, K., and Sturrock, R. D. (1997). MHC Class II alleles in ankylosing spondylitis. *Arthritis Rheum.* **40** (Suppl.), S211.

60. Serranorios, M., Lopez, M. D. G., Perezbravo, F., Martinez, M. T., Antona, J., Rowley, M., MacKay, I., and Zimmet, P. (1996). HLA DR, DQ and anti-GAD antibodies in first degree relatives of type I diabetes. *Diabetes Res. Clin. Pract.* **34**, (Suppl.), S133–139.

61. Gay, S., Gay, R. E., and Koopman, W. J. (1993). Molecular and cellular mechanisms of joint destruction in rheumatoid arthritis: Two cellular mechanisms explain joint destruction? *Ann. Rheum. Dis.* **52** (Suppl.), S39–S47.

62. Weyand, C. M., and Goronzy, J. J. (1994). Disease mechanisms in rheumatoid arthritis: Gene dosage effect of HLA-DR haplotypes. *J. Lab. Clin. Med.* **124**, 335–338.

63. Weyand, C. M., and Goronzy, J. J. (1995). Inherited and noninherited risk factors in rheumatoid arthritis. *Curr. Opin. Rheumatol.* **7**, 206–213.

64. Sany, J. (1994). Clinical and biological polymorphism of rheumatoid arthritis. *Clin. Exp. Rheumatol.* **12** (Suppl.), S59–S61.

65. Nichol, F. E., and Woodrow, J. C. (1981). HLA-DR antigens in Indian patients with rheumatoid athritis. *Lancet* **1**, 220–221.

66. Combes, B., Eliaou, J. F., Daures, J. P., Meyer, O., Clot, J., and Sany, J. (1995). Prognostic factors in rheumatoid arthritis. Comparative study of two subsets of patients according to severity of articular damage. *Br. J. Rheumatol.* **34**, 529–534.

67. Sanchez, B., Moreno, I., Magarino, R., Garzon, M., Gonzalez, M. F., Garcia, A., and Nunez-Roldan, A. (1990). HLA-DRw10 confers the highest susceptibility to rheumatoid arthritis in a Spanish population. *Tissue Antigens* **36**, 174–176.

68. Gao, X., Gazit, E., Livneh, M., and Stastny, P. (1991). Rheumatoid arthritis in Isreali Jews. Shared sequences in the third hypervariable region of DRB1 alleles are associated with susceptibility. *J. Rheumatol.* **18**, 801–803.

69. Wilkens, R. F., Nepom, G. T., Marks, C. R., Nettles, M., and Nepom, B. S. (1991). Association of HLA-Dw16 with rheumatoid arthritis in Yakima Indians. *Arthritis Rheum.* **34**, 43–47.

70. Gregersen, P. K., Silver, J., and Winchester, R. J. (1987). The shared epitope hypothesis. An approach to understanding the molecular genetics of susceptibility to rheumatoid arthritis. *Arthritis Rheum.* **30**, 1205–1213.

71. Albani, S., and Roudier, J. (1992). Molecular basis for the association between HLA DR4 and rheumatoid arthritis. From the shared epitope hypothesis to a peptidic model of rheumatoid arthritis. *Clin. Biochem.* **25**, 209–212.

72. Auger, I., Toussirot, E., and Roudier, J. (1997). Molecular mechanisms involved in the association of HLA-DR4 and rheumatoid arthritis. *Immunol. Res.* **16**, 121–126.

73. Perdriger, A., Chales, G., Semana, G., Guggenbuhl, P., Meyer, O.,

Quillivic, F., and Pawlotsky, Y. (1997). Role of HLA DR and DR DQ associations in the expression of extraarticular manifestations and rheumatoid factor in rheumatoid arthritis. *J. Rheumatol.* **24**, 1272–1276.

74. McDaniel, O., Reveille, J. D., and Pratt, P. W. (1994). The large majority of African-American patients with seropositive RA do not possess the rheumatoid epitope. *Arthritis Rheum.* **37**, S169.

75. Ollier, W., and Thompson, W. (1992). Population genetics of rheumatoid arthritis. *Rheum. Dis. Clin. North Am.* **18**, 741–746.

76. Ploski, R., Mellbye, O. J., Ronningen, K. S., Forre, O., and Thorsby, E. (1994). Seronegative and weakly seropositive rheumatoid arthritis differ from clearly seropositive rheumatoid arthritis. *J. Rheumatol.* **21**, 1397–1402.

77. Dizier, M. H., Eliaou, J. F., Babron, M. C., Combe, B., Sany, J., Clot, J., Clerget, and Darpoux, F. (1993). Investigation of the HLA component involved in rheumatoid arthritis (RA) by using the marker association seggregation X2 (MACS) method: Rejection of the unifying shared epitope hypothesis. *Am. J. Hum. Genet.* **53**, 715–721.

78. Nepom, B. S., Nepom, G. T., Mickelson, E., Schaller, J. G., Antonelli, P., and Hansen, J. A. (1984). Specific HLA-DR4-associated histocompatibility molecules characterize patients with juvenile rheumatoid arthritis. *J. Clin. Invest.* **74**, 287–291.

79. Weyand, C. M., Hicok, K. C., Conn, D. L., and Goronzy, J. J. (1992). The influence of HLA-DRB1 genes on disease severity in rheumatoid arthritis. *Ann. Intern. Med.* **117**, 801–806.

80. Williams, R. C., Jr., Malone, C. C., and Kao, K. J. (1996). IgM rheumatoid factors react with human class I HLA molecules. *J. Immunol.* **156**, 1684–1694.

81. Sarraux, A., Guedes, C., Allain, J., Devauchelle, V., Vallis, I., Baron, D., Youinou, P., and Legoff, P. (1997). Diagnostic value of HLA phenotype in inflammatory rheumatoid disease. *Presse Med.* **26**, 1040–1044.

82. Van Zeben, D., and Breedveld, F. C. (1996). Prognostic factors in rheumatoid arthritis. *J. Rheumatol.* **44** (Suppl.), 31–33.

83. Neidhart, M., Fehr, K., Pataki, F., and Michel, B. A. (1996). The levels of memory (CD45RA−, RO+) CD4+ and CD8+ peripheral blood T-lymphocytes correlate with IgM rheumatoid factors in rheumatoid arthritis. *Rheumatol. Int.* **15**, 201–209.

84. Das, P., Bradley, D. S., Griffiths, M. M., Luthra, H. S., Kurie, R., and David, C. S. (1997). An HLA-DRB1*0402 derived peptide (65–79) prevents the onset of CIA in HLA-DQ8 transgenic mice. *Arthritis Rheum.* **40** (Suppl.), S72.

85. Van der Horst-Bruinsma, J. F., de Vries, R. R. P., de Buck, P. D. M., van Schendel, P. W., Breedveld, P. C., Schreuder, G. M. T., and Hazes, J. M. W. (1997). The influence of HLA-class II incompatibility between mother and fetus on the onset and course of rheumatoid arthritis of the mother. *Arthritis Rheum.* **40** (Suppl.), S330.

86. Klouda, P. T., Corbin, S. A., Bidwell, J. L., Bradley, B. A., Ahern, M. J., and Maddison, P. J. (1986). Felty's syndrome and HLA-DR antigens. *Tissue Antigens* **27**, 112–113.

87. Hillarby, M. C., Hopkins, J., and Grennan, D. M. (1991). A re-analysis of the association between rheumatoid arthritis with and without extraparticular features, HLA-DR4 and DR4 subtypes. *Tissue Antigens* **37**, 39–41.

88. Meyer, J. M., Han, J., Singh, R., and Moxley, G. (1996). Sex influence on the penetrance of HLA shared-epitope genotypes for rheumatoid arthritis. *Am. J. Hum. Genet.* **58**, 371–383.

89. Jorgensen, C., and Sany, J. (1994). Modulation of the immune response by the neuro-endocrine axis in rheumatoid arthritis. *Clin. Exp. Rheumatol.* **12**, 435–441.

90. Jorgensen, C., Maziad, H., Bologna, C., and Sany, J. (1995). Kinetics of prolactin release in rheumatoid arthritis. *Clin. Exp. Rheumatol.* **13**, 705–709.

91. Brennan, P., Hajeer, A., Ong, K. R., Worthington, J., John, S., Thompson, W., Silman, A., and Ollier, B. (1997). Allelic markers

close to prolactin are associated with HLA-DRB1 susceptibility alleles among women with rheumatoid arthritis and systemic lupus erythematosus. *Arthritis Rheum.* **40**, 1383–1386.

92. Young, A., Jaraquemada, D., Awad, J., Festenstein, H., Corbett, M., Hay, F. C., and Roitt, I. M. (1984). Association of DR4/Dw4 and DR2/Dw2 with radiologic changes in a prospective study of patients with rheumatoid arthritis: Preferential relationship with HLA-Dw rather than HLA-DR specificities. *Arthritis Rheum.* **27**, 20–25.

93. Thomson, W., Pepper, L., Payton, A., Carthy, D., Scott, D., Ollier, W., Silman, A., and Symmons, D. (1993). Absence of an association between HLA-DRB1*04 and rheumatoid arthritis in newly diagnosed cases from the community. *Ann. Rheum. Dis.* **52**, 539–541.

94. Reveille, J. D., Alarcon, G. S., Fowler, S. E., Pillemer, S. R., Neuner, R., Clegg, D. O., Mikhail, I. S., Trethan, D. E., Leisen, J. C., Bluhm, G., Cooper, S. M., Duncan, H., Tuttleman, H., Heyse, S. P., Sharp, J. T., and Tilley, B. (1996). HLA-DRB1 genes and disease severity in rheumatoid arthritis. The MIRA trial group minocycline in rheumatoid arthritis. *Arthritis Rheum.* **39**, 1802–1807.

95. Snowden, N., Reynolds, I., Morgan, K., and Holt, L. (1997). T cell responses to human type II collagen in patients with rheumatoid arthritis and healthy controls. *Arthritis Rheum.* **40**, 1210–1218.

96. Jeng, K. C., Liu, M. T., Lan, J. L., and Peng, T. K. (1990). Collagen autoimmunity to rheumatoid arthritis. *Chung-hua Min Kuo Wei Shen Wu Chi Mien I Hsueh Tsa Chih* **23**, 239–247.

97. Neidhart, M., Hauser, N., Paulsson, M., DiCesare, P. E., Michel, B. A., and Häuselmann, H. J. (1997). Small fragments of cartilage oligomeric matrix protein in synovial fluid and serum as markers for cartilage degradation. *Br. J. Rheumatol.* **36**, 1151–1160.

98. Helbling, C., Marti, C., Seifert, B., Hauser, N., Caravatti, M., Michel, B. A., and Häuselmann, H. J. (1997). Cartilage oligomeric matrix protein: Signifikante Unterschiede im Serum bei RA-Patienten mit unterschiedlichem HLA-DRB1 allel status. *Schweiz. Med. Wochenschr.* **34** (Suppl. 90), 14S.

99. Albani, S., Carson, D. A., and Roudier, J. (1992). Genetic and environmental factors in the immune pathogenesis of rheumatoid arthritis. *Rheum. Dis. Clin. North Am.* **18**, 729–740.

100. David, C. S. (1990). Genes for MHC, TCR and Mls determine susceptibility to collagen-induced arthritis. *APMIS* **98**, 575–584.

101. Fugger, L., Rothbard, J. B., and Sonderstrup-McDevitt, G. (1996). Specificity of an HLA-DRB1 *0401-restricted T cell response to type II collagen. *Eur. J. Immunol.* **26**, 928–933.

102. Penzotti, J. E., Nepom, G. T., and Lybrand, T. P. (1997). Use of T cell receptor HLA DRB1*04 molecular modeling to predict site specific interactions for the DR shared epitope associated with rheumatoid arthritis. *Arthritis Rheum.* **40**, 1316–1326.

103. Wuorela, M., Jalkanen, S., Kirveskari, J., Laitio, P., and Granfors, K. (1997). *Yersinia enterocolica* serotype O:3 alters the expression of serologic HLA-B27 epitopes on human monocytes. *Infect. Immun.* **65**, 2060–2066.

104. Friede, T., Gnau, V., Jung, G., Keilholz, W., Stevanovic, S., and Rammensee, H. G. (1996). Natural ligand motif of closely related HLA-DR4 molecules predicts features of rheumatoid arthritis associated peptides. *Biochim. Biophys. Acta* **1316**, 85–101.

105. Signorelli, K. L., Watts, L. M., and Lambert, L. E. (1995). The importance of DR4Dw4 beta chain residues 70, 71, and 86 in peptide binding and T cell recognition. *Cell. Immunol.* **162**, 217–224.

106. Auger, I., and Roudier, J. (1997). A function for the QKRAA amino acid motif: Mediating binding of DNaJ to DNaK. Implication for the association of rheumatoid arthritis with HLA-DR4. *J. Clin. Invest.* **99**, 1818–1822.

107. Madden, D. R., Gorga, J. C., Strominger, J. L., and Wiley, D. C. (1991). The structure of HLA-B27 reveals nonamer self peptides bound in an extended conformation. *Nature* **353**, 321–325.

108. Liu, Z., Sun, Y. K., Xi, Y. P., Maffei, A., Reed, E., Harris, P., and

Suciu-Foca, N. (1993). Contribution of direct and indirect recognition pathways to T cell alloreactivity. *J. Exp. Med.* **177**, 1643–1650.

109. Roudier, J., Petersen, J., Rhodes, G. H., Luka, J., and Carson, D. A. (1989). Susceptibility to rheumatoid arthritis maps to a T cell epitope shared by the HLA-Dw4 DR beta 1 chain and the Epstein-Barr virus glycoprotein gp 110. *Proc. Natl. Acad. Sci. U.S.A.* **86**, 5104–5108.

110. LaCava, A., Nelson, J. L., Ollier, W. E. R., MacGregor, A., Keystone, E. C., Thorne, J. C., Scavulli, J. F., Berry C. C., Carson, D. A., and Albani, S. (1997). Genetic bias in immune responses to a cassette shared by different microorganisms in patients with rheumatoid arthritis. *J. Clin. Invest.* **100**, 658–663.

111. Fox, R. I., Luppi, M., Pisa, P., and Kang, H. I. (1992). Potential role of Epstein-Barr virus in Sjögren's syndrome and rheumatoid arthritis. *J. Rheumatol.* **32**, (Suppl.), 18–24.

112. Hirohata, S., Inoue, T., and Ito, K. (1992). Development of rheumatoid arthritis after chronic hepatitis caused by hepatitis C virus infection. *Intern. Med.* **31**, 493–495.

113. Harris, E. D., Jr. (1996). The rationale for combination therapy of rheumatoid arthritis based on pathophysiology. *J. Rheumatol.* **44** (Suppl.), 2–4.

114. Franz, J. K., Hummel, K. M., Lahrtz, F., Neidhart, M., Aicher, W. K., Gay, R. E., Fontana, A., and Gay, S. (1997). Rheumatoid synovial fibroblasts express interleukin 16—a potent chemoattractant factor for CD4+ T-cells. *Arthritis Rheum.* **40** (Suppl.), S197.

115. Petrow, P. K., Hummel, K. M., Franz, J. K., Kriegsmann, J., Prince, C., Gay, R. E., and Gay, S. (1997). Expression of osteopontin protein in the synovial membrane and cartilage-pannus junction in rheumatoid arthritis. Effects on the release of collagenase 1 from articular chondrocytes and synovial fibroblasts. *Arthritis Rheum.* **40** (Suppl.), S251.

116. Cornélis, F., Hardwick, I., Flipo, M., Martinez, M., Lasbleiz, S., Prud'Homme, J. F., Tran, T. H., Walsh, S., Delaye, A., Nicod, A., Loste, M. N., Lepage, V., Gibson, K., Pile, K., Djoulah S. *et al.* (1997). Association of rheumatoid arthritis with an amino acid allelic variation of the T cell receptor. *Arthritis Rheum.* **40**, 1387–1390.

117. Mu, I. I., Charmley, P., King, M. C., and Criswell, L. A. (1996). Synergy between T cell receptor β gene polymorphism and HLA-DR4 in susceptibility to rheumatoid arthritis. *Arthritis Rheum.* **39**, 931–937.

118. Theophilopoulos A. N. (1995). The basis of autoimmunity: Part II. Genetic predisposition. *Immunol. Today* **16**, 150–153.

119. Tan, F. K., Silvers, D. N., Foster, M. W., Chakraborty, R., Howard, R. F., Milewicz, D. M., and Arnett, F. C. (1997). Microsatellite markers flanking the fibrillin-1 gene on human chromosome 15q are associated with scleroderma in a native american population. *Arthritis Rheum.* **40** (Suppl.), S73.

120. Messer, G., Kick, G., Ranki, A., Koskimies, S., Reunala, T., and Meurer, M. (1994). Polymorphism of the tumor necrosis factor genes in patients with dermatitis herpetiformis. *Dermatology* **189** (Suppl. 1), 135–137.

121. Mulcahy, B., Waldron-Lynch, F., McDermott, M. F., Adams, C., Amos, C. I., Zhu, D. K., Ward, R. H., Clegg, D. O., Shanahan, F., Molloy, M. G., and O'Gara, F. (1996). Genetic variability in the tumor necrosis factor-lymphotoxin region influences susceptibility to rheumatoid arthritis. *Am. J. Hum. Genet.* **59**, 676–683.

122. Hajeer, A. H., Worthington, J., Silman, A. J., and Ollier, W. E. (1996). Association of tumor necrosis factor microsatellite polymorphisms with HLA-DRB1*04-bearing haplotypes in rheumatoid arthritis patients. *Arthritis Rheum.* **39**, 1109–1114.

123. Hajeer, A., John, S., Ollier, W. E., Silman, A. J., Dawes, P., Hassell, A., Mattey, D., Fryer, A., Strange, R., and Worthington, J. (1997). Tumor necrosis factor microsatellite haplotypes are different in male and female patients with RA. *J. Rheumatol.* **24**, 197–198.

124. Sullivan, K. E., Wooten, C., Schmeckpeper, B. J., Goldman, D., and Petri, M. A. (1997). A promoter polymorphism of tumor necrosis

factor alpha associated with systemic lupus erythematosus in African-Americans. *Arthritis Rheum.* **40**, 2207–2211.

125. Wilson, A. G., de Vries, N., Pociot, F., di Giovine, F. S., van de Putte, L. B. A., and Duff, G. W. (1993). An allelic polymorphism within the human tumor necrosis factor alpha promoter region is strongly associated with HLA-A1, B8 and DR3 alleles. *J. Exp. Med.* **177**, 577–580.

126. Criswell, L. A., Mu, H., Such, C. L., and KIang, M. C. (1997). Tumor necrosis factor microsatellite polymorphism is associated with long-term RA outcomes. *Arthritis Rheum.* **40** (Suppl.), S330.

127. Field, M., Gallagher, G., Ekdale, J., McGarry, F., Richards, S. D., Munro, R., Oh, H. H., and Campbell, C. (1997). Tumor necrosis factor locus polymorphisms in rheumatoid arthritis. *Tissue Antigens* **50**, 303–3077.

128. Hardwick, L. J., Walsh, S., Butcher, S., Nicod, A., Shatford, J., Bell, J., Lathrop, M., and Wordsworth, B. P. (1997). Genetic mapping of suscep-

tibility loci in the genes involved in rheumatoid arthritis. *J. Rheumatol.* **24**, 197–198.

129. Shiozawa, S., Hayashi, S., Tsukamoto, Y., Yasuda, N., Goko, H., Kawasaki, H., Wada, T., Shimizu, K., Takasugi, K., Tanaka, Y., Shiozawa, K., and Imura, S. (1997). Identification of the gene loci that predispose to rheumatoid arthritis. *Arthritis Rheum.* **40** (Suppl.), S329.

130. Cornélis, F., Fauré, S., Martinez, M., Prud'homme, J. F., Fritz, P., Dib, C., Alves, H., Barrera, P., de Vries, N., Balsa, A., Pascual-Salcido, D., Maenaut, K., and Westhoevens, R. (1997). Rheumatoid arthritis genome scan and putative autoimmune locus. *Arthritis Rheum.* **40** (Suppl.), S329.

131. John, S., Myerscough, A., Marlow, A., Hajeer, A., Silman, A., Ollier, W., and Worthington, J. (1997). Linkage of cytokine genes to rheumatoid arthritis. Evidence of genetic heterogeneity. *Arthritis Rheum.* **40** (Suppl.), S330.

CHAPTER 31

Body Fluid Markers of Cartilage Metabolism

EUGENE J.-M. A. THONAR   Departments of Biochemistry, Internal Medicine, and Orthopedic Surgery, Rush Medical College at Rush-Presbyterian-St. Luke's Medical Center, Chicago, Illinois 60612

MARY ELLEN LENZ   Department of Biochemistry, Rush Medical College at Rush-Presbyterian-St. Luke's Medical Center, Chicago, Illinois 60612

KOICHI MASUDA   Departments of Biochemistry and Orthopedic Surgery, Rush Medical College at Rush-Presbyterian-St. Luke's Medical Center, Chicago, Illinois 60612

DANIEL-HENRI MANICOURT   Laboratoire de Chimie Physiologique (Metabolic Research Group), Christian de Duve Institute of Cellular Pathology and Department of Rheumatology, Saint Luc University Hospital, University of Louvain in Brussels, 1200 Brussels, Belgium

I. ABSTRACT

The concept that levels of certain molecules, termed markers, in body fluids provide directly or indirectly a measure of anabolic and/or catabolic processes in cartilage is gaining popularity. *Direct* markers originate principally from cartilagenous structures and thus provide relatively specific information about alterations in cartilage matrix anabolism or catabolism. Marker molecules not derived principally from cartilage, but with the potential to influence the metabolism of the chondrocytes or the integrity of their matrix, qualify as *indirect* markers of cartilage metabolism. They include: (i) proteolytic enzymes and their inhibitors; (ii) growth factors; (iii) proinflammatory cytokines capable of mediating directly or indirectly the metabolism of the chondrocytes; and (iv) other molecules derived principally from noncartilagenous sources but whose concentrations in body fluids provide clues as to the state of health of cartilage. Because several of these molecules can influence the same metabolic process in cartilage, extreme caution should be exercised when attempting to relate their body fluid levels to the state of health of one or more cartilagenous structures in the body.

Many factors must be considered when selecting a body fluid for analysis. Joint fluid is preferred when the aim is to identify metabolic changes in articular cartilage within a single joint, whereas blood or urine is usually selected when

453

the goal is to identify changes occurring systemically. It is critical to use a well-characterized assay and to match study groups with respect to variables known to influence marker levels (e.g., age and sex, liver and kidney clearance, time and site of sampling, amount of load-bearing exercise, drugs, and intensity of inflammation).

II. INTRODUCTION

The 1990s have seen the emergence of assays capable of measuring molecules whose concentrations in body fluids (joint fluid, blood, or urine) provide information about specific metabolic processes occurring in cartilagenous tissues [1, 2]. The measurement of these "markers" of metabolic processes is enabling scientists and clinicians to address questions they had not been able to ask before. The quantification of such markers already has shed new light upon the etiology and pathogenesis of diseases affecting cartilage and has been useful in identifying among patients with osteoarthritis those most likely to exhibit rapid joint destruction [3, 4]. There also is emerging evidence that comparison of the levels of a specific marker in a body fluid before and after therapy can help assess the effects *in vivo* of various factors (growth factors, cytokines, drugs) and disease processes on a specific aspect of the metabolism of chondrocytes [1, 2]. Interestingly, some of these studies have helped demonstrate the need to exercise caution when extrapolating to the *in vivo* situation the results of *in vitro* studies of the effects of

cytokines, drugs, and physical forces on the chondrocytes and their extracellular matrix. A good example of this is the surprising observation that oral administration of piroxicam, a nonsteroidal anti-inflammatory drug with profound effects upon the metabolism of cartilage aggrecan *in vitro* [5], has no measurable effect on the serum level of antigenic keratan sulfate [6], a marker of one or more aspects of the metabolism of aggrecan *in vivo*.

In this review, markers of cartilage metabolism have been subdivided into two classes: direct and indirect markers. The direct markers all originate principally from the cartilagenous structures in which they are normally present. Some examples of commonly used direct markers are listed in Table I [7–44]. The indirect markers, on the other hand, are found in many tissues and are produced by many cell types (see Table II) [45–61]. In this brief report, we will discuss considerations that must be given when selecting markers for analysis. We will attempt to provide examples not only of their usefulness but also of their limitations.

III. SELECTION OF BODY FLUIDS FOR ANALYSIS

A. Joint Fluid

Joint fluid obtained either as undiluted synovial fluid or by lavage of a synovial joint offers a number of advantages when the goal is to identify changes or abnormalities in the

TABLE I.   Direct Markers of Cartilage Metabolism in Human Joint Fluid and Blood

Direct Marker[a]	Metabolic process measured[b]	Joint fluid (references)	Serum/Plasma (references)
Proteoglycans and related molecules			
Aggrecan core protein	Aggrecan degradation/synthesis	[7–9]	[10]
Aggrecan core protein (cleavage-induced neoepitopes)	Cleavage of the core protein of aggrecan at specific sites	[11, 12]	
Antigenic keratan sulfate	Aggrecan degradation/synthesis	[13–18]	[3, 13, 19–33]
Small nonaggregating PGs	Degradation of small proteoglycans (PGs)	[34]	
Chondroitin sulfate epitopes (3-B-3, 7-D-4, 846)	Synthesis of chondroitin sulfate chains with unusual structures	[16, 35–37]	[16, 38]
Chondroitin sulfate 6S/4S ratio	Degradation/synthesis of aggrecan molecules bearing chondroitin-6 or -4 sulfate chains	[39, 40]	
Collagen type II			
C-propeptide	Synthesis of collagen type II	[39, 41]	[42]
Fragments of α chain	Degradation of collagen type II	[43]	
Matrix proteins			
148 kDa protein	Degradation/turnover of the matrix of nonarticular cartilagenous tissues		[44]

Note. The list only provides examples; it is not meant to be a comprehensive review of published studies.

[a] Direct markers are defined as molecules or fragments thereof originating principally from cartilagenous structures.

[b] As outlined in this review, levels of direct markers can change following alterations in both degradation and synthesis.

TABLE II. Indirect Markers of Cartilage Metabolism in Human Joint Fluid and Blood

Indirect marker[a]	Metabolic process measured (relationship to cartilage integrity or metabolism)	Joint fluid (references)	Serum/Plasma (references)
Hyaluronan	Hypermetabolism of synovial and other connective tissue cells (a high serum level prognosticates rapid cartilage/joint destruction)		[3, 45, 46]
Cartilage oligomeric matrix protein	Degradation/synthesis of cartilage oligomeric matrix protein (a high serum level prognosticates rapid cartilage/joint destruction)	[47–49]	[50, 51]
Proteolytic enzymes and inhibitors			
Collagenase (MMP-1)	Synthesis and secretion of MMP-1	[9]	[30, 31, 52]
Stromelysin (MMP-3)	Synthesis and secretion of MMP-3	[9, 53]	[30, 31, 52, 54, 55]
TIMP-1	Synthesis and secretion of TIMP-1 (high ratios of MMP-1 and MMP-3 to TIMP-1 correlate with cartilage matrix degradation)	[9, 53]	[30, 31, 52, 54]
Proinflammatory cytokines			
Interleukin-1 and tumor necrosis factor-α	Synthesis and secretion of these proinflammatory cytokines (these cytokines promote cartilage matrix degradation and suppress cartilage matrix repair)	[56–60]	[27, 57, 59]
Interleukin-6	Synthesis and secretion of interleukin-6 (interleukin-6 promotes TIMP-1 synthesis and thus may help slow down cartilage matrix degradation)	[61]	[27, 61]
C-Reactive protein	Inflammation and/or tissue necrosis (elevated serum level prognosticates rapid cartilage/joint destruction in osteoarthritis)		[4]

Note. The list only provides examples; it is not meant to be a comprehensive review of published studies.

[a] Indirect markers are defined as molecules that do not originate principally from cartilagenous structures but that have the potential to influence the metabolism of the chondrocytes or the integrity of their matrix.

metabolism of articular cartilage. First, the concentration of a specific marker is usually higher in joint fluid than in other body fluids since the former lies in closer proximity to the articular surface [62]. It should be noted that the fact that most markers have much longer half-lives in joint fluid than in blood also contributes in part to this difference. Second, the level of a marker in joint fluid provides information about changes taking place in a single joint; levels of markers in blood or urine are often more difficult to put in perspective because these body fluids contain molecules/fragments derived from all cartilagenous tissues in the body [1]. Third, disease-related changes in marker levels are usually much greater in joint fluid than in other body fluids and thus are easier to assess. Such changes usually provide an amplified measure of altered metabolic processes occurring in articular cartilage within that joint. For example, the rapid but minor loss (less than 20%) of aggrecan from the articular surfaces of rabbit knees injected with a small amount of tumor necrosis factor-α is accompanied within twelve hours by a nearly 50-fold increase in the level of antigenic keratan sulfate in joint fluid [17]. Fourth, as markers can be further degraded in the joint or in the lymphatic system before they enter the blood circulation [62], joint fluid offers a much greater chance of identifying a high proportion of all fragments that have diffused out of the articular cartilage [2].

Analysis of joint fluid, however, offers some potential disadvantages when compared to analysis of blood or urine. First, joint fluid is much more difficult to obtain than blood or urine. Second, the concentration of the marker in synovial fluid depends on volume flux through the joint, which is not constant in disease [63, 64]. Because the volume of fluid may vary markedly with time, the concentration of a marker may not always give an accurate measure of the total amount of marker present. One way of circumventing this problem is to report the results of marker analyses as the ratio of one marker to another. Levick [64] has suggested that if the values for a marker in synovial fluid are to be reported as absolute concentrations, then the latter should be reexpressed after taking into consideration both the concentration of hyaluronan in the joint (to obtain a measure of available volume space) and fluid turnover. Lavage of the joint appears to help overcome this problem because it enables calculation of the total amount of marker present in the joint fluid [1, 62]. However, lavage may be inappropriate when it is performed repeatedly on the same joint; our own experience [E. J.-M. A. Thonar, unpublished data] suggests that lavage does affect the metabolic activities of chondrocytes in the joint studied. Finally, there remain some uncertainties as to the effect of inflammatory processes upon the kinetics of clearance of most cartilage markers from joint fluid. For example, certain investigators suggested that clearance from the joint might decrease when synovitis is present [65].

B. Blood

While a proportion of all marker molecules in a synovial joint may diffuse through capillary walls in the synovium and directly enter the blood circulation [64], most probably enter local lymph nodes where they can be further degraded and/or are altered (i.e. loss of antigenicity) before reentering the blood circulation via the thoracic duct. Hyaluronan, a marker of synovial proliferation with potential prognostic value in evaluating articular cartilage destruction (see below), is an exception; it goes through the lymphatic system relatively unscathed [66].

Markers in the blood circulation are eliminated via the liver and other organs of the reticuloendothelial system and/or by filtration though the kidney [62, 67]. The rate of clearance of cartilage-derived markers from the blood varies markedly from molecule to molecule. In the case of aggrecan-derived fragments, for example, the molecules that predominate in blood are small and have relatively long half-lives ($\approx$50 min) [68]. This probably reflects principally the fact that fragments of larger sizes bear more free terminal galactose residues on their carbohydrate side chains and are thus more rapidly cleared by liver cells bearing receptors for galactose [2]. There is some evidence that only the smallest aggrecan-related molecules are cleared by filtration through the basement membrane of the glomerulus [2, 68]. Given the complex nature of the clearance mechanisms, it is extraordinary that the level of a marker such as antigenic keratan sulfate is constant throughout the day and from week to week in normal human adults [1, 69]. This strongly suggests that the clearance pathways must be under close regulation.

In most cases, quantification of a cartilage-specific marker in serum or plasma provides a measure of the average metabolic activities taking place in all the cartilagenous tissues in the body rather than in a single joint [6, 67]. Because synovial joints contain no more than 20% of the total mass of cartilage in the body [70], an increase in the rate of loss of a marker molecule from the matrix of articular cartilage in a single synovial joint is unlikely to cause the blood level of that marker to rise, unless the joint is large and the loss is both pronounced and rapid [6, 71]. Measurements of markers in serum or plasma thus are most useful for identifying changes taking place systemically and involving all or most cartilagenous structures [72] (see also Thonar *et al.* [1, 2, 6, 67] for reviews on the subject). They can be used for monitoring responses of cartilage to drugs, growth factors, cytokines, and other agents or factors that circulate in the bloodstream and, from there, are able to reach the chondrocytes in all cartilagenous structures [6]. A major advantage of serum/plasma is that it is easy to obtain. In addition, its volume is relatively constant and it is independent of local joint volume flux [63].

A significant disadvantage is that some of the markers are present in normal serum or plasma at concentrations below the limit of detection of the assays available for quantification.

C. Urine

Because urine is a filtrate of blood, the level of a cartilage-derived marker in this body fluid also reflects the average of what is taking place in all the cartilagenous tissues in the body. As most peptides and peptidoglycans do not readily go through the negatively-charged basement membrane of the kidney, this body fluid does not contain as broad a spectrum of marker molecules as blood [2]. While urine is easy to obtain, the cartilage-derived markers are usually present in it at concentrations too low to measure. In some cases (e.g., keratan sulfate), the marker is present but in a modified form that is poorly recognized by the antibody used in the immunoassay.

Unlike most other markers of connective tissue metabolism, the pyridinium cross-links of collagen reach much higher levels in urine than in other body fluids [73, 74]. While analysis of these cross-links in urine is most commonly used to assess the rate of bone turnover, measurement of hydroxylysylpyridinoline, the pyridinium cross-link normally present in cartilage, has proved useful in detecting changes in the metabolism of cartilage in some animal studies [75]. However, as this is the major pyridinium cross-link found in many other connective tissues including bone, its potential as a direct marker of cartilage metabolism is somewhat limited.

IV. SELECTION OF MARKERS AND INTERPRETATION OF THE RESULTS OF ANALYSES

The cartilagenous tissues of normal human adults exhibit steady-state metabolism; i.e., each molecule that is proteolytically degraded during normal turnover is replaced by a new one. In these normal individuals, the level of a direct marker of cartilage metabolism in a body fluid thus provides a measure of the average rate of turnover of the parent molecules in the cartilage matrix within a joint (joint fluid) or in the body (blood and urine). In normal human adults, the markers appearing in body fluids are derived principally from (i) the turnover of the cell-associated matrix that surrounds each cell (or a group of cells in a chondron) (Fig. 1) [76] and (ii) the degradation of newly synthesized molecules as they are released extracellularly (77). Studies have suggested that aggrecan molecules in the more abundant interterritorial matrix compartment further removed from the cells have very long half-lives and thus contribute much less to the appearance of aggrecan fragments in body fluids [77, 78]. It is likely that most macromolecules in the extracellular matrix of normal adult cartilage exhibit similar compartment-related differences in their rates of turnover. Because the two

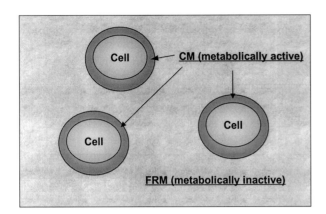

FIGURE 1   The two major compartments of the adult cartilage matrix are shown schematically. Each chondrocyte is surrounded by a thin rim of cell-associated matrix (CM), the metabolically active compartment of the matrix. In normal adult human articular cartilage, the chondrocytes and their CM occupy only approximately 5% of the total volume of the tissue [76]. The interterritorial matrix further removed from the cells (FRM) is thought to represent a compartment in which matrix macromolecules turn over much more slowly than in the cell-associated matrix [76].

compartments have different compositions, it is tempting to postulate that measurements of the concentrations of one or more markers predominating in the further removed matrix may help identify degradative changes occurring in this normally metabolically-inactive compartment in disease.

When the state of homeostasis is lost, as occurs in most disease states, the respective contributions of *catabolic* and *anabolic/repair* processes to the level of a specific direct marker are much more difficult to assess. At least one of the markers, e.g., the C-propeptide of the type II procollagen molecule, appears to provide a measure of the biosynthetic or repair processes since it is produced only by cleavage of the procollagen molecule as the latter is released into the extracellular matrix [39, 79–81]. This assumes, of course, that the majority of these propeptide molecules diffuse out of the matrix relatively rapidly after they are produced and do not accumulate with time in the matrix.

The significance of a high or low body fluid level of a marker is clearly not always easy to interpret. Because most direct markers of cartilage metabolism are products of the degradation of matrix molecules, most investigators consider that they provide a measure of degradative processes in cartilagenous tissues [2]. This interpretation is only valid, however, when cartilage matrix metabolism is at steady state and the rate of synthesis of a molecule is in balance with its rate of degradation. It is worth noting that under these conditions, the level of the degradation product also provides a measure of the rate of synthesis of the molecule from which this fragment is derived. When anabolic and catabolic processes are no longer in balance, such as during matrix repair, alterations in the rate of synthesis of the marker may actually become the major factor responsible for changes in marker levels. This contention is based on an observation that proteolytic

degradation of aggrecan molecules occurs predominantly in the rapidly turning over cell-associated matrix, close to the chondrocyte membrane. Aggrecan molecules that escape unharmed and reach the interterritorial areas further removed from the cells are degraded at a much slower rate [77, 78]. It is logical to assume, therefore, that the total number of aggrecan-derived fragments entering the body fluids will rise if the rate of synthesis of aggrecan increases (Fig. 2). It follows that the number of aggrecan-derived fragments entering the body fluids is likely to decrease markedly if one shuts down aggrecan synthesis.

Because most of the direct markers can be influenced by alterations in the rates of matrix degradation as well as synthesis/repair, extreme caution should be exercised when interpreting the results of marker measurements. This is particularly true for disease states involving loss of cartilage matrix homeostasis. It usually is more appropriate to interpret an abnormally high level of a direct marker as evidence of an alteration in the metabolism of the parent molecule in cartilage rather than an increase in its rate of degradation in the matrix. While the concern is sometimes raised that a change in the level of a serum marker may simply reflect a change in the rate of clearance of the marker from joint fluid and/or blood, there is no strong evidence at this time that this is a major influencing factor, especially if special care is taken to only study individuals with normal liver and kidney functions [31].

V. DIRECT VERSUS INDIRECT MARKERS

A. Direct Markers

Table I provides examples of direct markers of one or more aspects of the metabolism of different macromolecules in human cartilage. These markers are relatively easy to measure in human joint fluid (with the exception of the assay for the 148 kDa protein since it is not present in articular cartilage [82, 83]) but most can also be measured in serum or plasma. It is worth noting that several, if not most, of the direct markers listed in Table I can be quantified in the body fluids of several animal species.

B. Indirect Markers

Several types of molecules not derived principally from cartilage, but with the potential to influence the metabolism of the chondrocytes or the integrity of their matrix, qualify as indirect markers of cartilage metabolism. They include: (i) proteolytic enzymes (e.g., metalloproteinases [MMPs], "aggrecanase," etc.) capable of degrading one or more molecules in the matrix, and their inhibitors, such as tissue inhibitors of MMPs (TIMPs) [9, 31, 84–88]; (ii) growth factors (e.g., insulin-like growth factor-1) that can stimulate biosynthetic

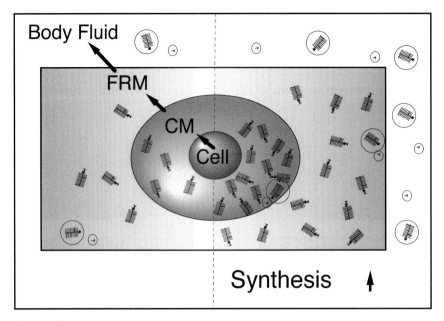

FIGURE 2 The effect of an increase in the rate of aggrecan synthesis on the level of keratan sulfate-bearing fragments of aggrecan in body fluids is shown schematically. Proteolytic degradation of aggrecan molecules occurs predominantly in the cell-associated matrix (CM) close to the chondrocyte membrane [77]. Keratan sulfate-bearing fragments of large size (large circles) that have lost their hyaluronan-binding region (small circles) rapidly diffuse out of the CM and, after a short time in the further-removed matrix (FRM), reach the body fluids. The scheme shows that the number of aggrecan-derived fragments appearing in body fluids rises measurably if the rate of aggrecan synthesis increases. In this example, the proportion of newly synthesized aggrecan molecules that are degraded remains constant, as one would expect to happen in the absence of an upregulation of the synthesis or activation of proteolytic enzymes.

processes [89, 90]; (iii) proinflammatory cytokines (e.g., interleukin-1, interleukin-6, tumor necrosis factor-α, etc.) capable of mediating directly or indirectly the metabolism of the chondrocytes [17, 27, 91, 92]; and (iv) other molecules, such as hyaluronan [3] and C-reactive protein [4], that originate principally from noncartilage sources and whose concentrations in body fluids provide clues as to the state of health of cartilage. As several of these molecules can mediate, directly or indirectly, the same metabolic process in chondrocytes, extreme caution should be exercised when attempting to relate their body fluid levels to the state of health of cartilagenous structures in a joint or in the body. The same caution should be applied when interpreting the results of the quantification of a proteolytic enzyme by an assay that can not distinguish between active and latent forms of the molecule.

VI. CHARACTERIZATION OF MARKER ASSAYS

ELISAs offer great sensitivity, are rapid, and, unlike radioimmunoassays, require little specialized equipment [2]. The fact that different studies of the same marker sometimes use different immunoassays, or at least different antibodies, makes comparisons among studies difficult. The lack of well-defined kits that can be used by all to quantify the various markers has therefore been a major hurdle to progress. Indirect inhibition ELISAs are popular because they require only minute amounts of a single specific antibody against an epitope on the marker of interest. An important advantage of this type of ELISA is its ability to detect the total number of epitopes present in a solution [2]. By comparison, sandwich ELISAs usually are more sensitive and yield binding curves that are linear over a much wider range of dilutions. However, they are more difficult to set up, and the results are sometimes more difficult to interpret because they can detect only marker molecules bearing at least two antigenic sites.

The development of an ELISA often takes a long time because it needs to be optimized with respect to precision (i.e., how reproducible is the measurement?), accuracy (i.e., is the amount of epitope detected a good measure of the molecule one is trying to quantify and does this change with age or in disease?), and sensitivity [93]. Some information about the intra- and interassay variation always should be provided. It is important to ascertain that the epitope detected is not hidden via interaction with other molecules present in the solution to be analyzed or denatured during freezing and thawing [67]. High-affinity antibodies usually are needed to gain the sensitivity required and to obtain sharp binding or inhibition curves that allow distinction between two similar concentrations [6]. Another possible problem, which applies for example to antibodies directed against antigenic keratan sulfate, is that not all monoclonal antibodies directed against the same epitope bind to it with equal affinity when the latter is present in the fluid phase on molecules/fragments of different sizes [6, 67, 94]. This creates a problem when it is important to detect all fragments bearing the epitope. Thus, antibodies that bind with greater affinities to molecules/fragments of larger size often are less suitable for the quantification of the smaller fragments present in blood and urine than of the larger fragments present in joint fluid. Researchers who modify a well-characterized immunoassay by replacing the well-defined specific antibody by one whose specificity, affinity, and other characteristics have not been as fully defined should be critical when assessing their results and comparing them to those generated by the better-characterized assay [1].

Other techniques also have proved useful to quantify certain markers. For example, high performance liquid chromatography methods have been shown to be very effective in quantifying with great sensitivity and precision some markers, such as the disaccharide repeating units of glycosaminoglycans [95, 96] and the hydroxylylpyridinoline cross-link of collagen [75, 97–99].

VII. INFLUENCE OF VARIOUS FACTORS AND PROCESSES ON MARKER LEVELS

The level of a marker of cartilage metabolism depends on the action of complex biochemical and biomechanical processes on the chondrocytes and the matrix. Some of the marker studies published have suggested that the metabolism of chondrocytes is highly regulated and not as readily altered *in vivo* as one may have anticipated based upon the results of some *in vitro* studies of the response of chondrocytes or cartilage explants in culture to stimulatory factors and/or mechanical stresses. This notwithstanding, a few factors previously shown capable of causing profound alterations in the metabolism of chondrocytes appear to be as effective in doing so *in vivo*. For example, a single dose of prednisolone, given orally or intraarticularly, causes a long lasting drop in the serum level of antigenic keratan sulfate [6] and probably of other markers as well.

Several of the marker studies have indicated the need to pay special attention to the selection of study designs and protocols designed to assess metabolic changes in patient populations. It is worth noting that conditions that may be critical when measuring a marker in serum or plasma may not necessarily be as important to control for when analyzing joint fluids. For example, because patients with liver or kidney disease may exhibit an altered rate of marker clearance from the blood, they should be excluded from studies of serum or plasma markers [31]. On the other hand, this is not as

significant a concern when one measures the level of a marker in joint fluid. It also should be noted that a parameter that has been documented to be critical for a specific marker might not necessarily be as important in the case of other markers.

Specific factors and metabolic processes that potentially can influence the levels of markers in body fluids are too numerous to list here. Their effects may not be as pronounced in the case of all markers and all body fluids analyzed. The following are particularly worth taking into consideration when measuring marker levels.

A. Hepatic or Renal Disease

Because the liver and kidney both contribute significantly to the normal clearance of marker molecules from the blood circulation [1], it is essential to exclude individuals with (i) abnormal findings on serum liver function tests and (ii) creatinine clearance rates ≤90 ml/minute [31] when measuring markers in serum, plasma, or urine. This, of course, is not an essential requirement in the case of analyses of joint fluids. The potential importance of the liver in the clearance of markers from the blood circulation is best exemplified by the observation that individuals with cirrhosis of the liver have abnormally high serum levels of hyaluronan [100]. This marker molecule normally has a very short half-life in the blood circulation (<3 minutes); its major mode of disappearance from this body fluid is thought to occur through binding to high-affinity receptors on liver cells [66].

B. Age and Sex

The body fluid levels of most markers of cartilage metabolism undergo tremendous changes during development and maturation, usually dropping at or near the time of epiphyseal plate closure [93]. These maturation-related changes reflect not only alterations in the metabolism of the chondrocytes but potentially also modifications to the structure/antigenic profile of the marker molecules themselves [94]. These changes may continue to develop, although much more slowly, as a consequence of normal aging. Consequently, all studies of patient populations should include a control population of age-matched individuals without disease affecting cartilage. Matching for sex also is recommended because some markers may show sex-related differences that may be more apparent at some ages (i.e. menopause) than at others [28].

C. Time of Sampling

The concentration of hyaluronan in serum undergoes a marked transient elevation after rising from bed and mobilization [100], reflecting the movement of this molecule out of the tissues and joint fluids in which they had accumulated during the night. Although there is no clear evidence at this time that this also occurs in the case of other markers, sampling of joint fluid and blood should not be performed until individuals (or animals) have been ambulatory for at least two hours. Because some markers have much longer half-lives in blood than hyaluronan, this waiting period may not be long enough for all markers. Studies of serum hyaluronan and antigenic keratan sulfate have suggested that diurnal variation in marker levels is relatively minimal over the remainder of the day [69, 100]; this, however, needs to be confirmed for other markers. Other potential contributors to fluctuations in marker levels with time include seasonal variation and menstruation. Their potential contributions are likely to vary from marker to marker and among species. For example, the very dramatic seasonal variation in the serum level of antigenic keratan sulfate observed in deer [101] does not occur in humans [E. J.-M. A. Thonar, unpublished observations]. In the case of measurement of pyridinium cross-links in urine, it is recommended that the first daily urine sample be discarded and that the levels be expressed relative to the concentration of creatinine [97].

D. Site of Blood Sampling

While investigators always note which knee they draw fluid from, most appear to have been under the impression that it is not important to be as critical when selecting the site of blood sampling. The results of a study of rabbits injected in one knee joint with a small amount of active chymopapain have shown that antigenic keratan sulfate and hyaluronan reach much higher concentrations in the popliteal vein draining the injected knee than in the one draining the noninjected knee [66]. When drawing blood from the cubital vein of patients with joint disease, it probably is worth noting, therefore, whether any of the joints in the hand or elbow drained by tributaries of that vein exhibit clinical signs of disease. In addition, if blood is to be drawn on multiple occasions from the same patient, it appears wise to select the same vein for sampling at all times.

E. Load-Bearing and Exercise

While cyclic loading of articular cartilage *in vitro* has a rapid and marked effect on the metabolism of chondrocytes, especially aggrecan synthesis [102], there is as yet no clear evidence that chondrocytes are as responsive to cyclic loading *in vivo*. Indeed, rigorous exercise, e.g., running a marathon [25], does not cause the serum level of antigenic keratan sulfate to change measurably in well-trained athletes. On the other hand, playing a soccer game [32] can cause markers such as antigenic keratan sulfate, TIMP-1, and procollagen II C-propeptide to rise modestly, although not significantly, in

joint fluid and, in the case of antigenic keratan sulfate, also in serum.

Patients confined to bed should not be included in study protocols because markers of articular cartilage metabolism accumulate in joint fluid during a night of bed rest; mobilization is required to pump these out of the joint. Mobilization also is needed to maintain the content of aggrecan in articular cartilage at a high level [103]. In this regard, it is worth noting that immobilization in bed, when sustained for several weeks, is accompanied by a slow progressive decrease in the serum level of antigenic keratan sulfate [104].

F. Inflammation

Clinical studies are beginning to provide evidence that products of inflammatory processes have negative effects on the state of health of cartilage in joint disease [105]. These effects contribute to the joint destruction not only in inflammatory joint diseases such as rheumatoid arthritis, but also in osteoarthritis, a condition in which inflammatory processes are much less active.

Marker studies have suggested that circulating proinflammatory cytokines (i.e., interleukin-1 and tumor necrosis factor-α) may be responsible, at least in part, for mediation of the chondrocytes' responses in these joint diseases (Fig. 3). These two cytokines have been shown to have profound influences on the metabolism of adult human articular chondrocytes *in vitro*; at low concentrations, they inhibit the synthesis of aggrecan and collagen type II, while at higher concentrations they also stimulate the cells to release proteolytic enzymes capable of degrading many matrix constituents [92]. Several marker studies have suggested that these cytokines, and possibly others, also exert those influences *in vivo*. In rheumatoid arthritis, for example, the serum level of tumor necrosis factor-α shows a strong positive correlation with the serum level of hyaluronan but a negative correlation with the serum level of keratan sulfate [27]. The positive correlation between serum levels of tumor necrosis factor-α and interleukin-1, on the one hand, and the serum level of hyaluronan, on the other [27], is not surprising given the ability of these cytokines to stimulate hyaluronan synthesis by synovial cells *in vitro* [106]. The negative relationship between the levels of these cytokines and antigenic keratan sulfate is interesting because it suggests that one or more of these mediators are capable of inhibiting aggrecan synthesis *in vivo*, as they do *in vitro* [76, 92]. If the cytokines had stimulated aggrecan degradation via chondrocytic chondrolysis, one would have expected the cytokines to cause a rise in the serum level of antigenic keratan sulfate. In retrospect, this is not surprising because studies have demonstrated that at the doses they are found in joint fluid from patients with osteoarthritis and rheumatoid arthritis, interleukin-1 and tumor necrosis factor-α are much more likely to inhibit matrix

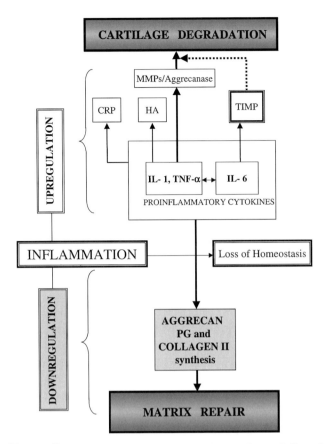

FIGURE 3 Effects of proinflammatory cytokines on the metabolism of chondrocytes and the state of cartilage matrix homeostasis. Proinflammatory cytokines appearing in body fluids in inflammation are thought to play a pivotal role in the loss of cartilage matrix homeostasis in joint diseases. Interleukin-1 (IL-1) and tumor necrosis factor-α (TNF-α) produced in inflammation are most effective in downregulating aggrecan and type II collagen synthesis [76, 92] and thus probably contribute significantly to the downregulation of cartilage matrix repair. At higher concentrations, these cytokines promote cartilage matrix degradation by upregulating the expression of proteolytic enzymes by chondrocytes and other connective tissue cells within affected joints [92]. These circulating cytokines also upregulate the synthesis of hyaluronan (HA) and C-reactive protein (CRP) by different tissues, possibly explaining why these two indirect markers prognosticate rapid joint destruction when present in serum in elevated amounts [3, 4]. The diagram also illustrates the complexity of the effects of inflammatory processes on the state of homeostasis in cartilage by showing that interleukin-6 (IL-6), produced in inflammation, may counteract some of these deleterious effects by promoting the synthesis of tissue inhibitor of metalloproteinases (TIMP), a major inhibitor of metalloproteinases (MMPs) and aggrecanase actions in the matrix.

formation or repair than to promote degradative processes [17, 27, 92].

Other marker studies have added further support for the contention that inflammatory processes have deleterious effects on cartilage matrix metabolism by showing that moderately elevated serum levels of either C-reactive protein [4] or hyaluronan [3] prognosticate rapid articular cartilage destruction in osteoarthritic joints. These results strongly suggest that investigators intent on measuring body fluid levels of markers of cartilage and/or joint metabolism in disease should also consider measuring one or, preferably, several markers of inflammatory processes.

VIII. CONCLUSIONS

The next few years will likely continue to offer a great challenge to investigators and clinicians interested in shedding more light on the potential usefulness of measuring body fluid markers of specific metabolic processes in cartilage. Progress has been limited in part because the significance of an abnormally high or low marker level often is difficult to interpret. In spite of this limitation, research has already led to important breakthroughs, such as the identification of serum hyaluronan, cartilage oligomeric matrix protein, and C-reactive protein as markers with prognostic value when assessing the rate of articular cartilage destruction in patients with osteoarthritis. Interest in the field of markers of cartilage metabolism is likely to gain momentum when more investigators enter the field and when the markers they develop begin to be used in the clinical setting.

Acknowledgments

The preparation of this manuscript was supported in part by grants AR39239 and AG04736 from the National Institutes of Health (U.S.A.), by the FDS of the UCL, the Greater Chicago Area Chapter of the Arthritis Foundation, the Fund for Medical Scientific Research (Belgium) (Grants 3.4547.95 and 3.4597.98), and the Arthritis and Orthopedics Institute at Rush-Presbyterian-St. Luke's Medical Center.

References

1. Thonar, E. J.-M. A., Shinmei, M., and Lohmander, L. S. (1993). Body fluid markers of cartilage changes in osteoarthritis. *In* "Rheumatic Disease Clinics of North America. Osteoarthritis" (R. W. Moskowitz, ed.), Vol. 19, No. 3, pp. 635–657. Saunders, Philadelphia.

2. Thonar, E. J.-M. A., Kuettner, K. E., and Williams, J. M. (1994). Markers of articular cartilage injury and healing. *In* "Sports Medicine and Arthroscopy Review: Chondral Injuries" (J. T. Andrish, ed.), Vol. 2, pp. 13–28. Raven Press, New York.

3. Sharif, M., George, E., Shepstone, L., Knudson, W., Thonar, E. J.-M. A., Cushnaghan, J., and Dieppe, P. (1995). Serum hyaluronic acid level as a predictor of disease progression in osteoarthritis of the knee. *Arthritis Rheum.* **38**, 760–767.

4. Spector, T. D., Hart, D. J., Nandra, D., Doyle, D. V., Mackillop, N., Gallimore, J. R., and Pepys, M. B. (1997). Low-level increases in serum C-reactive protein are present in early osteoarthritis of the knee and predict progressive disease. *Arthritis Rheum.* **40**, 723–727.

5. Bulstra, S. K., Kuijer, R., Buurman, W. A., Terwindt-Rouwenhorst, E., Guelen, P. J., and van der Linden, A. J. (1992). The effect of piroxicam on the metabolism of isolated human chondrocytes. *Clin. Orthop. Relat. Res.* **277**, 289–296.

6. Thonar, E. J.-M. A., Manicourt, D.-H., Williams, J. M., Fukuda, K., Campion, G. V., Sweet, M. B. E., Lenz, M. E., Schnitzer, T. J., and

Kuettner, K. E. (1992). Serum keratan sulfate: A measure of cartilage proteoglycan metabolism. *In* "Articular Cartilage and Osteoarthritis" (K. E. Kuettner, R. Schleyerbach, J. G. Peyron, and V. C. Hascall, eds.), pp. 429–445. Raven Press, New York.

7. Lohmander, L. S., Dahlberg, L., Ryd, L., and Heinegård, D. (1989). Increased levels of proteoglycan fragments in knee joint fluid after joint injury. *Arthritis Rheum.* **32**, 1434–1442.

8. Sandy, J. D., Flannery, C. R., Neame, P. J., and Lohmander, L. S. (1992). The structure of aggrecan fragments in human synovial fluid. Evidence for the involvement in osteoarthritis of a novel proteinase which cleaves the GLU 373-ALA 374 bond of the interglobular domain. *J. Clin. Invest.* **89**, 1512–1516.

9. Lohmander, L. S., Hoerrner, L. A., and Lark, M. W. (1993). Metalloproteinases, tissue inhibitor and proteoglycan fragments in knee synovial fluid in human osteoarthritis. *Arthritis Rheum.* **36**, 181–189.

10. Saxne, T., Hayford, J., Heinegård, D., Lenz, M. E., Thonar, E. J.-M. A., Wollheim, F. A., and Pachman, L. (1989). Serum levels of the proteoglycan core protein and keratan sulfate correlate in juvenile rheumatoid arthritis. *Arthritis Rheum.* **32** (Suppl.), S105 (abstr.).

11. Lohmander, L. S., Neame, P., and Sandy, J. D. (1993). The structure of aggrecan fragments in human synovial fluid: Evidence that aggrecanase mediates cartilage degradation in inflammatory joint disease, joint injury and osteoarthritis. *Arthritis Rheum.* **36**, 1214–1222.

12. Lark, M. W., Bayne, E. K., and Lohmander, L. S. (1995). Aggrecan degradation in osteoarthritis and rheumatoid arthritis. *Acta Orthop. Scand.* **66** (Suppl. 266), 92–97.

13. Campion, G. V., McCrae, F., Schnitzer, T. J., Lenz, M. E., Dieppe, P. A., and Thonar, E. J.-M. A. (1991). Levels of keratan sulfate in the serum and synovial fluid of patients with osteoarthritis of the knee. *Arthritis Rheum.* **34**, 1254–1259.

14. Carroll, G. J., Bell, M. C., Laing, B. A., McCapppin, S., Blumer, C., and Leslie, A. (1992). Reduction of the concentration and total amount of keratan sulphate in synovial fluid from patients with osteoarthritis during treatment with piroxicam. *Ann. Rheum. Dis.* **51**, 850–854.

15. Ongchi, D. R., Thonar, E. J.-M. A., Johnson, C., Williams, J. M., Bach, B., and Schnitzer, T. J. (1992). Keratan sulfate content of synovial fluid after knee injury. *In* "Articular Cartilage and Osteoarthritis" (K. E. Kuettner, R. Schleyerbach, J. G. Peyron, and V. C. Hascall, eds.), pp. 734–735. Raven Press, New York.

16. Poole, A. R., Ionescu, M., Swan, A., and Dieppe, P. A. (1994). Changes in cartilage metabolism in arthritis are reflected by altered serum and synovial fluid levels of the cartilage proteoglycan aggrecan—implications for pathogenesis. *J. Clin. Invest.* **94**, 25–33.

17. Paris, M. M., Friedland, I. R., Ehrett, S., Hickey, S. M., Olsen, K. D., Hansen, E., Thonar, E. J.-M. A., and McCracken, G. H., Jr. (1995). Effect of interleukin-1 receptor antagonist and soluble tumor necrosis factor receptor in animal models of infection. *J. Infect. Dis.* **171**, 161–169.

18. Cameron, M., Buchgraber, A., Passler, H., Vogt, M., Thonar, E. J.-M. A., Fu, F., and Evans, C. (1997). The natural history of the ACL deficient knee: Changes in synovial fluid cytokine and keratan sulfate concentrations. *Am. J. Sports Med.* **25**, 751–754.

19. Thonar, E. J.-M. A., Lenz, M. E., Klintworth, G. K., Caterson, B., Pachman, L. M., Glickman, P., Katz, R., Huff, J., and Kuettner, K. E. (1985). Quantification of keratan sulfate in blood as a marker of cartilage catabolism. *Arthritis Rheum.* **28**, 1367–1376.

20. Thonar, E. J.-M. A., Meyer, R. F., Dennis, R. F., Lenz, M. E., Maldonado, B., Hassell, J. R., Hewitt, A. T., Stark, W. J., Stock, E. L., Kuettner, K. E., and Klintworth, G. K. (1986). Absence of normal keratan sulfate in the blood of patients with macular corneal dystrophy. *Am. J. Ophthalmol.* **102**, 561–569.

21. Kliner, D. J., Gorski, J. P., and Thonar, E. J.-M. A. (1987). Keratan sulfate levels in sera of patients bearing cartilage tumors. *Cancer* **59**, 1931–1935.

22. Sweet, M. B. E., Coelho, A., Schnitzer, C. M., Schnitzer, T. J., Lenz, M. E., Jakim, I., Kuettner, K. E., and Thonar, E. J.-M. A. (1988).

Serum keratan sulfate levels in osteoarthritis patients. *Arthritis Rheum.* **31**, 648–652.

23. Campion, G. V., McCrae, F., Schnitzer, T. J., Lenz, M. E., Dieppe, P. A., and Thonar, E. J.-M. A. (1991). Levels of keratan sulfate in the serum and synovial fluid of patients with osteoarthritis of the knee. *Arthritis Rheum.* **34**, 1254–1259.

24. Mehraban, F., Finegan, C. K., and Moskowitz, R. W. (1991). Serum keratan sulfate—quantitative and qualitative comparisons in inflammatory versus noninflammatory arthritides. *Arthritis Rheum.* **34**, 383–392.

25. Sweet, M. B. E., Jakim, I., Coelho, A., Becker, P. J., and Thonar, E. J.-M. A. (1992). Serum keratan sulfate levels in marathon runners. *Int. J. Sports Med.* **13**, 348–350.

26. Spector, T. D., Woodward, L., Hall, G. M., Hammond, A., Williams, A., Butler, M. G., James, I. T., Hart, D. J., Thompson, P. W., and Scott, D. L. (1992). Keratan sulphate in rheumatoid arthritis, osteoarthritis, and inflammatory diseases. *Ann. Rheum. Dis.* **51**, 1134–1137.

27. Manicourt, D. H., Triki, R., Fukuda, K., Devogelaer, J.-P., Nagant de Deuxchaisnes, C., and Thonar, E. J.-M. A. (1993). Levels of circulating tumor necrosis factor alpha and interleukin-6 in patients with rheumatoid arthritis: Relationship to serum levels of hyaluronan and antigenic keratan sulfate. *Arthritis Rheum.* **36**, 490–499.

28. Lohmander, L. S., and Thonar, E. J.-M. A. (1994). Serum keratan sulfate concentrations are different in primary and posttraumatic osteoarthrosis of the knee. *Orthop. Res. Soc. Trans.* **19**, 459 (abstr.).

29. Haraoui, B., Thonar, E. J.-M. A., Martel-Pelletier, J., Goulet, J.-R., Raynauld, J.-P., Ouellet, M., and Pelletier, J.-P. (1994). Serum keratan sulfate levels in rheumatoid arthritis: Inverse correlation with radiographic staging. *J. Rheumatol.* **21**, 813–817.

30. Manicourt, D.-H., Fujimoto, N., Obata, K., and Thonar, E. J.-M. A. (1994). Serum levels of collagenase, stromelysin-1, and TIMP-1: Age- and sex-related differences in normal subjects and relationship to the extent of joint involvement and serum levels of antigenic keratan sulfate in patients with osteoarthritis. *Arthritis Rheum.* **37**, 1774–1783.

31. Manicourt, D.-H., Fujimoto, N., Obata, K., and Thonar, E. J.-M. A. (1995). Levels of circulating collagenase, stromelysin-1, and tissue inhibitor of matrix metalloproteinases I in patients with rheumatoid arthritis: Relationship to serum levels of antigenic keratan sulfate and systemic parameters of inflammation. *Arthritis Rheum.* **38**, 1031–1039.

32. Roos, H., Dahlberg, L., Hoerrner, L. A., Lark, M. W., Thonar, E. J.-M. A., Shinmei, M., Lindqvist, U., and Lohmander, L. S. (1995). Markers of cartilage matrix metabolism in human joint fluid and serum: The effect of exercise. *Osteoarthritis Cartilage* **3**, 7–14.

33. Vaitainen, U., Lohmander, L. S., Thonar, E. J.-M. A., Hongisto, T., Ägren, U., Ronkko, S., Jaroma, H., Kosma, V.-M., Tammi, M., and Kiviranta, I. (1998). Markers of cartilage matrix metabolism in synovial fluid and serum of patients with chondromalacia of the patella. *Osteoarthritis Cartilage* **6**, 115–128.

34. Witsch-Prehm, P., Miehlke, R., and Kresse, H. (1992). Presence of small proteoglycan fragments in normal and arthritic human cartilage. *Arthritis Rheum.* **35**, 1042–1052.

35. Hazell, P. K., Dent, C., Fairclough, J. A., Bayliss, M. T., and Hardingham, T. E. (1995). Changes in glycosaminoglycan epitope levels in knee joint fluid following injury. *Arthritis Rheum.* **38**, 953–959.

36. Slater, Jr., R. R., Bayliss, M. T., Lachiewicz, P. F., Visco, D. M., and Caterson, B. (1995). Monoclonal antibodies that detect biochemical markers of arthritis in human. *Arthritis Rheum.* **38**, 655–659.

37. Lohmander, L. S., Ionescu, M., and Poole, A. R. (1995). Changes in aggrecan structures and metabolism after knee injury and in osteoarthritis. *Trans. Orthop. Res. Soc.* **20**, 412 (abstr.).

38. Mansson, B., Carey, D., Alini, M., Ionescu, M., Rosenberg, L. C., Poole, A. R., Heinegård, D., and Saxne, T. (1995). Cartilage and bone metabolism in rheumatoid arthritis. Differences between rapid and slow progression of disease identified by serum markers of cartilage metabolism. *J. Clin. Invest.* **95**, 1071–1077.

39. Shinmei, M., Inamori, Y., Yoshiwara, Y., Kikuchi, T., Hayakawa, T., and Shimomura, Y. (1991). Molecular markers of joint disease:

Significance of the level of type II collagen C-propeptide, chondroitin sulfate and TIMP in joint fluid. *Trans. Annu. Meet. Jpn. Orthop. Soc.*, abstr., p. 443.

40. Shinmei, M., Miyauchi, S., Machida, A., and Miyazaki, K. (1992). Quantitation of chondroitin 4-sulfate and chondroitin 6-sulfate in pathologic joint fluid. *Arthritis Rheum.* **35**, 1304–1308.

41. Lohmander, L. S., Yoshihara, Y., Roos, H., Kobayashi, T., Yamada, H., and Shinmei, M. (1996). Procollagen II C-propeptide in joint fluid. Changes in concentrations with age, time after joint injury and osteoarthritis. *J. Rheumatol.* **23**, 1765–1769.

42. Carey, D. E., Alini, M., Ionescu, M., Hyams, J. S., Rowe, J. C., Rosenberg, L. C., and Poole, A. R. (1997). Serum content of the C-propeptide of the cartilage molecule type II collagen in children. *Clin. Exp. Rheumatol.* **15**, 325–328.

43. Hollander, A. P., Heathfield, T. F., Webber, C., Iwata, Y., Bourne, R., Rorabeck, C., and Poole, A. R. (1994). Increased damage to type II collagen in osteoarthritic cartilage detected by a new immunoassay. *J. Clin. Invest.* **93**, 1722–1732.

44. Saxne, T., and Heinegård, D. (1989). Involvement of nonarticular cartilage, as demonstrated by release of a cartilage-specific protein, in rheumatoid arthritis. *Arthritis Rheum.* **32**, 1080–1086.

45. Goldberg, R. L., Huff, J. P., Lenz, M. E., Glickman, P., Katz, P., and Thonar, E. J.-M. A. (1991). Elevated plasma levels of hyaluronate in patients with osteoarthritis and rheumatoid arthritis. *Arthritis Rheum.* **34**, 799–807.

46. Hedin, P.-J., Weitoft, T., Hedin, H., Engstrom-Laurent, A., and Saxne, T. (1991). Serum concentrations of hyaluronan and proteoglycan in joint disease. Lack of association. *J. Rheumatol.* **18**, 1601–1605.

47. Lohmander, L. S., Saxne, T., and Heinegård, D. (1994). Release of cartilage oligomeric matrix protein (COMP) into joint fluid after injury and in osteoarthrosis. *Ann. Rheum. Dis.* **53**, 8–13.

48. Saxne, T., and Heinegård, D. (1992). Cartilage oligomeric matrix protein: A novel marker of cartilage turnover detectable in synovial fluid and blood. *Br. J. Rheumatol.* **31**, 583–591.

49. Vilim, V., Lenz, M. E., Vytasek, R., Masuda, K., Pavelka, K., Kuettner, K. E., and Thonar, E. J.-M. A. (1997). Characterization of monoclonal antibodies recognizing different fragments of cartilage oligomeric matrix protein in human body fluids. *Arch. Biochem. Biophys.* **341**, 8–16.

50. Forslind, K., Eberhardt, K., Jonsson, A., and Saxne, T. (1992). Increase serum concentrations of cartilage oligomeric matrix protein. A prognostic marker in early rheumatoid arthritis. *Br. J. Rheumatol.* **31**, 593–598.

51. Sharif, M., Saxne, T., Shepstone, L., Kirwan, J. R., Elson, C. J., Heinegård, D., and Dieppe, P. A. (1995). Relationship between cartilage oligomeric matrix protein levels and disease progression in osteoarthritis of the knee joint. *Br. J. Rheumatol.* **34**, 306–310.

52. Manicourt, D., Iwata, K., and Thonar, E. J.-M. A. (1992). Serum levels of TIMP, MMP-1 and MMP-3 in OA patients. *Osteoarthritis Cartilage* **1**, 63 (abstr.).

53. Clark, I. M., Powell, L. K., Ramsey, S., Hazleman, B. L., and Cawston, T. E. (1993). The measurement of collagenase, tissue inhibitor of metalloproteinases (TIMP), and collagenase-TIMP complex in synovial fluids from patients with osteoarthritis and rheumatoid arthritis. *Arthritis Rheum.* **36**, 372–379.

54. Yoshihara, Y., Obata, K. I., Fujimoto, N., Yamashita, K., Hayakawa, T., and Shinmei, M. (1995). Increased levels of stromelysin-1 and tissue inhibitor of metalloproteinases-1 in sera from patients with rheumatoid arthritis. *Arthritis Rheum.* **38**, 969–975.

55. Zucker, S., Lysik, R. M., Zarrabi, M. H., Greenwald, R. A., Gruber, B., Tickle, S. P., Baker, T. S., and Docherty, A. J. (1994). Elevated plasma stromelysin levels in arthritis. *J. Rheumatol.* **21**, 2329–2333.

56. Wood, D. D., Ihrie, E. J., Dinarello, C. A., and Cohen, P. L. (1983). Isolation of interleukin-1 like factor from human joint effusions. *Arthritis Rheum.* **26**, 975–983.

57. Nordahl, S., Alstergren P., Eliasson, S., and Kopp, S. (1998). Interleukin-1 beta in plasma and synovial fluid in relation to radiographic changes in arthritic temperomandibular joints. *Eur. J. Oral Sci.* **106**, 559–563.

58. Kubota, E., Imamura, H., Kubota, T., Shibata, T., and Murakami, K. (1997). Interleukin-1 beta and stromelysin (MMP3) activity of synovial fluid as possible markers of osteoarthritis in the temperomandibular joint. *J. Oral Maxillofacial Surg.* **55**, 20–27.

59. Tetta, C., Camussi, G., Modena, V., DiVittorio, C., and Baglioni, C. (1990). Tumour necrosis factor in serum and synovial fluid samples of patients with active and severe rheumatoid arthritis. *Ann. Rheum. Dis.* **49**, 665–667.

60. Jeng, G.W., Wang, C. R., Liu, S. T., Su., C. C., Tsai, R. T., Yeh, T. S., Wen, C. L., Wu, Y. Q., Lin, C. Y., Lee, G. L., Chen, M. Y., Liu, M. F., Chuang, C. Y., and Chen, C. Y. (1997). Measurement of synovial fluid tumor necrosis factor-alpha in diagnosing emergency patients with bacterial arthritis. *Am. J. Emerg. Med.* **15**, 626–629.

61. Houssiau, F. A., Devogelaer, J. P., van Damme, J., Nagant de Deuxchaisnes, C., and van Snick, J. (1988). Interleukin-6 in synovial fluid and serum of patients with rheumatoid arthritis and other inflammatory arthritides. *Arthritis Rheum.* **31**, 784–788.

62. Lohmander, L. S., Lark, M. W., Dahlberg, L., Walakovits, L. A., and Roos, H. (1992). Cartilage matrix metabolism in osteoarthritis: Markers in synovial fluid, serum and urine. *Clin. Biochem.* **25**, 167–174.

63. Levick, J. R. (1990). The "clearance" of macromolecular substances such as cartilage markers from synovial fluid and serum. *In* "Methods in Cartilage Research" (A. Maroudas and K. E. Kuettner, eds.), pp. 352–357. Academic Press, San Diego, CA.

64. Levick, J. R. (1992). Synovial fluid. Determinants of volume turnover and material concentration. *In* "Articular Cartilage and Osteoarthritis" (K. E. Kuettner, R. Schleyerbach, J. G. Peyron, and V. C. Hascall, eds.), pp. 529–541. Raven Press, New York.

65. Myers, S. L., Brandt, K. D., and Eilam, O. (1995). Even low-grade synovitis significantly accelerates the clearance of protein from the canine knee. Implications for measurement of synovial fluid "marker" of osteoarthritis. *Arthritis Rheum.* **38**, 1085–1091.

66. Rayan, V., Thonar, E. J.-M. A., Chen, L.-M., Lenz, M. E., and Williams, J. M. (1998). Regional differences in the rise in blood levels of antigenic keratan sulfate and hyaluronan after chymopapain induced knee joint injury. *J. Rheumatol.* **25**, 521–526.

67. Thonar, E. J.-M. A., Williams, J. M., Maldonado, B. A., Lenz, M. E., Schnitzer, T. J., Campion, G. V., and Kuettner, K. E. (1991). Serum keratan sulfate concentration as a measure of the catabolism of cartilage proteoglycans. *In* "Monoclonal Antibodies, Cytokines, and Arthritis: Mediators of Inflammation and Therapy" (T. F. Kresina, ed.), pp. 373–398. Dekker, New York.

68. Maldonado, B. A., Williams, J. M., Otten, L. M., Flannery, M., Kuettner, K. E., and Thonar, E. J.-M. A. (1989). Differences in the rate of clearance of different KS-bearing molecules injected intravenously in rabbits. *Orthop. Res. Soc. Trans.* **14**, 161 (abstr.).

69. Block, J. A., Schnitzer, T. J., Andersson, G. B. J., Lenz, M. E., Jeffery, R., McNeill, T. W., and Thonar, E. J.-M. A. (1989). The effect of chemonucleolysis on serum keratan sulfate levels in humans. *Arthritis Rheum.* **32**, 100–104.

70. Attencia, L. J., McDevitt, C. A., Nile, W. B., and Sokoloff, L. (1989). Cartilage content of an immature dog. *Connect. Tissue Res.* **18**, 235–242.

71. Williams, J. M., Downey, C., and Thonar, E. J.-M. A. (1988). Increase in levels of serum keratan sulfate following cartilage proteoglycan degradation in the rabbit knee joint. *Arthritis Rheum.* **31**, 557–560.

72. Manicourt, D.-H., Lenz M. E., and Thonar, E. J.-M. A. (1991). Levels of serum keratan sulfate rise rapidly and remain elevated following anterior cruciate ligament transection in the dog. *J. Rheumatol.* **18**, 1872–1876.

73. Eyre, D. R., Dickson, I. R., and Van Ness, K. P. (1988). Collagen crosslinking in human bone and articular cartilage. Age-related changes in the content of mature hydroxypyridinium residues. *Biochem. J.* **252**, 495–500.

74. Seibel, M. J., Duncan, A., and Robins, S. P. (1989). Urinary hydrox-ypyridinium crosslinks provide indices of cartilage and bone involve-ment in arthritic disease. *J. Rheumatol.* **16**, 964–970.

75. Uebelhart, D., Thonar, E. J.-M. A., Pietryla, D. W., and Williams, J. M. (1993). Elevation in urinary levels of pyridinium cross-links of colla-gen following chymopapain-induced degradation of articular cartilage in the rabbit knee provides evidence of metabolic changes in bone. *Osteoarthritis Cartilage* **1**, 185–192.

76. Kuettner, K. E., and Thonar, E. J.-M. A. (1998). Osteoarthritis and related disorders: Cartilage integrity and homeostasis. *In* "Rheuma-tology" (J. H. Klippel and P. A. Dieppe, eds.), 2nd ed., pp. 6.1–6.15. Mosby, London.

77. Mok, S. S., Masuda, K., Häuselmann, H. J., Aydelotte, M. B., and Thonar, E. J.-M. A. (1994). Aggrecan synthesized by mature bovine chondrocytes suspended in alginate: Identification of two distinct metabolic matrix pools. *J. Biol. Chem.* **269**, 33021–33027.

78. Häuselmann, H. J., Fernandes, R. J., Mok, S. S., Schmid, T. M., Block, J. A., Aydelotte, M. B., Kuettner, K. E., and Thonar, E. J.-M. A. (1994). Phenotypic stability of bovine articular chondrocytes in long-term cul-tures of alginate. *J. Cell Sci.* **107**, 17–27.

79. Shinmei, M., Ito, K., Matsuyama, S., and Sakota, K. (1991). Type II procollagen C-peptide in the joint fluid. *Lab. Exam.* **35**, 1293–1298.

80. Shinmei, M., Nagaya, I., Miyanaga, Y., Iwata, H., Yamamoto, S., Tsorisu, T., Fujii, K., Fukubayashi, T., Kondo, M., Kurosaka, M., and Sekiguchi, S. (1992). Clinical usefulness of the measurement of Type-II procollagen carboxypeptide (C-II propeptide, pColl-II-C) in synovial fluid as a marker of collagen metabolism in cartilage. *Ryumaki* **32**, 453–460.

81. Shinmei, M., Ito, K., Matsuyama, S., Yoshihara, Y., and Matsuzawa, K. (1993). Carboxy-terminal Type II procollagen peptide levels in joint fluids as a marker of collagen biosynthesis of cartilage in joint diseases. *Osteoarthritis Cartilage* **1**, 121–128.

82. Heinegård, D., and Oldberg, A. (1989). Structure and biology of car-tilage and bone matrix noncollagenous macromolecules. *FASEB J.* **3**, 2042–2051.

83. Heinegård, D., and Pimentel, E. R. (1992). Cartilage matrix pro-teins. *In* "Articular Cartilage and Osteoarthritis" (K. E. Kuettner, R. Schleyerbach, J. G. Peyron, and V. C. Hascall, eds.), pp. 95–111. Raven Press, New York.

84. Okada, Y., Shinmei, M., Tanaka, O., Naka, K., Tomita, K., Nakanishi, I., Bayliss, M. T., Iwata, K., and Nagase, H. (1992). Localization of matrix metalloproteinase 3 (Stromelysin) in osteoarthritic cartilage and synovium. *Lab. Invest.* **66**, 680–690.

85. Walakovits, L. A., Moore, V. L., Bhardwaj, N., Gallick, G. S., and Lark, M. W. (1992). Detection of stromelysin and collagenase in synovial fluid from patients with rheumatoid arthritis and posttraumatic knee injury. *Arthritis Rheum.* **35**, 35–42.

86. Flannery, C. R., Lark, M. W., and Sandy, J. D. (1992). Identification of a stromelysin cleavage site within the interglobular domain of human aggrecan: Evidence for proteolysis at this site *in vivo* in human articular cartilage. *J. Biol. Chem.* **267**, 1008–1014.

87. Lohmander, L. S., Hoerrner, L. A., Dahlberg, L., Roos, H., Bjornsson, S., and Lark, M. W. (1993). Stromelysin, tissue inhibitor and proteo-glycan fragments in human knee joint fluid after injury. *J. Rheumatol.* **20**, 1362–1368.

88. Lohmander, L. S., Roos, H., Dahlberg, L., Hoerrner, L. A., and Lark, M. W. (1994). Temporal patterns of stromelysin-1, tissue inhibitor and proteoglycan fragments in human knee joint fluid after injury to the cruciate ligament or meniscus. *J. Orthop. Res.* **12**, 21–28.

89. Tyler, J. A. (1989). IGF1 can decrease degradation and promote syn-thesis of proteoglycan in cartilage exposed to cytokines. *Biochem. J.* **260**, 543–548.

90. Morales, T. I. (1992). Polypeptide regulators of matrix homeosta-sis in articular cartilage. *In* "Articular Cartilage and Osteoarthritis"

91. Tyler, J. A., Bolis, S., Dingle, J. T., and Middleton, J. F. S. (1992). Me-diators of matrix catabolism. *In* "Articular Cartilage and Osteoarthritis" (K. E. Kuettner, R. Schleyerbach, J. G. Peyron, and V. C. Hascall, eds.), pp. 251–264. Raven Press, New York.

92. Häuselmann, H. J., Flechtenmacher, J., Michal, L., Thonar, E. J.-M. A., Shinmei, M., Kuettner, K. E., and Aydelotte, M. B. (1996). The superficial layer of human articular cartilage is more susceptible to interleukin-1-induced damage than the deeper layers. *Arthritis Rheum.* **39**, 478–488.

93. Thonar, E. J.-M. A., Pachman, L. M., Lenz, M. E., Hayford, J., Lynch, P., and Kuettner, K. E. (1988). Age related changes in the concentration of serum keratan sulfate in children. *J. Clin. Chem. Clin. Biochem.* **26**, 57–63.

94. Thonar, E. J.-M. A., and Glant, T. T. (1992). Serum keratan sulfate—a marker of predisposition to polyarticular osteoarthritis. *Clin. Biochem.* **25**, 175–180.

95. Yoshida, K., Miyauchi, S., Kikuchi, H., Tawada, A., and Tokuyasu, A. (1989). Analysis of unsaturated disaccharides produced from chon-droitin sulfates in rabbit plasma by high performance liquid chromatog-raphy. *Anal. Biochem.* **177**, 327–332.

96. Shinmei, M., Inamori, Y., Yoshihara, Y., Kikuchi, T., and Hayakawa, T. (1992). The potential of cartilage markers in joint fluid for drug evaluation. *In* "Articular Cartilage and Osteoarthritis" (K. E. Kuettner, R. Schleyerbach, J. G. Peyron, and V. C. Hascall, eds.), pp. 597–609. Raven Press, New York.

97. Uebelhart, D., Gineyts, E., Chatpuy, M.-C., and Delmas, P. (1990). Urinary excretion of pyridinium crosslinks: A new marker of bone resorption in metabolic bone disease. *Bone Miner.* **8**, 87–96.

98. Robins, S. P., McLaren, A. M., Nicol, P., and Seibel, M. J. (1992). Pyridinium cross-link measurements in serum and synovial fluid of patients with osteoarthritis. *In* "Articular Cartilage and Osteoarthritis" (K. E. Kuettner, R. Schleyerbach, J. G. Peyron, and V. C. Hascall, eds.), pp. 738–739. Raven Press, New York.

99. Thompson, P. W., Spector, T. D., James, I. T., Henderson, E., and Hart, D. J. (1992). Urinary collagen cross-links reflect the radiographic severity of knee osteoarthritis. *Br. J. Rheumatol.* **31**, 759–761.

100. Tsutsumi, M., Urashima, S., Takase, S., Ueshima, Y., Tsuchishima, M., Shimananka, K., and Kawahara, H. (1997). Characteristics of serum hyaluronate concentration in patients with alcoholic liver disease. *Alcohol.: Clin. Exp. Res.* **21**, 1716–1721.

101. Dinsmore, C. E., Goss, R. J., Lenz, M. E., and Thonar, E. J.-M. A. (1986). Correlation between phases of deer antler regeneration and levels of serum keratan sulfate. *Calcif. Tissue Int.* **39**, 244–247.

102. Sah, R. L.-Y., Grodzinsky, A. J., Plaas, A. H. K., and Sandy, J. D. (1992). Effects of static and dynamic compression on matrix metabolism in cartilage explants. *In* "Articular Cartilage and Osteoarthritis" (K. E. Kuettner, R. Schleyerbach, J. G. Peyron, and V. C. Hascall, eds.), pp. 373–392. Raven Press, New York.

103. Palmoski, M., Perricone, E., and Brandt, K. D. (1979). Development and reversal of a proteoglycan aggregation defect in normal canine knee cartilage after immobilization. *Arthritis Rheum.* **22**, 508–517.

104. Sweet, M. B. E., Jakim, I., Coelho, A., Becker, P. J., and Thonar, E. J.-M. A. (1990). Serum keratan sulphate levels during prolonged rest. *S. Afr. Med. J.* **78**, 629–630.

105. Ledingham, J., Regan, M., Jones, A., and Doherty, M. (1995). Factors affecting radiographic progression of knee osteoarthritis. *Ann. Rheum. Dis.* **54**, 53–58.

106. Butler, D. M., Vitti, G. F., Leizer, T., and Hamilton, J. A. (1988). Stimulation of the hyaluronic acid levels of human synovial fibroblasts by recombinant human tumor necrosis factor α, tumor necrosis factor β(lymphotoxin), interleukin-1α, and interleukin-1β. *Arthritis Rheum.* **31**, 1281–1289.

CHAPTER 32

Laboratory Assessment of Postmenopausal Osteoporosis

PATRICK GARNERO   INSERM Research Unit 403, Lyon, France

PIERRE D. DELMAS   Université Claude Bernard, Lyon France; and INSERM Research Unit 403, Lyon, France

I. INTRODUCTION

The internationally agreed definition of osteoporosis is: "a progressive systemic skeletal disease characterized by low bone mass and microarchitectural deterioration of bone tissue, with a consequent increase in bone fragility and susceptibility to fracture" [1]. Osteoporosis is one of the most prevalent diseases associated with aging and because of its cost, it is viewed as a major health problem. The most common fractures include vertebral compression fractures and fractures of the distal radius and the proximal femur (hip fracture). In addition, osteoporotic patients commonly sustain fractures at several other sites including the pelvis, proximal humerus, distal femur, tibia, and ribs. Osteoporotic fractures occurring at the spine and the forearm are associated with significant morbidity, but the most serious consequences arise in patients with hip fracture, which is associated with a significant increase in mortality (15–20%), particularly in elderly men and women. In white women, the lifetime risk of hip fracture is 19%. It is 15.6% for vertebral fracture and 16% for distal forearm fracture. The lifetime risk of any fracture of the hip, spine, and forearm is almost 40% in white women from age 50 years onward [2].

The definition of osteoporosis captures the notion that a low bone mass is by far the most important risk factor for osteoporotic fractures. However, other factors must also be taken into account including age per se, family and personal history of fracture, some ill-defined structural parameters which influence the fragility of bone architecture, hip-axis length, and some factors unrelated to bone such as the propensity to fall in the elderly. Nevertheless, it is only bone mass, assessed by bone mineral density (BMD), that forms the basis for the diagnosis of osteoporosis. BMD in late postmenopausal women, at the time when fractures occur, depends on the peak bone mass achieved in adolescence and the subsequent rate of bone loss. Genetic factors have important effects on peak bone mass, while environmental factors may be more important in age-related bone loss. In women, there are some uncertainties about the age at which peak bone mass is achieved and starts to decline and about the magnitude of premenopausal bone loss according to the skeletal site. Women show an accelerated phase of bone loss after menopause which occurs for about 5 to 8 years and is followed by a sustained but somewhat smaller bone loss throughout life. Estrogen deficiency is the main determinant of early postmenopausal bone loss but there is good evidence that it also plays a role in bone loss occurring in the elderly. Other age-related changes in hormonal status, such as vitamin D deficiency and secondary hyperparathyroidism, are likely to play a role in bone loss in the elderly, both in men and in women [3, 4].

The prognostic assessment of fracture risk—which is important to optimize therapeutic strategies—is mainly based on the quantification of BMD and in some cases on the rate of bone loss that can be assessed indirectly by measurement of biochemical markers of bone turnover. Some laboratory tests, such as measurements of plasma PTH and 25 hydroxy-vitamin D, may be useful in the differential diagnosis of osteoporosis. Other tests, such as assessment of cytokine production, may provide insights in the pathogenesis of the disease. Repeated bone mass and turnover measurements are also useful to assess the efficacy of antiresorptive therapy. Bone mass measurements and biochemical markers of bone turnover, which have greatly improved in recent years, appear to be key methods to diagnose osteoporosis, predict future fracture, and monitor therapeutic regimens.

In this chapter we review the determinants of peak bone mass and rate of bone loss and then discuss the use of diagnostic techniques, including bone mineral density measurement and bone markers, in postmenopausal osteoporosis.

II. PEAK BONE MASS

Peak bone mass, which is attained in early adult life, depends primarily on genetic factors. However, it is also influenced by dietary calcium intake during adolescence—as suggested by intervention studies in prepubertal girls [5]—and by physical activity [6, 7]. The influence of genetic factors in regulating attainment of peak bone mass is obvious from twin and family studies; they have shown that these factors account for up to 60–80% of the interindividual variance of bone mass of young adults. Several studies have reported higher concordances of bone mineral density between monozygotic than dizygotic twins, indicating a greater importance of shared genes compared to shared environmental factors in determining bone mass [8, 9]. Supporting data have been obtained from family studies showing, for example, that premenopausal daughters of women with osteoporosis have reduced lumbar spine, femoral neck, and femoral shaft BMD compared to premenopausal women without a family history of osteoporosis [10]. The most important issue is the identification of genes involved in this heritability. This field has progressed mainly since the report of Morisson *et al.*

[11] showing that polymorphisms in the 3′ untranslated region of the vitamin D receptor gene (VDR) were associated with peak bone mineral density of the spine in twins, and that these polymorphisms accounted for most of the genetic effect on BMD. However, another group reported no association in a similar twin cohort [12], and subsequent studies have yielded conflicting results. In a large population-based cohort of French premenopausal women, no relationship was found between VDR polymorphisms and bone formation and resorption rate, as assessed by a panel of specific biochemical markers of bone turnover, nor with BMD measured at various skeletal sites by dual-energy X-ray absorptiometry (DXA) [13]. Morisson's group subsequently reported that reanalysis of the twin pairs did not confirm original findings in their twin population [14]. This does not imply that VDR genotypes are not linked to differences in bone metabolism, but rather that the effect of these polymorphisms is small, with differences between extreme genotypes of 2–3% as suggested by a recent meta-analysis [15]. The differences between the studies may be partly explained by age-related changes in the association between VDR genotypes and BMD, with probably a greater effect in younger ages [16]. There is also some evidence that the variability between studies may be related to interactions between VDR genotypes and environmental factors such as calcium intake. Thus, the effect of the VDR with BMD could be partly masked in conditions of high calcium intake and could be more pronounced in women with calcium-intake deficiency [17, 18]. Another possibility is that the VDR polymorphisms described originally by Morisson *et al.* [11] are, in certain populations, in linkage disequilibrium with functional polymorphism elsewhere in the gene or in neighboring genes. It should be noted that a second polymorphism in the VDR gene that creates an alternative initiation codon has been reported to be associated with BMD of postmenopausal women [19]. However, the association of this polymorphism with peak bone mass measured at different skeletal sites in a large cohort of French premenopausal women has not been confirmed [20], suggesting that the effect may also vary according to populations. More likely, the genetic influence on peak bone mass is mediated by several candidate genes (Table I). Isolated studies have found associations between BMD and polymorphisms of the estrogen receptor [21], interleukine-6 [22], and transforming growth factor beta (TGF β) [23] genes.

However, these observations need to be repeated in different populations and the mechanism which links these polymorphisms with differences in bone metabolism needs to be identified as, for most of them, DNA sequence interindividual variation is situated in noncoding regions. Also of interest are the polymorphisms of the genes encoding type I collagen (COLIA1 and COL1A2) because this protein is the major organic component of bone matrix and coding mutations of these genes have been shown to be associated with a severe osteoporotic phenotype in the disease osteogenesis

TABLE I.   Potential Candidate Genes for Regulation of Bone Mass

Hormones/hormone receptors	Growth factors/cytokines and their receptors	Bone matrix proteins	Enzymes
Vitamin D receptor (VDR[a] 3′ untranslated)	TGF β[a]	Type I collagen[a]	Matrix metalloproteases
VDR[a] (Start translational site)	IL-1[a]	Osteocalcin	
Estrogen receptor[a]	IL-1 ra[a]	Bone sialoprotein	Cathepsin K
Progesterone receptor	IL-6[a]	alpha 2 HS[a]	
Glucocorticoid receptor	IGF-1		
PTH/PTH rp[a] and PTH receptor			

[a] Shown to be associated with bone mineral density in some studies.

imperfecta. A G/T substitution polymorphism of an Sp1 binding site within the first intron of the COL1A1 gene has been shown to be associated with spine and femoral neck BMD and with risk of fracture in cohorts of mainly postmenopausal women from the UK [24], France [25] and the Netherlands [26]. In a large cohort of healthy premenopausal women (n = 220), this polymorphism was associated with height and peak bone mass in the spine and total body (with small differences between genotypes) but not with BMD of hip and forearm [27] (Fig. 1). This association of genotype with BMD was not significant after adjustment for anthropometric vari-

ables including height, suggesting that part of the effect of COL1A1 on BMD could be mediated by differences in body size. However, other studies have reported no significant association between COL1A1 genotypes and BMD, and although the polymorphism is situated at the transcription factor binding site, the potential molecular mechanisms linking the G/T substitution to osteoporosis needs to be established. At this stage, it can be concluded that no identified polymorphism of bone related genes can be used, alone or in combination, as a diagnostic test to predict the risk of osteoporosis in premenopausal women.

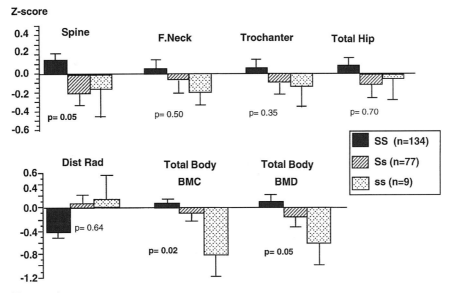

FIGURE 1   Peak bone mineral density in unrelated premenopausal women (220 women, mean age: 40 ± 6 year) in relation to COL1A1 Sp1 polymorphism. Results are expressed in number of standard deviations from the mean of the whole premenopausal cohort (Z-score). Bold p values indicate significant differences (at p < 0.05). After adjustment for height, which was significantly associated with genotypes (p = 0.03, with lowest values in ss), the differences between genotypes at the spine and total body decreased and were no longer significant (p = 0.08, 0.17, and 0.33 for spine BMD, total body BMD, and total body BMC, respectively). Adapted from *J. Bone Miner. Res.* (1998). Garnero *et al.* Collagen I alpha 1 Sp1 polymorphism, bone mass and bone turnover in healthy French premenopausal women: The OFELY study, **13**, 813–817, with permission of the American Society for Bone and Mineral Research.

III. POSTMENOPAUSAL BONE LOSS

A. Pattern of Bone Loss

Osteoporosis is much more prevalent in women than in men because of the major role that estrogen deficiency plays in the pathogenesis of bone loss. Numerous studies have shown that among women there is an accelerated bone loss that coincides temporally with menopause [28–30]. Although osteoporosis is a systemic disease affecting the whole skeleton (with the exception of the bones of the skull and face), the pattern of bone loss differs slightly according to skeletal envelopes. Because of a much slower rate of bone remodeling within cortical compared to trabecular envelopes, cortical bone loss may start later than cancellous bone loss, but the total amount of cortical bone loss in women in their eighties is probably similar to the loss of cancellous bone, i.e., from 30–50% of the peak bone mass achieved at adulthood. The loss of bone after menopause follows an exponential pattern [31–34] and varies markedly from one woman to another [35–37]. After the accelerated rate of bone loss, lasting 5 to 8 years following menopause, the rate decreases linearly to an average of about 0.5–1% per year, but it may accelerate again after age 75, at least at the hip [38]. The proportion of the overall bone loss related to menopause and estrogen-independent aging is still debated, but clearly bone loss in the elderly is still under the influence of estrogen deficiency [39].

B. Genetic Factors and Postmenopausal Bone Loss

In contrast to the established genetic influence on peak bone mass, whether the genetic pattern affects the rate of bone loss after menopause is still debated. Because the precise evaluation of the rate of bone loss in a single patient requires repeated bone mass measurements over a long period, very few studies have investigated the determinants of bone loss and conflicting results have been published concerning a potential genetic influence. In a population of male twins studied over a 16 year period, Christian *et al.* [40] found no significant genetic contribution to change in radial bone mass despite evidence of genetic effects on bone mass itself. However, the within-pair correlation for both twin types was significant, suggesting that factors common with twin pairs, such as environmental influences, may be important in determining age-related bone loss. In a population comprising male and pre and postmenopausal female twins between 25 and 75 years of age, Kelly *et al.* [41] suggested the existence of a genetic influence on BMD changes at the spine and Ward's triangle, but they were unable to demonstrate a significant effect at the femoral neck over a median 3 year follow-up. The rate of bone loss in postmenopausal women depends on the negative balance between resorption and formation. Some studies have shown that the rate of bone loss is correlated with the postmenopausal increase in bone turnover, i.e., that high turnover is associated with accelerated bone loss (see below). In order to determine whether or not a proportion of the variance of bone turnover in postmenopausal women is explained by genetic factors, Garnero *et al.* [42] have looked for a genetic influence on the levels of biochemical markers of bone turnover in a large group of postmenopausal twins. The study showed that genetic factors are probably not a major determinant of the large interindividual variance of the levels of bone turnover markers, especially of bone resorption, suggesting that environmental mechanisms are likely to play a large role in mediating postmenopausal bone turnover and thus postmenopausal bone loss. These data contrast with the well-documented genetic influence on premenopausal bone turnover and peak bone mass. Long-term prospective studies with repeated BMD measurements at various skeletal sites in postmenopausal twins are required to clarify the genetic influence on postmenopausal bone loss, if any.

C. Sex Hormone and Postmenopausal Bone Loss

Of the many factors influencing bone loss in postmenopausal women, sex hormone deficiency is by far the most important. This central role in the pathogenesis of postmenopausal bone loss is indeed strongly supported by the higher prevalence of osteoporosis in women than in men, the increase in the rate of bone loss after artificial or natural menopause [43], the existence of a relationship between estrogen levels and rates of bone loss [44], and the protective effect of estrogen replacement with respect to bone loss and fracture incidence [45–52]. The mechanism by which estrogen prevents bone loss is mainly related to its ability to block resorption, although stimulation of bone formation may also play a contributory role [53, 54]. Estrogen-dependent inhibition of bone resorption is due to both decreased osteoclastogenesis and diminished resorptive activity of mature osteoclasts. The mechanism of action of estrogen is still controversial. The discovery of estrogen receptors in osteoblasts, their stromal precursors, and mature osteoclasts suggests that a direct effect on bone or bone marrow may be involved [55]. However, it is not clear which of these cells are the primary targets for estrogen *in vivo*. There is evidence that estrogen may mediate its effects indirectly through the stimulation of the release of growth factors such as TGF β [56] (which has been shown in specific experimental conditions to decrease both osteoclastic resorptive activity and recruitment) and/or the inhibition of secretion of potent bone resorbing cytokines such as interleukins (IL)-1 and -6 and tumor necrosis factor (TNF) (reviewed in Chapter 7). Several studies have shown that natural and surgical menopause are associated with increased production of IL-1 and TNF from peripheral blood and bone marrow monocytes with a greater persistence of the increase in osteoporotic patients [57–59]. The culture media of monocytes from postmenopausal women have a higher *in vitro* bone resorption activity than that of either premenopausal women or estrogen-treated postmenopausal women, suggesting a direct link between increased monocytic production of cytokines and increased postmenopausal bone resorption [60]. However, the measurement of cytokines from peripheral blood or bone marrow monocytes can not be used as a diagnostic test to quantify the effects of estrogen deficiency on bone turnover. In addition, estrogen also has direct effects on osteoclasts and may promote osteoclast apoptosis. Also to be noted is the potential role of prostaglandin of the E series whose production is increased *in vivo* by estrogen deficiency.

D. Parathyroid Hormone, Vitamin D, and Postmenopausal Bone Loss

It is well established that parathyroid hormone (PTH) levels increase with advancing age, mainly after 65 years of age [61]. Aging is characterized by a decrease of calcium intake and intestinal absorption, a decrease of vitamin D intake and synthesis, and declining production of 1,25-dihydroxyvitamin D, resulting in secondary hyperparathyroidism. This is likely to increase bone turnover and may play a role in cortical bone loss with age, thus increasing the risk of fracture. However, in a large cohort of healthy postmenopausal women, no significant correlation between serum intact PTH and markers of bone turnover was found in women within 20 years of menopause, and only a modest contribution of serum PTH levels to bone turnover variance ($r^2 < 0.10$) was found in elderly women 20 years past menopause [62]. Thus, secondary hyperparathyroidism is probably not a major determinant of increased bone turnover in postmenopausal women and in osteoporosis. In a prospective study of the determinants of hip fracture, neither baseline serum 25-hydroxyvitamin D nor PTH levels were predictive of the subsequent risk of hip fracture [63]. Nevertheless, the identification of vitamin D deficiency and its correction by calcium and low doses of vitamin D in the elderly is important [4, 64].

E. Local Cytokines and Growth Factors

Histomorphometric studies of iliac crest biopsies suggest that postmenopausal bone loss is due to distinct abnormalities such as an imbalance between bone resorption and bone formation within a remodeling unit (due to increased osteoclastic activity and/or decreased osteoblastic activity) and to an increase in the activation frequency, i.e., in the number of remodeling units initiated per unit of time and space. Thus, the small negative bone balance within each remodeling unit is amplified by the overall increase in bone turnover, which is mainly due to estrogen deficiency. The imbalance results from abnormalities in the coupling mechanism that links resorption and formation. This coupling process is regulated by several local regulatory factors produced by cells of the microenvironment of the bone remodeling unit. Changes in the local production of these factors and/or abnormal responsiveness of cells to these factors are likely to be responsible for alterations in the coupling mechanism. In addition to the cytokines IL-I, IL-6, and TNF, these local factors include the growth regulatory factors which are stored in bone matrix, such as insulin-like growth factors (IGF) I and II, TGF β, fibroblast growth factors, and bone morphogenetic proteins. It should be recognized, however, that most of the data supporting a role of these factors are derived from animal models and there is little information about humans. Of special interest is the potential role of IGF-I. It has been shown that with aging in humans, there is a decrease in the levels of IGF-I in serum and cortical bone [65, 66]. Serum IGF-I correlated with spine, femoral neck, and radius BMD and decreased levels have been reported in postmenopausal women with vertebral fractures [67]. Studies of the role of IGF-I are obscured by the fact that its action may be modulated by binding proteins (IGFBP)—at least six different ones have identified—all of them synthesized by osteoblasts. Some of them, such as IGFBP-5, stimulate bone formation, whereas others are inhibitory, such as IGFBP-4 (see Chapter 6). In the circulation, IGF-I is bound to various IGFBPs, and a major part of bound IGF-I is connected to IGFBP-3, which has also been shown to be decreased in osteoporotic women [67]. Serum levels of IGF-I mainly reflect liver synthesis which is regulated by different systemic and local factors than IGF-I, which is synthesized by osteoblasts. Alternatively, skeletal IGF-I may be trapped into bone from the circulation. IGF-I stimulates osteoblasts *in vitro* and increases both resorption and formation *in vivo* [68, 69].

IV. MANAGEMENT OF POSTMENOPAUSAL OSTEOPOROSIS

The identification of postmenopausal women at risk for osteoporosis relies mainly on the quantification of the amount of bone and on the estimation of the rate of bone loss. Both of these parameters can be non-invasively assessed by diagnostic techniques such as dual X-ray absorptiometry and biochemical markers of bone turnover. Once women at high risk are identified and treatment is initiated, these techniques are also very useful in monitoring therapeutic efficacy.

A. Measurement of Bone Mineral Density with Dual Energy X-Ray Absorptiometry (DXA) and Ultrasound (US)

Dual X-ray absorptiometry (DXA) is the most reliable technique for measuring BMD and has several advantages, including low precision error, minimal radiation exposure, fast scanning, and the possibility of measuring virtually all skeletal sites. Osteoporosis is a systemic disease and loss of bone occurs at all sites. For this reason, bone scans for diagnostic purposes should normally be undertaken at any one site. Cross-sectional studies have shown that bone mass measurements performed at various anatomical sites correlate significantly with each other, though with a low correlation coefficient. This result indicates that bone mass at one site can not be used to predict BMD value at another site in a single individual and, therefore, assessment of the relevant biological site is preferable. BMD is usually measured at the lumbar spine and hip, but the spine should be avoided in the elderly because values are often overestimated because of osteoarthritis, which is highly prevalent. Smaller and cheaper DXA and SXA devices have been developed to measure the distal forearm and/or the calcaneum, and these peripheral densitometers may prove very helpful for screening purposes.

Several long-term prospective studies have demonstrated that women with a low bone mass, measured either at the forearm, heel, spine, proximal femur, or whole body, have an increased risk of vertebral, hip, and forearm fracture [70–73]. Clearly there is a gradient of risk; i.e., the lower BMD, the higher the risk of fracture. BMD can be measured at any skeletal site; however, fracture risk prediction is improved by performing site-specific measurements (e.g. by measuring hip BMD to predict hip fracture risk) [71]. The cost-effectiveness benefit of measuring BMD at two sites rather than at one is doubtful. The absolute risk of fracture depends not only on bone mass but also on life expectancy.

Ultrasound velocity (SOS) and broadband attenuation (BUA) measurements are rather inexpensive, radiation-free methods for estimating bone mass that may also provide insights into bone quality. These techniques have been applied to the patella, heel, tibia, and phalanx. The precision error of these measurements is variable. Several studies have shown significant but weak correlation between ultrasonographic parameters and BMD measurements, with correlation coefficients ranging from 0.34 to 0.72 for SOS and 0.32 to 0.87 for BUA [74, 75]. Several cross-sectional studies have shown that ultrasonography may discriminate normal from osteoporotic subject groups as reliably as DXA. Two prospective cohort studies have shown that heel ultrasound measurement of BMD predicts hip fracture risk with a relative risk comparable to that obtained with DXA and it does so independently of femoral neck BMD [76, 77]. However, whether or not combining ultrasound with DXA improves fracture prediction is still unclear and needs further study. To date, few studies have reported the usefulness of ultrasound to monitor treatment of osteoporosis; further longitudinal studies are required. Several issues need to be addressed before ultrasound can be used as a routine diagnostic test in clinical practice, such as normative data, cut off values for defining osteopenia

and osteoporosis, and quality control programs. Because the technical features vary substantially from one device to another, data obtained with one piece of equipment may not be extrapolated to others.

B. Measurement of Bone Turnover with Biochemical Markers

Postmenopausal bone loss results both from an imbalance between resorption and formation at the level of a bone remodeling unit and from an increase in the activation frequency, i.e., in the number of remodeling units initiated per unit of time and space. The increase in activation frequency after menopause is mainly dependent on estrogen deficiency, whereas the remodeling imbalance might be related to a combination of age-related factors, such as a decrease of IGF-I production. Biochemical markers (whose technical aspects are reviewed in detail in Chapters 19, 27, and 28) reflect the degree of increase in overall skeletal turnover and can not be used to give insight to the mechanism of imbalance at the level of a bone remodeling unit. Osteocalcin is a small protein specifically synthesized by the osteoblasts. The fraction of newly synthesized osteocalcin released into the circulation can be measured by immunoassay [78]. Measurement of both the intact molecule and the large N-Mid fragment, which is the main proteolytic degradation product of the intact molecule, results in improved stability and therefore sensitivity of the assay [79, 80]. Measurement of the circulating levels of the bone isoenzyme of alkaline phosphatase by direct immunoassays, which have been shown to have a small cross-reactivity with the liver isoenzyme [81], is an alternative to serum osteocalcin for assessing bone formation. Bone formation also can be assessed by measuring the procollagen I extension peptides. In general, the immunoassay of the carboxy-terminal peptide has been disappointing because of lack of sensitivity [82]. In contrast, a new immunoassay for the intact form of the circulating N-terminal extension peptide is available and it appears to be as sensitive as serum osteocalcin and bone alkaline phosphatase in osteoporosis [83]. The assessment of bone resorption has markedly improved in recent years. Currently, the best biochemical indices of bone resorption are the new immunoassays for the type I collagen pyridinoline cross-links and related peptides which advantageously substitute for the high performance liquid chromatography measurement of the total excretion of the pyridinoline crosslinks in hydrolyzed urine [84, 85]. These immunoassays comprise measurements of free pyridinoline and deoxypyridinoline (Pyrilinks and Pyrilink-D) [86] and measurement of related peptides in serum (ICTP) [87], in urine (N-telopeptide to helix, or NTx Osteomark) [88], or in both serum and urine (C-telopeptide to helix or CTx, Crosslaps) [89] (see Chapter 28).

C. Estimation of the Rate of Postmenopausal Bone Loss

Given the precision error of DXA measurements (1–1.5% on average, i.e., 2.8–4.2% in a single patient) and the magnitude of change in bone mass that is expected, the quantitation of bone loss in an osteoporotic patient would require measurement of BMD to be repeated after at least a 4 year interval. Such a strategy is not convenient when it is necessary to decide whether or not to treat at the time of initial assessment.

Several cross-sectional studies indicate that bone turnover increases rapidly after menopause. In contrast with what was originally thought, this increase in both bone formation and bone resorption is sustained long after the menopause, up to 40 years [62]. BMD measured at various skeletal sites correlated negatively with bone turnover assessed by various markers in postmenopausal women. The correlation between bone markers and BMD becomes much stronger with advancing age, so that in women more than 30 years after menopause, bone turnover accounts for 40–50% of the variance of bone mineral density of the whole skeleton [62]. These cross-sectional data suggest that a sustained increase of bone turnover in postmenopausal women induces a faster bone loss and therefore an increased risk of osteoporosis. Longitudinal studies, which are required to confirm that hypothesis, suffer from a methodological issue: indeed, when the rate of bone loss is assessed by annual measurement of bone mineral density at the spine, hip, or radius over 2–4 years, the amount of bone loss is on the same order of the magnitude of the precision error of repeated measurements in a single individual (i.e., 3–4%). This technical limitation greatly impairs a valid assessment of the relationship between bone turnover and the subsequent rate of bone loss in individual postmenopausal women, and it probably explains the conflicting results that have been published. When the precision error was reduced by performing nine bone mineral density measurements over 24 months at a highly precise skeletal site such as the radius, the ability of baseline bone markers to predict rate of loss was markedly improved, with correlation coefficients increasing from about 0.2 to 0.4 (when rate of loss is assessed from yearly bone mass measurements) to 0.7–0.8 [90]. Ultimately, the proof of evidence will come from long-term studies. Two such studies show that the assessment of bone turnover was correlated with the spontaneous rate of forearm and calcaneal bone loss over the 12–13 years following initial assessment [91, 92]. The first study showed that, despite identical bone mass at baseline, women who were classified as fast losers at the time of menopause, based on conventional bone markers including total alkaline phosphatase and urinary hydroxyproline, had lost 50% more bone 12 years later than those diagnosed as slow losers (total bone loss 26.6% versus 16.6%, p < 0.001). One study [92] in older women (mean age at baseline: 62) performed over

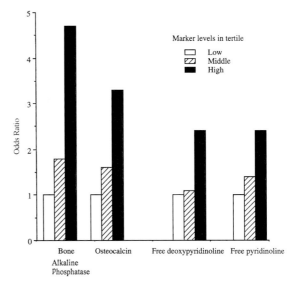

FIGURE 2   Association of high levels of biochemical markers with rapid calcaneal bone loss. Calcaneal bone loss was assessed in 354 postmenopausal women (mean age at baseline: 62) by up to eight measurements over 13 years. At the end of the follow-up period, biochemical markers were measured in the 100 women with the highest bone loss (mean: −2.2%/yr) and in the 100 women with the lowest bone loss (mean: −0.4%/yr). Women were categorized in tertiles of bone markers and the risk (odds ratio) of rapid bone loss was calculated in each group, the lowest tertile being used as a reference (odds ratio = 1). Adapted from *J. Bone Miner. Res.* (1998) **13**, 297–302 [92] with permission of the American Society for Bone and Mineral Research.

13 years, where calcaneal BMD loss was assessed by eight measurements, showed one standard deviation increase in new specific bone markers (such as osteocalcin, bone specific alkaline phosphatase, and free pyridinoline cross-links) was associated with a two-fold increased risk of rapid bone loss, defined as the upper tertile of rate of loss (Fig. 2). However, one of the limitations of that study is that bone markers were measured at the end of the follow-up period; although bone turnover is likely to be stable in postmenopausal women, long-term prospective studies are needed to evaluate the associations of bone marker levels with future loss. Such studies, with rates of loss assessed at different skeletal sites including spine, radius, and hip, and using the newly developed bone markers, have been initiated.

D. Biochemical Markers of Bone Turnover and Fracture Risk

Retrospective studies comparing bone marker levels in patients who had already sustained an osteoporotic fracture and in controls are inadequate to assess the relationship between bone turnover and fracture. Indeed, bone turnover can change after fracture because of immobilization, because of the callus formation, and/or because of a frequent regional activation of bone turnover.

TABLE II. Relative Risk (Odds Ratio) of a Fracture Causing Low Bone Mass at Menopause and/or a Fast Rate of Bone Loss

	+ Fracture n = 48	− Fracture n = 134	Odds ratio
Fast losers (n = 49)	18	31	2.0[a]
Normal losers (n = 133)	30	103	
Low bone mass (n = 55)	19	36	1.9[a]
Normal bone mass (n = 127)	29	98	
Fast loser/low bone mass (n = 17)	7	10	3.0[a]
Normal loser/normal bone mass (n = 95)	18	77	

[a] $p < 0.05$

Osteoporotic fractures (25 spinal, 23 peripheral) were registered during 15 year follow-up. A fast loser is defined by a rate of bone loss >3% per year over the first 2 years. A low bone mass is defined by a t score <−1 at baseline. Reprinted from [93] *Bone* **19**, Riis, S. B. J., Hansen, A. M., Jensen, K., Overgaard, K., and Christiansen, C. Low bone mass and fast rate of bone loss at menopause—equal risk factors for future fracture. A 15 year follow-up study. Pages 9–12, copyright 1996, with permission from Elsevier Science.

Relating bone marker levels measured prior to the fracture to the subsequent risk of fracture is the only valid methodology to assess their clinical utility. The predictive value of biochemical markers should be analyzed separately for hip, vertebral, and other osteoporotic fractures because of heterogeneity in the pathogenesis and potentially in underlying bone turnover abnormalities. Riis *et al.* [93] reported that within 3 years of menopause, women classified as "fast bone losers" had a two-fold higher risk of sustaining vertebral and peripheral fractures during a 15 year follow-up than women classified as "normal" or "slow" losers. Interestingly, bone mass and rate of bone loss predispose women to fractures to the same extent, with an odds ratio of about two. Women with both a low bone mass and a fast rate of bone loss after menopause had a higher risk of subsequently sustaining fractures than women with only one of the two risk factors (Table II). Concordant results have been obtained in two prospective studies of risk factors for hip fractures: The ROTTERDAM Study [94] and The EPIDOS Study [63]. In the latter study, markers of bone formation, including total osteocalcin and bone alkaline phosphatase, were not predictive. The EPIDOS-study showed that in those women who had a hip fracture during a 2 year follow-up, baseline measurements of urinary C-telopeptide breakdown products (CTx) and free deoxypyridinoline (free D-Pyr) were higher than in nonfractured controls. Increased CTx and free D-Pyr above the normal range of premenopausal women, which occurred in 25% of the women, was associated with a two-fold increase in the risk of hip fracture; this increase was still significant after adjusting for hip bone mineral density and mobility status, with a very similar odds ratio. Thus, the combination of bone mass and bone turnover measurements allows identification of a subgroup of elderly women that is at much higher risk of hip fracture than each test alone would have shown. Increased bone resorption was associated with in-creased risk only for values above the upper limit of premenopausal range, suggesting that bone resorption becomes deleterious for bone strength only when it exceeds the normal physiological threshold. Because bone resorption rate predicts fracture independently of bone mass, these data also suggest that increased bone resorption can lead to increased skeletal fragility by two independent mechanisms (Fig. 3). First, a prolonged increase in bone turnover will lead after several years to a lower bone mass, which is a major determinant of reduced bone strength. Second, increased bone resorption above the upper limit of the normal range may induce microarchitectural deterioration of bone tissue, a major component of bone strength; this is consistent with histological studies of bone remodeling showing a perforation of bone trabeculae by osteoclasts.

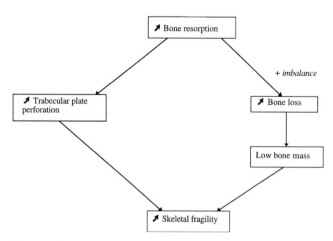

FIGURE 3 The two mechanisms by which increased bone resorption, assessed by relevant biochemical markers, could lead to increased skeletal fragility.

One of the main issues is whether or not the combination of bone markers and bone mass/structure measurements could be useful for the assessment of fracture risk of individual postmenopausal women. Using the data base of the EPIDOS-study, it was found that by defining patients at risk as those with both low BMD (T-score < −2.5) and high urinary CTx, who represented only 16% of the elderly population, the specificity of hip fracture prediction can be increased to a level better than that of either measurement alone [95] (Table III). That combination could be useful in identifying a subset of high-risk patients. Interestingly, this strategy appears to be more cost-effective than bone mineral density measurement alone, as indicated by the 37% lower number of patients to be treated to avoid one fracture per year (Table III). Such an analysis needs to be repeated in other populations of different ages, especially in women in their late 60s and early 70s; such a study would require an even larger population or a longer follow-up because of a lower fracture incidence. The predictive value of bone markers should also be investigated in men. In addition, it would be useful to know if the thresholds of increased bone resorption differ from one type of osteoporotic fracture to another one. Because of economical constraints on healthcare, it appears that effective (but somewhat expensive) treatments that have shown a marked reduction in the incidence of fractures should be targeted to those women that are at higher risk. In those women that are still asymptomatic (i.e., without fractures), combining measurement of a bone marker with a measurement of bone mineral density is likely to be helpful in improving the assessment of fracture risk.

E. Monitoring Treatment

The goal of therapy in a patient with osteoporosis is to prevent further bone loss in order to decrease fracture risk. After 2 years of antiresorptive therapy such as estrogen and bisphosphonate therapy, there is usually a small gain in bone mass on the order of 5–10% at the lumbar spine and less than 5% at the femoral neck and forearm. Given the 1–2% precision error of bone mass measurement of the lumbar spine by the most precise techniques (DXA and SXA) and the expected change in bone mass induced by antiresorptive treatment, it is usually necessary to wait 2 years after initiating therapy to determine, in a single patient, if treatment is effective, i.e., if it increases bone mass significantly. Thus, in most instances, repeating bone mass measurement at a shorter interval may not be helpful for the physician's decision making about treatment efficacy. Antiresorptive therapy induces a 30–60% decrease of markers of resorption and formation that fall within the premenopausal range within 3 to 6 months; the effect is seen earlier for resorption than for formation markers. In a study comparing various doses of intravenous injections of the bisphosphonate ibandronate, there was a clear dose-dependent decrease of urinary CTx after 1 month of treatment that reflected the dose-dependent increase of spinal bone

TABLE III. Combination of Diagnostic Tests for Predicting Hip Fracture

Models	Cutoff for high risk	Women at risk (%)	Sensitivity (%)	Specificity (%)	Odds ratio (95% CI)	Estimated number of women to be treated to avoid one fracture per year[a]
Without diagnostic test						364
A1: Hip BMD	Quartile I (T-score ≤ −2.9)	25	32	78	1.8 (1.0–3.1)	246
A2: Hip BMD	T score ≤ −3.1	16	23	86	1.9 (1.0–3.6)	220
B: CTX	Above premenopausal range (T-score ≥2)	23	36	81	2.4 (1.3–4.3)	196
C: Hip BMD and CTX	WHO definition of osteoporosis (T-score ≤ −2.5) (T-score ≥ 2)	16	30	88[b]	4.1 (2.2–7.2)	156
D: CTX and history of fracture	T-score ≥ +1.5 yes	12	28	94[b]	5.3 (2.5–11.1)	94

[a] Based on the annual incidence of hip fracture at this age (1.1%/yr), the assumption that treatment would reduce fracture risk by 50% and that compliance is 50%.

[b] $p < 0.01$ versus A1 and B.

Case-control analysis (75 hip fractures, 228 controls, two year follow-up) of the EPIDOS Prospective Study.

Thresholds and combinations for a strategy targeting treatment to a subset of high risk patients. At baseline, before fracture, women were classified at risk according to different cutoffs of hip BMD by DXA or urinary CTX. Cutoffs of high risk and combinations of tests were chosen to have a high specificity, at the expense of sensitivity. When the same proportion of women (16%, models A2 and C) were identified by BMD alone (model A2) and by the combination of BMD and CTX (model C), the sensitivity is significantly higher with the combination of both diagnostic tests resulting in a lower number of patients to be treateds to avoid one fracture compared to BMD alone. If DXA is not available, combining CTX with a history of previous fracture (model D), provides better results than using BMD alone. Reprinted from Garnero et al. [95], with permission.

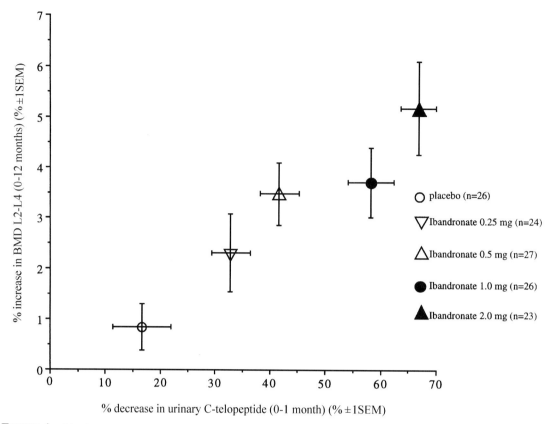

FIGURE 4   Bivariate dose–response curve with respect to changes of urinary C-telopeptide (CTX) after 1 month and changes in lumbar spine BMD after 1 year of treatment by bolus IV injection every 3 months of a placebo or the bisphosphonate ibandronate in osteoporotic women. Reprinted from *Am. J. Med.* **103**, Thiebaud, D., *et al.* Three monthly intravenous injections of ibandronate in the treatment of postmenopausal osteoporosis. Pp. 298–307, copyright 1997, with permission from Excerpta Medica Inc.

mineral density after 12 months of treatment [96] (Fig. 4). Several studies have also shown that the short-term decrease in bone markers correlates with the effects of estrogen [97, 98] and bisphosphonate [99] on bone mass over the subsequent 1–2 years. The rather low correlation between the percent change in bone markers and the percent change in BMD (around 0.4–0.6) indicates that bone markers can not accurately predict the late effect of therapy on BMD at the individual level. In other words, we can not say that if treatment decreases bone markers after 3–6 months by 40%, BMD will increase by 3% after 2 years in that particular patient. However, for the clinician, the primary concern is the identification of nonresponders (i.e., patients who will fail to demonstrate a significant increase of BMD after 1–2 years of treatment). Using a certain cutoff for a significant decrease in bone marker after 3 months of treatment (30–60%, depending on the precision error of the marker), Garnero *et al.* [99] have shown that bone markers are reliable predictors of treatment effect in a single patient. Predictive models, currently in development, using both the level of bone markers after 3–6 months of treatment and the percent change from baseline should improve the reliability of the early detection of nonresponders for whom treatment could be adapted.

V. CONCLUSIONS

Low peak bone mass and fast rate of postmenopausal bone loss, the two main determinants of postmenopausal osteoporosis, are determined by complex interactions of genetic and environmental factors which regulate bone cell activity and bone turnover. Peak bone mass is mainly under genetic influence, whereas estrogen deficiency plays the major role in determining postmenopausal bone loss. Although some polymorphisms in candidate genes, such as those encoding for the $\alpha 1$ chain of type I collagen, have been shown to be associated with BMD level, the differences between genotypes are generally small and not consistent in all studies. Thus, at the present time these polymorphisms can not be used to identify individual patients at risk of osteoporosis. On-going studies will identify polymorphisms in other candidate genes with greater effect and we can envisage a situation where testing a panel of few of these polymorphisms may be clinically useful. Decisions for therapeutic intervention are made in individual patients. The level of intervention will depend on the severity of bone loss measured by DXA, but also on age, the presence or absence of prevalent fractures, associated risk factors, and the benefit/risk ratio of the proposed therapeutic regimen.

For intermediate values (neither high or low) of BMD, the subsequent rate of bone loss is likely to be important in the assessment of risk. The rate of loss can be measured directly by performing a second BMD measurement 4 years later, or it can be estimated at the time of the first measurement by measuring specific biochemical markers of bone turnover. There is an increasing body of evidence suggesting that a high bone turnover rate is associated with increased risk of subsequent fracture, both at the spine and hip, with a predictive value similar to that obtained from bone mass assessment. Combining a measurement of bone mass and bone turnover is likely to improve the assessment of the risk of osteoporosis. Because of the relatively small change of bone mass (as compared to its long-term precision error) in patients treated with antiresorptive therapy, monitoring treatment efficacy by DXA in the individual patient is a challenge. Clearly, repeated bone marker measurement during treatment would be useful for the management of patients with osteoporosis.

References

1. World Health Organization. (1994). Assessment of fracture risk and its application to screening for postmenopausal osteoporosis. W.H.O. *Tech. Rep. Ser.* **843**.
2. Cooper, C., Atkinson, E. J., O'Fallon, W. M. *et al.* (1992). Incidence of clinically diagnosed vertebral fractures: A population-based study in Rochester Minnesota, 1985–1989. *J. Bone Miner. Res.* **7**, 221–227.
3. Gallagher, J. C., Kinyamu, H. K., Fowler, S. E. *et al.* (1998). Calciotropic hormones and bone markers in the elderly. *J. Bone Miner. Res.* **13**, 475–482.
4. Dawson-Hughes, B., Harris, S. S., Krall, E. A., and Dallal, G. E. (1997). Effect of calium and vitamin D supplementation on bone density in men and women 65 years of age or older. *N. Engl. J. Med.* **337**, 670–676.
5. Bonjour, J.-P., Carrie, A.-N., Ferrari, S., Clavien, H., Slosman, D., Theintz, G., and Rizzoli, R. (1997). Calcium-enriched foods and bone mass growth in prepubertal girls: A randomized, double-blind, placebo-controlled trial. *J. Clin. Invest.* **99**, 1287–1294.
6. Bouxsein, M. L., and Marcus, R. (1994). Overview of exercise and bone mass. *Rheum. Dis. Clin. North Am.* **20**, 787–802.
7. Ho, S. C., Wong, E., Chan, S. G., Lau, J., Chan, C., and Leung, P. C. (1997). Determinants of peak bone mass in Chinese women aged 21–40 years. Physical activity and bone mineral density. *J. Bone Miner. Res.* **12**, 1262–1271.
8. Pocock, N. A., Eisman, J. A., Hopper, J. L., Yeates, P. N., Sambrook, P. N., and Ebert, S. (1987). Genetic determinants of bone mass in adults: A twin study. *J. Clin. Invest.* **80**, 706–710.
9. Dequecker, J., Nijs, J., Verstraeten, A., Geusens, P., and Gevers, G. (1987). Genetic determinants of bone mineral content at the spine and radius: A twin study. *Bone* **8**, 207–209.
10. Seeman, E., Hopper, J. L., Bach, L. A., Cooper, M. E., Parkinson, E., McKay, J., and Wong, P. (1989). Reduced bone mass in daughters of women with osteoporosis. *N. Engl. J. Med.* **320**, 554–558.
11. Morisson, N. A., Qi, J. C., Tokita, A., Kelly, L., Crofts, L., Nguyen, T. V., Sambrook, P. N., and Eisman, J. A. (1994). Prediction of bone density from vitamin D receptor alleles. *Nature* **367**, 284–287.
12. Hustmyer, F. G., Peacock, M., Hui, S., Johnston, C. C., and Christian, J. (1994). Bone mineral density in relation to polymorphism at the vitamin D receptor gene locus. *J. Clin. Invest.* **94**, 2130–2134.
13. Garnero, P., Borel, O., Sornay-Rendu, E., and Delmas, P. D. (1995). Vitamin D receptor gene polymorphisms do not predict bone turnover and bone mass in healthy premenopausal women. *J. Bone Miner. Res.* **10**, 1283–1288.
14. Morisson, N. A., Qi, J. C., Tokita, A., Kelly, L., Crofts, L., Nguyen, T. V., Sambrook, P. N., and Eisman, J. A. (1997). Prediction of bone density from vitamin D receptor alleles. *Nature* **387**, 106.
15. Cooper, G. S., and Umbach, D. M. (1996). Are vitamin D receptor polymorphisms associated with bone mineral density? A meta analysis. *J. Bone Miner. Res.* **11**, 1841–1849.
16. Sainz, J., Van Tornout, J. M., Loro, M. L., Sayre, J., Roe, T., and Gilsanz, V. (1997). Vitamin D-receptor gene polymorphisms and bone mineral density in prepubertal American girls of Mexican descent. *N. Engl. J. Med.* **337**, 77–82.
17. Ferrari, S., Rizzoli, R., Chevalley, T., Slosman, D., Eisman, J. A., and Bonjour, J.-P. (1995). Vitamin-D-receptor-gene polymorphisms and change in lumbar-spine bone mineral density. *Lancet* **345**, 423–424.
18. Krall, E. A., Parry, P., Lichter, J. B., and Dawson-Hughes, B. (1995). Vitamin D receptor alleles and rates of bone loss: Influences of years since menopause and calcium intake. *J. Bone Miner. Res.* **10**, 978–984.
19. Gross, C., Eccleshall, R., Malloy, P. J., Villa, M. R., Marcus, R., and Feldman, D. (1996). The presence of a polymorphism at the translation site of the vitamin D receptor gene is associated with low mineral density in postmenopausal Mexican-American women. *J. Bone Miner. Res.* **11**, 1850–1855.
20. Eccleshall, T. R., Garnero, P., Gross, C., Delmas, P. D., and Feldman, D. (1998). Lack of correlation between start codon polymorphism of the vitamin D receptor gene and bone mineral density in premenopausal French women: The OFELY study. *J. Bone Miner. Res.* **13**, 31–35.
21. Kobayashi, S., Inoue, S., Hosoi, T., Ouchi, Y., Shiraki, M., and Orimo, H. (1996). Association of bone mineral density with polymorphism of the estrogen receptor gene. *J. Bone Miner. Res.* **11**, 306–311.
22. Murray, R. E., McGuigan, F., Grant, S. F. A., Reid, D. M., and Ralston, S. H. (1997). Polymorphisms of the interleukin-6 gene are associated with bone mineral density. *Bone* **21**, 89–92.
23. Langdahl, B. L., Knudsen, J. Y., Jensen, H. K., Gregersen, N., and Eriksen, E. F. (1997). A sequence variation: 713-8 delC in the transforming growth factor-beta 1 gene has higher prevalence in osteoporotic women than in normal women and is associated with very low bone mass in osteoporotic women and increased bone turnover in both osteoporotic and normal women. *Bone* **20**, 289–294.
24. Grant, S. F. A., Reid, D. M., Blake, G., Herd, R., Fogelman, I., and Ralston, S. H. (1996). Reduced bone density and osteoporosis associated with a polymorphic Sp1 binding site in the collagen type I α 1 gene. *Nat. Genet.* **14**, 203–205.
25. Roux, C., Dougados, M., Abel, L., Mercier, G., and Lucotte, G. (1998). Association of a polymorphism in the collagen I alpha 1 gene with osteoporosis in French women. *Arthritis Rheum.* **41**, 187–188.
26. Uitterlinden, A. G., Burger, H., Huang, Q., Yue, F., McGuigan, F. E. A., Grant, S. F. A., Hofman, A., van Leewen, J. P. T. M., Pols, H. A. P., Ralston, S. H. (1998). Relation of alleles of the collagen type Ia1 gene to bone density and the risk of osteoporotic fractures in postmenopausal women. *N. Engl. J. Med.* **338**, 1016–1021.
27. Garnero, P., Borel, O., Grant, S. F. A., Ralston, S. H., and Delmas, P. D. (1998). Collagen I alpha 1 Sp1 polymorphism, bone mass and bone turnover in healthy French premenopausal women: The OFELY study. *J. Bone Miner. Res.* **13**, 813–817.
28. Riggs, B. L., Wahner, H. W., Melton, L. J., III, Richelson, L. S., Judd, H. L., and Offord, K. P. (1985). Rates of bone loss in the appendicular and axial skeletons of women: Evidence of substantial bone loss prior menopause. *J. Clin. Invest.* **77**, 1487–1491.
29. Riggs, B. L., Wahner, H. W., Dunn, W. L., Seeman *et al.* (1982). Changes in bone mineral density of the proximal femur and spine with aging. *J. Clin. Invest.* **70**, 716–723.
30. Arlot, M. E., Sornay-Rendu, E., Garnero, P., Vey-Marty, B., and Delmas, P. D. (1997). Pre and postmenopausal bone loss evaluated by DXA at

different skeletal sites in healthy women: The OFELY cohort. *J. Bone Miner. Res.* **12**, 683–690.

31. Pouilles, J. M., Tremollières, F., and Ribot, C. (1993). The effects of menopause on longitudinal bone loss from the spine. *Calcif. Tissue Int.* **52**, 340–343.

32. Hui, S. L., Slemenda, W., Johnston, C. C., and Appledorn, C. R. (1987). Effects of age and menopause on vertebral bone density. *Bone Miner.* **2**, 141–146.

33. Ribot, C., Tremollières, F., Pouilles, J. M., Louvet, J. P., and Guiraud, R. (1988). Influence of the menopause and aging on spinal density in French women. *Bone Miner.* **5**, 89–97.

34. Heldlund, L. R., and Gallagher, J. C. (1989). The effect of age and menopause on bone mineral density of the proximal femur. *J. Bone Miner. Res.* **4**, 639–641.

35. Nordin, B. E. C., Need, A. G., Chatterton, B. E., Horowitz, M., and Morris, H. A. (1989). The relative contributions of age and years since menopause to postmenopausal bone loss. *J. Clin. Endocrinol. Metab.* **70**, 83–88.

36. Christiansen, C., Riis, B. J., and Rodbro, P. (1987). Prediction of rapid bone loss in postmenopausal women. *Lancet* **1**, 1105–1108.

37. Pouillès, J. M., Trémollière, F., and Ribot, C. (1996). Variability of vertebral and femoral postmenopausal bone loss. *Osteoporosis Int.* **6**, 320–324.

38. Jones, G., Nguyen, T., Sambrook, P., Kelly, P. J., and Eisman, J. A. (1994). Progressive loss of bone in the femoral neck in elderly people: Longitudinal findings from the Dubbo osteoporosis epidemiology study. *Br. Med. J.* **309**, 691–695.

39. Prestwood, K. M., Pilbeam, C. C., Burleson, J. A., Woodiel, F. N., Delmas, P. D., Deftos, L. J., and Raisz, L. G. (1994). The short-term effects of conjugated estrogen on bone turnover in older women. *J. Clin. Endocrinol. Metab.* **79**, 366–371.

40. Christian, J. C., Yu, P. L., Slemenda, C. W., and Johnston, C. C., Jr. (1989). Heritability of bone mass: A longitudinal study in aging male twins. *Am. J. Hum. Genet.* **44**, 429–433.

41. Kelly, P. J., Nguyen, T., Hopper, J., Pocock, N., Sambrook, P., and Eisman, J. (1993). Changes in axial bone density with age: A twin study. *J. Bone Miner. Res.* **8**, 11–17.

42. Garnero, P., Arden, N. K., Griffiths, G., Delmas, P. D., and Spector, T. D. (1995). Genetic influence on bone turnover in postmenopausal twins. *J. Clin. Endocrinol. Metab.* **81**, 140–146.

43. Genant, H. K., Cann, C. E., Ettinger, B., and Gordon, G. S. (1982). Quantitative computed tomography of vertebral spongiosa: A sensitive method for detecting early bone loss after oophorectomy. *Ann. Intern. Med.* **97**, 699–705.

44. Slemenda, C., Hui, S. L., Longcope, C., and Johnston, C. C. (1987). Sex steroids and bone mass: A study of changes about the time of menopause. *J. Clin. Invest.* **80**, 261–1269.

45. Gordan, G. S., Picchi, J., and Roof, B. S. (1973). Antifracture efficacy of long term estrogens for osteoporosis. *Trans. Assoc. Am. Physicians* **86**, 326–332.

46. Ettinger, B., Genant, H. K., and Cann, C. E. (1979). Long term estrogen replacement therapy. I. Metabolic effects. *Am. J. Obstet. Gynecol.* **133**, 525–536.

47. Hutchinson, T. A., Polansky, S. M., and Feinstein, A. R. (1979). Postmenopausal estrogens protect against fractures of hip and distal radius. *Lancet* 706–710.

48. Weiss, N. S., Ure, C. L., Ballard, J. H., Williams, A. R., and Dailing, J. R. (1980). Decreased risk of fractures of the hip and lower forearm with postmenopausal use of estrogens. *N. Engl. J. Med.* **303**, 1195–1198.

49. Johnson, R. E., and Specht, E. E. (1981). The risk of hip fracture in postmenopausal females with and without estrogen drug exposure. *Am. J. Public Health* **71**, 138–144.

50. Kreiger, N., Keysley, J. L., Holford, T. R., and O'Connor, T. (1982). An epidemiologic study of hip fracture in postmenopausal women. *Am. J. Epidemiol.* **116**, 141–148.

51. Williams, A. R., Weiss, N. S., Ure, C. L., Ballard, J., and Dailing, J. (1982). Effect of weight, smoking, and estrogen use on the risk of hip and forearm fractures in postmenopausal women. *Obstet. Gynecol.* **60**, 695–699.

52. Kanis, J. A., Johnell, O., Gulberg, B. *et al.* (1992). Evidence for efficacy of drugs affecting bone metabolism in preventing hip fracture. *Br. Med. J.* **305**, 1124–1128.

53. Chow, J., Tobias, J. H., Colston, K. W., and Chambers, T. J. (1992). Estrogen maintains trabecular bone volume in rats not only by suppression of bone resorption but also by stimulation of bone formation. *J. Clin. Invest.* **89**, 74–78.

54. Bain, S. D., Bailey, S. C., Celino, D. L., Lantry, M. M., and Edwards, M. W. (1993). High-dose estrogen inhibits bone resorption and stimulates bone formation in the ovariectomized mouse. *J. Bone Miner. Res.* **8**, 435–441.

55. Oursler, M. J., Kassem, M., Turner, R., Riggs, B. L., and Spelsberg, T. C. (1996). Regulation of bone cell function by gonadal steroids. *In* "Osteoporosis" R. Marcus, D. Feldman, and J. Kelsey. (eds.), pp. 237–260. Academic Press, San Diego, CA.

56. Oursler, M. J., Cortese, P., Keeting, P., Anderson, M. A., Bonde, S. K., Riggs, B. L., and Spelsberg, T. C. (1991). Modulation of transforming growth factor-beta production in normal osteoblast-like cells by 17 beta-estradiol and parathyroid hormone. *Endocrinology* **112**, 313–3320.

57. Pacifici, R., Rifas, L., McCracken, R. *et al.* (1989). Ovarian steroid treatment blocks a postmenopausal increase in blood monocyte interleukine 1 release. *Proc. Natl. Acad. Sci. U.S.A.* **86**, 2398–2402.

58. Pacifici, R., Vannice, J. L., Rifas, L., and Kimble, R. B. (1993). Monocytic secretion of interleukine-1 receptor antagonist in normal and osteoporotic women: Effects of menopause and estrogen/progesterone therapy. *J. Clin. Endocrinol. Metab.* **77**, 1135–1141.

59. McKane, Khosla, S., Peterson, J. M., Egan, K., and Riggs, B. L. (1994). Circulating levels of cytokines that modulate bone resorption. Effects of age and menopause in women. *J. Bone Miner. Res.* **9**, 1313–1318.

60. Cohen-Solal, M. E., Craulet, A. M., Denne, M. A., Gueris, D., Baylink, D., and de Vernejoul, M. D. (1993). Peripheral monocyte culture supernatants of menopausal women can induce bone resorption: Involvement of cytokines. *J. Clin. Endocrinol. Metab.* **77**, 1648–1653.

61. Epstein, S., Bryce, G., Hinnan, J. W. *et al.* (1986). The influence of age on bone mineral regulating hormones. *Bone* **7**, 421–425.

62. Garnero, P., Sornay-Rendu, E., Chapuy, M. C., and Delmas, P. D. (1996). Increased bone turnover in late postmenopausal women is a major determinant of osteoporosis. *J. Bone Miner. Res.* **11**, 337–349.

63. Garnero, P., Hausherr, E., Chapuy, M. C. *et al.* (1996). Markers of bone resorption predict hip fracture in elderly women: The EPIDOS Prospective study. *J. Bone Miner. Res.* **11**, 1531–1538.

64. Chapuy, M. C., Arlot, M. E., Duboeuf, F., Brun, J., Crouzet, B., Arnaud, S., Delmas, P. D., and Meunier, P. J. (1992). Vitamin D3 and calcium to prevent hip fractures in elderly women. *N. Engl. J. Med.* **327**, 1637–1642.

65. Hammerman, M. R. (1987). Insuline-like growth factors and aging. *Endocrinol. Metab. Clin. North Am.* **16**, 995–1008.

66. Nicolas, V., Prewett, V., Bettica, P., Mohan, P., Finfleman, R. D., Baylink, D. J., and Farley, J. T. (1994). Age-related decreases in IGF-I and transforming growth factor beta in femoral cortical bone from both men and women: Implications for loss in aging. *J. Clin. Endocrinol. Metab.* **78**, 1001–1016.

67. Sugimoto, T., Nishiyama, K., Kuribayashi, F., and Chihara, K. (1997). Serum levels of insulin-like growth factor (IGF) I and IGF-Biding protein (IGFBP)-2 and IGFBP-3 in osteoporotic patients with and without spinal fractures. *J. Bone Miner. Res.* **12**, 1272–1279.

68. Ebeling, P. R., Jones, J. D., O'Fallon, W. M., Janes, C. H., and Riggs, B. L. (1993). Short-term effects of recombinant human insulin-like growth factor I on bone turnover in normal women. *J. Clin. Endocrinol. Metab.* **77**, 1384–1387.

69. Grinspoo, S. K., Baum, H. B. A., Peterson, S., and Klibanski, A. (1995). Effects of rhIGF-I administration on bone turnover during short-term fasting. *J. Clin. Invest.* **96**, 900–906.

70. Black, D. J., Cummings, S. R., and Melton, L. J., III. (1992). Appendicular bone mineral and a woman's lifetime risk of hip fracture. *J. Bone Miner. Res.* **7**, 639–646.

71. Cummings, S. R., Black, D. M., Nevitt, M. C. *et al.* (1993). Bone density at various sites for prediction of hip fractures. *Lancet* **341**, 72–75.

72. Gardsell, P., Johnell, O., and Nilsson, B. E. (1989). Predicting fractures in women by using forearm bone densitometry. *Calcif. Tissue Int.* **44**, 235–242.

73. Schott, A. M., Cormier, C., Hans, D. *et al.* (1998). How hip and whole body bone mineral density predict hip fracture in elderly women: The EPIDOS prospective study. *Osteoporosis Int.* (in press).

74. Rosenthall, L., Tenenhouse, A., and Caminis, J. (1995). A correlative study of ultrasound calcaneal and dual-energy x-ray absorptiometry bone measurements of the lumbar spine and femur in 100 women. *Eur. J. Nucl. Med.* **22**, 402–406.

75. Schott, A. M., Weillengener, S., Hans, D., Duboeuf, F., Delmas, P. D., and Meunier, P. J. (1995). Ultrasound discriminates patients with hip fracture equally well as dual energy x-ray absorptiometry and independently of bone mineral density. *J. Bone Miner. Res.* **10**, 243–249.

76. Hans, D., Dargent-Molina, P., Schott, A. M. *et al.* (1996). Ultrasonic heel measurements to predict hip fracture in elderly women: The EPIDOS prospective study. *Lancet* **384**, 511–514.

77. Bauer, D. C., Gluer, C. C., Cauley, J. A. *et al.* (1997). Bone ultrasound predicts fractures strongly and independently of densitometry in older women. *Arch. Intern. Med.* **157**, 629–634.

78. Brown, J. P., Delmas, P. D., Malaval, L. *et al.* (1984). Serum bone Gla-protein: A specific marker for bone formation in postmenopausal osteoporosis. *Lancet* **1**, 1091–1093.

79. Garnero, P., Grimaux, M., Demiaux, B., Preaudat, C., Seguin, P., and Delmas, P. D. (1992). Measurement of serum osteocalcin with a human-specific two-site immunoradiometric assay. *J. Bone Miner. Res.* **7**, 1389–1398.

80. Garnero, P., Grimaux, M., Seguin, P., and Delmas, P. D. (1994). Characterization of immunoreactive forms of human osteocalcin generated in vivo and in vitro. *J. Bone Miner. Res.* **9**, 255–264.

81. Garnero, P., and Delmas, P. D. (1993). Assessment of the serum levels of bone alkaline phosphatase with a new immunoradiometric assay in patients with metabolic bone disease. *J. Clin. Endocrinol. Metab.* **77**, 1046–1053.

82. Hassager, C., Fabbri-Mabelli, G., and Christiansen, C. (1993). The effect of the menopause and hormone replacement therapy on serum carboxyterminal propeptide of type I collagen. *Osteoporosis Int.* **3**, 50–52.

83. Garnero, P., Vergnaud, P., and Delmas, P. D. (1997). Aminoterminal propeptide of type I collagen (PINP) is a more sensitive marker of bone turnover than C-terminal propeptide in osteoporosis. *J. Bone Miner. Res.* **12**(S1), S497.

84. Uebelhart, D., Gineyts, E., Chapuy, M. C., and Delmas, P. D. (1990). Urinary excretion of pyridinium crosslinks: A new marker of bone resorption in metabolic bone disease. *Bone Miner.* **8**, 87–96.

85. Delmas, P. D., Schlemmer, A., Gineyts, E., Riis, B., and Christiansen, C. (1991). Urinary excretion of pyridinoline crosslinks correlates with bone turnover measured on iliac crest biopsy in patients with vertebral osteoporosis. *J. Bone Miner. Res.* **6**, 639–644.

86. Robins, S. P., Woitge, H., Duncan, A., Seyedin, S., and Seibel, M. J. (1994). Immunoassay of deoxypyridinoline: A specific marker of bone resorption. *J. Bone Miner. Res.* **9**, 1643–1649.

87. Risteli, J., Elomaa, I., Niemi, S., Novamo, A., and Risteli, L. (1993). Radioimmunoassay for the pyridinoline cross-linked carboxy-terminal telopeptide of type I collagen: A new serum marker of bone collagen degradation. *Clin. Chem.* **39**, 635–640.

88. Hanson, D. A., Weis, M. A. E., Bollen, A.-M., Maslan, S. L., Singer, F. R., and Eyre, D. R. (1992). A specific immunoassay for monitoring human bone resorption: Quantitiation of type I collagen cross-linked N-teleopeptides in urine. *J. Bone Miner. Res.* **7**, 1251–1258.

89. Bonde, M., Qvist, P., Fledelius, C., Riis, B. J., and Christiansen, C. (1994). Immunoassay for quantifying type I collagen degradation products in urine evaluated. *Clin. Chem.* **40**, 2022–2025.

90. Uebelhart, D., Schlemmer, A., Johansen, J., Gineyts, E., Christiansen, C., and Delmas, P. D. (1991). Effect of menopause and hormone replacement therapy on the urinary excretion of pyridinium crosslinks. *J. Clin. Endocrinol. Metab.* **72**, 367–373.

91. Hansen, M. A., Kirsten, O., Riss, B. J., and Christiansen, C. (1991). Role of peak bone mass and bone loss in postmenopausal osteoporosis: 12 years study. *Br. Med. J.* **303**, 961–964.

92. Ross, P. D., and Knowlton, W. (1998). Rapid bone loss is associated with increased levels of biochemical markers. *J. Bone Miner. Res.* **13**, 297–302.

93. Riis, S. B. J., Hansen, A. M., Jensen, K., Overgaard, K., and Christiansen, C. (1996). Low bone mass and fast rate of bone loss at menopause—equal risk factors for future fracture. A 15 year follow-up study. *Bone* **19**, 9–12.

94. Van Daele, P. L., Seibel, M. J., Burger, H., Hofman, A., Grobbee, D. E., van Leeuwen, J. P., Birkenhäger, J. C., and Pols, H. A. P. (1996). Case control analysis of bone resorption markers, disability and hip fracture risk: The Rotterdam study. *Br. Med. J.* **312**, 482–483.

95. Garnero, P., Dargent-Molina, P., Hans, D., Schott, A.-M., Bréart, G., Meunier, P. J., and Delmas, P. D. (1998). Do markers of bone resorption add to bone mineral density or ultrasonography to predict hip fracture in elderly women: The EPIDOS Prospective Study. *Osteoporosis Int.* **8**, 563–569.

96. Thiébaud, D., Burckardt, P., Kriegbaum, H., Mulder, H., Juttmann, J. R., and Schöter, K. H. (1997). Three monthly intravenous injections of ibandronate in the treatment of postmenopausal osteoporosis. *Am. J. Med.* **103**, 298–307.

97. Riis, B. J., Overgaard, K., and Christiansen, C. (1995). Biochemical markers of bone turnover to monitor the bone mass response to postmenopausal hormone replacement therapy. *Osteoporosis Int.* **5**, 276–280.

98. Chesnut, C. H., Bell, N. H., Clark, G. Y. *et al.* (1997). Hormone replacement therapy in postmenopausal women: Urinary N-telopeptide of type I collagen monitors therapeutic effect and predicts response of bone mineral density. *Am. J. Med.* **102**, 29–37.

99. Garnero, P., Shih, W. J., Gineyts, E. *et al.* (1994). Comparison of new biochemical markers of bone turnover in late postmenopausal osteoporotic women in response to alendronate treatment. *J. Clin. Endocrinol. Metab.* **79**, 1693–1700.

CHAPTER 33

Age-Related Osteoporosis and Skeletal Markers of Bone Turnover

CLIFFORD J. ROSEN   Maine Center for Osteoporosis Research and Education, St. Joseph Hospital, Bangor, Maine 04401

I. INTRODUCTION

Advanced age represents a major risk factor for osteoporosis [1]. Although low bone density accounts for a significant proportion of the risk in older individuals, age is clearly an independent risk factor for fracture [1, 2]. Indeed, the overwhelming majority of osteoporotic fractures occur after age 65 [2, 3]. Therefore, as the general population ages, it is projected that there will be significantly more osteoporotic fractures [3].

The pathogenesis of age-related fractures is complex. A hip fracture in a 75-year-old woman can be related to profound changes in several organ systems. Whether these perturbations are part of the normal aging process, are genetically programmed, or are pathognomic of a larger subset of individuals susceptible because of environmental or hormonal determinants remains to be determined. Still, there is

strong evidence that there are certain phenotypic characteristics of individuals who sustain age-related fractures. This chapter will focus on the metabolic and biochemical changes in the skeleton that characterize age-related osteoporosis. By convention, the term osteoporosis will denote a bone mineral density more than 2.5 standard deviations below young normal mean values, irrespective of fracture history [4, 5]. Age-related osteoporotic fractures will refer to either hip or spine fractures, recognizing that other sites are also susceptible to fractures. No attempt will be made in this chapter to classify individuals based on a single biochemical measure (e.g., parathyroid hormone), because several factors, in concert, reduce skeletal strength. Still, there are final common pathways (e.g., increased bone resorption or decreased bone formation) which are activated by aging and which contribute to skeletal weakness. These pathways are examined in this chapter.

479

II. EPIDEMIOLOGY AND PATHOGENESIS OF AGE-RELATED OSTEOPOROSIS—RELATIONSHIP TO BONE TURNOVER

A. Scope and Severity of the Problem

Based on the WHO definition of osteoporosis (i.e., a bone mineral density [BMD] more than 2.5 standard deviations below mean for a young normal individual), 30% of all postmenopausal women likely have osteoporosis of the hip, spine, or distal forearm [6]. Age has a dramatic impact on the epidemiology of this disease. Although only about 4% of women in their sixth decade have low bone density, the figure for women 80 years or older is approximately 50% [7]. Age-related osteoporosis is manifested as fractures of the hip, wrist, and spine in older individuals. Hip fractures are by far the most dangerous and expensive manifestation of osteoporosis [8–12]. One year mortality from this event can range from 10–30% depending on several factors, including age, gender, nutritional status, body composition, and place of residence [13]. For survivors, 15–50% will require long-term institutional care after their injury [14]. Medical complications such as infections, venous thrombosis, atelectasis, pneumonia, and malnutrition all contribute to morbidity [14]. Even if individuals do return to their previous living situation, many will have impaired quality of life and functional disabilities which persist beyond the first year.

B. Pathogenesis of Age-Related Osteoporosis: Relationship to Bone Remodeling

1. FALLS AND FRACTURES

Older men and women fall frequently, and these events lead to osteoporotic fractures of the spine and hip. Forty percent of individuals over the age of 80 have sustained at least one fall within the last year [15]. Several studies have confirmed that gait, immobility, leg and foot dysfunction, and medications are the greatest risk factors for falling [16]. All of these factors are much more common in the elderly. However, not all falls result in fracture, even in the very old. Among hip fracture patients, falling directly on the hip or falls straight down increase the risk of a hip fracture up to 30-fold [17]. This is in sharp contrast to the relatively modest increased risk for fracture for every one standard deviation decline in BMD. In fact, analysis of case-control and cohort studies reveal that major risk factors for hip fracture, such as body weight (or weight loss after age 50), lower extremity strength, and mobility, are completely independent of BMD [18].

2. PROTEIN-CALORIE MALNUTRITION AND OSTEOPOROTIC FRACTURES

It is estimated that 20–30% of elderly individuals are malnourished [19]. This may be an underestimate because it is difficult to survey the most vulnerable populations. Irrespective of the magnitude of the problem, this is a particularly relevant problem in respect to age-related osteoporosis because many hip fracture patients are undernourished at the time of injury. Since all individuals become catabolic postfracture, poor dietary intake prior to a fracture is an ominous sign. Serum albumin, an indirect indicator of protein/calorie stores, is also a very good predictor of survival following hip fracture [20]. Protein supplementation for hip fracture patients has been shown to improve outcome and reduce hospital stays [21].

Whether there is a causal association between protein-calorie undernutrition and hip fractures is still speculative. However, weight loss, especially after age 50, is a major risk factor for hip fracture in women [22]. In addition, low serum albumin also has been associated with a greater risk of fracture [20]. Because poor muscle mass and impaired balance are important determinants of a subsequent hip fracture, and are also features of protein-calorie malnutrition, this may be one mechanism whereby nutritional status has a major effect on the skeletal response to trauma.

Another potential pathway whereby malnutrition may affect fracture risk is through the insulin-like growth factor (IGF) system. IGF-I is produced by osteoblasts and is a major anabolic factor for bone [23]. It enhances osteoblast proliferation and collagen matrix biosynthesis [23]. Serum and skeletal levels of IGF-I decline with advanced age and may contribute to the pathogenesis of age-related osteoporosis [24]. Serum IGF-I levels also drop dramatically during protein-calorie malnutrition [25]. With poor dietary intake, falling levels of serum IGF-I could contribute to an overall reduction in bone formation which, in turn, may lead to uncoupling of bone turnover. However, the major source of circulating IGF-I is the liver, and numerous hormones, cytokines, and other factors regulate hepatic synthesis of IGF-I [23]. Hence, even though it is relatively easy to extrapolate changes in serum IGF-I to a state of undernutrition, the evidence that poor nutrition alters the skeletal IGF regulatory system is incomplete. Also, there are no published studies in which recombinant IGF-I has been administered to malnourished elders. However, short courses of rhIGF-I to fasting young women and women with anorexia nervosa have led to a marked stimulation of markers of bone formation and bone resorption [26].

In addition to reduced bone formation, malnourished individuals also have high rates of bone resorption. The mechanisms responsible for such an effect are not known. There is evidence from at least one large epidemiological study in elderly women that increased bone resorption is an independent risk factor for fracture [27]. However, individuals who fracture often are vitamin D deficient, live in chronic care facilities, are on multiple medications, and suffer from several disease states simultaneously. Therefore, from a broad perspective, true cause and effect between malnutrition and rapid bone resorption is difficult to ascertain. Certainly secondary hyperparathyroidism, which results from calcium and vitamin D deficiency, can stimulate bone resorption and may be one pathway by which bone resorption is accentuated.

3. CALCIUM INTAKE AND AGE-RELATED OSTEOPOROTIC FRACTURES

Older individuals consume little calcium. Most studies estimate calcium intake in healthy elders to be between 400–600 mg/day [28]. In part, this can be related to reduced milk intake, although use of multiple medications, changes in appetite, taste alterations, and other factors contribute to poor dietary calcium consumption. In addition to minimal calcium intake, the compensatory mechanisms, which are so key to maintaining calcium homeostasis, change dramatically. The renal response to increased serum PTH is attenuated, the skin synthesizes less vitamin D, intestinal mucosal alterations reduce the capacity of the gastrointestinal tract to enhance calcium absorption, 1α-hydroxylase activity declines, and kidney function deteriorates [29]. Due to these age-related alterations, calcium balance studies have established that maintenance of calcium homeostasis in the elderly requires a dietary intake of approximately 1500 mg/day [30].

Bone turnover is accelerated in the elderly and is associated with bone loss. Although initially most investigators postulated that reduced bone formation led to uncoupling in the remodeling unit of very old individuals, it has now been established that bone resorption is markedly enhanced in both men and women beyond the eighth decade of life (31). Markers of bone resorption, such as deoxypyridinoline, have been shown to predict rapid bone loss in older postmenopausal women and this may be an independent risk factor for fracture (see Section IIIB1) [32].

There is probably no single cause for accelerated bone resorption in the elderly, but secondary hyperparathyroidism, which results from reduced calcium and vitamin D intake, must play an important role [33]. In fact, there is a marked rise in serum PTH with age that correlates with declining renal function [34]. This increase in PTH is also associated with several markers of bone turnover [35]. In one of the larger cohort studies of elders, the Baltimore Longitudinal Study of Aging, radial bone mineral density was found to be inversely related to serum PTH [36]. Similarly, in another study, a strong inverse relationship was noted between PTH and femoral bone density [37]. However, Chapuy et al. [38] found in elderly French women that only 4% of the variance in femoral BMD could be related to PTH. Other cross-sectional studies have shown that hip fracture patients have higher levels of serum PTH than age-matched controls but, because of design issues, this could reflect many age-related perturbations in other organ systems [39].

During calcium deficiency states, bone formation is suppressed, almost certainly to protect the supply of calcium in the circulation. However, it is unclear how this occurs within the skeleton. Older individuals are likely to be in a chronic and persistent calcium deficiency state which, in turn, can lead to secondary hyperparathyroidism. It has been noted that one of the IGF binding proteins (IGFBPs) that is synthesized by osteoblasts, IGFBP-4, is markedly increased in elderly individuals [40]. Furthermore, serum PTH levels correlate closely with IGFBP-4 [41]. In addition, PTH can increase IGFBP-4 expression in bone cells, and in one small cross-sectional study, IGFBP-4 binding intensity was significantly higher in hip fracture patients than in controls [42]. Because this binding protein is strongly inhibitory to IGF-I at all concentrations, it is conceivable that impaired bone formation during experimental calcium deficiency relates to increased IGFBP-4 production leading to reduced IGF-I bioactivity. In sum, bone turnover is markedly altered in the elderly when dietary calcium is limited. Clearly, bone resorption is increased by calcium deficiency, but at the same time, bone formation may also be suppressed. Hence, it is not surprising that bone loss could be dramatic in elders with calcium deficient diets.

The strongest evidence to support the thesis that chronic calcium deficiency in the elderly is a major risk factor for osteoporotic fractures is derived from case control and cohort studies. Most of these studies have shown that women consuming the greatest amount of calcium have the lowest risk of hip fracture [43, 44]. Prospective calcium intervention trials in older postmenopausal women also support that premise. In one study, women more than five years past menopause with calcium intakes below 450 mg/day who were randomized to calcium supplementation exhibited virtually no bone loss from three skeletal sites [45]. In another study, calcium supplementation to osteoporotic women with calcium intakes less than 1 gram/day resulted in a reduction in incident vertebral fractures [46]. Besides preserving bone mass and preventing spinal fractures, supplemental calcium in older postmenopausal women also has been shown to reduce the number of nonvertebral fractures [47]. The largest calcium intervention trial involved more than 3000 elderly French women (mean age 84) who were randomized to either 1200 mg of calcium phosphate plus 800 IU of vitamin D or a placebo for three years. Calcium-supplemented women showed a reduction in all nonvertebral fractures and a 30% decrease in hip fractures after only 18 months of treatment [38].

In virtually all the calcium intervention trials in the elderly, calcium (with or without vitamin D) not only preserves bone density but also leads to a reduction in serum PTH [43–47]. These findings suggest that calcium supplementation is effective because it can indirectly block bone resorption via suppression of PTH. However, it is not clear what threshold dose of calcium is required to suppress PTH. One study showed that 2400 mg/day of calcium reduced PTH values to young normal values [48]. Timing of calcium supplementation may also be critical because there is a strong diurnal variation in bone resorption that is more accentuated in the elderly [31, 49]. Further studies will be needed to determine whether calcium supplementation in the evening is more effective than calcium supplements consumed during meals.

In summary, calcium deficiency promotes a state of secondary hyperparathyroidism, which leads to an increase in calcium mobilization from bone stores but also results in suppression in bone formation [50]. Biochemical markers of bone resorption are increased while bone formation indices may be increased, unchanged, or reduced, depending on the surrogate marker. Serum IGF-I levels are low in age-related osteoporotic patients compared to controls, and growing evidence suggests there is a significant increase in serum IGFBP-4. These perturbations could further accentuate the uncoupling of bone turnover and lead to a marked decline in bone mineral density.

4. Vitamin D and Age-Related Osteoporosis

Adequate vitamin D is essential for increasing the efficiency of calcium absorption in the gut [51]. The presence of normal levels of vitamin D can enhance calcium absorption from 15–60% [51, 52]. Most elderly people consume very little calcium because they do not drink milk. Since the major dietary source of vitamin D in the United States is fortified milk, dietary vitamin D insufficiency is very common. It is estimated that upwards of 85% of elderly nursing home residents who do not receive a vitamin supplement have serum levels of 25-hydroxyvitamin D below 20 ng/ml [53]. Classically, a level of 12 ng/ml or lower of serum 25-hydroxyvitamin D is considered vitamin D deficiency [54]. Estimates for the number of chronic care residents who are vitamin D deficient range from 20–70% [54]. In part this can be explained by the fact that most circulating 25-hydroxyvitamin D is derived from percutaneous conversion of provitamin to previtamin D. Previtamin D is metabolically unstable and is converted within hours to vitamin D_3, where it subsequently undergoes 25 hydroxylation in the liver and 1,25 hydroxylation in the kidney. Lack of sunlight, skin coverings, or sunscreen, or living in a region where the apogee of the sun during winter is not high enough to permit the nonenzymatic conversion of provitamin D to previtamin D in the epidermis are all factors which lead to the number of elderly people who are vitamin D sufficient. Also, it should be noted that elderly individuals can only make approximately one-third the vitamin D_3 from skin that younger individuals can produce [55]. Thus, it is the sum of age, poor dietary intake, and limited solar exposure that contribute to the high rate of vitamin D deficiency in the elderly.

Lack of vitamin D reduces the efficiency of calcium absorption in the gut and leads to secondary hyperparathyroidism. A rise in PTH, which is triggered by a drop in serum 25-hydroxyvitamin D and low dietary calcium, can result in increased bone resorption and is the most likely explanation for bone loss in vitamin D insufficient elders. In addition to chronically low dietary calcium intake, PTH is also stimulated by seasonal changes in serum 25-hydroxyvitamin D. In both cross-sectional and longitudinal studies of healthy elderly women living in northern latitudes, serum 25-hydroxyvitamin D can drop by as much as 25% during the winter months [56–58]. This triggers PTH release which, in turn, can lead to an increase in bone turnover as measured by serum osteocalcin and urinary N-telopeptide excretion [59]. The seasonal rise in PTH as a result of a decline in serum 25 hydroxyvitamin D is also responsible for a rise in serum IGFBP-4 observed during the winter in northern New England women [59]. In a two year prospective placebo controlled trial with calcium carbonate, healthy elderly women given a placebo calcium pill demonstrated a 45% increase in urinary N-telopeptide and a 50% increase in osteocalcin during the winter months (Fig. 1a, b) [59]. These changes were directly related to a marked seasonal decline in 25-hydroxyvitamin D and a secondary increase in PTH secretion (Fig. 1c). Surprisingly, elderly women in that study lost nearly 3% of their femoral BMD over six winter months [59]. Based on these data, it is likely that this high rate of bone loss over a relatively short period of time in otherwise healthy elders was related to uncoupling of the bone remodeling cycle as a result of increased bone resorption and decreased bone formation.

Although vitamin D deficiency results in bone loss, it also has other effects which may contribute to increased bone fragility. Low vitamin D reduces mineralization of new bone and, in some cases, can lead to osteomalacia [61]. This may contribute to reduced bone strength. The percentage of elderly women who sustain hip fractures and have osteomalacia is likely to be about 10%, although this is only an estimate because few patients have bone biopsies to verify overt osteomalacia. In several studies, upwards of 30% of osteoporotic women with hip fractures were vitamin D deficient (<12 ng/ml) [62]. This proportion is highly dependent on the geographic site of the study, the origin of the patient (nursing home, hospital, or community), and the general nutritional status of the individual. In addition to reduced bone mineralization, osteomalacia is associated with proximal muscle weakness which is a risk factor for falls and subsequent fracture. Thus, vitamin D may play a major role in several pathophysiologic pathways leading to enhanced skeletal fragility.

5. Vitamin K Deficiency and Age-Related Osteoporosis

Vitamin K is a cofactor for enzymes involved in the post-translational modification of osteocalcin and other bone matrix proteins that bind to hydroxyapatite. In some elderly

A

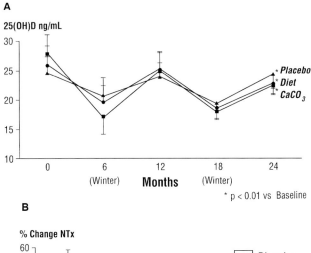

B

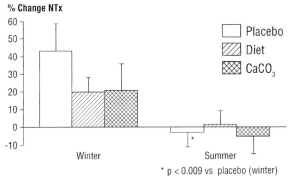

C

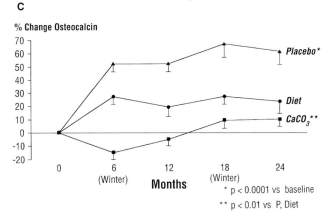

FIGURE 1   (A) Serial changes in serum 25OH vitamin D over a 24 month period in elderly women residing in northern New England. Three groups of women were followed: twenty women receiving placebo calcium, twenty women consuming four glasses of milk/day, and twenty women getting 1000 mg/day of calcium supplements. Baseline calcium intake was approximately 600 mg/day for each group. Mean summer serum 25OH vitamin D levels were statistically different than winter levels for each group at p < 0.01. (B) In the same three groups of women, the winter and summer urine NTX values were averaged for the two years of the study; bone turnover was greatest in the winter for the placebo group (mean 45% increase over baseline) consuming the lowest amount of calcium. During the summer months, bone turnover was negligible. A similar effect was noted for greater trochanteric BMD; winter loss for placebo women was −2.1% versus summer loss, which was negligible (−0.2%). (C) Serial changes in osteocalcin from baseline in three groups of healthy elderly women. Women consuming the least amount of calcium had the greatest increase in osteocalcin, all of which occurred during winter months (adapted from Storm et al. [59]).

patients with osteoporosis, undercarboxylated osteocalcin can be detected in the circulation, and these levels are suppressed by supplementary vitamin K [63]. Also, decreased serum levels of vitamin K (phyloquinone and the menaquinones) have been found in elders who have sustained a hip fracture [64]. In a prospective study of elderly institutionalized women, those women with high levels of undercarboxylated osteocalcin at baseline had a greater likelihood of hip fracture than women with high levels of any other biochemical marker or carboxylated osteocalcin [65]. However, the level of undercarboxylated osteocalcin also correlated with vitamin D status, suggesting that this may be a nonspecific marker of undernutrition.

It is not clear precisely how skeletal or serum vitamin K affects bone remodeling. In one study, urinary calcium loss in some patients with osteoporosis was reduced by vitamin K supplementation [66]. In another study, vitamin K supplementation reduced bone resorption [60]. On the other hand, it is possible that vitamin K may modulate bone formation via matrix biosynthesis. The only prospective fracture study with vitamin K supplementation involved a small cohort of patients with renal failure. That study demonstrated a relationship between vitamin K1 levels and fracture risk [67]. Longitudinal studies are currently underway to further assess the importance of vitamin K in age-related osteoporosis.

In summary, age-related osteoporotic fractures are closely linked to overall nutrition as well as calcium/vitamin D and vitamin K sufficiency. Lack of these dietary factors is associated with increased bone resorption and decreased bone formation. The end result of changes in nutrient intake is uncoupling of the bone remodeling process leading to rapid bone loss and increased skeletal fragility. Seasonal changes in 25-hydroxyvitamin D and PTH accelerate bone resorption and may suppress bone formation. From these perturbations, it is easy to see how accelerated bone loss in the elderly may lead to altered skeletal architecterure and subsequent fractures.

6. HORMONAL DEFICIENCY STATES AND BONE TURNOVER IN THE ELDERLY

a. Overview of Aging and Hormonal Factors   Aging is accompanied by major changes in every hormonal system. Decreased synthesis, altered feedback inhibition, enhanced catabolism, reduced receptor half-life, and postreceptor perturbations can lead to hormonal deficiency or resistance [68]. Such hormonal changes in older individuals are certain to affect bone remodeling. For example, diminution in gonadal steroid production in both males and females can lead to higher rates of bone resorption. Similarly, impaired growth hormone release can lower serum and skeletal IGF-I, thereby affecting bone formation. Age-related increases in PTH have already been examined in relation to calcium and vitamin D availability. Weak adrenal androgens such as DHEA and DHEA-S decline with age, are associated with low serum IGF-I, and may affect both bone resorption and formation

[69]. The major hormonal activators (or suppressors) of bone remodeling are discussed in the following sections.

b. Testosterone Deficiency and Turnover   In men there is a modest decline in total and free testosterone with age [70]. Although this drop is similar to the age-associated reduction in bone mineral density noted among males, cause and effect have never been firmly established. Several cross-sectional studies have indirectly linked testosterone to bone density [71]. However, larger studies have not been able to confirm such a relationship [72]. Certainly, males with frank hypogonadism have low bone mineral density and high rates of bone resorption. In response to parenteral testosterone replacement, these men have an increase in BMD and decreased bone resorption [73]. However, in the aging male without hypogonadism, the evidence that testosterone, or its metabolite dihydrotestosterone, is critical for the maintenance of bone mass is much less clear.

Theoretically, androgens can affect bone turnover in two ways. First, it has been shown that testosterone supplementation blocks cytokine release from osteoblasts, whereas androgen deficiency leads to upregulation of several cytokines including IL-6 [74]. These perturbations are associated with a profound alteration in the rate of bone resorption. Second, there are androgen receptors on osteoblasts, and there is some evidence that androgens can increase osteoblastic activity, independent of their effects on resorption [75]. However, *in vivo* studies with androgen replacement suggest that inhibition of bone resorption is the predominant mechanism of action [76]. Despite these lines of experimental evidence, data from the relatively few prospective studies in men reveal only a very weak relationship between serum testosterone (or free testosterone) and bone mineral density or future fracture [77, 78]. This is also true for postmenopausal women who produce some androgens, including testosterone. Several prospective studies have failed to demonstrate a significant relationship between testosterone and bone density [79]. However, there is preliminary evidence that levels of sex hormone binding globulin may be indirectly related to risk of a hip fracture [80].

c. Estrogen Deficiency and the Aging Skeleton   For more than a half a century the role of estrogen in controlling bone remodeling has been appreciated [81]. However, the effects of estrogens on the aging skeleton have only recently been examined. The conventional approach to the elderly individual with osteoporosis previously consisted exclusively of nonhormonal therapy. However, two recent trials with HRT in older postmenopausal osteoporotic women have established that the bone mineral density response to HRT in elderly women is vigorous and may actually exceed bone mineral density increments in younger women [82, 83]. This had led many investigators to postulate that estrogen deficiency contributes to the pathogenesis of age-related osteoporosis.

In part, an exaggerated skeletal response to estrogen can be traced to baseline indices of bone turnover. In both of the longitudinal trials, one with transdermal and one with oral estrogens, the women undergoing treatment were frankly osteoporotic [82, 83]. Although not measured in the original studies, subsequent evaluations of older osteoporotic women have demonstrated a very high rate of bone turnover accompanied by accelerated bone loss. These studies employed several markers of resorption to demonstrate an age-associated rise in bone turnover [31, 84]. Indeed, high turnover is the most likely explanation for the marked increase in bone density following antiresorptive therapy with estrogens. However, this does not mean that chronic estrogen deprivation causes age-related osteoporotic fractures. This disease is multifactorial and declining estrogen levels may be but one of several permissive factors that increase bone turnover. This hypothesis is reinforced by findings from a prospective study in which endogenous estradiol levels in postmenopausal women were directly correlated with femoral bone mineral density [85]. In sum, older postmenopausal women who are osteoporotic are likely to have relatively high rates of bone turnover and are more responsive to antiresorptive therapy such as estrogen supplementation.

Estrogen concentrations may play a crucial role in the pathogenesis of age-related bone loss in men. The report of a young male with osteoporosis who lacked the alpha estrogen receptor provided the impetus to further examine the relationship between endogenous estrogen production and bone mass in men [86]. The phenotype of that seminal case was a tall man with severe osteopenia whose epiphyses had not fused and who had high normal testosterone levels. Biochemical markers of bone turnover suggested a markedly increased rate of bone resorption, although histomorphometric analysis was not conclusive [86]. Two cases of selective aromatase deficiency in men with a similar phenotype as the estrogen receptor deficient male further support the hypothesis that absence of endogenous estrogen, or its receptor, is associated with low bone density and high bone turnover [87, 88]. In one of those cases, estrogen replacement led to a 25% increase in bone density after one year of treatment [J. Bilezikian, personal communication]. That response would be consistent with the antiresorptive properties of estrogen in patients with high bone turnover. These lines of evidence have pushed investigators to examine the role of endogenous estrogen in healthy men with and without low bone mass. One cross-sectional study has confirmed a very strong correlation between serum estradiol and bone mineral density [89].

In summary, estrogen production may play an important role in restraining bone resorption in males. Heritable or acquired disorders of estrogen synthesis or defects in the estrogen receptor are associated with very low bone mass and heightened bone turnover in men. Whether the gonadal steroids serve a dual function to maintain bone integrity (i.e., to restrict bone resorption but stimulate bone formation) will still need to be proved. However, this concept is relevant for age-related osteoporosis because estrogen levels in men decline with age. Also, the advent of second and third generation selective estrogen receptor modulators raises the possibility of treating high turnover bone loss in the elderly male with an agent such as raloxifene without causing other undue side effects.

d. The Growth Hormone/IGF-I Axis and Age-Related Osteoporosis Advanced age is associated with a decline in the magnitude and frequency of growth hormone surges from the pituitary [90]. This, in part, may be related to waning production of endogenous GH secretagogues or enhanced synthesis of somatostatin. Irrespective of the etiology, less growth hormone secretion means lower concentrations of serum and tissue IGF-I [91]. Although attempts have been made to link age-associated declines in IGF-I with bone loss due to aging, cause and effect have never been established.

Several lines of evidence, however, suggest that growth hormone deficiency could impact bone turnover, thereby affecting the overall rate of bone loss. First, it is recognized that adult growth hormone deficiency (GHD) is associated with low bone mass, and replacement with rhGH can increase bone density by upwards of 5% after three years [92]. Second, several cross-sectional studies have identified a correlation between serum IGF-I and bone density [93, 94]. In two large cohort studies, there is further evidence of an association between IGF-I and age-related osteoporosis. In the Study of Osteoporotic Fractures with over 9000 postmenopausal women, the lowest quartile of IGF-I was associated with the greatest risk of hip fracture [S. Cummings, personal communication]. Furthermore, in a subset of men and women from the Framingham cohort, there was a strong association between quartiles of serum IGF-I and bone mineral density at the spine, hip, and wrist [95]. Third, other components of the IGF regulatory system that are synthesized in the skeleton have been linked to age-related changes in growth hormone secretion. As noted previously, serum levels of IGFBP-4 are increased in older individuals and may be even higher among hip fracture patients [42]. Because this is an inhibitory binding protein which blocks IGF-I action and there is an age-related decline in bone formation, this protein may have pathophysiologic significance. Two IGF binding proteins which are agonists for IGF-I and are synthesized by osteoblasts, IGFBP-3 and IGFBP-5, are also affected by the aging process. IGFBP-3 is the major IGF carrier protein in the circulation and is modulated principally by growth hormone. Elderly individuals show a marked decrease in serum IGFBP-3 [92]. Because several cross-sectional studies have shown a relationship between serum IGFBP-3 and bone mineral density, changes in this binding protein, either locally or systemically, may be important [96, 97]. Similarly, IGFBP-5, an osteoblast-derived IGFBP that binds IGF-I to hydroxyapatite, also shows a decline with age both in the serum and in the skeleton [98].

Like IGFBP-3, IGFBP-5 enhances IGF bioactivity, is related to circulating GH, and increases during peak bone mass acquisition. Hence a combination of changes in several IGFBPs as a result of a relative GH deficiency could alter bone remodeling. Finally, studies in patients who survive a hip fracture reveal a marked decline in lean body mass, bone mineral content, and serum IGF-I in the immediate postoperative period [99]. These changes reflect not only the catabolic state which follows injury, but also the predisposing characteristics of the individuals who fracture. Use of rhGH, GH releasing analogs, or rhIGF-I to reverse some of those changes after surgical intervention are being investigated. These trials might provide important indirect evidence that GH deficiency could contribute to the etiology as well as the morbidity of fractures in the elderly.

In summary, declining skeletal levels of IGF-I, IGFBP-3, and IGFBP-5 due to growth hormone deficiency, and an increase in IGFBP-4 secondary to high PTH levels, may contribute to the process of age-related bone loss and the subsequent fractures which accompany low bone mass. However, because most, if not all, of the components of the IGF regulatory system are under multiple layers of control, it is difficult to assess how changes in a single regulatory component (e.g., growth hormone) perturb the system enough to cause a fracture. For example, nutritional deficiencies can affect not only IGF-I but also synthesis of IGFBPs -1, -3, -4, and -5 as well as IGF receptor expression [25]. Thus, the bioactivity of IGF-I could be affected at several different levels from the ligand all the way to the receptor. Clearly, changes in the hypothalamic-pituitary axis, which modulates GH secretion, could ultimately affect several IGF-rich tissues including bone. These hormonal alterations may ultimately turn out to be major etiologic factors in the pathogenesis of age-related osteoporosis.

7. Genetic Determinants of Age-Related Osteoporosis

Maternal history of a hip fracture is a major and independent risk factor for a future fracture [100]. This would suggest that there might be genetic determinants of fracture that are independent of bone mineral density "genes." Indeed, previous fracture and a maternal history of hip fracture are powerful predictors of subsequent fracture for elderly individuals [100]. However, assessing the genetic determinants of the hip fracture phenotype is daunting for several reasons. First, the onset of hip fractures is almost always after the seventh decade. This makes phenotyping extremely difficult. It also makes family and twin studies almost impossible to conduct. Second, hip fractures are multifactorial in origin. Several different structural, environmental, and hormonal factors contribute to fracture risk. These may include hip axis length, dietary intake of calcium, length of estrogen exposure, relative growth hormone production, serum IGF-I, and a host of other factors. Third, it is unclear that hip fracture represents a continuous variable like bone mineral density. Progress in defining the genetic aspects of osteoporosis has been successful, in part because the phenotype (i.e., bone mineral density) is so easy to characterize. These measurements have opened the door for more sophisticated twin, cohort, and population studies.

Notwithstanding the difficulties inherent in studying the genetic regulation of bone loss in the elderly, most investigators believe there are genetic programs that regulate the onset and severity of age-related osteoporosis. For example, it is possible that with advanced age, GH regulation at the pituitary or hypothalamus level is under the control of genetic determinants. Similarly, it conceivable that certain factors which control bone strength, and thereby contribute to overall skeletal fragility, are programmed for alterations during the aging process. Unfortunately, genetic studies in humans will have to overcome several barriers to isolate such factors. On the other hand, in healthy inbred mouse strains there are clear-cut differences in peak bone mass acquisition that are maintained throughout a lifetime. These differences have allowed investigators to search for bone density "genes" that contribute as much as 80% to the variance in BMD for male and female mice. Independent of estrogen status or environmental factors, some strains of inbred mice lose bone after their first year of life, while others maintain a constant density [101]. These differences are reflected in patterns of bone turnover in that the high density mouse strain has low bone turnover and the low density strain has markedly increased rates of bone resorption.

Mouse models may become particularly useful for studying genetic regulation of age-related bone loss for several reasons. First, inbred strains of mice produce innumerable sets of identical "twins". Second, the mouse genome has more than 9000 markers that facilitate genotyping and permit tracking of specific loci after breeding. Third, acquisition and maintenance of bone mass in mice parallel the same processes in humans. Fourth, the finite life span of a mouse (i.e., two years) makes it amenable to studies on genetic regulation of bone loss. Finally, there is a 65% sequence homology between mouse and man, supporting the notion that finding mouse "osteoporosis genes" will facilitate discovery of similar genes in humans.

III. MARKERS OF BONE TURNOVER AND AGE-RELATED OSTEOPOROSIS—CLINICAL IMPLICATIONS

A. Overview

Bone turnover is altered in patients with age-related osteoporosis. As noted previously, osteoporotic women have higher rates of bone turnover than age-matched controls. Similarly, elderly women with osteoporotic fractures have greater rates of bone turnover than elders without fracture, based on studies of biochemical markers such as urinary N-telopeptide, C-telopeptide, or deoxypyridinoline [31]. Such changes have been confirmed by bone histomorphometry. Although there is strong evidence that aging is associated with greater bone resorption than previously appreciated, the difference in bone formation markers between osteoporotic and nonosteoporotic elders is much less clear. Bone formation by histomorphometry is reduced in some elderly osteoporotic individuals while biochemical markers of formation are variable. Osteocalcin levels are increased in most elderly women with fractures, but this marker may reflect turnover as much as expression of osteoblast activity. Bone specific alkaline phosphatase and procollagen peptide concentrations can be high, normal, or low in most patients with age-related osteoporosis. Serum IGF-I, IGFBP-3, and IGFBP-5 are synthesized by osteoblasts, but serum levels of these peptides can not be used to extrapolate activity in the bone remodeling unit. Several other nonspecific skeletal parameters are altered in elderly women who sustain fractures, but these can not be used to determine how remodeling is altered. In addition, more longitudinal studies will be needed to assess the predictive value for fracture of these markers. Table I summarizes several variables that are altered in age-related osteoporosis and their relationships to bone loss and fracture prediction.

TABLE I.   Age-Related Osteoporosis: Markers of Bone Turnover and Calciotropic Hormones

Skeletal marker	Effects on remodeling	Bone loss	Fracture prediction
↓Serum 25OHD	↓formation; ↑resorption	++++	±
↓Serum Vit K	↓formation	+1/2	−
↑Serum PTH	↓formation; ↑resorption	++++	±
↓Serum albumin	no effect	−	±
↑Urine NTX	↑resorption	++++	±
↑Urine DPD	↑resorption	++++	++
↑Urine CTX	↑resorption	++++	++
↑Serum OC	↑turnover	+++	−
↑BSAP	↑turnover	+	−
↑PICP	↑turnover	+	−
↑IGF-I	?formation	−	?+
↑IGFBP-4	↓formation	−	?+
↓IGFBP-3, -5	↓formation	−	??

Abbreviations refer to the various markers as noted below; + means the strength of evidence that a marker can predict bone loss; − means no evidence; ± means possible; ? means that it is conceivable although there are no data. 25OHD, 25 hydroxyvitamin D; PTH, parathyroid hormone; NTX, N-telopeptide; DPD, free deoxypyridinoline; CTX, C-telopeptide; OC, osteocalcin; BSAP, bone specific alkaline phosphatase; PICP, procollagen peptide; IGF-I, insulin like growth factor-I; IGFBP-4, insulin-like growth factor binding protein-4; IGFBP-3, -5, insulin-like growth factor binding protein-3, -5.

B. Clinical Application of Biochemical Markers in the Elderly

Biochemical markers are potentially very useful in understanding the pathophysiology of age-related osteoporosis, as well as diagnosing and treating older individuals. In particular, there are three clinically relevant indications for utilizing bone markers in the older adult population: (1) to monitor bone loss in the postmenopausal period, (2) to assess overall fracture risk, and (3) to monitor response to therapy.

1. MONITORING BONE LOSS WITH BIOCHEMICAL MARKERS

Bone loss can be measured by repetitive bone density determinations. However, this does not provide immediate feedback to the patient and can be expensive as well as inconvenient. In general, women during and after menopause lose approximately 1% of their spine bone density per year. However, as many as one-third of postmenopausal women lose bone at a rate exceeding 1% a year during the immediate menopausal period [102]. Biochemical markers can detect those women who are considered "rapid losers" (i.e., those losing upwards of 3–5% of bone per year) and can predict those women most likely to respond to HRT [103].

Similar data are now available regarding bone turnover in elderly individuals. Rapid bone loss is common in many older men and women. Ensrud *et al.* [104] demonstrated, in the Study of Osteoporotic Fractures (SOF), that bone loss increases with advancing age. Rates of bone loss from the spine and hip can exceed 1% per year after age 70 and these changes can be detected by markers of bone turnover. In a cross-sectional study of 653 healthy European women, including many who were more than 20 years beyond menopause, the highest levels of OC, NTX, CTX, and BSAP were found in those individuals who were in the lowest tertile of BMD (Fig. 2) [31]. In fact, a combination of three biochemical markers accounted for more than 50% of the variance in BMD noted in elderly individuals (see Fig. 2, 3) [31]. Similarly, in one of the largest ongoing prospective studies of elderly postmenopausal women in Europe (EPIDOS), the bone markers osteocalcin, CTX, and BSAP all were significantly greater in older than younger women. Furthermore, those marker values were inversely related to hip BMD (27). It is now estimated that skeletal turnover rates may be as much as 85% higher in older women with low bone mass compared to elderly women with normal bone density.

Interpretation of biochemical markers of bone resorption has always been plagued by the relatively large noise to signal ratio, especially in comparison to DXA. This analytical variability has made single determinants of turnover to assess risk of bone loss in elderly subjects somewhat problematic. For resorption markers, the coefficient of variation for free deoxypyridinoline (DPD) is somewhat less than 15% and, similarly, N-telopeptide measurements in an established lab-

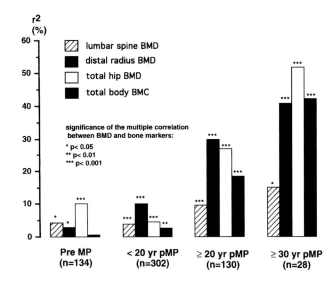

FIGURE 2   Contribution of the bone turnover rate to bone mass as a function of menopausal status and skeletal site. To explain the variation of BMC (total body) and BMD (total hip, distal radius, and lumbar spine), stepwise regression analyses including height, age, years since menopause, and bone markers (serum OC, serum B-ALP, serum PICP, urinary CTX, and urinary NTX) as independent variables were performed in premenopausal women (pre-MP) and in three postmenopausal groups: women within 20 years of menopause (<20 years pMP; mean age, 59 years), women 20 years since menopause and over (≥20 years pMP; mean age, 75 years), and women 30 years postmenopause and over (≥30 years pMP; mean age, 81 years). Each bar represents the square of the multiple correlation coefficient between bone markers that significantly contributed to BMD variance and BMD measured at several skeletal sites. Thus, each bar represents the percentage of BMC and BMD variation that is explained by the bone turnover rate (from Garnero *et al.* [31] with permission).

oratory have a coefficient of variation of approximately 20% [57, 103]. Bollen *et al.* [105] demonstrated that in elderly men and women (57 men, 69 women; mean age 73 years), urinary N-telopeptide values were consistent over time, as assessed by coefficient of concordance, which was 0.74 for women and 0.79 for men. In particular, among those subjects in the highest quartile for NTX at baseline, 82% of women and 64% of men remained within that quartile in the second year and 71% of both groups in the third year. In that same longitudinal study, smoking, physical activity, race, and BMI did not affect urine NTX values [105].

Still, there are several important variables that can affect bone turnover and relate to biologic variation in the test, independent of urinary collection or creatinine excretion. For example, osteocalcin and urinary cross-links exhibit diurnal variation with amplitudes of up to 30% [106]. Moreover, these changes are accentuated in the elderly [31]. However, probably one of the most important variables for people living in the northern hemisphere is the effect of seasonal variation. Several prospective studies have noted that turnover markers in the elderly increase during winter months [54–59]. This can be attributed to a decline in serum 25-hydroxyvitamin D levels as a result of reduced sunlight exposure. In turn, this leads to secondary hyperparathyroidism which may

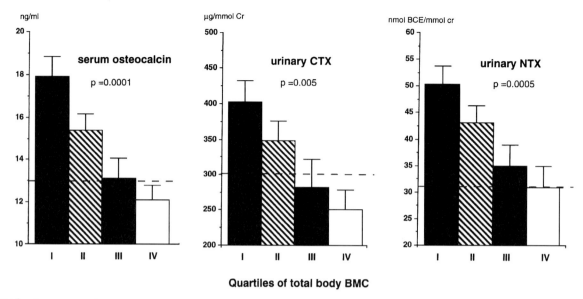

FIGURE 3   Bone turnover in elderly women as a function of quartiles of total body BMC. Whole body BMC measured with DXA was divided in quartiles with increasing value from quartile I to quartile IV. Bars represent the mean and 1 S.E.M. of bone marker levels in each quartile of BMC. NTX, cross-linked N-telopeptide of type I collagen; CTX, type I collagen C-telopeptide breakdown products. *p* values apply to the comparison of trend in bone marker levels for increasing total body BMC, assessed by analysis of variance. The dashed line represents the mean +1 S.D. of premenopausal women (from Garnero *et al.* [31] with permission).

accelerate bone turnover [54–59, 107]. In a cross-sectional study of nearly 600 European adults (50–81 years of age), Woitge *et al.* [57] noted that by multivariate regression analyses, seasonal variations accounted for more of the variability in biomarkers (up to 12%) than any of the other anthropometric or lifestyle factors except age. Thus, age-associated bone loss is related to increased bone turnover, which can be detected by several biochemical markers. Variability in bone turnover among elderly individuals depends on several factors besides age; these include calcium intake, seasonal effects, timing of urine and serum collection, and coexistence of other metabolic diseases. Still, use of one or more biochemical markers to predict subsequent bone loss remains both practical and acceptable.

2. ASSESSING FRACTURE RISK FROM BIOCHEMICAL MARKERS

For the same bone mineral density, older individuals have a much greater risk of fracture. In part, this may be due to the higher rates of bone turnover which lead to bone loss, disruption of trabecular networks, and reduced connectivity. Hence, a relationship between biochemical markers of bone turnover and fracture risk has been investigated. There is significant variation in biochemical markers among individual osteoporotic subjects. This limits, for the present time, definitive conclusions about relative risk based on a single biochemical marker. However, there are several provocative studies that are important. For example, in hip fracture patients sampled immediately after the injury, bone resorption markers were found to be markedly increased [108]. Although

this could be a function of other factors which affect hip fracture risk, including decreased mobility, weight loss, protein undernutrition, or acute trauma, there is certainly a suggestion that turnover might be increased in patients sustaining a hip fracture. Stronger data are available from prospective studies of older women in large cohorts. For example, in a 12 year follow-up study, Hansen *et al.* [109] reported that vertebral fractures occurred most commonly in those subjects with the highest rate of bone turnover as measured by osteocalcin. In one of the largest prospective study to date, EPIDOS, which includes more than 7500 women, baseline urinary C-telopeptide (CTX) and free deoxypyridinoline (DPD) in subsequent hip fracture patients were noted to be significantly greater than age-matched controls [27]. Moreover, for CTX values above the premenopausal range, there was a two-fold greater risk of hip fracture which was independent of femoral bone mineral density and mobility status. When the two risk factors were combined (i.e. low femoral BMD and high CTX), the relative risk of a hip fracture increased nearly five fold. On the other hand, in this cohort, markers of bone formation were not predictive of hip fracture risk. However, in a Swedish population study, a decrease in the carboxy-terminal propeptide of collagen (PICP) was associated with a greater risk of future fracture [110]. Results similar to those found in the EPIDOS study were earlier reported in the ROTTERDAM study [111], although in this study, no data on BMD measurements were provided.

In summary, elderly people, especially those who are calcium deficient, can suffer rapid bone loss. This is principally related to an increase in bone resorption. Increased bone turnover may be associated with a greater risk of vertebral and femoral fractures independent of bone density, although the mechanisms responsible for the structural changes which result from accelerated bone turnover have not been precisely delineated. These data would suggest that one mechanism whereby antiresorptive therapy may reduce fracture risk is through reduction in bone turnover. Whether this effect is more important than a secondary rise in bone mineral density remains to be determined.

3. MONITORING ANTIOSTEOPOROSIS THERAPY WITH MARKERS

The gold standard for assessing the effects of treatment on bone mass is follow-up bone density measurements. The timing and frequency of repeat determinations remain major issues not only scientifically but also from a cost-effectiveness standpoint. Because current therapy for osteoporosis centers on inhibiting bone turnover with agents such as calcium, calcitonin, estrogens, or bisphosphonates, baseline and follow-up biochemical markers of turnover could be particularly useful. In fact, almost all the antiosteoporotic agents cause a marked decrease in bone resorption which is detectable by conventional assays. In healthy early postmenopausal women, Rosen et al. [103] reported that the percent change in NTX from baseline to six months was the strongest predictor of subsequent spine BMD. Similarly, Riis et al. [112] reported that bone turnover markers declined by 50–100% in postmenopausal women treated with HRT for at least six months. For bisphosphonate-treated older postmenopausal women, urinary markers of resorption declined by at least 50% within three months of alendronate therapy. A marked decline in bone resorption indices has also been noted in women treated with nasal calcitonin [113]. Like resorption indices, formation markers are also suppressed by antiresorptive therapy. Garnero et al. [114] reported very significant correlations between the percent change in formation markers (BSAP, OC, and PICP) after three months of alendronate and spinal BMD at 24 months.

It should be noted that changes in biochemical markers in response to antiosteoporosis therapies may differ by treatment regimen and vary considerably even in the same individual. For example, bisphosphonates decrease urinary excretion of peptide-bound collagen products (NTX, CTX) without changing free cross-link excretion [115]. On the other hand, HRT suppresses both free and peptide-bound cross-links to the same extent. The problem of biologic variation for markers was alluded to earlier and remains a major concern for clinicians who want to use sequential markers as an indicator of therapeutic efficacy. Signal to noise ratios can be enhanced by reducing intrinsic variability in measurements. For example, either 24-hour sampling or collecting second void two hour morning samples (i.e. the time of peak excretion) reduces intersample variation. Bone turnover changes due to seasonal variation also should be considered. Still, most people exhibit more than a 50% decline in bone resorption markers during therapy with calcitonin, estrogen, or the bisphosphonates. Hence, some level of confidence can be attained in most situations if there is consistent suppression of bone resorption and the patient is compliant with the medication.

IV. SUMMARY

Bone turnover is increased in elderly individuals. In part this can be related to reduced calcium and vitamin D intake, as well as other environmental variables. Age is an independent predictor of an osteoporotic fracture, and now data suggest that accelerated bone turnover itself may predispose an individual to future fractures. Still, it is not clear yet that a single marker of bone turnover or a calciotropic hormone will be able to predict which elderly individual will sustain an osteoporotic fracture. Because this disorder is multifactorial in origin, there are a host of parameters which can be used to identify those patients at greatest risk. Some of these indices will help provide insight into the pathogenesis of this disease and could be useful in following patients undergoing treatment with antiresorptive drugs.

References

1. Hui, S. L., Slemenda, C. W., and Johnston, C. C. (1988). Age and bone mass as predictors of fracture in a prospective study. *J. Clin. Invest.* **81**, 1804–1809.
2. Kiel, D. P. (1995). The approach to osteoporosis in the elderly patient. *In* "Osteoporosis: Diagnostic and Therapeutic Principles" (C. J. Rosen, ed.), pp. 225–2388. Humana Press, Totowa, NJ.
3. Melton, L. (1993). Hip fractures. A worldwide problem today and tomorrow. *Bone* **14**, S1–S8.
4. Miller, P. R., Bonnick, S. M., and Rosen, C. J. (1996). Consensus of an international conference on the clinical utilization of bone mineral density measurements. *Calcif. Tissue Int.* **58**, 207–214.
5. Kanis, J., Melton, L., Christiansen, C. C., Johnston, C., and Khaltaev, N. (1994). The diagnosis of osteoporosis. *J. Bone Miner. Res.* **9**, 1137–1141.
6. Cummings, S. R., Kelsey, J., Nevitt, M., and O'Dowd, K. (1985). Epidemiology of osteoporosis and osteoporotic fractures. *Epidemiol. Rev.* **7**, 178–208.
7. Looker, A., Johnston, C. C., Wahner, H., Dunn, W., Calvo, M., Harris T., Heyse, S., and Lindsay, R. (1995). Prevalence of low femoral bone mineral density in older U.S. women. *J. Bone Miner. Res.* **10**, 796–802.
8. Cummings, S. R., Black, D., and Rubin, S. (1989). Lifetime risks of hip and vertebral fracture among postmenopausal women. *Arch. Intern. Med.* **149**, 2445–2448.
9. Cooper, C., Campion, G., and Melton, L. (1992). Hip fractures in the elderly: A worldwide projection. *Osteoporosis Int.* **2**, 285–289.
10. Melton, L. J. (1995). How many women have osteoporosis now? *J. Bone Miner. Res.* **10**, 175–177.
11. Wasnich, R. D., Davis, J. W., and Ross, P. D. (1995). Spine fracture risk is predicted by non-spine fractures. *Osteoporosis Int.* **4**, 1–5.
12. Ray, N. F., Chan, J. K., Thamer, M., and Melton, L. J. (1997). Medical

expenditures for the treatment of osteoporotic fractures in the U.S. in 1995: Report from the NOF. *J. Bone Miner. Res.* **12**, 24–35.

13. Parker, M., and Palmer, C. (1995). Prediction of rehabilitation after hip fracture. *Age Ageing* **24**, 96–98.

14. Keene, G., Parker, M., and Pryor, G. (1993). Mortality and morbidity after hip fractures. *Br. Med. J.* **307**, 1248–1250.

15. Campbell, A. J., Borrie, M. J., and Spears, G. F. (1989). Risk factors for falls in a community based prospective study of people 70 years of age and older. *J. Gerontol.* **44**, M112–M117.

16. Tinetti, M. E., Speechley, M., and Gunter, S. F. (1988). Risk factors for falls among elderly persons living in the community. *N. Engl. J. Med.* **319**, 1701–1707.

17. Nevitt, M. C., Cummings, S. R., and Hudes, E. S. (1991). Risk factors for injurious falls: A prospective study. *J. Gerontol.* **56M**, 164–171.

18. Greenspan, S. L., Myers, E. R., Maitland, L. A., Resnick, N. M., and Hayes, W. C. (1994). Fall severity and bone mineral density as risk factors for hip fracture in ambulatory elderly. *JAMA, J. Am. Med. Assoc.* **271**, 128–133.

19. Vellas, B., Baumgarter, S. J., Wayne, S. J., Concelcao, C., Lafont, J. L., Albarede, J. L., and Garry, P. J. (1992). Relationship between malnutrition and falls in the elderly. *Nutrition* **8**, 105–108.

20. Heaney, R. P. (1993). Nutritional factors in osteoporosis. *Annu. Rev. Nutr.* **13**, 287–316.

21. Bastow, M. D., Rawlings, J., and Allison, S. P. (1983). Benefits of supplementary tube feeding after fractured neck of femur. *Br. Med. J.* **287**, 1589–1592.

22. Ceder, L., Thorngren, K. G., and Wallden, B. (1980). Prognostic indicators and early home rehabilitation in elderly patients with hip fractures. *Clin. Orthop. Relat. Res.* **152**, 173–184.

23. Rosen, C. J., Donahue, L. R., and Hunter, S. J. (1994). IGFs and bone: The osteoporosis connection. *Proc. Soc. Exp. Biol. Med.* **206**, 83–102.

24. Donahue, L. R., Hunter, S. J., Sherblom, A. P., and Rosen, C. J. (1990). Age-related changes in serum IGF binding proteins in women. *J. Clin. Endocrinol. Metab.* **71**, 575–579.

25. Estivariz, C. F., and Ziegler, T. R. (1997). Nutrition and the IGF system. *Endocrine* **7**, 65–71.

26. Grinspoon, S. K., Baum, H. B. A., Peterson, S., and Klibanski, A. (1995). Effects of rhIGF-I adminsitration on bone turnover during short-term fasting. *J. Clin. Invest.* **96**, 900–905.

27. Garnero, P., Hausherr, E., Chapuy, M. C., Marcelli, C., Grandjean, H., Muller, C., Cormier, C., Bréart, G., Meunier, P. J., and Delmas, P. D. (1996). Markers of bone resorption predict hip fracture in elderly women: The EPIDOS prospective study. *J. Bone Miner. Res.* **11**, 1531–1538.

28. NIH Consensus Conference. (1995). Optimal calcium intake. Bethesda Med *JAMA, J. Am. Med. Assoc.* **272**, 1942–1948.

29. McKane, W., Khosla, S., Egan, K., and Riggs, B. L. (1996). Role of calcium intake in modulating age-related increases in PTH and bone resorption. *J. Clin. Endocrinol. Metab.* **81**, 1699–1703.

30. Heaney, R. P. (1991). Effects of calcium on skeletal development, bone loss and risk of fractures. *Am. J. Med.* **91**, 23S–28S.

31. Garnero, P., Sornay-Rendu, E., Chapuy, M. C., and Delmas, P. D. (1996). Increased bone turnover in late postmenopausal women is a major determinant of osteoporosis. *J. Bone. Miner. Res.* **11**, 337–349.

32. Ross, P. D., and Knowlton, W. (1998). Rapid bone loss is associated with increased levels of biochemical markers. *J. Bone. Miner. Res.* **13**, 297–302.

33. Dresner-Pollak, R., Parker, R. A., Poku, M., Thompson, J., Seibel, M. J., and Greenspan, S. L. (1996). Biochemical markers of bone turnover reflect femoral bone loss in elderly women. *Calcif. Tissue Int.* **59**, 328–333.

34. Orwoll, E., and Meier, D. (1986). Alterations in calcium, vitamin D and PTH physiology in normal men with aging. *J. Clin. Endocrinol. Metab.* **63**, 1262–1269.

35. Ledger, G., Burritt, M., Kao, P., O'Fallon, W., Riggs, B. L., and Khosla, S. (1994). Abnormalities of PTH secretion in elderly women that are reversible by short term therapy with 1,25 dihydroxyvitamin D. *J. Clin. Endocrinol. Metab.* **79**, 211–216.

36. Sherman, S., Hollis, B., and Tobin, J. (1990). Vitamin D status and related parameters in a healthy population: The effects of age, sex and season. *J. Clin. Endocrinol. Metab.* **71**, 405–413.

37. Compston, J., Silver, A., Croucher, P., Brown, R., and Woodhead, J. (1989). Elevated serum PTH in elderly patients with hip fracture. *Clin. Endocrinol.* **31**, 557–672.

38. Chapuy, M. C., Arlot, M. E., Duboeff, F., Brun, J., Crouzet, B., Arnaud, S., Delmas, P. D., and Meunier, P. J. 1992. Vitamin D and calcium to prevent hip fractures in elderly women. *N. Engl. J. Med.* **327**, 1637–1642.

39. Kamel, S., Brazier, M., Picar, C., Boitte, F., Sarzason, L., Desmet, G., and Sebert, J. L. (1994). Urinary excretion of pyridinoline cross-links measured by immunoassay and HPLC techniques in normal subjects and elderly patients with vitamin D deficiency. *Bone Miner.* **26**, 197–208.

40. Mohan, S., Farley, J. R., and Baylink, D. J. (1995). Age-related changes in IGFBP-4 and IGFBP-5 in human serum and bone; implications for bone loss with aging. *Prog. Growth Factor Res.* **6**, 465–473.

41. Mohan, S., and Baylink, D. J. (1997). Serum IGFBP-4 and IGFBP-5 in aging and age-associated diseases. *Endocrine* **7**, 87–91.

42. Rosen, C. J., Donahue, L. R., Hunter, S. J., Holick, M., Kavookjian, H., Kirschenbaum, A., Mohan, S., and Baylink, D. J. (1992). The 24/25 kDa serum IGFBP is increased in elderly women with hip and spine fractures. *J. Clin. Endocrinol. Metab.* **74**, 24–27.

43. Holbrook, T., Barrett-Connor, E., and Wingard, D. (1988). Dietary calcium and risk of hip fracture: A 14 year prospective study. *Lancet* **2**, 1046–1049.

44. Wickham, C., Walsh, K., Cooper, C., Barker, D., Margewatts, B., Morris, J., and Bruce, S. (1989). Dietary calcium, physical activity and risk of hip fracture: A prospective study. *Br. Med. J.* **299**, 889–892.

45. Dawson-Hughes, B., Dallal, G. E., Krall, E., Sadowski, L., Sahyoun, N., and Tannenbaum, S. (1990). A controlled trial of the effect of calcium supplementation on bone density in postmenopausal women. *N. Engl. J. Med.* **323**, 878–888.

46. Recker, R. R., Hinders, S., Davies, M., Heaney, R. P., Stegman, M. R., Lappe, J. M., and Kimmel, D. B. (1996). Correcting calcium nutritional deficiency prevents spine fractures in elderly women. *J. Bone. Miner. Res.* **11**, 1961–1966.

47. Dawson-Hughes, B., Harris, S. S., Krall, E. A., and Dallal, G. E. (1997). Effect of calcium and vitamin D supplementation on bone density in men and women 65 years of age and older. *N. Engl. J. Med.* **337**, 670–676.

48. McKane, W., Khosla, S., Egan, K., and Riggs, B. L. (1996). Role of calcium intake in modulating age-related increases in PTH and bone resorption. *J. Clin. Endocrinol. Metab.* **81**, 1699–1703.

49. Ju, H.-S. J., Leung, S., Brown, B., Stringer, M. A., *et al.* (1997). Comparison of analytic performance and biological variability of three bone resorption assays. *Clin. Chem.* **43**, 1570–1576.

50. Prince, R. l. (1997). Diet and the prevention of osteoporotic fractures. *N. Engl. J. Med.* **337**, 701–702.

51. Holick, M. F. (1994). Vitamin D: New horizons for the 21st century. *Am. J. Clin. Nutr.* **60**, 619–630.

52. Reichel, H., Koeffler, H. P., and Norman, A. W. (1980). The role of the vitamin D endocrine system in health and disease. *N. Engl. J. Med.* **320**, 981–991.

53. Gallagher, J. C., Riggs, B. L., and Eisman, J. (1996). Intestinal calcium absorption and serum vitamin D metabolites in normal subjects and osteoporotic patients. *J. Clin. Invest.* **64**, 729–736.

54. Webb, A. R., Pilbeam, D., Hanfin, N., and Holick, M. F. (1989). A one year study to evaluate the roles of exposure to sunlight and diet on

the circulating concentrations of 25OH D in an elderly population in Boston. *J. Clin. Nutr.* **125**, 1692–1697.

55. Holick, M. F., Matsuokoa, L. Y., and Wortsman, J. (1989). Age, vitamin D and solar ultraviolet radiation. *Lancet* **4**, 1104–1105.

56. Krall, E., Sahyoun, N., Tannenbaum, S., Dallal, G., and Dawson-Hughes, B. (1989). Effect of vitamin D intake on variations in PTH secretion in postmenopausal women. *N. Engl. J. Med.* **321**, 1777–1783.

57. Woitge, H. W., Schneidt-Nave, C., Kissling, C., Leidig-Bruckner, G., Meyer, K., Grauer, A., Scharla, S. H., Ziegler, R., and Seibel, M. J. (1998). Seasonal variation of biochemical indexes of bone turnover: Results of a population based study. *J. Clin. Endocrinol. Metab.* **83**, 68–75.

58. Rosen, C. J., Morrison, A., and Zhou, H. (1994). Elderly women in northern New England exhibit seasonal changes in bone mineral density and calciotropic hormones. *Bone Miner.* **25**, 83–92.

59. Storm, D., Eslin, R., Porter, E. S., Musgrave, K., Vereault, D., Patton, C., Kessenich, C., Mohan, S., Chen, T., Holick, M. F., and Rosen, C. F. (1998). Calcium supplementation prevents seasonal bone loss and changes in biochemical markers of bone turnover in elderly New England women: A randomized placebo-controlled trial. *J. Clin. Endocrinol. Metab.* **83**, 3817–3825.

60. Hara, K., Akiyama, Y., Nakamura, T., Murota, S., and Morita, I. (1995). The inhibitory effect of vitamin K2 on bone resorption may be related to its side chain. *Bone* **16**, 179–184.

61. Doppelt, S. H., Neer, R. M., Daly, M., Bourret, L., Schiller, A., and Holick, M. F. (1983). Vitamin D deficiency and osteomalacia in patients with hip fractures. *Orthop. Trans.* **7**, 512–513.

62. Holick, M. F. (1995). Vitamin D in health and prevention of metabolic bone disease. *In* "Osteoporosis: Diagnostic and Therapeutic Principles" (C. J. Rosen, ed.), pp. 29–35. Humana Press, Totowa NJ.

63. Szulc, P., Arlot, M., Chapuy, M. C., Duboeuf, F., Meunier, P. J., and Delmas, P. D. (1994). Serum undecarboxylated osteocalcin correlates with hip bone mineral density in elderly women. *J. Bone Miner. Res.* **9**, 1591–1595.

64. Hodges, S. J., Akesson, K., Vergnaud, P., Obrant, K., and Delmas, P. (1993). Circulating levels of vitamin K1 and K2 are decreased in elderly women with hip fractures. *J. Bone Miner. Res.* **8**, 1241–1245.

65. Szulc, P., Chapuy, M. C., Meunier, P. J., and Delmas, P. D. (1993). Serum underdecarboxylated osteocalcin is a marker of the risk of hip fracture in elderly women. *J. Clin. Invest.* **91**, 1769–1774.

66. Knapen, M. H. J., Jie, K. S. G., Hamulyak, K., and Vermeer, C. (1993). Vitamin K induced changes in markers for osteoblast activity and urinary calcium loss. *Calcif. Tissue Int.* **53**, 81–85.

67. Kohlmier, M., Saupe, J., Shearer, M. J., Shaefer, I. K., and Asmus, G. (1996). Bone fracture risk in hemodialysis patients is related to apolipoprotein E genotype, a modulator of vitamin K status. *Osteoporosis Int.* **6**(S1), 89.

68. Rosen, C. J. (1994). Growth hormone, IGFs and the senescent skeleton. *J. Cell. Biochem.* **58**, 346–348.

69. Yen, S. S., Morales, A. J., and Khorran, O. (1995). Replacement of DHEA in men and women: Potential beneficial effects. *Ann. N.Y. Acad. Sci.* **774**, 128–142.

70. Vanderschueren, D., (1991). Androgens in the aging male. *J. Clin. Endocrinol. Metab.* **73**, 221–224.

71. Jackson, J. J., Riggs, B., and Spiekerman, A. (1992). Testosterone deficiency as a risk factor for hip fractures in men: A case control study. *Am. J. Med. Sci.* **304**, 4–8.

72. Orwoll, E. S., and Klein, R. F. (1995). Osteoporosis in men. *Endocr. Rev.* **16**, 87–116.

73. Finkelstein, J., Klibanski, A., Neer, R., Greenspan, S., Rosenthal, D., and Crowley, W. (1987). Osteoporosis in men with idiopathic hypogonadotropic hypogonadism. *Ann. Intern. Med.* **106**, 354–360.

74. Manolagas, S. C., and Jilka, R. L. (1995). Bone marrow, cytokines and bone remodeling. *N. Engl. J. Med.* **332**, 305–311.

75. Wakley, G., Schutte, H., Hannon, K., and Turner, R. (1991). Androgen treatment prevents loss of cancellous bone in the orchidectomized rat. *J. Bone Miner. Res.* **6**, 325–330.

76. Devogelaaer, J., De Cooman, S., and Nagant de Deuxchaisnes, C. (1992). Low bone mass in hypogonadal lames: Effect of testosterone substitution therapy. *Maturitas* **15**, 17–23.

77. Meier, D. E., Orwoll, E. S., Keenan, E. J., and Fagerstrom, R. M. (1987). Marked decline in trabecular bone mineral content in healthy men with age: Lack of association with sex steroid levels. *J. Am. Geriatr. Soc.* **35**, 189–197.

78. Gray, A., Feldman, H., McKinlay, J., and Longcope, C. (1991). Age, disease and changing sex hormone levels in middle age men. *J. Clin. Endocrinol. Metab.* **73**, 1016–1025.

79. Greendale, G., Edelstein, S., and Barrett-Connor, E. (1997). Endogenous sex steroids and bone mineral density in older women and men. *J. Bone Miner. Res.* **12**, 1833–1843.

80. Davidson, B. J., Ross, R. K., Paganini-Hill, A., Hammond, G. D., Siiteri, P. K., and Judd, H. L. (1982). Total and free estrogens and androgens in postmenopausal women with hip fractures. *J. Clin. Endocrinol. Metab.* **54**, 115–120.

81. Albright, F., Smith, P. H., and Richardson, A. M. (1941). Postmenopausal osteoporosis. *JAMA, J. Am. Med. Assoc.* **116**, 2465–2474.

82. Lindsay, R., and Tohme, J. F. (1991). Estrogen treatment of patients with postmenopausal osteoporosis. *Obstet. Gynecol.* **76**, 290–295.

83. Lufkin, E. J., Wachner, H. W., and O'Fallon, W. M. (1992). Treatment of postmenopausal osteoporosis with transdermal estrogen. *Ann. Intern. Med.* **117**, 1–9.

84. Uebelhart, D., Schlemmer, A., Johansen, J. S., Gineyts, E., Christiansen, C., and Delmas, P. D. (1991). Effect of menopause and hormone replacement therapy on the urinary excretion of pyridinium cross-links. *J. Clin. Endocrinol. Metab.* **72**, 367–373.

85. Slemenda, C. C., Longcope, C., Peacock, M., Hui, S., and Johnston, C. C. (1996). Sex steroids, bone mass and bone loss: A prospective study of pre-peri and postmenopausal women. *J. Clin. Invest.* **97**, 14–21.

86. Smith, E. P., Boyd, J., Frank, G. R., Takahashi, H., Cohen, R. M., Specker, B., Williams, T. C., Lubahn, D. B., and Korach, K. S. (1994). Estrogen resistance caused by a mutation in the estrogen receptor gene in a man. *N. Engl. J. Med.* **331**, 1056–1061.

87. Morishima, A., Grumbach, M. M., Simpson, E. R., Fisher, C., and Qqin, K. (1995). Aromatase deficiency in male and female siblings caused by a novel mutation in the physiological role of estrogens. *J. Clin. Endocrinol. Metab.* **80**, 3689–3698.

88. Carani, C., Qin, K., Simoni, M., Faustini, M., Serpente, S., Boyd, J., Korach, K. S., and Simpson, E. R. (1997). Effect of testosterone and estradiol in a man with aromatase deficiency. *N. Engl. J. Med.* **337**, 91–95.

89. Riggs, B. L., Khosla, S., and Melton, L. J. (1998). A unitary model for involutional osteoporosis: Estrogen deficiency causes both type I and type II osteoporosis in postmenopausal women and contributes to bone loss in aging men. *J. Bone Miner. Res.* **13**, 763–773.

90. Veldhuis, J. D., Iranmanesh, A., and Weltman, A. (1997). Elements in the pathophysiology of diminished GH secretion in aging humans. *Endocrine* **7**, 41–48.

91. Jones, J., and Clemmons, D. R., (1995). IGFs and their binding proteins: Biological actions. *Endocr. Rev.* **16**, 3–34.

92. Marcus, R. (1997). Skeletal effects of GH and IGF-I in adults. *Endocrine* **7**, 53–55.

93. Boonen, S, Aerssnes, J., Dequeker, J., Nicholson, P., Cheng, X., Lowet, G., Verbeke, G., and Bouillon, R. (1997). Age associated decline in human femoral neck cortical and trabecular content of IGF-I: Potential implications for age-related osteoporotic fracture occurrence. *Calcif. Tissue Int.* **61**, 173–178.

94. Boonen, S., Lesaffre, E., Dequeker, J., Aerssens, J., Nijs, J., Pelemans, W., and Bouillon, R. (1996). Relationship between baseline IGF-I and femoral neck bone density in women aged over 70 years. *J. Am. Geriatr. Soc.* **44**, 1301–1306.

95. Gelato, M. C., and Frost, R. A. (1997). IGFBP-3 Functional and structural implications in aging and wasting sydromes. *Endocrine* **7**, 81–85.

96. Johansson, A., Forslund, A., Hambraeus, L., Blum, W., and Ljunghall, S. (1993). Growth hormone dependent IGFBP-3 is a major determinant of bone mineral density in healthy men. *J. Bone. Miner. res.* **9**, 915–921.

97. Benedict, M., Ayers, D., Calore, J., and Richman, R. (1994). Differential distribution of IGFs and IGFBPs within bone: Relationship to bone mineral density. *J. Bone. Miner. Res.* **9**, 1803–1811.

98. Mohan, S., and Baylink, D. J. (1997). Serum IGFBP-4 and IGFBP-5 in aging and age-associated diseases. *Endocrine* **7**, 87–91.

99. Cook, F., Rosen, C. J., Vereault, D., Steffens, C., Kessenich, C. R., Greenspan, S., Ziegler, T. R., Watts, N. B., Mohan, S., and Baylink, D. J. (1996). Major changes in the circulatory IGF regulatory system after hip fracture surgery. *J. Bone Miner. Res.* **11**, S327.

100. Slemenda, C. W., Christian, J. C., Williams, C. J., Norton, J. A., and Johnston, C. C. (1991). Genetic determinants of bone mass in adult women: a reevaluation of the twin model and the potential importance of gene interaction on heritability estimates. *J. Bone Miner. Res.* **6**, 561–567.

101. Beamer, W. G., Donahue, L. R., Rosen, C. J., and Baylink, D. J. (1996). Genetic variability in adult bone density among inbred strains of mice. *Bone* **18**, 397–403.

102. Christiansen, C., Riis, B. J., and Rodbro, P. (1987). Prediction of rapid bone loss in postmenopausal women. *Lancet* **1**, 1105–1108.

103. Rosen, C. J., Chesnut, C. H., and Mallinak, J. S. (1997). The predictive value of biochemical markers of bone turnover for bone mineral density in early postmenopausal women with hormone replacement or calcium supplementation. *J. Clin. Endocrinol. Metab.* **82**, 1904–1910.

104. Ensrud, K. E., Palermo, L., Black, D. M. *et al.* (1995). Hip and calcaneal bone loss increase with advancing of age: Longitudinal results from the study of osteoporotic fractures. *J. Bone Miner. Res.* **10**, 1778–1787.

105. Bollen, A. M., Kiyak, H. A., and Eyre, D. R. (1997). Longitudinal evaluation of a bone resorption marker in elderly subjects. *Osteoporosis Int.* **7**, 544–549.

106. Nielsen, H. K., Brixen, K., and Mosekilde, L. (1990). Diurnal rhythm and 24 hour integrated concentrations of serum osteocalcin in normals: Influence of age, sex, season and smoking habits. *Calcif. Tissue Int.* **47**, 284–290.

107. Chapuy, M. C., Schott, A. M., Garnero, P., Hans D., Delmas, P. D., Meunier, P. J., and Epidos Study Group. (1996). Healthy elderly French women living at home have secondary hyperparathyroidism and high bone turnover in winter. *J. Clin. Endocrinol. Metab.* **81**, 1129–1133.

108. Cheung, C. K., Panesar, N. S., Lau, E., Woo, J., and Swaminathan, R. (1995). Increased bone resorption and decreased bone formation in Chinese patients with hip fracture. *Calcif. Tissue Int.* **56**, 347–349.

109. Hansen, M. A., Overgaard, K., Riis, B. J., and Christiansen, C. (1991). Role of peak bone mass and bone loss in postmenopausal osteoporosis: 12 year study. *Br. Med. J.* **303**, 961–964.

110. Akesson, K., Vergnaud, P., Gineyts, E., Delmas, P. D., and O'Brant, K. (1993). Impairment of bone turnover in elderly women with hip fracture. *Calcif. Tissue Int.* **53**, 162–169.

111. Van Daele, P. L., Seibel, M. J., Burger, H., Hofman, A., Grobbee, D. E., van Leeuwen, J. P., Birkenhäger, J. C., and Pols, H. A. P. (1996). Case control analysis of bone resorption markers, disability and hip fracture risk: The Rotterdam study. *Br. Med. J.* **312**, 482–483.

112. Riis, B. J., Overgaard, K., and Christiansen, C. (1995). Biochemical markers of bone turnover to monitor the bone response to postmenopausal hormone replacement therapy. *Osteoporosis Int.* **5**, 276–280.

113. Kraenzlin, M. E., Seible, M. J., Trechsel, U., Boerlin, V., Axria, M., Kraenzlin, C. A., and Haas, H. G. (1996). The effect of intranasal calcitonin on postmenopausal bone turnover: Evidence for maximal effect after 8 weeks of continuous treatment. *Calcif. Tissue Int.* **58**, 216–220.

114. Garnero, P., Shih, W. J., Gineyts, E., Karpf, D. B., and Delmas, P. D. (1994). Comparison of new biochemical markers of bone turnover in late postmenopausal women in response to alendronate treatment. *J. Clin. Endocrinol. Metab.* **79**, 1693–1700.

115. Garnero, P., Gineyts, E., Arbault, P., Christiansen, C., and Delmas, P. (1995). Different effects of bisphosphonates and estrogen therapy on free and peptide bound bone crosslinks excretion. *J. Bone Miner. Res.* **10**, 641–649.

CHAPTER 34

Osteoporosis in Men

ERIC S. ORWOLL Oregon Health Sciences University and Portland Veterans Administration Medical Center, Portland, Oregon 97201

I. INTRODUCTION

The earliest reports of the epidemiology of fractures associated with osteoporosis revealed that the classical age-related increase in fractures seen in women is evident in men as well. Only since the early 1990s has it been recognized that the problem of osteoporosis in men represents an important public health issue, and that it also presents a unique array of scientific challenges and opportunities [1–3].

II. EPIDEMIOLOGY OF FRACTURES IN MEN

In women, the relationship between bone mass and fracture risk has become increasingly clear, and it is possible to confidently discuss the epidemiology of osteoporosis as defined either by the presence of atraumatic fractures or by low bone mass [4, 5]. In men there is less information available regarding the cause of fracture, and hence a discussion of osteoporosis epidemiology must be primarily related to fracture patterns.

The incidence of all fractures is higher in men than women early in life, probably as a result of serious trauma [6, 7]. At about age 40–50 years, there is a reversal of this trend with fractures in general, but in particular with those of the pelvis, humerus, forearm, and femur becoming much more common in women. Nevertheless, the incidence of fractures due to minimal to moderate trauma (particularly hip and spine) also increases rapidly with aging in men (Fig. 1) [7] and reflects an increasing prevalence of skeletal fragility. Some fractures are due to excessive trauma or local bone pathology, but in older men, most can not be attributed to these factors and are probably osteoporotic. The Dubbo Osteoporosis Epidemiology Project [8] has raised the possibility that low trauma fracture rates in men may be greater than previously recognized, and data from that study suggest that the lifetime risk of an atraumatic fracture is about 25% in an average 60 year old man.

III. DETERMINANTS OF FRACTURE IN MEN

A. Bone Mass

1. AGE-RELATED CHANGES IN BONE MASS IN MEN

The pattern of osteoporotic fractures is intimately related to aging, and changes in bone mass with age clearly contribute to that association. The decline in axial bone density was initially considered to be relatively slow in men, primarily because of the results of cross-sectional studies using techniques that assess total spinal bone mass (dual photon absorptiometry [DPA]). Vertebral cancellous bone density as measured by quantitative computed tomography (QCT), however, suggested a much more rapid rate of bone loss with aging in

493

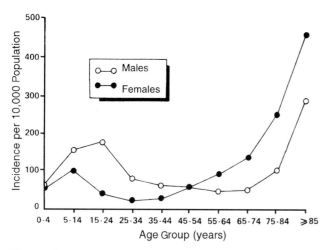

FIGURE 1 Average annual fracture incidence rate per 10,000 population in Leicester, United Kingdom, by age group and sex. Reproduced from Donaldson *et al.* [7], *J. Epidemiol. Comm. Health* **44**, 241–245, 1990; with permission from the BMJ Publishing Group.

2. SEX STEROID LEVELS

Clinical hypogonadism is a well-established cause of osteoporosis in men. Bone loss results from the appearance of hypogonadism in adults, and a failure to achieve peak bone mass is a consequence of hypogonadism before the onset of puberty [23, 24]. It has become quite clear that testosterone replacement therapy has beneficial effects on bone mass in men with established gonadal failure, sometimes to the extent that bone mass is normalized [25–28]. Because testicular and adrenal androgen concentrations decline in men with aging, an important issue is whether the decline in androgen levels with aging contributes to the decrease in bone mass and the increase in fracture risk that occur concomitantly. A number of studies have examined the relationship between androgen levels and bone mass in nonhypogonadal men, but the results have been inconclusive. In some, there has been a correlation (albeit weak) between androgen levels and measures of bone density [29–32], but in other reports, when age is considered in the statistical model, it is not possible to document a clear influence of androgen levels on bone [33–35]. Unfortunately, these studies have utilized small numbers of subjects and have been cross-sectional in design. There have been few attempts to more directly assess the influence of androgens in elderly men. In one notable report, Tenover [36] found that a three month period of testosterone supplementation in a small group of elderly men with low normal testosterone levels at baseline was associated with a significant decline in urinary hydroxyproline excretion (although there was no change in osteocalcin levels). In sum, the issue of whether declines in androgen activity with aging have a clear impact on skeletal health remains unresolved. Important questions include whether there is a threshold level of androgen activity which is necessary for the maintenance of skeletal health, whether some skeletal compartments are more affected than others by changes in androgen levels, whether androgens may affect the skeleton via indirect effects on other tissue (e.g., muscle or body composition), and whether androgen supplementation is capable of preventing or reversing age-related changes in skeletal mass.

Although attention has been traditionally focused on the role of androgens in men, reports of severe osteopenia in several men with estrogen deficiency (estrogen receptor abnormality or absent aromatase activity) [37] have raised the question of the role of estrogens in men. Aromatase activity is present in bone [38]. In transsexuals, estrogens are capable of maintaining bone mass in the absence of androgens [39], and two cross-sectional studies have suggested that bone density in older men may be more closely related to estrogen than to androgens [40, 41]. Studies in experimental animals and in osteoblastic cells *in vitro* indicate that nonaromatizable androgens are potent modulators of skeletal homeostasis [42–45], but the role of estrogens now must also be systematically evaluated.

normal men [9]. Subsequently, the results derived from DPA were shown to be influenced by artifacts introduced by extravertebral calcifications. If men with such calcifications are excluded, the relationship of spinal bone density to age is similar in men and women [10]. Longitudinal studies verify a more rapid rate of vertebral bone loss with aging in normal men [11]. In cross-sectional studies, the negative slope of density with age at proximal femoral sites is similar, albeit somewhat less, in men compared to women [12–14]. Moreover, bone volume in the iliac crest declines at very similar rates in both men and women. In both sexes the rate of bone loss appears to increase with increasing age [15].

In cortical bone, the pattern of age-related loss also affects eventual fracture risk. Cortical bone mass in young men is much greater than that in women, probably accounting in part for the lower incidence of cortical bone fractures in men. Cross-sectional studies suggest that age is associated with a fairly linear decrease in cortical bone mass [11, 14, 16–19], but some studies also indicate the BMD:age slope becomes more negative in men after 50 years [11, 18, 20, 21]. This slope is not quite as steep as that in women [19], thereby accentuating the sexual differences in cortical mass present in early adulthood. However, the rate of loss of cortical bone mass in men as reported in longitudinal studies is considerably more rapid (5–10% per decade) [11, 18, 20, 21] than previously estimated from cross-sectional studies (1–3% per decade) [12, 14, 17]. The differences noted in longitudinal vs cross-sectional studies may reflect the difficulty in adequately estimating time-dependent processes by cross-sectional methods, but also suggest that an increasingly greater rate of bone loss in men has taken place since the 1960s. This possibility is in accord with an apparent increase in fracture incidence [22].

3. OTHER CAUSES OF LOW BONE MASS IN MEN

Although important, age-related bone loss explains only part of the problem of osteoporosis in men. Weight contributes substantially to the variation in bone mass, with heavier men having greater bone mass [8, 46]. Weight loss seems to be associated with greater rates of bone loss in older men [8]. Tobacco smoking exerts a negative effect on bone [8, 47, 48]. Particularly in younger men, idiopathic osteoporosis represents an important fraction of the overall problem. Kelepouris *et al.* [49] found that approximately one third of osteoporotic men have idiopathic disease. A link between idiopathic osteoporosis and low levels of insulin like growth factor-1 (IGF-1) or IGF-1 binding protein 3 (IGFBP-3) levels has been postulated [50, 51], but the importance of those relationships is not understood.

Especially consequential are systemic diseases, medications and lifestyles that may increase the risk of bone loss (Table I). The frequency with which these conditions contribute to the etiology of osteoporosis in men is illustrated by several series in which the majority of men with osteoporotic fractures were found to have secondary causes of metabolic bone diseases [49, 52]. In clinical situations, success in the prevention and treatment of osteoporosis depends heavily upon the recognition of these conditions.

4. THE RELATIONSHIP BETWEEN BONE MASS AND FRACTURE IN MEN

The data available are consistent with an inverse relationship between bone mass and fracture. For instance, spinal fractures in men are related to femoral cortical area and

Singh grade [53], proximal femoral bone mass [8, 10], and vertebral bone mass [11, 54–56]. There are few specific data concerning the measurement of bone mass in men with hip fracture, although several studies have reported that hip and spine bone mass are clearly reduced in a series of men with hip fracture when compared with age-matched controls [57–59]. Moreover, in the Dubbo Osteoporosis Epidemiology Study, it was found that femoral bone density measures were quite predictive of subsequent atraumatic fractures (although spinal BMD was not) [59].

B. Falls

In addition to bone mass, the risk of falling has been identified as a major determinant of fracture in women. In men, there are few prospective data that directly relate fall propensity to subsequent fractures, but a variety of factors indirectly related to risk of falling are associated with fracture. For instance, Nguyen *et al.* [59] found that men who went on to experience a nontraumatic fracture exhibited more body sway and lower grip strength (as well as lower bone density) than nonfracture controls. These impressions were substantiated in an epidemiological study of the factors associated with hip fracture in men (Table II) [60]. The characteristics of falls may be different in men and women. Some [61], but not all [62, 63], studies suggest that falls are less common in older men than in women, and when they fall, women may more often fall on their hip [63].

C. Genetics

A major part of the determination of adult bone mass is under genetic control. The nature of the relationship is not well

TABLE I. Causes of Osteoporosis in Men

I. Primary
Aging
Idiopathic
Genetic
II. Secondary
Hypogonadism
Glucocorticoid excess
Alcoholism
Gastrointestinal disorders
Hypercalciuria
Anticonvulsants
Thyrotoxicosis
Immobilization
Osteogenesis imperfecta
Homocystinuria
Systemic mastocytosis
Neoplastic diseases
Rheumatoid arthritis

TABLE II. Some Factors Associated with Hip Fractures in Men

Metabolic Disorders
Thyroidectomy
Gastrectomy
Pernicious anemia
Chronic respiratory diseases
Disorders of movement and balance
Hemiparesis/hemiplegia
Parkinsonism dementia
Other neurological diseases
Vertigo
Alcoholism
Anemia
Blindness
Use of cane or walker

established in either sex, and the primary evidence comes from studies of bone mass and fracture prevalence in related individuals. Longitudinal twin studies document a substantial heritability of bone mass in men [20, 64]. Men who have osteoporotic parents have bone mineral density levels that are lower than those of control subjects [65, 66]. In the European Vertebral Osteoporosis Study, maternal history of hip fracture increased the risk of vertebral fracture in men (odds ratio 1.3, 95% confidence intervals 1.0–1.8) [67]. Although not extensively examined, some data indicate that there is not a significant effect of gender on the heritability of bone mass, suggesting the effect (whatever genes it may be due to) is equally strong in men and women [68–70]. The relationship between family history and fracture risk has not been established in prospective trials, and verification of the importance of family history in the determination of fracture risk in men should await those results. There has also been no specific gene(s) convincingly associated with bone mass or fracture in men, and so the mechanism by which family history influences bone mass or fracture risk in men is unknown. Several genes have been suggested to be of importance, including the vitamin D receptor [71, 72], unknown genes on chromosome 11 [73], and type I procollagen [72]. Not all of these results are reproducible [74].

D. Growth Factors and Cytokines

Growth factors are important in the regulation of bone metabolism in men as well as in women, but there is little information concerning the specific nature of their roles or their

usefulness in the clinical situation (see Chapter 6). Growth factors [75], or one of the growth factor binding proteins (IGFBP-3) (Fig. 2) [50], have been reported to be related to bone mass in normal men. In idiopathic osteoporosis in men, evidence has arisen that suggests insulin-like growth factor 1 (IGF-1) [51, 76], levels may also be reduced. These studies found that mean levels of IGF-1 were lower than in control populations but were nevertheless within the expected normal ranges. The idea that growth factors and bone mass are related is intriguing in view of the association between growth hormone deficiency and low bone mass in men [77], an association that may primarily reflect growth hormone deficiency during peak bone mass development [78]. There are also a number of reports that growth hormone administration may improve bone mass in deficient adults [79, 80]. The treatment of adults with growth hormone provokes an increase in biochemical markers of bone remodeling, and men have been reported to be more responsive to replacement therapy with growth hormone than women (Fig. 3) [81]. The etiologic role of growth factors in the genesis of osteoporosis in men is of great interest but clearly must be further examined. Unless there is other evidence of growth hormone deficiency, the measurement of growth factor levels can not be considered a routine part of the evaluation of osteoporosis in men.

E. Indices of Mineral Metabolism

Bone mass is, of course, intimately linked to mineral metabolism. On that basis, prominent relationships between indices of mineral homeostasis and metabolic bone disease should be expected. In fact, in men as in women, gross derangements in mineral physiology are associated with skeletal disorders. For instance, men with hyperparathyroidism, vitamin D deficiency, malignancies, hypercalciuria, etc. are at risk for osteopenia and fractures [52], and the differential diagnosis of osteopenic disorders should include the consideration of these diseases. Certainly, the prevalence of vitamin D deficiency appears to be high in both sexes and should be of particular concern to clinicians [82].

The issue of whether the immense increase in fracture rate that occurs with aging in men is related to concomitant alterations in mineral metabolism is more difficult to resolve. Increasing age is associated with slight but significant increases in parathyroid hormone levels and declines in 25(OH)D levels [83], and these changes have been linked to the gradual decrease in bone mass that accompanies aging [83–85]. Declines in calcium absorption also have been reported to occur in older men and possibly are related to reductions in the ability to produce 1,25(OH)2D [84]. This fall in 1,25(OH)2D levels seems to be limited to those men who have more severe reductions in renal function [83, 86]. Although there are no definite gender differences in these age-related changes, there have been some reports that older men have higher

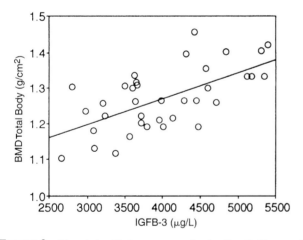

FIGURE 2   The relationship between serum levels of insulin like growth factor binding protein-3 (IGFBP-3) and bone mineral density (BMD) of the total body in healthy men. R = 0.63, p < 0.001. Reproduced from Johansson, A., *et al.* [75], Growth-hormone-dependent insulin-like growth factor binding protein is a major determinant of bone mineral density in healthy men. *J. Bone Miner. Res.* **9**, 915–921, 1994; © The Endocrine Society.

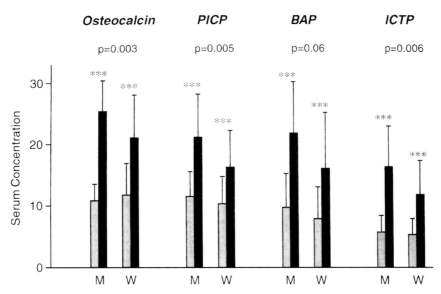

FIGURE 3   Concentrations of osteocalcin (μg/L), carboxyl-terminal cross-linked telopeptide of type 1 collagen (ICTP, μg/L), carboxyl-terminal propeptide of type 1 procollagen (PICP, μg/L $\times 10^{-1}$), and bone-specific alkaline phosphatase (bALP, μkat/L $\times 10^{-1}$) in 21 men and 15 women with growth hormone deficiency before and after nine months of treatment with recombinant human growth hormone. Results are shown as the mean + SD. **, $p < 0.001$. The p values refer to the difference in response to treatment between men and women. Filled bars = treatment, open bars = control. Reproduced from Burman, P., *et al.* [81], Growth hormone-deficient men are more responsive to GH replacement therapy than women. *J. Clin. Endocrinol. Metab.* **82**, 550–555, 1997; © The Endocrine Society.

25(OH)D levels than women [82, 85, 87]. Nevertheless, an improvement in bone mass is seen in normal older men with modest calcium and vitamin D supplementation [87], suggesting that alterations in mineral metabolism may contribute to age-related increases in fractures.

F. Bone Remodeling and Biochemical Markers of Bone Metabolism

The unequivocal decline in bone mass that occurs with aging in men is undoubtedly the result of trends in the remodeling process that result in excess bone resorption. Histological evaluations of cancellous bone indicate that there is trabecular plate thinning and dropout, and that these changes have expected biomechanical consequences [88]. In men, this process is similar to that which occurs in women, with the exception that at menopause women experience a particularly rapid rate of trabecular plate perforation and loss [88–90]. In cortical bones, aging men also are affected by bone resorption, loss of bone mass, and an increase in fragility. At endocortical sites, bone resorption occurs and results in cortical thinning. This happens to some extent in both men and women, but the biomechanical consequences are somewhat lessened in men by a simultaneous increase in periosteal bone accretion which yields larger bones which are more fracture resistant [91]. The specific remodeling imbalance that is re-

sponsible for the age-related decline in bone mass in men is unclear. In women, the postmenopausal period appears to be associated with an increase in bone remodeling rates with a particular excess of resorption, but there is no counterpart in men. The decline in bone mass may be less the result of absolute increases in bone resorption than reduction in the rate of osteoblastic bone formation [92–94]. Of course, disruptions of remodeling may be accelerated in overt disease states (hyperparathyroidism, immobilization, glucocorticoid excess, etc.), leading to more rapid bone loss and increasing fracture risk.

The histomorphometric changes in bone metabolism that are associated with aging in men may be reflected in alterations in biochemical indices of bone remodeling (see Chapter 29). The available literature is modest and somewhat inconsistent. Unfortunately, all studies in men are cross sectional. Delmas *et al.* [95] reported that there was a gradual increase in pyridinoline excretion with age in men starting in middle age, and Orwoll and Deftos [96] found an increase in osteocalcin levels with aging in normal men. Similar findings have been reported for bone alkaline phosphatase [97]. On the other hand, Wishart *et al.* [35] reported that a decrease in several markers of bone formation and resorption was associated with increasing age in men. Orwoll *et al.* [98] examined urinary N-telopeptide levels in a large group of men and found no change after the age of 30 years (Fig. 4). Although there was a tendency for N-telopeptide excretion to increase in the oldest men, the trend was not

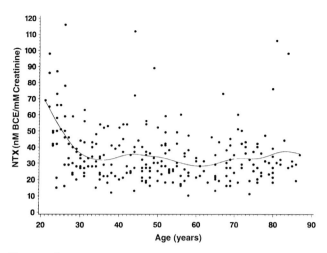

FIGURE 4   Urinary collagen N-telopeptide (NTx) excretion in normal men by age. Individual subject values are plotted as a function of age. Reproduced from Orwoll, E. S., *et al.* [98], Collagen N-telopeptide excretion in men: The effects of age and intra-subject variability. *J. Bone Miner. Res.* **83**, 3930–3935, 1998; © The Endocrine Society.

significant. In studies that concentrated on older men (rather than a spectrum of young to old), two groups have reported that there is a slight increase in biochemical indices with age [85, 99]. If a consensus can be reached from the existing literature, it is that there is little change in biochemical indices of resorption in men until the later stages of life, when slight increases occur. Markers of bone formation may increase with age.

An important finding reported by two groups is that markers of bone remodeling are higher in men during the third decade than in the rest of adult life [35, 98]. This is apparently a continuation of the process of peak bone mass development, as markers of remodeling are known to be increased during growth and adolescence [100, 101]. From a clinical perspective, it is important to recognize this phenomenon when attempting to use biochemical indices during this period of life. Another important finding has been the description of a diurnal variation in markers of bone metabolism in men and women [102, 103], which may be to some extent related to the diurnal variation in cortisol secretion [104].

The relationship between biochemical indices of remodeling and bone health is not well understood in men. For women, there are longitudinal data that support the usefulness of measuring biochemical indices as predictors of change in bone mass or of fracture risk; no such data are available for men. However, urinary levels of collagen N-telopeptide are apparently correlated with levels of bone mass in men (as in women) (Fig. 5) [99], and higher levels of serum osteocalcin are associated with higher parathyroid hormone concentrations [85]. Some researchers have described differences in indices of remodeling between normal and osteoporotic men [105], and low bone mass was related to high bone turnover in male long-distance runners [106]. Again, all of these studies have been cross-sectional, and longitudinal trials are neces-

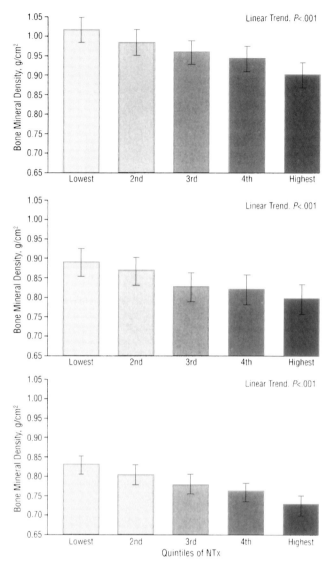

FIGURE 5   Total hip mean bone mineral density levels by quintiles of N-telopeptide (NTx) levels in 374 men (top), 223 estrogen-using women (center), and 364 nonestrogen-using women (bottom). The figures are adjusted for age, body mass index, total daily calcium, current smoking, alcohol use three or more days per week, exercise three or more times per week, limited physical health, noninsulin dependent, and current use of thiazide diuretics, thyroid hormone, and corticosteroids. Reproduced from Schneider and Barrett-Conner [99], *Arch. Intern. Med.* **157**, 1241–1245. Copyrighted 1997, American Medical Association.

sary to understand the real value of biochemical measures in men.

One area in which a reasonable experience with biochemical markers has accumulated is in the treatment of hypogonadal men with androgens. Hypogonadism in men is associated with an acceleration in bone remodeling and with increases in biochemical indices [23, 28, 107], a phenomenon quite similar to that seen in postmenopausal women. In a variety of studies, androgen replacement has been associated with changes in markers of bone metabolism (Fig. 6), with

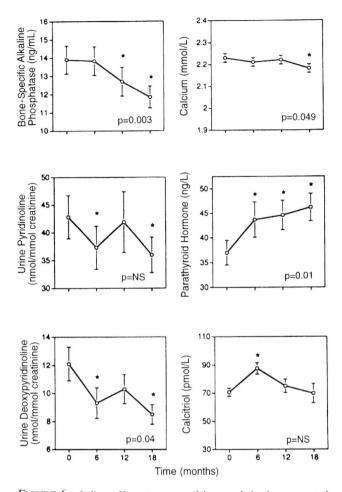

FIGURE 6   Indices of bone turnover, calcium regulating hormones, and calcium in hypogonadal men receiving testosterone replacement therapy. Data are expressed as the mean ± SEM. Statistical significance for analyses of the mean slope is shown in the bottom right-hand corner of each figure (NS = not significant). *, p < 0.05 compared to the baseline value, by paired t-test analysis. Reproduced from Katznelson, L., *et al.* [26], Increase in bone density and lean body mass during testosterone administration in men with acquired hypogonadism. *J. Clin. Endocrinol. Metab.* **81**, 4358–4365, 1996; © The Endocrine Society.

concomitant increases in bone density. Although most trials have reported a decline in both formation and resorption markers [26, 28], some have described an increase in formation parameters and have suggested that androgens (or the estrogens that result from aromatose activity) increase osteoblastic activity while reducing resorption [27, 108]. Similarly, in normal older men or eugonadal men with osteoporosis, treatment with testosterone has been noted to reduce indices of resorption, with smaller changes in markers of formation [36, 109]. These are interesting findings, but the meaning of the biochemical changes remains uncertain. It would be helpful to have a direct measure of bone remodeling in these situations to document authentic relationships between markers of formation and resorption and their respective morphological counterparts.

IV. THE EVALUATION OF OSTEOPOROSIS IN MEN

Guidelines for the most efficient, cost-effective approach for the evaluation of the patient with osteoporosis, or the patient suspected of having osteoporosis, are poorly validated for either sex. Recommendations are, therefore, based on existing knowledge of disease epidemiology and clinical characteristics [110, 111] rather than on models that have been carefully tested in prospective studies. Within these constraints, it is possible to formulate an approach to the male osteoporotic patient (Fig. 7).

There are several clinical situations in which the presence of osteoporosis should be considered likely. These include the occurrence of fractures with little trauma, the radiographic finding of low bone mass or vertebral deformity, and the presence of conditions known to be associated with osteoporosis. In these circumstances, further diagnostic steps are appropriate.

A. Differential Diagnosis

If a man is found to be osteopenic or osteoporotic, an evaluation should be considered to determine with reasonable certainty the cause of the disorder. In women with low trauma fractures, the vast majority have histological osteoporosis, but a small proportion are found to be osteomalacic [112–114]. Similarly, a fraction of men with fracture have osteomalacia [112–114]. Osteomalacia is estimated to be present in <4–47% of men with femoral fractures, with most reports being ≤ 20% [112–116]. Because food is fortified with vitamin D, occult osteomalacia may be less frequent in the United States than in other areas (e.g., Northern Europe). Increasing age is associated with an increasing prevalence of osteomalacia [114]. Thus far, the only patients who have been carefully surveyed are those with femoral fractures, and it is not known whether populations with other fractures (vertebral) would include similar proportions of osteoporotic and osteomalacic individuals. Some have suggested that women with femoral fracture are more frequently osteomalacic than men [112, 113], but others report no distinction [114]. Although the exact magnitude of the problem presented by osteomalacia in men is uncertain, it is clear that any differential diagnosis of low bone mass and fractures in men must consider the possibility. This becomes particularly imperative because the treatment for osteomalacia differs considerably from that of osteoporosis [117].

B. Initial Evaluation of Osteoporosis: History, Physical, and Routine Biochemical Measures

The history, physical, and routine biochemical profile can be very helpful in directing a focused evaluation of a man

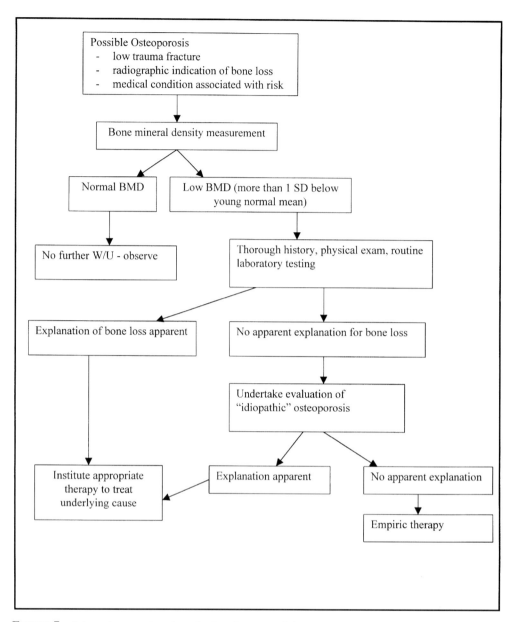

FIGURE 7   Schematic approach to the evaluation of osteoporosis in men.

with low bone mass. A variety of approaches for the differential diagnosis of low bone mass have been suggested
using standard clinical and biochemical information [113,
118, 119]. The goals of this stage of the evaluation should
be to determine the specific diagnosis (what is the cause of
the low bone mass—osteoporosis or osteomalacia?) and to
identify contributing factors in the genesis of the disorder. Of
particular importance in the history and physical, therefore,
are clinical signs of genetic, nutritional/environmental, so-
cial (alcohol, tobacco), medical, or pharmacological factors
that may be present to aid in these goals. Routine laboratory
testing should include levels of serum creatinine, calcium,
phosphorus, alkaline phosphatase, and liver function tests, as
well as a complete blood count. If, on the basis of these tests,

there is evidence for medical conditions associated with bone
loss (alcoholism, hyperparathyroidism, malignancy, Cushing's syndrome, thyrotoxicosis, malabsorption, etc.), a definitive diagnosis should be pursued with appropriate testing.

C. Evaluation of the Patient with "Idiopathic" Osteoporosis

In men with reduced bone mass in whom no clear pathophysiology is identified by routine methods, it has been considered appropriate to be diagnostically aggressive, primarily
because the potential for occult "secondary" causes of osteoporosis may be higher in men. However, the incidence

of occult causes of osteoporosis in men (or whether it is greater than in women) is poorly studied. The diagnostic yield and cost-effectiveness of extensive biochemical studies in the man with apparently "idiopathic" osteoporosis is thus unknown. Nevertheless, lacking this information, a reasonable evaluation of the man without a clear etiology for osteoporosis might include:

- 24-hour urine calcium and creatinine, to identify hypercalciuria
- 24-hour urine cortisol
- serum 25-hydroxyvitamin D level
- serum testosterone
- serum thyroid stimulating hormone level
- serum protein electrophoresis (in those >50 years old, to exclude multiple myeloma)

D. Histomorphometric Characterization

Transiliac bone biopsy is a safe and effective means of assessing skeletal histology and remodeling characteristics [120]. Some have suggested a transiliac bone biopsy is indicated in those men in whom a thorough biochemical evaluation has failed to reveal an etiology for osteoporosis [121]. The rationale for this approach is based on the need to accomplish several objectives: (1) ensure that occult osteomalacia is not present; (2) identify unusual causes of osteoporosis that may be revealed only by a histological analysis, such as mastocytosis [122, 123]; and (3) to yield information concerning the remodeling rate, which in turn may further direct the differential diagnosis (e.g., unappreciated thyrotoxicosis or secondary hyperparathyroidism suggested by the presence of increased turnover) or may be helpful in designing the most appropriate therapeutic approach. Considerable histological heterogeneity exists among men with osteoporosis. Whether distinct histological patterns represent different stages of a single disease entity, separate subtypes of the disease, or simply an arbitrary subdivision of a normal distribution of remodeling rates is unknown. Realistically, the cost and invasiveness of a bone biopsy, coupled with the uncertain likelihood of detecting useful information (in addition to that available from noninvasive testing), has relegated the procedure to only the most unusual situations.

E. Biochemical Indices of Bone Remodeling

A more reasonable approach to the evaluation of remodeling dynamics in men with osteoporosis may be to utilize the advantages of biochemical markers of bone turnover. In women, biochemical indices of remodeling have frequently been found to correlate with histological measures of bone turnover, rates of bone loss, and the risk of fracture. Although similar studies are not available in men, the presence

of an increase in biochemical indices of remodeling may indicate one of those conditions associated with higher bone turnover (early hypogonadism, thyrotoxicosis, mastocytosis, etc.). Even if no obvious etiology is discovered, the increase in biochemical markers can help judge the effectiveness of subsequent therapy. The presence of normal or low levels of markers is less helpful. Although these are reasonable recommendations based on the available evidence, it must be understood that the longitudinal trials necessary to be confident of the efficacy of these approaches are not yet available.

V. SUMMARY

Osteoporosis in men is a substantial public health problem. Although in many ways similar to the disease in women, the character and pathophysiology of osteoporosis in men is unique. Information concerning the risk factors for osteoporosis in men has begun to emerge, and it is finally possible to formulate some reasonable clinical approaches for its detection, evaluation, and prevention. The judicious use of biochemical parameters of mineral and bone metabolism is an essential part of the the evaluation and therapy of men with metabolic bone disease. However, many of the assumptions that are made about the clinical approach to osteoporosis in men are based on data derived from the experience in women. A substantial amount of work is needed to be more confident of the specific roles of many of the available approaches to osteoporosis in men.

References

1. Scane, A. C., Sutcliffe, A. M., and Francis, R. M. (1992). Osteoporosis in men. *Clin. Rheum.* **7**, 589–601.
2. Niewoehner, C. (1993). Osteoporosis in men: Is it more common than we think? *Postgrad. Med.* **93**, 59–60, 63–70.
3. Seeman, E. (1993). Osteoporosis in men: Epidemiology, pathophysiology, and treatment possibilities. *Am. J. Med.* **95**, 22S–28S.
4. World Health Organization. (1994). "Assessment of Fracture Risk and its Application to Screening for Postmenopausal Osteoporosis," Report of a WHO Study Group. W.H.O., Geneva.
5. Melton, L. J. I. (1995). How many women have osteoporosis now? *J. Bone Miner. Res.* **10**, 175–177.
6. Garraway, W. M., Stauffer, R. N., Kurland, L. T., and O'Fallon, W. M. (1979). Limb fractures in a defined population. I. Frequency and distribution. *Mayo Clin. Proc.* **54**, 701–707.
7. Donaldson, L. J., Cook, A., and Thomson, R. G. (1990). Incidence of fractures in a geographically defined population. *J. Epidemiol. Commun. Health* **44**, 241–245.
8. Nguyen, T. V., Eisman, J. A., Kelly, P. J., and Sambrook, P. N. (1996). Risk factors for osteoporotic fractures in elderly men. *Am. J. Epidemiol.* **144**, 258–261.
9. Meier, D. E., Orwoll, E. S., and Jones, J. M. (1984). Marked disparity between trabecular and cortical bone loss with age in healthy men: Measurement by vertebral computed tomography and radial photon absorptiometry. *Ann. Intern. Med.* **101**, 605–612.
10. Mann, T., Oviatt, S. K., Wilson, D., Nelson, D., and Orwoll, E. S. (1992). Vertebral deformity in men. *J. Bone Miner. Res.* **7**, 1259–1265.

11. Orwoll, E. S., Oviatt, S. K., McClung, M. R., Deftos, L. J., and Sexton, G. (1990). The rate of bone mineral loss in normal men and the effects of calcium and cholecalciferol supplementation. *Ann. Intern. Med.* **112**, 29–34.

12. Riggs, B. L., Wahner, H. W., Dunn, W. L., Mazess, R. B., Offord, K. P., and Melton, L. J. I. (1981). Differential changes in bone mineral density of the appendicular and axial skeleton with aging. *J. Clin. Invest.* **67**, 328–335.

13. Elliott, J. R., Gilchrist, N. L., Wells, J. E., Turner, J. G., Ayling, E., Gillespie, W. J., Sainsbury, R., Hornblow, A., and Donald, R. A. (1990). Effects of age and sex on bone density at the hip and spine in a normal Caucasian New Zealand population. *N. Z. Med. J.* **103**, 33–37.

14. Hannan, M. T., Felson, D. T., and Anderson, J. J. (1992). Bone mineral density in elderly men and women: Results from the Framingham osteoporosis study. *J. Bone Miner. Res.* **7**, 547–553.

15. Jones, G., Nguyen, T., Sambrook, P., Kelly, P. J., and Eisman, J. A. (1994). Progressive loss of bone in the femoral neck in elderly people: Longitudinal findings from the Dubbo osteoporosis epidemiology study. *Br. Med. J.* **309**, 691–695.

16. Gotfredsen, A., Hadberg, A., Nilas, L., and Christiansen, C. (1987). Total body bone mineral in healthy adults. *J. Lab. Clin. Med.* **110**, 362–368.

17. Mazess, R. B., Barden, H. S., Drinka, P. J., Bauwens, S. F., Orwoll, E. S., and Bell, N. H. (1990). Influence of age and body weight on spine and femur bone mineral density in U.S. white men. *J. Bone Miner. Res.* **5**, 645–652.

18. Davis, J. W., Ross, P. D., Vogel, J. M., and Wasnich, R. D. (1991). Age-related changes in bone mass among Japanese-American men. *Bone Miner.* **15**, 227–236.

19. Garn, S. M., Sullivan, T. V., Decker, S. A., Larkin, F. A., and Hawthorne, V. M. (1992). Continuing bone expansion and increasing bone loss over a two-decade period in men and women from a total community sample. *Am. J. Hum. Biol.* **4**, 57–67.

20. Slemenda, C. W., Christian, J. C., Reed, T., Reister, T. K., Williams, C. J., and Johnston, C. C. J. (1992). Long-term bone loss in men: Effects of genetic and environmental factors. *Ann. Intern. Med.* **117**, 286–291.

21. Tobin, J. D., Fox, K. M., and Cejku, M. L. (1993). Bone density changes in normal men: A 4–19 year longitudinal study. *J. Bone Miner. Res.* **8**, 102.

22. Elffors, I., Allander, E., Kanis, J. A., Gullberg, B., Johnell, O., Dequeker, J., Dilsen, G., Gennari, C., Lopes Vaz, A. A., Lyritis, G., Mazzuoli, G. F., Miravet, L., Passeri, M., Cano, R. P., Rapado, A., and Ribot, C. (1994). The variable incidence of hip fracture in Southern Europe: The MEDOS study. *Osteoporosis Int.* **4**, 253–263.

23. Stepan, J. J., Lachman, M., Zverina, J., Pacovsky, V., and Baylink, D. J. (1989). Castrated men exhibit bone loss: Effect of calcitonin treatment on biochemical indices of bone remodeling. *J. Clin. Endocrinol. Metab.* **69**, 523–527.

24. Finkelstein, J. S., Neer, R. M., Biller, B. M. K., Crawford, J. D., and Klibanski, A. (1992). Osteopenia in men with a history of delayed puberty. *N. Engl. J. Med.* **326**, 600–604.

25. Finkelstein, J. S., Klibanski, A., Neer, R. M., Doppelt, S. H., Rosenthal, D. I., Sergè, G. V., and Crowley, W. F. (1989). Increase in bone density during treatment of men with idiopathic hypogonadotropic hypogonadism. *J. Clin. Endocrinol. Metab.* **69**, 776–783.

26. Katznelson, L., Finkelstein, J. S., Schoenfeld, D. A., Rosenthal, D. I., Anderson, E. J., and Klibanski, A. (1996). Increase in bone density and lean body mass during testosterone administration in men with acquired hypogonadism. *J. Clin. Endocrinol. Metab.* **81**, 4358–4365.

27. Wang, C., Eyre, D. R., Clark, D., Kleinberg, C., Newman, C., Iranmanesh, A., Veldhuis, J., Dudley, R. E., Berman, N., Davidson, T., Barstow, T. J., Sinow, R., Alexander, G., and Swerdloff, R. S. (1996). Sublingual testosterone replacement improves muscle mass and strength, decreases bone resorption, and increases bone formation

28. Guo, C.-Y., Jones, H., and Eastell, R. (1997). Treatment of isolated hypogonadotropic hypogonadism effect on bone mineral density and bone turnover. *J. Clin. Endocrinol. Metab.* **82**, 658–665.

29. McElduff, A., Wilkinson, M., Ward, P., and Posen, S. (1988). Forearm mineral content in normal men: relationship to weight, height and plasma testosterone concentrations. *Bone* **9**, 281–283.

30. Kelly, P. J., Pocock, N. A., Sambrook, P. N., and Eisman, J. A. (1990). Dietary calcium, sex hormones, and bone mineral density in men. *Br. Med. J.* **300**, 1361–1364.

31. Rudman, D., Feller, A. G., Hoskote, S., Nagraj, S., Gergans, G. A., Lalitha, P. Y., Goldberg, A. F., Schlenker, R. A., Cohn, L., Rudman, I. W., and Mattson, D. E. (1990). Effects of human growth hormone in men over 60 years old. *N. Engl. J. Med.* **323**, 1–6.

32. Murphy, S., Khaw, K.-T., Cassidy, A., and Compston, J. E. (1993). Sex hormones and bone mineral density in elderly men. *Bone Miner.* **20**, 133–140.

33. Meier, D. E., Orwoll, E. S., Keenan, E. J., and Fagerstrom, R. M. (1987). Marked decline in trabecular bone mineral content in healthy men with age: Lack of association with sex steroid levels. *J. Am. Geriatr. Soc.* **35**, 189–197.

34. Drinka, P. J., Olson, J., Bauwens, S., Voeks, S., Carlson, I., and Wilson, M. (1993). Lack of association between free testosterone and bone density separate from age in elderly males. *Calcif. Tissue Int.* **52**, 67–69.

35. Wishart, J. M., Need, A. G., Horowitz, M., Morris, H. A., and Nordin, B. E. C. (1995). Effect of age on bone density and bone turnover in men. *Clin. Endocrinol.* **42**, 141–146.

36. Tenover, J. S. (1992). Effects of testosterone supplementation in the aging male. *J. Clin. Endocrinol. Metab.* **75**, 1092–1098.

37. Morishima, A., Grumbach, M. M., Simpson, E. R., Fisher, C., and Qin, K. (1995). Aromatase deficiency in male and female siblings caused by a novel mutation and the physiological role of estrogens. *J. Clin. Endocrinol. Metab.* **80**, 3689–3698.

38. Sasano, H., Uzuki, M., Sawai, T., Nagura, H., Matsunaga, G., Kashimoto, O., and Harada, N. (1997). Aromatase in human bone tissue. *J. Bone Miner. Res.* **12**, 1416–1423.

39. Van Kesteren, P., Lips, P., Deville, W., Popp-Snijders, C., Asscheman, H., Megens, J., and Gooren, L. (1996). The effect of one-year cross-sex hormonal treatment on bone metabolism and serum insulin-like growth factor-1 in transsexuals. *J. Clin. Endocrinol. Metab.* **81**, 2227–2232.

40. Greendale, G. A., Edelstein, S., and Barrett-Connor, E. (1997). Endogenous sex steroids and bone mineral density in older women and men: The Rancho Bernardo Study. *J. Bone Miner. Res.* **12**, 1833–1843.

41. Slemenda, C. W., Longscope, C., Zhou, I., Hui, S., Peacock, M., and Johnston, C. C. (1997). Sex steroids and bone mass in older men. Positive associations with serum estrogens and negative associations with androgens. *J. Clin. Invest.* **100**, 1755–1759.

42. Wakley, G. K., Schutte, H. D. J., Hannon, K. S., and Turner, R. T. (1991). Androgen treatment prevents loss of cancellous bone in the orchidectomized rat. *J. Bone Miner. Res.* **6**, 325–330.

43. Goulding, A., and Gold, E. (1993). Flutamide-mediated androgen blockade evokes osteopenia in the female rat. *J. Bone Miner. Res.* **8**, 763–769.

44. Mason, R. A., and Morris, H. A. (1997). Effects of dihydrotestosterone on bone biochemical markers in sham and oophorectomized rats. *J. Bone Miner. Res.* **12**, 1431–1437.

45. Wiren, K. M., Zhang, X., Chang, C., Keenan, E., and Orwoll, E. (1997). Transcriptional up-regulation of the human androgen receptor by androgen in bone cells. *Endocrinology* **138**, 2291–2300.

46. Felson, D. T., Zhang, Y., Hannan, M. T., Kiel, D. P., Wilson, P. W. F., and Anderson, J. J. (1993). The effect of postmenopausal estrogen therapy on bone density in elderly women. *N. Engl. J. Med.* **329**, 1141–1146.

markers in hypogonadal men—A clinical research center study. *J. Clin. Endocrinol. Metab.* **81**, 3654–3662.

47. Nguyen, T. V., Kelly, P. J., Sambrook, P. N., Gilbert, C., Pocock, N. A., and Eisman, J. A. (1994). Lifestyle factors and bone density in the elderly: Implications for osteoporosis prevention. *J. Bone Miner. Res.* **9**, 1339–1346.

48. Vogel, J. M., Davis, J. W., Nomura, A., Wasnich, R. D., and Ross, P. D. (1997). The effects of smoking on bone mass and the rates of bone loss among elderly Japanese-American men. *J. Bone Miner. Res.* **12**, 1495–1501.

49. Kelepouris, N., Harper, K. D., Gannon, F., Kaplan, F. S., and Haddad, J. G. (1995). Severe osteoporosis in men. *Ann. Intern. Med.* **123**, 452–460.

50. Johansson, A. G., Eriksen, E. F., Lindh, E., Langdahl, B., Blum, W. F., Lindahl, A., Ljunggren, O., and Ljunghall, S. (1997). Reductions in serum levels of the growth hormone-dependent insulin-like growth factor binding protein and a negative bone balance at the level of individual remodeling units in idiopathic osteoporosis in men. *J. Clin. Endocrinol. Metab.* **82**, 2795–2798.

51. Kurland, T. S., Rosen, C. J., Cosman, F., McMahon, D., Chan, F., Shane, E., Lindsay, R., Dempster, D., and Bilezikian, J. P. (1997). Insulin-like growth factor-I in men with idiopathic osteoporosis. *J. Clin. Endocrinol. Metab.* **82**, 2799–2805.

52. Orwoll, E. S., and Klein, R. F. (1995). Osteoporosis in men. *Endocr. Rev.* **16**, 87–116.

53. Francis, R. M., Peacock, M., Marshall, D. H., Horsman, A., and Aaron, J. E. (1989). Spinal osteoporosis in men. *Bone Miner.* **5**, 347–357.

54. Riggs, B. L., Wahner, H. W., Seeman, E., Offord, K. P., Dunn, W. L., Mazess, R. B., Johnson, K. A., and Melton, L. J. (1982). Changes in bone mineral density of the proximal femur and spine with aging. *J. Clin. Invest.* **70**, 716–723.

55. Genant, H. K., Gordan, G. S., and Hoffman, P. G. J. (1983). Osteoporosis. Part I. Advanced radiologic assessment using quantitative computed tomography—Medical Staff Conference, University of California, San Francisco. *West. J. Med.* **139**, 75–84.

56. Resch, A., Schneider, B., Bernecker, P., Battmann, A., Wergedal, J., Willvonseder, R., and Resch, H. (1995). Risk of vertebral fractures in men: relationship to mineral density of the vertebral body. *Am. J. Res.* **164**, 1447–1450.

57. Chevalley, T., Rizzoli, R., Nydegger, V., Slosman, D., Tkatch, L., Rapin, C.-H., Vasey, H., and Bonjour, J.-P. (1991). Preferential low bone mineral density of the femoral neck in patients with a recent fracture of the proximal femur. *Osteoporosis Int.* **1**, 147–154.

58. Karlsson, M. K., Johnell, O., Nilsson, B. E., Sernbo, I., and Obrant, K. J. (1993). Bone mineral mass in hip fracture patients. *Bone* **14**, 161–165.

59. Nguyen, T., Sambrook, P., Kelly, P., Jones, G., Lord, S., and Freund, J. (1993). Prediction of osteoporotic fractures by postural instability and bone density. *Br. Med. J.* **307**, 1111–1115.

60. Poor, G., Atkinson, E. J., O'Fallon, W. M., and Melton, J. L. (1995). Predictors of hip fractures in elderly men. *J. Bone Miner. Res.* **10**, 1902–1905.

61. Hindmarsh, J. J., and Estes, E. H. (1989). Falls in older persons: Causes and interventions. *Arch. Intern. Med.* **149**, 2217–2222.

62. Tinetti, M. E., Speechley, M., and Ginter, S. F. (1988). Risk factors for falls among elderly persons living in the community. *N. Engl. J. Med.* **319**, 1701–1707.

63. O'Neill, T. W., Varlow, J., Reeve, J., Reid, D. M., Todd, C., Woolf, A. D., and Silman, A. J. (1995). Fall frequeny and incidence of distal forearm fracture in the UK. *J. Epidemiol. Commun. Health* **49**, 597–598.

64. Christian, J. C., Yu, P.-L., Slemenda, C. W., and Johnston, C. C. J. (1989). Heritability of bone mass: A longitudinal study in aging male twins. *Am. J. Hum. Genet.* **44**, 429–433.

65. Evans, R. A., Marel, G. M., Lancaster, E. K., Kos, S., Evans, M., and Wong, S. Y. P. (1988). Bone mass is low in relatives of osteoporotic patients. *Ann. Intern. Med.* **109**, 870–873.

66. Soroko, S. B., Barrett-Connor, E., Edelstein, S. L., and Kritz-Silverstein, D. (1994). Family history of osteoporosis and bone mineral density at the axial skeleton: The Rancho Bernardo Study. *J. Bone Miner. Res.* **9**, 761–769.

67. Diaz, M. N., O'Neill, T. W., and Silman, A. J. (1997). The influence of family history of hip fracture on the risk of vertebral deformity in men and women: The European vertebral osteoporosis study. *Bone* **20**, 145–149.

68. Smith, D. M., Nance, W. E., Kang, K. W., Christian, J. C., and Johnston, C. C. (1973). Genetic factors determining bone mass. *J. Clin. Invest.* **52**, 2800–2808.

69. Krall, E. A., and Dawson-Hughes, B. (1993). Heritable and lifestyle determinants of bone mineral density. *J. Bone Miner. Res.* **8**, 1–9.

70. Gueguen, R., Jouanny, P., Guillemin, F., Kuntz, C., Pourel, J., and Siest, G. (1995). Segregation analysis and variance components analysis of bone mineral density in healthy families. *J. Bone Miner. Res.* **10**, 2017–2022.

71. Morrison, N. A., Qi, J. C., Tokita, A., Kelly, P. J., Crofts, L., Nguyen, T. V., Sambrook, P. N., and Eisman, J. A. (1994). Prediction of bone density from vitamin D receptor alleles. *Nature* **367**, 284–287.

72. Spolita, L. D., Caminis, J., Devoto, M., Shimoya, K., Sereda, L., Ott, J., Whyte, M. P., Tenenhouse, A., and Prockop, D. J. (1996). Osteopenia in 37 members of seven families: Analysis based on a model of dominant inheritance. *Mol. Med.* **2**, 313–324.

73. Johnson, M. L., Gong, G., Kimberling, W., Recker, S. M., Kimmel, D. B., and Recker, R. R. (1997). Linkage of a gene causing high bone mass to human chromosome 11 (11q12–13). *Am. J. Hum. Genet.* **60**, 1326–1332.

74. Uitterlinden, A. G., Pols, H. A. P., Burger, H., Huang, Q., Van Daele, P. L. A., Van Duijn, C. M., Hofman, A., Birkenhager, J. C., and Leeuwen, J. P. T. M. (1996). A large-scale population-based study of the association of vitamin D receptor gene polymorphisms with bone mineral density. *J. Bone Miner. Res.* **11**, 1241–1248.

75. Johansson, A., Forslund, A., and Hambraeus, L. (1994). Growth-hormone-dependent insulin-like growth factor binding protein is a major determinant of bone mineral density in healthy men. *J. Bone Miner. Res.* **9**, 915–921.

76. Ljunghall, S., Johansson, A. G., Burman, P., Kampe, O., Lindh, E., and Karlsson, F. A. (1992). Low plasma levels of insulin-like growth factor 1 (IGF-1) in male patients with idiopathic osteoporosis. *J. Intern. Med.* **232**, 59–64.

77. Inzucchi, S. E., and Robbins, R. J. (1996). Growth hormone and the maintenance of adult bone mineral density. *Clin. Endocrinol.* **45**, 665–673.

78. Toogood, A. A., Adams, J. E., O'Neill, P. A., and Shalet, S. M. (1997). Elderly patients with adult onset growth hormone deficiency are not osteopenic. *J. Clin. Endocrinol. Metab.* **82**, 1462–1466.

79. Marcus, R. (1997). Skeletal effects of growth hormone and IGF-1 in adults. *Endocrine* **7**, 53–55.

80. Kotzmann, H., Riedl, M., Bernecker, P., Clodi, M., Kainberger, F., Kaider, A., Woloszczuk, W., and Luger, A. (1998). Effects of long term growth hormone substitution therapy on bone mineral density and parameters of bone metabolism in adult patients with growth hormone deficiency. *Calcif. Tissue Int.* **62**, 40–46.

81. Burman, P., Johansson, A. G., Siegbahn, A., Vessby, B., and Karlsson, A. (1997). Growth hormone (GH)-deficient men are more responsive to GH replacement therapy than women. *J. Clin. Endocrinol. Metab.* **82**, 550–555.

82. Thomas, M. K., Lloyd-Jones, D. M., Thadhani, R. I., Shaw, A. C., Deraska, D. J., Kitch, B. T., Vamvakas, E. C., Dick, I. M., Prince, R. L., and Finkelstein, J. S. (1998). Hypovitaminosis D in medical inpatients. *N. Engl. J. Med.* **338**, 777–783.

83. Orwoll, E. S., and Meier, D. E. (1986). Alterations in calcium, vitamin D, and parathyroid hormone physiology in normal men with aging: Re-

lationship to the development of senile osteopenia. *J. Clin. Endocrinol. Metab.* **63**, 1262–1269.

84. Riggs, B. L., and Melton, L. J. (1986). Medical progress: Involutional osteoporosis. *N. Engl. J. Med.* **314**, 1676–1686.

85. Gallagher, J. C., Kinyamu, H. K., Fowler, S. E., Dawson-Hughes, B., Dalsky, G. P., and Sherman, S. S. (1998). Calciotropic hormones and bone markers in the elderly. *J. Bone Miner. Res.* **13**, 475–482.

86. Halloran, B. P., Portale, A. A., Lonergan, E. T., and Morris, R. C. J. (1990). Production and metabolic clearance of 1,25-dihydroxyvitamin D in men: Effect of advancing age. *J. Clin. Endocrinol. Metab.* **70**, 318–323.

87. Dawson-Hughes, B., Harris, S. S., Krall, E. A., and Dallal, G. E. (1997). Effect of calcium and vitamin D supplementation on bone density in men and women 65 years of age or older. *N. Engl. J. Med.* **337**, 670–702.

88. Mosekilde, L. (1989). Sex differences in age-related loss of vertebral trabecular bone mass and structure—biomechanical consequences. *Bone* **10**, 425–432.

89. Eriksen, E. F. (1986). Normal and pathological remodeling of human trabecular bone: Three dimensional reconstruction of the remodeling sequence in normals and in metabolic bone disease. *Endocr. Revi.* **7**, 379–408.

90. Mosekilde, L., and Mosekilde, L. (1990). Sex differences in age-related changes in vertebral body size, density and biomechanical competence in normal individuals. *Bone* **11**, 67–73.

91. Martin, R. B., and Atkinson, P. J. (1977). Age and sex-related changes in the structure and strength of the human femoral shaft. *J. Biomech.* **10**, 223–231.

92. Nordin, B. E. C., Aaron, J., Speed, R., Francis, R. M., and Makins, N. (1984). Bone formation and resorption as the determinants of trabecular bone volume in normal and osteoporotic men. *Scott. Med. J.* **29**, 171–175.

93. Marie, P. J., de Vernejoul, M. C., Donnes, D., and Hott, M. (1991). Decreased DNA synthesis by culture osteoblastic cells in eugonadal osteoporotic men with defective bone formation. *J. Clin. Invest.* **88**, 1167–1172.

94. Clarke, B. L., Ebeling, P. R., Jones, J. D., Wahner, H. W., O'Fallon, W. M., and Fitzpatrick, L. A. (1996). Changes in quantitative bone histomorphometry in aging healthy men. *J. Clin. Endocrinol. Metab.* **81**, 2264–2270.

95. Delmas, P. D., Gineyts, E., Bertholin, A., Garnero, P., and Marchand, F. (1993). Immunoassay of pyridinoline crosslink excretion in normal adults and in Paget's disease. *J. Bone Miner. Res.* **8**, 643–648.

96. Orwoll, E. S., and Deftos, L. J. (1990). Serum osteocalcin (BGP) levels in normal men: A longitudinal evaluation reveals an age-associated increase. *J. Bone Miner. Res.* **5**, 259–262.

97. Garnero, P., and Delmas, P. D. (1993). Assessment of the serum levels of bone alkaline phosphatase with a new immunoradiometric assay in patients with metabolic bone disease. *J. Clin. Endocrinol. Metab.* **77**, 1046–1053.

98. Orwoll, E. S., Bell, N. H., Nanes, M. S., Flessland, K. A., Pettinger, M. B., Mallinak, J. S., and Cain, D. F. (1998). Collagen N-telopeptide excretion in men: The effects of age and intra-subject variability. *J. Bone Miner. Res.* **83**, 3930–3935.

99. Schneider, D. L., and Barrett-Connor, E. L. (1997). Urinary N-telopeptide levels discriminate normal, osteopenic and osteoporotic bone mineral density. *Arch. Intern. Med.* **157**, 1241–1245.

100. Hanson, D. A., Weis, M. A. E., Bollen, A.-M., Maslan, S. L., Singer, F. R., and Eyre, D. R. (1992). A specific immunoassay for monitoring human bone resorption: Quantitation of Type I collagen cross-linked n-telopeptides in urine. *J. Bone Miner. Res.* **7**, 1251–1258.

101. Rico, H., Revilla, M., and Hernandez, E. R. (1992). Sex differences in the acquisition of total bone mineral mass peak assessed through dual-energy x-ray absorptiometry. *Calcif. Tissue Int.* **51**, 251–254.

102. Lakatos, P., Blumsohn, A., Eastell, R., Tarjan, G., Shinoda, H., and

103. Stern, P. H. (1995). Circadian rhythm of *in vitro* bone-resorbing activity in human serum. *J. Clin. Endocrinol. Metab.* **80**, 3185–3190.

103. Greenspan, S. L., Dresner-Pollack, R., Parker, R. A., London, D., and Ferguson, L. (1996). Diurnal variation of bone mineral turnover in elderly men and women. *Calcif. Tissue Int.* **60**, 419–423.

104. Nielsen, H. K., Brixen, K., Kassem, M., Charles, P., and Mosekilde, L. (1992). Inhibition of the morning cortisol peak abolishes the expected morning decrease in serum osteocalcin in normal males: Evidence of a controlling effect of serum cortisol on the circadian rhythm in serum osteocalcin. *J. Clin. Endocrinol. Metab.* **74**, 1410–1414.

105. Resch, H., Pietschmann, P., Woloszczuk, W., Krexner, E., Bernecker, P., and Willvonseder, R. (1992). Bone mass and biochemical parameters of bone metabolism in men with spinal osteoporosis. *Eur. J. Clin. Invest.* **22**, 542–545.

106. Hetland, M. L., Haarbo, J., and Christiansen, C. (1993). Low bone mass and high bone turnover in male long distance runners. *J. Clin. Endocrinol. Metab.* **77**, 770–775.

107. Goldwray, D., Weisman, Y., Jaccard, N., Merdler, C., Chen, J., and Matzkin, H. (1993). Decreased bone mineral density in elderly men treated with the gonadotropin-releasing hormone agonist decapeptyl (D-trp6-GnRH). *J. Clin. Endocrinol. Metab.* **76**, 288–290.

108. Morley, J. E., Perry, H. M., III, Kaiser, F. E., Kraenzel, D., Jensen, J., Houston, K., Mattammal, M., and Perry, H. M., Jr. (1993). Effects of testosterone replacement therapy in old hypogonadal males: A preliminary study. *J. Am. Geriatr. Soc.* **41**, 149–152.

109. Anderson, F. H., Francis, R. M., Peaston, R. T., and Wastell, H. J. (1997). Androgen supplementation in eugonadal men with osteoporosis: Effects of six months' treatment on markers of bone formation and resorption. *J. Bone Miner. Res.* **12**, 472–478.

110. Eastell, R., and Riggs, B. L. (1980). Diagnostic evaluation of osteoporosis. *Endocrinol. Metab. Clin. North Am.* **17**, 547–571.

111. Lane, J. M., and Vigorita, V. J. (1984). Osteoporosis. *Orthop. Clin. North Am.* **15**, 711–728.

112. Aaron, J. E., Stasiak, L., Gallagher, J. C., Longton, E. B., Nicholson, M., Anderson, J., and Nordin, B. E. C. (1974). Frequency of osteomalacia and osteoporosis in fractures of the proximal femur. *Lancet* **1**, 229–233.

113. Campbell, G. A., Hosking, D. J., Kemm, J. R., and Boyd, R. V. (1984). How common is osteomalacia in the elderly? *Lancet* **2**, 386–388.

114. Hordon, L. D., and Peacock, M. (1990). Osteomalacia and osteoporosis in femoral neck fracture. *Bone Miner.* **11**, 247–259.

115. Sokoloff, L. (1978). Occult osteomalacia in America (USA) patients with fracture of the hip. *Am. J. Surg. Pathol.* **2**, 21–30.

116. Wilton, T. J., Hosking, D. J., Pawley, E., Stevens, A., and Harvey, L. (1987). Osteomalacia and femoral neck fractures in the elderly patient. *J. Bone Jt. Surg. Br. Vol.* **69-B**, 388–390.

117. Marel, G. M., McKenna, M. J., and Frame, B. (1986). Osteomalacia. *Bone Miner. Res.* **4**, 335–413.

118. Johnston, C. C., Jr., Slemenda, C. W., and Melton, L. J., III. (1991). Clinical use of bone densitometry. *N. Engl. J. Med.* **324**, 1105–1109.

119. Looker, A. C., Johnston, C. C., Wahner, H. W. J., Dunn, W. L., Calvo, M. S., Harris, T. B., Heyse, S. P., and Lindsay, R. L. (1995). Defining low femur bone density levels in men. *17th Annu. Meet. Am. Soc. Bone Miner. Res.*, Baltimore, MD.

120. Klein, R. F., and Gunness, M. (1992). The transiliac bone biopsy: When to get it and how to interpret it. *Endocrinologist* **2**, 158–168.

121. Jackson, J. A., and Kleerekoper, M. (1990). Osteoporosis in men: Diagnosis, pathophysiology, and prevention. *Medicine* **69**, 137–152.

122. Chines, A., Pacifici, R., Avioli, L. V., Teitelbaum, S. L., and Korenblat, P. E. (1991). Systemic mastocytosis presenting as osteoporosis: A clinical and histomorphometric study. *J. Clin. Endocrinol. Metab.* **72**, 140–144.

123. Chines, A., Pacifici, R., Avioli, L. A., Korenblat, P. E., and Teitelbaum, S. L. (1993). Systemic mastocytosis and osteoporosis. *Osteoporosis Int.* **1**, S147–S149.

CHAPTER 35

Steroid-Induced Osteoporosis

IAN R. REID   Department of Medicine, University of Auckland, Auckland, New Zealand

I. ABSTRACT

Glucocorticoids in supraphysiological doses rapidly lead to a reduction in bone mass; up to 40% of trabecular bone is lost after several years of continuous therapy. This results in fractures in about one-third of patients treated long-term with these drugs. Histologically, the most consistent changes are a reduction in bone formation and a reduction in osteoblast proliferation. The former is probably mediated by direct glucocorticoid receptor effects on the transcription of genes coding for bone matrix proteins. Circulating concentrations of osteocalcin, a marker of bone formation, are very sensitive to glucocorticoid effects on the osteoblast; they are substantially reduced within hours of glucocorticoid exposure and recover within a day or two of its discontinuation. Changes in other specific osteoblast markers are much less consistent, and there is no clear evidence of glucocorticoid effects on biochemical indices of bone resorption. Markers have proven valuable in determining the mechanisms by which glucocorticoids impact bone but they are not, at the present time, established as having a role in the evaluation and management of individual patients requiring glucocorticoid therapy.

II. INTRODUCTION

Glucocorticoid drugs were introduced into clinical practice in the 1950s and have proved lifesaving in conditions such as asthma. They are able to substantially modify the course of many other conditions such as rheumatoid arthritis and inflammatory bowel disease. Their more widespread use is prevented by their side effects, which include the development of osteoporosis. Bone loss occurs rapidly following the introduction of these drugs; barely supraphysiological doses (e.g., prednisone 7.5 mg/day) reduce trabecular bone density by 8% over a 20 week period [1]. Cross-sectional studies in patients receiving treatment for several years typically show reductions of integral bone density in the spine and proximal femur of 10–20% [2] and of approximately twice this magnitude when predominantly trabecular bone is assessed [3, 4]. This results in approximately one-third of patients on long-term steroids showing evidence of vertebral fractures after 5–10 years of treatment [5–10]. The risk of hip fracture is also increased nearly threefold [11].

This chapter reviews the mechanisms by which glucocorticoids produce this dramatic bone loss and summarizes the changes that have been reported in biochemical markers of bone turnover. The potential role of markers in the management of steroid-treated subjects will then be discussed.

III. PATHOGENESIS OF STEROID-INDUCED OSTEOPOROSIS

Because of the widespread distribution of the glucocorticoid receptor, these agents are able to impact bone and calcium metabolism at many levels.

A. Osteoblasts

The most consistently demonstrated effects of glucocorticoids on bone are in the osteoblast. *In vitro*, glucocorticoids can be characterized as increasing osteoblast differentiation and decreasing their proliferation. The former effect may be partly attributable to increased production of bone morphogenic protein-6 [12] and the latter to reduced expression of cyclin-dependent kinases and cyclin-D3 together with enhanced transcription of inhibitors of cyclin-dependent kinases [13]. There is also evidence for glucocorticoid regulation of a number of important osteoblastic genes, including those for type I collagen, osteocalcin, osteopontin, fibronectin, β-1 integrin, bone sialoprotein, alkaline phosphatase, collagenase, and the nuclear proto-oncogenes c-myc, c-fos, and c-jun. In osteoblast precursor cells, gene expression is modulated to produce a more differentiated osteoblastic phenotype, whereas in the mature osteoblast cell proliferation and matrix synthesis are reduced with glucocorticoids. These effects may be biphasic with respect to both dose and time; inhibition of osteoblast proliferation and activity are evident at high hormone concentrations and with long exposure periods [14, 15].

Osteoblasts produce factors that act in an autocrine manner to regulate their own activity. Insulin-like growth factors (IGF)-1 and -2 act in this way, and their local synthesis is inhibited by glucocorticoids. Their local activity is modulated by the interplay of specific binding proteins and there is now evidence that glucocorticoids cause a reduction in the levels of the stimulatory binding proteins, IGFBP-3 and IGFBP-5 [16–18] and an increase in production of IGFBP-6, an inhibitor of IGF-2 activity [19]. However, blocking the effects of endogenous IGFs does not abrogate the effect of glucocorticoids on osteoblast proliferation and collagen synthesis [20]. Transforming growth factor-β is another important autocrine factor that is modulated by glucocorticoids [21, 22].

B. Osteoclasts

The effects of glucocorticoids on osteoclasts are contradictory. There is evidence that glucocorticoids increase osteoclast formation from precursor cells in bone marrow [23, 24] but also that they lead to apoptosis of mature osteoclasts [25, 26]. These opposing effects may account for the findings in organ culture that glucocorticoids can either increase or decrease bone resorption, depending on the culture conditions [27–29]. In organ culture, glucocorticoid effects may also be contributed to by their inhibition of local production of cytokines, such as interleukin-1 and the tumor necrosis factors, which themselves have potent effects on bone resorption.

C. Intestinal and Renal Handling of Calcium and Phosphate

Clinical studies have consistently demonstrated an inhibition of calcium absorption associated with glucocorticoid treatment. This is not mediated by changes in vitamin D metabolites and is therefore likely to represent a direct effect on the calcium transport system in the small intestine.

Within weeks of glucocorticoid treatment there is a substantial rise in urine calcium excretion [30, 31] which is not accounted for by changes in the serum ionized calcium or the glomerular filtration rate. This suggests that glucocorticoids directly regulate tubular resorption of calcium [32]. There is also evidence for malabsorption of phosphate in both the gut and renal tubule associated with glucocorticoid use, as demonstrated in Figures 1 and 2 [33].

D. Vitamin D

There is little evidence to support the contention that changes in vitamin D metabolism contribute significantly to the development of steroid-induced osteoporosis. Prospective studies of patients or normal subjects beginning steroid therapy have shown no changes in 25-hydroxyvitamin D or 24,25-dihydroxyvitamin D, but significant increases in 1,25-dihydroxyvitamin D have been observed 2–15 days after initiation of therapy (see Figs. 1 and 2) [33]. These effects are likely to be secondary to changes in parathyroid hormone and/or serum phosphate concentrations. There is no evidence for glucocorticoid effects on concentrations of vitamin D binding protein [34].

E. Parathyroid Hormone

A number of groups have found increases in circulating concentrations of parathyroid hormone within minutes to weeks of the initiation of steroid therapy (see Figs. 1 and 2) [33, 35], although this has not been universal. In cross-sectional studies of patients receiving chronic glucocorticoid therapy, elevations of parathyroid hormone levels of 50–100% above those of control subjects have been reported [35].

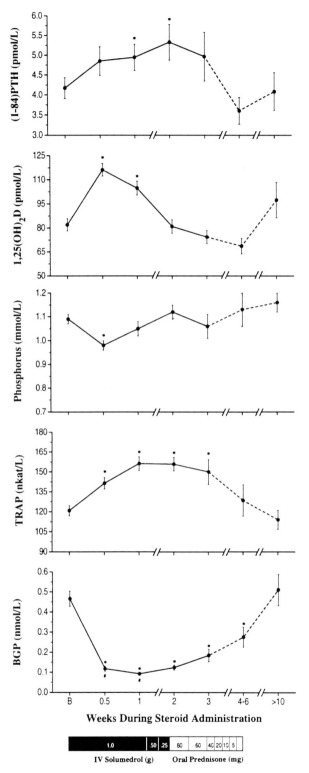

FIGURE 1 Effects of intravenous methylprednisolone and oral prednisone in the doses indicated on serum indices of bone and mineral metabolism. Asterisks denote a significant change from baseline. PTH, parathyroid hormone; TRAP, tartrate-resistant acid phosphatase; BGP, osteocalcin. Reproduced from [33] *J. Bone Miner. Res.* 1994; 1097–1105 with permission of the American Society for Bone and Mineral Research and the authors.

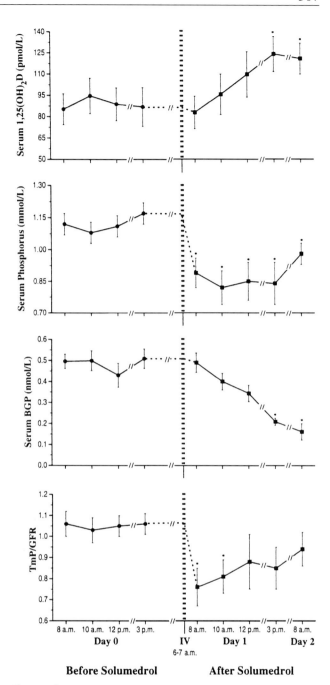

FIGURE 2 Changes in serum and urine indices after an intravenous infusion of 1 g methylprednisolone. Asterisks denote a significant change from baseline. BGP, osteocalcin; TmP/GFR, tubular maximum for phosphate reabsorption. Reproduced from [33] *J. Bone Miner. Res.* 1994; 1097–1105 with permission of the American Society for Bone and Mineral Research and the authors.

In vitro studies of parathyroid tissue from rats [36], cattle [37], and humans [38] suggest that hyperparathyroidism may result directly from the action of glucocorticoids on the parathyroid cell, though it is also possible that calcium malabsorption in both the gut and the renal tubule contributes. It is interesting to note that some groups have suggested circulating calcium levels are elevated in steroid-treated subjects [39, 40], though there are many studies which have not found this and some which have found the opposite [41]. In addition to studies of parathyroid hormone concentrations, there is a substantial literature suggesting an increase in osteoblast sensitivity to parathyroid hormone after glucocorticoid treatment [42–45], possibly as a result of increased G-protein expression [46].

F. Sex Hormones

Sex hormones are important regulators of bone metabolism, and hypogonadism in either sex is associated with the development of osteoporosis. Glucocorticoids acutely depress plasma levels of testosterone in men [47] and their chronic use is associated with a dose-dependent reduction in free testosterone concentrations of approximately 50% [48]. These changes appear to result from inhibition of gonadotropin secretion and a reduction in numbers of gonadotropin-binding sites in the testis. High-dose steroid therapy is associated with oligomenorrhea in women, suggesting a similar effect on the pituitary-gonadal axis.

IV. EFFECTS OF GLUCOCORTICOIDS ON HISTOLOGICAL INDICES OF BONE TURNOVER

The morphometric effects of glucocorticoids on bone have been reviewed by Dempster [49]. Such studies have sampled bone at different sites and studied patients with a variety of underlying conditions—these factors may account for the heterogeneity of findings. However, in general, osteoid thickness is reduced by glucocorticoids, as is the mineral apposition rate [50–53]. The rate of formation of mineralized bone per unit of osteoid surface is usually found to be reduced by glucocorticoids [51, 54]. Consistent with this is the finding that the amount of bone replaced within each osteoclast lacuna is diminished (i.e., the wall thickness is reduced) [54, 55]. Thus, there is clear histomorphometric evidence of reduced osteoblast activity during steroid treatment. Similar results have also been reported in elderly ewes [56].

The effects on histological assessments of bone resorption are less clear-cut. Eroded surfaces are increased by steroid treatment [50, 57]. However, much of this surface does not contain active osteoclasts, and some studies have actually shown osteoclast numbers to be decreased [56]. This has been interpreted as reflecting an inhibition of recruitment of osteoblasts to the eroded surface (leaving eroded surfaces unfilled for a greater time than normal) rather than an acceleration of bone resorption itself. This would be consistent with the data from biochemical markers of bone resorption, to be reviewed in the next section.

V. EFFECTS OF GLUCOCORTICOIDS ON MARKERS OF BONE TURNOVER

A. Osteocalcin

Shortly after this bone matrix protein was shown to be measurable in the circulation and to reflect bone formation rates, it was noted to be reduced by approximately 50% in subjects treated with glucocorticoids [58]. Circulating levels of osteocalcin were found to be inversely related to the current glucocorticoid dose and were positively related to circulating levels of 1,25-dihydroxyvitamin D. Subsequently, it was shown that circulating osteocalcin concentrations decline within 24 hours of the first steroid dose and rapidly return to normal following the discontinuation of steroid therapy [59]. These effects are demonstrated in Figures 1 and 2. The molecular basis of these observations has been provided by the work of Morrison et al. [60] who demonstrated that transcription of the osteocalcin gene was negatively regulated by the glucocorticoid receptor and positively by the calcitriol receptor. There appear to be multiple glucocorticoid receptor binding sites in the osteocalcin gene promoter [61]. Detailed studies in sheep have indicated that glucocorticoids reduce the plasma production rate of osteocalcin and that osteocalcin plasma clearance rates are unaffected by prednisone, though they are increased by high doses of deflazacort [62].

The sensitivity of circulating osteocalcin concentrations to glucocorticoids has been of great value in assessing the systemic bioavailability of topically-administered steroids. This has been extensively used in studies of the various inhaled glucocorticoids [63–65] as well as in demonstrating bone effects from glucocorticoids administered rectally [66] and by intra-articular injection [67]. However, studies of osteocalcin in steroid-treated patients need to be interpreted with caution because the patient's underlying condition, in some cases, will also influence circulating concentrations of this peptide. In rheumatoid arthritis, for example, osteocalcin levels are lower than normal even in those not receiving glucocorticoids [68].

B. Other Markers of Bone Formation

The sensitivity of osteocalcin to glucocorticoids is probably a reflection of the direct regulation of the osteocalcin gene by the glucocorticoid receptor, because other osteoblast markers show less consistent responses (see Table I). Thus, total alkaline phosphatase level (AP) has been found to be no different from control values when studied cross-sectionally [69], though in prospective studies of glucocorticoid administration some depression of this index is detectable in most [70–72], but not all, studies [73]. The bone isoenzyme of alkaline phosphatase has been studied in two prospective

TABLE I.   Prospective Studies of the Effects of Glucocorticoids on Biochemical Markers of Bone Turnover

	Study reference					
	Prummel *et al.* [70]	Morrison *et al.* [77]	Cosman *et al.* [33]	Lems *et al.* [73]	Lane *et al.* [71]	Wolthers *et al.* [74]
Underlying disease	EGO	COAD	MS	RA	Asthma	Nil
Treatment duration	12 weeks	4 weeks	5 weeks	8 days	5 days	3 days
Drug	Pred	Pred	Pred	Dexa	Pred	Pred
Daily dose	40 mg	20 mg	1 g → 5 mg	75 mg	40 mg	40 mg
Formation markers						
Osteocalcin	↓	→	↓↓	↓	↓	
Total AP	↓	↓		→	↓	
Bone AP	↓ (NS)				→	
PICP				↓		↓
Resorption markers						
ICTP				↓		↓
Pyridinoline			→	↓		→
Deoxypyridinoline				↓	→	→
Hydroxyproline	→	↑	→	→		
TRAP			↑		→	
Urine calcium	↑		↑	→		

Abbreviations: EGO, euthyroid Grave's opthalmopathy; COAD, chronic obstructive airways disease; MS, multiple sclerosis; RA, rheumatoid arthritis; pred, (methyl)prednis(ol)one; dexa, dexamethasone; AP, alkaline phosphatase; PICP, carboy-terminal propeptide of type I procollagen; ICTP, carboxy-terminal telopeptide of type I collagen; TRAP, tartrate-resistant acidphosphatase; NS, not significant; →, no change; ↑, increase; ↓, decrease. Copyright © 1998 I. R. Reid, used with permission.

studies, showing no change in one [71] and a nonsignificant decline in the other [70]. The carboxy-terminal propeptide of type I procollagen (PICP) is a circulating marker of type I collagen synthesis. This has been found to decrease following the introduction of glucocorticoids [73, 74]. Following cure of Cushing's syndrome, there is a prompt increase in markers of bone formation associated with substantial increases in bone mass [75, 76].

C. Resorption Markers

The short-term prospective studies reviewed in the preceding section have also assessed effects of glucocorticoids on biochemical markers of bone resorption. Across the studies, changes in urinary excretion of hydroxyproline, deoxypyridinoline, and pyridinoline have been assessed, as have serum levels of the cross-linked carboxy-terminal telopeptide of type I collagen (ICTP). None of these markers, except for hydroxyproline in one study [77], have shown increases in response to glucocorticoids; Some have, in fact, decreased. In a further prospective study of the administration of inhaled glucocorticoids, there was also evidence of increased hydroxyproline excretion [78]. Since these changes are not seen with the more specific indices of bone resorption, it is possible that this change represents an effect of glucocorticoids on

release of hydroxyproline from other sources (such as skin or complement) or an alteration in its metabolism or excretion. A further novel serum marker of osteoclast activity, tartrate-resistant acid phosphatase (TRAP), was found to increase in one prospective study (Fig. 1) but remained unchanged in another. The positive change in the study of Cosman *et al.* [33] could be interpreted as indicating a change in osteoclast function not resulting in increased bone resorption.

Fasting urine calcium excretion has, in the past, been used as a measure of bone resorption. In several studies, this index has been shown to rise following glucocorticoid use. However, urine calcium excretion will only reflect bone resorption when all other variables affecting it remain constant. There is clear evidence that glucocorticoids inhibit the tubular reabsorption of calcium [32]. This finding, coupled to the absence of any change in the much more specific markers of bone matrix breakdown, suggests that changes in urine calcium do not reliably reflect changes in bone resorption in subjects taking steroid treatment.

The biochemical data are fairly consistent in indicating that bone resorption is not accelerated during the first few months of steroid therapy, a time during which bone loss certainly occurs. These data have helped resolve some of the inconsistencies in the histomorphometric studies. Implicit in these conclusions is the assumption that glucocorticoids have no effect on the metabolism or clearance of the collagen fragments being studied. While this cannot be absolutely proven, the consistent lack of change over a range of different fragments suggests that changes in bone resorption rate are not a major contributor to steroid-induced bone loss.

Following cure of Cushing's syndrome, there is an increase in markers of bone resorption (ICTP and hydroxyproline) as well as those of bone formation [75, 76]. This may, to some extent, reflect the coupling of resorption and formation and may also result from a decline in the rate of osteoclast apoptosis. It does imply that direct stimulation of bone resorption is not a feature of the severe hypercortisolism seen in these patients prior to cure.

VI. EVALUATION OF STEROID-TREATED PATIENTS

The prediction of fractures from clinical characteristics or bone densitometry has only been studied extensively in postmenopausal women. In the absence of comprehensive data relating to steroid osteoporosis, most clinicians extrapolate from the data that are available in postmenopausal women to conclude that previous fractures after minimal trauma and low bone density are both substantial risk factors for future fracture. A clinical history and directed examination are important to determine past fracture history and the extent of trauma associated with each fracture, and also to assess other risk factors such as body weight, cigarette smoking, frequency of falls, alcohol intake, and the presence of other medical conditions.

In the absence of previous low trauma fractures, assessment of future fracture risk is based substantially on the current bone density. Bone loss is initially most marked in the spine, and assessment of spinal bone mass by quantitative computed tomography or dual-energy X-ray absorptiometry (DXA) is appropriate. DXA should preferably be undertaken in the lateral projection because this avoids measurement of the cortical bone of the posterior processes [3], though the antero-posterior projection is frequently used. There is preliminary evidence that ultrasound assessment of bone is as satisfactory as conventional bone densitometry [79].

The development of biochemical markers of bone turnover has been substantially driven by the hope that these would be useful in assessing an individual's fracture risk. There is little convincing evidence that this is so in steroid-treated subjects, though the available data are few. Baseline levels of osteocalcin and other markers, or their changes in the early months of therapy, have generally not been found to relate to subsequent bone loss either in adults [4, 68] or in children [80]. In a group of patients with rheumatoid arthritis, some of whom began hormone replacement therapy, there was a correlation (−0.37) between the change in the carboxy-terminal telopeptide of type I collagen at three months and the change in bone density at two years [68]. All this result is really show-

ing is that both techniques can detect the effects of hormone replacement therapy and it probably has little relevance for predicting outcomes in individuals.

In a study of patients undergoing heart transplantation, Shane [81] did show some correlations between the subsequent rates of bone loss and osteocalcin, urinary deoxypyridinoline, urinary hydroxyproline, and urinary calcium levels. However, these relationships varied from one bone density site to another and from time to time over the period of study. In general, they accounted for less than 10% of the variance in rates of bone loss, suggesting that they are unlikely to be of clinical utility in assessing individuals. This study also suggested that low levels of either serum 25-hydroxyvitamin D or serum testosterone three months after transplantation were related to more rapid bone loss, although the predictive value was, as for the turnover markers, relatively low. Sambrook et al. [82] have reported similar findings in their cardiac transplant patients in whom change in bone mass was related to concentrations of both osteocalcin (directly) and testosterone (inversely). It is of interest that in both of these studies bone loss was positively related to osteocalcin concentrations whereas the effect of glucocorticoids on osteocalcin is to depress it. However, in cardiac transplant patients, cyclosporin is administered in addition to steroids and this increases bone turnover. Thus, this relationship may be specific to this particular drug combination and is not necessarily generalizable to monotherapy with glucocorticoids.

VII. TREATMENT AND FOLLOW-UP

The principal treatments available for steroid osteoporosis are calcium supplementation, replacement of sex hormones in those with demonstrable deficiency, and administration of bisphosphonates, vitamin D and its metabolites, calcitonin, and fluoride. There is little evidence that measurements other than sex hormones and 25-hydroxyvitamin D are useful in selecting which therapy is most appropriate for a specific patient.

The need for calcium supplementation is usually based on the baseline dietary intake; a total intake of 1000–1500 mg/ day is the goal. There is some evidence that higher intakes reduce bone resorption [83], but the effect of this on bone loss is probably relatively small.

Sex hormone replacement is only appropriate for those who are hypogonadal. In postmenopausal women this is clearly the case; in premenopausal women, the presence of regular menstruation is presumptive evidence of adequate sex hormone levels. In amenorrheic premenopausal women and in men, measurement of estradiol or testosterone, respectively, is necessary to assess gonadal function.

Bisphosphonates appear to increase bone density in virtually all subjects. In the large studies carried out with these drugs in postmenopausal osteoporosis it has not been consistently demonstrated that baseline turnover markers are predictive of response.

Vitamin D supplementation with calciferol is appropriate in all individuals with demonstrable deficiency (i.e., those with low serum levels of 25-hydroxyvitamin D). The use of the metabolites of vitamin D has been associated with inconsistent results from clinical trials. In none of the randomized trials have these agents been used as an intervention targeted to individuals on the basis of their baseline vitamin D metabolite concentrations or their intestinal calcium absorption. Therefore, it is entirely speculative as to whether these agents should be targeted according to baseline biochemical values. Fluoride ion has similarly been used in an untargeted fashion in a number of trials.

In contrast, bone density measurement is important in determining to whom therapy should be offered and at what intensity. Thus, in the patient whose bone density is several standard deviations below the young normal range, multiple interventions are often used, such as sex hormone replacement together with a bisphosphonate, or a bisphosphonate together with calcitriol. Such a policy is based on the belief that these agents will work together to increase bone density more effectively than either would alone. While trial evidence supporting this contention is not available in steroid-induced osteoporosis, the experience of clinicians working in the area is that multiple therapies produce larger changes in bone density.

Monitoring of efficacy is based on bone density measurement and fracture occurrence. The latter is an uncommon event, and thus the absence of a new fracture does not necessarily reflect the success of a management regimen. Bone density is a much more sensitive end-point, and after 12 months of therapy with either hormone replacement therapy or a bisphosphonate, there is usually clear evidence of increased spinal bone density in the individual patient. Conversely, if a patient is continuing to suffer multiple fractures, this is a clear indication for review of the management of that individual's osteoporosis, whatever the bone densitometry indicates. However, in my own experience, it is unusual for new fractures to occur in patients in whom bone density has increased significantly.

References

1. Laan, R. F. J. M., Vanriel, P. L. C. M., Vandeputte, L. B. A., Vanerning, L. J. T. O., Vanthof, M. A., and Lemmens, J. A. M. (1993). Low-dose prednisone induces rapid reversible axial bone loss in patients with rheumatoid arthritis—a randomized, controlled study. *Ann. Intern. Med.* **119**, 963–968.

2. Reid, I. R., Evans, M. C., Wattie, D. J., Ames, R., and Cundy, T. F. (1992). Bone mineral density of the proximal femur and lumbar spine in glucocorticoid-treated asthmatic patients. *Osteoporosis Int.* **2**, 103–105.

3. Reid, I. R., Evans, M. C., and Stapleton, J. (1992). Lateral spine densitometry is a more sensitive indicator of glucocorticoid-induced bone loss. *J. Bone Miner. Res.* **7**, 1221–1225.

4. Reid, I. R., and Heap, S. W. (1990). Determinants of vertebral mineral density in patients receiving chronic glucocorticoid therapy. *Arch. Intern. Med.* **150**, 2545–2548.

5. Adinoff, A. D., and Hollister, J. R. (1983). Steroid-induced fractures and bone loss in patients with asthma. *N. Engl. J. Med.* **309**, 265–268.

6. Luengo, M., Picado, C., Del Rio, L., Guanabens, N., Montserrat, J. M., and Setoain, J. (1991). Vertebral fractures in steroid dependent asthma and involutional osteoporosis: A comparative study. *Thorax* **46**, 803–806.

7. Michel, B. A., Bloch, D. A., and Fries, J. F. (1991). Predictors of fractures in early rheumatoid arthritis. *J. Rheumatol.* **18**, 804–808.

8. Laan, R. F. J. M., van Riel, P. L. C. M., van Erning, L. J. T., Lemmens, J. A. M., Ruijs, S. H. J., and van de Putte, L. B. (1992). Vertebral osteoporosis in rheumatoid arthritis patients: Effect of low dose prednisone therapy. *Br. J. Rheumatol.* **31**, 91–96.

9. Spector, T. D., Hall, G. M., McCloskey, E. V., and Kanis, J. A. (1993). Risk of vertebral fracture in women with rheumatoid arthritis. *Br. Med. J.* **306**, 558.

10. Lems, W. F., Jahangier, Z. N., Jacobs, J. W. G., and Bijlsma, J. W. J. (1995). Vertebral fractures in patients with rheumatoid arthritis treated with corticosteroids. *Clin. Exp. Rheumatol.* **13**, 293–297.

11. Cooper, C., Coupland, C., and Mitchell, M. (1995). Rheumatoid arthritis, corticosteroid therapy and hip fracture. *Ann. Rheum. Dis.* **54**, 49–52.

12. Boden, S. D., Hair, G., Titus, L., Racine, M., McCuaig, K., Wozney, J. M., and Nanes, M. S. (1997). Glucocorticoid-induced differentiation of fetal rat calvarial osteoblasts is mediated by bone morphogenetic protein-6. *Endocrinology* **138**, 2820–2828.

13. Rogatsky, I., Trowbridge, J. M., and Garabedian, M. J. (1997). Glucocorticoid receptor-mediated cell cycle arrest is achieved through distinct cell-specific transcriptional regulatory mechanisms. *Mol. Cell. Biol.* **17**, 3181–3193.

14. Gallagher, J. A., Beresford, J. N., MacDonald, B. R., and Russell, R. G. G. (1984). Hormone target cell interactions in human bone. *In* "Osteoporosis" (C. Christiansen, ed.). Copenhagen.

15. Dietrich, J. W. Canalis, E. M., Maina, D. M., and Raisz, G. (1979). Effects of glucocorticoids on fetal rat bone collagen synthesis in vitro. *Endocrinology* **104**, 715–721.

16. Chevalley, T., Strong, D. D., Mohan, S., Baylink, D. J., and Linkhart, T. A. (1996). Evidence for a role for insulin-like growth factor binding proteins in glucocorticoid inhibition of normal human osteoblast-like cell proliferation. *Eur. J. Endocrinol.* **134**, 591–601.

17. Gabbitas, B., Pash, J. M., Delany, A. M., and Canalis, E. (1996). Cortisol inhibits the synthesis of insulin-like growth factor-binding protein-5 in bone cell cultures by transcriptional mechanisms. *J. Biol. Chem.* **271**, 9033–9038.

18. Okazaki, R., Riggs, B. L., and Conover, C. A. (1994). Glucocorticoid regulation of insulin-like growth factor-binding protein expression in normal human osteoblast-like cells. *Endocrinology* **134**, 126–132.

19. Gabbitas, B., and Canalis, E. (1996). Cortisol enhances the transcription of insulin-like growth factor-binding protein-6 in cultured osteoblasts. *Endocrinology* **137**, 1687–1692.

20. Kream, B. E., Tetradis, S., Lafrancis, D., Fall, P. M., Feyen, J. H. M., and Raisz, L. G. (1997). Modulation of the effects of glucocorticoids on collagen synthesis in fetal rat calvariae by insulin-like growth factor binding protein-2. *J. Bone Miner. Res.* **12**, 889–895.

21. Centrella, M., McCarthy, T. L., and Canalis, E. (1991). Glucocorticoid regulation of transforming growth factor beta 1 activity and binding in osteoblast-enriched cultures from fetal rat bone. *Mol. Cell. Biol.* **11**, 3390–3396.

22. Oursler, M. J., Riggs, B. L., and Spelsberg, T. C. (1993). Glucocorticoid-induced activation of latent transforming growth factor-beta by normal human osteoblast-like cells. *Endocrinology* **133**, 2187–2196.

23. Shuto, T., Kukita, T., Hirata, M., Jimi, E., and Koga, T. (1994). Dexamethasone stimulates osteoclast-like cell formation by inhibiting

granulocyte-macrophage colony-stimulating factor production in mouse bone marrow cultures. *Endocrinology* **134**, 1121–1126.

24. Kaji, H., Sugimoto, T., Kanatani, M., Nishiyama, K., and Chihara, K. (1997). Dexamethasone stimulates osteoclast-like cell formation by directly acting on hemopoietic blast cells and enhances osteoclast-like cell formation stimulated by parathyroid hormone and prostaglandin e-2. *J. Bone Miner. Res.* **12**, 734–741.

25. Tobias, J., and Chambers, T. J. (1989). Glucocorticoids impair bone resorptive activity and viability of osteoclasts disaggregated from neonatal rat long bones. *Endocrinology* **125**, 1290–1295.

26. Dempster, D. W., Moonga, B. S., Stein, L. S., Horbert, W. R., and Antakly, T. (1997). Glucocorticoids inhibit bone resorption by isolated rat osteoclasts by enhancing apoptosis. *J. Endocrinol.* **154**, 397–406.

27. Caputo, C. B., Meadows, D., and Frisz, L. G. (1976). Failure of estrogens and androgens to inhibit bone resorption in tissue culture. *Endocrinology* **98**, 1065–1068.

28. Lowe, C., Gray, D. H., and Reid, I. R. (1992). Serum blocks the osteolytic effect of cortisol in neonatal mouse calvaria. *Calcif. Tissue Int.* **50**, 189–192.

29. Gronowicz, G., McCarthy, M. B., and Raisz, L. G. (1990). Glucocorticoids stimulate resorption in fetal rat parietal bones in vitro. *J. Bone Miner. Res.* **5**, 1223–1230.

30. Welten, D. C., Kemper, H. C. G., Post, G. B., Vanmechelen, W., Twisk, J., Lips, P., and Teule, G. J. (1994). Weight-bearing activity during youth is a more important factor for peak bone mass than calcium intake. *J. Bone Miner. Res.* **9**, 1089–1096.

31. Gray, R. E. S., Doherty, S. M., Galloway, J., Coulton, L., de Broe, M., and Kanis, J. A. (1991). A double-blind study of deflazacort and prednisone in patients with chronic inflammatory disorders. *Arthritis Rheum.* **34**, 287–295.

32. Reid, I. R., and Ibberston, H. K. (1987). Evidence for decreased tubular reabsorption of calcium in glucorticoid-treated asthmatics. *Horm. Res.* **27**, 200–204.

33. Cosman, F., Nieves, J., Herbert, J., Shen, V., and Lindsay, R. (1994). High-dose glucocorticoids in multiple sclerosis patients exert direct effects on the kidney and skeleton. *J. Bone Miner. Res.* **9**, 1097–1105.

34. Braun, J. J., Juttman, J. R., Visser, T. J., and Birkenhager, J. C. (1982). Short-term effect of prednisone on serum 1,25-hydroxy-vitamin D in normal individuals an in hyper- and hypoparathyroidism. *Clin. Endocrinol.* **17**, 21–28.

35. Fucik, R. F., Kukreja, S. C., Hargis, G. K., Bowser, E. N., Hendersen, W. J., and Williams, G. A. (1975). Effect of glucocorticoids on function of the parathyroid glands in man. *J. Clin. Endocrinol. Metab.* **40**, 152–185.

36. Au, W. Y. W. (1976). Cortisol stimulation of parathyroid hormone secretion by rat parathyroid glands in organ culture. *Science* **193**, 1015–1017.

37. Sugimoto, T., Brown, A. J., Ritter, C., Morrissey, J., Slatopolsky, E., and Martin, K. J. (1989). Combined effects of dexamethasone and 1,25-dihydroxyvitamin D3 on parathyroid hormone secretion in cultured bovine parathyroid cells. *Endocrinology* **125**, 638–641.

38. Peraldi, M. N., Rondeau, E., Jousset, V., el M'Selmi, A., Lacave, R., Delarue, F., Garel, J. M., and Sraer, J. D. (1990). Dexamethasone increases preproparathyroid hormone messenger RNA in human hyperplastic parathyroid cells in vitro. *Eur. J. Clin. Invest.* **20**, 392–397.

39. Bikle, D. D., Halloran, B., Fong, L., Steinbach, L., and Shellito, J. (1993). Elevated 1,25-dihydroxyvitamin-D levels in patients with chronic obstructive pulmonary disease treated with prednisone. *J. Clin. Endocrinol. Metab.* **76**, 456–461.

40. Hattersley, A. T., Meeran, K., Burrin, J., Hill, P., Shiner, R., and Ibbertson, H. K. (1994). The effect of long- and short-term corticosteroids on plasma calcitonin and parathyroid hormone levels. *Calcif. Tissue Int.* **54**, 198–202.

41. Mahgoub, A., Hirsch, P. F., and Munson, P. L. (1997). Calcium-lowering action of glucocorticoids in adrenalectomized-parathyroidectomized rats—specificity and relative potency of natural and synthetic glucocorticoids. *Endocrine* **6**, 279–283.

42. Chen, T. L., and Feldman, D. (1979). Glucocorticoid receptors and actions in subpopulations of cultured rat bone cells. *J. Clin. Invest.* **63**, 750–758.

43. Hahn, T. J., and Halstead, L. R. (1979). Cortisol enhancement of PTH-stimulated cyclic AMP accumulation in cultured fetal rat long bone rudiments. *Calcif. Tissue Int.* **29**, 173–175.

44. Titus, L., Rubin, J. E., Lorang, M. T., and Catherwood, B. D. (1988). Glucocorticoids and 1,25-dihydroxyvitamin D3 regulate parathyroid hormone stimulation of adenosine 3'5'-monophosphate-dependent protein kinase in rat osteosarcoma cells. *Endocrinology* **123**, 1526.

45. Zajac, J. D., Livesey, S. A., Michelangeli, V. P., *et al.* (1986). Glucocorticoid treatment facilitates cyclic adenosine 3',5'-monophosphate-dependent protein kinase response in parathyroid hormone-responsive osteogenic sarcoma cells. *Endocrinology* **118**, 2059–2064.

46. Mitchell, J., and Bansal, A. (1997). Dexamethasone increases g-alpha (q-11) expression and hormone-stimulated phospholipase C activity in umr-106-01 cells. *Am. J. Physiol.—Endocrinol. Metab.* **36**, E528–E535.

47. Doerr, P., and Pirke, K. M. (1976). Cortisol-induced suppression of plasma testosterone in normal adult males. *J. Clin. Endocrinol. Metab.* **43**, 622–629.

48. Reid, I. R., France, J. T., Pybus, J., and Ibbertson, H. K. (1985). Low plasma testosterone levels in glucocorticoid-treated male asthmatics. *Br. Med. J.* **291**, 574.

49. Dempster, D. W. (1989). Bone histomorphometry in glucocorticoid-induced osteoporosis. *J. Bone Miner. Res.* **4**, 137–141.

50. Bressot, C., Meunier, P. J., Chapuy, M. C., Lejeune, E., Edouard, C., and Darby, A. J. (1979). Histomorphometric profile, pathophysiology and reversibility of corticosteroid-induced osteoporosis. *Metab. Bone Dis. Relat. Res.* **1**, 303–311.

51. Lund, B., Storm, T. L., Lund, B., Melsen, F., Mosekilde, L., Andersen, R. B., Egmose, C., and Sorensen, O. H. (1985). Bone mineral loss, bone histomorphometry and vitamin D metabolism in patients with rheumatoid arthritis on long-term glucocorticoid treatment. *Clin. Rheumatol.* **4**, 143–149.

52. Aaron, J. E., Francis, R. M., Peacock, M., and Makins, N. B. (1989). Contrasting microanatomy of idiopathic and corticosteroid-induced osteoporosis. *Clin. Orthop. Relat. Res.* **243**, 294–305.

53. Chavassieux, P., Pastoureau, P., Chapuy, M. C., Delmas, P. D., and Meunier, P. J. (1993). Glucocorticoid-induced inhibition of osteoblastic bone formation in ewes: A biochemical and histomorphometric study. *Osteoporosis Int.* **3**, 97–102.

54. Stellon, A. J., Webb, A., and Compston, J. E. (1988). Bone histomorphometry and structure in corticosteroid treated chronic active hepatitis. *Gut* **29**, 378–384.

55. Dempster, D. W., Arlot, M. A., and Meunier, P. J. (1983). Mean wall thickness and formation periods of trabecular bone packets in corticosteroid-induced osteoporosis. *Calcif. Tissue Int.* **35**, 410–417.

56. Chavassieux, P., Buffet, A., Vergnaud, P., Garnero, P., and Meunier, P. J. (1997). Short-term effects of corticosteroids on trabecular bone remodeling in old ewes. *Bone* **20**, 451–455.

57. Gallagher, J. C., Aaron, J., Horsman, A., Wilkinson, R., and Nordin, B. E. (1973). Corticosteroid osteoporosis. *Clin. Endocrinol. Metab.* **2**, 355–368.

58. Reid, I. R., Katz, J., Ibbertson, H. K., and Gray, D. H. (1986). The effects of hydrocortisone, parathyroid hormone and the bisphosphonate APD on bone resorption in neonatal mouse calvaria. *Calcif. Tissue Int.* **38**, 38–43.

59. Godschalk, M. F., and Downs, R. W. (1988). Effect of short-term glucocorticoids on serum osteocalcin in healthy young men. *J. Bone Miner. Res.* **3**, 113–115.

60. Morrison, N. A., Shine, J., Fragonas, J. C., Verkest, V., McMenemy, M. L., and Eisman, J. A. (1989). 1,25-dihydroxyvitamin D-responsive

element and glucocorticoid repression in the osteocalcin gene. *Science* **246**, 1158–1161.

61. Heinrichs, A. A. J., Bortell, R., Rahman, S., Stein, J. L., Alnemri, E. S., Litwack, G., Lian, J. B., and Stein, G. S. (1993). Identification of multiple glucocorticoid receptor binding sites in the rat osteocalcin Gene Promoter. *Biochemistry* **32**, 11436–11444.

62. Oconnell, S. L., Tresham, J., Fortune, C. L., Farrugia, W., McDougall, J. G., Scoggins, B. A., and Wark, J. D. (1993). Effects of prednisolone and deflazacort on osteocalcin metabolism in sheep. *Calcif. Tissue Int.* **53**, 117–121.

63. Hodsman, A. B., Toogood, J. H., Jennings, B., Fraher, L. J., and Baskerville, J. C. (1991). Differential effects of inhaled budesonide and oral prednisolone on serum osteocalcin. *J. Clin. Endocrinol. Metab.* **72**, 530–540.

64. Boulet, L. P., Giguere, M. C., Milot, J., and Brown, J. (1994). Effects of long-term use of high-dose inhaled steroids on bone density and calcium metabolism. *J. Allergy Clin. Immunol.* **94**, 796–803.

65. Doull, I., Freezer, N., and Holgate, S. (1996). Osteocalcin, growth, and inhaled corticosteroids—a prospective study. *Arch. Dis. Child.* **74**, 497–501.

66. Robinson, R. J., Iqbal, S. J., Whitaker, R. P., Abrams, K., and Mayberry, J. F. (1997). Rectal steroids suppress bone formation in patients with colitis. *Aliment. Pharmacol. Thert.* **11**, 201–204.

67. Emkey, R. D., Lindsay, R., Lyssy, J., Weisberg, J. S., Dempster, D. W., and Shen, V. (1996). The systemic effect of intraarticular administration of corticosteroid on markers of bone formation and bone resorption in patients with rheumatoid arthritis. *Arthritis Rheum.* **39**, 277–282.

68. Hall, G. M., Spector, T. D., and Delmas, P. D. (1995). Markers of bone metabolism in postmenopausal women with rheumatoid arthritis—Effects of corticosteroids and hormone replacement therapy. *Arthritis Rheum.* **38**, 902–906.

69. Reid, I. R., Chapman, G. E., Fraser, T. R. C., *et al.* (1986). Low serum osteocalcin levels in glucocorticoid-treated asthmatics. *J. Clin. Endocrinol. Metab.* **62**, 379–383.

70. Prummel, M. F., Wiersinga, W. M., and Lips, P. (1991). The course of biochemical parameters of bone turnover during treatment with corticosteroids. *J. Clin. Endocrinol. Metab.* **72**, 382–386.

71. Lane, S. J., Vaja, S., Swaminathan, R., and Lee, T. H. (1996). Effects of prednisolone on bone turnover in patients with corticosteroid resistant asthma. *Clin. Expe. Allergy* **26**, 1197–1201.

72. Ekenstam, E., Stalenheim, G., and Hallgren, R. (1988). The acute effect of high dose corticosteroid treatment on serum osteocalcin. *Metab., Clin. Exp.* **37**, 141–144.

73. Lems, W. F., Gerrits, M. I., Jacobs, J. W. G., Vanvugt, R. M., Vanrijn, H. J. M., and Bijlsma, J. W. J. (1996). Changes in (markers of) bone metabolism during high dose corticostereroid pulse treatment in patients with rheumatoid arthritis. *Ann. Rheum. Dis.* **55**, 288–293.

74. Wolthers, O. D., Heuck, C., Hansen, M., and Kollerup, G. (1997). Serum and urinary markers of types I and III collagen turnover during short-term prednisolone treatment in healthy adults. *Scand. J. Clin. Lab. Invest.* **57**, 133–139.

75. Hermus, A. R., Smals, A. G., Swinkels, L. M., Huysmans, D. A., Pieters, G. F., Sweep, C. F., Corstens, F. H., and Kloppenborg, P. W. (1995). Bone mineral density and bone turnover before and after surgical cure of Cushing's syndrome. *J. Clin. Endocrinol. Metab.* **80**, 2859–2865.

76. Sartorio, A., Conti, A., Ferrario, S., Passini, E., Re, T., and Ambrosi, B. (1996). Serum bone Gla protein and carboxyterminal cross-linked telopeptide of type I collagen in patients with Cushing's syndrome. *Postgrad. Med. J.* **72**, 419–422.

77. Morrison, D., Ali, N. J., Routledge, P. A., and Capewell, S. (1992). Bone turnover during short course prednisolone treatment in patients with chronic obstructive airways disease. *Thorax* **47**, 418–420.

78. Ali, N. J., Capewell, S., and Ward, M. J. (1991). Bone turnover during high dose inhaled corticosteroid treatment. *Thorax* **46**, 160–164.

79. Blanckaert, F., Cortet, B., Coquerelle, P., Flipo, R. M., Duquesnoy, B., Marchandise, X., and Delcambre, B. (1997). Contribution of calcaneal ultrasonic assessment to the evaluation of postmenopausal and glucocorticoid-induced osteoporosis. *Rev. Rhum. Mal. Osteo-Articulaires* **64**, 305–313.

80. Reeve, J., Loftus, J., Hesp, R., Ansell, B. M., Wright, D. J., and Woo, P. M. M. (1993). Biochemical prediction of changes in spinal bone mass in juvenile chronic (or rheumatoid) arthritis treated with glucocorticoids. *J. Rheumatol.* **20**, 1189–1195.

81. Shane, E., Rivas, M., McMahon, D. J., Staron, R. B., Silverberg, S. J., Seibel, M. J., Mancini, D., Michler, R. E., Aaronson, K., Addesso, V., and Lo, S. H. (1997). Bone loss and turnover after cardiac transplantation. *J. Clin. Endocrinol. Metab.* **82**, 1497–1506.

82. Sambrook, P. N., Kelly, P. J., Fontana, D., Nguyen, T., Keogh, A., Macdonald, P., Spratt, P., Freund, J., and Eisman, J. A. (1994). Mechanisms of rapid bone loss following cardiac transplantation. *Osteoporosis Int.* **4**, 273–276.

83. Reid, I. R., and Ibbertson, H. K. (1986). Calcium supplements in the prevention of steroid-induced osteoporosis. *Am. J. Clin. Nutr.* **44**, 287–290.

CHAPTER 36

Transplantation Osteoporosis

CAROLINA A. MOREIRA KULAK Department of Endocrinology, Federal University of Parana, Hospital de Clinicas, Curitiba, Brazil

ELIZABETH SHANE Department of Medicine, College of Physicians and Surgeons, Columbia University, New York, New York 10032

I. INTRODUCTION

Since the 1980s, organ transplantation has become established as effective therapy for end-stage renal, hepatic, cardiac, and pulmonary disease. The kidney is the most commonly transplanted organ, followed by liver, heart, pancreas, lung, and heart-lung. Overall, one-year patient survival is excellent, ranging from 97% for living donor kidney recipients to 63% for heart-lung recipients [1, 2]. Five-year survival is also quite good and many patients live more than ten years after transplantation. Unfortunately, however, many transplant recipients demonstrate a propensity to fracture, which has a negative impact upon their quality of life [3–6].

The pathogenesis of transplantation osteoporosis is complex and incompletely understood. Risk factors for osteoporosis (Caucasian race, older age, postmenopausal status, dietary calcium deficiency, vitamin D deficiency, physical inactivity, tobacco, and excessive use of alcohol) and exposure to medications associated with bone loss (loop diuretics, anticoagulants, glucocorticoids) are common among patients who are candidates for transplantation. Moreover, pretrans-

plant mineral homeostasis may also be influenced by the diseased organ, which is a particularly common circumstance in the case of renal or hepatic failure. However, it is generally considered that posttransplantation immunosuppressive therapy plays the pivotal role in the evolution of bone loss and the incidence of fracture in organ transplant recipients [6].

All transplant recipients require immunosuppressive therapy to prevent rejection of the transplanted organ. In the 1990s, the majority of patients have been managed with "triple" immunosuppressive therapy. Such regimens generally include glucocorticoids, cyclosporine A (CsA), or tacrolimus (FK506) (which suppress the immune response by inhibition of T-cell function) and azathioprine or mycophenolate mofetil. Glucocorticoids, notorious for causing osteoporosis (Chapter 35), are commonly prescribed in high doses (up to 120 mg of prednisone or its equivalent daily) immediately after transplantation and during episodes of severe rejection, with gradual reduction over several weeks. In addition, Epstein and colleagues [7–9] have demonstrated that administration of CsA to rats in doses comparable to those used after transplantation causes severe trabecular bone loss. In this animal model, bone turnover is accelerated, with histological evidence of increased bone resorption and bone formation. The bone loss is largely prevented by agents that inhibit bone resorption [10–12]. Biochemical changes in rats include elevated serum osteocalcin concentrations and increased renal 1-α hydroxylase activity and serum concentrations of 1,25(OH)$_2$D [13], whereas parathyroid hormone levels do not change. FK506 causes even greater bone loss in the rat than that observed with CsA [14]. In human subjects, whether CsA and FK506 contribute to the pathogenesis of transplantation osteoporosis remains controversial. Because both drugs are used in conjunction with glucocorticoids, it has been difficult to establish that CsA has specific effects on bone and mineral metabolism in the human model.

In this chapter, we will summarize the natural history of bone loss and fracture associated with kidney, heart, lung, liver, and bone marrow transplantation. The changes in calcitropic hormones and biochemical markers of bone turnover that follow various types of organ transplants will also be reviewed.

II. KIDNEY TRANSPLANTATION

A. Before Transplantation

Most patients undergoing kidney transplantation already have at least some evidence of renal osteodystrophy. This may include hyperparathyroidism (with or without osteitis fibrosa), osteomalacia, osteosclerosis, or adynamic or aplastic bone disease [15]. In some patients, more than one of these conditions may be present. In addition, patients with end-stage renal disease are commonly hypogonadal and many have received previous therapy with medications (glucocorticoids and/or CsA for immune complex disease, loop diuretics or aluminum-containing phosphate binders) that can affect bone and mineral metabolism.

B. After Transplantation

1. INDICES OF MINERAL METABOLISM

Restoration of renal function after kidney transplantation rectifies many of the disturbances that lead to renal osteodystrophy [15, 16]. With the presence of a functioning transplanted kidney, there is normalization of phosphate and 1,25(OH)$_2$D levels. The extremely high levels of PTH often observed in patients with end-stage renal disease decline rapidly after transplantation. However, because reversal of parathyroid hyperplasia may require months or years, parathyroid hormone levels frequently remain elevated throughout the immediate posttransplant period. In some patients, particularly those with severe pretransplant hyperparathyroidism, serum PTH may never become completely normal.

Hypercalcemia occurs commonly during the first few months after kidney transplantation [17, 18]. Its pathogenesis is related to persistent parathyroid hyperplasia, elevated parathyroid hormone levels, and increased calcitriol production by the renal allograft. Patients with severe hyperparathyroidism prior to transplantation are at greatest risk. In such patients, serum calcium generally ranges between 10.5 and 12.0 mg/dl, although more severe hypercalcemia (>13.0 mg/dl) may develop occasionally. In approximately 90% of patients, parathyroid-hormone dependent hypercalcemia is well tolerated and usually resolves within a year. Because severe hypercalcemia may be associated with allograft dysfunction, subtotal parathyroidectomy should be considered for patients with severe hypercalcemia (>14.0 mg/dl) and for those who still have moderate hypercalcemia (>12.5 mg/dl) more than one year after transplantation.

Hypophosphatemia also occurs commonly after renal transplantation [17, 18]. In the majority of patients, it is related to persistent parathyroid hyperplasia and decreased renal tubular reabsorption of phosphorous. Pharmacological doses of glucocorticoids also increase renal phosphate losses and may contribute to the hypophosphatemia. In a minority of patients, there may be a primary defect in renal phosphate handling. Mild hypophosphatemia is generally well tolerated. However, severe hypophosphatemia (<1.0 mg/dl) may be associated with proximal muscle weakness and fatigue and should be treated with oral phosphorus replacement.

2. BONE MASS

Immunosuppressive therapy constitutes an additional insult to a skeleton often already compromised with respect to bone mass. Prospective studies indicate that lumbar spine bone loss during the first three to 18 months following renal transplantation varies from 3–9%. Bone loss is greatest during the first six months after transplantation and predominantly affects cancellous bone [19–22]. Virtually all cross-sectional studies of renal transplant recipients demonstrate that bone mass is lower than in age- and sex-matched normal populations [22a–28]. One study of 20 young adults who received a renal transplant during childhood revealed that 14 had lumbar spine BMD T scores below -1.0, six of whom were below -2.0 [29]. Some [23, 27–29], but not all [19, 21, 22a, 24], studies demonstrate a direct relationship between glucocorticoid dose and bone mass and/or rates of bone loss. None have noted either increased or decreased rates of bone loss in cyclosporine-treated patients. In fact, one cross-sectional study of 165 kidney transplant recipients observed that daily CsA dose correlated in a positive manner with BMD at the femoral neck [29]. In the majority of studies, pre- and posttransplant PTH levels have not been related to the rates of bone loss [19, 20, 30]. There is also evidence for significant ongoing vertebral bone loss (approximately 2% per year) between eight and ten years after transplantation in patients followed longitudinally, [27].

3. FRACTURE

Fracture prevalence ranges from 7 to 11% in nondiabetic renal transplant recipients [22a, 31] but is considerably higher (45%) in patients transplanted because of diabetic nephropathy [31]. Fractures more commonly involve the long bones or metatarsals than the vertebral bodies or ribs and usually occur relatively late, usually more than three years after transplantation. This may be due, in part, to the catabolic effects of pretransplant hyperparathyroidism or persistent posttransplant hyperparathyroidism on cortical bone.

4. BONE TURNOVER

Markers of bone formation have been frequently assessed after renal transplantation. Julian and colleagues [19] observed that total serum alkaline phosphatase activity declined by 60% during the first 18 months after renal transplantation. In a cross-sectional study, Bagni and colleagues [23] measured serum osteocalcin in 44 renal transplant recipients 6–144 months after transplantation. Levels were markedly increased, on average, and directly correlated with intact PTH concentrations, which were also mildy elevated. Osteocalcin levels did not differ between patients taking CsA (n = 24) and patients not taking CsA (n = 20). Renal function was mildly compromised (mean creatinine clearance-66 ml/min and serum creatinine-1.5 mg/dl). Because serum osteocalcin levels have been shown to increase only after the creatinine clearance falls below 30 ml/min [32], it is unlikely that the increase in osteocalcin could be attributed to impaired clearance of this small molecule. Briner et al. [33] measured biochemical indices of mineral metabolism, including serum PTH, osteocalcin, and urinary hydroxyproline excretion, in 34 patients before and at six month intervals for two years after transplantation. They also performed bone biopsies in 20 patients, before transplantation and during the second posttransplant year. Serum total alkaline phosphatase activity declined in patients with elevated pretransplant levels and rose in those with normal or low pretransplant levels. Serum osteocalcin was markedly elevated before transplantation, fell by approximately 50% at six months, and remained stable for the next 18 months. However, despite the marked decrease in serum osteocalcin after transplantation, levels remained almost twice the upper limit of normal throughout the two years of observation. PTH also remained elevated and was correlated with serum osteocalcin and creatinine concentrations. Static parameters of bone formation and resorption were increased before transplantation and one year after transplantation. Unfortunately, no data were provided to correlate histologic and biochemical parameters of bone formation. Approximately one-third of the patients were managed with CsA monotherapy. However, there was no comparison of biochemical or histomorphometric parameters between patients on CsA monotherapy and those who also required prednisone. In another cross-sectional study, Boiskin et al. [34] measured serum alkaline phosphatase activity and osteocalcin and PTH (in a midmolecule assay) levels at various intervals and in varying numbers of patients before transplantation and during an eight month period after transplantation. All markers were elevated before transplantation and all declined after transplantation. Serum alkaline phosphatase and osteocalcin fell to slightly above the upper end of the normal range and remained there. Values of these markers were directly correlated with each other and with PTH. Pietschmann et al. [35] compared serum osteocalcin and intact PTH concentrations in 30 patients measured an average of two years after transplantation and 30 age- and sex-matched controls. All patients were receiving prednisone (7.5 mg/day on average) and CsA. PTH and osteocalcin were significantly higher in the renal transplant recipients, even those with creatinine clearances above 95 ml/min. Again, serum osteocalcin correlated with total alkaline phosphatase activity and PTH, but bore no relationship to serum creatinine, prednisolone dose, or CsA levels.

Bone-specific alkaline phosphatase (BSAP) is an enzyme located in the membrane of the osteoblastic cells and is considered to be a sensitive and specific marker of bone formation. Because total serum alkaline phosphatase activity also reflects contributions from liver, BSAP is a more specific marker of skeletal activity. BSAP is a large molecule which is not excreted by the kidney. Thus, when glomerular filtration is impaired, as it may frequently be after renal transplantation, serum BSAP may more closely reflect bone formation than would serum osteocalcin, a small molecule that is cleared by the kidney. BSAP concentrations have been reported after renal transplantation. Withold et al. [36] observed that total alkaline phosphatase and BSAP were normal and highly correlated prior to transplantation in 23 patients with end-stage renal disease. However, BSAP was often frankly elevated when total alkaline phosphatase activity was in the upper half of the normal range. Although there was a significant decrease in BSAP during the first week after transplantation, perhaps reflecting the high doses of glucocorticoids given during this period, the next six months were characterized by an approximate doubling of BSAP. Levels correlated highly with intact PTH both before and after transplantation. The authors concluded that BSAP is a useful marker of bone formation after renal transplantation. These same investigators also evaluated the carboxy-terminal extension peptide of type 1 procollagen (PICP) in 13 renal transplant recipients [37]. The concentration of circulating PICP is thought to be directly associated with type 1 collagen synthesis and hence, bone formation. PICP has been shown to correlate with histomorphometric parameters of bone formation in patients with renal osteodystrophy [38, 39]. BSAP and PICP were highly correlated with each other both before and after transplantation. There was an approximate 50% increase in both BSAP and PICP by three months after transplantation. BSAP and PICP correlated with PTH before, but not after transplantation. Gonzalez et al. [40] compared osteocalcin, BSAP, and PICP in 23 patients after renal transplantation. Despite a concomitant decline in intact PTH concentrations, there was a significant rise in all three markers of bone formation which became apparent by the third posttransplant month, with a further increase occurring by the sixth month.

In general, glucocorticoids suppress bone formation by inhibiting the transformation of preosteoblasts to osteoblasts and the synthesis of type 1 collagen and osteocalcin (Chapter 35). Because virtually all of the studies summarized above have been conducted in patients who were taking glucocorticoids, the mechanism of the increase in the biochemical and histomorphometric parameters of bone formation is not clear. One possibility is that serum parathyroid hormone concentrations, while usually lower than before transplantation, remain elevated in many renal transplant recipients for a significant period of time, sometimes years. PTH is a known stimulator of bone formation [41] and could conceivably overcome the suppressive effects of glucocorticoids on bone formation. In this regard, Lane and colleagues [42] have reported that intermittent injections of PTH significantly increase bone mass in patients on chronic glucocorticoid therapy. Also in support of this theory, most of the studies reviewed report significant correlations between biochemical markers of bone formation and PTH. The degree of posttransplant renal impairment may influence the situation by delaying the resolution of hyperparathyroidism, hence maintaining high bone turnover for longer periods of time. Also, osteocalcin [32], although not BSAP or PICP excretion, may be reduced when renal function is impaired. Another possible reason for the increase in bone formation markers is the use of CsA, which has been shown to increase both bone formation and resorption when administered to rats [6–9]. Some data suggest that CsA may stimulate bone formation, an effect opposite to that usually observed with glucocorticoids. Rambausek *et al.* [43] reported that total alkaline phosphatase activity was significantly higher in renal transplant recipients managed with prednisone and CsA than those managed with prednisone and azathioprine. In a histomorphometric study, Aubia and colleagues [44] reported that indices of both bone resorption and formation were significantly higher in patients receiving CsA and prednisone than those managed with prednisone and azathioprine. Wilmink *et al.* [45] compared three groups of patients: one managed with CsA alone, the second with CsA and prednisone, and the third with azathioprine and prednisone. Patients managed with CsA were significantly more likely to have an elevated alkaline phosphatase level. Furthermore, alkaline phosphatase activity decreased markedly after patients were switched from CsA to prednisone and azathioprine. However, Dumoulin and colleagues [46] compared two groups of long-term renal transplant recipients, one group receiving CsA and the other not. The groups were well matched with respect to gender, age, time since transplantation (4–5 years), doses of other immunosuppressive agents, and renal function, which was well preserved. Intact PTH was at the upper end of the normal range. Osteocalcin

levels were, on average, at the upper end of the normal range. No difference in osteocalcin levels was observed between the two groups. Moreover, the response to an oral calcium challenge was the same in both groups. Finally, no study has yet reported any relationship between CsA level or dose and any marker of bone formation. Thus, the balance of the evidence seems to implicate hyperparathyroidism rather than CsA as the cause of increased bone turnover in renal transplant recipients, as suggested by Amado and colleagues [47].

III. CARDIAC TRANSPLANTATION

A. Before Transplantation

In contrast to end-stage renal disease, congestive heart failure (CHF) has not been associated with a well-defined disorder of bone and mineral metabolism. However, mean bone mineral density (BMD) has been reported to be lower in patients before heart transplantation than in age- and sex-matched normal individuals [48–50]. A study of 101 patients with advanced CHF [50] (Fig. 1A) found that only 50% had normal lumbar spine BMD and 47% had normal total hip

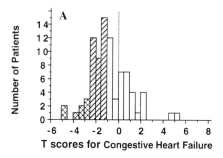

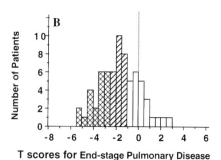

FIGURE 1   Frequency distribution of bone mineral density (BMD) measurements of the lumbar spine in patients with congestive heart failure (A) and in patients with end-stage pulmonary disease awaiting lung transplantation (B). The data are expressed as T scores which relate BMD measurements of individual patients to those of a young normal population of the same gender. T score measurements falling between -1 and -2.5 standard deviations below the mean (hatched bars) indicate low bone mass or osteopenia; those below -2.5 standard deviations below the mean (cross-hatched bars) indicate osteoporosis. Open bars are indicative of normal bone mass.

BMD (T score > -1.0). Frankly low serum concentrations of 25-hydroxyvitamin D (25-OHD) and $1,25(OH)_2D$ were quite common, occurring in 18% and 26% of the patients respectively. Moreover, vitamin D deficiency was significantly more common in the patients with more severe heart failure [50]. Secondary hyperparathyroidism, related primarily to prerenal azotemia, was observed in 30% of the patients. Markers of bone resorption (hydroxyproline, pyridinoline, and deoxypyridinoline) were elevated in the group as a whole and were significantly higher in patients with low 25-OHD and $1,25(OH)_2D$ concentrations. Despite mild prerenal azotemia, serum osteocalcin was normal in men and women. In contrast, Lee *et al.* [49] found both serum PTH and osteocalcin concentrations to be elevated in a smaller group of patients with CHF.

B. After Transplantation

1. BONE MASS AND FRACTURE

Osteoporosis and fractures are common in cardiac transplant recipients. Cross-sectional studies have documented that vertebral fracture prevalence ranges from 18 to 50% [48, 49, 51, 52]. A study of 40 cardiac transplant recipients evaluated an average of two years after transplantation found lumbar spine and femoral neck BMD to be ≥ 2 SD below values from age- and sex-matched individuals in 30% and 20% of the patients, respectively [51]. Ninety percent had elevated serum creatinine levels and 21% had elevated intact PTH concentrations. Serum osteocalcin was elevated in 60% of the patients, despite an average prednisone dose of 10 mg/day. In addition, serum osteocalcin was higher in the group of patients with elevated intact PTH levels but did not appear to be related to any index of renal function.

A longitudinal study [53] demonstrated that 36% of patients sustained one or more fractures during the first year following transplantation despite supplementation with calcium (1000 mg/day) and vitamin D (400 IU/day). The majority of fractures involved the spine with 85% of the fractures occurring during the first six months following transplantation. Although no pretransplant BMD or biochemical parameter was predictive of fracture after transplantation in the individual patient, lower pretransplant BMD was associated with a trend towards increased fracture risk. Moreover, women with low femoral neck BMD were significantly more likely to sustain posttransplant fractures. Fracture incidence was similar in a European study of 105 cardiac transplant recipients [54].

Several longitudinal studies describing the natural history and pattern of bone loss after cardiac transplantation have been published [55–59]. In general, lumbar spine BMD falls by approximately 6–10% during the first six months after transplantation, after which there is little further deterioration [59] (Fig. 2). In contrast, hip BMD declines throughout the first year, reaching 10–15% below pretransplant levels [59].

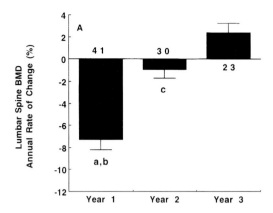

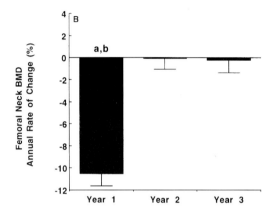

FIGURE 2   Annual rates of bone loss in percent during the first three years after cardiac transplantation. (A) Lumbar spine bone mineral density; (B) femoral neck bone mineral density. The numbers next to each bar indicate the "number" of patients included in the analysis. At the lumbar spine and the femoral neck, virtually all of the bone loss occurred during the first year. a: $p < 0.001$ compared to year 2; b: $p < 0.001$ compared to year 3; c: $p < 0.02$ compared to year 3.

Bone loss slows or stops in the majority of patients after the first year and lumbar spine BMD has been shown to increase slightly in the third year [58, 59].

2. INDICES OF MINERAL METABOLISM AND BONE TURNOVER

Biochemical changes after cardiac transplantation include sustained reductions in serum $1,25(OH)_2D$, transient declines in markers of bone formation (osteocalcin; Fig. 3A) and testosterone (in men), and increases in markers of bone resorption (Fig. 3B) with return to pretransplant concentrations by six months [59, 60]. Higher rates of bone loss were associated with greater exposure to prednisone, lower serum concentrations of vitamin D metabolites, higher levels of bone resorption markers [59], and in men, lower serum testosterne concentrations [59, 60]. Mean intact PTH concentrations were at the upper end of the normal range before transplantation and remained at that level throughout the three years of observation. Sambrook and colleagues [60] have reported

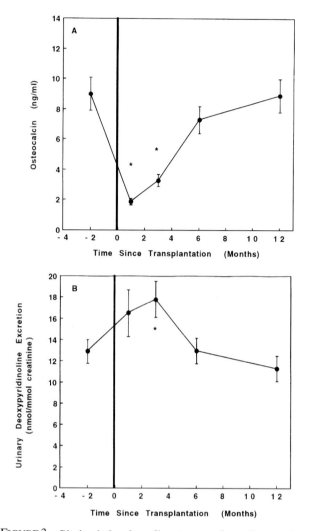

FIGURE 3   Biochemical markers of bone turnover after cardiac transplantation. (A) Serum osteocalcin concentration, a marker of bone formation. The early posttransplant period was characterized by suppression of serum osteocalcin and increases in hydroxyproline and deoxypyridinoline excretion, a biochemical pattern suggestive of uncoupling of bone remodeling. (B) Urinary excretion of deoxypyridinoline, a marker of bone resorption. *, $p < 0.05$ compared to baseline.

that serum osteocalcin, suppressed immediately after transplantation, increased markedly over the ensuing year. They observed that the change in osteocalcin correlated significantly with the daily doses of CsA and prednisolone and that the six month osteocalcin level correlated inversely with lumbar spine bone loss. Thiebaud *et al.* [61] have demonstrated progressive increases in serum osteocalcin and intact PTH concentrations during 18 months following cardiac transplantation, a pattern that differs both from our observations and from the suppression of osteocalcin concentrations observed in patients on glucocorticoids. Osteocalcin concentrations were directly correlated with PTH but unrelated to serum creatinine or doses of CsA or glucocorticoids [61]. Urinary

hydroxyproline excretion was elevated at all times after transplantation. Because many of these patients were withdrawn from glucocorticoids and maintained on CsA alone, this observation may reflect either an independent effect of CsA to increase bone formation or simply the withdrawal of steroids. Markers of bone resorption have been shown to increase transiently after cardiac transplantation [59, 60], a pattern which also differs from that reported in patients on glucocorticoids alone [62, 63]. Administration of bisphosphonates to cardiac transplant recipients was shown to suppress markers of bone resorption and to reduce rates of lumbar spine and femoral neck bone loss during the first year after transplantation [64] (Fig. 4)

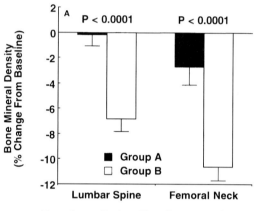

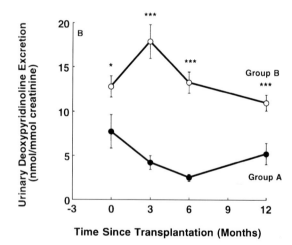

FIGURE 4   (A) Rates of lumbar spine and femoral neck bone loss during the first year after cardiac transplantation. Rates of bone loss are expressed as percent change from baseline Group A patients (black bars) received antiresorptive therapy after transplantation. Group B patients (white bars) received 1000 mg calcium and 400 IU vitamin D daily. Data are shown ±S.E.M. (B) Serial measurements of deoxypyridinoline, a marker of bone resorption, during the first year after cardiac transplantation. Group A patients (closed circles) received antiresorptive therapy after transplantation. Group B patients (open circles) received 1000 mg calcium and 400 IU vitamin D daily. Data are shown ±S.E.M. *, $p < 0.05$; ***, $p \leq 0.001$.

Eastell and colleagues [65] reported the results of a cross-sectional study of 50 male cardiac transplant recipients. The men were evaluated between two weeks and 47 months after transplantation with measurements of BMD, calciotropic hormones, and markers of bone formation (osteocalcin and BSAP) and resorption (urinary N-telopeptide excretion); the results were compared to those of a group of normal men. They observed that BMD was significantly decreased and markers of both formation and resorption were significantly increased. Bone turnover markers correlated with intact PTH, which in turn was related to the degree of renal impairment.

IV. LIVER TRANSPLANTATION

A. Before Transplantation

Osteoporosis and abnormal mineral metabolism have been described in association with alcoholic liver disease [66, 67], hemochromatosis [68], steroid-treated autoimmune chronic active hepatitis [69], and chronic cholestatic liver diseases such as biliary cirrhosis [70–72]. Therefore, candidates for liver transplantation frequently have significant pretransplant skeletal demineralization and fractures which place them at increased risk for fracture after surgery. A study of 58 patients with cirrhotic end-stage liver disease referred for liver transplantation has been reported [73]. When compared to age- and sex-matched controls, 43% had osteoporosis, which the authors defined as a BMD Z score >2 SD below control or the presence or vertebral fractures. Serum 25-OHD, $1,25(OH)_2D$, intact PTH, and osteocalcin were lower and urinary hydroxyproline excretion was higher in cirrhotic patients than in controls. Male patients had lower serum testosterone levels than controls. Other investigators have also observed low serum osteocalcin concentrations in patients with primary biliary cirrhosis [70, 74], and histomorphometric data have confirmed that bone formation is decreased in patients with primary biliary cirrhosis [70, 75, 76]. While the pathogenesis of the decrease in bone formation is not known, Riggs and colleagues [77] have reported that unconjugated hyperbilirubinemia causes impairment of osteoblast activity in jaundiced patients, but it is reversible after selective removal of bilirubin from plasma by photobleaching.

While serum osteocalcin appears to be a valid marker of bone formation in cholestatic liver disease, the utility of collagen-related markers of bone turnover has been called into question [74]. In fibrotic liver diseases, the synthesis of type I collagen is markedly increased. Guañabens et al. [74] evaluated collagen-related markers of bone formation (osteocalcin, carboxy-terminal and amino-terminal propeptides of type I collagen) and resorption (serum tartrate-resistant acid phosphatase, cross-linked carboxy-terminal telopeptide of type I collagen, and urinary excretion of pyridinium cross-links, hydroxyproline, N- and C-telopeptides) in 34 women

with primary biliary cirrhosis. Of these markers, serum osteocalcin was significantly lower in patients with the disease than in controls, and tartrate-resistant acid phosphatase (TRAP) did not differ from controls. In contrast, all of the collagen-related markers of bone turnover were significantly higher in patients with the disease than in controls, and all markers correlated with indices of liver fibrogenesis and disease severity rather than with osteocalcin and TRAP levels. Thus, these collagen-related markers appear influenced by liver-, rather than bone-, collagen metabolism.

B. After Transplantation

1. BONE MASS AND FRACTURE

The natural history of osteoporosis after liver transplantation is similar to that observed after cardiac transplantation, although rates of bone loss and fracture may be higher [78–83]. Lumbar spine BMD falls by 3.5–24%, primarily in the initial year. However, in patients with primary biliary cirrhosis, bone loss appears to stop after three months, with gradual improvement by the second and third posttransplant years [82]. Fracture incidence is also highest in the first year and ranges from 24–65%; the highest values are from a group of women with primary biliary cirrhosis [82]. The vertebrae and ribs are the most common fracture sites [78]. As with cardiac transplantation, no pretransplant indicator reliably predicts fracture risk in the individual patient. However, retransplanted patients, those with primary biliary cirrhosis, and those with previous fragility fractures are at increased risk [81]. In addition, Haagsma et al. [78] observed that patients with low urinary calcium excretion prior to transplantation were at increased risk for fracture.

2. INDICES OF MINERAL METABOLISM AND BONE TURNOVER

Studies of calciotropic hormone levels and bone turnover markers after liver transplantation are limited. Compston et al. [84] reported a significant increase in serum intact PTH during the first three months after liver transplantation. Others have found intact PTH levels to be within the normal range in liver transplant recipients [83, 85, 86]. In a cross-sectional study, markers of bone formation (osteocalcin and carboxy-terminal peptide of type I collagen) were found to be significantly higher in 120 liver transplant recipients than in a normal control population [86]. Similarly, serum osteocalcin was higher than age- and sex-matched controls in 18 men and nine postmenopausal women after liver transplantation; urinary hydroxproline excretion was also elevated [83]. Significant increases in serum osteocalcin were not observed in one study in which levels were obtained before and one month after transplantation [87]. However, in other studies of longer duration, serum osteoaclcin levels were found to increase substantially during the first posttransplant year [88, 89]. The balance of the data suggests that low bone turnover observed in many patients with liver failure converts to a high-turnover state that persists indefinitely after liver transplantation.

V. LUNG TRANSPLANTATION

A. Before Transplantation

Patients who undergo lung transplantation are at increased risk for osteoporosis even before surgery. Decreased mobility, hypoxemia, malnutrition, vitamin D deficiency, tobacco use, and prior glucocorticoid therapy are frequent attributes of candidates for lung transplantation, and all of these factors may contribute to pretransplant osteopenia. Cystic fibrosis, a common disease for which patients undergo lung transplantation, is itself associated with osteoporosis and fractures [90–92] due to pancreatic insufficiency, vitamin D deficiency [93], and calcium malabsorption and hypogonadism. A cross-sectional study revealed that 45% of 55 pretransplant patients and 73% of 45 posttransplant patients had BMD ≥ 2 SD below age- and sex-matched controls [94]. A similar study of 70 patients awaiting lung transplantation revealed that only 34% had normal spine BMD (Fig. 1B) and 22% had normal hip BMD [95]. In both studies, glucocorticoid exposure was inversely related to BMD. Fracture prevalence was 29% in patients with chronic obstructive pulmonary disease and 25% in patients with cystic fibrosis [95]. Serum 25-hydroxyvitamin D levels were at the low end of the normal range in the group as a whole, and 20% of the patients had frankly subnormal values [95].

B. After Transplantation

1. Bone Mass and Fracture

Relatively few studies have prospectively evaluated changes in bone mass and fracture incidence in patients who have received a lung transplant. However, a study of bone mass in 12 patients who underwent lung transplantation demonstrated an average 4% decrease in lumbar spine BMD during the first six months after transplantation despite supplementation with calcium and 400 IU of vitamin D [96]. Eight of the 12 patients had significant lumbar spine bone loss, seven sustained significant femoral neck bone loss, and two men sustained multiple vertebral fractures. On average, BMD at the femoral neck, femoral shaft, and whole body did not change significantly. In another study, researchers prospectively followed spine and hip BMD and fracture incidence in a group of 30 lung transplant recipients [97]. Despite the fact that all received antiresorptive therapy initiated shortly after transplantation, 37% of the patients suffered fragility fractures

during the first posttransplant year and approximately 50% sustained significant bone loss at either the spine or the hip. Risk factors for fracture included low pretransplant lumbar spine bone mass and pretransplant glucocorticoid therapy.

2. Indices of Mineral Metabolism and Bone Turnover

Few data are available on biochemical indices of mineral metabolism in lung transplant recipients. In the above referenced study [97], biochemical indices of mineral metabolism (serum and urinary calcium, intact PTH, vitamin D metabolites) were similar in patients who did and did not fracture. However, bone turnover (both resorption and formation), including six month serum bone alkaline phosphatase levels and 12 month urinary pyridinoline and deoxypyridinoline excretion, was higher in fracture patients. The 15 patients with significant bone loss at one or both sites did not differ from those with stable BMD with respect to any pretransplant demographic, densitometric, or biochemical parameter, or with exposure to glucocorticoids or tobacco. They also did not differ with respect to posttransplant exposure to glucocorticoids, number of rejection episodes, or type of osteoporosis therapy. At 12 months after transplantation, serum calcium was lower, serum PTH tended to be higher, and urinary deoxypyridinoline excretion was significantly higher than in patients with stable BMD. Thus, increased bone resorption, possibly due to secondary hyperparathyroidism, may have contributed to bone loss in these patients. The pathogenesis of the secondary hyperparathyroidism may have been related to urinary calcium losses which were greater in patients who lost bone mass and were directly related to intact PTH concentrations.

VI. BONE MARROW TRANSPLANTATION

Low BMD has also been reported in patients after bone marrow transplantation [98, 99]. Similar to solid organ transplantation, osteopenia is probably related to both pre- and posttransplant factors. In preparation for transplantation, patients receive myeloablative therapy (alkylating agents and/or total body irradiation). Such therapy commonly causes profound and frequently permanent hypogonadism, which almost certainly contributes to bone loss [100]. A prospective three month study of 24 patients undergoing bone marrow transplantation demonstrated a significant decrease in markers of bone formation (osteocalcin and bone alkaline phosphatase) at one, two, three, and twelve weeks after the marrow infusion; this pattern was accompanied by a simultaneous increase in bone resorption as measured by the carboxy-terminal cross-linked telopeptide of type I collagen [101]. Another prospective study of nine adults undergoing high dose glucocorticoid and cyclosporine therapy three months after marrow transplantation for chronic graft-versus-host disease found urinary hydroxyproline, magnesium, and calcium excretion to be elevated even before the immunosuppressive regimen was instituted [102]. Although urinary calcium and hydroxyproline excretion had normalized by the end of six months of immunosuppressive theapy, there was significant bone loss in two-thirds of the patients.

VII. CONCLUSIONS

Candidates for all types of transplantation have significant risk factors for osteoporosis and many have low bone mass, fractures, or evidence of abnormal mineral metabolism before transplantation. In the majority of cases, markers of both bone formation and resorption are increased before transplantation. The exception to this is cholestatic liver disease, in which bone turnover is low before transplantation. After transplantation, there is rapid bone loss in the majority of patients and fractures also occur commonly. These complications occur with the greatest frequency during the first six to twelve months. Early after transplantation, when glucocorticoid doses are highest, serum osteocalcin and bone alkaline phosphatase are suppressed and markers of resorption are elevated; these patterns provide biochemical evidence of uncoupled formation and resorption. However, by the middle of the first year after transplantation, bone formation markers recover. The balance of the evidence in organ transplant recipients evaluated after the first six months favors the notion that transplantation-related bone loss is a form of high turnover osteoporosis. As such, antiresorptive therapy is likely to be beneficial in the prevention of bone loss and fractures after transplantation. The majority [103–106], although not all, [107] published studies support this hypothesis.

Acknowledgments

This work was supported in part by Grants AR-41391 and RR-006645 from the National Institutes of Health.

References

1. United Network of Organ Sharing (UNOS) OPTN/SR. (1997). Annual Report-Graft/Patient Survival. Department of Health and Human Services, Health Resources and Services Administration.

2. Hosenpud, J. D., Bennett, L. E., Keck, B. M., Fiol, B., and Novick, R. J. (1997). The Registry of the International Society for Heart and Lung Transplantation: Fourteenth Official Report—1997. *J. Heart Lung Transplant.* **16**, 691–712.

3. Epstein, S., and Shane, E. (1996). Transplantation osteoporosis. *In* "Osteoporosis" R. Marcus, D. Feldman, and J. Kelsey, eds.), pp. 947–957. Academic Press, New York.

4. Shane, E., and Epstein, E. (1994). Immunosuppressive therapy and the skeleton. *Trends Endocrinol. Metab.* **4**, 169–175.

5. Rodino, M. A., and Shane, E. (1998). Osteoporosis after organ transplantation. *Am. J. Med.* **104**, 459–469.

6. Epstein, S. (1996). Post-transplantation bone disease: The role of immunosuppressive agents on the skeleton. *J. Bone Miner. Res.* **11**, 1–7.

7. Movsowitz, C., Epstein, S., Fallon, M., Ismail, F., and Thomas, S., (1988). Cyclosporin A in vivo produces severe osteopenia in the rat: Effect of dose and duration of administration. *Endocrinology* **123**, 2571–2577.

8. Movsowitz, C., Epstein, S., Ismail, F., Fallon, M., and Thomas, S. (1989). Cyclosporin A in the oophorectomized rat: Unexpected severe bone resorption. *J. Bone Miner. Res.* **4**, 393–398.

9. Schlosberg, M., Movsowitz, C., Epstein, S., Ismail, F., Fallon, M., and Thomas, S. (1989). The effect of cyclosporin A administration and its withdrawal on bone mineral metabolism in the rat. *Endocrinology* **124**, 2179–2184.

10. Joffe, I., Katz, I., Jacobs, T., Stein, B., Takizawa, M., Liu, C., Berlin, J., and Epstein, S. (1992). 17 Beta-estradiol prevents osteopenia in the oophorectomized rat treated with cyclosporin A. *Endocrinology* **130**, 578–586.

11. Stein, B., Takizawa, M., Katz, I., Joffe, I., Berlin, J., Fallon, M., and Epstein, S., (1991). Salmon calcitonin prevents cyclosporin A induced high turnover bone loss. *Endocrinology* **129**, 92–98.

12. Sass, D. A. Bowman, A. R., Marshall, I., Yuan, Z., Ma, Y. F., Jee, W. S. S., and Epstein, S. (1997). Alendronate prevents cyclosporin-induced osteopenia in the rat. *Bone* **21**, 65–70.

13. Stein, B., Halloran, B. P., Reinhardt, T., Engstrom, G. W., Bales, C. W., Drezner, M. K., Currie, K. L., Takizawa, M., Adams, J. S., and Epstein, S. (1991). Cyclosporin A increases synthesis of 1,25 dihydroxyvitamin D3 in the rat and mouse. *Endocrinology* **128**, 1369–1373.

14. Cvetkovic, M., Mann, G., Romero, D., Liang, X., Ma, Y., Jee, W., and Epstein, S. (1994). Deleterious effects of long term cyclosporine A, cyclosporine G, and FK506 on bone mineral metabolism in vivo. *Transplantation* **57**, 1231–1237.

15. Goodman, W. G., Coburn, J. W., Slatopolsky, E., and Salusky, I. (1996). Renal osteodystrophy in adults and children. *In* "Prime on the Metabolic Bone Diseases and Disorders of Mineral Metabolism" (M. J. Favus, ed.), 3rd ed., pp. 341–360. Lippincott-Raven, Philadelphia.

16. Hruska, K. A., and Teitelbaum, S. L. (1995). Renal osteodystrophy. *N. Engl. J. Med.* **333**, 166–174.

17. Conceicao, S. C., Wilkinson, R., Feest, T. J., Owen, J. P., Dewar, J., and Kerr, D. N. (1981). Hypercalcemia following renal transplantation: Causes and consequences. *Clin. Nephrol.* **16**, 235–244.

18. Deierhoi, M. H., and Diethelm, A. G. (1991). Management of hyperparathyroidism following renal transplantation. *Transplant. Manage.* **2**, 3–10.

19. Julian, B. A., Laskow, D. A., Dubovsky, J., Dubovsky, E. V., Curtis, J. J., and Quarles, L. D. (1991). Rapid loss of vertebral bone density after renal transplantation. *N. Engl. J. Med.* **325**, 544–550.

20. Horber, F. F., Casez, J. P., Steiger, U., Czerniak, A., Montandon, A., and Jaeger, P. H. (1994). Changes in bone mass early after kidney transplantation. *J. Bone Miner. Res.* **9**, 1–9.

21. Kwan, J. T. C., Almond, M. K., Evans, K., and Cunningham, J. (1992). Changes in total body bone mineral content and regional bone mineral density in renal patients following renal transplantation. *Miner. Electrolyte Metab.* **18**, 166–168.

22. Almond, M. K., Kwan, J. T. C., Evans, K., and Cunningham, J. (1994). Loss of regional bone mineral density in the first 12 months following renal transplantation. *Nephron* **66**, 52–57.

22a. Grotz, W. H., Mundinger, A., Gugel, B., Exner, V., Kirste, G., and Schollmeyer, P. J. (1994). Bone fracture and osteodensitometry with dual energy x-ray absorptiometry in kidney transplant recipients. *Transplantation* **58**, 912–915.

23. Bagni, B., Gilli, P., Cavallini, A., Bagni, I., Marzola, M. C., Orzincolo, C., and Wahner, H. W. (1994). Continuing loss of vertebral

mineral density in renal transplant recipients. *Eur. J. Nucl. Med.* **21**, 108–112.

24. Massari, P. U., Garay, G., and Ulla, M. R. (1994). Bone mineral content in cyclosporine-treated renal transplant patients. *Transplant Proc.* **26**, 2646–2648.

25. Kalef-Ezra, J. A., Karantanas, A. H., Hatzikonstantnou, I., Sferopoulos, G., Glaros, D. K., and Siampoulos, K. C. (1994). Bone mineral status after renal transplantation. *Invest. Radiol.* **29**, 127–133.

26. Grotz, W. H., Mundinger, F. A., Gugel, B., Exner, V. M., Kirste, G., and Schollmeyer, P. J. (1995). Bone mineral density after kidney transplantation. *Transplantation* **59**, 982–986.

27. Pichette, V., Bonnardeaux, A., Prudhomme, L., Gagne, M., Cardinal, J., and Ouimet, D. (1996). Long-term bone loss in kidney transplant recipients: A cross-sectional and longitudinal study. *Am. J. Kidney Dis.* **28**, 105–114.

28. Boot, A. M., Nauta, J., Hokken-Koelega, A. C. S., Pols, H. A. P., de Ridder, M. A. J., and Keizer-Schrama, S. M. P. F. (1995). Renal transplantation and osteoporosis. *Arch. Dis. Child.* **72**, 502–506.

29. Grotz, W., Mundinger, A., Gugel, B., Exner, V., Reichelt, A., and Schollmeyer, P. (1994). Missing impact of cyclosporine on osteoporosis in renal transplant recipients. *Transplant. Proc.* **26**, 2652–2653.

30. Yun, Y. S., Kim, B. J., Hong, T. W., Lee, C. G., and Kim, M. J. (1996). Changes of bone metabolism indices in patients receiving immunosuppressive therapy including low doses of steroids after transplantation. *Transplant. Proc.* **28**, 1561–1564.

31. Nisbeth, U., Lindh, E., Ljunghall, S., Backman, U., and Fellstrom, B. (1994). Fracture frequency after kidney transplantation. *Transplant. Proc.* **26**, 1764.

32. Delmas, P. D., Wilson, D. M., Mann, K. G., and Riggs, B. L. (1983). Effect of renal function on plasma levels of bone Gla-protein. *J. Clin. Endocrinol. Metab.* **57**, 1028–1030.

33. Briner, V. A., Thiel, G., Monier-Faugere, M.-C., Bognar, B., Landmann, J., Kamber, V., and Malluche, H. (1995). Prevention of cancellous bone loss but persistence of renal bone disease despite normal 1,25 vitamin D levels two years after kidney transplantation. *Transplantation* **59**, 1393–1400.

34. Boiskin, I., Epstein, S., Ismail, F., Thomas, S. B., and Raja, R. (1989). Serum osteocalcin and bone mineral metabolism following successful renal transplantation. *Clin. Nephrol.* **31**, 316–322.

35. Pietschmann, P., Vychtil, A., Woloszczuk, W., and Kovaril, J. (1991). Bone metabolism in patients with functioning kidney grafts: Increased serum levels of osteocalcin and parathyroid hormone despite normalization of kidney function. *Nephron* **59**, 533–536.

36. Withold, W., Degenhard, S., Castelli, D., Heins, M., and Grabensee, B. (1994). Monitoring of osteoblast activity with an immunoradiometric assay for determination of bone alkaline phosphatase mass concentration in patients receiving renal transplants. *Clin. Chim. Acta* **225**, 137–146.

37. Withold, W., Degenhard, S., Grabensee, B., and Reinauer, H. (1995). Comparison between serum levels of bone alkaline phosphatase and the carboxy-terminal propeptide of type I procollagen as markers of bone formation in patients following renal transplantation. *Clin. Chim. Acta* **239**, 143–151.

38. Coen, G., Mazzafero, S., Ballanti, P., Bonucci, E., Bondatti, F., Manni, M., Pasquali, M., Perruzzi, I., Sardella, D., and Spurio, A. (1992). Procollagen type I C-terminal extension peptide in predialysis chronic renal failure. *Am. J. Nephrol.* **12**, 246–251.

39. Hamdy, N. A. T., Risteli, J., Risteli, L., Harris, S., Beneton, M. N., Brown, C. B., and Kanis, J. A. (1994). Serum type I procollagen peptide: A non-invasive index of bone formation in patients on haemodialysis? *Nephrol. Dial. Transplant.* **9**, 511–516.

40. Gonzalez, M. T., Bonnin, R., Cruzado, J. M., Garcia, R., Moreso, F., Fulladosa, X., Alsina, J., Navarro, M. A., and Grino, J. M. (1995).

Course of three biochemical bone markers after kidney transplantation. *Transplant. Proc.* **27**, 2266–2271.

41. Dempster, D. W., Cosman, F., Parisien, M., Shen, V., and Lindsay, R. (1993). Anabolic actions of parathyroid hormone on bone. *Endocr. Rev.* **14**, 690–709.

42. Lane, N. E., Sanchez, S., Modin, G. W., Genant, H. K., and Arnaud, C. D. (1998). Parathyroid hormone treatment can reverse corticosteroid-induced osteoporosis. Results of a randomized controlled clinical trial. *J. Clin. Invest.* **102**, 1627–1633.

43. Rambausek, M., Ritz, E., Pomer, S., Mohring, K., and Rohl, L. (1988). Alkaline phosphatase levels in renal transplant recipients receiving cyclosporine or azathioprine/steroids. *Lancet,* **1**: 247.

44. Aubia, J., Masramon, J., Serrano, S., Lloveras, J., and Morinoso, L. L. (1988). Bone histology in renal transplant patients receiving cyclsoporin. *Lancet* **1**: 1048.

45. Wilmink, J. M., Bras, J., Surachno, S., Heyst, J. L. A. M., and vd Horst, JM. Bone repair in cyclosporin-treated renal transplant patients. *Transplant. Proc.* **21**, 1492–1494.

46. Dumoulin, G., Hory, B., Nguyen, N. U., Henriet, M.-T., Bresson, C., Regnard, J., and Saint-Hillier, Y. (1995). Lack of evidence that cyclosporine treatment impairs calcium-phosphorus homeostasis and bone remodeling in normocalcemic long-term renal transplant recipients. *Transplantation* **59**, 1690–1694.

47. Amado, J. A., Riancho, J. A., De Francisco, A. L. M., Cotorruelo, J. G., Feijanes, J., Arias, M., Napal, J., and Gonzalez-Macias, J. (1996). Hyperparathyroidism is responsible for the increased levels of osteocalcin in patients with normally functioning kidney grafts. Bone mass after renal transplantation. *Kidney Int.* **50**, 1726–1733.

48. Muchmore, J. S., Cooper, D. K. C., Ye, Y., Schlegel, V. J., and Zudhi, N. (1991). Loss of vertebral bone density in heart transplant patients. *Transplant. Proc.* **23**, 1184–1185.

49. Lee, A. H., Mull, R. L., Keenan, G. F., Callegari, P. E., Dalinka, M. K., Eisen, H. J., Manicini, D. M., DiSesa, V. J., and Attie, M. F. (1994). Osteoporosis and bone morbidity in cardiac transplant recipients. *Am. J. Med.* **96**, 35–41.

50. Shane, E., Mancini, D., Aaronson, K., Silverberg, S. J., Seibel, M. J., Addesso, V., and McMahon, D. J. (1997). Bone mass, vitamin D deficiency, and hyperparathyroidism in congestive heart failure. *Am. J. Med.* **103**, 197–207.

51. Shane, E., Rivas, M., Silverberg, S. J., Kim, T. S., Staron, R. B., and Bilezikian, J. P. (1993). Osteoporosis after cardiac transplantation. *Am. J. Med.* **94**, 257–264.

52. Rich, G. M., Mudge, G. H., Laffel, G. L., and LeBoff, M. S. (1992). Cyclosporine A and prednisone-associated osteoporosis in heart transplant recipients. *J. Heart Lung Transplant.* **11**, 950–958.

53. Shane, E., Rivas, M., Staron, R. B., Silverberg, S. J., Seibel, M. J., Kuiper, J., Mancini, D., Addesso, V., Michler, R. E., and Factor-Litvak, P. (1996). Fracture after cardiac transplantation: A prospective longitudinal study. *J. Clin. Endocrinol. Metab.* **81**, 1740–1746.

54. Leidig-Bruckner, G., Eberwein, S., Czeczatka, D., Dodidou, P., Schilling, T., Pritsch, M., Klose, C., Otto, G., Theilman, L., Zimmerman, R., Lange, R., and Ziegler, R. (1997). Incidence of osteoporosis fractures after liver and heart transplantation. *J. Bone Miner. Res.* **12** (Suppl. 1), S145.

55. Sambrook, P. N., Kelly, P. J., Keogh, A., MacDonald, P., Spratt, P., Freund, J., and Eisman, J. A. (1994). Bone loss after cardiac transplantation: A prospective study. *J. Heart Lung Transplant.* **13**, 116–121.

56. Van Cleemput, J., Daenen, W., Nijs, J., Geusens, P., Dequeker, J., and Vanhaecke, J. Timing and quantification of bone loss in cardiac transplant recipients. *Transplant. Int.* **8**, 196–200.

57. Berguer, D. G., Krieg, M.-A., Thiebaud, D., Burckhardt, P., Stumpe, F., Hurni, M., Sadeghi, H., Kappenberger, L., and Goy, J. J. (1994). Osteoporosis in heart transplant recipients: A longitudinal study. *Transplant. Proc.* **26**, 2649–2651.

58. Henderson, N. K., Sambrook, P. N., Kelly, P. J., Macdonald, P., Keogh, A. M., Stratt, P., and Eisman, J. A. (1995). Bone mineral loss and recovery after cardiac transplantation. *Lancet* **2**, 905.

59. Shane, E., Rivas, M., McMahon, D. J., Shane, E., Rivas, M., McMahon, D. J., Staron, R. B., Silverberg, S. J., Seibel, M. J., Mancini, D., Michler, R. E., Aaronson, K., Addesso, V., and Lo, S. H. (1997). Bone loss turnover after cardiac transplantation. *J. Clin. Endocrinol. Metab.* **82**, 1497–1506.

60. Sambrook, P. N., Kelly, P. J., Fontana, D., Nguyen, T., Keogh, A., MacDonald, P., Spratt, P., Freund, J., and Eisman, J. A. (1994). Mechanics of rapid bone loss following cardiac transplantation. *Osteoporosis Int.* **4**, 273–276.

61. Thiebaud, D., Kreig, M. A., Gillard-Berguer, D., Jacquet, A. F., Goy, J. J., and Burckhardt, P. (1996). Cyclosporine induces high bone turnover and may contribute to bone loss after heart transplantation. *Eur. J. Clin. Invest.* **26**, 549–555.

62. Prummel, M. F., Wiersinga, W. M., Lips, P., Sanders, G. T. P., and Sauerwein, H. P. (1991). The course of biochemical parameters of bone turnover during treatment with corticosteroids. *J. Clin. Endocrinol. Metab.* **72**, 382–386.

63. Lems, W. F., Gerrits, M. I., Jacobs, J. W. G., van Vugt, R. M., van Rijn, H. J. M., and Bijlsma, J. W. J. (1996). Changes in (markers of) bone metabolism during high dose corticosteroid pulse treatment in patients with rheumatoid arthritis. *Ann. Rheum. Dis.* **55**, 288–293.

64. Shane, E., Rodino, M. A., McMahon, D. J., Addesso, V., Staron, R. B., Seibel, M. J., Mancini, D. M., Michler, R. E., and Lo, S. H. (1998). Prevention of bone loss after cardiac transplantation with antiresorptive therapy: A pilot study. *J. Heart Lung Transplant.* **17**, 1089–1096.

65. Guo, C.-Y., Johnson, A., Locke, T. J., and Eastell, R. (1998). Mechanisms of bone loss after cardiac transplantation. *Bone* **22**, 267–271.

66. Bikle, D. D., Genant, M. D., Conn, C., Cann, C., Becker, R. R., Halloran, B. P., and Strewler, G. J. (1985). Bone disease in alcohol abuse. *Ann. Intern. Med.* **103**, 42–48.

67. Friday, K. E., and Howard, G. A. (1991). Ethanol inhibits human bone cell proliferation and function in vitro. *Metab., Clin. Exp.* **40**, 562–565.

68. Diamond, T., and Stiel, D. (1989). Osteoporosis in hemochromatosis. Iron excess, gonadal deficiency or other factors? *Ann. Intern. Med.* **110**, 430–436.

69. Stellon, A. J., Davies, A., and Compston, J. (1985). Bone loss in autoimmune chronic active hepatitis on maintenance corticosteroid therapy. *Gastroenterology* **89**, 1078–1083.

70. Hodgson, S. F., Dickson, E. R., Wahner, H. W., Johnson, K. A., Mann, K. G., and Riggs, B. L. (1980). Bone loss and reduced osteoblast function in primary biliary cirrhosis. *Ann. Intern. Med.* **103**, 855–860.

71. Floreani, A., Chiaramonte, M., Gianninni, S., Malvasi, L., Lodetti, M. G., Castrignano, R., Giacommmini, A., D'Angelo, A., and Naccarato, R. (1991). Longitudinal study on osteodystrophy in primary biliary cirrhosis and a pilot study on calcitonin treatment. *J. Hepatol.* **12**, 217–223.

72. Maddrey, W. C. (1990). Bone disease in patients with primary biliary cirrhosis. *Prog. Liver Dis.* **9**, 537–554.

73. Monegal, A., Navasa, M., Guañabens, N., Peris, P., Pons, F., Martinez de Osaba, M. J., Rimola, A., Rodes, J., and Munoz-Gomez, J. (1997). Osteoporosis and bone mineral metabolism in cirrhotic patients referred for liver transplantation. *Calcif. Tissue Int.* **60**, 148–154.

74. Guañabens, N., Pares, A., Alvarez, L., Martinez de Osaba, M. J., Monegal, A., Peris, P., Ballesta, A. M., and Rodes, J. (1998). Collagen-related markers of bone turnover reflect the severity of liver fibrosis in patients with primary biliary cirrhosis. *J. Bone Miner. Res.* **13**, 731–738.

75. Guañabens, N., Pares, A., Marinoso, L., Brancos, M. A., Piera, C., Serrano, S., Rivera, F., and Rodes, J. (1990). Factors influencing the development of metabolic bone disease in primary biliary cirrhosis. *Am. J. Gastroenterol.* **85**, 1356–1362.

76. Hodgson, S. F., Dickson, E. R., Eastell, R., Eriksen, E. F., Bryant, S. C., and Riggs, B. L. (1993). Rates of cancellous bone remodeling and turnover in osteopenia associated with primary biliary cirrhosis. *Bone* **14**, 819–827.

77. Janes, C. H., Dickson, E. R., Okazaki, R., Bonde, S., McDonagh, A. F., and Riggs, B. L. (1995). Role of hyperbilirubinemia in the impairment of osteoblast proliferation associated with cholestatic jaundice. *J. Clin. Invest.* **95**, 2581–2586.

78. Haagsma, E. B., Thijn, C. J. P., Post, J. G., Slooff, M. J. H., and Gisp, C. H. (1988). Bone disease after liver transplantation. *J. Hepatol.* **6**, 94–100.

79. Arnold, J. C., Hauser, R., Ziegler, R., Kommerelli, B., Otto, G., Theilmann, L., and Wuster, C. (1992). Bone disease after liver transplantation. *Transplant. Proc.* **24**, 2709–2710.

80. McDonald, J. A., Dunstan, C. R., Dilworth, P., Sherbon, K., Ross Sheil, A. G., Evans, R. A., and McCaughan, G. W. (1991). Bone loss after liver transplantation. *Hepatology* **14**, 613–619.

81. Navasa, M., Monegal, A., Guanabens, N., Peris, P., Rimola, A., Munoz-Gomez, J., Visa, J., and Rodes, J. (1994). Bone fracture in liver transplant patients. *Br. J. Rheumatol.* **33**, 52–55.

82. Eastell, R., Dickson, E. R., Hodgson, S. F., Wiesner, R. H., Porayko, M. K., Wahner, H. W., Cedel, S. L., Riggs, B. L., and Krom, R. A. (1991). Rates of bone loss before and after liver transplantation in women with primary biliary cirrhosis. *Hepatology* **14**, 296–300.

83. Meys, E., Fontanges, E., Fourcade, N., Thomasson, A., Pouyet, M., and Delmas, P. D. (1994). Bone loss after orthotopic liver transplantation. *Am. J. Med.* **97**, 445–450.

84. Compston, J. E., Greer, S., Skingle, S. J., Stirling, D. M., Price, C., Friend, P. J., and Alexander, G. (1996). Early increase in plasma parathyroid hormone levels following liver transplantation. *J. Hepatol.* **25**, 715–718.

85. Hawkins, F. G., Leon, M., Lopez, M. B., Larrodera, L., Garcia-Garcia, I., Loinaz, C., and Morena Gonzalez, E. (1994). Bone loss and turnover in patients with liver transplantation. *Hepatogastroenterology* **41**, 158–161.

86. Valero, M. A., Loinaz, C., Larrodera, L., Leon, M., Morena, E., and Hawkins, F. (1995). Calcitonin and bisphosphonates treatment in bone loss after liver transplantation. *Calif. Tissue Int.* **57**, 15–19.

87. Rabinowitz, M., Shapiro, J., Lian, J., Block, G. D., Merkel, I. S., and Van Thiel, D. H. (1992). Vitamin D and osteocalcin levels in liver transplant recipients. In osteocalcin a reliable marker of bone turnover in such cases? *J. Hepatol.* **16**, 50–55.

88. Watson, R. G., Coulton, L., Kanis, J. A., Lombard, M., Williams, R., Neuberger, J., and Elias, E. (1990). Circulating osteocalcin in primary biliary cirrhosis following liver transplantation and during treatment with ciclosporin. *J. Hepatol.* **11**, 354–358.

89. Abdelhadi, M., Eriksson, S. A., Ljusk Eriksson, S., Ericzon, B. G., and Nordenstrom, J. (1995). Bone mineral status in end-stage liver disease and the effect of liver transplantation. *Scand. J. Gasterenterol.* **30**, 1210–1215.

90. Grey, A. B., Ames, R. W., Matthews, R. D., and Reid, I. R. (1993). Bone mineral density and body composition in adult patients with cystic fibrosis. *Thorax* **48**, 589–593.

91. Bachrach, L. K., Loutit, C. W., Moss, R. B., and Marcus, R. (1994) Osteopenia in adults with cystic fibrosis. *Am. J. Med.* **96**, 27–34.

92. Aris, R. M., Renner, J. B., Winders, A. D., Buell, H. E., Riggs, D. B., Lester, G. E., and Ontjes, D. A. (1998). Increased rate of fractures and severe kyphosis: Sequelae of living into adulthood with cystic fibrosis. *Ann. Intern. Med.* **128**, 186–193.

93. Donovan, D. S., Papadopoulos, A., Staron, R. B., Addesso, V., Schulman, L., McGregor, C., Cosman, F., Lindsay, R., and Shane, E. (1998). Bone mass and vitamin D deficiency in adults with advanced cystic fibrosis lung disease. *Am. J. Respir. Crit. Care Med.* **157**, 1892–1899.

94. Aris, R. M., Neuringer, I. P., Weiner, M. A., Egan, and T. M., Ontjes, D. (1996). Severe osteoporosis before and after lung transplantation. *Chest* **109**, 1176–1183.

95. Shane, E., Silverberg S. J., Donovan, D., Papadopoulos, A., Staron, R. B., Addesso, V., Jorgeson, B., McGregor, C., and Schulman, L. (1996). Osteoporosis in lung transplantation candidates with end-stage pulmonary disease. *Am. J. Med.* **101**, 262–269.

96. Ferrari, S. L., Nicod, L. P., Hamacher, J., Spiliopoulos, A., Slosman, D. O., Rochat, T., Bonjour, J.-P., and Rizzoli, R. (1996). Osteoporosis in patients undergoing lung transplantation. *Eur. Respir. J.* **9**, 2378–2382.

97. Shane, E., Papodopoulos, A., Staron, R. B., Addesso, V., Donovan, D., McGregor, C., and Schulman, L. L. (1999). Bone loss and fracture after lung transplantation. *Transplantation* (in press).

98. Kelly, P., Atkinson, K., Ward, R. L., Sambrook, P. N., Biggs, J. C., and Eisman, J. A. (1990). Reduced bone mineral density in men and women with allogeneic bone marrow transplantation. *Transplantation* **50**, 881–883.

99. Castaneda, S., Carmona, L., Carvajal, I., Arranz, R., Diaz, A., and Garcia-Vadilla, A. (1997). Reduction of bone mass in women after bone marrow transplantation. *Calcif. Tissue Int.* **60**, 343–347.

100. Schubert, M. A., Sullivan, K. M., Schubert, M. M., Nims, J., Hansen, M., Sanders, J. E., O'Quigley, J., Witherspoon, R. P., Bickner, C. D., and Storb, R. (1990). Gynecologic abnormalities following allogeneic bonr marrow transplantation. *Bone Marrow Transplant.* **5**, 425–430.

101. Carlson, K., Simonsson, B., and Ljunghall, S. (1994). Acute effects of high dose chemotherapy followed by bone marrow transplantation on serum markers of bone metabolism. *Calcif. Tissue Int.* **55**, 408–411.

102. Stern, J. M., Chesnut, C. H., III, Bruemmer, B., Sullivan, K. M., Lenssen, P. S., Aker, S. N., and Sanders, J. (1996). Bone density loss during treatment of chronic GVHD. *Bone Marrow Transplant.* **17**, 395–400.

103. Shane, E., Rodino, M. A., McMahon, D. M., Addesso, V., Staron, R. B., Seibel, M. J., Mancini, D., Michler, R. E., and Lo, S. H. (1999). Prevention of bone loss after cardiac transplantation with anitresorptive therapy: A pilot study. *J. Heart Lung Transplant.* **17**, 1089–1096.

104. Fan, S., Almond, M. K., Ball, E., Evans, K., and Cunningham, J. (1996). Randomized prospective study demonstrating prevention of bone loss by pamidronate during the first year after renal transplantation. *J. Am. Soc. Nephrol.* **7**, A2717 (abstr.).

105. Van Cleemput, J., Daenen, W., Geusens, P., Dequeker, J., Van de Werf, E., and Vanhaecke, J. (1996). Prevention of bone loss in cardiac transplant recipients. A comparison of biphosphonates and vitamin D. *Transplantation* **61**, 1495–1499.

106. Valero, M. A., Loinaz, C., Larrodera, L., Leon, M., Moreno, E., and Hawkins, F. (1995). Calcitonin and bisphosphonate treatment and bone loss after liver transplantation. *Calcif. Tissue Int.* **57**, 15–19.

107. Riemens, S. C., Oostdijk, A., van Doormaal, J., Thijn, C. J., Drent, G., Piers, D. A., Groen, E. W., Meerman, L., Slooff, M. J., and Haagsma, E. B. (1996). Bone loss after liver transplantation is not prevented by cyclical etidronate, calcium and alpha calcidiol. *Osteoporosis Int.* **6**, 213–218.

CHAPTER 37

Secondary Osteoporosis

JEAN E. MULDER   Department of Medicine, College of Physicians and Surgeons, Columbia University, New York, New York 10032

CAROLINA A. MOREIRA KULAK   Department of Medicine, College of Physicians and Surgeons, Columbia University, New York, New York 10032; Department of Endocrinology, Federal University of Parana, Hospital de Clinicas, Curitiba, Brazil

ELIZABETH SHANE   Department of Medicine, College of Physicians and Surgeons, Columbia University, New York, New York 10032

I. INTRODUCTION

Osteoporosis is the most common metabolic bone disease worldwide. The term primary osteoporosis is generally used to describe the progressive bone loss which occurs with aging, in both men and women, but especially in postmenopausal women. Secondary osteoporosis may result from endocrine abnormalities such as hyperthyroidism, hypogonadism, Cushing's syndrome, and hyperparathyroidism (Table I). In addition, some chronic conditions, such as malabsorption, immobilization, hepatic disease, and renal disease, can result in bone loss. Finally, many drugs also cause secondary osteoporosis. In this chapter, we review the impact of some of these more commonly encountered disorders on the skeleton, with specific emphasis on bone mineral density and parameters of bone remodeling.

II. HYPERTHYROIDISM AND OSTEOPOROSIS

The relationship between hyperthyroidism and bone loss was described in the late 1800s, when a postmortem study in a thyrotoxic patient revealed excessive bone destruction [1]. Subsequent histomorphometric studies of bone in hyperthyroidism support this early observation. Reductions in the resorption and formation phases of the bone remodeling cycle have been noted, resulting in an overall increase in the activation frequency of the remodeling cycle. Both osteoblast and osteoclast activities are enhanced. Specifically, an increased calcification rate, increased resorption surface, and a decreased mineralization lag time have been described in cancellous bone of hyperthyroid patients. In cortical bone, increases in active resorption and cortical porosity have also been reported [2, 3]. Typical of the adult skeleton subjected to events associated with high bone turnover, untreated hyperthyroidism results in a net negative bone balance and reduced bone mass [4]. The mechanism of the deleterious effect of excessive thyroid hormone on bone has not been fully clarified. Stimulation of bone-resorbing cytokines, such as interleukin-6 and interleukin 1β, by thyroid hormone is one proposed mechanism [5, 6].

Hyperthyroidism is multifactorial in etiology and may result from autoimmune disease (Graves' disease), toxic nodular or multinodular goiter, thyroiditis, or excessive exogenous thyroid hormone intake. In addition, hyperthyroidism

527

TABLE I.   Secondary Osteoporosis

Hypogonadal states	Chapter 37
Turner's syndrome	
Athletic amenorrhea	
Anorexia nervosa	
Hyperprolactinemia	
GnRH therapy	
Hypothalamic amenorrhea	
Thyroid disorders	Chapter 37
Other endocrine disorders	
Hyperparathyroidism	Chapter 40
Diabetes mellitus	
Hemochromatosis	
Acromegaly	
Medications	
Glucocorticoids	Chapter 35
Anticonvulsant drugs	Chapter 37
Cyclosporin	Chapter 36
Diuretics	
Anticoagulants	
Methotrexate	
Renal disorders	Chapter 39
Gastrointestinal disorders	
Primary biliary cirrhosis	
Inflammatory bowel disease	
Celiac disease and sprue	
Hepatic diseases	
Hematologic disorders	
Multiple myeloma	Chapter 42
Systemic mastocytosis	
Lymphoproliferative disorders	
Rheumatologic disorders	Chapter 44
Immobilization	
Genetic disorders	
Osteogenesis imperfecta	Chapter 43
Vitamin D resistant osteomalacia	Chapter 38
Hypophosphatasia	
Marfan syndrome	
Ehlers-Danlos	
Glycogen storage diseases	

can vary in severity, from severe thyrotoxicosis to subclinical hyperthyroidism. Osteoporosis is also multifactorial in etiology and is influenced by genetic, hormonal, nutritional, and lifestyle factors. Therefore, the impact of hyperthyroidism on bone loss and its long-term consequences are variable, depending on the nature and severity of the thyroid disease as well as on individual bone health and the presence of other risk factors for osteoporosis. The increased availability of bone densitometry and biochemical markers of bone remodeling has resulted in a greater understanding of thyroid-related bone loss. In this section, we will review the impact of hyperthyroidism on bone remodeling, with special emphasis on changes in bone mineral density (BMD) and parameters of bone remodeling.

A. Hyperthyroidism (Endogenous)

BMD is decreased both in premenopausal and in post-menopausal women with thyrotoxicosis [7–11]. Values 10–30% lower than age-matched controls have been reported [7–11]. Normalization of thyroid function results in improvement in BMD. Lupoli *et al.* [10] reported a 26% increase in spinal bone density (measured by dual energy x-ray absorptiometry—DEXA) in premenopausal women treated with antithyroid drugs for 12 months and an 18.6% increase in postmenopausal patients treated with antithyroid drugs plus hormone replacement therapy (HRT). However, final BMD in these patients was still lower than BMD in the control group matched for age and menopausal status. Interestingly, both pre- and postmenopausal patients treated with alendronate, in addition to antithyroid drugs and HRT (postmenopausal women only), achieved greater increases in spinal BMD after 12 months. Final BMD in this subgroup was not significantly different from that of the control population. It is unclear whether BMD would have normalized in the patients treated solely with antithyroid drugs with longer follow-up. In this regard, a five year evaluation of lumbar spine BMD in a very small group of men and women with treated hyperthyroidism has demonstrated complete restoration of vertebral bone density after antithyroid therapy [12]. The single postmenopausal woman in the study experienced a 9.8% increase in lumbar spine BMD over five years. Most studies report an increase in BMD of 1–11% in women after resolution of hyperthyroidism [7–9, 11, 12]. Of note, intranasal calcitonin has not been shown to improve BMD beyond the improvement noted with correction of thyroid function [11].

Few studies have addressed the effects of thyrotoxicosis on bone mass in men [7, 13–15]. A single prospective study addressing the effect of Graves' disease on radial BMD in men revealed a lower baseline BMD in hyperthyroid patients compared with age-matched controls [14]. Treatment with either radioactive iodine or antithyroid drugs resulted in an initial decrease in BMD followed by a return to baseline after two years. Radial BMD (assessed by single photon absorptiometry—SPA) in men with Graves' disease remained lower than that of controls after two years. In a cross-sectional study of BMD (assessed by dual photon absorptiometry—DPA) that included a very small number of men with untreated Graves' disease, there was no difference in vertebral or hip BMD in the men with Graves' disease compared with age-matched controls [15]. Overall, there is insufficient data on the deleterious effects of thyrotoxicosis on BMD or on the extent of recovery after treatment in men.

The decrease in BMD associated with hyperthyroidism is secondary to an increase in bone remodeling, with bone resorption exceeding bone formation. Well-documented increases in serum and urinary markers of bone turnover in thyrotoxic patients support this premise (Fig. 1). Urinary markers

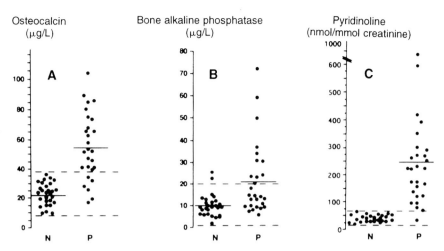

FIGURE 1   (A) Serum osteocalcin, (B) bone-specific alkaline phosphatase, and (C) urinary pyridinoline crosslinks in patients with endogenous hyperthyroidism. N—age-matched normal subjects; P—patients. Dotted lines represent the normal ranges ± 2 SD. Reprinted from Garnero *et al.* [19]. Markers of bone turnover in hyperthyroidism and the effects of treatment. *J. Clin. Endocrinol. Metab.* **78(4)**, 955–959, 1994, © The Endocrine Society, with permission.

of bone resorption (hydroxyproline, pyridinium cross-links) are increased in both pre- and postmenopausal women with untreated Graves' disease [16, 17] and in patients with hyperthyroidism in general [18]. Pyridinium cross-link levels, whether measured by HPLC [17, 18] or by direct immunoassay [19], are elevated in nearly all thyrotoxic patients and correlate well with free thyroxine (T4) and free triiodothyronine (T3) levels [17, 19]. Urinary assays which measure type I collagen C-telopeptide also correlate well with free T3 and T4 levels [20]. Elevated serum markers of bone formation (total and bone specific alkaline phosphatase, osteocalcin, or PICP, the carboxyterminal propeptide of type 1 procollagen) have also been reported in Graves' disease [9, 15, 16, 19, 21] and in patients with toxic nodular goiter and amiodarone-induced hyperthyroidism [19]. Osteocalcin [16, 19] and PICP [16] levels correlate well with free T3 [19, 21], total T4 [21], and free T4 levels [16]. Osteocalcin levels have also been reported to correlate negatively with BMD Z scores at the spine, femoral neck, and trochanter [15]. However, Garnero *et al.* [19] demonstrated three-fold higher elevations in bone resorption markers than in formation markers, supporting the hypothesis of an imbalance between resorption and formation that favors bone loss.

Beta receptor antagonists, frequently used in the therapy of Graves' disease, do not appear to alter the rise in pyridinium cross-links and therefore probably do not inhibit thyroid hormone-mediated bone resorption [17]. In one study, radioactive iodine therapy resulted in a prompt reduction in pyridinium cross-links, with normalization by approximately 10–12 weeks. Osteocalcin levels remained unchanged during this time interval [17]. In contrast, Garrel *et al.* [21] demonstrated normalization of osteocalcin levels by 16 weeks after treatment of hyperthyroidism in the 70% of patients (men

and women) with elevated baseline levels. In premenopausal women, euthyroidism after six months of methimazole therapy was associated with significant reductions in serum PICP and urinary hydroxyproline excretion. There was a nonsignificant decrease in osteocalcin and total alkaline phosphatase activity [16]. In contrast, Garnero *et al.* [19] observed that osteocalcin, measured by ELISA, decreased significantly by one month after therapy with antithyroid drugs, radioactive iodine, or surgery in 11 of 27 patients evaluated. In the same study, the pattern of change of bone specific alkaline phosphatase differed, increasing after one month of therapy and decreasing four months after therapy. The discrepancy between normalization of osteocalcin, bone specific alkaline phosphatase, and PICP, all markers of bone formation, may be explained by differences in assay technique, osteoblast function, release from bone, and clearance of the markers [16, 19]. Given that bone specific alkaline phosphatase values were elevated in <50% of hyperthyroid patients studied and that levels did not correlate with the degree of hyperthyroidism, it appears to be a less sensitive marker of hyperthyroid-induced bone turnover than osteocalcin or PICP [19].

Other biochemical changes documented in hyperthyroid patients include elevated serum and urinary calcium levels and decreased intact parathyroid hormone (PTH) levels, although these values generally remain within the normal range. Treatment with methimazole results in significant reductions in serum and urinary calcium and an increase in intact PTH [16]. In general, 25-hydroxyvitamin D levels are normal, whereas 1,25-dihydroxyvitamin D levels may be decreased [22], reflecting decreased PTH concentrations.

In summary, the decrease in bone mineral density and the elevation of markers of bone remodeling in patients with overt hyperthyroidism supports the histologic findings of increased cortical porosity and increased cancellous resorption surfaces and calcification rates, indicating accelerated bone turnover and net loss of bone. The increase in BMD and improvement of markers of bone remodeling with normalization of thyroid function suggest that the bone loss is, at least in part, reversible. However, complete recovery, especially in postmenopausal women, is not documented consistently. Furthermore, Franklyn [23] and others [24, 25] have demonstrated that a previous history of thyrotoxicosis in postmenopausal women conferred an increased risk of low BMD, even in patients who had been euthyroid for many years. In contrast, premenopausal women with a history of thyrotoxicosis did not have an increased risk of low BMD [23]. Thus, estrogen may protect premenopausal women from the deleterious effects of excess endogenous thyroxine production on BMD. Further prospective longitudinal studies are needed to determine if bone loss is completely reversible in all patients and whether intervention with antiresorptive drugs is of benefit when recovery is not complete.

B. Subclinical Hyperthyroidism (Endogenous)

Patients with multinodular goiter with autonomy or solitary autonomous functioning nodules often develop thyroid hormone abnormalities characterized by a suppressed TSH level with a normal T4 level, a pattern which has been designated subclinical hyperthyroidism. Endogenous subclinical hyperthyroidism has also been associated with a decrease in bone mineral density in pre- and postmenopausal women [26], although the data in premenopausal women are conflicting. Faber *et al.* [27] observed no change in bone mineral density of the distal forearm or lumbar spine over two years in premenopausal women with goiter and subclinical hyperthyroidism. Similarly, in a cross-sectional study of 39 premenopausal women with autonomously functioning thyroid nodules and subclinical hyperthyroidism, Foldes *et al.* [28] reported no significant difference in Z scores at any site compared with the control group. In contrast, 52 postmenopausal women with subclinical hyperthyroidism had significantly lower Z scores at both the femoral neck and radius, but not at the lumbar spine, compared with the postmenopausal control group (Fig. 2). Osteopenia was present, but osteoporosis was rarely detected. In this study, spine and femoral neck bone density were measured by DEXA; radial bone density was measured by SPA [28].

The cross-sectional study design prohibits the assessment of the impact of the duration of subclinical hyperthyroidism on bone density. In addition, there are often large individual variations in BMD values within patient subgroups. Therefore, it is difficult to conclude from the Foldes *et al.* study [28] whether postmenopausal women had lower bone density Z scores at the femoral neck and radius because they had a longer duration of subclinical hyperthyroidism, whether bone loss due to estrogen deficiency was accelerated by the

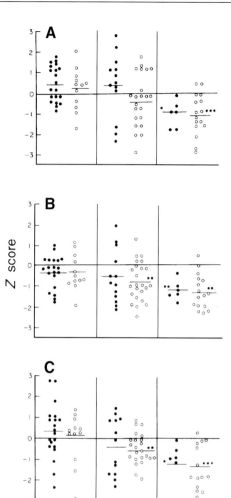

FIGURE 2 Z-scores for (A) vertebral, (B) femoral neck, and (C) midshaft radial BMD values in premenopausal (closed circles) and postmenopausal (open circles) women with nodular goiter and either normal thyroid function (left panel), endogenous subclinical hyperthyroidism (middle panel), or endogenous overt hyperthyroidism (right panel). The horizontal bars represent the mean values of the groups. Asterisks denote significant differences from a sex and age-matched population. *p < 0.05, **p < 0.01, ***p < 0.001. Reprinted from Foldes *et al.* [28], with permission.

presence of subclinical hyperthyroidism, or whether some women had suboptimal peak bone densities earlier in life, independent of thyroid dysfunction. Mudde *et al.* [29] have reported an increase in distal radial BMD (predominantly cancellous bone), but not proximal radial BMD (predominantly cortical bone), in eight postmenopausal women with multinodular goiter and subclinical hyperthyroidism who received treatment with antithyroid drugs for two years. These data suggest that subclinical hyperthyroidism in postmenopausal women can result in bone loss which may be reversible with normalization of thyroid function.

Studies of markers of bone remodeling in patients with endogenous subclinical hyperthyroidism are conflicting. Faber *et al.* [30] demonstrated elevated osteocalcin levels in 6 of 44 patients with nontoxic goiter. Osteocalcin levels correlated negatively with TSH levels both in pre- and in postmenopausal women [30]. However, Foldes et al. [28] did not report a significant difference in osteocalcin levels in pre- or postmenopausal women with subclinical hyperthyroidism compared with an appropriately matched control population. In Mudde's study [29], there was also no difference in serum osteocalcin or urinary hydroxyproline levels in the group treated with antithyroid drugs compared to the untreated group, even though the treated group experienced a small increase in distal radial BMD. In contrast, another study has demonstrated increased urinary deoxypyridinoline (DPD) excretion, a more sensitive and specific marker of bone resorption, in postmenopausal patients with subclinical hyperthyroidism compared with age-matched controls, indicating excessive bone resorption [31].

The discrepancies among these reports may be related to the duration of subclinical hyperthyroidism or to the impact of excessive thyroid hormone on bone in the presence of estrogen deficiency. It is also possible that other local growth factors, such as insulin-like growth factor (IGF-1), may be involved in mediating the effects of thyroid hormone on the skeleton. IGF-1 has stimulatory effects on osteoblasts and is a known stimulator of bone formation. IGF-1 levels have been measured in both pre- and postmenopausal women with hyperthyroidism [31]. Whereas premenopausal women with overt hyperthyroidism had elevated IGF-1 levels, postmenopausal women with either subclinical or overt hyperthyroidism did not. This relative IGF-1 deficiency may contribute to the reduced bone mass observed in postmenopausal women. Taken together, the above data suggest that endogenous subclinical hyperthyroidism can result in increased bone resorption and a decrease in bone mineral density in postmenopausal women. However, premenopausal women with endogenous subclinical hyperthyroidism appear to be at lower risk.

C. Hyperthyroidism (Exogenous)

Overt hyperthyroidism (elevated T4 and/or T3 with suppressed TSH) secondary to excessive levothyroxine (L-T4) therapy occurs infrequently, given the advent of ultrasensitive TSH assays and an increased awareness of the potential adverse effects of excess exogenous L-T4 on BMD and cardiac function. The data suggest that exogenous L-T4, in doses sufficient to cause hyperthyroidism, results in decreased BMD and an increased risk of fractures [32]. Histomorphometric analysis of bone in such patients has revealed increased cancellous and cortical bone turnover similar to that reported in endogenous hyperthyroidism [3, 32].

D. Subclinical Hyperthyroidism (Exogenous)

Suppressive therapy with L-T4 is often used in the treatment of nodular thyroid disease and in thyroid cancer. Bio-

chemical testing in these patients often reveals subclinical hyperthyroidism. Results on the effects of excess exogenous thyroid hormone on bone mineral density are conflicting, with some studies demonstrating a decrease in bone density [24, 25, 33–38] and others suggesting no effect [39–42]. The relationship between L-T4 suppressive therapy and biochemical markers of bone remodeling is similarly controversial [36, 37, 39–43]. These discrepancies are explained, in part, by the heterogeneity of the patient populations studied, the heterogeneity of the underlying thyroid disease, differences in methodology and site of bone density determination, and by the small sample size and cross-sectional design of many of the studies. There is also great variability in the TSH assays (second or third generation assays), the degree of suppression of TSH levels, the duration and type of thyroid hormone suppressive therapy, and the frequency of past endogenous hyperthyroidism in the patients studied. Finally, other factors that impact BMD are not controlled for in many studies, such as calcium and vitamin D intake, physical activity, sun exposure, and ethnicity and race.

Cross-sectional studies have suggested that exogenous subclinical hyperthyroidism does not significantly alter BMD when patients are compared with controls matched for age, menopausal status, height, and weight. Giannini et al. [41] evaluated 25 women (12 premenopausal) who were treated with suppressive doses of L-T4 for thyroid cancer for a mean of 7.6 years. TSH levels were below normal in all patients. There was no difference in lumbar spine Z scores (DEXA) between the premenopausal patients and controls nor between the postmenopausal patients and controls [41]. Similarly, Franklyn et al. [40] reported no effect of L-T4 suppressive therapy on femoral or vertebral BMD in pre- or postmenopausal women treated for thyroid cancer for a mean of 7.9 years.

In contrast, Kung et al. [37] evaluated 34 postmenopausal Chinese women treated with suppressive doses of L-T4 for a mean of 12.2 years, after thyroidectomy for thyroid cancer. Patients had lower BMD (DEXA) at the lumbar spine, femoral neck, Ward's triangle, and trochanter compared to the control population. In addition, two patients in the treated group had a history of fracture (femoral neck, wrist). The differences among these studies may be accounted for by the longer duration of L-T4 use or by ethnic differences. In support of this, Ross et al. [33] have demonstrated that premenopausal women treated with suppressive doses of L-T4 for more than ten years had the most significant reduction in cortical BMD, suggesting that duration of suppressive therapy is an important factor in predicting bone mass. However, Franklyn et al. [40] did not find any correlation between duration of L-T4 suppressive therapy and BMD. Finally, two meta-analyses evaluating the effect of exogenous subclinical hyperthyroidism on bone mass revealed no significant change in bone mineral density in premenopausal women with suppressed TSH levels. However, a small but significant decrease in BMD was noted in postmenopausal women [44, 45].

Cross-sectional studies evaluating biochemical markers of bone remodeling in exogenous subclinical hyperthyroidism have been similarly conflicting. Total alkaline phosphatase activity has been either elevated [37] or unchanged [39, 40] in postmenopausal women with suppressed TSH levels. Elevated levels of bone specific alkaline phosphatase have been reported in both pre- and postmenopausal women taking suppressive doses of L-T4 compared to controls matched for age and menopausal status [41]. Elevated osteocalcin levels have been reported in pre- and postmenopausal women with suppressed TSH levels by some [36, 37], but not all [39, 42, 43], investigators. Elevated urinary hydroxyproline levels have been reported in both premenopausal [41] and postmenopausal women with suppressed TSH levels [37]. More specific urinary markers of bone resorption, such as urinary DPD and pyridinoline (PYD) excretion, have been demonstrated to be elevated in postmenopausal women with subclinical hyperthyroidism, but not in premenopausal women with similarly suppressed TSH levels [42, 46]. Many studies have reported no significant change in PTH, calcitriol, or calcitonin levels [37, 41, 42].

There are few longitudinal studies assessing the impact of suppressive L-T4 therapy on BMD and markers of bone remodeling [42, 47, 48]. In one very small study involving older premenopausal women, there was no change in radial BMD assessed by SPA, but mean spinal BMD, assessed by DPA, decreased over a three year interval compared to age-matched controls [47]. This decrease may have been related to subtle changes in estrogen levels during the perimenopausal period, although all women continued to have regular menses during the study. Guo et al. [48] evaluated longitudinal changes in BMD and markers of bone turnover in a homogeneous group of postmenopausal women on suppressive (n = 41) or replacement (n = 23) doses of levothyroxine, compared with age-matched healthy postmenopausal women (n = 36). There was no difference in mean BMD (DEXA: lumbar spine, femoral neck, or total body) or markers of bone turnover in any of the groups at baseline or at the end of the two-year observation period. However, two years after the dose of L-T4 was decreased in the subgroup of patients with primary hypothyroidism who were inappropriately taking suppressive doses (n = 18), there was a significant increase in BMD in the lumbar spine and femoral neck and a significant decrease in all three markers of bone turnover compared with the women who remained on suppressive therapy for thyroid cancer (n = 23) and the healthy control population (Fig. 3). Therefore, it appears that suppressive L-T4 therapy can increase bone turnover, but bone markers in this study remained within the normal range for age. Furthermore, bone loss was not accelerated over a two-year observation period. However, a reduction in L-T4 dose resulted in a decrease in bone turnover and an increase in BMD [48].

Taken together, the above data suggest that suppressive doses of L-T4 can increase bone remodeling in a subset of

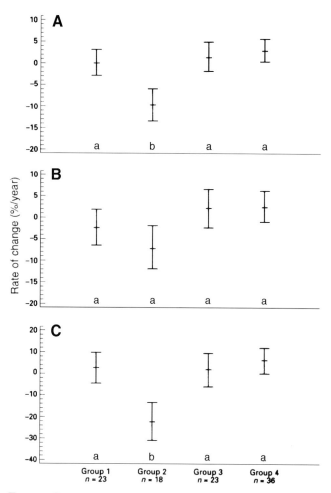

FIGURE 3   The rate of change of serum (A) osteocalcin, (B) bone-specific alkaline phosphatase, and (C) urinary NTX/Cr in three groups of postmenopausal women taking L-thyroxine. Group 1—hypothyroidism with normal TSH levels, Group 2—hypothyroidism with previously suppressed TSH levels. The dose of L-thyroxine was reduced after the baseline measurement, and TSH levels normalized 1–4 months later. Group 3—thyroid cancer with persistently suppressed TSH levels, and Group 4—a control group with normal TSH levels. The middle horizontal lines represent the mean values. The upper and lower horizontal lines represent the 95% confidence interval. The decrease in serum osteocalcin and urinary NTX/Cr in Group 2 was significantly different from the other groups (p < 0.05). Groups with the same letters were not different from each other. From Guo et al. Longitudinal changes of bone mineral density and bone turnover in postmenopausal women on thyroxine. Clin. Endocrinol. 46, 305, 1997 [48], with permission.

pre- and postmenopausal women with exogenous subclinical hyperthyroidism. Thus, these patients are predisposed to an excessive increase in bone resorption relative to bone formation, and subsequently are at a higher risk of decreased BMD. The risk of decreased BMD appears to be greater in postmenopausal women. However, BMD in patients on suppressive L-T4 therapy is not only dependent on the degree of TSH suppression, but perhaps also on the duration of use, as well as on lifestyle, hormonal, nutritional, genetic, and other factors. Consequently, patients on suppressive L-T4 do

TABLE II. Hyperthyroidism and Osteoporosis

	Hyperthyroidism (endogenous)		Subclinical hyperthyroidism (endogenous)		Hyperthyroidism (levothyroxine treatment)		Subclinical hyperthyroidism (levothyroxine treatment)	
	Menopausal status		Menopausal status		Menopausal status		Menopausal status	
	Pre	Post	Pre	Post	Pre	Post	Pre	Post
BMD	Decreased	Decreased	No change	Decreased	Decreased	Decreased	No change	Decreased or No change
Bone turnover	Increased	Increased	No change	Variable	Insufficient data	Insufficient data	Variable	Variable

not necessarily develop osteopenia or osteoporosis. Cross-sectional studies of BMD and subclinical hyperthyroidism often fail to account for individual variation in BMD as a result of these other factors. A definitive understanding of the relationship between suppressive dose L-T4 and BMD requires longitudinal studies of greater duration.

Given the potential risk of bone loss, patients expected to continue long-term L-T4 suppressive therapy, especially patients with other risk factors for osteoporosis, require a careful evaluation of BMD and markers of bone remodeling. Postmenopausal patients and those with elevated markers of bone remodeling require long-term monitoring of BMD. If BMD declines, the dose of L-T4 should be reduced. If not possible, antiresorptive therapy should be considered. One cross-sectional study revealed that postmenopausal women taking both high dose thyroid hormone and estrogen had BMD levels similar to women taking only estrogen. In contrast, women taking high dose thyroid hormone without estrogen had lower BMD values in the spine, hip, and forearm [38]. These data suggest that estrogen protects against thyroid hormone-related bone loss. There are insufficient data to determine whether all postmenopausal women treated with suppressive doses of L-T4 should also receive estrogen or other antiresorptive agents. Measuring biochemical markers of bone remodeling may serve to identify an "at risk" population that may benefit from antiresorptive therapy, although this strategy has not been rigorously evaluated in patients with subclinical hyperthyroidism.

E. Conclusions

Women with thyrotoxicosis secondary to Graves' disease or thyroid autonomy have increased bone remodeling and decreased bone density, which is at least partially reversible with correction of thyroid function. Simultaneous treatment with bisphosphonates resulted in a more rapid normalization of BMD in one study [10]. Further studies are required to evaluate whether bisphosphonates confer additional long-term benefit beyond that achieved with normalization of thyroid function. Subclinical hyperthyroidism in postmenopausal women with toxic multinodular goiter or solitary autonomous nodules appears to be a risk factor for osteoporosis and should be evaluated and treated in the context of other osteoporosis risk factors. Premenopausal women with similar thyroid dysfunction are at lower risk, possibly because of a protective effect of estrogen. Subclinical hyperthyroidism secondary to L-T4 suppressive therapy is associated with an increase in markers of bone remodeling and a decrease in BMD in some women. Again, postmenopausal women appear to be at greater risk than premenopausal women (Table II). Longitudinal studies are required to determine if estrogen replacement therapy or other antiresorptive therapy diminishes this risk in postmenopausal women. In the interim, patients requiring thyroid hormone replacement therapy should be treated with the lowest dose of L-T4 to maintain a normal TSH level. The utility of biochemical markers of bone remodeling in identifying the subset of patients at greatest risk for L-T4 related bone loss requires further investigation.

III. OSTEOPOROSIS SECONDARY TO HYPOGONADISM

The effects of gonadal steroids on bone and mineral metabolism are relatively well known. Gonadal hormones, particularly estradiol, play a crucial role in the achievement of peak bone mass [49–51]. In addition, they are of fundamental importance in maintaining bone mass [50]. In later life, bone mass depends on both peak bone density attained at an earlier age as well as on the rate of bone loss. Therefore, hypogonadism at any time in life may increase the risk of osteoporosis and fractures.

The beneficial effects of gonadal hormones on bone at the cellular level are not completely understood. In adults, the major effect of estrogen on bone remodeling is to decrease resorption rather than to affect bone formation [52]. Estrogen receptors and postreceptor signaling in response to estrogen administration have been demonstrated in osteoblasts, osteoclasts, and bone marrow stromal cells in culture. Osteoblasts and stromal cells produce cytokines, such as interleukin-1, interleukin-6, tumor necrosis factor, and macrophage-colony stimulating factor, that regulate osteogenesis. Estrogen appears to modulate the production of osteoclastogenic cytokines and hence prevents bone resorption [53, 54]. Estrogen deficiency, on the other hand, results in increased production of bone resorbing cytokines leading to an increase in osteoclast activity and consequently greater bone resorption. In this section, we will review the consequences of hypogonadism on bone mineral density and indices of bone remodeling.

A. Turner's Syndrome

Turner's syndrome is characterized by total or partial X-chromosome monosomy, which is associated with gonadal dysgenesis and diminished or absent ovarian estrogen production [55]. Skeletal abnormalities, including short stature, cubitus valgus, delayed skeletal maturation, and osteoporosis, are commonly described in patients with Turner's syndrome [56–59]. BMD values from 19–27% below control values have been reported in patients with Turner's syndrome [57, 58, 60]. However, earlier studies are limited by less sophisticated bone densitometry technology, heterogeneity in the patient population studied, and variability in treatment regimens with respect to the timing and dose of estrogen or growth hormone therapy and use of anabolic steroids, such as oxandrolone, all of which may significantly impact BMD. Finally, an appropriate control population is difficult to identify. Girls and women with Turner's syndrome have short stature and weigh less than other females. BMD is an areal rather than a volumetric measurement, and therefore BMD is often underestimated in smaller individuals. Thus, height and weight-matched controls are preferable to age-matched controls when comparing BMD values in Turner's patients to those in a normal control population.

Although early studies failed to account for the small stature of Turner's patients, there are studies that address this issue [61, 62]. For example, Ross *et al.* [61] evaluated BMD, assessed by SPA and DPA, in 78 prepubertal girls with Turner's syndrome. Bone density of the wrist was decreased compared to a prepubertal control group matched for chronological age, but wrist BMD was similar to the control group after adjusting for height in a multiple regression analysis. BMD of the spine did not differ between girls with Turner's syndrome and the age-matched prepubertal control population.

There are only two longitudinal studies that evaluate BMD in girls with Turner's syndrome [62, 63]. Shaw *et al.* [63] measured lumbar spine BMD sequentially for two years in 18 girls with Turner's syndrome. BMD values, assessed by DEXA, were compared with two separate reference data populations, an age-matched control group and a control group matched for body weight and pubertal status. At baseline, mean standard deviation scores (SDS) were lower in the girls with Turner's syndrome compared with age-matched con-

trols. In contrast, mean SDS scores in Turner's girls were normal when compared with the reference population matched for weight and pubertal status. Subsequently, fourteen girls had BMD evaluations 2.5 years later. Only 11% of the 11- to 13-year-old girls had normal increments in BMD for age, whereas 63% of the 5- to 11-year-old girls had normal age-related increases in BMD. One possible hypothesis to account for the observation that bone accretion slowed as the girls reached pubertal age is that the dose, type, or pattern of exogenous estrogen replacement therapy, traditionally initiated at age 12 years, may not mimic normal puberty sufficiently to allow girls with Turner's syndrome to achieve optimal peak bone density. In this study, there was no correlation between growth hormone or estrogen dose and increments in BMD. However, all girls received similar doses of ethinyl estradiol. An estrogen regimen that more closely replicates normal physiology may enable girls with Turner's syndrome to achieve appropriate age-related increases in BMD.

In contrast to prepubertal girls, adults with Turner's syndrome have consistently demonstrated low BMD compared both with age-matched controls [64, 65] and with controls matched for height [57]. Davies *et al.* [57] evaluated lumbar spine BMD in 40 women with Turner's syndrome. Mean vertebral BMD, assessed by DEXA, was more than two standard deviations below the age-matched control population. Furthermore, when vertebral BMD was controlled for height and weight, it remained similarly low compared to the normal population. There was no relationship between duration of estrogen use and vertebral BMD in women with Turner's syndrome. Taken together, these data suggest that prepubertal girls with Turner's syndrome have similar lumbar spine and wrist BMD values compared with age-matched girls when BMD values are adjusted for height and weight. In contrast, women with Turner's syndrome have lower BMD than age-matched controls, regardless of correction for height and weight.

Osteopenia in adult women with Turner's syndrome appears to be related primarily to estrogen deficiency during the critical period of bone acquisition in the teenage years [57, 65, 66]. In cross-sectional studies, adult women with Turner's syndrome on estrogen replacement therapy invariably have higher BMD values than untreated patients [58, 64–66]. In addition, girls who begin estrogen therapy before 11 years of age have been shown to have better radial bone mineral content than girls started on therapy after 12 years of age [59]. Furthermore, BMC of spine and forearm have been demonstrated to correlate positively with duration of estrogen treatment [67]. The results of small longitudinal studies evaluating the effects of estrogen therapy on radial BMC [58, 59], radial BMD [68], or vertebral BMD [69] suggest that BMC or BMD may increase slightly [59, 69] or remain unchanged [58, 68] with estrogen therapy. BMD does not typically reach a normal range for age and height, even with estrogen replacement therapy [59, 68].

Because BMD does not completely normalize with estrogen treatment, some authors have hypothesized that an intrinsic bone defect related to the chromosomal abnormality, rather than estrogen deficiency, may contribute to bone loss in patients with Turner's syndrome [58, 59]. However, it is unlikely that a primary defect in bone structure contributes to low bone mass in this syndrome [57]. First, patients with Turner's syndrome have been shown to have similar BMD values when compared to patients with pure gonadal dysgenesis who have estrogen deficiency but normal karyotypes, suggesting that the chromosomal abnormality *per se* does not result in an intrinsic structural defect [65]. Secondly, a difference in BMD between Turner's patients with mosaicism or a 45,X karyotype has not been reported [57, 59, 67]. Finally, prepubertal girls appear to have BMD values similar to those of control populations when matched for height [63]. An intrinsic structural defect would result in lower BMD values in prepubertal children, but the decrease in BMD does not become apparent until after puberty. Therefore, it appears that low bone density in patients with Turner's syndrome results from a failure to achieve an optimal peak bone density secondary to estrogen deficiency. In addition, untreated adults with Turner's syndrome have continued bone loss. The observation that Turner's patients who experience spontaneous vaginal bleeding have higher BMD values than typical Turner's patients who require estrogen treatment to induce puberty [57, 68] supports the premise the endogenous estrogen production allows for normal bone acquisition, but that the current method of replacing estrogen may not.

Bone histomorphometric studies support the hypothesis that increased bone resorption secondary to estrogen deficiency is the primary cause of osteopenia in Turner's patients. In 1974, Brown *et al.* [70], described bone morphology in eight girls (9–19 years of age) with Turner's syndrome. None were treated with estrogen, despite the fact that many were past the normal age of puberty. The predominant histomorphometric feature was an increase in the percentage of bone surface undergoing resorption, with evidence of normal bone formation.

Reports of biochemical markers of bone remodeling in Turner's syndrome are conflicting. Saggese *et al.* [71] reported normal total alkaline phosphatase levels in 14 untreated females with Turner's syndrome, aged 4.2–21.0 years. However, elevated total [64, 70] and bone-specific alkaline phosphatase [65] were reported in 5 of 8 untreated adolescent girls [70] and in estrogen-treated adults with Turner's syndrome [64, 65]. In contrast, osteocalcin levels have been elevated in untreated adults with Turner's syndrome, but not in estrogen-treated women [64, 65, 72]. In addition, Saggese *et al.* [71] have reported that serum osteocalcin concentrations increase after $1,25(OH)_2$ D administration in untreated patients (4.2–21.0 years of age), demonstrating that osteoblasts respond normally to physiologic stimulus in patients with Turner's syndrome.

Markers of bone resorption in patients with Turner's syndrome vary with age and estrogen therapy. Urinary hydroxyproline levels have been normal in prepubertal girls with Turner's syndrome compared with controls matched for chronologic age [74] or bone age [75]. However, urinary hydroxyproline levels were elevated in girls older than 14 years and in women who were not receiving estrogen therapy, compared with age-matched controls [65, 74]. Stepan *et al.* [65] also reported increased urinary hydroxyproline levels in estrogen treated adults with Turner's syndrome. However, the values were lower than in the untreated group. Interestingly, urinary pyridinium cross-links level, a more specific marker of bone resorption, has been demonstrated to be mildly elevated in prepubertal girls (4.6–14.8 years) with Turner's syndrome compared with controls matched for bone age, suggesting that bone resorption may be increased even in some young girls with Turner's syndrome [75]. However, whether rising pyridinium cross-links values in the oldest girls, who were entering puberty and not receiving estrogen therapy, accounted for the mild elevation was not addressed in the study. Taken together, these data suggest that markers of bone remodeling in Turner's patients increase around the time of puberty, supporting the histomorphometric finding of increased bone resorption surfaces. Markers remain elevated in patients who are not treated with estrogen. However, because estrogen therapy does not consistently normalize markers, estrogen replacement alone may not be sufficient to reduce remodeling rates, at least in currently prescribed doses. Alternatively, other mechanisms of bone loss may be involved.

Abnormal growth hormone (GH) secretory dynamics may also contribute to low bone mass in patients with Turner's syndrome [76–78]. Although abnormal patterns of GH secretion have been observed in this syndrome, most patients are not GH deficient, as classically defined by provocative testing [76]. Serum levels of IGF-1, as well as IGF binding protein-3 (IGFBP3), have been reported to be normal in this syndrome. However, *in vitro* studies have shown that despite normal IGF-1 plasma levels, the autocrine/paracrine actions of this growth factor are reduced [77]. Many therapeutic trials of supraphysiologic doses of recombinant human growth hormone have shown an increase in height velocity in girls with Turner's syndrome [79]. Further studies are required to elucidate the relationship between low bone mass, growth factors, and cytokines in Turner's syndrome.

B. Athletes with Amenorrhea

The relationship between exercise and BMD is complex and incompletely understood. In general, exercise is associated with increased BMD. In women, however, the beneficial effect of physical activity on bone mineral density can be lost if the amount of exercise is so intensive that it is associated with menstrual disturbances. The prevalence of amenorrhea among runners ranges from 25–50%. In contrast, only 12% of swimmers and cyclists have amenorrhea [80, 81]. Young girls who begin intensive athletic training before menarche often demonstrate delayed puberty, which may also be associated with lower bone mass [82].

The pathogenesis of exercise-induced amenorrhea is unclear. Risk factors include a prior history of menstrual irregularity, weight loss, and a low caloric intake. The absence of regular menses in exercising women is related to a disruption of the pulsatile release of gonadotropin releasing hormone from the hypothalamus, resulting in low levels of gonadotropins and secondary reduction of estrogen and progesterone secretion [83].

Women who have missed 50% of their expected menstrual periods by 20 years of age are likely to have reduced bone mineral density as compared to normal controls. The most severe reductions in bone mass have been documented in the lumbar spine [83–86]. However, BMD is also lower at the femoral neck, trochanter, Ward's triangle, and tibia (Fig. 4) [87]. In contrast, bone mineral density of the radius is generally normal [83–86]. Therefore, as in postmenopausal women, cancellous bone appears to be more severely affected by exercise-induced hypoestrogenism than cortical bone [88].

The effect of exercise on the growing skeleton also depends on the type of physical activity, the region of the skeleton involved [89], body weight, and dietary calcium intake. For example, gymnasts have been noted to have higher bone mineral density at the femoral neck than runners, despite similar past and current menstrual cycle patterns [90]. Similarly, Slemenda and Johnston [90a] demonstrated that ice skaters with oligoamenorrhea and amenorrhea had only a minimal (2%) decrease in bone mineral density compared to controls. Such data suggest that the mechanical forces associated with impact loading and muscular contraction during gymnastics and skating training have powerful osteogenic effects, which may counteract the deleterious effects of estrogen deficiency on the skeleton. Therefore, the type of exercise is an important factor in predicting bone loss in this young population.

The effect of physical activity on serum concentrations of calcitropic hormones and biochemical markers of bone remodeling has not been extensively studied. In rodents, exercise training promotes a positive calcium and phosphorus balance, increased serum concentrations of $1,25(OH)_2$ D, increased intestinal absorption of calcium, and an increase in bone mass [91]. Grimston *et al.* [92] evaluated the effects of 45 minutes of submaximal running on calcitropic hormone concentrations in trained female long distance runners with normal or low BMD, compared with a control group of sedentary women with normal bone mineral density. In all groups, serum calcium levels rose, with a larger increment occurring after the oral calcium load. In the runners with normal BMD, the rise in serum calcium was accompanied by a decrease in PTH and an increase in calcitonin. In the runners with low BMD, there was a significant increase in PTH and a decrease in calcitonin levels, despite the significant increase in serum calcium. The rise in PTH and fall in calcitonin levels observed in exercising women with low bone mass may result in an increased rate of bone turnover and, in turn, decreased bone density. Serum osteocalcin levels were higher in the osteopenic runners and were also inversely correlated with BMD.

Few other studies have evaluated markers of bone turnover in exercising women. In one study of amenorrheic dancers, serum osteocalcin levels were elevated and inversely related to age, Tanner stage, bone density, and weight [93]. Osteocalcin declined with return of menses but not with estrogen therapy, suggesting that either exogenous therapy was inadequate or that factors other than estrogen deficiency are operative in the increased bone turnover in this group.

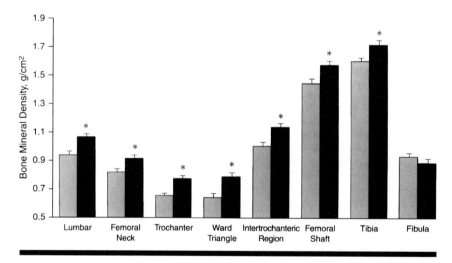

FIGURE 4   Bone mineral density of amenorrheic (gray bars) and eumenorrheic (black bars) athletes (*p < 0.01). Reprinted from Rencken *et al. JAMA* **276**, 239 [87]. Copyright 1996, American Medical Association, with permission.

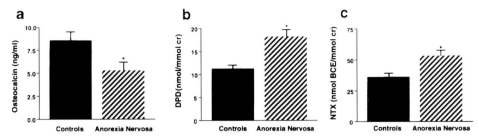

FIGURE 5   Comparison of baseline bone turnover in women with anorexia nervosa (n = 22) and normal controls. (A) osteocalcin (*p < 0.001); (B) deoxypyridinoline (*p < 0.001); (C) N-telopeptide (*p < 0.01). From Grinspoon *et al.* [108]. Effect of short-term recombinant human insulin-like growth factor-1 administration on bone turnover in osteopenic women with anorexia nervosa. *J. Clin. Endocrinol. Metab.* **81(11)**, 3864–3870, 1996, © The Endocrine Society, with permission.

In summary, exercise-induced amenorrhea is a risk factor for osteoporosis. Although estrogen deficiency is an important cause of the bone loss, there may be other mechanisms for bone loss in these women which require further study.

C. Eating Disorders

Anorexia nervosa (AN) and bulimia affect 5–10% of women. The onset may be during early or late adolescence or in the third and fourth decades of life. These eating disorders are often chronic and resistant to treatment, resulting in significant morbidity and even mortality.

Osteopenia and osteoporosis have been described in association with anorexia nervosa [94–103]. While the etiology of osteoporosis in AN remains unclear, several metabolic consequences of AN may adversely affect skeletal mass. These include estrogen deficiency, secondary hyperparathyroidism due to low dietary calcium or vitamin D deficiency, endogenous cortisol excess, reduced IGF-1 levels, and protein-energy malnutrition. Osteopenia has been reported in both cancellous [95–100] and cortical [94, 97, 101, 102] bone. However, cancellous bone loss is more frequent and more severe. Fifty percent of anorectic patients have bone density values of the lumbar spine that are more than two SD below those of age-matched normal controls [98, 100].

Histomorphometric studies in patients with anorexia report conflicting results [104, 105]. Kaplan *et al.* [104] reported a markedly reduced rate of bone formation and a concomitant increase in parameters of bone resorption in one patient with anorexia. In general, the level of bone remodeling activity was reduced, suggesting inactive or low turnover osteoporosis. In contrast, Joyce *et al.* [105] reported a high turnover pattern in two anorectic women and three patients with other types of eating disorders.

Data on markers of bone remodeling in anorectic women are similarly conflicting. For example, total alkaline phosphatase activity was reported to be elevated in women with eating disorders [106]. However, other liver enzymes were also elevated, suggesting hepatic dysfunction as the etiology of the elevated alkaline phosphatase levels. Moreover, the majority of studies have not demonstrated any elevation in this enzyme [94, 96, 99, 101, 102]. Osteocalcin, a more specific marker of osteoblast function, has been noted to be very low in some studies of women with AN [107, 108] (Fig. 5). Furthermore, a significant correlation between serum osteocalcin and body mass index has been demonstrated, suggesting a link between nutritional status and decreased rates of bone formation [108]. In contrast, other reports have shown normal [99, 102] or elevated [109] levels of osteocalcin.

With respect to markers of bone resorption, urinary hydroxyproline was normal in one study of anorectic patients [99]. However, measurements of more specific markers of bone resorption, such as deoxypyridinoline and N-telopeptide excretion, have revealed increased levels, which were inversely correlated with bone mineral density (Fig. 5) [108]. Moreover, in this study, serum osteocalcin was very low, thus supporting the hypothesis that uncoupling of bone remodeling with decreased bone formation and increased resorption contributes to bone loss in some young women with anorexia.

Other factors may also contribute to metabolic bone disease in patients with anorexia. Serum vitamin D concentrations are highly variable in patients with eating disorders. Serum levels can be affected by reduced dietary intake and diminished hepatic synthesis or binding capacity of vitamin D binding protein in patients with estrogen deficiency. Total 25-hydroxyvitamin D levels are normal in the majority of AN patients [99, 101, 104, 109], but not in all [106].

Elevated serum and urinary cortisol levels are common in women with AN [98, 99, 110, 111]. In a group of 53 women with eating disorders, hypercortisolism was present in 55% of the anorectic patients but in just 6% of the bulimic women [99]. Hypercortisolism results both from increased production and from decreased clearance of cortisol, secondary to enhanced activity of the hypothalamic–pituitary–adrenal axis. High cortisol levels may contribute to the severe bone loss seen in patients with AN. In this regard, Biller *et al.* [98] reported elevated urinary cortisol levels in 26 amenorrheic women with AN compared with the control group.

Moreover, urinary cortisol levels correlated inversely with vertebral bone density, supporting the hypothesis that endogenous hypercortisolism is important in the development of osteopenia in women with AN.

In addition to hypercortisolism, elevated GH and suppressed IGF-1 levels have been described in patients with AN. It has been hypothesized that prolonged nutritional deprivation in AN induces downregulation of the GH receptor or its postreceptor processing, resulting in reduced production of IGF-1 and elevated GH levels. IGF-1 is a nutritionally-dependent bone factor that stimulates collagen formation by osteoblasts. Therefore, deficiency of IGF-1 may contribute to decreased bone formation and bone loss in women with AN. Counts et al. [112] evaluated the GH-IGF-1 axis in ten women with anorexia nervosa. Serum levels of GH, IGFBP1, and IGFBP2 were increased, whereas those of IGF-1, IGFBP3, and growth hormone binding protein (GHBP) were decreased. All the alterations were reversible with refeeding. Furthermore, Klibanski et al. [100] have demonstrated that IGF-1 levels were predictive of the change in vertebral bone mass in untreated patients with AN. In addition, Grinspoon et al. [108] evaluated the effects of short term recombinant IGF-1 (rhIGF-1) administration on bone turnover in ten women with AN. Markers of bone remodeling were stimulated in a dose dependent manner. The highest dose of rhIGF-1 stimulated markers of both bone formation (osteocalcin, PICP) and resorption (DPD), whereas the lower dose stimulated only a single marker of bone formation (PICP). These data support the hypothesis that low bone mass in AN is related, at least in part, to disturbances in the GH-IGF-1 axis. Further studies evaluating the long term effect of rhIGF-1 on bone density in women with anorexia are required.

In summary, bone loss associated with anorexia nervosa is multifactorial in etiology and may be related to estrogen deficiency, vitamin D deficiency, cortisol excess, reduced IGF-1 levels, and malnutrition. Biochemical markers of bone resorption are usually elevated. Markers of bone formation may be elevated or depressed and may vary with the severity or duration of the disease. It is unclear whether markers of bone remodeling will be useful in identifying patients who are most at risk for osteoporosis and future fracture.

D. Hyperprolactinemia

Hyperprolactinemia commonly occurs secondary to pituitary or hypothalamic diseases, as well as in some physiological conditions such as pregnancy and lactation. High levels of prolactin inhibit gonadotropin releasing hormone (GnRH) and consequently cause hypogonadotropic hypogonadism. As many as 25–30% of premenopausal women with amenorrhea have hyperprolactinemia [113]. Decreased bone mass has been reported in patients with hyperprolactinemia [114–118]. Cross-sectional studies have demonstrated BMD

values 4–23% lower at appendicular sites [118, 121, 119] and 8–23% lower at axial sites [119–121] in patients with hyperprolactinemia, compared with age-matched controls.

The importance of hypogonadism in the pathogenesis of bone loss in these patients has been well documented [115, 119–122]. Ciccarelli et al. [116] demonstrated that there was a positive correlation between BMC and estrogen levels in a group of women with hyperprolactinemia. Furthermore, Kayath et al. [115] reported that men and women with a history of prolactinoma and hypogonadism for more than ten years had lower BMD values than patients who were more recently diagnosed. Similarly, Biller et al. [118] reported lower BMD in hyperprolactinemic women with amenorrhea than in those with hyperprolactinemia and oligoamenorrhea or normal menses. These findings suggest that the severity of bone loss in patients with hyperprolactinemia is related to the presence and duration of hypogonadism, emphasizing the significant role of estrogen deficiency in the pathogenesis of osteoporosis associated with this condition.

Few studies have addressed the reversibility of osteopenia in hyperprolactinemic amenorrheic patients [118, 122a]. In Biller's study [118], vertebral BMD, assessed by computerized tomography, declined progressively in untreated hyperprolactinemic amenorrheic women followed for a mean of 1.7 years. In contrast, 56% of treated patients, who had resumption of menstrual function, had improvement in BMD. The authors concluded that menstrual function is the most important predictor of progressive bone loss in hyperprolactinemic women. However, 44% of women did not have an increase in BMD, despite restoration of their menstrual function, suggesting that other factors may play a role in the bone loss seen in these women.

One such factor may be PTH related peptide (PTHrP), a potent stimulator of bone resorption. A significant elevation in serum levels of PTHrP has been reported in patients with hyperprolactinemia [123, 124]. Kovacs and Chik [124] evaluated 33 lactating women and 16 patients with prolactin-secreting pituitary adenomas. Both groups had higher levels of PTHrP than sex- and age-matched controls. Repeat measurements in four patients after therapy with either bromocriptine, surgery, or octreotide revealed a decrease in PTHrP levels. Furthermore Stiegler et al. [125] reported lower vertebral BMD Z scores in hyperprolactinemic patients with high PTHrP levels compared with hyperprolactinemic patients with normal levels. There was a significant negative correlation between PTHrP and BMD Z scores. In addition, patients with higher PTHrP levels had significantly higher mean serum calcium, total alkaline phosphatase, and osteocalcin levels and lower mean serum phosphorous levels. Urinary calcium and phosphorus excretion were also higher in the group with the high PTHrP levels. Therefore, PTHrP may play a role in bone loss associated with hyperprolactinemia.

Few studies have evaluated biochemical markers of bone remodeling in patients with hyperprolactinemia. In Ciccarelli's study [116], there was no difference in urinary hydroxyproline levels between the hyperprolactinemic women with or without amenorrhea. Similarly, total alkaline phosphatase levels have been reported to be normal in several studies [115, 117, 118, 120]. However, measurements of more specific markers of bone remodeling, such as osteocalcin and N-telopeptide, have revealed important changes. For example, Sartorio et al. [126] reported low osteocalcin levels in 29 hyperprolactinemic women with prolactinomas compared with age-matched controls. After 12 months of therapy with dopamine agonists, osteocalcin levels significantly increased and prolactin levels decreased. Similarly, Di Somma et al. [117] reported low osteocalcin levels in 20 men with pituitary adenoma, compared with controls matched for age and BMI. In contrast, urinary N-telopeptide levels were increased. BMD of the lumbar spine correlated positively with serum osteocalcin and inversely with urinary N-telopeptide excretion. Furthermore, a significant inverse correlation was observed between serum prolactin and osteocalcin levels. After 18 months of treatment with dopamine agonists, osteocalcin levels significantly increased and N-telopeptide levels decreased [117]. Taken together, these findings suggest that an uncoupling of bone remodeling, with an increase in bone resorption and a decrease in bone formation, occurs in patients with hyperprolactinemia. Further studies are needed to confirm these findings.

E. Conclusions

In conclusion, patients with hypogonadism from any cause are at risk for developing osteoporosis. The decrease in bone mass is primarily due to deficiency of gonadal steroids. However, disturbances in nutrition and other hormonal factors, such as IGF-1, PTHrP, and cortisol, may also contribute. The utility of biochemical indices of bone remodeling in the evaluation and treatment of patients with osteoporosis secondary to hypogonadism remains unclear. Further evaluation within each patient subgroup, particularly longitudinal studies, are required to determine whether markers of bone turnover predict rates of bone loss and fracture in affected individuals.

IV. ANTICONVULSANT DRUGS AND OSTEOPOROSIS

Metabolic bone disease may complicate the management of patients receiving several of the commonly used anticonvulsant drugs [127–131]. Diphenylhydantoin, phenobarbital, carbamazepine, and sodium valproate have all been implicated in anticonvulsant bone disease. Anticonvulsant bone disease occurs more frequently with long-term, high-dose, multi-drug regimens (Table III). Anticonvulsant-induced bone disease [127, 128] may present as overt osteomalacia or rickets, with fractures, proximal muscle weakness, frank

TABLE III.   Anticonvulsant Bone Disease Risk Factors

Long-term therapy
High-dose therapy
Multiple drug regimens
Reduced physical activity levels
Low vitamin D intake
Chronic illness
Elderly or institutionalized patients
Limited sun exposure
Concomitant therapy with drugs that induce hepatic enzymes

hypocalcemia, and hypophosphatemia. However, in the more common modern presentation [130, 131], patients may present with an asymptomatic decrease in bone mineral density [132–135].

The majority of anticonvulsant drugs are thought to affect bone and mineral metabolism indirectly by causing abnormal metabolism of vitamin D. Diphenylhydantoin, phenobarbital, and carbamazepine stimulate hepatic mixed function oxidase activity [131, 136] and therapy with these drugs is associated with increased degradation of steroid hormones. In contrast, another antiepileptic agent, sodium valproate, is not thought to affect vitamin D metabolism directly [137]. However, this drug has been reported to cause renal toxicity, which could indirectly affect bone and mineral metabolism [138].

The data on serum 25-hydroxyvitamin (25-OHD) levels in patients on anticonvulsant drugs are conflicting. Hahn et al. [135] have clearly demonstrated increases in both the disappearance of vitamin D and 25-OHD from the circulation and the appearance of inactive polar metabolites of vitamin D in the bile and urine during chronic administration of anticonvulsant drugs. In several studies conducted in the United States, serum levels of 25-OHD were decreased in patients with longstanding epilepsy [136, 139, 140]. Similarly, a Finnish study found serum levels of 25-OHD to be lower in patients on various combinations of diphenylhydantoin, phenobarbital, and carbamazepine [141]. However, two other studies found serum 25-OHD levels in patients on diphenylhydantoin to be no different from normal controls [142, 143]. These discrepancies may be attributed to geographic differences in the study populations, because the studies in which low 25-OHD levels were found were conducted in more northern latitudes where there is less sunlight exposure [131, 141]. Thus, lack of vitamin D may be particularly likely to cause anticonvulsant bone disease in patients who are from northern climates or are institutionalized, where access to ultraviolet light may be diminished [130].

In addition to the actions of anticonvulsant drugs on hepatic vitamin D metabolism, direct effects on cellular metabolism have been described. Diphenylhydantoin, which interferes with cation transport in many tissues, directly inhibits intestinal calcium transport [144], and together with phenobarbital, has been shown to inhibit vitamin D-mediated calcium absorption [145]. Furthermore, Hahn and Halstead [132] demonstrated that higher levels of vitamin D metabolites are required to maintain normal intestinal calcium absorption in patients taking anticonvulsant drugs. In addition, both phenobarbital and diphenylhydantoin inhibit parathyroid hormone-mediated bone resorption *in vitro*, which could cause secondary increases in circulating parathyroid hormone levels [146, 147]. Diphenylhydantoin, which appears to exert this effect by inhibition of hormone-sensitive adenylate cyclase activity, is the more potent of the two drugs. Other actions of diphenylhydantoin on the skeleton include direct inhibition of collagen synthesis and lysozomal enzyme release by bone explants [148].

Two excellent histomorphometric studies by Mosekilde and Melsen [149] and Weinstein *et al.* [143] and have contributed in a major way to our current understanding of the skeletal effects of anticonvulsant drugs. Mosekilde and Melsen [149] evaluated a group of 20 adults all treated with diphenylhydantoin for at least ten years, some of whom were also taking other anticonvulsant drugs. Compared to a group of normal controls, these patients had significantly reduced serum and urinary calcium levels and elevated serum total alkaline phosphatase activity. Analysis of transiliac crest bone biopsies revealed normal cancellous bone volume and increases in osteoid volume, active osteoid surface, mineralizing surface, and resorption surface. Although osteoid seams were slightly thicker than those in a control population, the mineral apposition rate was normal. Weinstein *et al.* [143] evaluated bone biopsies in 20 of 120 epileptic patients who had taken anticonvulsants for 18 years. The biopsied patients had decreased serum ionized calcium, increased parathyroid hormone levels, and low cortical bone mineral density. Although cancellous bone volume was normal, cortical bone was thin and porous. Osteoid volume and surface were increased, osteoid width was normal, and the mineralization rate was normal or increased. Their findings were essentially in agreement with those of Mosekilde and Melsen [149], thus establishing anticonvulsant bone disease as a disorder of high remodeling rather than abnormal mineralization.

Although the hypothesis that low 25-OHD levels could result in decreased intestinal calcium absorption, secondary hyperparathyroidism, and increased bone remodeling activity is consistent with the observed histomorphometric alterations [143, 149], routine serum measurements of indices of bone and mineral metabolism are frequently unremarkable in patients on anticonvulsant drugs. Biochemical evaluation may reveal normal or minimally depressed serum calcium and phosphate levels, and serum total alkaline phosphatase activity may be normal or only slightly elevated. However, the more sensitive biochemical techniques now available may reveal abnormalities in many patients in whom routine as-

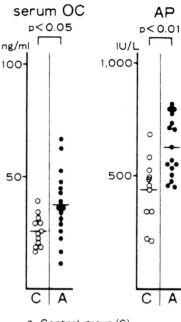

FIGURE 6   Serum levels of osteocalcin (OC) and alkaline phosphatase (AP) in subjects treated with anticonvulsant drugs (closed circles) and in control subjects (open circles). Reprinted from Takeshita *et al.* [150], with permission.

says show normal levels [130, 131]. Serum 25-OHD levels are frequently reduced in anticonvulsant-treated patients and there may be mild elevations of parathyroid hormone [132, 141, 143]. Serum, 1,25-dihydroxyvitamin D levels may be normal, high, or low. Markers of bone formation such as osteocalcin [141, 150, 151], serum total [150, 152] and bone-specific alkaline phosphatase [141, 151], and procollagen carboxy-terminal peptide [141, 151] have been reported to be elevated in children and adults taking anticonvulsant drugs (Fig. 6). With respect to markers of resorption, Ohishi *et al.* [153] documented that urinary hydroxyproline, pyridinoline, and deoxypyridinoline excretion were increased in 15 premenopausal women taking anticonvulsant drugs compared with 211 healthy age- and sex-matched controls. Elevated urinary excretion of hydroxyproline [150, 152] and cross-linked carboxy-terminal peptide of type I collagen [141] have also been reported in patients on antiepileptic drugs. Thus, the available data suggest that biochemical markers of bone turnover are elevated in patients on anticonvulsant drugs; this finding is consistent with the histomorphometric studies that have established this disorder as a state of increased bone remodeling [143, 149].

Data on bone mineral density in children and adults taking anticonvulsant drugs are also conflicting. In a cross-sectional study of 226 free-living patients with epilepsy, radial bone mass was significantly reduced and, in 18% of the patients, was more than two SD below young normal controls [154]. Similarly, Hahn *et al.* [135] found radial BMD to be 10% below normal in 22 children on anticonvulsant drugs. In contrast, Valimaki *et al.* [141] measured spine and hip bone density in 38 men and women between the ages of 20 and 49 who were taking diphenylhydantoin, carbamazepine, or both. BMD was abnormal only in women and only at the hip site. Sheth and colleagues [155] evaluated both axial and appendicular bone mass by DEXA in 26 children who had been taking sodium valproate or carbamezepine for more than 18 months. While BMD was normal in patients on carbamazepine, those receiving sodium valproate had reduced BMD at both the lumbar spine and the radius. Thus, although bone turnover is frequently elevated in patients on anticonvulsant drugs, bone mass is not necessarily reduced.

Risk factors for the development of anticonvulsant bone disease include high dose, multiple drug regimens, long duration of therapy, institutionalization, vitamin D deficiency either due to inadequate dietary intake or reduced sunlight exposure, physical inactivity, use of ketogenic diets or acetazolamide to induce chronic metabolic acidosis, and concomitant therapy with other drugs that induce hepatic enzymes [131]. Evidence for anticonvulsant bone disease should be sought in individuals with a history of chronic long-term therapy and one or more of the risk factors discussed above. A routine biochemical evaluation may reveal hypocalcemia, hypophosphatemia, and increased alkaline phosphatase activity. More specialized testing may reveal reduced urinary calcium excretion and serum 25-OHD levels as well as mild elevations of intact parathyroid hormone. Both serum osteocalcin concentrations and urinary pyridinium cross-link excretion may be increased. However, any or all of these biochemical parameters may be normal, and decreased bone mineral density may be the only manifestation. Alternatively, bone density may be normal in the face of clear-cut biochemical abnormalities. In difficult cases, bone biopsy may be helpful in establishing the diagnosis.

Management of patients on chronic anticonvulsant drug therapy should include routine prophylaxis with a daily vitamin supplement that contains at least 400 IU of vitamin D. This is particularly important in the case of elderly or institutionalized patients. Barden *et al.* [156] have demonstrated that this approach will prevent bone loss in institutionalized adults. The amount of vitamin D required to correct low 25-OHD levels both in institutionalized and in noninstitutionalized patients on anticonvulsant drugs may vary from 400 to 4000 IU daily for 12 to 15 months [157]. The common side effects of vitamin D therapy, hypercalciuria and hypercalcemia, are unlikely to occur at the relatively small doses (usually <2000 IU) that have been shown to be effective. Treatment of established anticonvulsant bone disease by therapy with 2000–4000 IU of vitamin D daily has been demonstrated to result in improved calcium absorption, decreases in parathyroid hormone and urinary hydroxyproline excretion, and increases in bone mineral content [156]. All of these approaches should prove relatively cost-effective, particularly when contrasted with medical costs associated with fractures.

References

1. Allain, T. J., and McGregor, A. M. (1993). Thyroid hormones and bone. *J. Endocrinol.* **139**, 9–18.
2. Mosekilde, L., Flemming, M., Bagger, J. P., Myhre-Jensen, O., and Sorensen, N. S. (1976). Bone changes in hyperthyroidism: Interrelationships between bone morphometry, thyroid function and calcium-phosphorous metabolism. *Acta Endocrinol.* **85**, 515–525.
3. Mosekilde, L., Eriksen, E. F., and Charles, P. (1990). Effects of thyroid hormones on bone and mineral metabolism. *Endocrinol. Metab. Clin. North Am.* **19**, 35–63.
4. Eriksen, E. F., Mosekilde, L., and Melsen, F. (1985). Trabecular bone remodeling and bone balance in hyperparathyroidism. *Bone* **6**, 421–428.
5. Bisbocci, D., Gallo, V., Damiano, P., Sidoli, L., Cantoni, R., Aimo, G., Priolo, G., Pagni, R., and Chiandussi, L. (1996). Spontaneous release of interleukin 1b from human blood monocytes in thyrotoxic osteodystrophy. *J. Endocrinol. Invest.* **16**, 511–515.
6. Lakatos, P., Foldes, J., Horvath, C., Kiss, L., Tatrai, A., Takacs, I., Tarjan, G., and Stern, P. H. (1997). Serum interleukin-6 and bone metabolism in patients with thyroid function disorders. *J. Clin. Endocrinol. Metab.* **82**, 78–81.
7. Linde, J., and Friis, T. (1979). Osteoporosis in hyperthyroidism estimated by photon absorptiometry. *Acta Endocrinol.* **91**, 437–448.
8. Krolner, B., Jorgensen, J. V., and Nielsen, S. P. (1983). Spinal bone mineral content in myxoedema and thyrotoxicosis: Effects of thyroid hormones and antithyroid treatment. *Clin. Endocrinol.* **18**, 439–446.
9. Diamond, T., Vine, J., Smart, R., and Butler, P. (1994). Thyrotoxic bone disease in women: A potentially reversible disorder. *Ann. Intern. Med.* **120**, 8–11.
10. Lupoli, G., Nuzzo, V., Di Carlo, C., Affinito, P., Vollery, M., Vitale, G., Cascone, E., Arlotta, F., and Nappi, C. (1996). Effects of alendronate on bone loss in pre- and postmenopausal hyperthyroid women treated with methimazole. *Gynecol. Endocrinol.* **10**, 343–348.
11. Jodar, E., Munoz-Torres, M., Escobar-Jimenez, F., Quesada, M., Luna, J. D., and Olea, N. (1997). Antiresorptive therapy in hyperthyroid patients: Longitudinal changes in bone and mineral metabolism. *J. Clin. Endocrinol. Metab.* **82**, 1989–1994.
12. Rosen, C. J., and Adler, R. A. (1992). Longitudinal changes in lumbar bone density among thyrotoxic patients after attainment of euthyroidism. *J. Clin. Endocrinol. Metab.* **75**, 1531–1534.
13. Fraser, S. A., Anderson, J. B., Smith, D. A., and Wilson, G. M. (1971). Osteoporosis and fractures following thyrotoxicosis. *Lancet* **1**, 981–983.
14. Toh, S. H., Claunch, B. C., and Brown, P. H. (1985). Effect of hyperthyroidism and its treatment on bone mineral content. *Arch. Intern. Med.* **145**, 883–886.
15. Lee, M. S., Kim, S. Y., Lee, M. C., Cho, B. Y., Lee, H. K., Koh, C., and Min, H. K. (1990). Negative correlation between the change in bone mineral density and serum osteocalcin in patients with hyperthyroidism. *J. Clin. Endocrinol. Metab.* **70**, 766–770.
16. Legovini, P., De Menis, E., Da Rin, G., Roiter, I., Breda, F., Artuso, V., Di Virgilio, R., and Conte, N. (1994). Increased serum levels of carboxyterminal propeptide of type I collagen (PICP) in hyperthyroidism. *Horm. Metab. Res.* **26**, 334–337.
17. MacLeod, J. M., McHardy, K. C., Harvey, R. D., Duncan, A., Reid,

I. W., Bewsher, P. D., and Robins, S. P. (1993). The early effects of radioiodine therapy for hyperthyroidism on biochemical indices of bone turnover. *Clin. Endocrinol.* **38**, 49–53.

18. Ohishi, T., Kushida, K., Takahashi, M., Kawana, K., Yagi, K., Kawakami, K., Horiuchi, K., and Inoue, T. (1994). Urinary bone resorption markers in patients with metabolic bone disorders. *Bone* **15**, 15–20.

19. Garnero, P., Vassy, V., Bertholin, A., Riou, J. P., and Delmas, P. D. (1994). Markers of bone turnover in hyperthyroidism and the effects of treatment. *J. Clin. Endocrinol. Metab.* **78**, 955–959.

20. Garnero, P., Gineyts, E., Riou, J. P., and Delmas, P. D. (1994). Assessment of bone resorption with a new marker of collagen degradation in patients with metabolic bone disease. *J. Clin. Endocrinol. Metab.* **79**, 780–785.

21. Garrel, D. R., Delmas, P. D., Malaval, L., and Tourniaire, J. (1986). Serum bone Gla protein: A marker of bone turnover hyperthyroidism. *J. Clin. Endocrinol. Metab.* **62**, 1052–1055.

22. Auwerx, J., and Bouillon, R. (1986). Mineral and bone metabolism in thyroid disease: A review. *Q. J. Med.* **60**, 737–752.

23. Franklyn, J., Betteridge, J., Holder, R., Daykin, J., Lilley, J., and Sheppard, M. (1994). Bone mineral density in thyroxine treated female with or without a previous history of thyrotoxicosis. *Clin. Endocrinol.* **41**, 425–432.

24. Adlin, E. V., Maurer, A. H., Marks, A. D., and Channick, B. J. (1991). Bone mineral density in postmenopausal women treated with L-thyroxine. *Am. J. Med.* **90**, 360–366.

25. Greenspan, S. L., Greenspan, F. S., Resnick, N. M., Block, J. E., Friedlander, A. L., and Genant, H. K. (1991). Skeletal integrity in premenopausal and postmenopausal women receiving long-term L-thyroxine therapy. *Am. J. Med.* **91**, 5–14.

26. Mudde, A. H., Reijnders, F. J. S., and Kruseman, A. C. N. (1992). Peripheral bone density in women with untreated multinodular goiter. *Clin. Endocrinol.* **37**, 35–39.

27. Faber, J., Overgaard, K., and Jarlow, A. (1992). Bone mineral content in premenopausal women with nontoxic goiter and reduced serum TSH. *Proc. 66th Meet., Am. Thyroid Assoc.*, Rochester, MN, Abstr. 1.

28. Foldes, J., Tarjan, G., Szathmari, M., Varga, F., Krasznai, I., and Horvath, Cs. (1993). Bone mineral density in patients with endogenous subclincal hyperthyroidism: Is this thyroid status a risk factor for osteoporosis? *Clin. Endocrinol.* **39**, 521–527.

29. Mudde, A. H., Houben, A. J. H. M., and Kruseman, A. C. N. (1994). Bone metabolism during anti-thyroid drug treatment of endogenous subclinical hyperthyroidism. *Clin. Endocrinol.* **41**, 421–424.

30. Faber, J., Perrild, H., and Johansen, J. S. (1990). Bone Gla protein and sex-hormone-binding globulin in nontoxic goiter: Parameters for metabolic status at the tissue level. *J. Clin. Endocrinol. Metab.* **70**, 49–55.

31. Foldes, J., Lakatos, P., Zsadanyi, J., and Horvath, Cs. (1997). Decreased serum IGF-I and dehydroepiandrosterone sulphate may be risk factors for the development of reduced bone mass in postmenopausal women with endogenous subclinical hyperthyroidism. *Eur. J. Endocrinol.* **136**, 277–281.

32. Fallon, M. D., Perry, H. M., Bergfeld, M., Droke, D., Teitelbaum, S. L., and Avioli, L. V. (1983). Exogenous hyperthyroidism with osteoporosis. *Arch. Intern. Med.* **143**, 442–444.

33. Ross, D. S., Neer, R. M., Ridgway, E. C., and Daniels, G. H. (1987). Subclinical hyperthyroidism and reduced bone density as a possible result of prolonged suppression of the pituitary-thyroid axis with L-thyroxine. *Am. J. Med.* **82**, 1167–1170.

34. Paul, T. L., Kerrigan, J., Kelly, A. M., Braverman, L. E., and Baran, D. T. (1988). Long-term L-thyroxine therapy is associated with decreased hip bone density in premenopausal women. *J. Am. Med. Assoc.* **259**, 3137–3175.

35. Staff, G. M., Harris, S., Sokoll, L. J., and Dawson-Hughes, B. (1990).

36. Diamond, T., Nery, L., and Hales, I. (1990). A therapeutic dilemma: Suppressive doses of thyroxine significantly reduce bone mineral measurements in both premenopausal and postmenopausal woman with thyroid carcinoma. *J. Clin. Endocrinol. Metab.* **72**, 1184–1188.

37. Kung, A. W. C., Lorentz, T., and Tam, S. C. F. (1993). Thyroxine suppressive therapy decreases bone mineral density in post-menopausal women. *Clin. Endocrinol.* **39**, 535–540.

38. Schneider, D. L., Barrett-Connor, E. L., and Morton, D. J. (1994). Thyroid hormone use and bone mineral density in elderly women. *JAMA, J. Am. Med. Assoc.* **271**, 1245–1249.

39. Gam, A. N., Jensen, G. F., Hasselstrom, K., Olsen, M., and Nielsen, K. S. (1991). Effect of thyroxine therapy on bone metabolism in substituted hypothyroid patients with normal or suppressed levels of TSH. *J. Endocrinol. Invest.* **14**, 451–455.

40. Franklyn, J. A., Betteridge, J., Daykin, J., Holder, R., Oates, G. D., Parle, J. V., Lilley, J., Heath, D. A., and Sheppard, M. C. (1992). Long-term thyroxine treatment and bone mineral density. *Lancet* **340**, 9–13.

41. Giannini, S., Nobile, M., Sartori, L., Binotto, P., Ciuffreda, M., Gemo, G., Pelizzo, M. R., D'Angelo, A., and Crepaldi, G. (1994). Bone density and mineral metabolism in thyroidectomized patients treated with long-term L-thyroxine. *Clin. Sci.* **87**, 593–597.

42. Garton, M., Reid, I., Loveridge, N., Robins, S., Murchison, L., Beckett, G., and Reid, D. (1994). Bone mineral density and metabolism in premenopausal women taking L-thyroxine replacement therapy. *Clin. Endocrinol.* **41**, 747–755.

43. Ross, D. S., Ardisson, L. J., Nussbaum, S. R., and Meskell, M. J. (1990). Serum osteocalcin in patients taking L-thyroxine who have subclinical hyperthyroidism. *J. Clin. Endocrinol. Metab.* **72**, 507–509.

44. Faber, J., and Galloe, A. M. (1994). Changes in bone mass during prolonged subclinical hyperthyroidism due to L-thyroxine treatment: A meta-analysis. *Eur. J. Endocrinol.* **130**, 350–356.

45. Uzzan, B., Campos, J., Cucherat, M., Nony, P., Boissel, J. P., and Perret, G. Y. (1996). Effects on bone mass of long term treatment with thyroid hormones: A meta-analysis. *J. Clin. Endocrinol. Metab.* **81**, 4278–4289.

46. Harvey, R. D., McHardy, K. C., Reid, I. W., Paterson, F., Bewsher, P. D., Duncan, A., and Robins, S. P. (1991). Measurement of bone collagen degradation in hyperthyroidism and during thyroxine replacement therapy using pyridinium cross-links as specific urinary markers. *J. Clin. Endocrinol. Metab.* **72**, 1189–1194.

47. Pioli, G., Pedrazzoni, M., Palummeri, E., Sianesi, M., Del Frate, R., Vescovi, P. P., Preisco, M., Ulietti, V., Costi, D., and Passeri, M. (1992). Longitudinal study of bone loss after thyroidectomy and suppressive thyroxine therapy in premenopausal women. *Acta Endocrinol.* **126**, 238–242.

48. Guo, C. Y., Weetman, A. P., and Eastell, R. (1997). Longitudinal changes of bone mineral density and bone turnover in postmenopausal women on thyroxine. *Clin. Endocrinol.* **46**, 301–307.

49. Dhuper, S., Warren, M. P., Brooks-Gunn, J., and Fox, R. (1990). Effects of hormonal status on bone density in adolescent girls. *J. Clin. Endocrinol. Metab.* **71**, 1083–1088.

50. Holmes, S. J., and Shalet, S. M. (1996). Role of growth hormone and sex steroids in achieving and maintaining normal bone mass. *Horm. Res.* **45**, 86–93.

51. Burckardt, P., and Michel, C. (1989). The peak bone mass concept. *Clin. Rheumatol.* **8** (Suppl. 2), 16–21.

52. Turner, R. T., Riggs, B. L., and Spesberg, T. C. (1994). Skeletal effects of estrogen. *Endocr. Rev.* **15**, 275–300.

53. Ernst, M., Parkert, M. G., and Rodan, G. A. (1991). Functional estrogen receptors in osteoblastic cells demonstrated by transfection with a reporter gene containing an estrogen response element. *Mol. Endocrinol.* **5**, 1597–1606.

Accelerated bone loss in hypothyroid patients overtreated with L-thyroxine. *Ann. Intern. Med.* **113**, 265–269.

54. Horowitz, M. C. (1993). Cytokines and estrogen in bone: Anti-osteoporotic effects. *Science* **260**, 626–627.

55. Ford, C. E., Jones, K. W., Polani, P. E., de Almeida, J. C., and Briggs, J. H. (1959). A sex-chromosome anomaly in a case of gonadal dysgenesis (Turner's Syndrome). *Lancet* 711–713.

56. Beal, R. K. (1973). Orthopedic aspects of the XO (Turner's) syndrome. *Clin. Orthop. Relat. Res.* **97**, 19–30.

57. Davies, M. C., Gulekli, B., and Jacobs, H. S. (1995). Osteoporosis in Turner's syndrome and other forms of primary amenorrhoea. *Clin. Endocrinol.* **43**, 741–746.

58. Shore, R. M., Chesney, R. W., Mazess, R. B., Rose, P. B., and Bargman, G. J. (1982). Skeletal demineralization in Turner's syndrome. *Calcif. Tissue Int.* **34**, 519–522.

59. Mora, S., Weber, G., Guarneri, M. P., Nizzoli, G., Pasolini, D., and Chiumello, G. (1992). Effect of estrogen replacement therapy on bone mineral content in girls with Turner's syndrome. *Obstet. Gynecol.* **79**, 747–751.

60. Smith, M. A., Wilson, J., and Price, W. H. (1982). Bone demineralisation in patients with Turner's syndrome. *J. Med. Genet.* **19**, 100–103.

61. Ross, J. L., Long, L. M., Feuillan, P., Cassorla, F., and Cutler, G. B. (1991). Normal bone density of the wrist and spine and increased wrist fractures in girls with Turner's syndrome. *J. Clin. Endocrinol. Metab.* **73**, 355–359.

62. Neely, E. K., Marcus, R., Rosenfeld, R. G., and Bachrach, L. K. (1993). Turner's syndrome adolescents receiving growth hormone are not osteopenic. *J. Clin. Endocrinol. Metab.* **76**, 861–866.

63. Shaw, N. J., Rehan, V. K., Husain, S., Marshall, T., and Smith, C. S. (1997). Bone longitudinal density in turner's syndrome—a longitudinal study. *Clin. Endocrinol.* **47**, 367–370.

64. Kurabayashi, T., Yasuda, M., Fujimaki, T., Yamamoto, Y., Oda, K., and Tanaka, K. (1993). Effect of hormone replacement therapy on spinal bone mineral density and T lymphocyte subsets in premature ovarian failure and Turner's syndrome. *Int. J. Gynecol. Obstet.* **42**, 25–31.

65. Stepan, J. J., Musilova, J., and Pacovsky, V. (1989). Bone demineralization, biochemical indices of bone remodeling, and estrogen replacement therapy in adults with Turner's syndrome. *J. Bone Miner. Res.* **4**, 193–198.

66. Louis, O., Devroey, P., Kalender, W., and Osteaux, M. (1989). Bone loss in young hypoestrogenic women due to primary ovarian failure: Spinal quantitative computed tomography. *Fertil. Steril.* **52**, 227–231.

67. Naeraa, R. W., Brixen, K., Hansen, R. M., Hasling, C., Mosekilde, L., Andersen, J. H., Charles, P., and Nielsen, J. (1991). Skeletal size and bone mineral contend in Turner's syndrome: Relation to karyotype, estrogen treatment, physical fitness and bone turnover. *Calcif. tissue Int.* **49**, 77–83.

68. Emans, S. J., Grace, E., Hoffer, F. A., Gundberg, C., Ravnikar, V., and Woods, E. R. (1990). Estrogen deficiency in adolescents and young adults: Impact on bone mineral content and effects of estrogen replacement therapy. *Obstet. Gynecol.* **76**, 585–592.

69. Gulekli, B., Davies, M. C., and Jacobs, H. S. (1994). Effect of treatment on established osteoporosis in young women with amenorrhoea. *Clin. Endocrinol.* **41**, 275–281.

70. Brown, D. M., Jowsey, J., Phil, D., and Bradford, D. S. (1974). Osteoporosis in ovarian dysgenesis. *J. Pediatr.* **84**, 816–820.

71. Saggese, G., Federico, G., Bertelloni, S., and Baroncelli, G. I. (1992). Mineral metabolism in Turner's syndrome: Evidence for impaired renal vitamin D metabolism and normal osteoblast function. *J. Clin. Endocrinol. Metab.* **75**, 998–1001.

72. Zseli, J., Bosze, P., Lakatos, P., Vargha, P., Tarjan, G., Kollin, E., Horvath, C., Laszlo, J., and Hollo, I. (1991). Serum bone Gla protein in streak gonad sydrome. *Calcif. Tissue. Int.* **48**, 387–391.

74. Jakubowski, L. (1981). Urinary total hydroxiproline excretion in patients with Turner's syndrome and Klinefelter's syndrome. *Horm. Metab. Res.* **13**, 399–403.

75. Rauch, F., Seibel, M., Woitge, H., Kruse, K., and Schonau, E. (1995). Increased urinary excretion of collagen crosslinks in girls with Ullrich-Turner syndrome. *Acta Paediatr.* **84**, 66–69.

76. Holl, R. W., Kunze, D., Blum, W. F., Benz, R., Etzrodt, H., and Heinze, E. (1993). The somatotropin-somatomedin axis in adult patients with Turner syndrome: Measurements of stimulated GH, GH-BP, IGF-I, IGF-II and IGFBP-3 in 25 patients. *Horm. Res.* **39**, 30–35.

77. Barreca, A., Larizza, D., Damonte, G., Arvigo, M., Ponzani, P., Cesarone, A., Curto, F., Severi, F., Giordano, G., and Minuto, F. (1997). Insulin-like growth factors (IGF-I and IGF-II) and IGF-binding protein-3 production By fibroblasts of patients with Turner's syndrome in culture. *J. Clin. Endocrinol. Metab.* **82**, 1041–1046.

78. Saggese, G., Federico, G., and Cinquanta, L. (1995). Plasma growth hormone-binding protein activity, insulin like growth factor I, and its binding protein levels in patients with Turner's syndrome: Effects of short- and longterm recombinant growth hormone administration. *Pediatr. Res.* **37**, 106–111.

79. Rosenfeld, R. G. (1992). Growth hormone therapy in Turner's syndrome: An update on final heights. *Acta Paediatr. Scand., Suppl.* **383**, 3–6.

80. Shangold, M. M., and Levine H. S. (1979). The effect of marathon training upon menstrual function. *Am. J. Obstet. Gynecol.* **54**, 47.

81. Sanborne, C. F., Martin, B. J., and Wagner, W. W. (1982). Is athletes amenorrhea specific to runners? *Am. J. Obstet. Gynecol.* **143**, 882–886.

82. Warren, M. P. (1980). The effect of exercise on pubertal progression and reproductive functions in girls. *J. Clin. Endocrinol. Metab.* **51**, 1150–1157.

83. Fisher, E. C., Nelson, M. E., Fronteira, W. R., Turksoy, R. N., and Evans, W. J. (1986). Bone mineral content and levels of gonadotropins and estrogens in amenorrheic running women. *J. Clin. Endocrinol. Metab.* **62**, 1232–1236.

84. Drikwater, B. L., Nilson, K., Chesnut, C. H., Bremner, W. J., Shainholtz, S., and Southworth, M. B. (1984). Bone mineral content of amenorrheic and eumenorrheic athletes. *N. Engl. J. Med.* **311**, 277–281.

85. Myerson, M., Gutin, B., Warren, M. P., Wang, J., Lichtman, S., and Pierson, R. N. (1992). Total body bone density in amenorrheic runners. *Obstet. Gynecol.* **79**, 973–978.

86. Marcus, R., Cann, C., Madvig, P., Minkoff, J., Goddard, M., Bayer, M., Martin, M., Gaudiani, L., Haskell, W., and Genant, H. (1985). Menstrual function and bone mass in elite women distance runners. *Ann. Intern. Med.* **102**, 158–163.

87. Rencken, M. L., Chesnut, C. H., and Drinkwater, B. L. (1996). Bone density at multiple skeletal sites in amenorrheic athletes. *J. Am. Med. Assoc.* **276**, 238–240.

88. Seeman, E., Wahner, H. W., Offord, K. P., Johnson, W. J., and Riggs, B. L. (1982). The differential effects of endocrine dysfunction on the axial and appendicular skeleton. *J. Clin. Invest.* **69**, 1302–1309.

89. Young, N., Formica, C., Szmukler, G., and Seeman, E. (1994). Bone density at weight-bearing and nonweight-bearing sites in ballet dancers: The effect of exercise, hypogonadism, and body weight. *J. Clin. Endocrinol. Metab.* **78**, 449–454.

90. Robinson, T. L., Snow-Harter, C., Taaffe, D. R., Gillis, D., Shaw, J., and Marcus, R. (1995). Gymnasts exhibit higher bone mass than runners despite similar prevalence of amenorrhea and oligomenorrhea. *J. Bone. Miner. Res.* **10**, 26–35.

90a. Slemenda, C. W., and Johnston, C. C. (1993). High intensity activities in young women: Site specific bone mass effects among female figure skaters. *Bone Miner. Res.* **20**, 125–132.

91. Yek, J. K., and Aloia, J. F. (1990). Effect of physical activity on calciotropic hormones and calcium balance in rats. *Am. J. Physiol.* **258**, E263–E268.

92. Grimston, S. K., Tanguay, K. E., Gundberg, C. M., and Hanley, D. A.

(1993). The calcitriopic hormone response to changes in serum calcium during exercise in female long distance runners. *J. Clin. Endocrinol. Metab.* **76**, 867–872.

93. Takacs, C., Solidum, A. A., Zimmerli, E. J., and Warren, M. P. (1997). Osteocalcin in young women with secondary amenorrhea. Society for Gynecologic Investigation, Annual Meeting, San Diego, CA, March 1997: #131.

94. Rigotti, N. A., Nussbaum, S. R., Herzog, D. B., and Neer, R. M. (1984). Osteoporosis in women with anorexia nervosa. *N. Engl. J. Med.* **311**, 1601–1606.

95. Andersen, A. E., Woodward, P. J., and LaFrance, N. (1995). Bone mineral density of eating disorder subgroups. *Intl. J. Eat. Disord.* **18**, 335–342.

96. Poet, J. L., Pujol, A. G., Serabian, I. T., Devolx, B. C., and Roux, H. (1993). Lumbar bone mineral density in anorexia nervosa. *Clin. Rheumatol.* **12**, 236–239.

97. Davies, K. M., Pearson, P. H., Huseman, C. A., Greger, N. G., Kimmel, D. K., and Recker, R. R. (1990). Reduced bone mineral in patients with eating disorders. *Bone* **11**, 143–147.

98. Biller, B. M. K., Saxe, V., Herzog, D. B., Rosenthal, D. I., Holzman, S., and Klibansk, A. (1989). Mechanisms of osteoporosis in adult and adolescent women with anorexia nervosa. *J. Clin. Endocrinol. Metab.* **68**, 548–554.

99. Carmichael, K. A., and Carmichael, D. H. (1995). Bone metabolism and osteopenia in eating disorders. *Medicine* **74**, 254–267.

100. Klibanski, A., Biller, B. M. K., Schoenfeld, D. A., Herzog, D. B., and Saxe, V. C. (1995). The effects of estrogen administration on trabecular bone loss in young women with anorexia nervosa. *J. Clin. Endocrinol. Metab.* **80**, 898–904.

101. Rigotti, N. A., Neer, R. M., Skates, S. J., Herzog, D. B., and Nussbaum, S. R. (1991). The clinical course of osteoporosis in anorexia nervosa. A longitudinal study of cortical bone mass. *JAMA, J. Am. Med. Assoc.* **265**, 1133–1138.

102. Maugars, Y. M., Berthelot, J. M. M., Forestier, R., Mammar, N., Ladande, S., Venisse, J. L., and Prost, A. M. (1996). Follow up of bone mineral density in 27 cases of anorexia nervosa. *Eur. J. Endocrinol.* **135**, 591–597.

103. Bachrach, L. K., Katzman, D. K., Litt, I. F., Guido, D., and Marcus, R. (1991). Recovery from osteopenia in adolescent girls with anorexia nervosa. *J. Clin. Endocrinol. Metab.* **72**, 602–606.

104. Kaplan, F. S., Pertschuck, M., Fallon, M., and Haddad, J. (1986). Osteoporosis and hip fracture in a young woman with anorexia nervosa. *Clin. Orthop.* **212**, 250–254.

105. Joyce, J. M., Warren, D. L., Humphries, L. L., Smith, A. J., and Coon, J. S. (1990). Osteoporosis in women with eating disorders: Comparison of physical parameters, exercise, and menstrual status with SPA and DPA evaluation. *J. Nucl. Med.* **31**, 325–331.

106. Mira, M., Stewart, P. M., Vizzard, J., and Abraham, S. (1987). Biochemical abnormalities in anorexia nervosa and bulimia. *Ann. Clin. Biochem.* **24**, 29–35.

107. Fonseca, V. A., D'Souza, V., Houlder, S., Thomas, M., Wakeling, A., and Dandona, P. (1988). Vitamin D deficiency and low osteocalcin concentrations in anorexia nervosa. *J. Clin. Pathol.* **41**, 195–197.

108. Grinspoon, S., Baum, H., Lee, K., Anderson, E., Herzog, D., and Klibanski, A. (1996). Effects of short-term recombinant human insulin-like growth factor I administration on bone turnover in osteopenic women with anorexia nervosa. *J. Clin. Endocrinol. Metab.* **81**, 3864–3870.

109. Maugars, Y., and Prost, A. (1989). Osteoporose trabeculaire compliquant une anorexie mentale meconnue. *Rev. Rhum. Mal. Osteo-Articulaires* **56**, 159–161.

110. Boyar, R. M., Hellman, L. D., Roffwarg, H., Kartz, J., Zumoff, B., O'Connor, J., Bradlow, H. L., and Fukushima, D. K. (1977). Cortisol secretion and metabolism in anorexia nervosa. *N. Engl. J. Med.* **296**, 190–193.

111. Kontula, K., Mustajoki, and P., Pelkonen, R. (1984). Development of Cushing's disease in a patient with anorexia nervosa. *J. Endocrinol. Invest.* **7**, 35–40.

112. Counts, D. R., Gwirtsman, H., Carlsson, L. M., Lesem, M., and Cutler, G. B. (1992). The effect of anorexia nervosa and refeeding on growth hormone-binding protein, the insulin-like growth factors (IGFs), and the IGF-binding proteins. *J. Clin. Endocrinol. Metab.* **75**, 762–767.

113. Petersson, F., Fries, H., and Nillius, S. J. (1973). Epidemiology of secondary amenorrhea. Incidence and prevalence rates. *Am. J. Obstet. Gynecol.* **117**, 80–86.

114. Klibanski, A., and Greenspan, S. L. (1986). Increase in bone mass after treatment of hyperprolactinemic amenorrhea. *N. Engl. J. Med.* **315**, 542–546.

115. Kayath, M. J., Lengyel, A. M. J., and Vieira, J. G. H. (1993). Prevalence and magnitude of osteopenia in patients with prolactinoma. *Braz. J. Med. Biol. Res.* **26**, 933–941.

116. Ciccarelli, E., Savino, L. Carlevatto, V., Bertagna, A., Isaia, G. C., and Camanni, F. (1988). Vertebral bone density in non amenorrhoeic hyperprolactinaemic women. *Clin. Endocrinol.* **28**, 1–6.

117. Di Somma, C., Colao, A., Di Sarno, A., Klain, M., Landi, M. L., Facciollo, G., Pivonello, R., Panza, N., Salvatore, M., and Lombardi, G. (1998). Bone marker and bone density responses to dopamine agonist therapy in hyperprolactinemic males. *J. Clin. Endocrinol. Metab.* **83**, 807–813.

118. Biller, B. M. K., Baum, H. B. A., Rosenthal, D. I., Saxe, V. C., Charpie, P. M., and Klibanski, A. (1992). Progressive trabecular osteopenia in women with hyperprolactinemic amenorrhea. *J. Clin. Endocrinol. Metab.* **75**, 692–697.

119. Schlechte, J., El-Khoury, G., Kathol, M., and Walkner, L. (1987). Forearm and vertebral bone mineral in treated and untreated hyperprolactinemia amenorrhea. *J. Clin. Endocrinol. Metab.* **64**, 1021–1026.

120. Koppelman, M. C. S., Kurtz, D. W., Morrish, K. A., Bou, E., Susser, J. K., Shapiro, J. R., and Loriax, D. L. (1994). Vertebral body bone mineral content in hyperprolactinemic women. *J. Clin. Endocrinol. Metab.* **59**, 1050–1053.

121. Klibanski, A., Biller, B. M. K., Rosenthal, D. I., Schoenfeld, D. A., and Saxe, V. (1988). Effects of prolactin and estrogen deficiency in amenorrheic bone loss. *J. Clin. Endocrinol. Metab.* **67**, 124–130.

122. Greenspan, S. L., Oppenheim, D. S., and Klibanski, A. (1989). Importance of gonadal steroids to bone mass in men with hyperprolactinemic hypogonadism. *Ann. Intern. Med.* **110**, 526–531.

122a. Schlechte, J., Walkner, L., and Kathol, M. (1992). A longitudinal analysis of premenopausal bone loss in healthy women and women with hyperprolactinemia. *J. Clin. Endocrinol. Metab.* **75**, 698–703.

123. Suva, L. J., Winslow, G. A., Wettenhall, R. E. H., Hammonds, R. G., Mosely, J. M., Diefenbach-Jagger, H., Rodda, C. P., Kemp, B. E., Rodriguez, H., and Chen, E. Y. (1987). A parathyroid hormone-related protein implicated in malignant hypercalcemia: Cloning and expression. *Science* **237**, 893–896.

124. Kovacs, C. S., and Chik, C. L. (1995). Hyperprolactinemia caused by lactation and pituitary adenomas is associated with altered serum calcium, phosphate, parathyroid hormone (PTH), and PTH-related peptide levels. *J. Clin. Endocrinol. Metab.* **80**, 3036–3042.

125. Stiegler, C., Leb, G., Kleinert, R., Warnkross, H., Ramschak-Schwarzer, S., Lipp, R., Clarici, G., Krejs, G. J., and Dobnig, H. (1995). Plasma levels of parathyroid hormone-related peptide are elevated in hyperprolactinemia and correlated to bone density status. *J. Bone Miner. Res.* **10**, 751–759.

126. Sartorio, A., Conti, A., Ambrosi, B., Muratori, M., and Faglia, G. (1990). Osteocalcin levels in patients with microprolactinoma before and during medical treatment. *J. Endocrinol. Invest.* **13**, 419–422.

127. Schmid, F. (1967). Osteopathien bei antiepileptischer dauerbehandlung. *Fortsch. Med.* **85**, 381.

128. Kruse, R. (1968). Osteopathien bei antiepiliptscher langzeit-therapie. *Monatsschr. Kinderheilkd.* **116**, 378–380.

129. Hahn, T. J., and Avioli, L. V. (1984). Anticonvulsant-drug-induced mineral disorders. In Drugs and Nutrients: The interactive effects. *Drugs Pharm. Sci.* **21**, 409–427.

130. Marcus, R. (1992). Secondary forms of osteoporosis. *In* "Disorders of Bone and Mineral Metabolism" (F. L. Coe and M. J. Favus, eds.), pp. 902–903. Raven Press, New York.

131. Hahn, T. J. (1993). Steroid and drug-induced osteopenia. *In* "Primer on the Metabolic Bone Diseases and Disorders of Mineral Metabolism" (M. J. Favus, ed.), pp. 252–255. Raven Press, New York.

132. Hahn, T. J., and Halstead, L. R. (1979). Anticonvulsant drug induced osteomalacia: Alterations in mineral metabolism and response to vitamin D$_3$ administration. *Calcif. Tissue Int.* **27**, 13–18.

133. Christiansen, C., Rodbro, P., and Lund, P. (1973). Incidence of anticonvulsant osteomalacia and effect of vitamin D: Controlled therapeutic trial. *Br. Med. J.* **4**, 695–701.

134. Christiansen, C., Rodbro, P., and Nielsen, C. T. (1975). Iatrogenic osteomalacia in epileptic children: A controlled therapeutic trial. *Acta Paediatr. Scand.* **64**, 219–224.

135. Hahn, T. J., Hendin, B. A., Scharp, C. R., Boisseau, V. C., and Haddad, J. G. (1975). Serum 25-hydroxycholecalciferol levels and bone mass in children on chronic anticonvulsant therapy. *N. Engl. J. Med.* **292**, 550–554.

136. Hahn, T. J., Birge, S. J., Scharp, C. R., and Avioli, L. V. (1972). Phenobarbital induced alterations in vitamin D metabolism. *J. Clin. Invest.* **51**, 741–748.

137. Tjellesen, L., Nilas, L., and Christiansen, C. (1983). Does carbamazepine cause disturbances in calcium metabolism in epileptic patients? *Acta Neurol. Scand.* **68**, 13–19.

138. Hawkins, E., and Brewer, E. (1993). Renal toxicity induced by valproic acid (Depakene). *Pediatr. Pathol.* **13**, 863–868.

139. Hahn, T. J., Hendin, B. A., Scharp, C. R., and Haddad, J. G. (1972). Effect of chronic anticonvulsant therapy on serum 25-hydroxycholecalciferol levels in adults. *N. Engl. J. Med.* **287**, 900–904.

140. Stamp, T. C. B., Round, J. M., Rowe, D. J. F., and Haddad, J. G. (1972). Plasma levels and therapeutic effect of 25-hydroxycholecalciferol in epileptic patients taking anticonvulsant drugs. *Br. Med. J.* **4**, 9–12.

141. Valimaki, M. J., Tiihonen, M., Laitinen, K., Tahtela, R., Karkkainen, M., Lamberg-Allardt, C., Makela, P., and Tunninen, R. (1994). Bone mineral density measured by dual-energy X-ray absorptiometry and novel markers of bone formation and resorption in patients on antiepileptic drugs. *J. Bone Miner. Res.* **9**, 631–637.

142. Wark, J. D., Larkins, R. G., Perry-Keene, D., Peter, C. T., Ross, D. L., and Sloman, J. G. (1979). Chronic diphenylhydantoin therapy does not reduce plasma 25-hydroxy-vitamin D. *Clin. Endocrinol.* **11**, 267–274.

143. Weinstein, R. S., Bryce, G. F., Sappington, L. J., King, D. W., and Gallagher, B. B. (1984). Decreased serum ionized calcium and normal vitamin D metabolite levels with anticonvulsant drug treatment. *J. Clin. Endocrinol. Metab.* **58**, 1003–1009.

144. Koch, H. C., Kraft, D., and von Herrath, D. (1972). Influence of diphenylhydantoin and phenobarbital on intestinal calcium transport in the rat. *Epilepsia* **13**, 829–841.

145. Harrison, H. C., and Harrison, H. E. (1976). Inhibition of vitamin D-stimulated active transport of calcium of rat intestine by diphenylhydantoinphenobarbital treatment. *Proc. Soc. Exp. Biol. Med.* **153**, 220–224.

146. Jenkins, M. V., Harris, M., and Willis, M. R. (1974). The effect of phenytoin on parathyroid extract and 25-hydroxycholecalciferol-induced bone resorption: Adenosine 3'5'-cyclic monophosphatase production. *Calcif. Tissue Res.* **16**, 163–167.

147. Hahn, T. J., Scharp, C. R., Richardson, C. A., Halstead, L. R., Kahn, A. J., and Teitelbaum, S. T. (1978). Interaction of dyphenylhydantoin (phenytoin) and phenobarbital with hormonal mediation of fetal rat bone reasorption in vivo. *J. Clin. Invest.* **62**, 406–414.

148. Dietrich, J. W., and Duffield, R. (1980). Effects of diphenylhydantoin on synthesis of collagen and noncollagen protein in tissue culture. *Endocrinology* **106**, 606–610.

149. Mosekilde, L., and Melsen, F. (1980). Dynamic differences in trabecular bone remodeling between patients after jejuno ileal by pass for obesity and epileptic patients receiving anticonvulsant therapy. *Metab. Bone Dis. Relat. Res.* **2**, 77–82.

150. Takeshita, N., Seino, Y., Ishida, H., Tanaka, H., Tsutsumi, C., Ogata, K., Kiyohara, K., Kato, H., Nozawa, M., Akiyama, Y., Hara, K., and Imura, H. (1989). Increased circulating levels of y-carboxyglutamic acid-containing protein and decreased bone mass in children on anticonvulsant therapy. *Calcif. Tissue Int.* **44**, 80–85.

151. Lau, K. H. W., Nakade, O., Barr, B., Taylor, A. K., Houchin, K., and Baylink, D. J. (1995). Phenytoin increases markers of osteogenesis for the human species in vitro and in vivo. *J. Clin. Endocrinol. Metab.* **80**, 2347–2353.

152. Tjellesen, L., Hummer, L., Christiansen, C., and Rodbro, P. (1986). Different metabolism of vitamin D2/D3 in epileptic patients treated with phenobarbital/phenytoin. *Bone* **7**, 337–342.

153. Ohishi, T., Kushida, K., Takahashi, M., Kawana, K., Yagi, K., Kwakami, K., Horiuchi, K., and Inoue, T. (1994). Urinary bone resorption markers in patients with metabolic bone disorders. *Bone* **15**, 15–20.

154. Christiansen, C., Rodbro, P., and Lund, P. (1973). Incidence of anticonvulsant osteomalacia and effect of vitamin D: Controlled therapeutic trial. *Br. Med. J.* **4**, 695–701.

155. Sheth, R. D., Wesolowski, C. A., Jacob, J. C., Penney, S., Hobbs, G. R., Riggs, J. E., and Bodensteiner, J. B. (1995). Effect of carbamazepine and valproate on bone mineral density. *J. Pediatr.* **127**, 256–262.

156. Barden, H. S., Mazess, R. B., Rose, P. G., and McSweeney. (1980). Bone mineral status measured by direct photon absorptiometry in institutionalized adults receiving long-term anticonvulsant therapy and multivitamin supplementation. *Calcif. Tissue Int.* **31**, 117–121.

157. Collins, N., Maher, J., Cole, M., Baker, M., and Callaghan, N. (1991). A prospective study to evaluate the dose of vitamin D required to correct low 25-hydroxyvitamin D levels, calcium and alkaline phosphatase in patients at risk of developing antiepileptic drug-induced osteomalacia. *Q. J. Med.* **78**, 113–122.

CHAPTER 38

Osteomalacia and Rickets

MARC K. DREZNER Duke University Medical Center, Durham, North Carolina 27710

I. DEFINITION

Rickets and osteomalacia are diseases characterized by defective bone and cartilage mineralization in children and bone mineralization in adults. The abnormal calcification of cartilage occurs at epiphyseal growth plates and contributes to an associated delayed maturation of the cartilage cellular sequence and disorganization of cell arrangement [1]. The resultant profusion of disorganized, nonmineralized, degenerating cartilage leads to widening of the epiphyseal plates with flaring or cupping, irregularity of the epiphyseal-metaphyseal junctions, attendant skeletal abnormalities, and possibly retardation of growth. Abnormal calcification of bone is limited to the newly formed organic matrix deposited at the bone-osteoid interfaces of remodeling tissue. This defect results in an increase in the bone forming surface covered by incompletely mineralized osteoid, an enhanced osteoid volume and thickness, a decrease in the mineralizing surface (the percentage of bone surface undergoing calcification), and likely a heightened susceptibility to fractures and/or bone deformities [2].

The various rachitic and osteomalacic disorders recognized to date include more than 30 subtypes, which may be divided into disease forms characterized by calciopenia, phosphopenia, or normal mineral availability (Table I). The calciopenic forms of the disease embrace disorders that affect the availability of calcium and/or vitamin D or its active metabolite. In general, these forms of the disease are marked by a low or marginally normal serum calcium level [3, 4], (secondary) hyperparathyroidism, and consequent increased bone turnover. While many of these calciopenic diseases are acquired or secondary to renal or gastrointestinal dysfunction, a subgroup of the disorders are due to genetic abnormalities of vitamin D metabolism [5, 6].

The phosphopenic disorders usually develop from a primary abnormality of transepithelial phosphate transport in the nephron, resulting in phosphate wasting. Often the underlying abnormality is due to a genetic defect which directly or indirectly influences renal phosphate handling. As a rule, patients with these disorders maintain a normal serum calcium concentration, whereas hypophosphatemia is characteristic. In contrast to the calciopenic disorders, parathyroid hormone levels and bone turnover are often normal in phosphopenic forms of the disease.

In those disorders marked by normal mineral availability, the abnormal calcification of cartilage and bone most often results from the presence of a circulating inhibitor of bone mineralization (often a drug) or a genetic defect causing abnormal bone collagen or matrix. In general, these disease states are characterized by normal or low bone turnover and a variable predisposition to fracture.

Although the phenotypic expression of the defective bone and cartilage mineralization is similar in this wide variety of disease forms, the associated genetic, hormonal, and biochemical abnormalities, as well as the resultant bone turnover, differ according to the pathogenetic defect. Therefore,

547

TABLE I. The Rickets and Osteomalacia Syndromes

Calciopenic disorders	Phosphopenic disorders	Normal mineral availability
Nutritional	Nutritional	Primary mineralization defect
Calcium deficiency	Low phosphate intake	Hereditary
Vitamin D deficiency	Ingestion of phosphate binding agents	Hypophosphatasia
Vitamin D malabsorption	Impaired renal tubular phosphate transport	Perinatal
Gastrointestinal disorders	Hereditary	Infantile
Partial/Total gastrectomy	X-linked hypophosphatemia	Childhood
Small bowel disease	Hereditary hypophosphatemic rickets	Adult-onset
Intestinal bypass	with hypercalciuria	Odontohypophosphatasia
Pancreatic insufficiency	X-linked recessive hypophosphatemia	Pseudohypophosphatasia
Hepatobiliary disease	Autosomal dominant hypophosphatemia	Acquired
Biliary atresia	Acquired	Drug-induced
Biliary obstruction	Tumor-induced osteomalacia	Fluoride
Biliary fistula	Mesenchymal, epidermal, endodermal tumors	Aluminum
Cirrhosis	Fibrous dysplasia of bone	Bisphosphonates
Loss of vitamin D metabolites	Neurofibromatosis	Abnormal matrix synthesis
Nephrotic syndrome	Linear nevus sebaceous syndrome	Fibrogenesis imperfecta ossium
Peritoneal dialysis	Light chain nephropathy	Axial osteomalacia
Abnormal vitamin D metabolism	Sporadic hypophosphatemic osteomalacia	Metabolic acidosis
Impaired hepatic 25-hydroxylation	General renal tubular disorders	
Liver disease	Fanconi's syndrome, type I	
Anticonvulsant therapy	Hereditary	
Impaired renal 1α-hydroxylation	Familial idiopathic	
Vitamin D-dependent rickets, type I	Cystinosis	
Chronic renal failure	Galactosemia	
Hypoparathyroidism	Glycogen storage disease	
Pseudohypoparathyroidism	Wilson's disease	
Vitamin D resistance	Lowe's syndrome	
Vitamin D-dependent rickets, type 2	Acquired	
Hormone binding negative	Renal transplantation	
Defective hormone binding capacity	Multiple myeloma	
Abnormal hormone binding affinity	Intoxication	
Deficient nuclear localization	Cadmium	
Decreased hormone-receptor affinity	Lead	
Anticonvulsant therapy	Fanconi's syndrome, type 2	

identification of rickets and/or osteomalacia demands systematic analysis to determine cause and thereby appropriate therapeutic approaches for the disorder. Traditionally complete characterization of bone turnover in a rachitic or osteomalacic disorder and monitoring of therapeutic response and patient compliance required histomorphometric analysis of bone biopsies. However, the development of specific and sensitive biochemical markers reflecting the overall rate of bone formation and bone resorption provides relatively noninvasive measurements of potential value in assessing the rachitic/osteomalacic diseases. Reports on the use of these markers in such disorders are unfortunately quite limited. Nevertheless, expected changes in markers of bone resorption and formation in these variable diseases are predictable for the most part, because changes in the biochemical markers reflect alterations in skeletal metabolism which may vary with the underlying cause. With these considerations in mind, an understanding of the etiology of the rachitic/osteomalacic diseases, with specific attention to the complex mineralization processes influencing cartilage and bone, should permit prediction of alterations in the bone markers in the calciopenic, phosphopenic, and normal mineral variants of these disorders and potentially provide new insight to their pathogenesis.

II. NORMAL AND ABNORMAL MINERALIZATION

Mineralization of cartilage and bone is a complex process in which the calcium-phosphorus inorganic mineral phase is deposited in an organic matrix in a highly ordered fashion. Such mineralization depends primarily on the availability of sufficient calcium and phosphorus at mineralization sites. Other requisite conditions necessary for normal calcification include [7]: (1) adequate metabolic and transport function of chondrocytes and osteoblasts to regulate the concentration of calcium, phosphorus, and other ions at the mineralization sites; (2) maintenance of an optimal pH (approximately 7.6) for deposition of calcium-phosphorus complexes; (3) a low concentration of calcification inhibitors (e.g., pyrophosphates, proteoglycans) in the circulation or bone matrix; and (4) the presence of collagen with unique type, number, and distribution of cross-links, remarkable patterns of hydroxylation and glycosylation, and abundant phosphate content, which collectively permit and facilitate deposition of mineral at gaps, "hole zones," between the distal ends of collagen molecules (see Chapters 11 and 17).

Bone mineral consists of Ca^{2+}, PO_4^{3-}, OH^-, and CO_3^{2-} ions arranged in space in accordance with the crystal lattice of hydroxyapatite [8]. The mineralizing potential of extracellular fluid (ECF) depends on the free ionic activity or effective concentration of Ca^{2+}, HPO_4^{2-} and H^+ ions. For both calcium and phosphorus, ionic concentrations differ from the total concentrations because of protein binding and ion complexing, both of which are affected by pH. At sites of mineralization, the successive addition of Ca^{2+} and HPO_4^{2-} ions present in ECF and the simultaneous removal of protons generate a series of compounds beginning with secondary calcium phosphate or brushite ($CaHPO_4 \cdot 2H_2O$), the first solid phase formed, and ending with hydroxyapatite [$Ca_{10}(PO_4)_6(OH)_2$] [9]. Mechanisms to accomplish initial mineral deposition include concentration gradients between mineralizing and nonmineralizing sites maintained by cells and by the ion binding and releasing properties of macromolecules synthesized by cells, sequestration and subsequent release of calcium by mitochondria, and heterogeneous nucleation by outside agents or substances [7, 9]. In contrast, mechanisms to retard the growth of hydroxyapatite crystals include the precise spatial relationships between mineral and matrix, the presence at critical locations of calcium chelators and inhibitors of mineralization (such as pyrophosphate and albumin), and the cellular and biochemical characteristics of the quiescent bone surface, the site of reversible mineral exchange [7].

A. Cartilage

Within this general framework, mineral is deposited in growth plate cartilage in the form of spherical clusters of randomly oriented crystals of varying size [10]. The clusters, called calcospherulites, are spatially associated with matrix vesicles, which are small membrane-bound particles that are derived from chondrocytes by an unknown mechanism. The vesicles serve as nucleation sites and are distributed with highest density in the resting and hypertrophic zones and lowest density in the proliferative and calcifying zones of cartilage. The mineral is deposited in discrete patches which aggregate to form a single longitudinal septum, 50 μm in width, extending across the growth plate [11]. Deposition of mineral is delayed approximately 24 hours after synthesis and secretion of matrix, likely reflecting changes in gene expression in chondrocytes [12]. Accumulation of uncalcified tissue in rachitic disorders is due entirely to a profound delay in this mineralization process, accompanied by structural disorganization of the metaphysis secondary to mechanical effects and a markedly altered pattern of vascular invasion. Inadequate mineralization is confined to the maturation zone of the cartilage, whereas the resting and proliferative zones of the epiphyses exhibit normal histologic features. In the maturation zone, the height of the cells columns is increased and the cells are closely packed and irregularly aligned. Moreover, calcification in the interstitial regions of this hypertrophic zone is defective. These changes result in increased thickness of the epiphyseal plate, accompanied by an increase in transverse diameter, which may extend beyond the ends of the bone causing characteristic cupping or flaring. The cause of this defective mineralization varies depending on the subtype of rickets in question. However, in general, defective mineralization is secondary to decreased mineral availability or a combination of mineral and/or vitamin D dependent or genetically impaired chondrocyte function.

B. Bone

In contrast, the mineralization of bone is marked by a paucity of matrix vesicles. Indeed, in lamellar bone, which is invariably formed in apposition to an existing surface, the matrix is compact in texture and the collagen fibrils are long and highly ordered. Mineral crystals are aligned with their long axis parallel to the collagen fibrils and are initially deposited within the hole zones by heterogeneous nucleation, but longer and wider crystals are subsequently formed on and between the fibrils [8, 10]. The deposition of mineral is, however, continuous and sharply demarcated, but delayed for approximately two weeks after matrix deposition. The delay likely reflects necessary maturation of the matrix which includes completion of collagen fibril cross-linking and the development of precise orientation, conformation, and aggregation of a variety of noncollagenous proteins and proteoglycans [7, 13]. Abnormal mineralization results in accumulation of excess osteoid, a *sine qua non* for the diagnosis of osteomalacia in most instances. The accumulation of unmineralized osteoid in bone is generally due to a prolongation of the mineralization lag time and is manifest by an increase in the forming surface covered by incompletely mineralized osteoid and an increase in osteoid volume and thickness [14]. The mineralization process is likely influenced by the availability of mineral and vitamin D dependent and/or genetic influences on osteoblast function. In this scenario, the osteoblast probably functions by a direct effect on matrix maturation and by its effects on mineral transport. In any case, the evident difference in the mineralization processes in cartilage and bone accounts for the differences, under some circumstances, in severity and response to treatment of rickets and osteomalacia.

III. INCIDENCE, EPIDEMIOLOGY, AND CLINICAL FINDINGS

Although vitamin D deficiency was a common form of calciopenic rickets/osteomalacia early in this 1900s, the therapeutic use of vitamin D and supplementation of foods with vitamin D has severely curtailed the occurrence of this disease form. Nevertheless, deficiency of vitamin D does persist in Asian populations, as well as in a growing number of elderly patients, vegans, children on macrobiotic diets, and black children in the Western World [15–17], and vitamin D deficiency secondary to malabsorptive disorders continues to occur with relative frequency. Regardless, with the virtual disappearance of vitamin D deficiency, attention became focused on the remaining subtypes of rickets/osteomalacia, which are characterized in general by a failure to respond to physiologic doses of vitamin D. These are related, for the most part, to calciopenic disorders due to primary vitamin D abnormalities (defective metabolism or postreceptor resistance) or a deficient calcium supply (especially in many African countries) and phosphopenic diseases due to genetic abnormalities or acquired defects in renal phosphate transport (tumor-induced osteomalacia). In addition, primary mineralization defects also occur, albeit infrequently, and they can be genetic (as in hypophosphatasia) or acquired (excess, fluoride, aluminum, or bisphosphonate).

The clinical manifestations of rickets are primarily related to skeletal pain and deformity, bone fractures, slipped epiphyses, and abnormalities of growth. In addition, hypocalcemia, when present, may be sufficiently severe to produce tetany, laryngeal spasm, or seizures [18, 19]. In infants and young children, features include listlessness, irritability, profound hypotonia, and proximal muscle weakness. By age 6 months,

frontal bossing with flattening at the back is evident. Later, a lateral collapse of both chest walls (Harrison's sulcus) and rachitic rosary may appear. If untreated, progressive bony deformities result in bowing and fractures in the long bones. In addition, dental eruption may be delayed and, in those forms of the disease with hypocalcemia or hereditary hypophosphatemia, enamel defects and inadequate dentin calcification occur, respectively.

Clinical signs of osteomalacia in adults are vague. Often the skeletal abnormalities are overlooked and features of an underlying disorder, such as malabsorption, may dominate. Nevertheless, diffuse skeletal pain and generalized muscular weakness are generally present [20]. Pain may be localized about the hips and result in an antalgic gait, and muscle weakness is primarily proximal and often is associated with wasting and hypotonia. Myopathy is present in virtually all forms of osteomalacia, with the exception of X-linked hypophosphatemia. In adults with a history of rickets, evidence of inactive rachitic abnormalities is often apparent.

The radiographic and metabolic abnormalities characteristic of rickets/osteomalacia vary according to the presence of calciopenic (high turnover) or phosphopenic (normal to low turnover) disease, as well as disorders secondary to primary mineralization defects. Markers of bone turnover may be the discriminant factors that permit categorization and guide investigation of the disease. Moreover, serial evaluation of such markers may permit a simple means to judge efficacy of therapy. Common radiographic abnormalities in rickets are evident at the growth plate, which is increased in thickness, is cupped, and displays an irregular, hazy appearance at the diaphyseal line secondary to uneven invasion of the recently calcified cartilage by adjacent bone tissue. In osteomalacia, there is usually a mild decrease in bone density associated with a coarsening of trabeculae and a blurring of their margins. Looser's zones (or pseudofractures), ribbon-like zones of rarefaction oriented perpendicular to the bone surface, are a more specific radiographic abnormality in osteomalacia.

IV. CALCIOPENIC RICKETS AND OSTEOMALACIA

A. General Features

Currently recognized forms of calciopenic rickets/osteomalacia include a group of disorders in which the availability of calcium or vitamin D and/or its active metabolite is compromised (Table I). These disorders are due to a nutritional deficiency, gastrointestinal malabsorption, abnormal vitamin D metabolism, or resistance to the effects of calcitriol. In general, the biochemical hallmarks of the disease (Table II)

TABLE II.   Metabolic Abnormalities in the Rachitic and Osteomalacic Disorders

	Serum						Urinary		
	Calcium	Phosphorus	Alkaline phosphatase	25(OH)D	1,25(OH)$_2$D	PTH	Calcium	Phosphorus	Amino acids
Calciopenic disorders									
Nutritional									
Calcium deficiency	⇓	⇓, N	⇑, N	N	N, ⇑	⇑	⇓	⇑, N	⇑, N
Vitamin D deficiency	⇓, N	⇓, N	⇑, N	⇓	N, ⇑	⇑	⇓	⇑, N	⇑, N
Vitamin D malabsorption	⇓, N	⇓, N	⇑, N	⇓	N, ⇑	⇑	⇓	⇑, N	⇑, N
Abnormal vitamin D metabolism									
Impaired 25-hydroxylation	⇓, N	⇓, N	⇑, N	⇓	⇓	⇑	⇓	⇑, N	⇑, N
Impaired 1-hydroxylation	⇓	⇓, N	⇑	N, ⇑	⇓	⇑	⇓	⇑, N	⇑, N
Vitamin D resistance									
Vitamin D-dependent rickets type II	⇓, N[1]	⇓, N	⇑	N, ⇑	⇑	⇑	⇓	⇑, N	⇑, N
Phosphopenic disorders									
Nutritional									
Phosphate deficiency	N	⇓	⇑, N	N	⇑	N	⇑	⇓	N
Hereditary									
X-linked hypophosphatemia	N	⇓	⇑, N	N	⇓[2]	N, ⇑	⇓, N	⇑[3]	N, ⇑
Hypophosphatemic rickets/ hypercalciuria	N	⇓	⇑, N	N	⇑	N	⇑	⇑[3]	N
X-linked recessive hypophosphatemia	N	⇓	⇑, N	N	⇑	⇓, N	⇑	⇑[3]	N
Autosomal dominant hypophosphatemia	N	⇓	⇑, N	N	⇓[2]	N	⇓, N	⇑[3]	N
Acquired									
Tumor-induced osteomalacia	N	⇓	⇑, N	N	⇓	N	⇓, N	⇑[3]	⇑, N
Renal tubular disorders	N	⇓	⇑, N	N	⇓[2]	N	⇑	⇑[3]	⇑
Normal mineral availability									
Primary mineralization defect									
Hypophosphatasia	N, ⇑[4]	N, ⇑[5]	⇓	N	N	N	N, ⇑[6]	N	N
Drug-induced	N, ⇓	N, ⇓	⇑, N	N, ⇓	N	N, ⇑	N, ⇓	N	N
Abnormal matrix synthesis									
Fibrogenesis imperfecta ossium	N	N	⇑, N	N	N	N	N	N	N

[1] Although the serum concentration in affected patients in generally low, in subjects with late presentation of disease the serum calcium level is normal.

[2] The serum 1,25(OH)$_2$D levels are low relative to the presence of hypophosphatemia, which should increase the circulating concentration.

[3] The 24 hour urinary excretion of phosphorus is increased relative to the serum phosphorus concentration and the renal TmP/GFR is decreased.

[4] Increased serum calcium concentrations occur frequently in patients with perinatal and infantile hypophosphatasia, apparently due to dyssynergy between gastrointestinal calcium absorption and defective skeletal growth and mineralization.

[5] Approximately 50% of patients are frankly hyperphosphatemic secondary to an increased TmP/GFR.

[6] Patients with hypercalcemia often exhibit hypercalciuria.

are a low or marginally normal serum calcium level, a decreased serum phosphorus concentration, and (secondary) hyperparathyroidism. Commensurately, urinary calcium is decreased and urinary phosphorus increased due to diminished gastrointestinal absorption of calcium and/or the influence of an increased circulating level of parathyroid hormone on renal function. In addition, serum 25-hydroxyvitamin D levels are decreased in states of vitamin D deficiency, usually to levels less than 3 ng/ml. In contrast, in these disorders, the serum 1,25(OH)$_2$D concentration is not overtly decreased, and may be elevated, secondary to the prevailing hyperparathyroidism and the stimulatory effects of parathyroid hormone on calcitriol production. Alternatively, a defect in vitamin D metabolism (impaired 1α-hydroxylation) results in an isolated deficiency of 1,25(OH)$_2$D, whereas end-organ resistance to this active vitamin D metabolite increases the circulating level of calcitriol. Generally, alkaline phosphatase is elevated in all forms of calciopenic rickets/osteomalacia,

TABLE III. Expected Alterations in Bone Density and Histomorphometry in the Rachitic and Osteomalacic Diseases

	Bone density	Bone histomorphometry			
		OS/BS	Md.S/BS	Ob.Pm/B.Pm	Oc.Pm/B.Pn
Calciopenic disorders					
Nutritional					
Calcium deficiency	⇓	⇑	⇓	⇑	⇑
Vitamin D deficiency	⇓	⇑	⇓	⇑	⇑
Vitamin D malabsorption	⇓	⇑	⇓	⇑	⇑
Abnormal vitamin D metabolism					
Impaired 25-hydroxylation	⇓	⇑	⇓	⇑	⇑
Impaired 1-hydroxylation	⇓	⇑	⇓	⇑	⇑
Vitamin D resistance					
Vitamin D-dependent rickets type II	⇓	⇑	⇓	⇑	⇑
Phosphopenic disorders					
Nutritional					
Phosphate deficiency	⇓	⇑	⇓	N	N,⇑[1]
Hereditary					
X-linked hypophosphatemia	⇓,⇑[2]	⇑	⇓	⇓,N	N,⇑[3]
Hypophosphatemic rickets/hypercalciuria	⇓	⇑	⇓	N	N,⇑[1]
X-linked recessive hypophosphatemia	⇓	⇑	⇓	⇓,N	N,⇑
Autosomal dominant hypophosphatemia	⇓[1]	⇑	⇓	N	N
Acquired					
Tumor-induced osteomalacia	⇓	⇑	⇓	⇓,N	N,⇑[4]
Renal tubular disorders	⇓	⇑	⇓	⇓,N	⇑,N
Normal mineral availability					
Primary mineralization defect					
Hypophosphatasia	⇓	⇑	⇓	N	N
Drug-induced	⇓	⇑	⇓	N	N
Abnormal matrix synthesis					
Fibrogenesis imperfecta ossium	⇓	⇑	⇓	N	N

OS/BS, osteoid covered bone surface; Md.S/BS, mineralizing bone surface; Ob.Pm/B.Pm, osteoblast covered bone perimeter; Oc.Pm/B.Pm, osteoclast covered bone perimeter.

[1] The increased serum 1,25(OH)$_2$D levels in this syndrome may contribute to a modest increase in osteoclast activity.

[2] Although the bone density in untreated patients is characteristically decreased, long term disease often results in increased density in the lumbar spine.

[3] A minimal increase in the number of osteoclasts along the bone margin is often observed but may represent the diminished mineralized trabecular bone surface.

[4] In the subgroup of patients with elevated urinary cyclic AMP, the circulating factor may increase osteoclast activity.

although affected adults may manifest normal circulating levels.

Unique radiographic and bone histomorphometric abnormalities of the calciopenic diseases reflect not only the presence of impaired mineralization but also that of increased parathyroid hormone. In this regard, x-rays often display not only decreased bone density but also subperiosteal resorption and bone cysts as evidence of long-standing secondary hyperparathyroidism. Concurrently, bone biopsies reveal the expected mineralization disorder, marked by increased osteoid surface and decreased mineralized surface, as well as the unambiguous sign of increased bone turnover, an increased number of osteoclasts, and osteoblasts along the bone surface (Table III).

B. Markers of Bone Resorption

Commensurate with the increased bone turnover due to secondary hyperparathyroidism in these calciopenic diseases, markers of bone resorption should be elevated (Table IV). However, few reports documenting such abnormalities are available. Nevertheless, in concert with the appearance of radiological rickets in the calciopenic disorders, documented

TABLE IV. Expected Levels of Bone Turnover Markers in the Rachitic and Osteomalacic Disorders

| | Bone formation markers | | | Bone resorption markers | | | | |
| | Serum | | | Serum | | Urinary | | |
	OC	PICP	PINP	ICTP	TRAP	OHP	PYD	DPD
Calciopenic disorders								
Nutritional								
Calcium deficiency	N[1]	⇑	⇑	⇑	⇑	⇑	⇑	⇑
Vitamin D deficiency	N[1]	⇑	⇑	⇑	⇑	⇑	⇑	⇑
Vitamin D malabsorption	N[1]	⇑	⇑	⇑	⇑	⇑	⇑	⇑
Abnormal vitamin D metabolism								
Impaired 25-hydroxylation	N[1]	⇑	⇑	⇑	⇑	⇑	⇑	⇑
Impaired 1-hydroxylation	N[1]	⇑	⇑	⇑	⇑	⇑	⇑	⇑
Vitamin D resistance								
Vitamin D dependent rickets, type 2	N[1]	⇑	⇑	⇑	⇑	⇑	⇑	⇑
Phosphopenic disorders								
Nutritional								
Phosphate deficiency	⇓,N	N,⇑	N,⇑	N,⇓	N,⇓	N,⇓	N,⇓	N,⇓
Hereditary								
X-linked hypophosphatemia	N,⇑[2]	N,⇑	N,⇑	N,⇓	N,⇓	N,⇓	N,⇓	N,⇓
Hypophosphatemic rickets/hypercalciuria	N	N,⇑	N,⇑	N[3]	N	N	N[3]	N[3]
X-linked recessive hypophosphatemia	N	N,⇑	N,⇑	N[3]	N	N	N[3]	N[3]
Autosomal dominant hypophosphatemia	N	N,⇑	N,⇑	N,⇓	N,⇓	N,⇓	N,⇓	N,⇓
Acquired								
Tumor induced osteomalacia	N	N,⇑	N,⇑	N,⇑[4]	N,⇑[4]	N,⇑[4]	N,⇑[4]	N,⇑[4]
Renal tubular disorders	N,⇑[2]	N,⇑	N,⇑	N,⇑[5]	N,⇑[5]	N,⇑[5]	N,⇑[5]	N,⇑[5]
Normal mineral availability								
Primary mineralization defect								
Hypophosphatasia	N	N	N	N,⇓[6]	N	N	N,⇓[6]	N,⇓[6]
Drug-Induced	N	N,⇓,⇑[7]	N,⇓,⇑[7]	N	N,⇓[8]	N	N,⇓[8]	N,⇓[8]
Abnormal matrix synthesis								
Fibrogenesis imperfecta ossium	N	N	N	N	N	N	N	N

OC, osteocalcin; PICP, C-terminal procollagen I extension peptides; PINP, N-terminal procollagen I extension peptides; ICTP, carboxy-terminal telopeptide of type I collagen; TRAP, tartrate resistant acid phosphatase; OHP, hydroxyproline; PYD, pyridinoline cross-links, DPD, deoxypyridinoline cross-links.

[1] Osteocalcin measurements are generally normal to low in untreated patients; however, in early stages of the disease elevation of serum $1,25(OH)_2D$ levels, commensurate with increased parathyroid hormone, is associated with above normal concentrations.

[2] Although the serum osteocalcin is generally normal, in a select few an increased concentration has been observed; whether this elevation corresponds to the infrequent hyperparathyroidism encountered in subjects with this disease remains unknown.

[3] The possibility that a sensitive marker of resorption will be decreased is less in these disorders since the serum $1,25(OH)_2D$ concentration is elevated which may increase osteoclast number/activity to a limited degree.

[4] An increased level of a resorption marker may occur in the limited subset of patients with elevated urinary cyclic AMP.

[5] The elevated serum parathyroid hormone concentration that occurs in some affected subjects may increase the resorption markers.

[6] In the subset of patients with hypercalcemia and suppressed parathyroid hormone secretion, bone resorption markers may be decreased.

[7] Collagen production and the markers reflecting this process may be quite variable in drug-induced disease, with a decrease realized secondary to aluminum and an increase due to fluoride.

[8] Sensitive markers of bone resorption may be decreased in drug-induced disease secondary to agents such as bisphosphonates.

elevations of biochemical markers have been reported. In this regard, many studies have revealed that the commonly used and well established measure of bone turnover, urinary hydroxyproline, is elevated in a wide variety of calciopenic rachitic/osteomalacic disorders [21]. However, as a consequence of the varied tissue origin and metabolism of hydroxyproline, this marker is poorly correlated with bone resorption assessed by bone histomorphometry or calcium kinetics [22]. Quantitation of the collagen pyridinium cross-links, pyridinoline (hyroxylysylpyridinoline) and deoxypyridinoline (lysylpyridinoline), has provided relatively specific markers of bone resorption (see Chapters 2 and 28). Indeed, these measurements correlate exceptionally well with rates of bone resorption and do so far better than hydroxyproline [23, 24]. Not surprisingly, therefore, measurement of this variable in patients with vitamin D deficiency osteomalacia showed hydroxypyridinium levels to be elevated [25]. In addition, several studies describe an increase in serum concentrations of pyridinoline cross-linked carboxy-terminal telopeptide of type 1 collagen (ICTP) in children with rickets [26, 27]. Although urinary hydroxylysine and plasma tartrate-resistant acid phosphatase are additional sensitive markers of bone resorption and osteoclast activity, respectively, their value in assessment of the calciopenic rachitic/osteomalacic diseases has not been evaluated.

C. Markers of Bone Formation

Because bone resorption and formation are generally tightly coupled, both in health and in disease states, the high turnover calciopenic disorders should manifest elevated levels of formation markers. However, reports of these measurements have demonstrated significant variability and, most notably, disparate ability to document a high turnover state. In this regard, assays of the N- and C-terminal procollagen I extension peptides (PINP, PICP), as well as the N-terminal propeptide of type III collagen (PIIINP), have revealed significant elevations of these peptides in patients with calciopenic disease [27–29]. Because the release of PICP and PINP into the circulation correlates with the incorporation of collagen into the bone matrix, the elevated levels likely reflect augmented deposition of poorly mineralized osteoid at the increased number of bone resorptive sites created by secondary hyperparathyroidism. In contrast, measurements of osteocalcin in the calciopenic disorders, albeit variable, have largely shown osteocalcin to be decreased to normal levels [30]. Because osteocalcin synthesis marks the matrix maturation and subsequent mineralization [31, 32], this finding implies a loss of, or an altered metabolic coupling between, aspects of matrix production and mineralization in affected patients. Hence, as expected, elevated PINP and PICP marks increased bone turnover/matrix production whereas normal or decreased osteocalcin may reflect a disturbed osteoblastic/matrix maturation and the consequent characteristic bone mineralization defect. A subset of patients with osteomalacia due to vitamin D deficiency have elevated circulating levels of osteocalcin [33]. The occurrence of this increase correlates with an elevation of the serum $1,25(OH)_2D$ concentration, which is found in early stages of vitamin D deficiency when increased circulating levels of parathyroid hormone enhance production of this active vitamin D metabolite. With progression of the disease and progressive decline of serum 25(OH)D levels, the serum osteocalcin returns to normal, again reflecting poor mineralization of the collagen.

D. Summary

Assay of bone markers may play an important role in the diagnosis and treatment of the calciopenic rachitic/osteomalacic disorders. In many cases, establishing a diagnosis of vitamin D deficiency osteomalacia presents formidable problems. Often the 25-hydroxyvitamin D level is not overtly decreased but remains in the low normal range. Similarly, evidence for secondary hyperparathyroidism is marginal. Documentation of increased bone turnover, therefore, may facilitate diagnosis and certainly place the disease amongst the calciopenic disorders. Moreover, successful treatment of these diseases may be easily tracked not only by following various biochemistries, such as serum calcium, phosphorus, 25(OH)D, and PTH, but also by serial determination of bone markers to assure that therapeutic intervention has normalized bone turnover. In addition, with normal mineralization, the measurement of serum osteocalcin will likewise exhibit normalization or, in some cases, overt elevation.

V. PHOSPHOPENIC RICKETS AND OSTEOMALACIA

A. General Features

Rickets and osteomalacia occur in association with a variety of disorders in which phosphate depletion predominates (Table I). Most typically, these disease have in common abnormal proximal renal tubular function, which results in an increased renal clearance of inorganic phosphorus and hypophosphatemia. However, the biochemical abnormalities characteristic of these disorders are quite variable (Table II). Typically, these disorders are marked by a normal serum calcium concentration, a decreased serum phosphorus level secondary to renal phosphate wasting, and normal parathyroid function. In addition, the urinary calcium is decreased or low normal and the gastrointestinal absorption of calcium and phosphorus is mildly compromised. Affected children often manifest substantial elevations of alkaline phosphatase activity as well, whereas this variable is often, but not unvaryingly, normal in affected adults. In all forms of the disease, the serum 25(OH)D concentration remains normal, heralding the absence of vitamin D deficiency. However, secondary to an aberration of vitamin D metabolism, the serum $1,25(OH)_2D$ level is often overtly decreased or inappropriately normal in the presence of hypophosphatemia. In contrast, rachitic/osteomalacic disease due to nutritional phosphate deficiency, X-linked recessive hypophosphatemia, or hypophosphatemic rickets with hypercalciuria occurs despite an elevated serum calcitriol level.

Because secondary hyperparathyroidism is not a part of the phosphopenic rachitic/osteomalacic disorders, the radiographic abnormalities and bone histomorphometry of these diseases are distinctly different than those of the calciopenic diseases. In this regard, while aberrant mineralization of cartilage in X-linked hypophosphatemia is marked by widening of the growth plate and diminished calcification of the metaphysis, the metaphyseal margin is more distinct than it is in vitamin D deficiency rickets and there is less expansion in the width of the metaphysis. Indeed, in some cases rachitic changes are not radiographically apparent [34]. In concert, bone X-rays generally display decreased bone density, but there is no subperiosteal resorption or bone cysts. In addition, patients with phosphopenic disorders of long duration often display Looser's zones in sites different than those affected in calciopenic diseases. Most commonly such defects are present in the outer cortex of the bowed femur but they may occur along the medial cortex of the shaft. However, Looser's zones in the ribs and pelvis are rare. While these pseudofractures may heal with appropriate treatment, as they do in vitamin D deficiency, often long-term defects persist despite therapy, due most likely to fibrous tissue deposition. In any case, although untreated patients with phosphopenic disease consistently demonstrate these radiographic abnormalities, which are distinctly different from those encountered in calciopenic rickets/osteomalacia, long-term treatment with large doses of phosphate, alone or in combination with vitamin D or calcitriol, may induce secondary hyperparathyroidism. Under these circumstances, the X-ray picture of incompletely healed rickets/osteomalacia may be confused by subperiosteal erosions in the hand [35].

Genetic phosphopenic disorders such as X-linked hypophosphatemia also manifest a variety of unique radiographic findings. Although there is defective mineralization of osteoid in this disease, the long-term accumulation of unmineralized tissue on bone surfaces (and the absence of secondary hyperparathyroidism) results in increased bone mass and, commonly, a paradoxically increased bone density with a coarse and prominent trabecular pattern [36]. This appearance is not related to treatment and is most evident in the axial skeleton. Additionally, in this disease, the bones display developmental abnormalities such as decreased length and widening of the shafts in long bones.

The histologic appearance of trabecular bone in children and adults with phosphopenic disease reflects the presence of a low turnover osteomalacia [37–41]. In this regard, patients with X-linked hypophosphatemia have bone biopsies that display a marked reduction in the osteoblastic calcification rate, which results in prolongation of the mineralization lag time and increased duration of the formation period. In addition, a severe reduction of the extent of osteoid with osteoblasts and of the tetracycline double-labeled areas shows that the number of active bone-forming centers is decreased, indicating that the birth rate of new bone metabolic units is profoundly depressed in the trabecular bone envelope. In contrast, the osteoclastic surface and the osteoclast number are normal or slightly increased, but this likely relects a prolongation of the resorption period rather than an increase in osteoclastic activity. Indeed, the normal to increased calcified bone volume present in affected patients indicates that the observed low bone formation rate is associated with an even more reduced rate of bone resorption. Hence, with a normal to increased extent of osteoclastic surface, the duration of the resorption phase must be as prolonged as the formation phase in order to maintain reasonably normal bone volume. A similar histomorphometric appearance characterizes the bone biopsies in a majority of patients with tumor-induced osteomalacia [42, 43]. However, a few patients with this syndrome have tumors that secrete a nonparathyroid hormone factor(s) which activates adenylate cyclase, increases urinary cyclic AMP, and increases bone turnover, resulting in changes similar to those encountered due to secondary hyperparathyroidism [44–46]. Similarly, patients with acquired forms of the phosphopenic rickets/osteomalacia, such as those with Fanconi's syndrome, may exhibit increased bone resorption on bone biopsy; in this case it is secondary to moderate renal failure, which may be part of their primary disease [47].

B. Markers of Bone Resorption

Available data regarding bone markers in the phosphopenic disorders are remarkably sparse. However, for the majority of these diseases, the expected levels of the various markers seem reasonably predictable. In this regard, the normal or decreased bone turnover reflected both in roentgenograms of affected patients and in histomorphometric analysis of bone biopsies suggests that serum and urine markers of bone resorption should be normal or mildly decreased. Measurement of urinary hydroxyproline excretion in children and adults with X-linked hypophosphatemia and tumor-induced osteomalacia confirms this expectation [M. K. Drezner, unpublished observations]. However, sensitivity of this variable as a marker of bone resorption is limited. Similar assessment of urinary pyridinoline and deoxypyridinoline cross-links likewise reveals normal values [unpublished observations]. However, data using assays for serum ICTP and TRAP are not available.

In a small subset of patients with phosphopenic disease, evidence of increased bone turnover is expected. Shane et al. [44] have reported frankly elevated pyridinium cross-link excretion in a patient with tumor-induced osteomalacia secondary to a nonparathyroid hormone factor which increases urinary cyclic AMP excretion. Similar data are expected, but not available, in three other patients with this disease and coincident elevation of urinary cyclic AMP [45, 46]; one patient has coexistent hyperparathyroidism [48]. The presence of secondary hyperparathyroidism in patients with renal failure and various forms of Fanconi's syndrome would likewise predispose researchers to expect evidence of increased bone resorption and, consequently, elevated urinary levels of markers such as hydroxyproline and pyridinoline cross-links. Somewhat surprisingly, a similar increment in indices of bone resorption is not expected in patients with hereditary hypophosphatemic rickets with hypercalciuria. In these patients, who have significantly elevated serum $1,25(OH)_2D$ levels, increased osteoclast activity secondary to the effects of the circulating calcitriol seems reasonable. However, extensive histomorphometric analysis of bone biopsies in affected patients clearly documents normal osteoclast activity, possibly because of the counter-balancing effects of suppressed parathyroid function [49].

Documentation of normal bone turnover in the majority of patients with phosphopenic rickets/osteomalacia provides a valuable diagnostic tool in establishing the presence of such a disorder. Hypophosphatemia is a common abnormality in patients with calciopenic and phosphopenic disease, whereas a calcium abnormality is often marginal in vitamin D deficient disorders. Hence, the ability to detect normal bone resorption may support the diagnostic impression of a phosphopenic disease. Alternatively, the rare variant of increased bone turnover in a phosphopenic disorder may direct study of patients and lead to diagnosis of tumor-induced osteomalacia and/or lead to the discovery of paraneoplastic factors with the potential to increase bone turnover and impact renal function through parathyroid hormone receptors.

C. Markers of Bone Formation

The expected levels of bone markers reflecting bone formation in the phosphopenic diseases is decidedly less certain than levels expected for bone resorption. While the rate of bone formation seems undeniably decreased upon histomorphometric exam of bone biopsies of affected patients, several factors preclude the certainty that appropriate markers will mirror this status. The presence of decreased bone turnover should result in decreased/normal serum levels of PICP and PINP, markers of collagen deposition. However, the potential that insufficient mineralization of bone matrix may increase the turnover of collagen [50] raises the possibility that these markers may be elevated in the phosphopenic disorders. While data are not available in untreated patients to substantiate such an elevation, Saggese *et al.* [51] reported an approximately five-fold elevation in PICP in patients with active rachitic/osteomalacic disease despite treatment with calcitriol and phosphorus. While this may have reflected a relatively enhanced bone formation secondary to the combination therapy in use, this seems unlikely because poor mineralization of bone matrix persisted. Nevertheless, further data are clearly necessary to substantiate that PINP and PICP are elevated in these diseases.

In contrast, the limited data available regarding another measure of collagen turnover (serum PIIINP levels) and hence potentially of bone formation, indicate a significant reduction

of this marker in patients with X-linked hypophosphatemia [49]. This aminoterminal propeptide of type II procollagen, however, is released by soft connective tissue and may reflect information about somatic growth, most particularly growth rate [50]. Thus, the depressed level observed in youths with X-linked hypophosphatemia might not represent a decreased bone formation rate but rather it might mark the poor growth of the affected patients.

Limited data are available regarding serum osteocalcin levels in untreated patients with phosphopenic disease. However, in a limited number of children with X-linked hypophosphatemia, Whyte [personal communication] has found normal serum calcitonin, consistent with the poor mineralization and the normal to decreased bone formation rate associated with this disease. Regulation of osteocalcin in X-linked hypophosphatemia, however, is a matter of debate. In *hyp-*mice, the murine homologue of the human disorder, serum osteocalcin levels are invariably elevated and are inappropriately decreased in response to $1,25(OH)_2D$ administration [52]. While these findings suggest that osteoblastic activity in this mutation is abnormal, the absence of a similar marker of osteoblast dysfunction in affected humans remains poorly understood.

The effects of treatment on expression of these bone markers in patients with phosphopenic disease are unknown. Traditional therapy includes use of oral phosphate supplements and calcitriol. A common complication is secondary hyperparathyroidism, which is likely due to phosphate-mediated transient reductions in the serum calcium concentration. The occurrence of this abnormality, however, depends on whether the calcitriol administered is sufficient to suppress parathyroid function and/or maintain the serum calcium levels. In any case, the hyperparathyroidism, when present, is generally expressed as a biochemical phenomenon manifest by an elevated concentration of parathyroid hormone without hypercalcemia. Moreover, bone biopsies from such affected patients do not exhibit overt evidence of increased bone turnover. Thus, it is difficult to predict if therapy will reveal evidence of increased bone resorption. Nevertheless, future studies to determine this possibility are extremely important because they will provide important information regarding the potential negative impact of the traditional therapeutic intervention.

Similar confusion surrounds the effects of therapy on bone formation markers. In fact, the increased circulating level of $1,25(OH)_2D$, which occurs upon treatment, adds further doubt to the potential alterations in these markers, since osteocalcin may increase in response to such a stimulus. In any case, identification of the panorama of changes in bone markers that do occur upon successful therapy for phosphopenic rickets/osteomalacia is evidently of considerable importance because it will provide a relatively noninvasive means to judge therapeutic efficacy in diseases which generally are remarkably refractory to treatment.

VI. NORMAL MINERAL RICKETS AND OSTEOMALACIA

A. General Features

Rickets and osteomalacia occur infrequently in the absence of a reduced serum calcium and/or phosphorus concentration. Typically, abnormal mineralization in these disorders is due to an intrinsic bone defect (in which apparently abnormal matrix is produced) or to a circulating inhibitor of mineralization. Matrix abnormalities result from production of disordered collagen or other proteins in the matrix or expression of enzyme activity aberrant from that essential for normal mineralization. Fibrogenesis imperfecta ossium and axial osteomalacia are examples of diseases marked by abnormal collagen production (Table I). The former is a rare, sporadically occurring disorder characterized by the gradual onset of intractable skeletal pain in middle-aged men and women. Pathologic fractures are a prominent clinical feature, and patients typically become bedridden. Although the serum calcium and phosphorus levels are normal, alkaline phosphatase is invariably elevated. The bones have a dense, amorphous, mottled appearance radiologically and a disorganized arrangement of collagen with decreased birefringence histologically. Biopsy sections reveal no evidence of increased bone resorption.

Axial osteomalacia generally affects only middle-aged men and the majority of patients present with vague, dull, chronic axial discomfort that usually affects the cervical region most severely. Abnormal radiographic findings are limited to the pelvis and spine, where the coarsened trabecular pattern is characteristic of osteomalacia. Although the alkaline phosphatase level may be increased, histopathologic studies reveal a normal lamellar pattern of collagen and no increased resorption. However, the osteoblasts appear flat and inactive, suggesting that an osteoblastic defect and perhaps attendant abnormal matrix inhibit normal mineralization.

Hypophosphatasia is an inheritable disorder in which a deficiency of the tissue nonspecific (liver/bone/kidney) isoenzyme of alkaline phosphatase results in the mineralization defect characteristic of rickets and osteomalacia. The severity of clinical expression is remarkably variable and spans intrauterine death from profound skeletal hypomineralization at one extreme to lifelong absence of symptoms at the other. As a consequence, six clinical disease types are distinguished (Table I). The age at which skeletal disease is initially noted delineates, in large part, the perinatal (lethal), infantile, childhood, and adult variants of the disorder. However, affected children and adults may manifest only the unique dental abnormalities of the syndrome and accordingly are classified as having odontohypophosphatasia. Finally, patients with the rare variant, pseudohypophosphatasia, have the clinical/radiologic/biochemical features of the classic disease without a decrease in the circulating levels of alkaline phosphatase. These individuals have defects in cellular localization and substrate specificity of the enzyme. Affected infants exhibit hypercalcemia, hypercalciuria, and often hyperphosphatemia, as well as enlarged sutures of the skull, craniostenosis, delayed dentition, enlarged epiphyses, and prominent costochondral junctions. Genu valgum or varum may develop subsequently. In older children, disease may be limited to rickets. Surprisingly, the disorder in adults is mild despite the presence of osteopenia. Nevertheless, 50% of patients have a history of early exfoliation of deciduous teeth and/or rickets. The physiologic basis for the bone disease likely relates to the role of alkaline phosphatase in cleaving pyrophosphate, an inhibitor of bone mineralization. Failure to hydrolyze this physiologic substrate results in inorganic pyrophosphate elevated to levels sufficiently high to inhibit the mineralization process. The consequence of this pathophysiological process is a block of the vectorial spread of mineral from initial nuclei within matrix vesicles outwards into the matrix of growth cartilage and bone. However, bone histomorphometry reveals no evidence of abnormal resorption or formation.

Among the circulating inhibitors of bone mineralization responsible for rickets/osteomalacia are bisphosphonates, fluoride, and aluminum. The bone diseases that result from exposure to these agents are highly variable, reflecting decreased resorption and formation secondary to aluminum and increased formation due to fluoride. The serum calcium and phosphorus are routinely normal, but the alkaline phosphatase is invariably elevated.

B. Markers of Bone Turnover

Because the majority of rachitic/osteomalacic disorders that occur without a reduced serum calcium or phosphorus concentration are marked by normal rates of bone turnover, investigators anticipate that markers of bone resorption and formation will fluctuate in the normal range. Thus, such tests can serve as supportive in efforts to ascertain the cause of a bone mineralization disorder. However, virtually no data are available to support such anticipation. Indeed, in select forms of normal mineral rickets/osteomalacia, abnormalities occur which may variably influence bone marker levels. For example, the hypercalcemia often seen in children with hypophosphatasia may suppress parathyroid hormone secretion and decrease bone resorption, thereby depressing levels of urinary pyridinoline cross-links. Similarly, aluminum sequestration in parathyroid glands may limit parathyroid hormone secretion, and effects on osteoblasts reduce collagen production. The net effect is likely the low turnover osteomalacia characteristically associated with aluminum exposure. Under such conditions, profound decreases in markers of resorption and formation are anticipated, provided that the often associated renal failure does not influence serum levels of these measures. In contrast, osteomalacia secondary to fluoride ingestion is marked by increased osteoblast activity. Thus, the possibility of increased levels of PINP and PICP are likely, correlating with enhanced incorporation of collagen into the bone matrix. However, the attendant defective mineralization may result in depressed serum osteocalcin levels, similar to that seen in calciopenic disorders in particular. The current availability of measurement for the bone markers should provide valuable tools to better understand the heterogeneous group of disorders that comprise the normal mineral rachitic and osteomalacic disorders.

References

1. Park, E. A. (1939). Observations on the pathology of rickets with particular reference to the changes at the cartilage-shaft junctions of the growing bones. *Bull. N. Y. Acad. Med.* **15**, 495–543.

2. Baylink, D., Stauffer, M., Wergedal, J., and Rich, C. (1970). Formation, mineralization and resorption of bone in vitamin D-deficient rats. *J. Clin. Invest.* **49**, 1122–1134.

3. Stanbury, S. W., and Mawer, E. B. (1990). Metabolic disturbances in acquired osteomalacia. *In* "The Metabolic and Molecular Basis of Acquired Disease" (R. D. Cohen, B. Lewis, K. G. M. M. Alberti, and A. M. Denman, eds.), pp. 1717–1782. Baillière Tindall, London.

4. Rao, D. S., Villanueva, A., Mathews, M., Bumo, B., Frame, B., Kleerekoper, M., and Parfitt, A. M. (1983). Histologic evolution of vitamin depletion in patients with intestinal malabsorption or dietary deficiency. *In* "Clinical Disorders of Bone and Mineral Metabolism" (B. Frame and J. T. Potts, eds.), pp. 224–226. Excerpta Medica, Amsterdam.

5. Fraser, D., Kooh, S. W., Kind, H. O., Holick, M. F., Tanaka, Y., and DeLuca, H. F. (1973). Pathogenesis of hereditary vitamin D dependent rickets: An inborn error of vitamin D metabolism involving defective conversion of 25-hydroxyvitamin D to 1,25-dihydroxyvitamin D. *N. Engl. J. Med.* **289**, 817–822.

6. Marx, S. J., Liberman, U. A., Eil, C., Gamblin, G. T., DeGrange, D. A., and Balsan, S. (1984). Hereditary resistance to 1,25-dihydroxyvitamin D. *Recent Prog. Horm. Res.* **40**, 589–620.

7. Robey, P. G., and Boskey, A. L. (1996). The biochemistry of bone. *In* "Osteoporosis" (R. Marcus, D. Feldman, and J. Kelsey, eds.), pp. 95–183. Academic Press, San Diego, CA.

8. Glimcher, M. J. (1992). The nature of the mineral component of bone and the mechanism of calcification. *In* "Disorders of Bone and Mineral Metabolism" (F. L. Coe and M. J. Favus, eds.), pp. 265–286. Raven Press, New York.

9. Neuman, W. F. (1980). Bone material and calcification mechanisms. *In* "Fundamental and Clinical Bone Physiology" (M. R. Urist, ed), pp. 83–107. Lippincott, Philadelphia.

10. Christoffersen, J., and Landis, W. J. (1991). A contribution with review to the description of mineralization of bone and other calcified tissues *in vivo. Anat. Rec.* **230**, 435–450.

11. Thorngren, K. G., Hansson, L. I., Menander-Sellman, K., and Stenstrom, A. (1973). Effect of hypophysectomy on longitudinal bone growth in the rat. *Calcif. Tissue Res.* **11**, 281–300.

12. Caplan, A. I., and Boyan, B. D. (1994). Endochondral bone formation: The lineage cascade. *In* "Bone: A Treatise" (B. K. Hall, ed.), Vol. 8, pp. 1–46. CRC Press, Boca Raton, FL.

13. Boskey, A. L. (1990). Mineral-matrix interactions in bone and cartilage. *Clin. Orthop. Relat. Res.* **281**, 244–274.

14. Parfitt, A. M. (1997). Vitamin D and the pathogenesis of rickets and osteomalacia. *In* "Vitamin D" (D. Feldman, F. H. Glorieux, and J. W. Pike, eds.), pp. 645–662. Academic Press, San Diego, CA.

15. Rudolf, M., Arulanantham, K., and Greenstein, R. M. (1980). Unsuspected nutritional rickets. *Pediatrics* **66**, 72–76.

16. Edidin, D. V., Levitsky, L. L., Schey, W., Dumbuvic, N., and Campos, A. (1980). Resurgence of nutritional rickets associated with breastfeeding and special dietary practices. *Pediatrics* **65**, 232–235.

17. Bachrach, S., Fisher, J., and Parks, J. S. (1979). An outbreak of vitamin D deficiency rickets in a susceptible population. *Pediatrics* **64**, 871–877.

18. Bonnici, F. (1978). Functional hypoparathyroidism in infantile hypocalcaemic stage I vitamin D deficiency rickets. *S. Afr. Med. J.* **54**, 611–612.

19. Buchanan, N., Pettifor, J. M., Cane, R. D., and Bill, P. L. A. (1978). Infantile apnoea due to profound hypocalcaemia associate with vitamin D deficiency. *S. Afr. Med. J.* **54**, 766–767.

20. Schott, G. D., and Wills, M. R. (1976). Muscle weakness in osteomalacia. *Lancet* **1**, 626–629.

21. Kruse, K. (1995). Pathophysiology of calcium metabolism in children with vitamin D-deficiency rickets. *J. Pediatr.* **126**, 736–741.

22. Delmas, P. D. (1990). Biochemical markers of bone turnover for the clinical assessment of metabolic disease. *Endocrinol. Metab. Clin. North Am.* **19**, 1–18.

23. Eastell, R., Hampton, L., Colwell, A., Green, J. R., Assiri, A. M. A., Hesp, R., Russell, R. G. G., and Reeve, J. (1990). Urinary collagen crosslinks are highly correlated with radioisotopic measurement of bone resorption. *In* "Osteoporosis 1990," Vol. 2, (C. Christiansen and K. Overqaard, eds.), pp. 469–470. Osteopress, Aalborg, Denmark.

24. Delmas, P. D., Schenmer, A., Gineyts, E., Riis, B., and Christiansen, C. (1991). Urinary excretion of pyridinoline crosslinks correlates with bone turnover measured on iliac crest biopsy in patients with vertebral osteoporosis. *J. Bone Miner. Res.* **6**, 639–644.

25. Robins, S. P., Black, D., Paterson, C. R., Reid, D. M., Duncan, A., and Seibel, M. J. (1991). Evaluation of urinary hydroxypyridinium crosslink measurements as resorption markers in metabolic bone disease. *Eur. J. Clin. Invest.* **21**, 310–315.

26. Scariano, J. K., Walter, E. A., Glew, R. H., Hollis, B. W., Henry, A., Ocheke, I., and Isichei, C. O. (1995). Serum levels of the pyridinoline crosslinked carboxyterminal telopeptide of type I collagen (ICTP) and osteocalcin in rachitic children in Nigeria. *Clin. Biochem.* **28**, 541–545.

27. Sharp, C. A., Oginni, L. M., Worsfold, M., Oyelami, O. A., Risteli, L., Risteli, J., and Davie, M. W. J. (1997). Elevated collagen turnover in Nigerian children with calcium-deficiency rickets. *Calcif. Tissue Int.* **61**, 87–94.

28. Saggese, G., Bertelloni, S., Baroncelli, G. I., and Di Nero, G. (1992). Serum levels of carboxyterminal propeptide of type I procollagen in healthy children from 1st year of life to adulthood and in metabolic bone diseases. *Eur. J. Pediatr.* **151**, 764–768.

29. Li, F., Iqbal, J., Wassif, W., Kaddam, I., and Moniz, C. (1994). Carboxyterminal propeptide of type I procollagen in osteomalacia. *Calcif. Tissue Int.* **55**, 90–93.

30. Abitbol, V., Roux, C., Chaussade, S., Guillemant, S., Kolta, S., Dougados, M., Couturier, D., and Amor, B. (1995). Metabolic bone assessment in patients with inflammatory bowel disease. *Gastroenterology* **108**, 417–422.

31. Price, P. A. (1983). The osteoblast. *In* "Primer on the Metabolic Bone Diseases and Disorders of Mineral Metabolism" (M. J. Favus, ed.), pp. 15–21. Princeton University, Princeton, NJ.

32. Heinrichs, A. A. J., Bortell, R., Bourke, M., Lian, J. B., Stein, G. S., and Stein, J. L. (1995). Proximal promoter binding protein contributes to developmental tissue-restricted expression of the rat osteocalcin gene. *J. Cell. Biochem.* **57**, 90–100.

33. Delmas, P. D. (1990). Biochemical markers of bone turnover for the clinical assessment of metabolic bone disease. *In* "Metabolic Bone Disease (R. D. Tiegs, ed.), Part 2, pp. 1–8, Saunders, Philadelphia.

34. Econs, M. J., Samsa, G. P., Monger, M., Drezner, M. K., and Feussner, J. R. (1994). X-linked hypophosphatemic rickets: A disease often unknown to affected patients. *Bone Miner.* **24**, 17–24.

35. Steinbach, H. L., Kolb, F. O., and Crane, J. T. (1959). Unusual roentgen manifestations of osteomalacia. *Am. J. Roentgenol.* **82**, 875–886.

36. Rivkees, S. A., el-Hajj-Fuleihan, G., Brown, E. M., and Crawford, J. D. (1992). Tertiary hyperparathyroidism during high phosphate therapy of familial hypophosphatemic rickets. *J. Clin. Endocrinol. Metab.* **76**, 1514–1518.

37. Marie, P. J., and Glorieux, F. H. (1982). Bone histomorphometry in asymptomatic adults with hereditary hypophosphatemic vitamin D-resistant osteomalacia. *Metab. Bone Dis. Relat. Res.* **4**, 249–253.

38. Lyles, K. W., Burkes, E. J., Jr., McNamara, C. R., Harrelson, J. M., Pickett, J. P., and Drezner, M. K. (1985). The concurrence of hypoparathyroidism provides new insights to the pathophysiology of X-linked hypophosphatemic rickets. *J. Clin. Endocrinol. Metab.* **60**, 711–717.

39. Drezner, M. K., Lyles, K. W., and Harrelson, J. M. (1980). Vitamin D resistant osteomalacia: Evaluation of vitamin D metabolism and response to therapy. *In* "Hormonal Control of Calcium Metabolism" (D. V. Choh, R. V. Talmage, and J. L. Matthews, eds.), pp. 243–251. Excerpta Medica, Amsterdam.

40. Lyles, K. W., Harrelson, J. M., and Drezner, M. K. (1982). The efficacy of vitamin D_2 and oral phosphorus therapy in X-linked hypophosphatemic rickets and osteomalacia. *J. Clin. Endocrinol. Metab.* **54**, 307–315.

41. Drezner, M. K., Lyles, K. W., Haussler, M. R., and Harrelson, J. M. (1980). Evaluation of a role for 1,25-dihydroxyvitamin D_3 in the pathogenesis and treatment of X-linked hypophosphatemic rickets and osteomalacia. *J. Clin. Invest.* **66**, 1020–1032.

42. Drezner, M. K. and Feinglos, M. N. (1977). Osteomalacia due to 1,25-dihydroxycholecalciferol deficiency: Association with a giant cell tumor of bone. *J. Clin. Invest.* **60**, 1046–1053.

43. Lyles, K. W., Berry, W. R., Haussler, M., Harrelson, J. M., and Drezner, M. K. (1980). Hypophosphatemic osteomalacia: Association with prostatic carcinoma. *Ann. Intern. Med.* **93**, 275–278.

44. Shane, E., Parisien, M., Henderson, J. E., Dempster, D. W., Feldman, F., Hardy, M. A., Tohme, J. F., Karaplis, A. C., and Clemens, T. L. (1997). Tumor-induced osteomalacia: Clinical and basis studies. *J. Bone Miner. Res.* **12**, 1502–1511.

45. Miller, M. J., Marel, G., and Frame, B. (1982). Adult acquired vitamin D and PTH-resistant hypophosphatemic osteomalacia with multiple skeletal lesions. *In* "Vitamin D-Chemical, Biochemical and Clinical Endocrinology of Calcium Metabolism" (A. W. Norman, K. Schaefer, D. V. Herrath, and H. G. Grigoleit, eds.), pp. 993–995. de Gruyter, New York.

46. Leicht, E., Biro, G., and Langer, H.-J. (1990). Tumor-induced osteomalacia: Pre- and post-operative biochemical findings. *Horm. Metab. Res.* **22**, 640–643.

47. Clarke, B. L., Wynne, A. G., Wilson, D. M., and Fitzpatrick, L. A. (1995). Osteomalacia associated with adult Fanconi's syndrome: Clinical and diagnostic features. *Clin. Endocrinol.* **43**, 479–490.

48. Reid, I. R., Teitelbaum, S. L., Dusso, A., and Whyte, M. P. (1987). Hypercalcemic hyperparathyroidism complicating oncogenic osteomalacia: Effect of successful tumor resection on mineral homeostasis. *Am. J. Med.* **83**, 350–354.

49. Gazit, D., Tieder, M., Liberman, U. A., Passi-Even, L., and Bab, I. A. (1991). Osteomalacia in hereditary hypophosphatemic rickets with hypercalciuria: A correlative clinical-histomorphometric study. *J. Clin. Endocrinol. Metab.* **71**, 229–235.

50. Saggese, G., Baroncelli, G. I., Bertelloni, S., and Perri, G. (1995). Long-term growth hormone treatment in children with renal hypophosphatemic rickets: Effects on growth, mineral metabolism and bone density. *J. Pediatr.* **127**, 395–402.

51. Saggese, G., Baroncelli, G. I., Bertelloni, S., Cinquanta, L., and Di Nero, G. (1994). Twenty-four-hour osteocalcin, carboxyterminal propeptide of type I procollagen and aminoterminal propeptide of type III procollagen rhythms in normal and in growth retarded children. *Pediatr. Res.* **35**, 409–415.

52. Gundberg, C. M., Clough, M. E., and Carpenter, T. O. (1992). Development and validation of a radioimmunoassay for mouse osteocalcin: Paradoxical response in the *hyp*-mouse. *Endocrinology* **130**, 1909–1915.

CHAPTER 39

Assessment of Bone and Joint Diseases: Renal Osteodystrophy

ESTHER A. GONZÁLEZ AND KEVIN J. MARTIN

Division of Nephrology, Saint Louis University School of Medicine, St. Louis, Missouri 63110

I. INTRODUCTION

The majority of patients with end-stage renal disease (ESRD) have abnormal bone histology. These skeletal abnormalities, generically termed renal osteodystrophy, encompass the manifestations of hyperparathyroidism on bone (osteitis fibrosa), a disorder of low bone turnover (adynamic bone), abnormalities of bone mineralization (osteomalacia), and combinations of these abnormalities (mixed renal osteodystrophy), together with the accumulation of retained ions such as aluminum, iron, cadmium, oxalate, as well as the deposition of proteins such as β_2 microglobulin [1]. It is also important to consider that the final manifestations in bone may be tempered by prior therapy for specific renal diseases (e.g., corticosteroids), inactivity as a consequence of chronic renal disease, ovarian failure (either due to drug therapy or uremia), as well as advancing age. These confounding factors may complicate the final pattern of bone histology and, in addition, may influence the changes over time and the responses to therapeutic interventions. The spectrum of histologic abnormalities found in patients with chronic renal failure is,

therefore, broad and is generally classified according to the major abnormalities seen on bone histology [2, 3]. The prevalence of the various types of renal osteodystrophy found in patients with end-stage renal failure is shown in Table I; the data are divided according to the type of dialysis therapy being administered. Thus, hyperparathyroid bone disease is the most common abnormality in patients on hemodialysis whereas the adynamic bone lesion is the most common finding in patients on peritoneal dialysis. Some patients have mixed patterns of bone histology that are intermediate between these two extremes, and some have only mild abnormalities [2].

Abnormalities in bone histology occur early in the course of renal insufficiency [4]. The earliest findings are those of hyperparathyroid bone disease resulting from high levels of parathyroid hormone in serum, which arise as a consequence of phosphate retention and decreased calcitriol production by the diseased kidney [5]. As renal disease progresses, other factors such as hypocalcemia, acidosis, intrinsic alterations of parathyroid function, and skeletal resistance to the actions of PTH all contribute to aggravate the hypersecretion of parathyroid hormone [6]. The finding of osteomalacia is a

TABLE I. Prevalence of Renal Osteodystrophy
in Patients with End Stage Renal
Disease (ESRD)

	Hemodialysis	Peritoneal dialysis
Osteitis fibrosa	38	9
Adynamic	36	60
Mixed ROD	11	4
Osteomalacia	2	6
Mild/Normal	13	21

The numbers shown represent the percentage of patients with each type of renal osteodystrophy according to dialysis modality. There were 117 patients in the hemodialysis group and 142 in the peritoneal dialysis group. Modified from Sherrard *et al.* [2].

diminishing feature of skeletal disease in chronic renal failure [7] and, when present, it is usually accompanied by the accumulation of aluminum at the mineralization front [8, 9]. The major sources of aluminum in this setting include the water used for hemodialysis and the administration of aluminum containing phosphate binders which may be used in the treatment of secondary hyperparathyroidism. With careful monitoring of the water and the use of alternative phosphate binders, aluminum-induced osteomalacia is becoming less of a problem [7]. The pathogenesis of adynamic bone disease, which is being increasingly recognized, remains unclear [10, 11]. It may be the result of over-aggressive therapy for hyperparathyroidism in some cases, but it could also represent the accumulation of inhibitors of osteoblast function occurring as a consequence of renal failure or a deficiency of stimulators of osteoblast growth or differentiation.

The symptoms and signs of renal osteodystrophy are generally vague and nonspecific (Table II). Bone pain, often presenting as vague aches particularly in the feet and legs, is common. Muscular aches and muscle weakness are also very common complaints. Occasional spontaneous fractures can

TABLE II. Clinical Features of
Renal Osteodystrophy

Bone pain

Fractures

Skeletal deformities

Growth retardation

Muscle weakness

Extraskeletal calcifications

Pruritus

Periarthritis

Spondyloarthropathy

occur, particularly in the ribs, as a result of minimal trauma or coughing. Additional manifestations include skeletal deformities, particularly in children who also demonstrate impaired growth, pruritus, joint pains, carpel tunnel syndrome, and occasional extraskeletal calcifications.

Because of the nonspecific nature of the symptoms, it becomes important to utilize biochemical and radiological diagnostic techniques to clarify or to confirm the precise diagnosis, and to serve as a guide for administration of specific therapy. The overall framework for the assessment of the factors involved in renal osteodystrophy is depicted in Figure 1. Thus, in the setting of renal failure, a series of events takes place, the most important being phosphorus retention and calcitriol deficiency, which lead to the development of hyperparathyroidism. The high levels of PTH serve to alter the cellular events involved in the process of skeletal remodeling with the resultant adverse consequences which lead to osteitis fibrosa. Osteitis fibrosa is characterized by an increase in bone remodeling, with increased osteoblast and osteoclast activities, and excess fibrous tissue deposition in the peritrabecular areas of the bone marrow. Accordingly, assessment of parathyroid activity is of paramount importance in the evaluation and therapy of renal osteodystrophy. PTH also regulates the serum concentrations of calcium and phosphorus, the disturbances of which may also provide information regarding PTH activity. Because PTH acts on osteoblast precursors as well as on mature osteoblasts, it would appear useful to measure parameters of osteoblast activity to assess the cellular consequences of the prevailing parathyroid activity. Thus, osteoblast markers such as alkaline phosphatase and osteocalcin are useful in this regard. In addition, osteoblast secretory products such as IL-6 and IL-11 produced in response to PTH interact with the osteoclast pathway to produce an increase in osteoclast number and activity and an increase in bone resorption. These intermediary substances may also be useful targets for measurement to gauge the cellular activity of the skeleton. Osteoclasts resorb bone and the products of resorption may be released into the circulation and provide an index of osteoclast activity. Likewise, other osteoclast markers such as tartrate resistant acid phosphatase (TRAP) may be released into the peripheral circulation where it can be measured. The histology may be modified by other systemic factors such as acidosis, which is common in advanced renal insufficiency and leads to mobilization of bone mineral as the hydrogen ion is buffered by bone carbonate. In addition, aluminum may accumulate at the mineralization front and impair mineralization. β_2-microglobulin may also accumulate in bones and joint ligaments. Assessment of the validity of these diagnostic aids requires relating the abnormalities to the "gold standard" for the diagnosis of renal osteodystrophy, which is the histologic examination of undecalcified sections of bone [12]. Bone biopsy is a minimally invasive technique that is not widely utilized in clinical practice; nonetheless, it is an important tool to demonstrate the validity of noninvasive

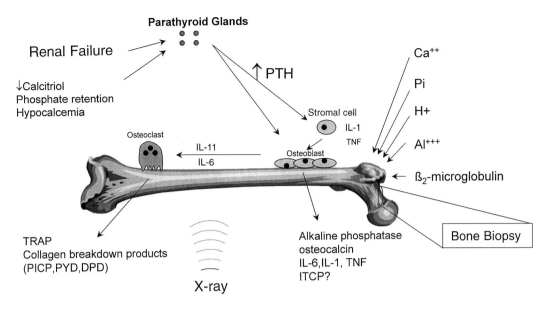

FIGURE 1   Diagrammatic representation of a framework for the assessment of the factors involved in renal osteodystrophy. See text for complete description.

diagnostic techniques and is essential in selected cases. Non-invasive radiographic techniques may also provide information with regard to the overall density and integrity of various parts of the skeleton.

II. BIOCHEMICAL ASSESSMENT OF RENAL OSTEODYSTROPHY

A. Measurements of Calcium and Phosphorus in Serum

Levels of serum calcium, particularly ionized calcium, are usually normal in mild to moderate renal insufficiency and tend to fall with advanced renal insufficiency; levels only decrease below the normal range in a minority of patients [13, 14]. The maintenance of normal values, during the course of renal insufficiency, is the result of compensatory secondary hyperparathyroidism. Decreases in total serum calcium are more common in patients with proteinuric renal diseases in whom hypoalbuminemia is present, but ionized calcium may be normal. The occurrence of frank hypocalcemia is even less common if calcium-containing antacids are used as phosphate binders; however, if hypocalcemia is present, it is a powerful stimulus for PTH secretion and should be corrected. Hypercalcemia is uncommon in mild or moderate renal failure but may occur in advanced renal failure or end stage renal disease. It may occur as a consequence of the ingestion of large amounts of calcium-containing antacids (used as phosphate binders), severe (tertiary) hyperparathyroidism, states of abnormally low bone turnover such as adynamic bone, or overtreatment with vitamin D or vitamin D analogs [1,

15, 16]. The diagnosis of the precise cause of hypercalcemia is extremely important because the therapy required differs greatly depending on the cause. Occasionally, hypercalcemia may be due to the overproduction of calcitriol or coexistent granulomatous diseases such as sarcoidosis or tuberculosis [17, 18].

The levels of serum phosphorus are usually normal or slightly decreased in early to moderate renal failure [13, 14]. Hyperphosphatemia does not become evident until renal function has declined to less than 20% of normal. Again, the maintenance of normal serum phosphorus concentration is due to the development of secondary hyperparathyroidism [19]. Efforts are usually made to prevent the development of hyperphosphatemia during the course of renal insufficiency by dietary phosphorus restriction and the use of phosphate-binding antacids. Hyperphosphatemia may aggravate hyperparathyroidism by decreasing the levels of ionized calcium, decreasing the production of calcitriol, and by a direct effect on the parathyroid gland to increase PTH secretion and regulate the growth of parathyroid cells [20–25]. Hyperphosphatemia is common when glomerular filtration rate (GFR) falls to very low levels unless treatment for hyperphosphatemia is pursued aggressively. In some instances, increased resorption of phosphorus from bone as a consequence of severe hyperparathyroidism may contribute to the development of hyperphosphatemia.

Apart from the frequent development of hypercalcemia (especially after the administration of low doses of calcitriol), which is suggestive of a low bone turnover syndrome, the levels of serum calcium do not have specific diagnostic value as to the precise nature of the underlying osteodystrophy. Likewise, measurements of serum phosphorus do not indicate specific abnormalities in bone histology. These measurements should be considered in conjunction with direct measurements of PTH.

B. Measurement of PTH

Because hyperparathyroidism is a major component of renal osteodystrophy, the accurate measurement of PTH in serum is important, not only as a diagnostic tool but also as a guide to therapy. Difficulties with different assays for PTH directed towards different regions of the PTH molecule, complicated by the dependance of the kidney for removal of hormone fragments from the circulation [26], have largely been obviated by the advent of two-site assays for intact PTH by immunoradiometric (IRMA) or immunochemiluminescence (ICMA) techniques [27, 28] (see also Chapter 26). Such assays give reliable information and can easily be compared from laboratory to laboratory. The use of such assays provides an accurate assessment of the current state of parathyroid activity and correlates well with the predominant type of osteodystrophy on bone histology, as illustrated in Figure 2. Thus, elevated PTH levels are the hallmark of osteitis fibrosa, whereas PTH values are much lower in the low bone turnover syndromes of adynamic bone or osteomalacia [29].

Hyperparathyroidism occurs early in the course of renal insufficiency, and PTH levels are often increased with histological evidence of hyperparathyroidism on bone. Precise guidelines for correlation of PTH levels with histological parameters of bone in early renal failure are relatively scarce, and most such correlations have been made in patients with end-stage renal disease. The correlations of PTH values with bone histology in patients with end-stage renal disease also have shown that there is a resistance of the skeleton to PTH in renal failure, because supranormal levels appear to be required to maintain bone turnover in the normal range [30, 31].

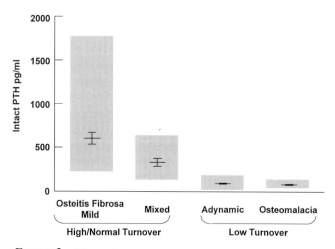

FIGURE 2   Diagnostic separation of the major types of renal bone disease by the measurement of intact PTH. Modified from Coburn and Salusky [29], with permission.

Thus, it has been found that PTH values of 2–3 times the upper limit of normal are necessary to achieve normal values for bone turnover. In view of these data, it is felt that values of intact PTH within 150 and 250 pg/ml are generally associated with normal bone turnover in patients with end-stage renal disease. The implications of these findings are that these values for PTH should be the target values to be achieved with therapy. Thus, values below this range are often associated with abnormally low bone turnover, and conversely, levels above this range are generally associated with histologic evidence of hyperparathyroidism. The correlations, however, are far from perfect, and other diagnostic tools, as well as the use of serial measurements of PTH, may be helpful in improving the diagnostic utility.

C. Measurement of Vitamin D Metabolites

Abnormalities of vitamin D metabolism play a major role in the development of secondary hyperparathyroidism characteristic of chronic renal disease [as a result of impaired production of calcitriol from the diseased kidney as renal mass decreases [32].] Accordingly, levels of calcitriol in blood progressively decline as renal function declines [14]. Levels are maintained within the normal range in mild to moderate renal insufficiency because high levels of PTH stimulate the production of calcitriol by the kidney. Thus, even normal levels of calcitriol could be considered inappropriately low for the prevailing levels of PTH. When GFR fall below 30% of normal, however, the reduction in renal mass limits the ability to produce sufficient amounts of calcitriol and, in spite of hyperparathyroidism, the levels of calcitriol in blood decline. Although the decrease in the levels of calcitriol is important as a pathogenetic factor for renal osteodystrophy, its measurement in chronic renal disease offers little diagnostically unless extrarenal production of calcitriol is suspected (e.g., in sarcoidosis).

Measurement of 25-hydroxyvitamin D provides the best index of vitamin D status and is useful if vitamin D deficiency is suspected (see also Chapter 26). During the course of renal failure, levels of this metabolite may decline, especially in proteinuric renal diseases, as a result of the loss of vitamin D binding protein in the urine. In certain circumstances, such as in patients who are malnourished, have intestinal disorders, or have little exposure to sunlight, vitamin D deficiency may occur. In general, vitamin D deficiency is felt to be a rare cause of osteomalacia in patients with renal failure in the United States.

D. Measurement of Serum Aluminum

Although the definitive diagnosis of aluminum-related osteodystrophy requires a bone biopsy, the use of noninvasive tests may be helpful in this regard. The measurement of basal serum aluminum levels is not a useful test in identifying patients with aluminum bone disease [33]. Increments in serum aluminum following the administration of the metal chelator deferoxamine (DFO) reflect total aluminum accumulation in the body and may be useful in evaluating the tissue burden of aluminum, however, such assays are not specific for bone [34]. The accuracy of this test in the diagnosis of aluminum bone disease increases when it is interpreted in conjunction with PTH values [35]. Thus, an increment in plasma aluminum of 150 μg/L following the administration of DFO in the presence of PTH values of less than 100 pg/ml is strongly suggestive of significant aluminum accumulation in bone. These criteria may require modification because the use of aluminum-containing antacids has markedly decreased. Bone biopsy and the use of specific staining are required to show the presence of aluminum at the mineralization front.

E. Measurements of Alkaline Phosphatase in Serum

Serum alkaline phosphatase is derived from intestine, liver, kidney, and bone (see also Chapter 27). Nevertheless, measurements of total alkaline phosphatase in blood provide an approximate index of osteoblast activity in patients with renal failure because elevations in alkaline phosphatase are often due to an increase in the bone isoenzyme (an index of osteoblast function) in cases of hyperparathyroidism. Conversely, alkaline phosphatase values tend to be reduced in cases of low bone turnover osteodystrophy [36]. Serial measurements of alkaline phosphatase activity in a given patient may provide useful information regarding the progression of skeletal disease as well as an index of response to therapy for hyperparathyroidism. Most studies of the correlation of alkaline phosphatase with PTH and parameters of bone histomorphometry show wide variation. For these reasons, as well as the prevalence of hepatic abnormalities in patients with renal failure, efforts have been made to develop specific measurements of the bone alkaline phosphatase isoenzyme with the hope of improving its diagnostic utility [37–39]. While such measurements eliminate the confusion with alkaline phosphatase from other tissues and show slightly better correlations with PTH and other parameters of bone histology than measurements of total alkaline phosphatase, they remain adjuncts to other parameters of skeletal metabolism. While elevated values are seen in states of high bone turnover, the inability to reliably distinguish normal from abnormally low bone turnover on an individual basis remains.

F. Measurements of Osteocalcin

Osteocalcin is a vitamin K-dependent protein produced by the osteoblast and, accordingly, is a potential marker of osteoblast activity (see also Chapter 27). Levels of osteocalcin may be elevated in patients with renal failure because of decreased renal clearance of the protein from the circulation. In spite of this, it has been suggested that osteocalcin might be a useful marker to separate patients with high bone turnover from those in whom bone turnover is abnormally low. In general, however, correlations of osteocalcin values with parameters of bone histomorphometry do not appear to be superior to measurements of bone alkaline phosphatase [40].

G. Other Markers of Bone Metabolism

There has been increasing interest in measurements of several new markers of bone metabolism, among which are markers of collagen synthesis (such as procollagen type IC-terminal extension peptide [PICP]) and markers of collagen degradation (such as collagen type IC-terminal cross-linked telopeptide [ICTP], pyridinoline [PYD], and deoxypyridinoline [DPD] cross-links) [40–42]. PICP is a 100 kDa glycoprotein procollagen cleavage product generated after secretion of procollagen by osteoblasts; an additional N-terminal peptide, PINP, is also liberated. In basal conditions, PICP in the circulation is mainly derived from bone and is metabolized by the liver; thus, its levels in serum are not directly influenced by the level of renal function (see also Chapter 27). ICTP is a 12 kDa peptide that is produced when collagen fibrils undergo degradation. PYD and DPD are also liberated as collagen is degraded. Due to their size, these substances are filtered by the kidney and excreted in the urine and would be expected to accumulate in serum when renal function is reduced (see also Chapters 2 and 28).

When these markers were studied in patients with renal osteodystrophy who were on dialysis, PICP did not correlate with histological evidence of bone formation. ICTP, PYD, and DPD all correlated with the other humoral markers, such as alkaline phosphatase, osteocalcin, and PTH [40]. At present, assays for these collagen synthesis and degradation products remain investigational, but they do not appear to offer any major advantage over the currently utilized markers of bone metabolism.

H. Cytokines

Cytokines and growth factors are important regulators of bone turnover and many are regulated by the major calciotropic hormones, PTH and calcitriol, and thus, derangements in uremia may affect the actions of these cytokines in bone [43] (see also Chapters 6 and 7). Chronic renal failure is associated with abnormalities in cytokine production. There is evidence for increased levels of IL-1, IL-6, and TNF-α, as well as other cytokines and growth factors, such as IGF-1 that may affect bone turnover [44–46]. In addition, the levels of cytokine antagonists and soluble receptors, such as IL-1 receptor antagonist and IL-6 soluble receptors, may also be elevated in uremia [47, 48]. Thus, the final effect of these factors in bone turnover represents an integration of the various components involved in the different systems. The role of cytokines in the pathogenesis of renal osteodystrophy is not clear at present. Ferreira *et al.* [47] found elevated levels of IL-1 and IL-1 receptor antagonist in patients on hemodialysis, and there was an inverse relationship between the plasma levels of IL-1 receptor antagonist and osteoblast surface. In the same study, elevated levels of IL-6 and IL-6 soluble receptors were found, and there was an inverse relationship between the levels of IL-6 receptor and osteoclast surface [47]. This study suggests that the relative imbalance between the different cytokine systems would influence the development of high versus low turnover bone disease. Studies by Langub *et al.* [49] have demonstrated the presence of IL-6 and IL-6 receptor mRNA *in vivo* using *in situ* hybridization in bone biopsies from patients with secondary hyperparathyroidism; the expression of IL-6 receptor paralleled bone resorbing activity. Levels of IGF-I have been found to correlate with bone formation rate in patients on hemodialysis [46]. Although considerable understanding of cytokines and growth factors in uremia has been gained their relationship with the different histologic types of renal osteodystrophy has not been well characterized. Further study will be required to define the roles of these factors in the skeletal abnormalities and to the define the utility of the assay for these mediators in serum for the diagnosis and management of renal bone disease.

I. β_2 Microglobulin

The syndrome of β_2 microglobin amyloidosis, characterized by carpal tunnel syndrome, destructive arthropathies, and juxta articular radiolucent cysts, is related to the accumulation of β_2 microglobulin due to impaired elimination of this protein by the diseased kidney. The manifestations of this disorder result from the deposition of β_2 microglobulin in the tissues in the form of amyloid fibrils [50]. However, measurements of the serum levels of β_2 microglobulin, although universally elevated in patients with advanced renal failure, do not correlate with the presence of amyloid deposits, and, therefore, are not clinically useful.

III. SKELETAL IMAGING IN RENAL OSTEODYSTROPHY

A. X-Ray

Subperiosteal erosions are the most consistent findings in secondary hyperparathyroidism. Radiographs, however, are quite insensitive and can appear virtually normal in patients who have histologic evidence of severe hyperparathyroidism on bone biopsy. The radiological features of secondary hyperparathyroidism are best detected on hand X-rays. The use of fine grain film and magnification techniques facilitates the detection of abnormalities [51]. Subperiosteal erosions may also be seen at the distal ends of the clavicles, the pelvis, and in the region of the sacroiliac joints. While subperiosteal erosions usually represent hyperparathyroidism, it is important to emphasize that the findings may not necessarily be current and may represent prior hyperparathyroidism that has now been replaced by osteomalacia, such as might occur with aluminum intoxication. Skull X-rays may show a ground glass appearance, focal radiolucencies, and areas of sclerosis. Patchy areas of osteosclerosis in the vertebrae lead to the characteristic appearance of the "rugger jersey spine." In children, there may be evidence of growth retardation and rickets. Cystic lesions and spondyloarthropathy may represent dialysis-related β_2 microglobulin amyloidosis [52, 53]. The presence of aluminum-related bone disease is suggested by the finding of Looser's zones, or pseudofractures.

B. Bone Scintiscans

Bone scanning using 99-technitium diphosphonate has been used to evaluate renal osteodystrophy and may also be used to assess the response to therapy [54–56]. Uptake of tracer tends to be diffusely increased in states of high bone turnover, such as in patients with hyperparathyroidism. Patients with low bone turnover and osteomalacia showed decreased uptake, with possible focal areas of increased activity representing microfractures. Ectopic calcification may also become apparent by bone scan. The sensitivity of bone scan studies to differentiate between the various kinds of renal osteodystrophy is not high and mixed renal osteodystrophy can not be identified.

C. Pet Scan

Efforts to characterize bone metabolic activity by positron emission tomography with ^{18}F have been described and appear capable of differentiating low bone turnover from high bone turnover lesions of renal osteodystrophy [57]. Excellent correlations of fluoride uptake with values of PTH and alkaline phosphatase were obtained. Although this technique has potential value for serial studies of bone metabolism, it is not widely utilized.

D. Measurement of Bone Density

While measurement of bone density has been shown to be a reliable indicator of fracture risk in patients without renal disease, the use of such techniques in patients with renal disease is less well defined. Single and dual photon absorptiometry have largely been replaced by dual energy X-ray absorptiometry (DEXA) [58]. Quantitative CT is less commonly used, although this technique can separate cortical from trabecular bone [11]. This method uses considerably more radiation than DEXA. Nonetheless, a noninvasive means of assessment of renal osteodystrophy, especially with regard to risk of fracture, would be extremely useful. Early studies of bone density, in general, showed that renal osteodystrophy was associated with a decrease in cortical bone. Axial bone mass measurements were more heterogeneous [37, 58, 59]. Some studies demonstrated a gradual loss or no bone loss overtime whereas other studies actually demonstrated a gain of bone. Other investigators found some patients who had a relatively rapid loss of bone. From the heterogeneity of bone histology, it is perhaps not surprising that a composite measurement of bone density would not have a specific diagnostic value in this patient population. In addition, there are many technical difficulties in this group of patients, because many may have vascular and ligament calcifications which may affect the results. Data on fracture risk in this patient population is limited and prospective data would be useful. Thus, the clinical utility of measurements of bone mineral density in renal osteodystrophy appears to be limited at the present time.

IV. SUMMARY

Renal osteodystrophy represents a complex disorder of bone metabolism resulting from the many derangements that occur during the course of chronic renal failure. The patterns of bone disease revealed by histological examination of bone lead to useful classifications of the disorder and provide specific diagnostic information. The many noninvasive tools that may be utilized for the assessment of bone metabolism are clinically useful when considered together, especially when serial measurements are available. An understanding of the pathogenesis of renal osteodystrophy and early therapy directed at these pathogenetic factors are important to minimize the significant morbidity that occurs as a result of this complication of chronic renal disease.

References

1. Llach, F., and Bover, J. (1996). Renal osteodystrophy. In "The Kidney" (B. Brenner, ed.), 5th ed., Vol. 2, pp. 2187–2273. Saunders, Philadelphia.
2. Sherrard, D. J., Hercz, G., Pei, Y., Maloney, N. A., Greenwood, C., Manuel, A., Saiphoo, C., Fenton, S. S., and Segré, G. V. (1993). The spectrum of bone disease in end-stage renal failure—an evolving disorder. Kidney Int. 43, 436–442.
3. Malluche, H., and Faugere, M. C. (1990). Renal bone disease 1990: An unmet challenge for the nephrologist. Kidney Int. 38, 193–211.
4. Malluche, H., Ritz, E., and Lange, H. (1976). Bone histology in incipient and advanced renal failure. Kidney Int. 9, 355–362.
5. Slatopolsky, E., and Delmez, J. A. (1994). Pathogenesis of secondary hyperparathyroidism. Am. J. Kidney Dis. 23, 229–236.
6. González, E., and Martin, K. (1995). Renal osteodystrophy: Pathogenesis and management. Nephrol. Dial. Transplant. 10 (Suppl. 3), 13–21.
7. González, E., and Martin, K. (1992). Aluminum and renal osteodystrophy: A diminishing clinical problem. Trends Endocrinol. Metab. 3, 371–375.
8. Goodman, W., Henry, D., Horst, R., Nudelman, R., Alfrey, A., and Coburn, J. (1984). Parenteral aluminum administration in the dog. II. Induction of osteomalacia and effect on vitamin D metabolism. Kidney Int. 25, 370–375.
9. Cournot-Witmer, G., Zingraff, J., Plachot, J. J., Escaig, F., Lefevre, R., Boumati, P., Bourdeau, A., Garabedian, M., Galle, P., Bourdon, R., Drueke, T., and Balsan, S. (1981). Aluminum localization in bone from hemodialyzed patients: Relationship to matrix mineralization. Kidney Int. 20, 375–378.
10. Hutchison, A. J., Whitehouse, R. W., Freemont, A. J., Adams, J. E., Mawer, E. B., and Gokal, R. (1994). Histological, radiological, and biochemical features of the adynamic bone lesion in continuous ambulatory peritoneal dialysis patients. Am. J. Nephrol. 14, 19–29.
11. Hutchison, A. J., Whitehouse, R. W., Boulton, H. F., Adams, J. E., Mawer, E. B., Freemont, T. J., and Gokal, R. (1993). Correlation of bone histology with parathyroid hormone, vitamin D3, and radiology in end-stage renal disease. Kidney Int. 44, 1071–1077.
12. Malluche, H., and Monier-Faugere, M. (1994). The role of bone biopsy in the management of patients with renal osteodystrophy. J. Am. Soc. Nephrol. 4, 1631–1642.
13. Kates, D., Sherrard, D., and Andress, D. (1997). Evidence that serum phosphate is independently associated with serum PTH in patients with chronic renal failure. Am. J. Kidney Dis. 30, 809–813.
14. Martinez, I., Saracho, R., Montenegro, J., and Llach, F. (1997). The importance of dietary calcium and phosphorous in the secondary hyperparathyroidism of patients with early renal failure. Am. J. Kidney Dis. 29, 496–502.
15. Hercz, G., Kraut, J. A., Andress, D. A., Howard, N., Roberts, C., Shinaberger, J. H., Sherrard, D. J., and Coburn, J. W. (1986). Use of calcium carbonate as a phosphate binder in dialysis patients. Miner. Electrolyte Metab. 12, 314–319.
16. Slatopolsky, E., Weerts, C., Lopez-Hilker, S., Norwood, K., Zink, M., Windus, D., and Delmez, J. (1986). Calcium carbonate as a phosphate binder in patients with chronic renal failure undergoing dialysis. N. Engl. J. Med. 315, 157–161.
17. Delmez, J. A., Dusso, A. S., Slatopolsky, E., and Teitelbaum, S. L. (1995). Modulation of renal osteodystrophy by extrarenal production of calcitriol. Am. J. Nephrol. 15, 85–89.
18. Barbour, G. L., Coburn, J. W., Slatopolsky, E., Norman, A. W., and Horst, R. L. (1981). Hypercalcemia in an anephric patient with sarcoidosis: Evidence for extrarenal generation of 1,25-dihydroxyvitamin D. N. Engl. J. Med. 305, 440–443.
19. Slatopolsky, E., Caglar, S., Gradowska, L., Canterbury, J., Reiss, E., and Bricker, N. S. (1972). On the prevention of secondary hyperparathyroidism in experimental chronic renal disease using "proportional reduction" of dietary phosphorus intake. Kidney Int. 2, 147–151.
20. Slatopolsky, E., and Bricker, N. S. (1973). The role of phosphorus restriction in the prevention of secondary hyperparathyroidism in chronic renal disease. Kidney Int. 4, 141–145.
21. Slatopolsky, E., Finch, J., Denda, M., Ritter, C., Zhong, M., Dusso, A., MacDonald, P. N., and Brown, A. J. (1996). Phosphorus restriction prevents parathyroid gland growth. High phosphorus directly stimulates PTH secretion in vitro. J. Clin. Invest. 97, 2534–2540.
22. Almaden, Y., Canalejo, A., Hernandez, A., Ballesteros, E., Garcia-Navarro, S., Torres, A., and Rodriguez, M. (1996). Direct effect of

phosphorus on PTH secretion from whole rat parathyroid glands in vitro. *J. Bone Miner. Res.* **11**, 970–976.

23. Tanaka, Y., and Deluca, H. F. (1973). The control of 25-hydroxyvitamin D metabolism by inorganic phosphorus. *Arch. Biochem. Biophys.* **154**, 566–574.

24. Denda, M., Finch, J., and Slatopolsky, E. (1996). Phosphorus accelerates the development of parathyroid hyperplasia and secondary hyperparathyroidism in rats with renal failure. *Am. J. Kidney Dis.* **28**, 596–602.

25. Naveh-Many, T., Rahamimov, R., Livni, N., and Silver, J. (1995). Parathyroid cell proliferation in normal and chronic renal failure rats. The effects of calcium, phosphate, and vitamin D. *J. Clin. Invest.* **96**, 1786–1793.

26. Martin, K. J., Hruska, K. A., Lewis, J., Anderson, C., and Slatopolsky, E. (1977). The renal handling of parathyroid hormone. Role of peritubular uptake and glomerular filtration. *J. Clin. Invest.* **60**, 808–814.

27. Brown, R. C., Aston, J. P., Weeks, I., and Woodhead, J. S. (1987). Circulating intact parathyroid hormone measured by a two-site immunochemiluminometric assay. *J. Clin. Endocrinol. Metab.* **65**, 407–414.

28. Nussbaum, S. R., Zahradnik, R. J., Lavigne, J. R., Brennan, G. L., Nozawa-Ung, K., Kim, L. Y., Keutmann, H. T., Wang, C. A., Potts, J. T., Jr., and Segre, G. V. (1987). Highly sensitive two-site immunoradiometric assay of parathyrin, and its clinical utility in evaluating patients with hypercalcemia. *Clin. Chem.* **33**, 1364–1367.

29. Coburn, J., and Salusky, I. (1994). Hyperparathyroidism in renal failure: Clinical features, diagnosis and management. *In* "The Parathyroids: Basic and Clinical Concepts" (J. Bilezikian, M. Levine, and R. Marcus, eds.), pp. 721–745. Raven Press, New York.

30. Qi, Q., Monier-Faugere, M. C., Geng, Z., and Malluche, H. H. (1995). Predictive value of serum parathyroid hormone levels for bone turnover in patients on chronic maintenance dialysis. *Am. J. Kidney Dis.* **26**, 622–631.

31. Wang, M., Hercz, G., Sherrard, D. J., Maloney, N. A., Segre, G. V., and Pei, Y. (1995). Relationship between intact 1–84 parathyroid hormone and bone histomorphometric parameters in dialysis patients without aluminum toxicity. *Am. J. Kidney Dis.* **26**, 836–844.

32. Slatopolsky, E., Lopez-Hilker, S., Delmez, J., Dusso, A., Brown, A., and Martin, K. J. (1990). The parathyroid-calcitriol axis in health and chronic renal failure. *Kidney Int., Suppl.* **29**, S41–S47.

33. Malluche, H. H., Smith, A. J., Abreo, K., and Faugere, M. C. (1984). The use of deferoxamine in the management of aluminium accumulation in bone in patients with renal failure. *N. Engl. J. Med.* **311**, 140–144.

34. Milliner, D. S., Nebeker, H. G., Ott, S. M., Andress, D. L., Sherrard, D. J., Alfrey, A. C., Slatopolsky, E. A., and Coburn, J. W. (1984). Use of the deferoxamine infusion test in the diagnosis of aluminum-related osteodystrophy. *Ann. Intern. Med.* **101**, 775–779.

35. Pei, Y., Hercz, G., Greenwood, C., Sherrard, D., Segre, G., Manuel, A., Saiphoo, C., and Fenton, S. (1992). Non-invasive prediction of aluminum bone disease in hemo- and peritoneal dialysis patients. *Kidney Int.* **41**, 1374–1382.

36. Couttenye, M. M., D'Haese, P. C., Van Hoof, V. O., Lemoniatou, E., Goodman, W., Verpooten, G. A., and De Broe, M. E. (1996). Low serum levels of alkaline phosphatase of bone origin: a good marker of adynamic bone disease in haemodialysis patients. *Nephrol. Dial. Transplant.* **11** (6), 1065–1072.

37. Fletcher, S., Jones, R. G., Rayner, H. C., Harnden, P., Hordon, L. D., Aaron, J. E., Oldroyd, B., Brownjohn, A. M., Turney, J. H., and Smith, M. A. (1997). Assessment of renal osteodystrophy in dialysis patients: Use of bone alkaline phosphatase, bone mineral density and parathyroid ultrasound in comparison with bone histology. *Nephron* **75**, 412–419.

38. Jarava, C., Armas, J. R., Salgueira, M., and Palma, A. (1996). Bone alkaline phosphatase isoenzyme in renal osteodystrophy. *Nephrol. Dial. Transplant.* **11** (Suppl. 3), 43–46.

39. Urena, P., Hruby, M., Ferreira, A., Ang, K. S., and de Vernejoul, M. C. (1996). Plasma total versus bone alkaline phosphatase as markers of bone turnover in hemodialysis patients. *J. Am. Soc. Nephrol.* **7**, 506–512.

40. Mazzaferro, S., Pasquali, M., Ballanti, P., Bonucci, E., Costantini, S., Chicca, S., De Meo, S., Perruzza, I., Sardella, D., Taggi, F., and Coen, G. (1995). Diagnostic value of serum peptides of collagen synthesis and degradation in dialysis renal osteodystrophy. *Nephrol. Dial. Transplant.* **10**, 52–58.

41. De la Piedra, C., Diaz Martin, M. A., Diaz Diego, E. M., Lopez Gavilanes, E., Gonzalez Parra, E., Caramelo, C., and Rapado, A. (1994). Serum concentrations of carboxyterminal cross-linked telopeptide of type I collagen (ICTP), serum tartrate resistant acid phosphatase, and serum levels of intact parathyroid hormone in parathyroid hyperfunction. *Scand. J. Clin. Lab. Invest.* **54**, 11–15.

42. Ibrahim, S., Mojiminiyi, S., and Barron, J. L. (1995). Pyridinium crosslinks in patients on haemodialysis and continuous ambulatory peritoneal dialysis. *Nephrol. Dial. Transplant.* **10**, 2290–2294.

43. González, E., and Martin, K. (1996). Bone cell response in uremia. *Semin. Dial.* **9**, 339–346.

44. Herbelin, A., Urena, P., Nguyen, A. T., Zingraff, J., and Deschamps-Latscha, B. (1991). Elevated circulating levels of interleukin-6 in patients with chronic renal failure. *Kidney Int.* **39**, 954–960.

45. Herbelin, A., Nguyen, A. T., Zingraff, J., Urena, P., and Deschamps-Latscha, B. (1990). Influence of uremia and hemodialysis on circulating interleukin-1 and tumor necrosis factor alpha. *Kidney Int.* **37**, 116–125.

46. Andress, D. L., Pandian, M. R., Endres, D. B., and Kopp, J. B. (1989). Plasma insulin-like growth factors and bone formation in uremic hyperparathyroidism. *Kidney Int.* **36**, 471–477.

47. Ferreira, A., Simon, P., Drueke, T. B., and Deschamps-Latscha, B. (1996). Potential role of cytokines in renal osteodystrophy. *Nephrol. Dial. Transplant.* **11**, 399–400.

48. Moutabarrik, A., Nakanishi, I., Namiki, M., and Tsubakihara, Y. (1995). Interleukin-1 and its naturally occurring antagonist in peritoneal dialysis patients. *Clin. Nephrol.* **43**, 243–248.

49. Langub, M. C., Jr., Koszewski, N. J., Turner, H. V., Monier-Faugere, M. C., Geng, Z., and Malluche, H. H. (1996). Bone resorption and mRNA expression of IL-6 and IL-6 receptor in patients with renal osteodystrophy. *Kidney Int.* **50**, 515–520.

50. Gejyo, F., Yamada, T., Odani, S., Nakagawa, Y., Arakawa, M., Kunitomo, T., Kataoka, H., Suzuki, M., Hirasawa, Y., Shirahama, T., Cohen, A. S., and Schmid, K. (1985). A new form of amyloid protein associated with chronic hemodialysis was identified as beta 2-microglobulin. *Biochem. Biophys. Res. Commun.* **129**, 701–706.

51. Meema, H. E., Rabinovich, S., Meema, S., Lloyd, G. J., and Oreopoulos, D. G. (1972). Improved radiological diagnosis of azotemic osteodystrophy. *Radiology* **102**, 1–10.

52. Murphey, M. D., Sartoris, D. J., Quale, J. L., Pathria, M. N., and Martin, N. L. (1993). Musculoskeletal manifestations of chronic renal insufficiency. *Radiographics* **13**, 357–379.

53. Moriniere, P., Marie, A., el Esper, N., Fardellone, P., Deramond, H., Remond, A., Sebert, J. L., and Fournier, A. (1991). Destructive spondyloarthropathy with beta 2-microglobulin amyloid deposits in a uremic patient before chronic hemodialysis. *Nephron* **59**, 654–657.

54. Karsenty, G., Vigneron, N., Jorgetti, V., Fauchet, M., Zingraff, J., Drueke, T., and Cournot-Witmer, G. (1986). Value of the 99mTc-methylene diphosphonate bone scan in renal osteodystrophy. *Kidney Int.* **29**, 1058–1065.

55. Vanherweghem, J. L., Schoutens, A., Bergman, P., Dhaene, M., Goldman, M., Fuss, M., and Kinnaert, P. (1985). Usefulness of 99mTc pyrophosphate bone scintigraphy in the survey of dialysis

osteodystrophy. *Proc. Eur. Dial. Transplant. Assoc.—Eur. Renal Assoc.* **21**, 431–434.

56. Olgaard, K., Heerfordt, J., and Madsen, S. (1976). Scintigraphic skeletal changes in uremic patients on regular hemodialysis. *Nephron* **17**, 325–334.

57. Messa, C., Goodman, W. G., Hoh, C. K., Choi, Y., Nissenson, A. R., Salusky, I. B., Phelps, M. E., and Hawkins, R. A. (1993). Bone metabolic activity measured with positron emission tomography and [18F] fluoride

ion in renal osteodystrophy: Correlation with bone histomorphometry. *J. Clin. Endocrinol. Metab.* **77**, 949–955.

58. Erlichman, M., and Holohan, T. V. (1996). Bone densitometry: Patients with end-stage renal disease. *Health Technol. Assess.* **8**, 1–27.

59. Asaka, M., Iida, H., Entani, C., Fujita, M., Izumino, K., Takata, M., Seto, H., and Sasayama, S. (1992). Total and regional bone mineral density by dual photon absorptiometry in patients on maintenance hemodialysis. *Clin. Nephrol.* **38**, 149–153.

CHAPTER 40

Primary Hyperparathyroidism

SHONNI J. SILVERBERG Department of Medicine, College of Physicians and Surgeons, Columbia University, New York, New York 10032

JOHN P. BILEZIKIAN Departments of Medicine and Pharmacology, College of Physicians and Surgeons, Columbia University, New York, New York 10032

I. INTRODUCTION

Primary hyperparathyroidism, one of the most common endocrine disorders, is characterized by hypercalcemia in the presence of elevated parathyroid hormone levels. The disease today bears little resemblance to the symptomatic disorder of "stones, bones, and groans" described by Fuller Albright and others in the 1930s [1–6]. Nephrocalcinosis was present in most patients, and neuromuscular dysfunction with muscle weakness was common. *Osteitis fibrosa cystica* was the skeletal hallmark of classic primary hyperparathyroidism. This condition was characterized by brown tumors of the long bones, subperiosteal bone resorption, distal tapering of the clavicles and phalanges, and "salt and pepper" appearance of the skull on radiograph [7]. With the advent of the automated serum chemistry autoanalyzer in the 1970s, diagnosis of primary hyperparathyroidism in the absence of typical features became common [8–10]. In the 1990s, more than three-quarters of patients have no signs or symptoms attributable to their primary hyperparathyroidism. Nephrolithiasis is still seen, although less frequently than in the past. However, radiologically evident bone disease is rare. This chapter presents the clinical picture of primary hyperparathyroidism as it presents in the 1990s in the United States and the current status of bone markers in the investigation and management of this disorder.

II. ETIOLOGY

The most common lesion found in patients with primary hyperparathyroidism is the solitary parathyroid adenoma, which accounts for 80% of cases [11]. Identifiable risk factors in the development of parathyroid adenoma include a history of neck irradiation [12] and prolonged use of lithium therapy for affective disorders [13–16]. Research has begun to elucidate the molecular pathogenesis of the parathyroid adenoma. The work of Arnold and others has demonstrated that most parathyroid adenomas are monoclonal in origin [17–20]. The molecular abnormalities identified include rearrangement of the PRAD 1 protooncogene, also known as cyclin D1, which places this gene in proximity to the strong tissue-specific enhancer elements of the parathyroid hormone gene [7, 17–19]. The realignment associates a growth promoter (cyclin D1) with a regulatory element that normally controls only a hormonal function (i.e. parathyroid hormone synthesis). The rearrangement of a growth promoting gene next to a gene that controls a homeostatic function provides a facile explanation for the genesis of an abnormal parathyroid cell and its subsequent progeny. As attractive as this mechanism is, clear-cut rearrangements of this sort are documented in only a small number of parathyroid adenomas. However, research assessing actual cyclin D1 protein levels suggests that cyclin D1 may be overexpressed in up to 20% of parathyroid adenomas [8].

The molecular pathogenesis of parathyroid adenomas includes other potential mechanisms. Loss of heterozygosity in chromosome 11q13 has been found in some adenomas, implying involvement of parathyroid tumor supressor genes in the processes associated with parathyroid neoplasia [20–22]. The multiple endocrine neplasia type 1 (MEN1) gene, located at that site, has been identified [9, 10] and is of particular interest because primary hyperparathyroidism is one of the clinical features of MEN type 1. It has long been considered a strong possibility that the tumor suppressor gene identified in MEN type 1 would be involved in sporadic cases of primary hyperparathyroidism. In support of this expectation, allelic loss of chromosome 11 markers has been observed in approximately 25–30% of sporadic parathyroid adenomas [11–13, 23]. More direct examination of the MEN 1 gene in primary hyperparathyroidism has confirmed this expectation, with mutations detected in 17% of parathyroid adenomas [24].

Other tumor suppressor genes are likely to be involved in parathyroid adenomas. Chromosomal regions of interest include 1p [15, 16], 1q [15], 6q, 9p, and 15q [14, 18]. Allelic loss on chromosome 1p is most commonly seen [16, 25].

The vast majority of cases of primary hyperparathyroidism remain idiopathic. In approximately 15% of cases, all four parathyroid glands are involved in a hyperplastic process. There are no clinical features that differentiate primary hyperparathyroidism due to adenoma vs hyperplasia. The etiology of parathyroid hyperplasia is multifactorial. In nearly one-half of cases, it is associated with a familial hereditary syndrome, such as multiple endocrine neoplasia types 1 and 2a.

III. CLINICAL PRESENTATION

At the time of diagnosis, 80% of patients with primary hyperparathyroidism have neither symptoms nor signs referable to their disease [7]. History of previous neck irradiation is obtained in 10–15% of cases. Diseases epidemiologically associated with primary hyperparathyroidism include hypertension [8, 26–28], peptic ulcer disease, pancreatitis, gout, or pseudogout [29, 30], but no causal relationship has been

established between primary hyperparathyroidism and these other disorders. Nonspecific complaints include weakness, easy fatigability, depression, and a sense of intellectual weariness. Neuropsychiatric features have been quantified in several small studies [31–34]. Physical examination is generally unremarkable.

A. Biochemical Profile

The diagnosis of primary hyperparathyroidism is made by the demonstration of hypercalcemia in the presence of elevated parathyroid hormone levels. Improved means of measuring intact parathyroid hormone, by immunoradiometric and immunochemiluminometric assays, offer far greater utility than previously available assays. Even using the newer assays, however, parathyroid hormone is frankly elevated in only 85–90% of patients at the time of diagnosis [7]. In the rest, the circulating parathyroid hormone concentration is in the upper range of normal, which is inappropriately high given the patient's hypercalcemia. It should be noted also that in younger individuals with primary hyperparathyroidism (45 yrs old), the normal range is actually lower than the given commerical laboratory normal range of 10–65 pg/ml. In those younger individuals, the normal range is more accurately defined as approximately 10–45 pg/ml. Thus, a parathyroid hormone level of 50 pg/ml in a 40 year old woman with hypercalcemia should be regarded as elevated. Any patient with hypercalcemia should have suppressed levels of parathyroid hormone unless they have primary hyperparathyroidism. The only exceptions to this rule are those with familial hypocalciuric hypercalcemia and those who are taking thiazide diuretics or lithium.

Other biochemical features of primary hyperparathyroidism include serum phosphorus concentration in the low normal range. Frankly low levels in primary hyperparathyroidism are present in less than one-quarter of patients. Serum 25-hydroxyvitamin D levels tend to be in the lower end of the normal range. While mean values of 1,25-dihydroxyvitamin D3 are usually in the high normal range, approximately one-third of patients have frankly elevated levels [35].

B. Extraskeletal Manifestations of Primary Hyperparathyroidism

Although the incidence of nephrolithiasis has declined since the 1960s, kidney stones remain the most common manifestation of symptomatic primary hyperparathyroidism. Klugman *et al.* place the incidence of kidney stones at 15–20% of all patients [36]. Other renal manifestations of primary hyperparathyroidism include hypercalciuria, which is seen in approximately 40% of patients, and nephrocalcinosis, the frequency of which is unknown [37]. Classical primary hyperparathyroidism used to be associated with a distinct neuromuscular syndrome, characterized by type II muscle cell atrophy [38, 39]. This is no longer seen [40]. The neurobehavioral manifestations noted above have yet to be thoroughly characterized or defined as an extraskeletal component of primary hyperparathyroidism [31–34].

C. The Skeleton in Primary Hyperparathyroidism

Osteitis fibrosa cystica is rarely seen. However, newer, more sensitive techniques have demonstrated that skeletal involvement in primary hyperparathyroidism is common. In this section, we review the profile of the skeleton in primary hyperparathyroidism as it is reflected by bone densitometry and bone histomorphometry.

1. Bone Densitometry

Bone densitometry is particularly well suited to the investigation of the skeleton in primary hyperparathyroidism. In addition to features such as sensitivity, accuracy, and precision, it is a noninvasive test that can be applied to sites containing different amounts of cortical and cancellous bone. Parathyroid hormone has long been thought to affect cortical bone more than cancellous bone. Consistent with this idea, measurement of bone mass in primary hyperparathyroidism typically shows reduced bone density at the distal radius, which is composed primarily of cortical bone [41, 42]. Studies have also shown bone density to be relatively preserved at the lumbar spine, a site containing a preponderance of cancellous bone. The femoral neck, a more even mixture of cortical and cancellous bone, is intermediate in bone density between the lumbar spine and the distal radius (see Fig. 1). These data support two different actions of parathyroid hormone: a catabolic effect in cortical bone and an anabolic effect in cancellous bone [43–45]. It should be noted that this pattern is also seen when bone mass is measured in postmenopausal women with primary hyperparathyroidism [43],

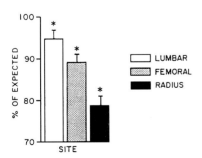

FIGURE 1   Bone densitometry in primary hyperparathyroidism. Data are shown in comparison to age and sex matched normal subjects. Divergence from expected values is different at each site (p = 0.0001). Reproduced from *J. Bone Miner. Res.* 1989; **4**, 283–291 [41] with permission of the American Society for Bone and Mineral Research.

this is a reversal of the pattern usually associated with postmenopausal bone loss, in which cancellous bone is lost first.

2. Bone Histomorphometry

Investigations at a histological level have supported and extended the data obtained by bone densitometry. Histomorphometric analysis of an iliac crest bone biopsy specimen showed cortical thinning consistent with the reduction of cortical bone suggested by densitometric evaluation [46–48]. Histomorphometric studies, however, have contributed most by elucidating the nature of cancellous bone in this disease. Cancellous bone volume is not only relatively preserved in primary hyperparathyroidism, it is actually increased as compared to normal subjects [46, 49, 50]. In primary hyperparathyroidism, there is an increase in trabecular number and a decrease in trabecular separation [46]. Using a histomorphometric technique called "strut analysis," it has been determined further that cancellous bone is preserved in primary hyperparathyroidism through the maintenance of well-connected trabecular plates [46, 51].

Thus, despite the absence of radiologically evident bone disease, skeletal involvement can actually be readily detected by bone densitometry in modern day primary hyperparathyroidism. If one can safely extrapolate from epidemiologic data correlating bone mass measurements with fracture risk, it would appear that patients with primary hyperparathyroidism may have increased risk of cortical bone fracture. However, the data are uncertain because the numbers of patients studied in this regard are small, and the studies have produced conflicting results [52, 53].

IV. TREATMENT OF PRIMARY HYPERPARATHYROIDISM

A. Surgery

Parathyroidectomy remains the only option for cure of primary hyperparathyroidism. As the clinical profile has changed, however, reasonable questions have been raised concerning the need for surgery in all asymptomatic patients. At the National Institutes of Health Consensus Development Conference on the Management of Asymptomatic Primary Hyperparathyroidism in 1991, this question was thoroughly discussed with regard to the data available at that time. Emerging from that conference were guidelines for patients with primary hyperparathyroidism who should be considered for parathyroidectomy [54]. These include patients with:

a. serum calcium >12 mg/dl
b. marked hypercalciuria (>400 mg/day)
c. any overt manifestation of primary hyperparathyroidism (nephrolithiasis, *osteitis fibrosa cystica*, classic neuromuscular disease)

d. markedly reduced cortical bone density (Z Score < −2)

e. reduced creatinine clearance in the absence of other cause

f. age <50 years

Using these criteria, approximately 50% of patients presenting with primary hyperparathyroidism in 1999 meet one or more of the guidelines for surgery. Less than half of these patients are symptomatic. Thus, in approximately two-thirds of the surgical group, guidelines such as hypercalciuria, serum calcium over 12 mg/dl, or reduced cortical density are met in asymptomatic patients. After parathyroidectomy, hypercalcemia resolves rapidly [55]. Surgery is also of clear benefit in reducing the incidence of recurrent nephrolithiasis [36, 56]. Parathyroidectomy also leads to a major improvement in bone mineral density [55], averaging 12% at the lumbar spine and femoral neck (see Fig. 2). This increase is sustained over a four year period after surgery. The increase in bone density after successful parathyroidectomy might be expected to reduce fracture incidence. This would be the case if improvements in bone mass are associated with reduction in fracture incidence in this disease, as they are in some therapies for postmenopausal osteoporosis. However, no studies of fracture incidence after successful parathyroid surgery are large enough to provide this information in a definitive way.

B. No Intervention

Many patients with asymptomatic hypercalcemia do not meet any of the National Institutes of Health Consensus Conference Guidelines for surgery and choose to be followed without parathyroidectomy. Data from our group and others have shown stability in patients with mild primary hyperparathyroidism followed over time [57–59]. In a large, prospective study of patients followed without surgery, annual measurements for seven years showed no change in serum calcium, phosphorus, parathyroid hormone, vitamin D, or alkaline phosphatase levels and no change in urinary calcium, hydroxyproline, or hydroxypyridinium cross-link excretion [59]. In sharp contrast to the change in bone mineral density seen in patients after parathyroidectomy, lumbar spine, femoral neck, and radius bone mineral density also showed stability in this group.

V. BONE MARKERS IN PRIMARY HYPERPARATHYROIDISM

Abundant histomorphometric evidence indicates that even in asymptomatic primary hyperparathyroidism, bone turnover is increased. Indices reflecting increased bone formation and bone resorption are readily demonstrable. Such direct observations would be expected to be demonstrable in the measurement of circulating and urinary markers of bone turnover. Both bone resorption and bone formation are increased by parathyroid hormone. Bone markers would be expected to accurately reflect skeletal metabolism in patients with primary hyperparathyroidism. Bone markers should also be helpful in the longitudinal assessment of bone turnover in those patients who undergo parathyroidectomy as well as those who are monitored without surgery.

A. Bone Formation Markers

Bone formation is reflected by products of osteoblast activity, including the enzyme alkaline phosphatase, osteocalcin, and the procollagen peptide of type I collagen [60]. Total alkaline phosphatase activity, readily available on routine multichannel panels, continues to be a useful marker in

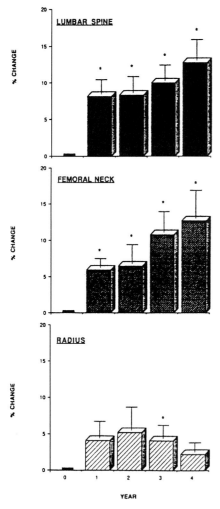

FIGURE 2   Bone density by site following parathyroidectomy. Data are presented as percentage change from preoperative baseline bone density measurement. *denotes significant change at p < 0.05. Reprinted with permission from Silverberg *et al.* [55], *J. Clin. Endocrinol. Metab.* **80**, 729–734, 1995; © The Endocrine Society.

primary hyperparathyroidism [61]. Concentrations of alkaline phosphatase are typically elevated, but in asymptomatic individuals they are usually no more than 15–20% above normal. It seemed promising to consider the potential usefulness of the isoenzyme of alkaline phosphatase specific for osteoblastic action because total alkaline phosphatase reflects not only bone activity but also activity from other tissues such as the liver. Bone-specific alkaline phosphatase activity is clearly elevated in patients with mild primary hyperparathyroidism [62, 63]. In a limited study, bone specific alkaline phosphatase correlated with parathyroid hormone levels and bone mineral density at the lumbar spine and femoral neck [62], but it was no more useful than the total alkaline phosphatase level. Osteocalcin is also generally increased in patients with primary hyperparathyroidism [63–66]. Osteocalcin correlates with other indices of bone formation [63–66]. However, in our patients, we found no correlation of this marker with parathyroid hormone levels or with bone mineral density at any site. Although carboxy- and aminoterminal extension peptides of procallagen reflect osteoblast activation and bone formation, they have not been shown to have significant predictive or clinical utility in primary hyperparathyroidism [67]. In a small study of patients with primary hyperparathyroidism, carboxy-terminal propeptide of human type 1 procollagen (PICP) levels were higher than in control subjects, but the deviations from the norm were much less impressive than those seen for alkaline phosphatase, osteocalcin, or even hydroxyproline [68] (see below).

B. Bone Resorption Markers

Bone resorption is reflected in a product of osteoclast activity, tartrate-resistant acid phosphatase (TRAP), and in collagen breakdown products such as hydroxyproline, hydroxypyridinium cross-links of collagen, and the small N- and C-telopeptides of collagen metabolism [60]. The oldest marker of bone resorption [69–71], urinary hydroxyproline excretion, is frankly elevated in patients with *osteitis fibrosa cystica*. However, in asymptomatic patients with mild, asymptomatic primary hyperparathyroidism, values of urinary hydroxyproline are often entirely normal. In addition, hydroxyproline does not reflect bone resorption exclusively, because its measurement can be influenced by diet, and assays for this imino acid have never been simplified for clinical convenience. The hydroxypyridinium cross-links of collagen have replaced hydroxyproline excretion as markers of bone resorption in primary hyperparathyroidism. These cross-links of collagen (pyridinoline and deoxypyridinoline) are clearly elevated in primary hyperparathyroidism [72]. The increase in deoxypyridinoline excretion in primary hyperparathyroidism is greater than that of pyridinoline, yet levels of both correlate with parathyroid hormone concentrations. The fact that urinary concentrations of pyridinoline

and deoxypyridinoline seem to correlate closely with disease activity, coupled with their usefulness in longitudinal follow-up, make the hydroxypyridinium cross-links of collagen an attractive choice as a bone resorptive marker in primary hyperparathyroidism. Assays for collagen cross-linked N-telopeptide levels have yet to be systematically explored in this disease. In the case of pyridinoline cross-linked telopeptide domain of type 1 collagen (ICTP), pooled data from patients with high turnover diseases (i.e., primary hyperparathyroidism as well as hyperthyroidism) suggest that this marker may reflect calcium kinetics [73] and histomorphometric indices [74]. Unfortunately, data on primary hyperparathyroidism alone are not available.

Other reports of newer bone resorption markers in primary hyperparathyroidism abound. Studies of the TRAP in primary hyperparathyroidism are limited, although levels have been shown to be elevated [75]. One study reported a correlation between levels of parathyroid hormone and tartrate-resistant acid phosphatase in primary hyperparathyroidism [76]. Bone sialoprotein is a phosphorylated glycoprotein which makes up approximately 5–10% of the noncollagenous protein of bone. It is elevated in high turnover states and reflects, in part, bone resorption. In primary hyperparathyroidism, bone sialoprotein levels are elevated and correlate with levels of urinary pyridinoline and deoxypyridinoline [77].

It is clear from the reports summarized in this section that markers of bone formation and resorption tend to be elevated, even in asymptomatic primary hyperparathyroidism. Thus, sensitive assays reflecting bone formation and bone resorption show both processes to be increased in mild primary hyperparathyroidism. It is not certain, however, whether quantification of these markers is useful to predict the extent of parathyroid hormone-dependent skeletal tumors or whether they are useful predictors of the course of the skeletal involvement. With more complete information, such expectations might well be documented.

C. Longitudinal Bone Markers in Prospective Studies of Primary Hyperparathyroidism

Measurements of bone markers hold promise in primary hyperparathyroidism not only as indices of disease activity when the patient is first evaluated, but also as a means by which patients can be followed after surgery. It could be expected that after successful surgery, these indices of disease activity would decline.

Studies of bone markers in the longitudinal follow-up of patients with primary hyperparathyroidism are limited. However, those which have been done offer some interesting results. Seibel *et al.* [72], Guo *et al.* [78], and Tanaka *et al.* [79] all report declining levels of bone markers following surgery. The kinetics of change in bone resorption versus bone formation markers following parathyroidectomy have

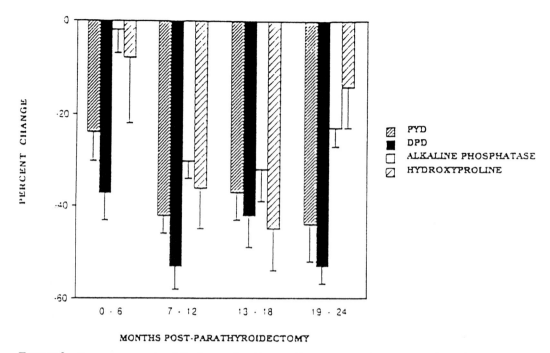

FIGURE 3   Bone turnover markers following parathyroidectomy. Data are presented as percentage change from preoperative baseline measurement. PYD is pyridinoline, DPD is deoxypyridinoline, *denotes significant change at p < 0.05. Reprinted with permission from Seibel *et al.* [72], *J. Clin. Endocrinol Metab.* **74**, 481–486, 1992; © The Endocrine Society.

provided insight into the nature of postoperative anabolic skeletal effects observed by a number of researchers. Seibel *et al.* [72] have found that markers of bone resorption decline rapidly following successful surgery, whereas indices of bone formation follow a slower decline. Urinary pyridinoline and deoxypyridinoline decline significantly as early as two weeks following parathyroidectomy, preceding the onset of reductions in alkaline phosphatase (see Fig. 3). Tanaka *et al.* [79] reported similar data which showed a discrepancy between changes in urinary N-telopeptide excretion (reflecting bone resorption) and osteocalcin (reflecting bone formation) following parathyroidectomy. Minisola *et al.* [68] reported a drop in bone resorptive markers but no significant change in alkaline phosphatase activity or osteocalcin. Several short-term studies reported a brief increase in PICP immediately following parathyroidectomy, whereas bone resorptive markers fell promptly [68, 80]. Such differences in the time course between the postoperative activities in bone resorption markers (rapid) and bone formation markers (slow) shift the dynamics of bone remodelling toward anabolic results. Over time, all indices of bone turnover fell. The return of resorption and formation markers to normal also favors an ultimate anabolic effect of parathyroid surgery, because in the adult, when bone turnover is reduced, bone formation proceeds. Elsewhere in this book, it is shown that reductions in bone turnover markers are independent predictors of gains in bone mass. With respect to the postoperative changes in

primary hyperparathyroidism, it is likely that the reduction in bone turnover is associated with a mineralization of the enlarged remodelling space seen so commonly in the preoperative state.

VI. CYTOKINES IN PRIMARY HYPERPARATHYROIDISM

In addition to studies of bone markers that have helped to clarify the skeletal dynamics of primary hyperparathyroidism, other investigations have sought to elucidate the mechanisms underlying these changes in bone markers. To this end, potential mediators of parathyroid hormone action in this disease have been identified. Candidate cytokine molecules such as interleukin-1 (IL-1), IL-6, and IL-II, TGF-alpha, EGF, and Tumor Necrosis Factor all stimulate bone resorption. Other factors, including IL-4, IGF-1, TGF-beta, and interferons, may be anabolic for bone. Measuring changes in the activity of some, or all, of these cytokines, may help elucidate the mechanism of bone loss in primary hyperparathyroidism.

Attention has focused on interleukin-6 and tumor necrosis factor-alpha as possible mediators of bone resorption in primary hyperparathyroidism. *In vitro* and *in vivo* studies support the hypothesis that parathyroid hormone induces production of IL-6, which leads to increased osteoclastogenesis

[81–83]. Antibodies to IL-6 prevent parathyroid hormone-mediated bone resorption. Reports from Rusinko *et al.* [84] and Grey *et al.* [81] have shown IL-6 and TNF-alpha levels to be elevated in primary hyperparathyroidism, to correlate well with parathyroid hormone levels, and to fall following parathyroidectomy. Although cytokine levels did not correlate with bone density measurements in this report, it should be noted that bone density was not assessed at the site containing most cortical bone (the radius), where the catabolic effects of excess parathyroid hormone would be expected to be seen. Although this seems a promising avenue of investigation, more data are needed. The above data require confirmation with appropriate control subjects. Furthermore, little is known about the effect of primary hyperparathyroidism on other bone resorptive cytokines.

Ongoing research efforts are also considering which cytokines might mediate, or potentiate, the anabolic effect of primary hyperparathyroidism on bone. One such factor is insulin-like growth factor-1 (IGF-1), which is known to be a direct mediator of parathyroid hormone action in bone [85–88]. Preliminary data have shown that IGF-1 and IGFBP3 (the major binding protein for IGF-1) change after parathyroidectomy in primary hyperparathyroidism. The alteration in the ratios of these cytokines supports enhanced delivery of IGF-1 to the tissues following surgery, resulting in an increase in IGF-1 that is inversely proportional to the observed rise in lumbar spine and femoral neck bone density. Further work is needed to document the relationship between these changes and the effects of parathyroid hormone excess in the hyperparathyroid state, and to document the effect of its withdrawal after parathyroidectomy.

VII. SUMMARY

Despite the absence of radiologically evident bone disease, modern day primary hyperparathyroidism has a clearly defined pattern of skeletal involvement. The diminution of cortical bone and preservation of cancellous bone documented in bone mineral density studies and histomorphometry are associated with increases in bone turnover. Increases in both bone formation and resorption are reflected in increased levels of bone turnover markers. New data on the genetics of primary hyperparathyroidism and the role of certain cytokines as potential mediators of skeletal effect in primary hyperparathyroidism are providing new insights into the pathogenesis of this important metabolic bone disease.

Acknowledgments

This work was supported in part by National Institutes of Health Grants NIDDK 32333 and RR 00645.

References

1. Albright, F., and Reifenstein, E. C. (1948). "The Parathyroid Glands and Metabolic Bone Disease." Williams & Wilkins, Baltimore, MD.
2. Cope, O. (1966). The story of hyperparathyroidism at the Massachusetts General Hospital. *N. Engl. J. Med.* **21**, 1174–1182.
3. Bauer, W. (1933). Hyperparathyroidism: Distinct disease entity. *J. Bone. Jt. Surg.* **15**, 135–141.
4. Bauer, W., and Federman, D. D. (1962). Hyperparathyroidism epitomized: Case of Captain Charles E. Martell. *Metab. Clin. Exp.* **11**, 21–22.
5. Mandl, F. (1925). Therapeutische Versuch bei Ostitis fibrosa generalisata mittels Extirpation lines Epithelkoperchentumon. *Wien. Klin. Wochenschr.* **50**, 1343–1344.
6. Albright, F., Aub, J. C., and Bauer, W. (1934). Hyperparathyroidism common and polymorphic condition as illustrated by seventeen proved cases from one clinic. *JAMA, J. Am. Med. Assoc.* **102**, 1276–1287.
7. Silverberg, S. J., Fitzpatrick, L. A., and Bilezikian, J. P. (1995). Primary hyperathyroidism. *In* "Principles and Practice of Endocrinology and Metabolism" K. L. Becker, (ed.), pp. 512–519. Lippincott, Philadelphia.
8. Heath, H., Hodgson, S. F., and Kennedy, M. A. (1980). Primary hyperparathyroidism: Incidence, morbidity, and economic impact in a community. *N. Engl. J. Med.* **302**, 189–193.
9. Mundy, G. R., Cove, D. H., and Fisken, R. (1980). Primary hyperparathyroidism: Changes in the pattern of clinical presentation. *Lancet* **1**, 1317–1320.
10. Scholz, D. A., and Purnell, D. C. (1981). Asymptomatic primary hyperparathyroidism. *Mayo Clin. Proc.* **56**, 473–478.
11. Bilezikian, J. P., Silverberg, S. J., Gartenberg, F. *et al.*, (1994). Clinical presentation of primary hyperparathyroidism. *In* "The Parathyroids: Basic and Clinical Concepts" J. P. Bilezikian, (ed.), pp. 457–470. Raven Press, New York.
12. Rao, S. D., Frame, B., Miller, M. J., Kleerekoper, M., Block, M. A., and Parfitt, A. M. (1980). Hyperparathyroidism following head and neck irradiation. *Arch. Intern. Med.* **140**, 205–207.
13. Seely, E. W., Moore, T. J., LeBoff, M. S., and Brown, E. M. (1989). A single dose of lithium carbonate acutely elevates intact parathyroid hormone levels in humans. *Acta Endocrinol.* **121**, 174–176.
14. Nordenstrom, J., Strigard, K., Perbeck, L., Willems, J., Bagedahl-Strindlund, M., and Linder, J. (1992). Hyperparathyroidism associated with treatment of manic-depressive disorders by lithium. *Eur. J. Surg.* **158**, 207–211.
15. McHenry, C. R., Rosen, I. B., Rotstein, L. E., Forbath, N., and Walfish, P. G. (1989). Lithiumogenic disorders of the thyroid and parathyroid glands as surgical disease. *Surgery* **108**, 1001–1005.
16. Krivitzky, A., Bentata-Pessayre, M., Sarfati, E., Gardin, J. P., Callard, P., and Delzant, G. (1986). Multiple hypersecreting lesions of the parathyroid glands during treatment with lithium. *Ann. Med. Intern.* **137**, 118–122.
17. Arnold, A., Staunton, C. E., Kim, H. G., Gaz, R. D., and Kronenberg, H. M. (1988). Monoclonality and abnormal parathyroid hormone genes in parathyroid adenomas. *N. Engl. J. Med.* **318**, 658–662.
18. Arnold, A., and Kim, H. G. (1989). Molecular cloning and chromosomal mapping of DNA rearranged with the parathyroid hormone gene in a parathyroid adenoma. *J. Clin. Invest.* **83**, 2034–2040.
19. Friedman, E., Bale, A. E., Marx, S. J. *et al.* (1990). Genetic abnormalities in sporadic parathyroid adenoma. *J. Clin. Endocrinol. Metab.* **71**, 293–297.
20. Arnold, A., and Kim, H. G. (1989). Clonal loss of one chromosome 11 in a parathyroid adenoma. *J. Clin. Endocrinol. Metab.* **69**, 496–499.
21. Cryns, V. L., Yi, S. M., Tahara, H., Gaz, R. D., and Arnold, A. (1995). Frequent loss of chromosome arm 1p in parathyroid adenomas. *Genes Chromosomes Cancer* **13**, 9–17.

22. Tahara, H., Smith, A. P., Gaz, R. D., Cryns, V. L., and Arnold, A. (1996). Genomic localization of novel candidate tumor suppressor gene loci in human parathyroid adenomas. *Cancer Res.* **56**, 599–605.

23. Carling, T., Correa, P., Hessman, O., Hedberg, J., Skogseid, B., Lindberg, D., Rastad, J., Westin, G., and Akerstrom, G. (1999). Parathyroid MEN1 gene mutations in relation to clinical characteristics of nonfamilial primary hyperparathyroidism. *J. Clin. Endocrinol. Metab.* **83**, 2960–2963.

24. Brown, E. M., Gardner, D. G., Brennan, M. F. *et al.* (1979). Calcium-regulated parathyroid hormone release in primary hyperparathyroidism. Studies in vitro with dispersed parathyroid cells. *Am. J. Med.* **66**, 923–931.

25. Lloyd, H. M., Parfitt, A. M., Jacobi, J. M. *et al.* (1989). The parathyroid glands in chronic renal failure: A study of their growth and other properties made on the basis of findings in patients with hypercalcemia. *J. Lab. Clin. Med.* **114**, 358–367.

26. Ringe, J. D. (1984). Reversible hypertension in primary hyperparathyroidism: Pre- and postoperative blood pressure in 75 cases. *Klin. Wochenschr.* **62**, 465–469.

27. Broulik, P. D., Horky, K., and Pacovsky, V. (1985). Blood pressure in patients with primary hyperparathyroidism before and after parathyroidectomy. *Exp. Clin. Endocrinol.* **86**, 346–352.

28. Rapado, A. (1986). Arterial hypertension and primary hyperparathyroidism. *Am. J. Nephrol.* **6** (Suppl. 1); 46–50.

29. Bilezikian, J. P., Aurbach, G. D., Connor, T. B. *et al.* (1973). Pseudogout following parathyroidectomy. *Lancet* **1**, 445–447.

30. Geelhoed, G. W., and Kelly, T. R. (1989). Pseudogout as a clue and complication in primary hyperparathyroidism. *Surgery* **106**, 1036–1041.

31. Joborn, C., Hetta, J., Johansson, H. *et al.* (1988). Psychiatric morbidity in primary hyperparathyroidism. *World J. Surg.* **12**, 476–481.

32. Joborn, C., Hetta, J., Frisk, P., Palmer, M., Akerstrom, G., and Ljunghall, S. (1986). Primary hyperparathyroidism in patients with organic brain syndrome. *Acta Med. Scand.* **219**, 91–98.

33. Alarcon, R. D., and Franceschini, J. A. (1984). Hyperparathyroidism and paranoid psychosis case report and review of the literature. *Br. J. Psychiatry* **145**, 477–486.

34. Brown, G. G., Preisman, R. C., and Kleerekoper, M. D. (1987). Neurobehavioral symptoms in mild primary hyperparathyroidism: Related to hypercalcemia but not improved by parathyroidectomy. *Henry Ford Med. J.* **35**, 211–215.

35. Vieth, R., Bayley, T. A., Walfish, P. G., Rosen, I. B., and Pollard, A. (1991). Relevance of vitamin D metabolite concentrations in supporting the diagnosis of primary hyperparathyroidism. *Surgery* **110**, 1043–1046.

36. Klugman, V. A., Favus, M., and Pak, C. Y. C. (1994). Nephrolithiasis in primary hyperparathyroidism. *In* "The Parathyroids: Basic and Clinical Concepts" J. P. Bilezikian, (ed.), pp. 505–518. Raven Press, New York.

37. Silverberg, S. J., Shane, E., Jacobs, T. P. *et al.* (1990). Nephrolithiasis and bone involvement in primary hyperparathyroidism. *Am. J. Med.* **89**, 327–334.

38. Aurbach, G. D., Mallette, L. E., Patten, B. M., Heath, D. A., Doppman, J. P., and Bilezikian, J. P. (1973). Hyperparathyroidism: Recent studies. *Ann. Intern. Med.* **79**, 566–581.

39. Patten, B. M., Bilezikian, J. P., Mallette, L. E., Prince, A., Engel, W. K., and Aurbach, G. D. (1989). The neuromuscular disease of hyperparathyroidism. *Ann. Intern. Med.* **80**, 182–194.

40. Turken, S. A., Cafferty, M., Silverberg, S. J., *et al.* (1989). Neuromuscular involvement in mild, asymptomatic primary hyperparathyroidism. *Am. J. Med.* **87**, 553–557.

41. Silverberg, S. J., Shane, E., De La Cruz, L. *et al.* (1989). Skeletal disease in primary hyperparathyroidism. *J. Bone Miner. Res.* **4**, 283–291.

42. Bilezikian, J. P., Silverberg, S. J. Shane, E., Parisien, M., and Dempster, D. W. (1991). Characterization and evaluation of asymptomatic primary hyperparathyroidism. *J. Bone Miner. Res.* **6** (Suppl. I), 585–589.

43. Dempster, D. W., Cosman, F., Parisien, M., Shen, V., and Lindsay, R. (1993). Anabolic actions of parathyroid hormone on bone. *Endocr. Rev.* **14**, 690–709.

44. Canalis, E., Hock, J. M., and Raisz, L. G. (1994). Anabolic and catabolic effects of parathyroid hormone on bone and interactions with growth factors. *In* "The Parathyroids: Basic and Clinical Concepts" J. P. Bilezikian, (ed.), pp. 65–82. Raven Press, New York.

45. Slovik, D. M., Rosenthal, D. I., Doppelt, S. H., Potts, J. T., Daly, M. A., and Neer, R. M. (1986). Restoration of spinal bone in osteoporotic men by treatment with human parathyroid hormone (1–34) and vitamin D. *J. Bone Miner. Res.* **1**, 377–381.

46. Parisien, M., Silverberg, S. J., Shane, E. *et al.* (1990). The histormorphometry of bone in primary hyperparathyroidism: Preservation of cancellous bone structure. *J. Clin. Endocrinol. Metab.* **70**, 930–938.

47. Parfitt, A. M. (1986). Accelerated cortical bone loss: Primary and secondary hyperparathyroidism. *In* "Current Concepts of Bone Fragility" (H. Uhthoff and E. Stahl, eds.), pp. 279–285. Springer-Verlag, Berlin.

48. Parfitt, A. M. (1989). Surface specific bone remodeling in health and disease. *In* "Clinical Disorders of Bone and Mineral Metabolism" (M. Kleerekoper, ed.), pp. 7–14. Mary Ann Liebert, New York.

49. van Doorn, L., Lips, P., Netelenbos, J. C., and Hackengt, W. H. L. (1989).Bone histomorphometry and serum intact parathyroid hormone (1-84) in hyperparathyroid patients. *Calcif. Tissue Int.* **44S**, N36.

50. Parisien, M., Dempster, D. W., Shane, E., Silverberg, S., Lindsay, R., and Bilezikian, J. P. (1988). Structural parameters of bone biopsies in primary hyperparathyroidism. *In* "Bone Morphometry" (H. E. Takahashi, ed.,) pp. 228–231. Smith-Gordon, New York.

51. Christiansen, P., Steiniche, T., Vesterby, A., Mosekilde, L., Hessov, I., and Melsen, F. (1992). Primary hyperparathyroidism: Iliac crest trabecular bone volume, structure, remodeling, and balance evaluated by histomorphometric methods. *Bone* **13**, 41–49.

52. Dauphine, R. T., Riggs, B. L., and Scholz, D. A. (1975). Back pain and vertebral crush fractures: An unrecognized mode of presentation for primary hyperparathyroidism. *Ann. Intern. Med.* **83**, 365–367.

53. Melton, L. J., 3rd, Atkinson, E. J., O'Fallon, W. M., and Heath, H. (1992). Risk of age-related fractures in patients with primary hyperparathyroidism. *Arch. Intern. Med.* **152**, 2269–2273.

54. National Institutes of Health. (1991). Consensus development conference statement on primary hyperparathyroidism. *J. Bone Miner. Res.* **6**, s9–s13.

55. Silverberg, S. J., Gartenberg, F., Jacobs, T. P., Shane, E., Siris, E., Staron, R. B., McMahon, D. J., and Bilezikian, J. P. (1995). Increased bone mineral density following parathyroidectomy in primary hyperparathyroidism. *J. Clin. Endocrinol. Metab.* **80**, 729–734.

56. Deaconson, T. F., Wilson, S. D., and Lemann, J. (1987). The effect of parathyroidectomy on the recurrence of nephrolithiasis. *Surgery* **215**, 241–251.

57. Rao, D. S., Wilson, R. J., Kleerekoper, M., and Parfitt, A. M. (1988). Lack of biochemical progression or continuation of accelerated bone loss in mild asymptomatic primary hyperparathyroidism. *J. Clin. Endocrinol. Metab.* **67**, 1294–1298.

58. Parfitt, A. M., Rao, D. S., and Kleerekoper, M. (1991). Asymptomatic primary hyperparathyroidism discovered by multichannel biochemical screening: Clinical course and considerations bearing on the need for surgical intervention. *J. Bone Miner. Res.* **6** (Suppl. 2), s97–s101.

59. Silverberg, S. J., Gartenberg, F., Jacobs, T. P., Shane, E, Siris, E, Staron, R. B., and Bilezikian, J. P. (1995). Longitudinal measurements of bone density and biochemical indices in untreated primary hyperparathyroidism. *J. Clin. Endocrinol. Metab.* **80**, 723–728.

60. Deftos, L. J. (1994). Markers of bone turnover in primary hyperparathyroidism. *In* "The Parathyroids: Basic and Clinical Concepts" (J. P. Bilezikian, ed.), pp. 485–492. Raven Press, New York.

61. Moss, D. W. (1992). Perspectives in alkaline phosphatase research. *Clin. Chem.* **38**, 2486–2492.

62. Silverberg, S. J., Deftos, L. J., Kim, T., and Hill, C. S. (1991). Bone alkaline phosphatase in primary hyperparathyroidism. *J. Bone. Miner. Res.* **6**, A624.

63. Duda, R. J., O'Brien, J. F., Katzman, J. A., Paterson, J. M., Mann, K. G., and Riggs, B. L. (1988). Concurrent assays of circulating bone Gla-protein and bone alkaline phosphatase: Effects of sex, age, and metabolic bone disease. *J. Clin. Endocrinol. Metab.* **5**, 1–7.

64. Price, P. A., Parthemore, J. G., and Deftos, L. J. (1980). New biochemical marker for bone metabolism. Measurement by radioimmunoassay of bone Gla-protein in the plasma of normal subjects and patients with bone disease. *J. Clin. Invest.* **66**, 878–883.

65. Deftos, L. J., Parthemore, J. G., and Price, P. A. (1982). Changes in plasma bone Gla-protein during treatment of bone disease. *Calcif. Tissue Int.* **34**, 121–124.

66. Eastell, R., Delmas, P. D., Hodgson, S., Eriksen, E. F., Mann, K. M., and Riggs, B. L. (1988). Bone formation rate in older normal women: Concurrent assessment with bone histomorphometry, calcium kinetics, and biochemical markers. *J. Clin. Endocrinol. Metab.* **67**, 741–748.

67. Ebeling, P. R., Peterson, J. M., and Riggs, B. L. (1992). Utility of type 1 procollagen propeptide assays for assessing abnormalities in metabolic bone diseases. *J. Bone Miner. Res.* **7**, 1243–1250.

68. Minisola, S., Romagnoli, E., Scarnecchia, L., Rosso, R., Pacitti, M. T., Scarda, A., and Mazzuoli, G. (1994). Serum CITP in patients with primary hyperparathyroidism: Studies in basal conditions and after parathyroid surgery. *Eur. J. Endocrinol.* **130**, 587–591.

69. Deftos, L. J. (1991). Bone protein and peptide assays in the diagnosis and management of skeletal disease. *Clin. Chem.* **37**, 1143–1148.

70. Delmas, P. H. (1991). Biochemical markers of bone turnover: Methodology and clinical use in osteoporosis. *Am. J. Med.* **91**, 169–174.

71. Parfitt, A. M. (1991). Serum markers of bone formation in parenteral nutrition patients. *Calcif. Tissue Int.* **49**, 143–145.

72. Seibel, M. J., Gartenberg, F., Silverberg, S. J., Ratcliffe, A., Robins, S. P., and Bilezikian, J. P. (1992). Urinary hydroxypyridinium cross-links of collagen in primary hyperparathyroidism. *J. Clin. Endocrinol. Metab.* **74**, 481–486.

73. Charles, P., Mosekilde, L., Risteli, L., and Eriksen, E. F. (1994). Assessment of bone remodeling using biochemical indicators of type 1 collagen synthesis and degradation: Relation to calcium kinetics. *Bone Miner.* **24**, 81–94.

74. Eriksen, E. F., Charles, P., Melsen, F., Mosekilde, L., Ristei, L., and Risteli, J. (1993). Serum markers of type 1 collagen formation and degradation in metabolic bone diseases: Correlation with bone histomorphometry. *J. Bone Miner. Res.* **8**, 127–132.

75. Kraenzlin, M. E., Lau, K. H. W., Liang, L. *et al.* (1990). Development of an immunoassay for human serum osteoclastic tartrate-resistant acid phosphatase. *J. Clin. Endocrinol. Metab.* **71**, 442.

76. De La Piedra, C., Diaz Martin, M. A., Diaz Diego, E. M., Lopez Gavilanes, E., Gonzalez Parra, E., Carmelo, C., and Rapado, A. (1994). Serum ICTP, serum tartrate resistant acid phosphatase, and serum levels of intact PTH in parathyroid hyperfunction. *Scand. J. Clin. Lab. Invest.* **54**, 11–15.

77. Seibel, M. J., Woigte, H. W., Pecherstorfer, M., Karmatschek, M., Horn, E., Ludwig, M., Armbruster, F. P., and Ziegler, R. (1996). Serum immunoreactive bone sialoprotein as a new marker of bone turnover in metabolic and malignant diseases. *J. Clin. Endocrinol. Metab.* **81**, 3289–3294.

78. Guo, C. Y., Thomas, W. E. R., Al-Dehaimi, A. W., Assiri, A. M. A., and Eastell, R. (1996). Longitudinal changes in bone mineral density and bone turnover in women with primary hyperparathyroidism. *J. Clin. Endocrinol. Metab.* **81**, 3487–3491.

79. Tanaka, Y., Funahashi, H., Imai, T., Tominga, Y., and Takagi, H. (1997). Parathyroid function and bone metabolic markers in primary and secondary hyperparathyroidism. *Semin. Surg. Oncol.* **13**, 125–133.

80. Hoshino, H., Kushida, K., Takahashi, M., Denda, M., Yamazaki, K., Yamanashi, A., and Inoue, T. (1997). Short term effect of parathyroidectomy on biochemical markers in primary and secondary hyperparathyroidism. *Miner. Electrolyte Metab.* **23**, 93–99.

81. Grey, A., Mitnick, M., Shapses, S., Gundberg, C., and Insogna, K. (1996). Circulating levels of IL-6 and TNF-alpha are elevated in primary hyperparathyroidism and correlate with markers of bone resorption. *J. Clin. Endocrinol. Metab.* **81**, 3450–3454.

82. Roodman, G. D. (1992). Interleukin-6: An osteotropic factor? *J. Bone Miner. Res.* **7**, 475–478.

83. Greenfield, E. M., Shaw, S. M., Gornik, S. A., and Banks, M. A. (1995). Adenyl cyclase and interleukin 6 are downstream effectors of PTH resulting in stimulation of bone resorption. *J. Clin. Invest.* **96**, 1238–1244.

84. Rusinko, R., Yin, J. J., Yee, J., and Saad, G. R. (1995). PTH excess is associated with increased IL-6 and soluble IL-6 receptor production. *J. Bone Miner. Res.* **10** (Suppl. 1), T585A.

85. Jones, J. I., and Clemmons, D. R. (1995). Insulin-like growth factors and their binding proteins. *Endocr. Rev.* **15**, 3–34.

86. Spencer, E. M., Si, E. C., Liu, C. C., and Howard, G. A. (1989). PTH potentiates the effect of IGF-1 on bone formation. *Acta Endocrinol.* **121**, 435–442.

87. McCarthy, T. L., Centrella, M. C., and Canalis, E. (1989). PTH enhances the transcript and polypetide levels of IGF-1 in osteoblast enriched cultures from fetal rat bone. *J. Clin. Endocrinol. Metab.* **124**, 1247–1253.

88. Pfeilschifter, J., Laukhuf, F., Muller-Beckmann, B., Blum, W. F., Pfister, T., and Ziegler, R. (1995). PTH increases the concentration of IGF-1 and TGF-B1 in rat bone. *J. Clin. Invest.* **96**, 767–774.

CHAPTER 41

Paget's Disease of Bone

ANDREAS GRAUER Institute for Endocrinology and Nuclear Medicine, Frankfurt, Germany

ETHEL SIRIS Department of Medicine, Columbia University College of Physicians and Surgeons, New York, New York 10032

I. INTRODUCTION

Paget's disease of bone is a chronic, localized disease which can be monostotic or polyostotic. It is characterized by increased bone remodelling, bone hypertrophy, and abnormal bone structure. Patients may suffer from bone pain and deformity. Complications involve fractures, osteoarthritis, nerve compression syndromes, and neoplastic transformation [1]. The disorder rarely presents before the age of 40. Thereafter it is found with increasing prevalence with advancing age. Large autopsy [2] or radiographic studies [3] suggest a prevalence of approximately 3% in the population over 40 years old, which increases up to 10% by the age of 95. Interestingly, there is a marked geographic variation. The disorder is particularly common in Great Britain, where the prevalence of the disease among hospital patients is 5% of the population over 50 [4]. In other parts of western and central Europe, and in regions of the world influenced by European migration, including the United States, Australia and New Zealand, Argentina, and South Africa, the prevalence of the disease is estimated to be 1–3% of the population over 50 [5]. The disorder seems to be extremely rare in Nordic countries [4], the Middle East, China, and Japan, and most of sub-Saharan Africa.

II. ETIOLOGY AND PATHOGENESIS

The demographics of Paget's disease of bone, together with an increasing awareness of the presence of Paget's disease in multiple members of affected families, indicate that genetic, infectious, or environmental factors probably play an important role in its etiology.

A. Genetics of Paget's Disease

In an epidemiologic study of Paget's disease of bone from the United States, using data from 788 cases and 387 spouse controls, a positive family history in parents or siblings was reported in 12.3% of cases and 2.1% of controls. The rate of Paget's disease was approximately seven times as high in relatives of patients with the disease as in relatives of controls, and this increased rate did not differ according to gender of case or control or gender of relatives. The risk was especially high if affected family members were young when diagnosed with the deforming bone disease [6]. In another study from Spain, up to 40% of patients had affected first-degree relatives; however, the locus (loci) and gene(s) involved are unknown [7]. In some families, an autosomal dominant trait of transmission appears to be evident, with high penetrance by the sixth decade [8]. Another bone disorder, familial expansile osteolysis (FEO), although extremely rare, also is characterized by similar osteoclast abnormalities but has an earlier age at onset and a more aggressive clinical progression. The causative gene for FEO has been localized to a region of human chromosome 18q21–22 [9]. On the basis of the presence of similar clinical findings and of viral-like nuclear inclusions in osteoclasts, it has been hypothesized that FEO and Paget's disease are allelic versions of the same locus. Eight large kindreds with a high incidence of Paget's disease were examined to determine whether Paget's disease was linked to genetic markers in the same region of chromosome 18 as FEO. The analysis provided evidence for genetic linkage to region 18q21–22 in five families, but not in the other three suggesting a genetically heterogeneous background. Multipoint linkage analysis in the five linked families showed lodscores of 3.50 over the whole susceptibility region and a maximum summated lodscore of 3.89 at the marker D182465 [10]. In an independent study with a large kindred, a two-point lodscore of 3.4 could be identified for the marker D18S42, a marker tightly linked to the FEO locus. This demonstrates that the gene(s) responsible for FEO and for Paget's disease are either closely linked or the same locus [11].

Other studies have explored the possibility of linkage of Paget's disease with the HLA complex on chromosome 6. In 25 pagetic patients, HLA-DR2 was more frequent compared to 57 healthy controls of the same ethnic origin [12]. Also, in Ashkenazi Jews with Paget's disease, the frequency of HLA DRB1 (1104 gene) was signficantly increased [13]. It has been hypothesized that linkage of Paget's disease to the HLA locus, where genes regulating the immune function are encoded, suggests involvement of some immune defect, possibly predisposing the bone cells to viral infection that could lead osteoclasts to cell fusion. There are, however, conflicting reports. In summary, the HLA studies have been inconclusive [14].

B. Role of a Viral Infection in the Etiology of Paget's Disease

Paget's disease is characterized by an exuberant increase in metabolic activity of bone. Bone remodelling normally occurs in 10% or less of the bone surface. In Paget's disease the activation frequency of bone remodelling units is markedly increased, so that up to 100% of the bone surface can be occupied by active events. The number of osteoclasts in pagetic bone may be increased up to 100-fold, coupled with an increase in osteoclast size and an excessive number of nuclei [15], containing virus-like nuclear and cytoplasmic inclusions [16, 17]. Subacute sclerosing panencephalitis is associated with similar inclusions in the nuclei and cytoplasm of

brain cells, which have been identified as viral nucleocapsids. These findings have led to the speculation that Paget's disease may be due to a slow viral infection affecting osteoclasts. Although very typical, these lesions are not totally specific for Paget's disease; they have also been found in the osteoclasts of a few patients with osteopetrosis [18]. Candidate viruses are the measles virus, the respiratory syncytial virus, and the canine distemper virus. For all antigens, positive results have been obtained using immunofluorescence, in situ hybridization, and reverse transcriptase polymerase chain reaction (RT-PCR) analysis, not only in pagetic osteclasts but also in mononucleated osteoclasts in bone marrow and peripheral blood [19–21]. In one study, four of five patients showed evidence for a mutated measles virus [22]. The evidence that the measles virus infection, possibly causative for Paget's disease, is present in systemically circulating blood cells, suggests that the pagetic marrow microenvironment plays a critical role in maintaining the highly localized nature of the lesions in Paget's disease.

In England, the paramyxovirus canine distemper virus (CDV) was considered a cancidate virus in Paget's disease because of epidemiological studies which suggested that English Paget's patients were more likely to have had a dog in the past [23]. This theory has been supported by some [24] and questioned by others [25]. An English group employing antisense probes and fusion genes of the canine distemper virus similarly revealed hybridization with the pagetic osteoclast. They did not, however, detect any hybridization for measles virus RNA [26]. Infection of canine bone marrow mononuclear cells with CDV, both in vitro and in vivo, produces a dose-dependent increase in the number and size of osteoclast-like cells, concomitant with an induction of interleukin-6 and c-fos mRNA in these cells.

Conflicting positive and negative results with respect to identifiying the putative virus have emerged from several studies applying advanced molecular biology tools. Using the technique of reverse transcription and polymerase chain reaction (PCR), Ralston et al. [27] found no evidence of viral products in RNA extracts of affected bone from ten consecutive patients with Paget's disease. In an extended study it was impossible to detect any of the expected viral products in four strains of human bone cells outgrown from pagetic bone and one strain derived from an uninvolved site of a patient with Paget's disease [28]. These studies fail to support the hypothesis that active infection with one of these or a related paramyxovirus is involved in the pathogenesis of Paget's disease. In juvenile Paget's disease, a possibly distinct entity of Paget's disease, no paramyxovirus transcripts can be detected [29].

C. Pathogenetic Considerations

The role of a viral infection as an etiologic agent in the pathogenesis of Paget's disease is still in question. The conflicting groups have agreed on the need for a blinded multipopulation study to assess the problem; it has yet to be initiated. Numerous questions remain to be answered. Can a variety of paramyxoviruses trigger the initial osteolytic process? If a paramyxovirus is the initiating event, what are the molecular and cellular events accounting for the evolution of the disease?

Osteoclast precursor cells obtained from pagetic marrow aspirations form multinucleated cells in culture with lower concentrations of $1,25(OH)_2D_3$ than comparable cells of normal patients [30]. This could be explained by the higher concentration of interleukin-6 (IL-6) found in plasma and conditioned media from pagetic marrow cultures [31]. Using *in situ* hybridization, the spatial localization of expression of IL-6, IL-6 receptor (IL-6R), and the transcription factor (NF-IL-6) in pagetic bone was investigated. Osteoblasts in the normal remodeling bone of osteoarthritis (controls) and in Paget's disease expressed IL-6, IL-6R, and NF-IL-6 genes, with higher levels of IL-6 and IL-6R mRNA in pagetic bone. Osteoclasts both in osteoarthritic and in pagetic bone expressed IL-6R mRNA and NF-IL-6, but only pagetic osteoclasts expressed IL-6, suggesting that in Paget's disease IL-6 can act as an autocrine factor on osteoclasts. These results suggest a major role of the IL-6 regulatory pathway in the phenotype of the pagetic osteoclasts and lead us to suggest a model linking possible paramyxovirus infection and IL-6 regulation in the pagetic osteoclast [32]. Of additional importance may be the role of the c-fos oncogene, a gene normally associated with osteosarcomas. It is greatly elevated in osteoclasts of patients with Paget's disease. Immunohistochemical staining with c-fos antibodies also shows increased protein in pagetic osteoclasts. In light of transgenic mouse experiments showing a key role for c-fos in bone resorption, elevated c-fos gene expression in pagetic osteoclasts may be an important component in producing the pagetic phenotype. Levels of c-fos gene and protein expression in pagetic osteoblasts are lower than those detected in osteoclasts but are still higher than in nonpagetic osteoblasts [33]. This may provide an explanation for the increased incidence of osteosarcomas in patients with Paget's disease, because overexpression of c-fos in osteoblasts of transgenic mice induces osteosarcoma formation.

III. DIAGNOSIS

Besides the typical clinical features of Paget's disease (Table I), which are evident only in a relatively small subset of patients with the disease, the diagnosis is based on typical radiographic abnormalities linked to areas of increased bone turnover in the bone scan, on characteristic histopathologic changes, and on elevation of the bone formation marker alkaline phosphatase (AP).

TABLE I. Typical Clinical Features of Paget's Disease of Bone

Bone pain
  hypervascularity due to disease activity
  bowing due to mechanical imcompetence
  joint dysfunction due to secondary osteoarthritis

Enlarging bones
  danger of nerve compression symptoms, if the base of the skull or the vertebral column is affected

Impaired hearing
  predominantly due to sensineural hearing loss
  rarely due to involvement of the internal auditory canal

A. Radiological Changes

Characteristic features of Paget's disease include a localized enlargement of bone, cortical thickening, sclerotic changes, osteolytic areas such as V-shaped lesions in long bones, and osteoporosis circumscripta in the skull [34]. Radionuclide bone scanning is a very sensitive method used to identify lesions with increased bone turnover, which is typical for Paget's disease, and should be performed at the time of diagnosis to screen clinically unaffected parts of skeleton for previously undetected manifestations [35].

B. Role of Biochemical Markers in the Diagnosis of Paget's Disease

Of the biochemical markers of bone metabolism, serum AP is usually, but not always, elevated in patients with Paget's disease. In approximately 15% of the symptomatic patients, AP values are within the statistical limits of the normal range. There is a strong relationship between the extent of the disease, measured by bone scan, and the AP activity [36]. It is important to note, however, that for the individual patient, even a statistically normal AP activity may be elevated and can be lowered by successful treatment [37]. In patients with concomittant liver or biliary disease, an elevation of the bone-specific isoenzyme of AP (BAP) may be masked when total AP is measured. In these cases, the determination of BAP is more useful [38].

Using samples from 51 patients with Paget's disease, Alvarez *et al.* [40] determined the levels of a variety of markers of bone formation. These include total alkaline phosphatase (AP), bone-specific alkaline phosphatase (BAP), carboxyterminal propeptide of type I procollagen (PICP), aminoterminal propeptide of type I procollagen (PINP), and osteocalcin. They also studied a group of markers of bone resorption, including hydroxyproline (OHP), pyridinoline (PYD), deoxypyridinoline (DPD), C-terminal telopeptide of type I collagen (CTx), N-terminal telopeptide of type I collagen (NTx), serum-tartrate-resistant acid phosphatase (TRAP), and serum-carboxyterminal telopeptide of type I collagen (TCIP). All biochemical markers except osteocalcin correlated with the disease activity and the disease extent. Serum PINP, BAP, and total AP showed the highest proportions of increased values among the bone formation markers (94%, 82%, and 76%, respectively). Among the bone resorption markers, urinary NTx showed the highest proportion of increased values in patients with Paget's disease (96%), compared with PYD (69%), DPD (71%), CTx (65%), and OHP (64%). In patients with mild disease activity, serum PINP was the marker with the highest proportion of increased values (71%) [39]. When the activity of the disease is high (AP values >500 U/l), most biochemical markers reveal values above the upper limit of normal [40]. However, when the disease activity is low, markers like PINP or BAP (as formation markers) and NTx (as a resorption marker) may improve the diagnostic sensitivity over the standard markers AP and DPD-cross-links.

IV. TREATMENT

The increasing potency of newer bisphosphonates has shifted the emphasis of treatment from simply reducing bone turnover towards a complete suppression of the pathologically increased bone turnover for prolonged periods of time [41]. The aim of this strategy is to relieve symptoms and to prevent long-term complications such as deformity, fracture, and neurological sequelae [42]. Effective treatment will

TABLE II. Potential Parameters to Assess Response to Treatment in Paget's Disease

symptoms
findings at examination
biochemical markers of bone turnover
radiological features
histological features

eventually lead to normal lamellar bone formation rather than the woven bone characteristic of Paget's disease [43]. In an observational study, 41 patients with Paget's disease of bone were followed over 12 years of treatment. In this study, only four of the twelve patients whose bone metabolism could be normalized during treatment developed long-term complications; however, 13 of 29 patients, for whom complete normalization of the disease activity was not possible, developed long-term complications [44].

How do we assess response to bisphosphonate treatment and determine the duration of the response? The biochemical markers of bone turnover appear to be clearly superior to other established parameters (Table II, III). Biochemical markers are more objective and reproducible than historical and clinical changes and they are readily available and more practical for clinical use than serial radiographs, bone scans, or bone biopsies [41]. Due to the development of detection systems for new parameters, the number of biochemical markers of bone metabolism available has increased. In Paget's disease, however, there is no clear evidence that any of the newer markers is of greater benefit in clinical decision making than

TABLE III. Biochemical Markers in the Assessment of Paget's Disease

Bone formation		
AP	total alkaline phosphatase	serum
BAP	bone-specific alkaline phosphatase	serum
PICP	carboxyterminal propeptide of type I procollagen	serum
PINP	aminoterminal propeptide of type I procollagen	serum
OC	osteocalcin	
Bone resorption		
PYD	pyridinolin	urine
DPD	deoxypyridinolin	urine/serum
tDPD	total DPD	urine
fDPD	free DPD	urine
CTx	C-telopeptide of alpha 1 chain of type I collagen	urine/serum
ICTP	C-terminal telopeptide of type I collagen	urine/serum
NTx	N-telopeptide of alpha 1 chain of type I collagen	urine
TRAP	tartrate-resistant acid phosphatase	serum
BSP	bone sialoprotein	serum

total serum alkaline phosphatase (AP) or the excretion of urinary hydroxyproline (OHP) [45–47]. However, major advantage of the newer markers of bone resorption over OHP is that they are largely independent of dietary influences, and therefore are not as prone to errors due to patient's malcompliance.

How can we use the information given by the magnitude of change of the biochemical markers in a meaningful way? There are two different issues to address: the assessment of response to treatment and the attempt to predict the duration of remission.

A. Assessing the Response to Treatment

The determination of total AP is inexpensive, accurate, and readiliy available. In daily practice, the determination of AP before and three to six months after initiation of any kind of antiresorptive treatment will provide sufficient information to assess the treatment response in an individual patient.

1. ROLE OF BONE RESORPTION MARKERS

Antiresorptive agents lead to a significant reduction of biochemical markers of bone resorption, such as OHP or pyridinium cross-links, with two to three days after initiation of treatment [48] (Fig. 1). The reduction is maximal after ten days [49]. Bone formation markers such as AP take longer to reveal the treatment response, usually three to four weeks or longer, reaching a minimum activity approximately three to six months after treatment (Fig. 2) [48, 50]. After three months, the bone formation and resorption markers follow mostly parallel curves (Fig. 2). The difference in the dynamics of marker changes, however, raises the question of whether we can utilize the fast response of the resorption markers for an optimal steering of our treatment. One study

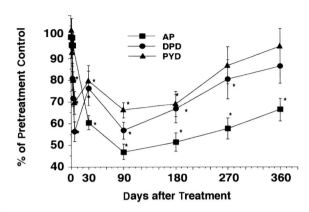

FIGURE 2   Long term effects of bisphosphonate treatment on bone resorption and bone formation markers in Paget's disease of bone. Serum total alkaline phosphatase (AP) activity, pyridinoline, and deoxypyridinoline cross-links (DPD) in % of pretreatment values (mean ± S.E.M.) after treatment with 2 mg ibandronate i.v. After three months the curves for bone formation and bone resorption markers become parallel. Therefore, there is no specific advantage of bone resorption over bone formation markers three or more months after treatment. Data from [50].

has addressed this question [49]. 21 patients were treated with daily infusions of two different aminobisphosphonates. Four different markers of bone resorption (OHP, total deoxypyridinoline cross-links (tDPD), free deoxypyridinoline cross-links (fDPD), and the cross-linked N-telopeptide of collagen type I (NTx) were compared. All markers showed a rapid decrease in urinary excretion within a few days. The reductions in urinary excretion of NTx and of the excess in OHP were nearly identical and more pronounced than the reduction of tDPD and fDPD. All patients who had a reduction in NTx >75% after ten days achieved a total AP within the normal range after one year. This preliminary study suggests that there may be a role in determining biochemical markers of bone resorption in the first ten days after the initiation of the treatment to predict treatment response in an individual patient. This interesting concept needs to be further evaluated.

2. PERFORMANCE OF OTHER BONE RESORPTION MARKERS

An increasing number of studies compares the performance of varius bone resorption markers to assess the response to bisphosphonate treatment in patients with Paget's disease. One study compared the response of different biochemical markers of bone resorption to bisphosphonate therapy (400 mg of etidronate daily for six months) in 14 patients with mild Paget's disease. Urinary markers included hydroxyproline (OHP), total and free pyridinolines (PYDs) determined by HPLC, immunoreactive fPYDs, immunoreactive tPYDs, and the N- and C-terminal telopeptides of type I collagen (NTx, CTx). Serum measurements included tartrate-resistant acid phosphatase (TRAP) and the C-terminal telopeptide of type I collagen (ICTP). ICTP and TRAP showed a minimal response to therapy (% change at six months, -13.1 ± 6.8 and -6.7 ± 3.4, respectively). The

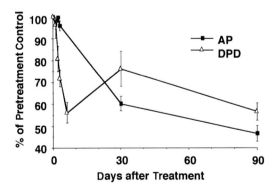

FIGURE 1   Short term effects of bisphosphonate treatment on bone resorption and bone formation markers in Paget's disease of bone. Serum total alkaline phosphatase (AP) activity and deoxypyridinoline cross-links (DPD) in % of pretreatment values (mean ± S.E.M.) after treatment with 2 mg ibandronate i.v. Note the sharp decline of the resorption marker, DPD, within a few days after treatment, whereas the formation marker, AP, reaches its minimum after three months. Data from [50].

response was greatest for urinary telopeptides (NTx and CTx; % change -75.7 ± 7.5 and -73.4 ± 8.9, respectively). The response was greater for total PYD than for free PYD [51]. These data suggest that oligopeptide-bound PYDs and telopetide fragments of type I collagen in urine show a somewhat greater response to therapy than do free PYDs and may be more sensitive indicators of bone resorption. They also confirm earlier observations that ICTP [47] and also TRAP are unreliable indicators of changes in bone turnover in Paget's disease.

In Paget's disease of bone, the normal lamellar bone is replaced by a woven structure with an irregular arrangement of collagen fibers. One study investigated whether the degree of beta-isomerization within the C-telopeptide of the $\alpha 1$ chain of type I collagen was altered in Paget's disease compared with other bone diseases with no alteration of bone structure (such as primary hyperparathyroidism or hyperthyroidism). The researchers found the urinary excretion of nonisomerized (α) fragments derived from degradation of type I collagen C-telopeptide (CTx) markedly increased compared with β-isomerized CTx (13-fold vs 3.5-fold over controls), resulting in a urinary αCTx/βCTx ratio 3-fold higher than in controls (2.6 ± 1.0 vs 0.8 ± 0.3, $p < 0.001$). In five pagetic patients in complete remission, as demonstrated by normal total alkaline phosphatase activity, the αCTx/βCTx ratio was normal. The immunohistochemistry of normal and pagetic human bone sections showed a preferential distribution of αCTx within woven structure, whereas lamellar bone was intensely stained with an anti-βCTx antibody, suggesting a lower degree of β-isomerization of type I collagen in the woven pagetic bone. In collagenase digest of human bone specimens, a lower proportion of β-isomerized type I collagen molecules was found in pagetic bone (40% of βCTx) compared to normal bone taken from trabecular (68%) and cortical compartments (71%). In Paget's disease, the αCTx/βCTx ratio in bone and in urine is markedly increased. This altered β-isomerization can be accurately detected *in vivo* by measuring urinary degradation products arising from bone resorption. Whether or not this defect of posttranslational modifcation of collagen is specific for pagetic bone or is a general characteristic of woven bone found in other disease states remains to be investigated [52].

3. BONE RESORPTION MARKERS IN SERUM

Most bone resorption markers are determined in urine. Recently, several markers of bone resorption in human serum have been developed (see Chapter 28).

a. Pyridinium Cross-links Determination of cross-links (DPD and PYD) in human serum yielded a correlation of 0.84 (DPD) with the urinary cross-link excretion [53].

b. CTx Using an ELISA for an isomerized form of an 8 amino acid sequence of the C-telopeptide of type I collagen, a system for measuring type I collagen degradation products in serum was developed. Values in untreated patients with Paget's disease were 6- to 8-fold higher than those of postmenopausal women, and patients with primary hyperparathyroidism had even higher levels. Intravenous pamidronate treatment for three days in Paget's disease patients was reflected in the S-ELISA by a decrease in collagen degradation products of 55% when compared with values before treatment ($n = 15$); similar results were obtained after a six month oral treatment with 20 mg alendronate/day. The assay appears to be a sensitive and specific index of bone resorption and may prove useful in the follow up of treatment of patients with metabolic bone diseases [54].

c. Bone Sialoprotein Another interesting marker of bone metabolism, bone sialoprotein (BSP), is also measurable in human serum. It is a phosphorylated glycoprotein with a M(r) of 70–80 kDa that accounts for approximately 5–10% of the noncollagenous proteins of bone. Due to its relatively restricted distribution to mineralized tissues, BSP may serve as a potential marker of bone metabolism. Compared to levels in healthy controls, serum BSP levels were significantly higher in patients with Paget's disease and other bone disorders with high turnover, such as pHPT or metastatic bone disease [55]. As early as 24 h after treatment with 2 mg of bisphosphonate ibandronate, BSP was significantly reduced compared to pretreatment levels, reaching a minimum after 30 days. This time course suggests that BSP primarily reflects bone resorption [56] and may be an interesting serum marker of bone resorption.

d. ICTP and TRAP The bone resorption markers ICTP [47] and TRAP measured in serum are unreliable indicators of changes in bone turnover in Paget's disease [51]. No evidence suggests that these markers are substantially better predictors of the clinical response to therapy than serum total AP or urinary OHP. There are several problems with the interpretation of these measurements in Paget's disease and the clinical utility of these measurements remains uncertain.

4. ROLE OF BONE FORMATION MARKERS

e. Total Alkaline Phosphatase (AP) Three months after initiation of a bisphosphonate treatment, the curves of resorption and formation markers synchronize, and so far there is no evidence suggesting a specific advantage for anything more complicated than the determination of a total AP. A commonly used method is to express the decrease in AP as a percentage of pretreatment AP (% decrease in AP), or the percent decrease of the pretreatment AP in relation to the upper limit of the reference range of a normal population (% decrease in excess AP). Although useful, this approach is limited by the inverse relationship between these percentage changes and the pretreatment AP. The greatest change in percentage is usually seen in those with the lowest pretreatment AP. To achieve a 50% reduction in AP, activity could either take a reduction from 800 to 400 or from 300 to 150

[57]. Moreover, the posttreatment AP is also affected by the pretreatment AP. Patients with active disease are less likely to be suppressed into the normal range [58, 59]. Therefore, unless matched for pretreatment AP, these methods are of limited use in the comparison between patients and studies of the efficacy of various bisphosphonates. A possible solution may be to assess the rate of AP decrease. It has been shown to be exponential and can be easily expressed as a half-life on a log-linear plot [60]. Using this method, the half-life of AP has been shown to be independent of pretreatment AP [41], which would suggest the AP half-life is a superior expression of response compared with percentage decrease. There is also a marked interindividual variation between patients with similar pretreatment AP who have been administered the same dose of intravenous bisphosphonate [57]; Here also the half-life of AP seems to give an indication of bone-cell sensitivity within an individual. The AP half-life may, therefore, be a good predictor of fair and poor response to bisphosphonate treatment and provide an opportunity to modify therapy in the hope of a better outcome [41]. This interesting concept needs to be evaluated in prospective clinical trials.

5. PERFORMANCE OF OTHER MARKERS OF BONE FORMATION

a. Bone-Specific Alkaline Phosphatase (BAP) Whether or not the bone-specific enzyme of alkaline phosphatase (BAP) is advantageous over the total AP in the assessment of treatment response in Paget's disease is a matter of debate. Although the decrease in its serum level was larger than that in total AP after treatment with the bisphosphonate pamidronate (-58% vs -43%; $p < 0.03$) [38], it is unlikely that this difference is clinically meaningful. In patients with various liver diseases, BAP was slightly increased but stayed within the normal range (mean ± 2 SD) until total AP was markedly increased.

b. Osteocalcin Several studies show that there is no significant relationship between osteocalcin levels, disease activity in Paget's disease, or any of the established markers of bone resorption or formation [46, 61, 62].

B. Predicting the Duration of Remission

The goal of a bisphosphonate treatment in Paget's disease of bone is to achieve prolonged suppression of bone turnover and reduced complications. Patients with a short AP half-life after bisphosphonate treatment tend to have a longer duration of remission, possibly indicating their increased sensitivity to the treatment [41]. The determinants of the duration of the response have been examined and shown to be dependent on both pre- and posttreatment AP. The greater the AP value before therapy and the lesser the degree of AP suppression after

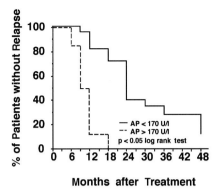

FIGURE 3 Effect of minimal AP on the duration of remission. After treatment with intravenous pamidronate, the duration of remission was significantly longer in those patients, where the minimal total AP after treatment reached the the statistical normal range (AP < 170 U/l). Data from [58].

treatment, the shorter the period during which bone turnover will be suppressed (Fig. 3). Interestingly, this seems also to apply when the posttreatment AP is within the population reference range [58, 59]. This highlights the difficulty of applying population ranges to individuals. A posttreatment AP of 150 U/l may be within the population range of 50–170 U/l but may still be clearly elevated if the individual's natural AP is 100 U/l. The difficulty in converting this finding into a treatment concept is that the individual's natural AP is usually not known. The observation suggests, however, that the AP should not only be "normalized" but also suppressed well within the population reference range to achieve a prolonged remission [63]. Again, this is a hypothesis which needs to be evaluated in prospective studies.

References

1. Delmas, P. D., and Meunier, P. J. (1997). The management of Paget's disease of bone. *N. Engl. J. Med.* **336**, 558–566.
2. Schmorl, G. (1932). Über Osteitis deformans Paget. *Virchow's Arch. A; Pathol. Anat.* **283**, 694–751.
3. Pygott, F. (1957). Paget's disease of bone: The radiological incidence. *Lancet* **1**, 1170–1171.
4. Detheridge, F. M., Guyer, P. B., and Barker, D. J. (1982). European distribution of Paget's disease of bone. *Br. Med. J.* **285**, 1005–1008.
5. Siris, E. S. (1996). Seeking the elusive etiology of Paget disease: A progress report. *J. Bone Miner. Res.* **11**, 1599–1601.
6. Siris, E. S., Ottman, R., Flaster, E., and Kelsey, J. L. (1991). Familial aggregation of Paget's disease of bone. *J. Bone Miner. Res.* **6**, 495–500.
7. Morales Piga, A. A., Rey Rey, J. S., Corres Gonzalez, J., Garcia Sagredo, J. M., and Lopez Abente, G. (1995). Frequency and characteristics of familial aggregation of Paget's disease of bone. *J. Bone Miner. Res.* **10**, 663–670.
8. Kim, G. S., Kim, S. H., Cho, J. K., Park, J. Y., Shin, M. J., Shong, Y. K., Lee, K. U., Han, H., Kim, T. G., Teitelbaum, S. L., Reinus, W. R., and Whyte, M. P. (1997). Paget bone disease involving young adults in 3 generations of a Korean family. *Medicine* **76**, 157–69.
9. Hughes, A. E., Shearman, A. M., Weber, J. L., Barr, R. J., Wallace, R. G., Osterberg, P. H., Nevin, N. C., and Mollan, R. A. (1994). Genetic

linkage of familial expansile osteolysis to chromosome 18q. *Hum. Mol. Genet.* **3**, 359–361.

10. Haslam, S. I., van Hul, W., Morales-Piga, A., Balemans, W., San-Millan, J. L., Nakatsuka, K., Willems, P., Haites, N. E., and Ralston, S. H. (1998). Paget's disease of bone: Evidence for a susceptibility locus on chromosome 18q and for genetic heterogeneity. *J. Bone Miner. Res.* **13**, 911–917.

11. Cody, J. D., Singer, F. R., Roodman, G. D., Otterund, B., Lewis, T. B., Leppert, M., and Leach, R. J. (1997). Genetic linkage of Paget disease of the bone to chromosome 18q. *Am. J. Hum. Genet.* **61**, 1117–1122.

12. Foldes, J., Shamir, S., Brautbar, C., Schermann, L., and Menczel, J. (1991). HLA-D antigens and Paget's disease of bone. *Clin. Orthop.* **266**, 301–303.

13. Singer, F. R., Siris, E., Knierim, A., Giertson, D., and Terasaki, P. I. (1996). The HLA DRβ1*1104 gene frequency is increased in Ashkenazi Jews with Paget's disease of bone. *J. Bone Miner. Res.* **11** (Suppl. 1), M752.

14. Siris, E. S. (1998). Paget's disease of bone. *J. Bone Miner. Res.* **13**, 1061–1065.

15. Meunier, P. J., Coindre, J. M., Edouard, C. M., and Arlot, M. E. (1980). Bone histomorphometry in Paget's disease. Quantitative and dynamic analysis of pagetic and nonpagetic bone tissue. *Arthritis Rheum.* **23**, 1095–1103.

16. Rebel, A., Malkani, K., and Basle, M. (1974). Anomalies nucléaires des ostéoclastes de la maladie osseuse de Paget. *Nouv. Presse Med.* **3**, 1299–1301.

17. Mills, B. G., and Singer, F. R. (1976). Nuclear inclusions in Paget's disease of bone. *Science* **194**, 201–202.

18. Mills, B. G., Yabe, H., and Singer, F. R. (1988). Osteoclasts in human osteopetrosis contain viral-nucleocapsid-like nuclear inclusions. *J. Bone Miner. Res.* **3**, 101–106.

19. Mills, B. G., Singer, F. R., Weiner, L. P., Suffin, S. C., Stabile, E., and Holst, P. (1984). Evidence for both respiratory syncytial virus and measles virus antigens in the osteoclasts of patients with Paget's disease of bone. *Clin Orthop.* **183**, 303–311.

20. Basle, M. F., Fournier, J. G., Rozenblatt, S., Rebel, A., and Bouteille, M. (1986). Measles virus RNA detected in Paget's disease bone tissue by in situ hybridization. *J. Gen. Virol.* **67**, 907–913.

21. Reddy, S. V., Singer, F. R., Mallette, L., and Roodman, G. D. (1996). Detection of measles virus nucleocapsid transcripts in circulating blood cells from patients with Paget disease. *J. Bone Miner. Res.* **11**, 1602–1607.

22. Reddy, S. V., Singer, F. R., and Roodman, G. D. (1995). Bone marrow mononuclear cells from patients with Paget's disease contain measles virus nucleocapsid messenger ribonucleic acid that has mutations in a specific region of the sequence. *J. Clin. Endocrinol. Metab.* **80**, 2108–2111.

23. O'Driscoll, J. B., and Anderson, D. C. (1985). Past pets and Paget's disease. *Lancet* **2**, 919–921.

24. Khan, S. A., Brennan, P., Newman, J., Gray, R. E., McCloskey, E. V., and Kanis, J. A. (1996). Paget's disease of bone and unvaccinated dogs. *Bone* **19**, 47–50.

25. Siris, E. S., Kelsey, J. L., Flaster, E., and Parker, S. (1990). Paget's disease of bone and previous pet ownership in the United States: dogs exonerated. *Int. J. Epidemiol.* **19**, 455–458.

26. Gordon, M. T., Anderson, D. C., and Sharpe, P. T. (1991). Canine distemper virus localised in bone cells of patients with Paget's disease. *Bone* **12**, 195–201.

27. Ralston, S. H., Digiovine, F. S., Gallacher, S. J., Boyle, I. T., and Duff, G. W. (1991). Failure to detect paramyxovirus sequences in Paget's disease of bone using the polymerase chain reaction. *J. Bone Miner. Res.* **6**, 1243–1248.

28. Birch, M. A., Taylor, W., Fraser, W. D., Ralston, S. H., Hart, C. A., and Gallagher, J. A. (1994). Absence of paramyxovirus RNA in cultures of pagetic bone cells and in pagetic bone. *J. Bone Miner. Res.* **9**, 11–16.

29. Whyte, M. P., Leelawattana, R., Reddy, S. V., and Roodman, G. D. (1996). Absence of paramyxovirus transcripts in juvenile Paget bone disease. *J. Bone Miner. Res.* **11**, 1041.

30. Demulder, A., Takahashi, S., Singer, F. R., Hosking, D. J., and Roodman, G. D. (1993). Abnormalities in osteoclast precursors and marrow accessory cells in Paget's disease. *Endocrinology* **133**, 1978–1982.

31. Roodman, G. D., Kurihara, N., Ohsaki, Y., Kukita, A., Hosking, D., Demulder, A., Smith, J. F., and Singer, F. R. (1992). Interleukin 6. A potential autocrine/paracrine factor in Paget's disease of bone. *J. Clin. Invest.* **89**, 46–52.

32. Hoyland, J. A., Freemont, A. J., and Sharpe, P. T. (1994). Interleukin-6, IL-6 receptor, and IL-6 nuclear factor gene expression in Paget's disease. *J. Bone Miner. Res.* **9**, 75–80.

33. Hoyland, J., and Sharpe, P. T. (1994). Upregulation of c-fos protooncogene expression in pagetic osteoclasts. *J. Bone Miner. Res.* **9**, 1191–1194.

34. Grauer, A., and Wüster, C. (1996). Morbus Paget. *In* "Klinische Endokrinologie" (B. Allolio and H. M. Schulte, eds.), pp. 336–341. Urban & Schwarzenberg, München.

35. Grauer, A. (1997). Seltene Osteopathien: Morbus Paget und Osteogenesis imperfecta. *In* "Syllabus, IV. Intensivkurs für Klinische Endokrinologie" (B. Allolio, M. Grussendorf, O. A. Müller, T. Olbricht and H. M. Schulte, eds.), pp. 67–76. Bundesdruckerei, Neu-Isenburg.

36. Meunier, P. J., Salson, C., and Methieu, L. (1987). Skeletal distribution and biochemical parameters of Paget's disease. *Clin. Orthop.* **217**, 37–44.

37. Grauer, A. (1998). Therapie des Morbus Paget: Indikationen und Strategien. *Osteologie* **7** (Suppl. 1), 85–86.

38. Garnero, P., and Delmas, P. D. (1993). Assessment of the serum levels of bone alkaline phosphatase with a new immunoradiometric assay in patients with metabolic bone disease. *J. Clin. Endocrinol. Metab.* **77**, 1046–1053.

39. Alvarez, L., Peris, P., Pons, F., Guanabens, N., Herranz, R., Monegal, A., Bedini, J. L., Deulofeu, R., Martinez de Osaba, M. J., Munoz Gomez, J., and Ballesta, A. M. (1997). Relationship between biochemical markers of bone turnover and bone scintigraphic indices in assessment of Paget's disease activity. *Arthritis Rheum.* **40**, 461–468.

40. Alvarez, L., Guanabens, N., Peris, P., Monegal, A., Bedini, J. L., Deulofeu, R., Martinez de Osaba, M. J., Munoz Gomez, J., Rivera Fillat, F., and Ballesta, A. M. (1995). Discriminative value of biochemical markers of bone turnover in assessing the activity of Paget's disease. *J. Bone Miner. Res.* **10**, 458–465.

41. Patel, S. (1995). Treatment response in Paget's disease. *Ann. Rheum. Dis.* **54**, 783–784.

42. Kanis, J. A., and Gray, R. E. (1987). Long-term follow-up observations on treatment in Paget's disease of bone. *Clin. Orthop. Relat. Res.* **217**, 99–125.

43. Meunier, P. J. (1994). Bone histomorphometry and skeletal distribution of Paget's disease of bone. *Semin. Arthritis Rheum.* **23**, 219–221.

44. Meunier, P. J., and Vignot, E. (1995). Therapeutic strategy in Paget's disease of bone. *Bone* **17**, 489S–491S.

45. Hamdy, N. A., Papapoulos, S. E., Colwell, A., Eastell, R., and Russell, R. G. (1993). Urinary collagen crosslink excretion: A better index of bone resorption than hydroxyproline in Paget's disease of bone? *Bone Miner.* **22**, 1–8.

46. Kaddam, I. M., Iqbal, S. J., Holland, S., Wong, M., and Manning, D. (1994). Comparison of serum osteocalcin with total and bone specific alkaline phosphatase and urinary hydroxyproline:creatinine ratio in patients with Paget's disease of bone. *Ann. Clin. Biochem.* **31**, 327–330.

47. Filipponi, P., Pedetti, M., Beghe, F., Giovagnini, B., Miam, M., and Cristallini, S. (1994). Effects of two different bisphosphonates on Paget's disease of bone: ICTP assessed. *Bone* **15**, 261–267.

48. Grauer, A., Klar, B., Scharla, S. H., and Ziegler, R. (1994). Long-term efficacy of intravenous pamidronate in Paget's disease of bone. *Semin. Arthritis Rheum.* **23**, 283–284.

49. Papapoulos, S. E., and Frolich, M. (1996). Prediction of the outcome of treatment of Paget's disease of bone with bisphosphonates from short-term changes in the rate of bone resorption. *J. Clin. Endocrinol. Metab.* **81**, 3993–3997.

50. Woitge, H. W., Grauer, A., Oberwittler, H., Heichel, S., Ziegler, R., and Seibel, M. J. (1999). Long term effects of ibandronate treatment on biochemical markers of bone turnover in patients with Paget's disease of bone. *J. Clin. Endocrinol. Metab.* (in press).

51. Blumsohn, A., Naylor, K. E., Assiri, A. M., and Eastell, R. (1995). Different responses of biochemical markers of bone resorption to bisphosphonate therapy in Paget disease. *Clin. Chem.* **41**, 1592–1598.

52. Garnero, P., Fledelius, C., Gineyts, E., Serre, C. M., Vignot, E., and Delmas, P. D. (1997). Decreased beta-isomerization of the C-terminal telopeptide of type I collagen alpha 1 chain in Paget's disease of bone. *J. Bone Miner. Res.* **12**, 1407–1415.

53. Sinigaglia, L., Varenna, M., Binelli, L., Beltrametti, P., Zucchi, F., Arrigoni, M., Frignani, S., and Abbiati, G. (1997). Serum levels of pyridinium crosslinks in postmenopausal women and Paget's disease of bone. *Calcif. Tissue Int.* **61**, 279–284.

54. Bonde, M., Garnero, P., Fledelius, C., Qvist, P., Delmas, P. D., and Christiansen, C. (1997). Measurement of bone degradation products in serum using antibodies reactive with an isomerized form of an 8 amino acid sequence of the C-telopeptide of type I collagen. *J. Bone Miner. Res.* **12**, 1028–1034.

55. Seibel, M. J., Woitge, H. W., Pecherstorfer, M., Karmatschek, M., Horn, E., Ludwig, H., Armbruster, F. P., and Ziegler, R. (1996). Serum immunoreactive bone sialoprotein as a new marker of bone turnover in metabolic and malignant bone disease. *J. Clin. Endocrinol. Metab.* **81**, 3289–3294.

56. Woitge, H. W., Seibel, M. J., Heichel, S., Grauer, A., and Ziegler, R. (1997). Serum immunoreactive bone sialoprotein in Paget's disease of bone treated with ibandronate. *J. Bone Miner. Res.* **12**, T676.

57. Patel, S., Coupland, C. A., Stone, M. D., and Hosking, D. J. (1995). Comparison of methods of assessing response of Paget's disease to bisphosphonate therapy. *Bone* **16**, 193–197.

58. Grauer, A., Knaus, J., Klar, B., and Ziegler, R. (1995). Relapse free interval after pamidronate treatment in Paget's disease of bone. *J. Bone Miner. Res.* **10** (Suppl. 1), 510.

59. Patel, S., Stone, M. D., Coupland, C., and Hosking, D. J. (1993). Determinants of remission of Paget's disease of bone. *J. Bone Miner. Res.* **8**, 1467–1473.

60. Fenton, A. J., Gutteridge, D. H., Kent, G. N., Price, R. I., Retallack, R. W., Bhagat, C. I., Worth, G. K., Thompson, R. I., Watson, I. G., Barry Walsh, C., and Matz, L. R. (1991). Intravenous aminobisphosphonate in Paget's disease: clinical, biochemical, histomorphometric and radiological responses. *Clin. Endocrinol.* **34**, 197–204.

61. Randall, A. G., Kent, G. N., Garcia Webb, P., Bhagat, C. I., Pearce, D. J., Gutteridge, D. H., Prince, R. L., Stewart, G., Stuckey, B., Will, R. K., Retallack, R. W., Price, R. I., and Ward, L. (1996). Comparison of biochemical markers of bone turnover in Paget disease treated with pamidronate and a proposed model for the relationships between measurements of the different forms of pyridinoline cross-links. *J. Bone Miner. Res.* **11**, 1176–1184.

62. de la Piedra, C., Rapado, A., Diaz Diego, E. M., Diaz Martin, M. A., Aguirre, C., Lopez Gavilanes, E., and Diaz Curiel, M. (1996). Variable efficacy of bone remodeling biochemical markers in the management of patients with Paget's disease of bone treated with tiludronate. *Calcif. Tissue Int.* **59**, 95–99.

63. Grauer, A. (1997). Morbus Paget. *In* "Metabolische Osteopathien" (M. J. Seibel and H. G. Stracke, eds.), pp. 288–300. Schattauer, Stuttgart and New York.

CHAPTER 42

Metastatic Bone Disease

JEAN-JACQUES BODY Supportive Care Clinic and Bone Diseases Clinic, Institut Jules Bordet,
Université Libre de Bruxelles, Brussels, Belgium

I. ABSTRACT

The skeleton is the most common site of metastatic disease and the most common site of first distant relapse in breast and in prostate cancer. Osteolytic bone disease is responsible for a considerable morbidity which also makes major demands on resources for health care provision. Increased bone resorption in tumor bone disease (bone metastases and myeloma) is mediated by the osteoclasts and not directly by the tumor cells themselves, explaining why bisphosphonates have been so successfully used for the treatment of tumor-induced osteolysis. Hypercalcemia occurs in about 20% of the patients with advanced cancer, and the uncoupling between bone resorption and bone formation is easily demonstrated by the measurement of bone markers. The differential diagnosis between tumor-induced hypercalcemia (TIH) and primary hyperparathyroidism has been much simplified since the discovery of assays specifically measuring intact PTH and now PTHrP. Commercially available assays can now detect increased PTHrP levels in at least 80% of patients with TIH. The diagnosis of bone metastases is often easy when the patient is symptomatic. The diagnostic usefulness of bone markers is limited and available data indicate that bone markers are so far unsuitable for an early diagnosis of neoplastic skeletal involvement. However, by combining bone-specific alkaline phosphatase (BAP), or maybe modern bone resorption markers, with specific tumor markers, such as PSA or CA15.3, the diagnostic sensitivity could be improved. On the other hand, biochemical markers of bone turnover have the unique potential to simplify and to improve the monitoring of metastatic bone disease, which remains a continuous challenge for the oncologist. Peptide-bound cross-links could be quite useful to discriminate between patients progressing early on treatment from those with longer disease control. Also, the diagnostic efficiency of a 50% increase in these markers could identify imminent progression. On the other hand, the optimal therapeutic schemes of bisphosphonate are largely unknown, and markers of bone resorption could be especially useful to monitor their effects. More importantly, the individual biochemical response can predict for pain relief and future work will have to determine if adjusting bisphosphonate dosage according to the levels of specific bone markers could enhance their efficiency.

II. INTRODUCTION

A. Clinical and Pathogenic Aspects of Tumor-Induced Bone Disease: A Brief Overview

1. CLINICAL ASPECTS

According to the series, 30–90% of patients with advanced cancer will develop skeletal metastases. Carcinomas of the

591

breast (47–85%), prostate (33–85%), and lung (32–60%) are the tumors most commonly associated with skeletal metastases. At the other end of the spectrum, tumors of the digestive tract are rarely (3–13%) complicated by metastatic involvement of bone [1]. The skeleton is, in fact, the most common site of metastatic disease in breast cancer and the most common site of first distant relapse [2, 3]. These patients have a relatively long survival after the diagnosis of bone metastases compared to patients with extraosseous metastases only. Their median survival is usually beyond 20 months and about 10% of these patients are still alive five to ten years after the first diagnosis of bone metastases [2].

Osteolytic bone disease can be responsible for a considerable morbidity and can markedly decrease the quality of life. Because of the long clinical course breast cancer may follow, morbidity from bone metastases also makes major demands on resources for health care provision. Besides the complications of bone marrow invasion, pain and functional disability occur in 45–75% of the cases [1, 4]. Major complications will be observed in up to one-third of the patients whose first relapse is in bone [2, 5]. Hypercalcemia occurs in 10–15% of the cases and, when long bones are invaded, fractures will occur in 10–20% of the cases [6].

Metastatic bone pain is traditionally attributed to various factors, notably the release of chemical mediators, the increased pressure within the bone, microfractures, the stretching of periosteum, reactive muscle spasm, and nerve root infiltration and/or compression [7]. However, as suggested by the clinical and biochemical effects of bisphosphonates, the dramatic increase in bone resorption, which is easily seen with bone turnover markers, probably plays an important contributory role as well. Pathological fractures constitute a major cause of prolonged disability in breast cancer, whereas pathological fracture is relatively unusual in prostatic cancer, with its predominantly sclerotic picture. The majority of bone metastases from breast cancer are osteolytic, but about one-fifth is purely or essentially osteosclerotic, as classically observed in prostate cancer.

It is not rare that metastatic breast cancer remains confined to the skeleton for a long time. Sherry et al. [8] studied 86 such patients who developed extraskeletal metastases after a mean delay of two years. Compared to patients who initially had metastases to other sites, these patients had a prolonged survival (median of 48 months vs 17 months) but presented even more often with major complications of their skeletal disease. Thus, 21% developed pathological fractures of the long bones and 15% had spinal cord compression [8]. This relatively slow evolution of breast cancer metastasizing in bone suggests some peculiar biological properties of these tumor cells. Indeed, breast cancers metastasizing to the skeleton are more frequently estrogen receptor-positive and well differentiated than the tumors metastasizing to lungs or liver [2, 9]. The presence of sclerotic lesions has been associated with a better prognosis than lytic lesions [10].

2. PATHOPHYSIOLOGY OF TUMOR-INDUCED OSTEOLYSIS

The osteotropism of breast and prostate neoplasms remains poorly understood. Preferential access of prostate cancer cells to the axial skeleton has been attributed to a passage through the vertebral venous plexus of Batson, which is a low-pressure, high-volume system of vertebral veins running adjacent to the spine. On the other hand, various properties of cancer cells, such as the production of proteolytic enzymes and the loss of specific cell adhesion molecules, can enhance their metastatic potential. More specifically, deposits into the skeleton can be due to the attraction of tumor cells by chemotactic factors released by the normal remodeling of bone matrix. These factors include fragments of type I collagen and of osteocalcin, and several growth factors [11, 12].

Once breast cancer cells colonize the bone marrow, they are probably attracted to bone surfaces by the products of resorbing bone and destroy bone via osteoclast stimulation. The importance of direct osteolytic effects of metastatic cancer cells, including the effects of collagenases, is uncertain although they may play a role in the late stages of tumor-induced osteolysis (TIO). They appear to induce osteoclast differentiation of hematopoietic stem cells and/or activate mature osteoclasts already present in bone. An increased osteoclast number has been particularly well demonstrated in the biopsies of 65 normocalcemic women with breast cancer and predominantly lytic bone metastases. Osteoclast number was high in biopsies from bone adjacent to the tumor and directly in the invaded bone, indicating that increased bone resorption in metastatic breast cancer is mediated by the osteoclasts and not directly by the tumor cells themselves [13]. Osteoblasts could be important target cells for tumor secretory products. Siwek et al. [14] have observed that breast cancer cells secrete factors that can inhibit the proliferation of osteoblast-like cells and normal human osteoblasts, and can increase their second messenger response to osteolytic agents. Osteoblasts could thus, in the process of TIO, keep the central role that they have in the physiological regulation of osteoclast resorption activity.

The nature of the tumor-derived factor(s) responsible for osteoclastic activation remains unknown, but data indicate that PTHrP could play an important role. PTHrP-like substances are expressed by about 60% of human breast cancers, and breast tumors which spread to the skeleton produce PTHrP more frequently than tumors metastasizing to nonosseous sites; however, these data have to be confirmed in larger studies [15, 16]. PTHrP and other factors would stimulate osteoclastic bone resorption, leading to the release of bone matrix degradation products which may be chemotactic for cancer cells. Tumor-associated factors, such as TGF-α, could also increase the end-organ effects of PTHrP.

The propensity of breast cancer cells to metastasize and proliferate in bone could be explained by a "seed and soil" concept [17]. Breast cancer cells (the "seed") appear to secrete factors, such as PTHrP, that potentiate the development of metastases in the skeleton, which constitutes a fertile "soil" rich in cytokines and growth factors that stimulate breast cancer cell growth, including insulin-like growth factors [18]. Local production of PTHrP and of other osteolytic factors such as TGF-α by cancer cells in bone would stimulate osteoclastic bone resorption, partly through the osteoblasts, the proliferation of which may also be inhibited. Such factors probably induce osteoclast differentiation from hematopoietic stem cells and activate mature osteoclasts already present in bone. Increased osteoclast number and activity would then cause local foci of osteolysis, which could further stimulate cancer cell proliferation [17].

Prostate cancer cells probably also stimulate osteoclast activity through the osteoblasts. The precise nature of the responsible factor is unknown and various substances have been implicated, notably TGF-β, bone morphogenetic proteins, IGFs, urokinase, and PTHrP [19].

Multiple myeloma is characterized by a marked increase in osteoclast activity and proliferation. This excessive resorption of bone could by itself play a contributory role to the growth of myeloma cells in bone through the release of growth factors from resorbed bone matrix and the secretion of interleukin-6 by bone cells. Using established cell lines, it has been shown that through direct cell-to-cell contact, myeloma cells can downregulate osteocalcin production but upregulate IL-6 secretion, supporting the concept of the importance of the bone microenvironment in the genesis of myeloma-induced osteolysis [20]. Much of this reasoning is still speculative, but the data summarized here indicate that bone-resorbing cells are a logical target for the treatment and perhaps the prevention of TIO.

B. Classical Methods for the Monitoring of Metastatic Bone Disease

The diagnosis of bone metastases is often easy when patients are symptomatic, and a bone biopsy is rarely necessary. However, the assessment of the response to therapy remains a continuous challenge. Quantitative pain assessment is performed too rarely by the oncologist. Although none of the available pain measuring instruments have been specifically developed for metastatic bone pain and the evident psychosocial influences on pain perception, pain intensity can be quickly assessed by visual analog scales.

The radionuclide bone scan remains the most widely used method for diagnosis and surveillance of bone metastatic involvement. The bone scan is more sensitive than X-rays for the early detection of bone metastases. However, the relative lack of specificity of the bone scan is well known and at least one-third of solitary abnormalities detected in cancer patients are due to benign diseases [21]. In one study, the appearance of one or two new abnormalities on the bone scan in cancer patients without known metastases was later confirmed to be of metastatic origin in only 11% and 24% of the cases, respectively [22], but the presence of multiple focal hot spots is more specific for metastatic bone disease. Increasing scintigraphic activity does not always correspond to progressive disease. Besides our inability to quantify these changes, which constitutes a major problem, one must be aware of the so-called flare phenomenon. This apparent worsening of the bone scan (increased scintigraphic activity in bone lesions or even the appearance of previously invisible lesions) represents the initial healing of osteolytic lesions and can thus be misinterpreted as evidence of tumor progression [23]. It is unknown if bone markers could be useful in such cases.

Radiographic methods remain the essential tool for the diagnosis and the characterization of bone metastases. Computed tomography (CT) or magnetic resonance imaging (MRI) are particularly useful to diagnose early metastatic involvement of bone when hot spots are detected on the radionuclide scan but corresponding X-rays are normal. MRI is especially helpful in detecting early bone marrow involvement in asymptomatic disease that shows no relationship with bone scan positivity or alkaline phosphatase increase [24].

The assessment of the response of skeletal metastases to therapy remains a daily challenge for the oncologist [6]. For example, a complete response to antineoplastic therapy of a bone metastasis requires the reversal of abnormal radiographic findings, which is highly subjective and almost impossible to achieve. On the other hand, development of new blastic lesions does not necessarily mean progression, because they can appear in previously lytic areas that were not detected on X-rays. All of the imaging techniques actually aim to detect recalcification of lytic areas, which is evidently not an early phenomenon. Symptom evaluation and measurement of biochemical parameters should definitely be further investigated for early assessment. A combination of pain assessment (with a score for analgesic consumption), performance status, and an assay for a bone resorption marker certainly deserves to be studied.

Markers of bone turnover could essentially be used as diagnostic tests and to assess response to treatment. Their role in predicting skeletal complications has not been well examined so far and will not be reviewed.

III. USE OF MARKERS OF BONE TURNOVER FOR THE DIAGNOSIS OF TUMOR-INDUCED BONE DISEASE

Available markers are reviewed elsewhere in the book; here they will briefly be reviewed as they pertain to the cancer field. Total alkaline phosphatase (TAP) is still the marker most often used in routine oncological practice. However, to exclude contribution from the liver and other organs, the measurement of the bone isoenzyme of alkaline phosphatase (BAP) is required. Reproducible assays for direct BAP determination are now commercially available with a cross-reactivity for liver AP between 7 and 13% [25]. Osteocalcin (or bone-GLA protein, BGP or OC) is a protein specifically made by the osteoblasts; its measurement appears to reflect the late phases of bone formation but its usefulness in oncology remains quite obscure [26]. Assays for the peptides released during the extracellular processing of collagen, referred as the procollagen carboxy-terminal propeptide (PICP) and the amino-terminal propeptide (PINP), might represent useful markers of bone formation because collagen is by far the most abundant organic component of bone matrix. However, preliminary results obtained with available assays appear to be disappointing, at least in patients with nonneoplastic diseases, and data from cancer patients are scanty.

On the bone resorption side, the fasting urinary excretion of calcium and of hydroxyproline are still the classical markers used in oncology. Urinary excretion of calcium is, however, not a true marker of bone resorption; rather it reflects the net effects of bone formation and resorption. It lacks sensitivity and specificity for diagnostic use. For example, in a study of 153 patients with various cancers, urinary calcium measurement could not differentiate patients with and without bone metastases [27]. Hydroxyproline is derived from the various forms of collagen and is influenced by dietary gelatin intake, but it remains a conventional and widely available parameter to assess bone resorption. When measured in fasting urine samples, it is a reasonably valid estimate of the bone resorption rate [28–30].

New parameters of bone resorption have been introduced that will probably be more helpful because of their increased specificity for bone matrix destruction. The intermolecular cross-linking compounds of mature collagen, pyridinoline (PYD) and deoxypyridinoline (DPD), could be particularly well suited to monitor the breakdown of bone matrix by cancer cells, especially because they are independent of dietary intake. Their measurement traditionally required the HPLC technique, but HPLC analysis already tend to be replaced by direct, commercially available, assays. Cross-links exist in both free (40%) and peptide-bound (60%) forms, and enzyme-linked immunoassays (ELISA) have been developed to measure the protein-bound cross-linking molecule at either the N-terminal part (NTX) or the C-terminal part (CTX), or the free portions of both PYD and DPD. However, there are no extensive face-to-face comparisons between the classical HPLC assay and these direct telopeptide assays [31]. Each of these immunoassays for free PYD and related peptides may reflect different aspects of bone resorption. For example, increased bone turnover is associated with a preferential increase of the peptide bound/total fraction and a decrease of the free/total fraction, at least in benign conditions [32].

There is also great interest in developing a reliable serum assay for cross-links. At present, the only largely available serum assay is a C-telopeptide cross-links assay which recognizes elements from the helical part of the collagen chain (ICTP). However, the clinical value of this assay is uncertain because it appears to be an index of collagen turnover [33] but not a specific marker of bone resorption, especially in cancer patients. New methods are being developed to measure NTX or CTX in serum and limited data indicate that they should be quite useful.

Lastly, bone sialoprotein (BSP) is a noncollagenous protein of the bone extracellular matrix accounting for 5–10% of the noncollagenous proteins of the bone matrix. It is found mainly in osteoblasts but also in osteoclasts. An assay has been developed for BSP which indicates that BSP measurement is more a marker of bone resorption than of bone formation [34, 35].

Markers are quite useful in the context of clinical research but much work remains to be done to prove their interest for the management of individual patients. One has to realize that this is a new field, especially for the new markers described above, which can explain the small number of good studies.

A. Tumor-Induced Hypercalcemia

Tumor-induced hypercalcemia (TIH) is one of the most frequent paraneoplastic syndromes. The prevalence of hypercalcemia is quite variable in the literature; this complication can affect 8–40% of cancer patients at some time during the course of their disease. TIH can complicate any type of cancer, but breast and lung carcinomas and multiple myeloma represent more than 50% of the cases. Most often, TIH complicates advanced cancer and the median survival varies between one and 4.5 months [11].

Secretion of humoral and paracrine factors by the tumor markedly stimulates osteoclast activity and proliferation, often with inhibition of osteoblastic activity, causing an uncoupling between bone resorption and bone formation, and thus a rapid rise in serum calcium [36]. In contrast, in primary hyperparathyroidism, bone formation is stimulated in parallel to bone resorption and serum calcium is much more stable. This has been confirmed by studies with biochemical markers of bone turnover; in TIH there is a marked increase in cross-link levels but quite variable concentrations of OC, often with very low values (Fig. 1), whereas both markers are increased in primary hyperparathyroidism [26, 37]. The ratio between DPD and OC is normal in primary hyperparathyroidism but markedly increased in both types of TIH, whether of humoral or local osteolytic origin (Fig. 2) [38]. Body et al. [39] measured BAP and other markers of bone turnover in 46 patients with TIH. Mean ($\pm$SD) BAP concentrations were slightly higher in patients with TIH than in healthy subjects (15.5 $\pm$ 8.5 versus 12.4 $\pm$ 3.5 mg/L; p < 0.05). However, the scatter of the data was quite marked (Fig. 3). Increased BAP values (22%) occurred only in patients with bone metastases [39]. BAP levels also correlated with the extent of bone uptake at scintigraphy ($r_s = 0.54$; p < 0.01) but this was not the

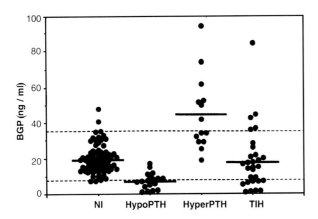

FIGURE 1   Serum osteocalcin (BGP) concentrations (measured by an immunoradiometric assay) in 61 healthy subjects (NI), 29 patients with tumor-induced hypercalcemia (TIH), 14 patients with primary hyperparathyroidism (HyperPTH), and 18 hypoparathyroid patients (HypoPTH). Note the scatter of the BGP values in patients with TIH. Horizontal lines indicate the lower and upper limits of the normal range (2.5th–97.5th percentiles). From Dumon *et al.* [26], with permission.

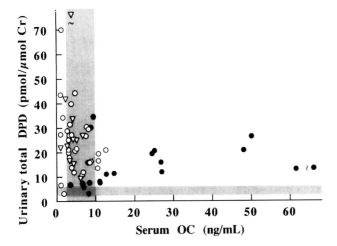

FIGURE 2   Relationship between total deoxypyridinoline (DPD) and osteocalcin (OC) in 20 patients with primary hyperparathyroidism (●), 31 patients with humoral hypercalcemia of malignancy (○), and 11 patients with hypercalcemia and bone metastases (△). Dotted areas indicate the normal ranges. Note the suppressed OC values in many hypercalcemic patients. Reproduced from Nakayama, K., *et al.* [38], Differences in bone and vitamin D metabolism between primary hyperparathyroidism and malignancy-associated hypercalcemia, *J. Clin. Endocrinol. Metab.* **81**, 607–611, 1996, © The Endocrine Society.

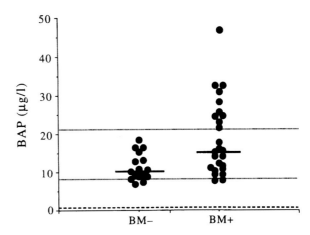

FIGURE 3   Serum concentrations of the bone isoenzyme of alkaline phosphatase (BAP) in 46 patients with TIH, divided according to the presence (BM+) or the absence (BM−) of bone metastases. Bars represent the median values. Note that increased values (22%) occurred only in the group BM+. Reprinted from *Eur. J. Cancer* **33**, Body, J. J., *et al.* [39], The bone isoenzyme of alkaline phosphatase in hypercalcaemic cancer patients, pp. 1578–1582, Copyright 1997, with permission from Elsevier Science.

case for TAP or OC. These data confirm the existence of an uncoupling in bone turnover in TIH and indicate that cancer hypercalcemia is another pathological condition characterized by a discordance between BAP and OC concentrations (as are glucocorticoid-induced osteoporosis and Paget's disease of bone) [39].

Bone resorption is classically considered to be greatly increased in TIH [28]. However, it is interesting to note that urinary pyridinium cross-links are not significantly higher in hypercalcemic patients than in normocalcemic patients with bone metastases (see last two series of data of Fig. 4) [27]. This finding suggests that the inhibition of osteoblast activity could have an important causal role in the development of TIH.

Several studies have established the essential role of parathyroid hormone-related protein (PTHrP) in most types of cancer hypercalcemia. The kidneys may also contribute to the pathogenesis and maintenance of TIH through a decrease in the glomerular filtration rate and an increase in the tubular reabsorption of calcium which result from the decreased circulating volume and the specific renal effects of PTHrP. The protein has been purified to homogeneity, sequenced, and cloned [40]. PTHrP effects are autocrine or paracrine in nature and its only known endocrine effect is its role in the pathophysiology of TIH. Animal models of humoral hypercalcemia of malignancy (HHM) constitute a useful means to assess the importance of hypercalcemic factors and, in nude mice transplanted with human PTHrP-producing tumors, passive immunization with anti-PTHrP monoclonal antibodies can correct hypercalcemia, decrease osteoclastic bone resorption, and markedly prolong the survival time of the tumor-bearing animals [41].

The differential diagnosis between TIH and primary hyperparathyroidism has been much simplified since the discovery of assays specifically measuring intact parathyroid hormone (PTH). These assays permit a complete separation of PTH levels in the two conditions. Serum PTH concentrations are indeed elevated, or at least are in the upper part of the normal range, in hyperparathyroid patients, whereas they are suppressed in patients with TIH [42]. Primary hyperparathyroidism is not a rare disease, however, and both conditions can coexist. An elevated intact PTH level in a hypercalcaemic

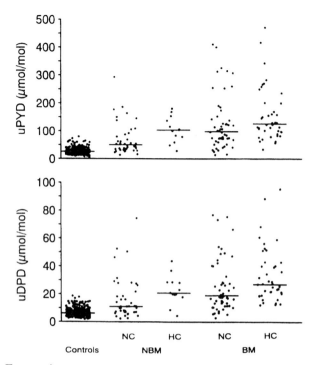

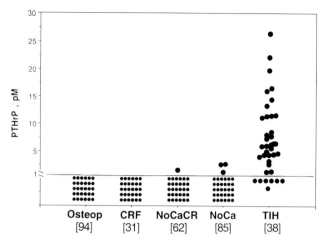

FIGURE 5   Individual PTHrP concentrations are undetectable in 94 patients with osteopenia or osteoporosis (Osteop.) and in 31 patients with chronic renal failure (CRF), detectable in 1 of 62 (2%) patients in complete remission from their cancer (NoCaCR) and in 4 of 85 (5%) normocalcemic patients with an active cancer (NoCa), and increased (detectable) in 31 of 38 (82%) hypercalcemic cancer patients (TIH). The assay detection limit is 1 pM. From Dumon *et al.* [47].

FIGURE 4   Urinary pyridinium cross-link levels in 153 healthy controls, 55 patients without bone metastases (NBM); 42 of them had a normal serum calcium level = NC and 13 were hypercalcemic = HC), and 98 patients with bone metastases (BM; 56 of them had a normal serum calcium level = NC and 42 were hypercalcemic = HC). Reproduced from Pecherstorfer, M., *et al.* [27], The diagnostic value of urinary pyridinium cross-links of collagen, serum total alkaline phosphatase and urinary calcium excretion in neoplastic bone disease, *J. Clin. Endocrinol. Metab.* **80**, 97–103, 1995, © The Endocrine Society.

cancer patient is a strong indicator for the presence of hyperparathyroidism and does not imply at all that the tumour is secreting PTH [43]. Several immunoassays have been developed to measure levels of circulating PTHrP. According to the published series, 45–100% of patients with TIH have increased circulating PTHrP concentrations [11, 44]. Virtually all hypercalcemic patients without bone metastases (humoral hypercalcemia of malignancy, or HHM) have elevated PTHrP levels but, with a sensitive assay, Grill *et al.* [45] showed that this is also the case in two-thirds of the patients with hypercalcaemia and bone metastases. Two-site assays including the measurement of large N-terminal regions appear to be optimal for TIH evaluation [46]. Dumon *et al.* [47] evaluated a commercial IRMA (Diasorin) for circulating PTHrP which utilizes two antibodies specific to separate regions of the protein. PTHrP levels were detectable in 31 of 38 patients with TIH (82%) and we found significant correlations between the concentrations of PTHrP and Pi ($r_s = -0.52$; p < 0.05), TmP/GFR ($r_s = -0.51$; p < 0.05), and an index of the tubular reabsorption of Ca ($r_s = 0.38$; p < 0.05). PTHrP was only rarely increased in normocalcemic cancer patients and was undetectable in all patients with benign diseases [47] (Fig. 5). If confirmed over the long run, this commercially available

PTHrP IRMA should be quite useful for routine assessments but also for research laboratories.

Circulating PTHrP concentrations do not change after successful therapy of TIH with bisphosphonates, implying that elevated PTHrP levels indeed constitute a primary phenomenon and that PTHrP secretion is not regulated *in vivo* by serum calcium, at least in hypercalcemic subjects [44]. On the contrary, PTH secretion rapidly recovers when serum calcium levels decrease, and circulating PTH levels are normalized as soon as calcium enters the normal range [48], implying that blood sampling for diagnostic purposes must preferably be done before starting bisphosphonate therapy.

B. Metastatic Bone Disease

The diagnostic usefulness of biochemical markers for the diagnosis of bone metastases is so far limited. Data in hypercalcemic cancer patients indicate that BAP levels appear to better reflect bone metastatic involvement than TAP or OC [39]. In breast cancer, the sensitivity of BAP determinations (whether by lectin precipitation, EIA, or IRMA) does not appear to be better than that of TAP [49]. Some data indicate that the diagnostic sensitivity of BAP for the diagnosis of bone metastases from breast cancer could be superior to that of CA15.3 but more data are needed [50]. Compared to TAP, the main advantage of measuring BAP in prostate cancer appears to be a higher positive predictive value for the diagnosis of bone metastatic involvement [51], probably due to a higher diagnostic specificity, as suggested by the study of Zaninotto *et al.* [52]. In 65 patients with metastatic prostate cancer, they found specificities of 57%

TABLE I. Sensitivity, Specificity, Positive Predictive Value, Negative Predictive Value, and Clinical Effectiveness of Bone Alkaline Phosphatase Enzyme and Prostate-Specific Antigen (PSA) Cutoff for Bone Metastasis in 150 Controls, 100 Patients with Benign Prostatic Hyperplasia, and 100 Patients with Prostate Cancer (48 metastatic)

	% Sensitivity	% Specificity	% Pos. predictive value	% Neg. predictive value	% Clin. effectiv.
Bone alkaline phosphatase enzyme more than 30 ng/ml	87.5	100	100	89.6	93.7
PSA more than 100 ng/ml	79.1	84.6	82.6	81.5	81.8
Bone alkaline phosphatase enzyme more than 30 ng/l and/or PSA more than 100 ng/ml	95.8	100	100	95.6	97.9

From Lorente *et al.* [56], with permission.

and 90% for TAP and BAP, respectively [52]. Highest levels are seen in patients with multiple blastic metastases [53]. BAP definitely has a better sensitivity than TAP in patients with metastatic prostate cancer when TAP is in the range of normal to twice-normal [54]. Limited data indicate that BAP could be superior to prostate-specific antigen (PSA) as a marker for bone metastases [55] and that the combination of both markers has a better diagnostic sensitivity than either marker alone [56]. Compared to the upper limit of normal, BAP could detect 88% of the patients with bone metastases with a specificity of 100%. By combining BAP with PSA, the sensitivity in detecting bone metastases increased to 96% (Table I) [56]. An enzyme immunoassay has also been described that could have an even better specificity for the bone isoenzyme than the IRMA mentioned above [57]. PICP levels typically correlate with BAP, especially in patients with blastic metastases [53].

Increased OC levels are frequently observed in patients without bone metastases [26, 58]. In a series of 60 patients with recurring breast cancer, less than 50% of patients with bone involvement had elevated OC levels [59]. OC also is less sensitive than PSA or prostatic acid phosphatase (PAP) for the detection of bone metastases in prostate cancer [60]. OC levels are nevertheless significantly increased in metastatic bone disease from breast and prostate cancers [61], but not in multiple myeloma. Bataille *et al.* [62] have shown that a subgroup of patients with multiple myeloma (around 12%) had increased OC levels with a more indolent disease and a lower osteolytic potential, whereas patients with decreased OC values had a more severe disease [62]. More generally, however, a large study showed that OC was a poor marker of the severity of multiple myeloma and that it did not correlate with survival; however, the study confirmed the good correlation of OC levels with histomorphometric parameters of bone formation (and not bone resorption) in this typical condition of bone uncoupling [63]. OC levels also do not correlate with BAP [64]. Preliminary results obtained with propeptide assays of type 1 collagen also appear to be disappointing, at least in patients with nonneoplastic diseases, because their sensitivity appears to be lower than that of OC or BAP [65]. It has been claimed that PICP has a greater

diagnostic specificity than PSA, PAP or TAP for the diagnosis of bone metastases in prostate cancer, but the superiority of PICP for diagnostic purposes was not convincing. In the ROC analysis, the areas under the curves were actually quite similar for all four markers, whereas the separation between patients with or without bone metastases was the greatest for PSA [66]. However, limited data suggest that PICP could be of value to separate patients who respond to therapy from patients who progress after therapy [66].

Urinary calcium is a poor diagnostic marker for bone metastases, whereas urinary hydroxyproline is typically increased in patients with advanced metastatic bone disease. In patients with bone metastases from breast cancer, levels of hydroxyproline, PYD, and DPD are significantly increased compared to normal values, but the proportionate increase is higher for PYD and DPD (Fig. 6). In a review of six studies, elevated levels of PYD and DPD have been found in 58–88% and 60–80% of the patients, respectively [67]. Lipton *et al.* [68] found elevated PYD and DPD in 66% of patients with bone metastatic involvement; however, elevated values were also found in 42% of cancer patients without documented bone metastases. This surprisingly high percentage in patients without bone metastases probably reflects an excellent sensitivity, but it could also reflect a very poor specificity of the pyridinoline cross-links. Similar results have been reported by Pecherstorfer *et al.* [27], who found significantly higher values in patients with bone metastases, but the discrimination was poor (Fig. 4) [27]. This could indicate a subclinical metastatic involvement, but more likely it is due to a subclinical osteolysis in advanced cancer patients without overt bone metastases under the influence of PTHrP or other unknown bone-mobilizing humoral tumor products or to the release of pyridinium cross-links from extraosseous tissues, as suggested by the slight increase in the ratio PYD/DPD [27]. Part of the increase can also be due to artificial menopause induced by antineoplastic treatments. In any case, these data indicate that these markers are unsuitable for an early diagnosis of neoplastic skeletal involvement.

NTX (urine N-telopeptide assay) has been reported to have the highest discriminatory power and to be the most

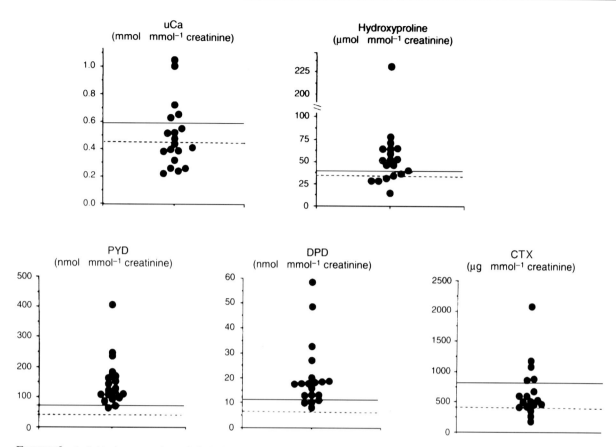

FIGURE 6   Individual concentrations of uCa, hydroxyproline, PYD, DPD, and CTX in 19 normocalcemic patients with breast cancer metastatic to bone. Cross-links were measured by HPLC. Values are compared to the upper limit of normal values in premenopausal (---) or postmenopausal (—) women. Note the larger effect of menopause on the direct peptide-bound CTX assay than on the classical measurement of cross-links. From Body *et al.* [70], with permission.

predictive biochemical marker of bone metastases when comparing groups of patients, but it appears to be less useful on an individual basis [69]. When cutoff values are chosen to give specificities between 90–100%, the NTX showed a sensitivity of around 30%, implying that 70% of subjects with bone metastases would be missed. We also found that the diagnostic sensitivity of the CTX assay was poor when the values were compared to those of healthy postmenopausal women. The diagnostic sensitivity was actually the highest for the collagen cross-links when measured by the classical HPLC method (see Fig. 6) [70]. The biological variability of telopeptide assays is also higher than that of the free DPD assay [71]. A direct ELISA for the measurement of urinary free DPD has been commercialized. The correlation with HPLC determination is excellent and preliminary results indicated that 14 of 17 (82%) patients with breast cancer and bone metastases had increased DPD levels [72]. Patients with bone metastases had significantly higher levels of DPD than patients without bone metastases, but DPD excretion was again often elevated in these patients, suggesting a higher rate of bone turnover in breast cancer patients without bone metastases. This result indicates that the diagnostic efficiency for bone metastatic

involvement for this marker will be similar to what has been described before [73].

Collagen cross-link metabolites are also increased in patients with bone metastases from prostate cancer, underscoring the existence of increased bone resorption even in blastic disease. These metabolites permit a better separation from patients with localized disease than does hydroxyproline, but the correlation with a bone scan score is similar for all three resorption markers [74]. Increased values of ICTP have been associated with a poor prognosis in prostate cancer, perhaps reflecting the lytic component of the metastases [75]. All of these data indicate that there is a great deal of scope for the development of more sensitive and specific markers to provide diagnostic tests.

Urinary galactosyl-hydroxylysine, another marker of bone matrix resorption, is a better predictor of bone metastatic involvement than urinary hydroxyproline or serum AP [76]. Bone sialoprotein (BSP) has been evaluated as a new marker of bone turnover in various conditions. BSP serum levels predominantly reflect processes related to bone resorption. BSP levels decreased in a manner similar to that of DPD after bisphosphonate therapy [34]. The diagnostic sensitivity of BSP for discriminating patients with and without bone metastases appeared to be inferior to that of BAP [77]. A homologous RIA has been described but its performance in cancer patients is unknown [78].

IV. USE OF MARKERS OF BONE TURNOVER FOR THE MONITORING OF TUMOR-INDUCED BONE DISEASE

Measurement of serum calcium (corrected for protein levels) remains the easiest and most efficient way to monitor hypercalcemic patients after successful therapy. Biochemical markers of bone turnover could be useful to assess the response of bone metastases to antineoplastic therapy and to monitor the effects of bisphosphonates.

A. Response Assessment of Bone Metastases

Biochemical markers of bone turnover have the potential to simplify and to improve the monitoring of metastatic bone disease, especially because it is notoriously difficult to rapidly evaluate the bone response to cancer therapy. There is, however, an urgent need for large-scale studies with the new markers.

Coleman et al. [79] have shown a decrease in urinary calcium (uCa) one month after therapy in patients subsequently classified as "partial responders." In the same patients, these authors also showed a transient increase in BAP and in osteocalcin levels [79]. The few available studies indicate that the BAP assay could be more useful for the follow-up of bone metastases than for an early diagnosis. Cooper et al. [80] have reported some patients in whom BAP levels increased before the elevation of a specific tumor marker. The measurement of osteoblastic products in the serum, such as OC, or the newly developed assay for the procollagen extension peptide, could be useful to monitor the regression of osteoblastic foci or the healing of osteolytic lesions. Limited results indicate that BAP measurement could be useful in monitoring bone metastases [64] and that BAP levels correlate with pain [52]. However, in prostate cancer, BAP and PSA changes were concordant only in 69% of 49 patients with metastatic disease [54], and the clinical potential of BAP for monitoring is still uncertain.

In myeloma patients, an increase in OC levels during treatment was initially reported to be a good indicator of treatment efficacy, whereas decreasing levels appeared to be correlated with disease progression [62]. However, the clinical interest of OC for follow-up remains unclear because both falling and rising serum levels are seen, notably in patients with progressive multiple myeloma [81].

Concerning the bone resoption markers, a preliminary report of PYD and DPD measurement in breast cancer patients receiving endocrine treatment has shown that cross-link excretion increased during progressive disease but remained stable or decreased in responders [82]. In prostate cancer, effective endocrine treatment led to normal levels of DPD, but in 13 out of 15 patients with progressive disease, increasing levels of DPD were found [83]. Another preliminary report of 37 well-evaluated patients suggests that NTX could be quite useful to discriminate reliably between patients progressing early on in treatment from those with longer disease control [84]. In patients with progressive disease, NTX levels steadily rose and the diagnostic efficiency of a 50% increase in NTX for identifying imminent progression was 78% [85]. Lastly, ICTP has been reported to be a sensitive and convenient way to monitor osteoclastic activity in patients with multiple myeloma [86] and maybe in patients with prostate cancer [87]. In any case, biochemical markers of bone turnover appear to be better suited for the monitoring of TIO than for the detection of metastatic bone involvement.

Calciotropic hormones levels could also be related to bone disease progression. It has been shown that serum 1,25-dihydroxyvitamin D may be inversely related to disease activity in breast cancer patients with bone metastases [88]. Patients with bone metastases had lower levels of 1,25-dihydroxyvitamin D than early breast cancer patients. The authors observed that mean serum 1,25-dihydroxyvitamin D levels decreased in the patients whose metastatic bone disease progressed, whereas they remained stable in the patients whose bone disease did not progress [88]. This is, of course, due to a slight increase in serum calcium levels and a subsequent decrease in PTH and then serum 1,25-dihydroxyvitamin D levels.

B. Monitoring of Bisphosphonate Therapy

Bisphosphonates constitute one of the most important therapies for the supportive care of the cancer patient. Bisphosphonates successfully reverse hypercalcemic episodes, relieve bone pain, may lead to recalcification of lytic metastases, protect the skeleton from new lesions, and can exert favorable effects on the quality of life. Prolonged use of clodronate or pamidronate decreases the frequency of skeletal-related events in breast cancer patients with metastatic bone disease. The mean skeletal morbidity rate can be reduced by more than one-third by adding regular pamidronate infusions to chemotherapy. Moreover, placebo-controlled trials, with clodronate and with pamidronate, indicate that bisphosphonates in addition to chemotherapy are superior to chemotherapy alone in patients with multiple myeloma. However, optimal therapeutic schemes are unknown and markers of bone resorption could be especially useful in monitoring the effects of bisphosphonate therapy.

Markedly increased levels of PYD and DPD, and even more elevated levels of NTX and CTX, have been found in hypercalcemic cancer patients, with a reduction of 80–90% after pamidronate therapy for NTX and CTX [28, 89]. In normocalcemic patients, Coleman *et al.* [90] reported a significant decline in these markers after oral pamidronate therapy, although the decline was of a lesser magnitude than the fall in fasting urinary calcium excretion. Body *et al.* [70] found that parameters of bone matrix resorption markedly fell after one pamidronate infusion and that they correlated with each other. However, uCa overestimates the activity of bisphosphonates because the decrease in uCa is exaggerated by the PTH surge following the slight decrease in serum calcium. The fall in CTX was particularly impressive and larger than that of hydroxyproline or DPD, indicating the potential of such new markers for delineating the optimal therapeutic schemes of bisphosphonates, especially the optimal frequency of the infusions [70] (Fig. 7).

Moreover, such markers could predict the analgesic response to bisphosphonate therapy. Vinholes *et al.* [91] showed that patients with NTX levels ≥2 times the upper limit of normal responded infrequently to intravenous pamidronate (13%) compared to patients with a baseline NTX level <2 times the normal upper limit (63% response) (Fig. 8). In addition, an analgesic response was much more frequent in the patients in whom NTX, CTX, or free DPD remained in the normal range or returned to normal values (53–63%, dependent on the marker) than in the patients whose markers did not return to normal values (0–20% of clinical response). A high rate of bone resorption appears to be one of the factors underlying resistance to bisphosphonates. It will be extremely important to determine if the frequency of other skeletal events due to bone metastases is similarly influenced by the rate of bone resorption and its inhibition, as estimated by biochemical markers of bone turnover. One could thus individualize

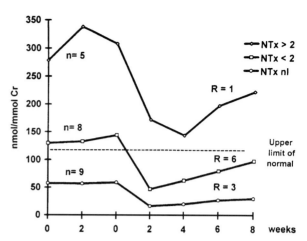

FIGURE 8   Analgesic response to intravenous pamidronate according to the baseline values of NTX in 22 patients with painful bone metastases from breast cancer. From Vinholes *et al.* [91], with permission.

the therapeutic scheme and optimize the efficiency of bisphosphonate therapy.

V. PREDICTION OF THE DEVELOPMENT OF BONE METASTASES

An important future role for bisphosphonate treatment will be the prevention of the development of bone metastases. Trials in patients with established bone metastases suggest that long-term administration of bisphosphonates could indeed fulfill this major objective, and initial prevention trials support this view.

It will be essential to select the patients at high risk of developing bone metastases before recommending a general primary preventive use of bisphosphonates. Breast cancer is a heterogeneous disease with a large variation in growth rate and in metastatic potential. The most powerful prognostic factor for long-term survival is the nodal status; patients with positive axillary nodes have a greater likelihood of recurrence and death than node-negative patients. The latter group, however, still has a risk of death from metastatic disease of approximately 30%. The identification of new prognostic factors that would be independent from these conventional variables would be of great value [11].

More specifically, concerning the risk for the development of bone metastases, data indicate that breast tumors metastasizing to the skeleton produce PTHrP more frequently than the tumors metastasizing to nonosseous sites, suggesting a role for PTHrP in the genesis of (TIO) [92]. This has been confirmed by *in situ* hybridization techniques that can demonstrate the production of PTHrP mRNA by primary breast tumors and by their metastatic cells [93]. Similarly, increased PTHrP gene expression, as quantified by PCR, has

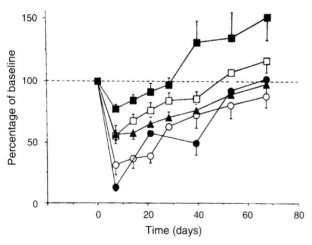

FIGURE 7   Relative changes in markers of bone resorption after a single infusion of pamidronate in 19 normocalcaemic patients with breast cancer metastatic to bone. Changes are shown for urinary DPD (□), PYD (■), CTX (●), hydroxyproline (▲) and calcium (○). From Body *et al.* [70].

been shown in the primary tumors of patients whose cancer subsequently recurs in bone as compared to patients without metastases or with extraskeletal metastases [16]. The expression of PTHrP in primary breast tumors could be a useful tool for selecting patients at high risk of developing bone metastases and thus those patients most likely to benefit from adjuvant bisphosphonate therapy.

Bone sialoprotein (BSP) could be another interesting marker because it is expressed by almost 90% of breast cancers, whereas normal mammary glands express undetectable or barely detectable amounts of BSP [94]. The expression of this protein in bone coincides with the appearance of hydroxyapatite crystals during bone development, but the significance of this observation remains to be demonstrated. The expression of BSP by most breast carcinomas has been postulated to be linked to the preferential homing of breast cancer cells to bone [94]. In a limited series of 39 patients, the degree of BSP expression by the primary tumor (immunoperoxidase score) was significantly higher in the patients who developed bone metastases, and there was no association with the presence of axillary lymph node metastases or the hormone receptor status [95]. In another study, however, the same authors reported an association between BSP expression by breast cancer cells and the axillary lymph node status. The prediction of future bone metastases did not reach statistical significance, but BSP expression was associated with a poor prognosis. However, the possible confounding effect of lymph node invasion was not examined and the possible prognostic influence of BSP expression thus needs further studies [96]. An increased BSP expression by lung cancer cells, which can be viewed as another osteotropic cancer, relative to ovarian cancer, which only rarely invades bone, has also been found (61% vs 21%) [97]. BSP could actually play a critical role in the interaction between bone cells and the mineralized matrix. The primary structure of BSP contains an RGD domain that confers to BSP its cell binding activity. The RGD sequence is an integrin-recognition motif and it is known that osteoclasts bind to BSP via an $\alpha v \beta 3$ integrin-type receptor. Bellahcène et al. [97] speculate that such an interaction may represent a mechanism by which circulating breast cancer cells bind to bone. Moreover, data suggest that serum BSP levels before surgery could be predictive of the future development of bone metastases [98]. The full publication is awaited and, if confirmed, this could be a major discovery. It probably reflects more than increased bone turnover due to subclinical disease, but other more sensitive markers of bone resorption should be measured.

References

1. Galasko, C. S. B. (1986). Skeletal metastases. *Clin. Orthop. Relat. Res.* **210**, 18–30.
2. Coleman, R. E., and Rubens, R. D. (1987). The clinical course of bone metastases from breast cancer. *Br. J. Cancer* **55**, 61–66.
3. Kamby, C., Vejborg, I., Daugaard, S., Guldhammer, B., Dirksen, H., Rossing, N., and Mouridsen, H. T. (1987). Clinical and radiologic characteristics of bone metastases in breast cancer. *Cancer* **60**, 2524–2531.
4. Body, J. J., Lossignol, D., and Ronson, A. (1997). The concept of rehabilitation of cancer patients. *Curr. Opin. Oncol.* **9**, 332–340.
5. Elte, J. W. F., Bijvoet, O. L. M., Cleton, F. J., van Oosterom, A. T., and Sleeboom, H. P. (1986). Osteolytic bone metastases in breast carcinoma: Pathogenesis, morbidity and bisphosphonate treatment. *Eur. J. Cancer Clin. Oncol.* **22**, 493–500.
6. Body, J. J. (1998). Bone metastases. *In* "Handbook of Supportive Care in Cancer" (J. Klastersky, S. C. Schimpff, and H. J. Senn, eds.), 2nd ed., pp. 453–481. Dekker, New York.
7. Mercadante, S. (1997). Malignant bone pain: Pathophysiology and treatment. *Pain* **69**, 1–18.
8. Sherry, M. M., Greco, F. A., Johnson, D. H., and Hainsworth, J. D. (1986). Metastatic breast cancer confined to the skeletal system. An indolent disease. *Am. J. Med.* **81**, 381–386.
9. Kamby, C., Rasmussen, B. B., and Kristensen, B. (1989). Oestrogen receptor status of primary breast carcinomas and their metastases. Relation to pattern of spread and survival after recurrence. *Br. J. Cancer* **60**, 252–257.
10. Yamashita, K., Koyama, H., and Inaji, H. (1995). Prognostic significance of bone metastasis from breast cancer. *Clin. Orthop. Relat. Res.* **312**, 89–94.
11. Body, J. J., Coleman, R. E., and Piccart, M. (1996). Use of bisphosphonates in cancer patients. *Cancer Treat. Rev.* **22**, 265–287.
12. Mundy, G. R. (1997). Mechanisms of bone metastasis. *Cancer* **80**, 1546–1556.
13. Taube, T., Elomaa, I., Blomqvist, C., Beneton, M. N. C., and Kanis, J. A. (1994). Histomorphometric evidence for osteoclast-mediated bone resorption in metastatic breast cancer. *Bone* **15**, 161–166.
14. Siwek, B., Lacroix, M., de Pollak, C., Marie, P., and Body, J. J. (1997). Secretory products of breast cancer cells affect human osteoblastic cells: Partial characterization of active factors. *J. Bone Miner. Res.* **12**, 552–560.
15. Vargas, S. J., Gillespie, M. T., Powell, G. J., Southby, J., Danks, J. A., Moseley, J. M., and Martin, T. J. (1992). Localization of parathyroid hormone-related protein mRNA expression in breast cancer and metastatic lesions by in situ hybridization. *J. Bone Miner. Res.* **7**, 971–979.
16. Bouizar, Z., Spyratos, F., Deytieux, S., de Vernejoul, M. C., and Jullienne, A. (1993). Polymerase chain reaction analysis of parathyroid hormone-related protein gene expression in breast cancer patients and occurence of bone metastases. *Cancer Res.* **53**, 5076–5078.
17. Guise, T. A., and Mundy, G. R. (1995). Breast cancer and bone. *Curr. Opin. Endocrinol.* **2**, 548–555.
18. Cullen, K. J., Yee, D., Sly, W. S., Perdue, J., Hampton, B., Lippman, M. E., and Rosen, N. (1990). Insulin-like growth factor receptor expression and function in human breast cancer. *Cancer Res.* **50**, 48–53.
19. Goltzman, D., and Rabbani, S. A. (1998). Pathogenesis of osteoblastic metastases. *In* "Tumor Bone Diseases and Osteoporosis in Cancer Patients" (J. J. Body, ed.). Dekker, New York.
20. Barillé, S., Collette, M., Bataille, R., and Amiot, M. (1995). Myeloma cells upregulate interleukin-6 secretion in osteoblastic cells through cell-to-cell contact but downregulate osteocalcin. *Blood* **86**, 3151–3159.
21. Gold, R. I., Seeger, L. L., Bassett, L. W., and Steckel, R. J. (1990). An integrated approach to the evaluation of metastatic bone disease. *Radiol. Clin. North Am.* **28**, 471–483.
22. Jacobson, A. F., Cronin, E. B., Stomper, P. C., and Kaplan, W. D. (1990). Bone scans with one or two new abnormalities in cancer patients with no known metastases: Frequency and serial scintigraphic behavior of benign and malignant lesions. *Radiology* **175**, 229–232.

23. Coleman, R. E., Mashiter, G., Whitaker, K. B., Moss, D. W., Rubens, R. D., and Fogelman, I. (1988). Bone scan flare predicts successful systemic therapy for bone metastases. *J. Nucl. Med.* **29**, 1354–1359.

24. Sanal, S. M., Flickinger, F. W., Caudell, M. J., and Sherry, R. M. (1994). Detection of bone marrow involvement in breast cancer with magnetic resonance imaging. *J. Clin. Oncol.* **12**, 1415–1421.

25. Price, C. P., Milligan, T. P., and Darte, C. (1997). Direct comparison of performance characteristics of two immunoassays for bone isoform of alkaline phosphatase in serum. *Clin. Chem.* **43**, 2052–2057.

26. Dumon, J. C., Wantier, H., Mathieu, F., Mantia, M., and Body, J. J. (1996). Technical and clinical validation of a new immunoradiometric assay for human osteocalcin. *Eur. J. Endocrinol.* **135**, 231–237.

27. Pecherstorfer, M., Zimmer-Roth, I., Schilling, T., Woitge, H. W., Schmidt, H., Baumgartner, G., Thiebaud, D., Ludwig, H., and Seibel, M. J. (1995). The diagnostic value of urinary pyridinium cross-links of collagen, serum total alkaline phosphatase and urinary calcium excretion in neoplastic bone disease. *J. Clin. Endocrinol. Metab.* **80**, 97–103.

28. Body, J. J., and Delmas, P. D. (1992). Urinary pyridinium cross-links as markers of bone resorption in tumor-associated hypercalcemia. *J. Clin. Endocrinol. Metab.* **74**, 471–475.

29. Body, J. J., and Dumon, J. C. (1994). Treatment of tumor-induced hypercalcaemia with the bisphosphonate pamidronate: Dose-response relationship and influence of the tumour type. *Ann. Oncol.* **5**, 359–363.

30. Body, J. J., Dumon, J. C., Piccart, M., and Ford, J. (1995). Intravenous pamidronate in patients with tumor-induced osteolysis: A biochemical dose-response study. *J. Bone Miner. Res.* **10**, 1191–1196.

31. Fermo, I., Arcelloni, C., Casari, E., and Paroni, R. (1997). Urine pyridinium cross-links determination by Beckman Cross Links kit. *Clin. Chem.* **43**, 2186–2187.

32. Garnero, P., Gineyts, E., Arbault, P., Christiansen, C., and Delmas, P. D. (1995). Different effects of bisphosphonate and estrogen therapy on free and peptide-bound crosslinks expression. *J. Bone Miner. Res.* **10**, 641–649.

33. Hassager, C., Jensen, L. T., Podenphant, J., Thomsen, K., and Christiansen, C. (1994). The carboxyterminal pyridinoline cross-linked telopeptide of type I collagen in serum as a marker of bone resorption: The effect of Nandrolone decanoate and hormone replacement therapy. *Calcif. Tissue Int.* **54**, 30–33.

34. Seibel, M. J., Woitge, H. W., Pecherstorfer, M., Karmatschek, M., Horn, E., Ludwig, H., Armbruster, F. P., and Ziegler, R. (1996). Serum immunoreactive bone sialoprotein as a new marker of bone turnover in metabolic and malignant bone disease. *J. Clin. Endocrinol. Metab.* **81**, 3289–3298.

35. Withold, W., Armbruster, F. P., Karmatschek, M., and Reinauer, H. (1997). Bone sialoprotein in serum of patients with malignant bone diseases. *Clin. Chem.* **43**, 85–91.

36. Stewart, A. F., Vignery, A., Silverglate, A., Ravin, N. D., Livolsi, V., Broadus, A. E., and Baron, R. (1982). Quantitative bone histomorphometry in humoral hypercalcemia of malignancy: Uncoupling of bone cell activity. *J. Clin. Endocrinol. Metab.* **55**, 219–227.

37. Dumon, J. C., and Body, J. J. (1995). Circulating osteocalcin in hypercalcemic cancer patients—A comparative evaluation of two immunoassays. *Diagn. Oncol.* **4**, 170–173.

38. Nakayama, K., Fukumoto, S., Takeda, S., Takeuchi, Y., Ishikawa, T., Miura, M., Hata, K., Hane, M., Tamura, Y., Tanaka, Y., Kitaoka, M., Obara, T., Ogata, E., and Matsumoto, T. (1996). Differences in bone and vitamin D metabolism between primary hyperparathyroidism and malignancy-associated hypercalcemia. *J. Clin. Endocrinol. Metab.* **81**, 607–611.

39. Body, J. J., Dumon, J. C., Blocklet, D., and Darte, C. (1997). The bone isoenzyme of alkaline phosphatase in hypercalcaemic cancer patients. *Eur. J. Cancer* **33**, 1578–1582.

40. Suva, L. J., Winslow, G. A., Wettenhall, R. E. H., Hammonds, R. G., Moseley, J. M., Diefenbach-Jagger, H., Rodda, C. P., Kemp, B. E.,

Rodriguez, H., Chen, E. Y., Hudson, P. J., Martin, T. J., and Wood, W. I. (1987). A parathyroid hormone-related protein implicated in malignant hypercalcemia: Cloning and expression. *Science* **237**, 893–896.

41. Sato, K., Yamakawa, Y., Shizume, K., Satoh, T., Nohtomi, K., Demura, H., Akatsu, T., Nagata, N., Kasahara, T., Ohkawa, H., and Ohsumi, K. (1993). Passive immunization with anti-parathyroid hormone-related protein monoclonal antibody markedly prolongs survival time of hypercalcemic nude mice bearing transplanted human PTHrP-producing tumors. *J. Bone Miner. Res.* **8**, 849–860.

42. Endres, D. B., Villanueva, R., Sharp, C. F., Jr., and Singer, F. R. (1991). Immunochemiluminometric and immunoradiometric determinations of intact and total immunoreactive parathyrin: Performance in the differential diagnosis of hypercalcemia and hypoparathyroidism. *Clin. Chem.* **37**, 162–168.

43. Walls, J., Ratcliffe, W. A., Howell, A., and Bundred, N. J. (1994). Parathyroid hormone and parathyroid hormone-related protein in the investigation of hypercalcaemia in two hospital populations. *Clin. Endocrinol.* **41**, 407–413.

44. Body, J. J., Dumon, J. C., Thirion, M., and Cleeren, A. (1993). Circulating PTHrP concentrations in tumor-induced hypercalcemia: Influence on the response to bisphosphonate and changes after therapy. *J. Bone Miner. Res.* **8**, 701–706.

45. Grill, V., Ho, P., Body, J. J., Johanson, N., Lee, S. C., Kukreja, S. C., Moseley, J. M., and Martin, T. J. (1991). Parathyroid hormone-related protein: Elevated levels in both humoral hypercalcemia of malignancy and hypercalcemia complicating metastatic breast cancer. *J. Clin. Endocrinol. Metab.* **73**, 1309–1315.

46. Burtis, W. J. (1992). Parathyroid hormone-related protein: Structure, function and measurement. *Clin. Chem.* **38**, 2171–2183.

47. Dumon, J. C., Jensen, T., Lueddecke, B., Spring, J., Barlé, J., and Body, J. J. (1999). Validation of a new immunoradiometric assay for circulating parathyroid hormone-related protein. Unpublished data.

48. Body, J. J., Dumon, J. C., Seraj, F., and Cleeren, A. (1992). Recovery of parathyroid hormone secretion during correction of tumor-associated hypercalcemia. *J. Clin. Endocrinol. Metab.* **74**, 1385–1388.

49. Woitge, H. W., Seibel, M. J., and Ziegler, R. (1996). Comparison of total and bone-specific alkaline phosphatase in patients with nonskeletal disorders or metabolic bone diseases. *Clin. Chem.* **42**, 1796–1804.

50. Marchei, P., Santini, D., Bianco, V., Chiodini, S., Reale, M. G., Simeoni, F., Marchei, G. G., and Vecchione, A. (1995). Serum ostase in the follow-up of breast cancer patients. *Anticancer Res.* **15**, 2217–2222.

51. Van Hoof, V. O., Van Oosterom, A. T., Lepoutre, L. G., and De Broe, M. E. (1992). Alkaline phosphatase isoenzyme patterns in malignant disease. *Clin. Chem.* **38**, 2546–2551.

52. Zaninotto, M., Secchiero, S., and Rubin, D. (1995). Serum bone alkaline phosphatase in the follow-up of skeletal metastases. *Anticancer Res.* **15**, 2223–2228.

53. Berruti, A., Piovesan, A., Torta, M., Raucci, C. A., Gorzegno, G., Paccotti, P., Dogliotti, L., and Angeli, A. (1996). Biochemical evaluation of bone turnover in cancer patients with bone metastatses: Relationship with radiograph appearances and disease extension. *Br. J. Cancer* **73**, 1581–1587.

54. Cooper, E. H., Whelan, P., and Purves, D. (1994). Bone alkaline phosphatase and prostate-specific antigen in the monitoring of prostate cancer. *Prostate* **25**, 236–242.

55. Wolff, J. M., Ittel, T., Boeckmann, W., Reinike T., Habib, F. K., and Jakse, G. (1996). Skeletal alkaline phosphatase in the metastatic workup of patients with prostate cancer. *Eur. Urol.* **30**, 302–306.

56. Lorente, J. A., Morote, J., Raventos, C., Encabo, G., and Valenzuela, H. (1996). Clinical efficacy of bone alkaline phosphatase and prostate specific antigen in the diagnosis of bone metastasis in prostate cancer. *J. Urol.* **155**, 1348–1351.

57. Gomez, B., Jr., Ardakani, S., Ju, J., Jenkins, D., Cerelli, M. J., Daniloff, G. Y., and Kung, V. T. (1995). Monoclonal antibody assay for measuring

bone-specific alkaline phosphatase activity in serum. *Clin. Chem.* **41**, 1560–1566.

58. Body, J. J., Cleeren, A., Pot, M., and Borkowski, A. (1986). Serum osteocalcin (BGP) in tumor-associated hypercalcemia. *J. Bone Miner. Res.* **1**, 523–527.

59. Kamby, C., Egsmose, C., Söletormos, G., and Dombernowsky, P. (1993). The diagnostic and prognostic value of serum bone GLA protein (osteocalcin) in patients with recurrent breast cancer. *Scand. J. Clin. Lab. Invest.* **53**, 439–446.

60. Shih, W. J., Wierzbinski, B., Collins, J., Magoun, S., Chen, I. W., and Ryo, U. Y. (1990). Serum osteocalcin measurements in prostate carcinoma patients with skeletal deposits shown by bone scintigram: Comparison with serum PSA/PAP measurements. *J. Nucl. Med.* **31**, 1486–1489.

61. Coleman, R. E., Mashiter, G., Fogelman, I., and Rubens, R. D. (1988). Osteocalcin: A marker of metastatic bone disease. *Eur. J. Cancer* **24**, 1211–1217.

62. Bataille, R., Delmas, P. D., Chappard, D., and Sany, J. (1990). Abnormal serum bone Gla protein levels in multiple myeloma. *Cancer* **66**, 167–172.

63. Mejjad, O., Le Loët, X., Basuyau, J. P., Ménard, J. F., Jego, P., Grisot, C., Darangon, A., Grosbois, B., Euller-Ziegler, L., Monconduit, M., and le Groupe d'Etude et de Recherche sur le Myélome (GERM). (1996). Osteocalcin is not a marker of progress in multiple myeloma. *Eur. J. Hematol.* **56**, 30–34.

64. Burlina, A., Rubin, D., Secchiero, S., Sciacovelli, L., Zaninotto, M., and Plebani, M. (1994). Monitoring skeletal cancer metastases with the bone isoenzyme of tissue unspecific alkaline phosphatase. *Clin. Chim. Acta* **226**, 151–158.

65. Ebeling, P. R., Peterson, J. M., and Riggs, B. L. (1992). Utility of type I procollagen propeptide assays for assessing abnormalities in metabolic bone diseases. *J. Bone Miner. Res.* **7**, 1243–1250.

66. Nakashima, J., Sumitomo, M., Miyajima, A., Jitsukawa, S., Saito, S., Tachibana, M., and Murai, M. (1997). The value of serum carboxyterminal propeptide of type 1 procollagen in predicting bone metastases in prostate cancer. *J. Urol.* **157**, 1736–1739.

67. Vinholes, J., Coleman, R., and Eastell, R. (1996). Effects of bone metastases on bone metabolism: Implications for diagnosis, imaging and assessment of response to cancer treatment. *Cancer Treat. Rev.* **22**, 289–331.

68. Lipton, A., Demers, L., Daniloff, Y., Curley, E., Hamilton, C., Harvey, H., Witters, L., Seaman, J., Van der Giessen, R., and Seyedin, S. (1993). Increased urinary excretion of pyridinium cross-links in cancer patients. *Clin. Chem.* **39**, 614–618.

69. Demers, L. M., Costa, L., Chinchilli, V. M., Gaydos, L., Curley, E., and Lipton, A. (1995). Biochemical markers of bone turnover in patients with metastatic bone disease. *Clin. Chem.* **41**, 1489–1494.

70. Body, J. J., Dumon, J. C., Gineyts, E., and Delmas, P. D. (1997). Comparative evaluation of markers of bone resorption in patients with breast cancer-induced osteolysis before and after bisphosphonate therapy. *Br. J. Cancer* **75**, 408–412.

71. Ju, H. S. J., Leung, S., Brown, B., Stringer, M. A., Leigh, S., Scherrer, C., Shepard, K., Jenkins, D., Knudsen, J., and Cannon, R. (1997). Comparison of analytical performance and biological variability of three bone resorption assays. *Clin. Chem.* **43**, 1570–1576.

72. Robins, S. P., Woitge, H., Hesley, R., Ju, J., Seyedin, S., and Seibel, M. J. (1994). Direct, enzyme-linked immunoassay for urinary deoxypyridinoline as a specific marker for measuring bone resorption. *J. Bone Miner. Res.* **9**, 1643–1649.

73. Nguyen-Pamart, M., Bonneterre, J., and Hecquet, B. (1995). Urinary excretion of deoxypyridinoline in patients with breast cancer. *Anticancer Res.* **15**, 1601–1604.

74. Miyamoto, K. K., McSherry, S. A., Robins, S. P., Besterman, J. M., and Mohler, J. L. (1994). Collagen cross-link metabolites in urine as markers of bone metastases in prostatic carcinoma. *J. Urol.* **151**, 909–913.

75. Kylmälä, T., Tammela, T. L. J., Risteli, L., Risteli, J., Kontturi, M., and Elomaa, I. (1995). Type I collagen degradation product (ICTP) gives information about the nature of bone metastases and has prognostic value in prostate cancer. *Br. J. Cancer* **71**, 1061–1064.

76. Moro, L., Gazzarrini, C., Crivellari, D., Galligioni, E., Talamini, R., and de Bernard, B. (1993). Biochemical markers for detecting bone metastases in patients with breast cancer. *Clin. Chem.* **39**, 131–134.

77. Withold, W., Armbruster, F. P., Karmatschek, M., and Reinauer, H. (1997). Bone sialoprotein in serum of patients with malignant bone diseases. *Clin. Chem.* **43**, 85–91.

78. Karmatschek, M., Maier, I., Seibel, M. J., Woitge, H. W., Ziegler, R., and Armbruster, F. P. (1997). Improved purification of human bone sialoprotein and development of a homologous radioimmunoassay. *Clin. Chem.* **43**, 2076–2082.

79. Coleman, R. E., Whitaker, K. D., Moss, D. W., Mashiter, G., Fogelman, I., and Rubens, R. D. (1988). Biochemical monitoring predicts response in bone to systemic treatment. *Br. J. Cancer* **58**, 205–210.

80. Cooper, E. H., Forbes, M. A., Hancock, A. K., Parker, D., and Laurence, V. (1992). Serum bone alkaline phosphatase and CA 549 in breast cancer with bone metastases. *Biomed. Pharmacother.* **46**, 31–36.

81. Williams, A. T., Shearer, M. J., Oyeyi, J., Aitchison, R. G., Newland, A. C., and Schey, S. A. (1992). Serum osteocalcin in the management of myeloma. *Eur. J. Cancer* **29A**, 140–142.

82. Downey, S., Walls, J., Ratcliffe, W. A., Assiri, A. M. A., Howell, A., Eastell, R., and Bundred, N. J. (1994). Pyridinoline excretion can monitor bone metastases in breast cancer. *Breast Cancer Res. Treat.* **32** (Suppl. 1), 83.

83. Ikeda, I., Miura, T., and Kondo, I. (1996). Pyridinium cross-links as markers of bone metastases in patients with prostate cancer. *Br. J. Urol.* **77**, 102–106.

84. Coleman, R. E. (1998). Monitoring of bone metastases. *Eur. J. Cancer* **34**, 252–259.

85. Vinholes, J., Coleman, R., Lacombe, D., Mignolet, F., Rose, C., Leonard, R., Nortier, J., Tubiana-Hulin, M., and EORTC Breast Group. (1996). Assessment of bone response to systemic therapy in an EORTC trial of oral pamidronate. *Eur. J. Cancer* **32A** (Suppl. 2), 50.

86. Elooma, I., Virkkunen, P., Risteli, L., and Risteli, J. (1992). Serum concentration of the cross-linked carboxyterminal telopeptide of type I collagen (ICTP) is a useful prognostic indicator in multiple myeloma. *Br. J. Cancer* **66**, 337–341.

87. Kylmälä, T., Tammela, T., Risteli, L., Risteli, J., Taube, T., and Elomaa, I. (1993). Evaluation of the effect of oral clodronate on skeletal metastases with type 1 collagen metabolites. A controlled trial of the Finnish Prostate Cancer Group. *Eur. J. Cancer* **29A**, 821–825.

88. Mawer, E. B., Walls, J., Howell, A., Davies, M., Ratcliffe, W. A., and Bundred, N. J. (1997). Serum 1,25-dihydroxyvitamin D may be related inversely to disease activity in breast cancer patients with bone metastases. *J. Clin. Endocrinol. Metab.* **82**, 118–122.

89. Vinholes, J., Guo, C. Y., Purohit, O. P., Eastell, R., and Coleman, R. (1997). Evaluation of new bone resorption markers in a randomized comparison of pamidronate or clodronate for hypercalcemia of malignancy. *J. Clin. Oncol.* **15**, 131–138.

90. Coleman, R. E., Houston, S., James, I., Rodger, A., Rubens, R. D., Leonard, R. C. F., and Ford, J. (1992). Preliminary results of the use of urinary excretion of pyridinium crosslinks for monitoring metastatic bone disease. *Br. J. Cancer* **65**, 766–768.

91. Vinholes, J. J. F., Purohit, O. P., Abbey, M. E., Eastell, R., and Coleman, R. E. (1997). Relationships between biochemical and symptomatic response in a double-blind randomised trial of pamidronate for metastatic bone disease. *Ann. Oncol.* **8**, 1243–1250.

92. Bundred, N. J., Walker, R. A., Ratcliffe, W. A., Warwick, J., Morrison, J. M., and Ratcliffe, J. G. (1992). Parathyroid hormone related protein and skeletal morbidity in breast cancer. *Eur. J. Cancer* **28**, 690–692.

93. Vargas, S. J., Gillespie, M. T., Powell, G. J., Southby, J., Danks, J. A., Moseley, J. M., and Martin T. J. (1992). Localization of parathyroid hormone-related protein mRNA expression in breast cancer and metastatic lesions by in situ hybridation. *J. Bone Miner. Res.* **7**, 971–979.

94. Bellahcène, A., Merville, M. P., and Castronovo, V. (1994). Expression of bone sialoprotein, a bone matrix protein, in human breast cancer. *Cancer Res.* **54**, 2823–2826.

95. Bellahcène, A., Kroll, M., Liebens, F., and Castronovo, V. (1996). Bone sialoprotein expression in primary human breast cancer is associated with bone metastases development. *J. Bone Miner. Res.* **11**, 665–670.

96. Bellahcène, A., Menard, S., Bufalino, R., Moreau, and L., Castronovo, V. (1996). Expression of bone sialoprotein in primary human breast cancer is associated with poor survival. *Int. J. Cancer* **69**, 350–353.

97. Bellahcène, A., Maloujahmoum, N., Fisher, L. W., Pastorino, H., Tagliabue, E., Menard, S., and Castronovo, V. (1997) Expression of bone sialoprotein in human lung cancer. *Calcif. Tissue Int.* **61**, 183–188.

98. Diel, I. J., Solomayer, E. F., Meisenbacher, H., Gollan, C., Conradi, R., Wallwiener, D., and Bastert, G. (1998). Elevated serum bone sialoprotein in primary breast cancer patients is a potent marker for bone metastases. *J. Clin. Oncol.* **17** (Suppl.), 122a.

CHAPTER 43

Rare Bone Diseases

MICHAEL P. WHYTE Metabolic Research Unit, Shriners Hospital for Children, St. Louis, Missouri 63131;
and Division of Bone and Mineral Diseases, Washington University School of Medicine,
St. Louis, Missouri 63110

I. INTRODUCTION

Rare bone diseases are inherently challenging for physicians. Lack of familiarity with their myriad clinical, radiographic, laboratory, and histopathological features make diagnosing difficult, and new skeletal disorders continue to be discovered. Little personal or cumulative experience with their management renders treatment uncertain. Understanding these entities is important for a number of reasons. First, although several rare bone diseases are mere radiological curiosities, most are maladies that pose significant lifelong problems and lack effective medical treatments. Second, many of the rare bone diseases are heritable so that more than one individual or future pregnancies in a family can be at risk. Third, there is a significant number of such disorders, and their cumulative prevalence in any population worldwide is not negligible. Finally, elucidation of the etiology and pathogenesis of these conditions can offer important insight into skeletal development and the dynamics of bone and cartilage metabolism in humans. Although a specific disorder may be encountered just once in a medical career, the individual patient with a rare bone disease is usually the subject of considerable interest, often representing an "experiment-of-nature," and is always memorable.

This chapter summarizes information concerning genetic as well as local and systemic factors involved in the etiology and pathogenesis of rare bone diseases where results from assays of biochemical markers of skeletal remodeling have been accumulating. For such disorders, bone turnover assessed biochemically can shed light on the nature of the skeletal pertubation and help to evaluate response to treatment. The conditions discussed are grouped into four categories: osteopenia, osteosclerosis and hyperostosis, ectopic calcification, and "other" disturbances.

II. OSTEOPENIA

Systemic or focal derangements in bone growth, modeling, and remodeling can cause generalized or regional osteopenia. Therefore, measurement of biochemical markers of formation or resorption of osseous tissue using blood or urine specimens can reflect either a global skeletal disturbance or the impact of a localized bone problem. Accordingly, the extent and severity of the pathologic process (i.e. the abnormal source of markers) might warrant consideration when interpreting results from such assays in individual osteopenic patients.

A. Osteogenesis Imperfecta

Osteogenesis imperfecta (OI) is a heritable disorder of connective tissue [1]. The pathogenesis in nearly all patients involves quantitative and often qualitative abnormalities of

605

TABLE I. Clinical Heterogeneity and Biochemical Defects in Osteogenesis Imperfecta[a]

OI type	Clinical features	Inheritance[b]	Biochemical defects
I	Normal stature, little or no deformity; blue scleras; hearing loss in about 50% of individuals; dentinogenesis imperfecta rare and may distinguish a subset	AD	Decreased production of type I procollagen; substitution for residue other than glycine in triple helix of $\alpha 1(I)$
II	Lethal in the perinatal period; minimal calvarial mineralization; beaded ribs; compressed femurs; marked long bone deformity; platyspondyly	AD (new mutation) AR (rare)	Rearrangements in the COL1A1 and COL1A2 genes; substitutions for glycyl residues in the triple-helical domain of the $\alpha 1(I)$ $\alpha 2(I)$ chain; small deletion in $\alpha 2(I)$ on the background of a null allele
III	Progressively deforming bones, usually with moderate deformity at birth; scleras variable in hue, often lighten with age; dentinogenesis common; hearing loss common; stature very short	AD AR	Point mutation in the $\alpha 1(I)$ or $\alpha 2(I)$ chain Frameshift mutation that prevents incorporation of pro$\alpha 2(I)$ into molecules (noncollagenous defects)
IV	Normal scleras, mild to moderate bone deformity; variable short stature; dentinogenesis common; hearing loss occurs in some	AD	Point mutations in the $\alpha 2(I)$ chain; rarely, point mutations in the $\alpha 1(I)$ chain; small deletions in the $\alpha 2(I)$ chain

[a] Reproduced from Byers [1], "The metabolic and molecular bases of inherited disease," Copyright 1995 by McGraw-Hill, with permission of The McGraw-Hill Companies.

[b] AD, autosomal dominant; AR, autosomal recessive.

the most abundant protein present in bone (i.e. type I collagen) [2]. Consequently, the clinical hallmark of OI is generalized osteopenia associated with recurrent fracture and skeletal deformity [3]. However, type I collagen is also found in dentin, ligaments, skin, and sclerae; hence, many patients with OI have additional disturbances involving the teeth (dentinogenesis imperfecta) and other tissues that normally contain this major structural protein [1, 3]. Severity of OI is, however, extremely variable among patients and ranges from stillbirth to perhaps lifelong absence of symptoms. The classification scheme for this disorder proposed by Sillence in 1979, according to clinical and radiographic features and perceived patterns of inheritance, provided a framework for prognostication and a foundation for further biochemical/genetic investigations (Table I). Understandably, however, this nosology (despite later modifications) has limitations and recombinant DNA studies were subsequently the source of significant advances in our knowledge concerning this disorder [1–3]. Such progress included clarification of the genetic basis for most severe cases of OI and elucidation of the clinical variability of this prototypic collagenopathy [1–3].

Type I OI features sclerae with bluish discoloration that is especially striking during childhood, relatively mild osteopenia with infrequent fractures (deformity is uncommon or mild), and deafness that typically manifests during early adulthood (30% incidence). Stature is usually normal. Type I OI has been subclassified into forms I-A and I-B depending upon the absence or (more rarely) the presence, respectively, of dentinogenesis imperfecta.

Type II OI is typically fatal within the first few days or weeks of life due to respiratory compromise from thoracic insufficiency. Affected newborns are often premature, small for gestational age, and have short, bowed limbs, numerous fractures, markedly soft skulls, and small chests.

Type III OI is characterized by progressive skeletal deformity due to recurrent fracture as well as short stature that results, in part, from fragmentation of growth plates (Fig. 1).

Type IV OI used to be considered rare. This type of OI often explains multigenerational disease. The sclerae have normal color, but other typical features include moderate deformity, dental defects, and hearing loss.

In the OI patient population worldwide, more than 150 distinctive abnormalities have been identified within the two genes that encode the two large protein chains that intertwine to become the type I collagen heterotrimer [2]. The genetic basis for nearly all cases of OI is a mutation involving one allele of either the COL1A1 or the COL1A2 genes [1–3]. These genes direct the biosynthesis of the proα_1(I) and the proα_2(I) chains that undergo posttranslational modification and combine in a 2:1 ratio to form the triple-helical domain of the type I collagen fibril [2]. Diminished synthesis of type I collagen (often associated with a structurally defective heterotrimer) is the principal biochemical abnormality in OI [1]. Molecular aberrations in one of these four alleles, causing functional loss of about 50% of either the proα_1(I) or the proα_2(I) chains, are responsible for mild OI [1–3]. Point mutations leading to substitution of one of the many critical glycyl residues in the triple-helical domain of a proα_1(I) or a proα_2(I) chain (or deletion of single exons) generally cause severe disease [1–3]. Altered amino acid sequences lead to posttranslational overmodification of the triple-helical region. Subsequently, most heterotrimer molecules form defectively, and dominant-negative effects stemming from a single abnormal collagen gene allele become an important pathogenetic

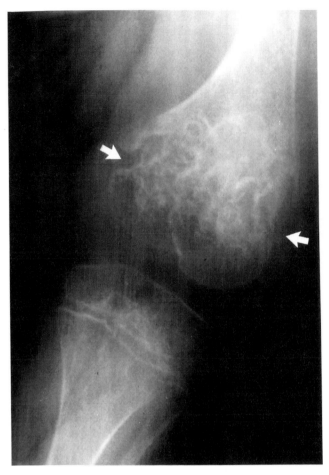

FIGURE 1   Osteogenesis imperfecta. Progressively deforming (type III) OI in this $4\frac{1}{2}$-year-old girl manifests with osteopenia and fragmentation of the distal growth plate of her left femur forming characteristic "popcorn calcifications" (arrows).

factor in OI. OI represents the archetypical disorder in which one defective allele encoding a structurally complex protein causes a dominantly-inherited disease [3]. The large size of the COL1A1 or COL1A2 gene explains, however, why nearly all families with OI differ from one another due to "private mutations" [2]. Nevertheless, approximately one-third of patients with type I OI reflect new dominant mutations, and the approximately 6% recurrence risk for type II OI within a sibship seems to be explained by gonadal mosaicism [1].

Bone histology in OI often reveals an abnormal skeletal matrix, especially in severely affected patients. Polarized-light microscopy shows disorganized "woven" bone where there should be predominantly lamellar osseous tissue. Irregular architecture of the fibrillar network of collagen is a characteristic histopathologic feature. Furthermore, individual reports indicate that the diameter of single collagen fibers can be either reduced [4] or increased [5]. Early studies of the OI skeleton were interpreted as showing low bone turnover [6, 7]. In 1983, however, Baron and colleagues [8] reported that dynamic histomorphometry of iliac crest specimens from

nine children with mild (tarda) OI suggested increased bone remodeling at the tissue level, although there was decreased bone formation by individual osteoblasts. The apparent defect in matrix synthesis by single osteoblasts seemed to be compensated for by increased numbers of these bone-forming cells. As a remnant of this pathologic process, many osteocytes were observed in cortical bone from patients [8]. Interpretation of the results of this investigation was limited, however, because there was little information available from control subjects. In 1984, Ste-Marie and colleagues [7] also noted decreased activity of individual osteoblasts, despite the fact that many cells were simultaneously forming osseous tissue. In 1991, Vetter and associates showed that apatite crystal size was relatively small in OI patient bone [9] and that the noncollagenous proteins were also altered [10]. Other studies confirm that the noncollagenous components of bone matrix are indeed disturbed in OI [4, 9–13]. In 1992, Fedarko *et al.* [4] found reduced amounts of several bone matrix glycoproteins including osteonectin, biglycan, and decorin. In 1995, they observed elevated levels of thrombospondin, fibronectin, and hyaluronan [14].

OI bone cells *in vitro* have also produced important findings. In 1992, Mörike *et al.* [15] reported that osteoblast-like cells in culture from all clinical forms of OI produce low extracellular levels of type I collagen irrespective of the absence or (more frequently) the presence of structural abnormalities within the heterotrimer itself. However, there were also important differences among the clinical types of OI. Diminished production versus aberrant secretion, processing, and pericellular accumulation of type I procollagen distinguished type I from types III and IV OI, respectively [15]. Types III and IV OI featured intracellular retention of the nascent protein. In 1993, Mörike and colleagues [16] also showed that OI bone cells in culture nevertheless express markers of osteoblast activity correctly (alkaline phosphatase, 1,25-dihydroxyvitamin D_3-stimulated osteocalcin, and PTH-induced cAMP). Their findings indicated that osteoblast differentiation is not altered in OI bone cells [16]. In 1995, overhydroxylation of lysyl and prolyl residues was confirmed using OI patient fibroblasts in culture, and the degree of this posttranslational overmodification was found to correlate with the clinical phenotype [17].

Despite quantitative and qualitative defects in bone tissue in OI, routine biochemical parameters of mineral homeostasis are typically unremarkable in patients, although hypercalciuria was documented in 36% of affected children followed in St. Louis, Missouri [18]. The magnitude of the hypercalciuria in this pediatric OI population reflected the clinical severity of the skeletal disease [18, 19] but was not associated with renal dysfunction [19]. In 1979, Neilsen *et al.* [20] reported normal serum calcitonin levels in OI patients. In 1993, Marini and co-workers [21] found no evidence of growth hormone deficiency in children with OI, although some patients had blunted serum IGF-1 level responses after growth hormone challenge. Since 1969, there has been evidence that inorganic pyrophosphate (PPi) accumulates endogenously in the OI population. Nevertheless, PPi levels measured in blood and urine do not reflect disease severity or change with magnesium oxide therapy [22].

Among the rare bone diseases, biochemical markers of bone turnover have been investigated most thoroughly in OI. Elevations in some patients of serum alkaline phosphatase (AP) activity and urinary levels of hydroxyproline (OHP) have been documented [6, 23]. In 1986, Castells et al. [24] found that plasma osteocalcin levels were increased in OI. However, the following year, Rico [25] reported that circulating osteocalcin levels were low. Furthermore, in 1991, Rico and colleagues [26] observed that serum tartrate-resistant acid phosphatase (TRAP) activity was reduced in patients with types I and III OI, suggesting that bone turnover is quiescent in these clinical subtypes and, therefore, consistent with an osteoblast defect. In 1993, Brenner et al. [27] found that serum levels of type I procollagen C-terminal propeptide were also generally low in OI (especially type I). They concluded that quantitation of this biochemical marker would be especially useful in the clinical management and assessment of future therapeutic interventions for OI [27]. They also noted increased serum osteocalcin levels, but only during childhood [27]—an observation that was in keeping with findings using OI bone itself (10). In 1994, Minisola and coworkers [28] reported a family with type I-A OI whose serum levels of type I procollagen C-terminal propeptide were indeed low, yet other biochemical parameters of skeletal remodeling were normal. The finding was probably due to decreased production of type I procollagen. In 1994, Brenner et al. [29] discovered generous urinary levels of type I collagen cross-linked N-telopeptides in children and adolescents with OI which correlated positively with urinary calcium excretion. They concluded that the synthesis and turnover of mature, cross-linked type I collagen is disturbed in OI, thereby providing evidence for increased bone remodeling rates in patients [29].

In summary, biochemical markers of bone remodeling in OI reflect the characteristic reduction in type I procollagen production and, in general, seem to support histomorphometric studies of osseous tissue showing enhanced rates of bone turnover despite quiescent activity of individual osteoblasts within an osteopenic skeleton.

B. Idiopathic Juvenile Osteoporosis

Osteoporosis in the pediatric population is usually unmasked when radiographs taken for fracture sustained during play also show generalized hypomineralization of the skeleton (i.e. osteopenia) but no evidence of rickets or excessive bone resorption (e.g. osteitis fibrosa). Corticosteroid therapy is the most common cause of acquired osteoporosis in childhood and adolescence, but a number of disorders comprise the differential diagnosis for this problem in the pediatric population [30].

Idiopathic juvenile osteoporosis (IJO) refers to a rare condition that is usually observed before puberty, but it can also trouble young children, especially those who are growing rapidly [31]. The term IJO was coined by Dent and Friedman in 1965 [32]. Since first described by Schippers in 1938 [33], fewer than 100 cases have been reported in the medical literature [30].

The patient with IJO is typically prepubertal and otherwise healthy [31]. Family history has been regarded as negative, but recent studies indicate that some cases may reflect a heritable disorder. Both sexes are affected with equal prevalence. Symptoms generally begin with discomfort in the lower back and difficulty walking. Knee and ankle pain and fractures of the lower extremities are usually present. Physical examination can be unremarkable or reveal thoracolumbar kyphosis or kyphoscoliosis, pigeon chest, reduced upper-segment to lower-segment ratio, long bone deformity, loss of height, and a limp. Radiographic studies show osteopenia and fractures, especially in the spine and metaphyses of the lower limbs (Fig. 2). IJO can resolve spontaneously with the onset of puberty. Generally, physical deformities are reversible [34, 35]. In 1995, in a longitudinal follow-up study of 21 affected children, Smith [34] reported that most patients "substantially or completely recovered," but several developed crippling deformities leaving them wheelchair bound with cardiopulmonary compromise as adults. However, the techniques used to investigate the patients as adults were not detailed in this report [34]. Because spontaneous recovery from IJO does occur, Smith [34] concluded that it was "impossible to assess the many forms of treatment given."

The clinical onset of IJO, usually just before puberty, may reflect the fact that one-half of adult skeletal mass is acquired during the adolescent years. Early on, investigation of a limited number of patients suggested that IJO develops from negative or inappropriately neutral mineral balance at this critical time. Recovery is heralded by improvement in calcium balance [32].

Few studies of bone tissue have been reported in IJO. Jowsey and Johnson [35] and Cloutier et al. [36] published histologic and microradiographic evidence of increased skeletal resorption, speculating that excessive dietary phosphorus stimulated PTH-mediated bone resorption. Conversely, Smith [34] reported similarly indirect evidence for decreased bone formation from static histomorphometry of iliac crest specimens. Using double tetracycline labeling techniques, Evans and colleagues [37] suggested that severe IJO in one boy likely resulted from a reduction in bone formation.

There are no biochemical abnormalities characteristic of IJO [34]. Case reports involve seemingly isolated disturbances. Descriptions of deficiency of $1,25(OH)_2D$ or

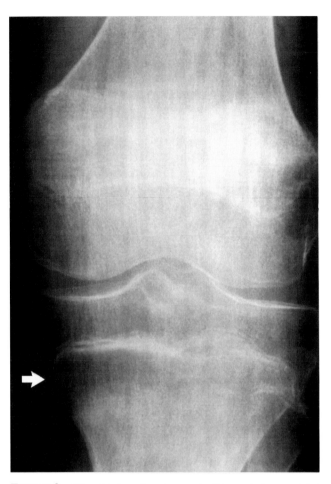

FIGURE 2 Idiopathic juvenile osteoporosis. Osteopenia is present, but there is no evidence of rickets or hyperparathyroidism, in this $10\frac{1}{2}$-year-old girl. Characteristic "neo-osseous osteoporosis" is noted in the metaphysis of the proximal left tibia (arrow).

calcitonin and beneficial response to treatment with these hormones have been published [38, 39]. However, in a relatively large study, circulating 25(OH)D and 1,25(OH)$_2$D levels were normal [34]. Increased urinary excretion of OHP as well as hypercalcemia and suppressed serum PTH levels have been observed in some patients with IJO. The secondary hypoparathyroidism could, in turn, reduce 1,25(OH)$_2$D synthesis and decrease intestinal calcium absorption, perhaps contributing to the negative calcium balance.

In 1992, Bertelloni et al. [40] reported normal osteoblast function in six patients after using a stimulation test that measured serum osteocalcin levels after 1,25(OH)$_2$D$_3$ challenge. In 1995, Smith [34] reported that most patients with IJO manifest no abnormality of collagen in specimens of their skin or in collagen synthesized by dermal fibroblasts in culture. That same year, however, Pocock and coworkers [41] reported that qualitative and quantitative abnormalities of type I collagen may occur in a minority of IJO patients who represent a subpopulation of this disorder.

C. Cleidocranial Dysplasia

Cleidocranial dysplasia (dysostosis) is an autosomal dominant disorder characterized by large cranial fontanelles, aplasia or hypoplasia of the clavicles, delayed skeletal development, and a variety of dental anomalies (Fig. 3) [42]. To some investigators, the clinical phenotype has suggested a defect in ossification.

In 1997, mutations were identified in the CBFA1 gene [43] that encodes the transcriptional activator of osteoblast differentiation, OSF2/CBFA1 [44]. In 1992, Moore et al. [45] reported in a preliminary communication that serum AP activity was low in several affected individuals—a finding in keeping with decreased osteoblast function. Other biochemical markers of skeletal remodeling in this condition await investigation.

III. OSTEOSCLEROSIS AND HYPEROSTOSIS

Osteosclerosis and hyperostosis refer to trabecular and cortical bone thickening, respectively [46]. Focal or generalized osteosclerosis and/or hyperostosis are caused by many rare (primarily hereditary) dysplastic diseases, as well as by a variety of dietary, metabolic, endocrine, hematologic, infectious, and neoplastic conditions (Table II). Several of the unusual dysplastic disorders are discussed here because they can be especially informative with regard to skeletal development and the dynamics of bone and cartilage metabolism [42, 46]. One wonders if increased skeletal mass per se from focal or generalized osteosclerosis or hyperostosis can account for increments in blood or urinary levels of markers of bone formation or resorption; if so, increases in these markers might not necessarily indicate rapid turnover of osseous tissue.

A. Osteopetrosis

Osteopetrosis (marble bone disease) was first described in 1904 by Albers-Schönberg. More than 300 cases have been reported in the medical literature and there now appear to be at least eight types of this disorder in humans (Table III) [47]. Two major clinical forms are well delineated: the autosomal dominant adult ("benign") type that is associated with few or no symptoms and the autosomal recessive infantile ("malignant") type that, if untreated, typically kills during infancy or early childhood. In the latter form of osteopetrosis, patients suffer from leukoerythroblastic anemia due to myelophthisis, cranial nerve compression, and infection. A rarer autosomal recessive "intermediate" form of osteopetrosis presents during childhood with some of the signs and symptoms of the malignant disease, but its impact on life expectancy is not

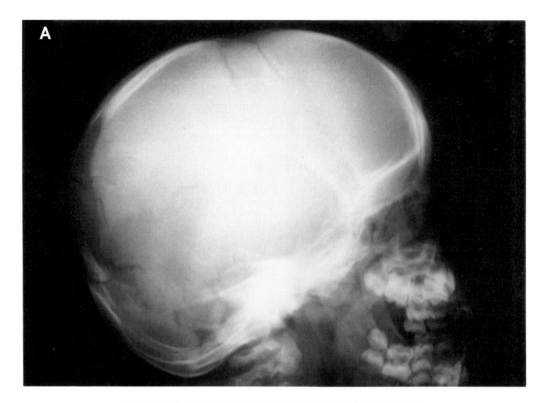

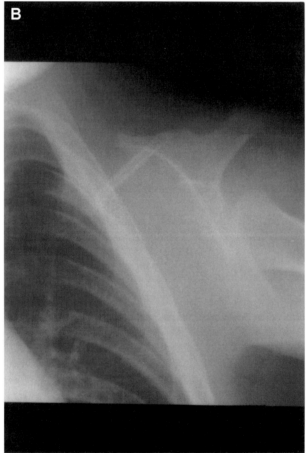

FIGURE 3   Cleidocranial dysplasia. (A) Open cranial sutures are readily apparent in this 4-year-old boy. (B) At 5 2/12 years of age, a chest radiograph shows characteristic clavicular hypoplasia.

TABLE II.   Disorders That Cause High Bone Mass[a]

Dysplasias and dysostoses
   Autosomal dominant osteosclerosis
   Central osteosclerosis with ectodermal dysplasia
   Craniodiaphyseal dysplasia
   Craniometaphyseal dysplasia
   Dysosteosclerosis
   Endosteal hyperostosis (van Buchem disease/sclerosteosis)
   Frontometaphyseal dysplasia
   Infantile cortical hyperostosis (Caffey disease)
   Lenz-Majewski syndrome
   Melorheostosis
   Metaphyseal dysplasia (Pyle disease)
   Mixed-sclerosing bone dystrophy
   Oculodento-osseous dysplasia
   Osteodysplasia of Melnick and Needles
   Osteoectasia with hyperphosphatasia (hyperostosis corticalis)
   Osteopathia striata
   Osteopetrosis
   Osteopoikilosis
   Pachydermoperiostosis
   Progressive diaphyseal dysplasia (Engelmann disease)
   Pycnodysostosis
   Tubular stenosis (Kenny-Caffey syndrome)

Metabolic
   Carbonic anhydrase II deficiency
   Fluorosis
   Heavy metal poisoning
   Hepatitis C-associated osteosclerosis
   Hypervitaminosis A, D
   Hyper-, hypo-, and pseudohypoparathyroidism
   Hypophosphatemic osteomalacia
   Milk-alkali syndrome
   Renal osteodystrophy
   X-linked hypophosphatemia
Other
   Axial osteomalacia
   Diffuse idiopathic skeletal hyperostosis (DISH)
   Erdheim-Chester disease
   Fibrogenesis imperfecta ossium
   Hypertrophic osteoarthropathy
   Ionizing radiation
   Leukemia
   Lymphoma
   Mastocytosis
   Multiple myeloma
   Myelofibrosis
   Osteomyelitis
   Osteonecrosis
   Paget's disease
   Polycythemia vera
   Sarcoidosis
   Sickle cell disease
   Skeletal metastases
   Tuberous sclerosis

[a] Updated from Whyte [46].

well characterized (Fig. 4). A fourth clinical type, inherited as an autosomal recessive trait, was formerly called the syndrome of "osteopetrosis with renal tubular acidosis (RTA) and cerebral calcification," but the disorder is now understood

TABLE III.   Types of Osteopetrosis in Humans

Type	Inheritance[a]
Benign (adult)	AD
Type I?	
Type II	
Malignant	AR
Carbonic anhydrase II deficiency	AR
Intermediate	AR
Lethal	AR
Malignant with neuronal storage disease	AR
Transient infantile	?
Postinfectious	—

[a] From Whyte [47], "Connective tissue and its heritable disorders," (P. M. Royce and B. Steinmann, eds.), copyright © 1993. Reprinted by permission of Wiley-Liss, Inc., a subsidiary of John Wiley & Sons, Inc.
AD, autosomal dominant; AR, autosomal recessive.

to be an inborn error of metabolism (carbonic anhydrase II (CA II) deficiency) [48]. Neuronal storage disease with malignant osteopetrosis has been reported in several infants and seems to reflect a distinct phenotype. There also appear to be especially rare "lethal," "transient infantile," and "postinfectious" forms (Table III) [47].

In infantile osteopetrosis, serum calcium levels generally reflect dietary mineral intake [46]. Hypocalcemia can occur and may be severe enough to cause rachitic changes on radiographic study of the skeleton [49]. Secondary hyperparathyroidism with elevated serum levels of $1,25(OH)_2D$ is commonly present [49]. In adult osteopetrosis, standard biochemical indices of mineral homeostasis are usually unremarkable. Description of nearly 50 cases of CA II deficiency has revealed considerable clinical variability among families [48]. Typically, diagnostic investigation is undertaken in infancy or early childhood because of failure to thrive, fracture, developmental delay, or short stature. Metabolic acidosis, however, occurs as early as the neonatal period. Both proximal and distal (types II and I, respectively) RTA have been reported, although distal RTA seems to be better documented [48]. The RTA, occasionally associated with hypokalemia, may explain the apathy, hypotonia, and muscle weakness that troubles some patients.

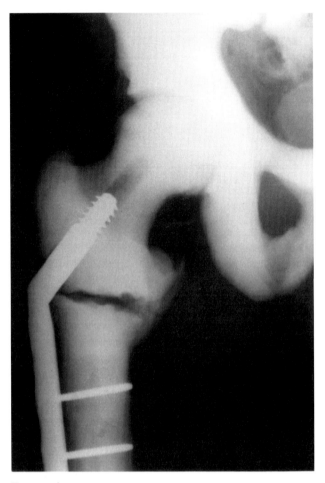

FIGURE 4 Osteopetrosis (intermediate severity). Skeletal mass of this 35-year old man with osteopetrosis is remarkably increased, yet his bone is of poor quality and led to a subtrochanteric fracture. The medullary space has not formed, because of diffuse thickening of cortical and trabecular bone, and he has profound anemia.

The pathogenesis of all true forms of osteopetrosis centers on a failure of osteoclast-mediated resorption of the skeleton [46]. This is certain because histological studies show that primary spongiosa (calcified cartilage deposited during endochondral bone formation) is not removed by bone remodeling. However, the diversity of clinical/hereditary forms of this disorder makes it apparent that several different gene defects and biological disturbances cause osteopetrosis in humans. The potential sources of osteoclast failure are numerous and complex and are illustrated by the relatively large number of animal models for this condition [50]. Abnormalities in the osteoclast stem cell microenvironment, osteoclast progenitor cells, mature osteoclasts, or the bone matrix itself could be at fault [50].

Although most forms of human osteopetrosis appear to be transmitted as autosomal traits (Table III), the molecular defects are unknown, except for CA II deficiency in which a variety of aberrations have been documented within

the candidate CA II gene [48]. In 1997, adult osteopetrosis was localized to chromosome 1p21 where the macrophage colony stimulating factor (M-CSF) gene (defective in the *op/op* mouse with osteopetrosis) maps outside the candidate region [51]. In fact, serum levels of M-CSF are normal in patients with severe osteopetrosis [52]. Other forms of marble bone disease in man have not been genetically mapped; nevertheless, there are potential clues concerning their pathogenesis. The especially rare cases of osteopetrosis with neuronal storage disease (characterized by accumulation of ceroid lipofuscin) may involve a lysosomal defect. In 1982, Marcucci *et al.* [53] reported elevated levels of acid mucopolysaccharides (primarily heparan sulfate) in the urine of two patients with severe osteopetrosis, providing evidence for a deficiency of hydrolytic enzyme activity within these intracellular structures. Viral-like inclusions have been found in osteoclasts in a few sporadic cases of benign osteopetrosis, but their significance is uncertain [46]. Defective production of interleukin-2 or superoxide (factors necessary for bone resorption) or synthesis of an abnormal PTH may also be pathogenetic defects [54]. In 1996, Lajeunesse and coworkers [55] published evidence implicating osteoblast dysfunction in two cases of malignant osteopetrosis, suggesting aberrant interaction between abnormal osteoblasts and osteoclasts. Indeed, one year earlier, the role of cytokines in bone resorption was reviewed by Key *et al.* [50, 54] who provided a theoretical basis for therapy with M-CSF and interferon gamma. Findings from a number of important animal models for osteopetrosis were also summarized [50].

A variety of "peripheral" defects have also been characterized in patients with osteopetrosis. In 1994, Danielsen and colleagues [56] studied the thermal stability of cortical bone collagen in affected adults and reported that an increased proportion of this protein was aged. Diminished remodeling of woven bone to compact bone and impaired bone resorption increase skeletal fragility because few collagen fibers properly connect osteons. Leukocyte function studies in the infantile form of osteopetrosis have revealed abnormalities in circulating monocytes and granulocytes, helping to explain the predisposition of patients to infection [54].

Markers of bone turnover have been reported in surprisingly few individuals with osteopetrosis. In the infantile form, TRAP activity is often increased in serum despite the osteoclast failure; however, urinary OHP levels can be low [49, 57]. There is decreased bone resorption, although secondary hyperparathyroidism occurs and the number of osteoclasts is characteristically increased [49]. In adult osteopetrosis, serum TRAP activity and immunoreactive PTH levels are often increased, and urinary OHP is decreased [58]. In all genuine forms of osteopetrosis in humans, the brain isoenzyme of creatine kinase (BB-CK) seems to be aberrantly present in serum [59]. Both TRAP and BB-CK appear to originate from the inactive osteoclasts.

B. Pycnodysostosis

Pycnodysostosis is the skeletal dysplasia that is believed to have affected the French impressionist painter Henri de Toulouse-Lautrec (1864–1901) [46]. More than 100 cases from 50 kindreds have been described since the condition was delineated in 1962. The disorder is transmitted as an autosomal recessive trait, and parental consanguinity has been reported for approximately 30% of patients. Most case descriptions have come from Europe or the United States, but the dysplasia has also been diagnosed in Israel, Indonesia, India, and Africa and appears to be especially common in Japan [46].

Pycnodysostosis is generally discovered during infancy or early childhood because of disproportionate short stature and dysmorphic physical features that include fronto-occipital prominence, relative macrocephaly, obtuse mandibular angle, small facies and chin, high-arched palate, dental malocclusion with retained deciduous teeth, proptosis, bluish sclerae, and a beaked and pointed nose. In addition, the anterior fontanelle and other cranial sutures are usually open, fingers are short and clubbed from acro-osteolysis or aplasia of terminal phalanges, hands are small and square, fingernails are hypoplastic, and the thorax is narrow. There may also be pectus excavatum, kyphoscoliosis, and increased lumbar lordosis. Mental retardation affects about 10% of cases [46]. Adult height ranges from 4 ft 3 in to 4 ft 11 in. Recurrent fractures typically involve the lower limbs and cause genu valgum deformity. Patients are, however, usually able to walk independently. Visceral manifestations and rickets have also been described. Recurrent respiratory tract infections and right heart failure (from chronic upper airway obstruction due to micrognathia) occur in some affected individuals. Anemia is generally not a problem.

Histopathologic study shows cortical bone structure that appears to be normal despite possibly decreased osteoclastic and osteoblastic activity and slowed skeletal turnover [60]. Both the rate of bone accretion and the size of the exchangeable calcium pool may be reduced. Diminished rates of skeletal resorption may explain the osteosclerosis. Electron microscopy of bone from two patients suggested that degradation of collagen could be defective, perhaps from an abnormality in the skeletal matrix or in the osteoclasts themselves [61]. In fact, abnormal inclusions in the osteoclasts, consisting of collagen-containing vacuoles, have been described. Virus-like inclusions were also found in the osteoclasts of two affected brothers [46].

Serum calcium and inorganic phosphate levels and AP activity are usually unremarkable in pycnodysostosis. Absorption of dietary calcium has been reported to be markedly increased. In 1993, the killing activity and IL-1 secretion of circulating monocytes was found to be low [62]. In 1996, defective growth hormone secretion and low serum IGF-1 levels were reported in five of six affected children [63]. That same year, however, the genetic basis for pycnodysostosis was found to involve defects within the cathepsin K gene [64]. Cathepsin K, a lysosomal cysteine protease, is highly expressed in osteoclasts. Impaired bone resorption from diminished collagen degradation appears to be the fundamental pathogenetic feature of this disorder.

C. Progressive Diaphyseal Dysplasia

Progressive diaphyseal dysplasia was characterized by Cockayne in 1920. Camurati discovered that the disorder was heritable and Engelmann described the severe typical form in 1929. Progressive diaphyseal dysplasia is transmitted as an autosomal dominant disease. Descriptions of more than 100 cases show that the clinical and radiological penetrance is quite variable [42, 65]. The defining feature is new bone formation that occurs gradually on both the periosteal and endosteal surfaces of long bone diaphyses (Fig. 5). In severe cases, osteosclerosis is widespread and the skull and

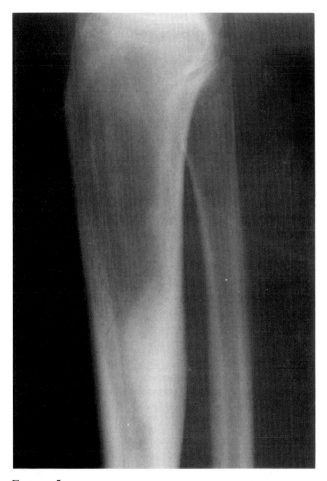

FIGURE 5   Progressive diaphyseal dysplasia. Cortical bone thickening partly envelops the proximal diaphyseal shaft of the tibia of this 17-year-old girl, but characteristically does not extend to the metaphysis or epiphysis.

axial skeleton are also involved. Some carriers have no radiographic changes, but bone scintigraphy is abnormal [46, 66].

The disorder typically presents during childhood with limping or a broad-based and waddling gait, leg pain, muscle wasting, and decreased subcutaneous fat in the extremities; it may be mistaken for a form of muscular dystrophy [67]. Severely affected patients have a characteristic body habitus that includes an enlarged head with prominent forehead, proptosis, and thin limbs with palpably thickened and tender bones and little muscle mass. Some affected individuals have hepatosplenomegaly, Raynaud's phenomenon, or other findings suggestive of vasculitis [68]. Cranial nerve palsies and raised intracranial pressure can occur when the skull is involved. Puberty is sometimes delayed. Although radiological studies typically show progressive disease, the clinical course is variable, and remission of symptoms seems to occur in some patients during the adult years. Bone scanning generally reveals focally increased radionuclide accumulation in affected areas [66]. Clinical, radiographic, and scintigraphic findings are generally concordant but, in some patients, bone scans can be unremarkable despite considerable abnormality on X-ray examination. This picture seems to reflect advanced, but quiescent, disease. Markedly increased radioisotope accumulation with minimal radiographic findings can reflect early and active skeletal pathology [46]. Cranial involvement has been assessed with magnetic resonance imaging and computed tomography.

Hyperostosis, both periosteal and endosteal, along diaphyses is the radiographic hallmark of progressive diaphyseal dysplasia (Fig. 5). Peripheral to the bony cortex, newly formed woven bone undergoes centripetal maturation and then incorporation into the histologically mature cortex. Electron microscopy of muscle has shown myopathic changes and vascular abnormalities [46].

Progressive diaphyseal dysplasia is caused by an autosomal gene defect that has not been mapped and characterized. Some especially mild cases were assumed to reflect recessive inheritance (i.e., "Ribbing disease") [42]. However, sporadic cases do occur, and mild disease can be transmitted as an autosomal dominant trait with variable penetrance [65]. In 1997, investigation of 18 affected individuals in a three-generation family indicated that males who inherited progressive diaphyseal dysplasia from their fathers perhaps reflected a dynamic mutation with repeat expansion that was enhanced by father-to-son transmission [65].

Some of the clinical and laboratory features of progressive diaphyseal dysplasia, together with its well-documented responsiveness to glucocorticoid treatment, have led several investigators to suggest that the disorder is a systemic condition (i.e. an inflammatory connective tissue disease) [46]. In fact, mild anemia and leukopenia and an elevated erythrocyte sedimentation rate may be detected in some patients [66]. Aberrant differentiation of monocytes/macrophages to fibroblasts and to osteoblasts has been discussed as a fundamental pathogenetic feature [46].

Routine biochemical parameters of bone and mineral metabolism are typically normal in progressive diaphyseal dysplasia, although serum AP activity and urinary OHP levels can be increased [69]. Modest hypocalcemia and significant hypocalciuria can occur in individuals with severe disease, apparently reflecting markedly positive calcium balance [70].

In 1997, investigation of many biochemical markers of bone remodeling in four cases in one affected family showed increased levels for both indices of bone formation and resorption. The magnitude of the disturbance generally reflected disease activity determined by bone scanning [69]. The findings were interpreted as indicative of rapid skeletal remodeling and showed utility for assaying certain biochemical parameters to evaluate response to therapy [69].

D. Endosteal Hyperostosis

Endosteal hyperostosis refers to several disorders featuring increased skeletal mass due to cortical bone thickening at endosteal surfaces [46]. Van Buchem disease (hyperostosis corticalis generalisata) is an autosomal recessive form of endosteal hyperostosis characterized also by enlargement of the jaw and thickening of the skull, which sometimes causes cranial nerve compression. Sclerosteosis has similar characteristics, but also includes gigantism and syndactyly. The two conditions may prove to be allelic disorders [42]. In 1998, van Buchem disease was mapped to chromosome 17q12–q21 [71]. Limited histological and biochemical investigation of skeletal remodeling suggests that osteoblast activity is excessive, with a secondary increase in bone turnover [72].

E. Hepatitis C-Associated Osteosclerosis

Hepatitis C-associated osteosclerosis refers to a syndrome that was discovered in 1992 [73]. The principal radiographic feature is severe, acquired, generalized osteosclerosis and hyperostosis [46]. Ten cases have been reported worldwide. Infection from parenteral transmission with hepatitis C virus has been common to all patients [74].

In hepatitis C-associated osteosclerosis, forearms and legs are painful, perhaps from subperiosteal new bone formation. Periosteal, endosteal, and trabecular bone thickening occurs throughout the skeleton. Densitometric studies of the hip and spine reveal bone mass that may be 200–300% above mean values for age and sex. Skeletal formation can be accelerated as shown by dynamic histomorphometry and implied by elevated serum AP activity and osteocalcin levels and enhanced radionuclide uptake on bone scanning [73]. Increased urinary OHP and deoxypyridinoline levels suggest that skeletal resorption is also rapid [73]. This enhanced bone turnover responds to calcitonin or bisphosphonate therapy in some patients [74]. However, gradual spontaneous remission in pain and normalization of bone remodeling may occur. A disturbance in the IGF system was identified that could be the cause of the high bone mass in these interesting patients [75].

F. Fibrogenesis Imperfecta Ossium

Fibrogenesis imperfecta ossium was first described in 1950. Fewer than ten cases have been reported in the medical literature [46]. Although radiographic studies show that there is generalized osteopenia, the coarse and dense appearance of areas of trabecular bone explains why this condition is included among the osteosclerotic disorders (Table II).

This acquired disease typically presents during or after middle age. Either sex can be affected. Intractable skeletal pain that rapidly progresses is the characteristic symptom. Subsequently, there is a debilitating course with progressive immobility. Spontaneous fracture is also a prominent feature. Patients generally become bedridden. Physical examination typically shows marked bony tenderness. Acute agranulocytosis and macroglobulinemia have been reported [46].

The bony lesion of fibrogenesis imperfecta ossium is a form of osteomalacia, although the amount of affected bone varies considerably from area to area. Cortical bone in the shaft of the femora and tibiae demonstrates the least abnormality. Aberrant collagen is found in regions with abnormal mineralization patterns but is unremarkable in other tissues. Osteoid seams are thick and osteoblasts and osteoclasts can be abundant. Polarized-light microscopy shows that collagen fibrils lack birefringence in the areas of abnormal bone. Electron microscopy reveals that the collagen fibrils are thin and randomly organized in a tangled pattern. In some regions, peculiar circular matrix structures of 300–500 nm diameter have been noted. Unless bone specimens are viewed with polarized-light or electron microscopy, this disorder can be mistaken for osteoporosis or another form of osteomalacia [46].

The etiology of fibrogenesis imperfecta ossium is unknown. Genetic factors have not been implicated because only sporadic cases have been reported. It seems to be an acquired disorder of collagen synthesis in lamellar bone. Serum calcium and inorganic phosphate levels are normal, but AP activity is increased. OHP levels in urine may be normal or supranormal. Typically, there is no aminoaciduria or other evidence of renal tubular dysfunction.

G. Pachydermoperiostosis

Pachydermoperiostosis (primary hypertrophic osteoarthropathy) is a rare autosomal dominant disorder characterized by thick skin, periosteal new bone formation, and clubbing

of the fingers and toes [42, 46]. Autosomal recessive forms also exist [76]. Patients suffer from arthralgias. An abnormality of blood flow to affected skeletal regions has been reported. In one affected individual, skin fibroblasts in culture were found to synthesize decreased amounts of collagen whereas formation of the proteoglycan, decorin, was strongly increased [77].

IV. ECTOPIC CALCIFICATION

A significant number and variety of disorders cause extraskeletal deposition of calcium and phosphate (Table IV) [78]. In some, mineral is precipitated as amorphous calcium phosphate or as hydroxyapatite crystals; in others, bone tissue is formed. The pathogenesis of the ectopic mineralization in these conditions is generally ascribed to one of three mechanisms: metastatic calcification, dystrophic calcification, or ectopic ossification.

A. Fibrodysplasia (Myositis) Ossificans Progressiva

Fibrodysplasia ossificans progressiva is a heritable disorder of connective tissue characterized by congenital mal-

TABLE IV. Disorders Associated with Extraskeletal Calcification or Ossification

Metastatic calcification
Hypercalcemia
Milk-alkali syndrome
Hypervitaminosis D
Sarcoidosis
Hyperparathyroidism
Renal failure
Hyperphosphatemia
Tumoral calcinosis
Hyperparathyroidism
Pseudohypoparathyroidism
Cell lysis following chemotherapy for leukemia
Renal failure
Dystrophic calcification
Calcinosis (universalis or circumscripta)
Childhood dermatomyositis
Scleroderma
Systemic lupus erythematosis
Posttraumatic
Ectopic ossification
Myositis ossificans (posttraumatic)
Burns
Surgery
Neurologic injury
Fibrodysplasia (myositis) ossificans progressiva

Reproduced with permission from Whyte [78].

formations of the great toes and recurrent episodes of painful soft-tissue swelling that evolve to become heterotopic ossification. More than 600 cases have been reported involving all ethnic groups. Autosomal dominant transmission with variable expressivity is established [42].

This rare disease can be suspected at birth, before soft-tissue lesions occur, if the typical congenital malformations are recognized. The hallmark on physical examination throughout life is shortening and deviation (hallux valgus) of the big toes due to defective formation of the cartilaginous anlages of the first metatarsals and proximal phalanges. Nevertheless, the digital anomalies are not pathognomonic. Usually, the disorder is diagnosed when soft-tissue swellings and radiologic evidence of heterotopic ossification are discovered [46].

Episodes of soft-tissue swelling typically begin during the first decade of life. Painful, tender, and rubbery lesions appear spontaneously, or they may appear to be precipitated by minor trauma. Usually, swellings occur in paraspinal muscles or in the limb girdle and may last for several weeks. Most lesions mature and then contain true heterotopic bone. Gradually, the bony masses immobilize joints and cause contractures and deformity, particularly in the neck and shoulders. Ankylosis of the spine and rib cage often imperil cardiopulmonary function. A remarkable radiographic feature is developmental fusion of cervical vertebrae; scoliosis is also common [46].

Radiographic studies of the abnormal bone suggest normal modeling and remodeling of the heterotopic skeleton. Bone scans are abnormal before ossification can be demonstrated by conventional radiographs. Computerized tomography and magnetic resonance imaging of early lesions has been described.

The soft-tissue masses are initially composed of one or more edematous skeletal muscles. Edema of fascial planes is one of the earliest findings. Immunostaining with a monoclonal antibody that recognizes bone morphogenetic protein 2/4 is intense. Subsequently, endochondral ossification is the major pathway for heterotopic bone formation. Mature osseous lesions have haversian systems and cancellous bone contains hematopoietic tissue [79]. Routine biochemical studies of mineral metabolism are usually normal, although AP activity in serum may be increased, especially during disease flare-ups.

B. Juvenile Dermatomyositis

Dermatomyositis is a multisystem connective tissue disorder caused by small vessel vasculitis and features a nonsuppurative inflammatory process of, especially, the skin and striated muscle. Dystrophic calcification often follows episodes of inflammation. There are more female than male patients and two peak ages when the disorder occurs: childhood (5 to 15 years) and adulthood (50 to 60 years). When dermato-

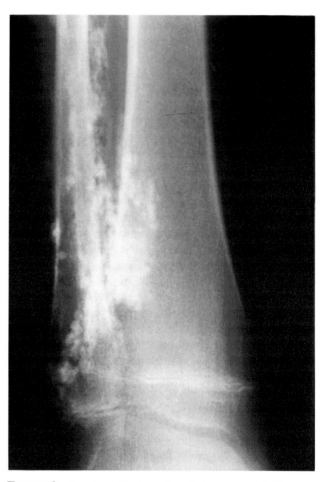

FIGURE 6   Ectopic calcification in juvenile dermatomyositis. Numerous radiopaque areas of calcification are present above the ankle of this 16-year-old boy with a 6-year history of juvenile dermatomyositis.

myositis manifests before age 16, it is called the juvenile or the childhood form. The adult form is associated with malignancy [46].

Juvenile dermatomyositis is being better controlled due to vigorous pharmacologic treatment; consequently, the prevalence of calcinosis may be decreasing. The patient's sex and the age-of-onset of symptoms do not, however, appear to influence the severity of calcinosis, which is generally noted one to three years after diagnosis and is usually subsequent to the acute phase (Fig. 6). Mineral deposits develop over one to three years. The dystrophic calcification then typically remains stable, although some regression may occur [80].

In calcinosis universalis, mineral deposition occurs throughout the subcutaneous tissues, but it primarily occurs in periarticular regions or in areas that are subject to trauma. In calcinosis circumscripta, these deposits are more localized and typically are noted around joints. The ectopic calcification can cause pain, ulcerate the skin, limit mobility, and predispose the patient to abscess formation. Radiographic studies delineate four types of dystrophic calcification in juvenile dermatomyositis: (i) superficial masses; (ii) deep, discrete, subcutaneous, nodular masses; (iii) deep, linear, sheet-like deposits within intramuscular fascial planes (calcinosis universalis); and (iv) lacy, reticular, subcutaneous deposits that encase the torso to form a generalized "exoskeleton" [80]. Children with severe disease that is refractory to medical therapy seem to be especially prone to developing an exoskeleton, which in turn is associated with severe calcinosis and poor physical function.

Juvenile dermatomyositis appears to be a form of complement-mediated microangiopathy. The precise cause of the dystrophic calcification, however, is unknown. Prior to especially agressive medical therapies, mineral deposition seemed to occur in the majority of long-term survivors and reflected a scarring process. This hypothesis is supported by the observation that calcification is found primarily in the muscles that are most severely affected during the acute phase of the disease. Electron microscopy shows that the mineralization consists of hydroxyapatite crystals [46].

A variety of mechanisms have been considered for the dystrophic calcification, including release of AP or discharge of free fatty acids from diseased muscle that, in turn, directly precipitates calcium or first binds acid mucopolysaccharides. Increased urinary levels of gamma-carboxylated peptides suggest that calcium-binding proteins may be responsible for the mineral deposition. In 1994, Perez *et al.* [81] reported dual-tracer stable isotope studies of 12 affected children and concluded that they are also at risk of significant loss of bone mineral due, in part, to decreased calcium absorption, especially in the acute phase of their disease when they are receiving glucocorticoid therapy. Hypercalcemia with hypercalciuria and hyperphosphaturia may occur.

V. OTHER DISORDERS

Fibrous dysplasia, including the McCune-Albright syndrome, and systemic mastocytosis are among the rare bone diseases for which researchers are interested in assays of biochemical markers of skeletal remodeling.

A. Fibrous Dysplasia and McCune-Albright Syndrome

Fibrous dysplasia is a sporadic developmental disorder characterized by a unifocal or multifocal expanding fibrous lesion of bone-forming mesenchyme that often results in fracture and/or deformity. McCune-Albright syndrome refers to patients with fibrous dysplasia (generally polyostotic) and patches of skin pigmentation, called café-au-lait spots, who also have hyperfunction of one or more endocrine glands. Both sexes are affected [42].

Monostotic fibrous dysplasia characteristically develops during the second or third decade of life; polyostotic disease

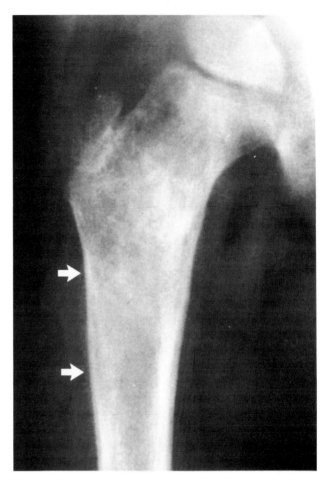

FIGURE 7   Fibrous dysplasia in McCune-Albright syndrome. Heterogenous areas of osteopenia and osteosclerosis with cortical thinning (arrows) are present in the proximal right femur of this $3\frac{1}{2}$-year-old girl.

typically manifests before 10 years of age. The monostotic form is more common. Generally, an expansile bony lesion causes fracture or deformity and may occasionally entrap nerves. The skull and long bones are affected most often (Fig. 7). Sarcomatous degeneration of involved skeletal sites occurs with somewhat increased frequency (incidence <1%), especially when the facial bones or femora are involved. Pregnancy may "reactivate" previously quiescent lesions.

In the McCune-Albright syndrome, café-au-lait spots are hyperpigmented macules with rough borders, compared to the smooth borders of the cutaneous lesions of neurofibromatosis (i.e., "Coast-of-Maine" versus "Coast-of-California," respectively). Most often, the endocrinopathy is pseudoprecocious puberty in girls due to ovarian activity. Less commonly, there is thyrotoxicosis, Cushing's syndrome, acromegaly, hyperprolactinemia, hyperparathyroidism, or pseudoprecocious puberty in boys. Some patients with widespread skeletal lesions have renal phosphate wasting that causes hypophosphatemic rickets or osteomalacia.

Both monostotic and polyostotic bone lesions have a similar histological appearance. They are anatomically well defined but are not encapsulated. Characteristically, spindle-shaped fibroblasts form "swirls" within the marrow space. Haphazardly arranged trabeculae are composed of woven bone. Cartilage is found within the lesions, more often when there is polyostotic involvement. Cystic regions that are lined by multinucleated giant cells may occur. The cumulative findings resemble the histopathology of hyperparathyroid bone disease (osteitis fibrosa cystica), but an important distinction is that characteristic osteoblasts are few in fibrous dysplasia. The skeletal lesion results from the formation of woven bone and fibrotic matrix, apparently because mesenchymal cells proliferate rapidly but do not fully differentiate to osteoblasts. Endocrine hyperfunction in the McCune-Albright syndrome is generally due to end-organ hyperactivity.

Somatic mosaicism for activating mutations in the gene that encodes the Gsα subunit of the receptor/adenylate cyclase-coupling G protein causes fibrous dysplasia and the McCune-Albright syndrome [82]. In 1991, such mutations were first discovered in McCune-Albright syndrome patients [83]. The mutations disturb the pathway for transmembrane signaling, leading to overactivity of adenyl cyclase [83]. In 1996, increased IL-6 secretion by fibroblasts in culture from these bone lesions was reported [84]. In 1997, monostotic and polyostotic fibrous dysplasia were also associated with these activating mutations [82, 84]. The fibrotic areas in fibrodysplastic bone were shown to consist of an excess of cells with phenotypic features of preosteogenic cells, and the lesional bone was produced by mature, but abnormal, osteoblasts with peculiar shape. Furthermore, there was production of bone matrix rich and poor in certain antiadhesion and proadhesion molecules, respectively [85]. Additionally, the synthesis of osteocalcin was diminished [84].

Although serum AP activity may be elevated, calcium and inorganic phosphate levels are usually normal in this group of disorders. Some studies, which explored the potential efficacy of bisphosphonates for these conditions, suggest that bone remodeling in the lesions is accelerated [86].

B. Mastocytosis

Systemic mastocytosis is charactrized by increased numbers of mast cells in the viscera. The skin can also contain many hyperpigmented macules that reflect dermal mast cell accumulation, a feature called urticaria pigmentosa. Bone marrow is typically involved, causing the skeletal pathology. The etiology, however, is unknown. Persistence of mast cell disease following successful bone marrow transplantation suggested that a defective myeloid precursor cell is not involved in the pathogenesis [46].

Symptoms of systemic mastocytosis result primarily from release of mediator substances by the mast cells and include generalized pruritus, urticaria, flushing, episodic hypo-

tension, syncope, diarrhea, weight loss, and peptic ulcer. Skeletal manifestations are relatively infrequent but include bone pain or tenderness from deformity resulting from fracture [46].

Radiographic abnormalities of the skeleton are common in systemic mastocytosis (about 70% of patients). Typically, there are diffuse, poorly-demarcated, sclerotic and lucent areas where red marrow is normally present (i.e., the axial skeleton in adults). However, circumscribed lesions can occur, especially in the skull and in the extremities. Lytic areas are often small and have a surrounding rim of osteosclerosis. Generalized osteopenia alone is also a common radiographic presentation of systemic mastocytosis. Urinary levels of methylimidazoleacetic acid, a metabolite of histamine and an indicator of mast cell mass, correlate positively with bone mineral density [87].

The histopathological findings of systemic mastocytosis in the skeleton are also well characterized. In fact, examination of undecalcified sections of bone can be a particularly effective way to establish the diagnosis. Iliac crest biopsy may be superior to bone marrow aspiration or biopsy. Multiple nodules, 150 to 450 microns in diameter, that resemble granulomas are found in the marrow space. Within these cellular aggregations are eosinophils, plasma cells, lymphocytes, and characteristic oval or spindle-shaped cells. The spindle-shaped cells superficially resemble histiocytes or fibroblasts, but they contain granules that stain metachromatically and are actually a type of mast cell. In addition, the marrow space houses increased numbers of these mast cells individually or in smaller aggregates [46].

Histomorphometric studies following tetracycline labeling show that skeletal remodeling is usually normal or rapid in systemic mastocytosis. Evaluation of biochemical markers of bone remodeling revealed elevations in serum AP activity and TRAP activity and in osteocalcin levels in some patients [87].

References

1. Byers, P. H. (1995). Disorders of collagen biosynthesis and structure. *In* "The Metabolic and Molecular Bases of Inherited Disease" (C. R. Scriver, A. L. Beaudet, W. S. Sly, and D. Valle, eds.), pp. 4029–4077. McGraw-Hill, New York.

2. Prockop, D. J., Kuivaniemi H., and Tromp, G. (1994). Molecular basis of osteogenesis imperfecta and related disorders of bone. *Clin. Plast. Surg.* **21**, 407–413.

3. Rowe, D. W., and Shapiro, J. R. (1995). Osteogenesis imperfecta. *In* "Metabolic Bone Disease" (L.V. Avioli and S. M. Krane, eds.), pp. 651–695. Academic Press, San Diego, CA.

4. Fedarko, N. S., Mörike, M., Brenner, R., Robey, P. G., and Vetter, U. (1992). Extracellular matrix formation by osteoblasts from patients with osteogenesis imperfecta. *J. Bone Miner. Res.* **7**, 921–930.

5. Cassella, J. P., and Ali, S. Y. (1992). Abnormal collagen and mineral formation in osteogenesis imperfecta. *Bone Miner.* **17**, 123–128.

6. Doty, S. B., and Mathews, R. S. (1971). Electron microscopic and

histochemical investigation of osteogenesis imperfecta tarda. *Clin. Orthop.* **80**, 191–201.

7. Ste-Marie, L. G., Charhon, S. A., Edouard, C., Chapuy, M. C., and Meunier, P. J. (1984). Iliac bone histomorphometry in adults and children with osteogenesis imperfecta. *J. Clin. Pathol.* **37**, 1081–1089.

8. Baron, R., Gertner, J. M., Lang, R., and Vignery, A. (1983). Increased bone turnover with decreased bone formation by osteoblasts in children with osteogenesis imperfecta tarda. *Pediatr. Res.* **17**, 204–207.

9. Vetter, U., Eanes, E. D., Kopp, J. B., Termine, J. D., and Robey, P. G. (1991). Changes in apatite crystal size in bones of patients with osteogenesis imperfecta. *Calcif. Tissue Int.* **49**, 248–250.

10. Vetter, U., Fisher, L. W., Mintz, K. P., Kopp, J. B., Tuross, N., Termine, J. D., and Robey, P. G. (1991). Osteogenesis imperfecta: Changes in noncollagenous proteins in bone. *J. Bone Miner. Res.* **6**, 501–505.

11. Dickson, I. R., Millar, E. A., and Veis, A. (1975). Evidence for abnormality of bone-matrix proteins in osteogenesis imperfecta. *Lancet* **2**, 586–587.

12. Riley, F. C., Jowsey, J., and Brown, D. M. (1973). Osteogenesis imperfecta: Morphologic and biochemical studies of connective tissue. *Pediatr. Res.* **7**, 757–768.

13. Shoenfeld, Y. (1975). Osteogenesis imperfecta. Review of the literature with presentation of 29 cases. *Am. J. Dis. Child.* **129**, 679–687.

14. Fedarko, N. S., Robey, P. G., and Vetter, U. K. (1995). Extracellular matrix stoichiometry in osteoblasts from patients with osteogenesis imperfecta. *J. Bone Miner. Res.* **10**, 1122–1129.

15. Mörike, M., Brenner, R. E., Bushart, G. B., Teller, W. M., and Vetter, U. (1992). Collagen metabolism in cultured osteoblasts from osteogenesis imperfecta patients. *Biochem. J.* **286**, 73–77.

16. Mörike, M., Schulz, M., Brenner, R. E., Bushart, G. B., Teller, W. M., and Vetter, U. (1993). In vitro expression of osteoblastic markers in cells isolated from normal fetal and postnatal human bone and from bone of patients with osteogenesis imperfecta. *J. Cell. Physiol.* **157**, 439–444.

17. Lehmann, H. W., Rimek, D., Bodo, M., Brenner, R. E., Vetter, U., Wörsörfer, O., Karbowski, A., and Müller, P. K. (1995). Hydroxylation of collagen type I: Evidence that both lysyl and prolyl residues are overhydroxylated in osteogenesis imperfecta. *Eur. J. Clin. Invest.* **25**, 306–310.

18. Chines, A., Petersen, D. J., Schranck, F. W., and Whyte, M. P. (1991). Hypercalciuria in children severely affected with osteogenesis imperfecta. *J. Pediatr.* **119**, 51–57.

19. Chines, A., Boniface, A., McAlister, W., and Whyte, M. (1995). Hypercalciuria in osteogenesis imperfecta: A follow-up study to assess renal effects. *Bone* **16**, 333–339.

20. Nielsen, H. E., Pedersen, U., Hansen, H. H., and Elbrond, O. (1979). Serum calcitonin and bone mineral content in patients with osteogenesis imperfecta. *Acta Orthop. Scand.* **50**, 639–643.

21. Marini, J. C., Bordenick, S., Heavner, G., Rose, S., Hintz, R., Rosenfeld, R., and Chrousos, G. P. (1993). The growth hormone and somatomedin axis in short children with osteogenesis imperfecta. *J. Clin. Endocrinol. Metab.* **76**, 251–256.

22. Granda, J. L., Falvo, K. A., and Bullough, P. G. (1977). Pyrophosphate levels and magnesium oxide therapy in osteogenesis imperfecta. *Clin. Orthop.* **126**, 228–231.

23. Cropp, G. J., and Myers, D. N. (1972). Physiological evidence of hypermetabolism in osteogenesis imperfecta. *Pediatrics* **49**, 375–391.

24. Castells, S., Yasumura, S., Fusi, M. A., Colbert, C., Bachtell, R. S., and Smith, S. (1986). Plasma osteocalcin levels in patients with osteogenesis imperfecta. *J. Pediatr.* **109**, 88–91.

25. Rico, H. (1987). Osteocalcin levels in osteogenesis imperfecta. *J. Pediatr.* **111**, 634.

26. Rico, H., Revilla, M., Iritia, M., Arribas, I., and Villa, L. F. (1991). Total body bone mineral and tartrate-resistant acid phosphatase levels in type I and III osteogenesis imperfecta. *Miner. Electrolyte Metab.* **17**, 396–398.

27. Brenner, R. E., Schiller, B., Vetter, U., Ittner, J., and Teller, W. M. (1993). Serum concentrations of procollagen I C-terminal propeptide, osteocalcin and insulin-like growth factor-I in patients with non-lethal osteogenesis imperfecta. *Acta Paediatr.* **82**, 764–767.

28. Minisola, S., Piccioni, A. L., Rosso, R., Romagnoli, E., Pacitti, M. T., Scarnecchia, L., and Mazzuoli, G. (1994). Reduced serum levels of carboxy-terminal propeptide of human type I procollagen in a family with type I-A osteogenesis imperfecta. *Metab., Clin. Exp.* **43**, 1261–1266.

29. Brenner, R. E., Vetter, U., Bollen, A. M., Mörike, M., and Eyre, D. R. (1994). Bone resorption assessed by immunoassay of urinary cross-linked collagen peptides in patients with osteogenesis imperfecta. *J. Bone Miner. Res.* **9**, 993–997.

30. Norman, M. E. (1996). Idiopathic juvenile osteoporosis. *In* "Primer on the Metabolic Bone Diseases and Disorders of Mineral Metabolism" (M. Favus, ed.), pp. 275–278. Lippincott-Raven, New York.

31. Smith, R. (1980). Idiopathic osteoporosis in the young. *J. Bone Jt. Surg., Br. Vol.* **62-B**, 417–427.

32. Dent, C. E., and Friedman, M. (1965). Idiopathic juvenile osteoporosis. *Q. J. Med.* **34**, 177–210.

33. Schippers, J. C. (1938). Spontaneous generalized osteoporosis in girl 10 years old. *Maandschr. Kindergeneeskd.* **8**, 108–116.

34. Smith, R. (1995). Idiopathic juvenile osteoporosis: Experience of twenty-one patients. *Br. J. Rheumatol.* **34**, 68–77.

35. Jowsey, J., and Johnson, K. A. (1972). Juvenile osteoporosis: Bone findings in seven patients. *J. Pediatr.* **81**, 511–517.

36. Cloutier, M. D., Hayles, A. B., Riggs, B. L., Jowsey, J., and Bickel, W. H. (1967). Juvenile osteoporosis: Report of a case including a description of some metabolic and microradiographic studies. *Pediatrics* **40**, 649–655.

37. Evans, R. A., Dunstan, C. R., and Hills, E. (1983). Bone metabolism in idiopathic juvenile osteoporosis: A case report. *Calcif. Tissue Int.* **35**, 5–8.

38. Jackson, E. C., Strife, F., Tsang, R. C., and Marder, H. K. (1988). Effect of calcitonin replacement therapy in idiopathic juvenile osteoporosis. *Am. J. Dis. Child.* **142**, 1237–1239.

39. Saggese, G., Bertelloni, S., Baroncelli, G. I., Perri, G., and Calderazzi, A. (1991). Mineral metabolism and calcitriol therapy in idiopathic juvenile osteoporosis. *Am. J. Dis. Child.* **145**, 457–462.

40. Bertelloni, S., Baroncelli, G. I., Di Nero, G., and Saggese, G. (1992). Idiopathic juvenile osteoporosis: Evidence of normal osteoblast function by 1,25-dihydroxyvitamin D_3 stimulation test. *Calcif. Tissue Int.* **51**, 20–23.

41. Pocock, A. E., Francis, M. J., and Smith, R. (1995). Type I collagen biosynthesis by skin fibroblasts from patients with idiopathic juvenile osteoporosis. *Clin. Sci.* **89**, 69–73.

42. McKusick, V. A. (1998). "Mendelian Inheritance in Man: A Catalog of Human Genes and Genetic Disorders," 12th ed. Johns Hopkins University Press, Baltimore, MD.

43. Mundlos, S., Otto, F., Mundlos, C., Mulliken, J. B., Aylsworth, A. S., Albright, S., Lindhout, D., Cole, W. G., Henn, W., Knoll, J. H. M., Owen, M. J., Mertelsmann, R., Zabel, B. U., and Olsen, B. R. (1997). Mutations involving the transcription factor CBFA1 cause cleidocranial dysplasia. *Cell* **89**, 773–779.

44. Otto, F., Thornell, A. P., Crompton, T., Denzel, A., Gilmour, K. C., Rosewell, I. R., Stamp, G. W., Beddington, R. S., Mundlos, S., Olsen, B. R., Selby, P. B., and Owen, M. J. (1997). Cbfa1, a candidate gene for cleidocranial dysplasia syndrome, is essential for osteoblast differentiation and bone development. *Cell* **89**, 765–771.

45. Moore, C. A., Ayangade, G., Okolo, P., Bull, M. J., Whyte, M. P., and Bixler, D. (1992). Cleidocranial dysplasia: A natural history study

including evaluation of a five generation family. *Proc. Greenwood Genet. Cent.* **10**, 91 (abstr.).

46. Whyte, M. P. (1997). Skeletal disorders characterized by osteosclerosis and hyperostosis. *In* "Metabolic Bone Disease" (L. V. Avioli and S. M. Krane, eds.), pp. 697–738. Academic Press, San Diego, CA.

47. Whyte, M. P. (1993). Osteopetrosis and the heritable forms of rickets. *In* "Connective Tissue and Its Heritable Disorders" (P. M. Royce and B. Steinmann, eds.), pp. 563–589. Wiley-Liss, New York.

48. Sly, W. S., and Hu, P. Y. (1995). The carbonic anhydrase II deficiency syndrome: Osteoporosis with renal tubular acidosis and cerebral calcification. *In* "The Metabolic and Molecular Bases of Inherited Disease" (C. R. Scriver, A. L. Beaudet, W. S. Sly, and D. Valle, eds.), pp. 4113–4124. McGraw-Hill, New York.

49. Reeves, J., Arnaud, S., Gordon, S., Subryan, B., Block, M., Huffer, W., Arnaud, C., Mundy, G., and Haussler, M. (1981). The pathogenesis of infantile malignant osteopetrosis: Bone mineral metabolism and complications in five infants. *Metab. Bone Dis. Relat. Res.* **3**, 135–142.

50. Key, L. L., Jr., Rodriguiz, R. M., and Wang, W. C. (1995). Cytokines and bone resorption in osteopetrosis. *Int. J. Pediatr. Hematol./Oncol.* **2**, 143–149.

51. Van Hul, W., Bollerslev, J., Gram, J., Van Hul, E., Wuyts, W., Benichou, O., Vanhoenacker, F., and Willems, P. J. (1997). Localization of a gene for autosomal dominant osteopetrosis (Albers-Schönberg disease) to chromosome 1p21. *Am. J. Hum. Genet.* **61**, 363–369.

52. Naffakh, N., Le Gall, S., Danos, O., Heard, J. M., Cournot, G., Motoyoshi, K., and Vilmer, E. (1993). Macrophage colony-stimulating factor: Serum levels and cDNA structure in malignant osteopetrosis. *Blood* **81**, 2817–2818.

53. Marcucci, F., Rufini, S., and Sensi, L. (1982). Abnormal urinary excretion of glycosaminoglycans in Albers-Schönberg disease. *Clin. Chim. Acta* **120**, 161–170.

54. Key, L. L., Jr., Rodriguiz, R. M., Willi, S. M., Wright, N. M., Hatcher, H. C., Eyre, D. R., Cure, J. K., Griffin, P. P., and Ries, W. L. (1995). Long-term treatment of osteopetrosis with recombinant human interferon gamma. *N. Engl. J. Med.* **332**, 1594–1599.

55. Lajeunesse, D., Busque, L., Mènard, P., Brunette, M. G., and Bonny, Y. (1996). Demonstration of an osteoblast defect in two cases of human malignant osteopetrosis. Correction of the phenotype after bone marrow transplant. *J. Clin. Invest.* **98**, 1835–1842.

56. Danielsen, C. C., Mosekilde, L., Bollerslev, J., and Mosekilde, L. (1994). Thermal stability of cortical bone collagen in relation to age in normal individuals and in individuals with osteopetrosis. *Bone* **15**, 91–96.

57. Key, L. L., Jr., Ries, W. L., Rodriguiz, R. M., and Hatcher, H. C. (1992). Recombinant human interferon gamma therapy for osteopetrosis. *J. Pediatr.* **121**, 119–124.

58. Bollerslev, J. (1989). Autosomal dominant osteopetrosis: Bone metabolism and epidemiological, clinical, and hormonal aspects. *Endocr. Rev.* **10**, 45–67.

59. Whyte, M. P., Chines, A., Silva, D. P., Landt, Y., and Ladenson, J. H. (1996). Creatine kinase brain isoenzyme (BB-CK) presence in serum distinguishes osteopetroses among the sclerosing bone disorders. *J. Bone Miner. Res.* **11**, 1438–1443.

60. Soto, R. J., Mautalen, C. A., Hojman, D., Codevilla, A., Piquè, J., and Pángaro, J. A. (1969). Pycnodysostosis: Metabolic and histologic studies. *Birth Defects, Orig. Artic. Ser.* **5**, 109–116.

61. Everts, V., Aronson, D. C., and Beertsen, W. (1985). Phagocytosis of bone collagen by osteoclasts in two cases of pycnodysostosis. *Calcif. Tissue Int.* **37**, 25–31.

62. Karkabi, S., Reis, N. D., Linn, S., Edelson, G. Tzehoval, E., Zakut, V., Dolev, E., Bar-Meir, E., and Ish-Shalom, S. (1993). Pyknodysostosis: Imaging and laboratory observations. *Calcif. Tissue Int.* **53**, 170–173.

63. Soliman, A. T., Rajab, A., AlSalmi, I., Darwish, A., and Asfour, M. (1996). Defective growth hormone secretion in children with pycnodysostosis and improved linear growth after growth hormone treatment. *Arch. Dis. Child.* **75**, 242–244.

64. Gelb, B. D., Shi, G. P., Chapman, H. A., and Desnick, R. J. (1996). Pycnodysostosis, a lysosomal disease caused by cathespin K deficiency. *Science* **273**, 1236–1238.

65. Saraiva, J. M. (1997). Progressive diaphyseal dysplasia: A three-generation family with markedly variable expressivity. *Am. J. Med. Genet.* **71**, 348–352.

66. Sty, J. R., Babbitt, D. P., and Starshak, R. J. (1978). Bone scintigraphy demonstrating Engelmann's disease. *Clin. Nucl. Med.* **3**, 69–70.

67. Low, L. C., Stephenson, J. B., and Stuart-Smith, D. A. (1985). Progressive diaphyseal dysplasia mimicking childhood myopathy: Clinical and biochemical response to prednisolone. *Aust. Paediatr. J.* **21**, 193–196.

68. Naveh, Y., Alon, U., Kaftori, J. K., and Berant, M. (1985). Progressive diaphyseal dysplasia: Evaluation of corticosteroid therapy. *Pediatrics* **75**, 321–323.

69. Hernandez, M. V., Peris P., Guanabens, N., Alvarez, L., Monegal, A., Pons, F., Ponce, A., and Munoz-Gomez, J. (1997). Biochemical markers of bone turnover in Camurati-Engelmann disease: A report on four cases in one family. *Calcif. Tissue Int.* **61**, 48–51.

70. Smith, R., Walton, R. J., Corner, B. D., and Gordon, I. R. (1977). Clinical and biochemical studies in Englemann's disease (progressive diaphyseal dysplasia). *Q. J. Med.* **46**, 273–294.

71. Van Hul, W., Balemans, W., Van Hul, E., Dikkers, F. G., Obee, H., Stokroos, R. J., Hildering, P., Vanhoenacker, F., Van Camp, G., and Willems, P. J. (1998). Van Buchem disease (hyperostosis corticalis generalisata) maps to chromosome 17q12–q21. *Am. J. Hum. Genet.* **62**, 391–399.

72. Stein, S. S., Witkop, C., Hill, S., Fallon, M. D., Viernstein, L., Gucer, G., McKeever, P., Long, D., Altman, J., Miller, N. R., Teitelbaum, S. L., and Schlesinger, S. (1983). Sclerosteosis: Neurogenetic and pathophysiologic analysis of an American kinship. *Neurology* **33**, 267–277.

73. Villareal, D. T., Murphy, W. A., Teitelbaum, S. L., Arens, M. Q., and Whyte, M. P. (1992). Painful diffuse osteosclerosis after intravenous drug abuse. *Am. J. Med.* **93**, 371–381.

74. Shaker, J. L., Reinus, W. R., and Whyte, M. P. (1998). Hepatitis C-associated osteosclerosis: Late onset after blood transfusion in an elderly woman. *J. Clin. Endocrinol. Metab.* **84**, 93–98.

75. Khosla, S., Hassoun, A. A. K., Baker, B. K., Liu, F., Zien, N. N., Whyte, M. P., Reasner, C. A., Nippoldt, T. B., Tiegs, R. D., Hintz, R. L., and Conover, C. A. (1998). Insulin-like growth factor system abnormalities in hepatitis C-associated osteosclerosis: A means to increase bone mass in adults? *J. Clin. Invest.* **101**, 2165–2173.

76. Sinha, G. P., Curtis, P., Haigh, D., Lealman, G. T., Dodds, W., and Bennett, C. P. (1997). Pachydermoperiostosis in childhood. *Br. J. Rheumatol.* **36**, 1224–1227.

77. Wegrowski, Y., Gillery, P., Serpier, H., Georges, N., Combemale, P., Kalis, B., and Maquart, F. X. (1996). Alteration of matrix macromolecule synthesis by fibroblasts from a patient with pachydermoperiostosis. *J. Invest. Dermatol.* **106**, 70–74.

78. Whyte, M. P. (1996). Extraskeletal (ectopic) calcification and ossification. *In* "Primer on Metabolic Bone Diseases and Disorders of Mineral Metabolism" (M. Favus, S. Christakos, R. F. Gagel, M. Kleerekoper, C. B. Langman, E. Shane, A. F. Steward, and M. P. Whyte, eds.), pp. 421–430. Lippincott-Raven Press, New York.

79. Shafritz, A. B., and Kaplan, F. S. (1998). Differential expression of bone and cartilage related genes in fibrodysplasia ossificans progressiva, myositis ossificans progressiva, myositis ossificans traumatica, and osteogenic sarcoma. *Clin. Orthop. Relat. Res.* **346**, 46–52.

80. Eddy, M. E., Leelawattana, R., McAlister, W. H., and Whyte, M. P. (1997). Calcinosis universalis complicating juvenile dermatomyositis:

Resolution during probenecid therapy. *J. Clin. Endocrinol. Metab.* **82**, 3536–3542.

81. Perez, M. D., Abrams, S. A., Koenning, G., Stoff, J. E., O'Brien, K. O., and Ellis, K. J. (1994). Mineral metabolism in children with dermatomyositis. *J. Rheumatol.* **21**, 2364–2369.

82. Marie, P. J., de Pollak, C., Chanson, P., and Lomri, A. (1997). Increased proliferation of osteoblastic cells expressing the activating Gs alpha mutation in monostotic and polyostotic fibrous dysplasia. *Am. J. Pathol.* **150**, 1059–1069.

83. Weinstein, L. S., Shenker, A., Gejman, P. V., Merino, M. J., Friedman, E., and Spiegel, A. M. (1991). Activating mutations of the stimulatory G protein in the McCune-Albright syndrome. *N. Engl. J. Med.* **325**, 1688–1695.

84. Yamamoto, T., Ozono, K., Kasayama, S., Yoh, K., Hiroshima, K., Takagi, M., Matsumoto, S., Michigami, T., Yamaoka, K., Kishimoto, T., and Okada, S. (1996). Increased IL-6-production by cells isolated from the fibrous bone dysplasia tissues in patients with McCune-Albright symdrome. *J. Clin. Invest.* **98**, 30–35.

85. Riminucci, M., Fisher, L. W., Shenker, A., Spiegel, A. M., Bianco, P., and Gehron-Robey, P. (1997). Fibrous dysplasia of bone in the McCune-Albright syndrome: Abnormalities in bone formation. *Am. J. Pathol.* **151**, 1587–1600.

86. Chapurlat, R. D., Delmas, P. D., Liens, D., and Meunier, P. J. (1997). Long-term effects of intravenous pamidronate in fibrous dysplasia of bone. *J. Bone Miner. Res.* **12**, 1746–1752.

87. Johansson, C., Roupe, G., Lindstedt, G., and Mellström, D. (1996). Bone density, bone markers and bone radiological features in mastocytosis. *Age Ageing* **25**, 1–7.

CHAPTER 44

Rheumatoid Arthritis and Other Inflammatory Joint Pathologies

STEVEN R. GOLDRING AND MARY B. GOLDRING

Department of Medicine, Rheumatology Division, Beth Israel Deaconess Medical Center, Harvard Medical School, Boston, Massachusetts 02215; New England Baptist Bone and Joint Institute, Boston, Massachusetts 02215

I. ABSTRACT

The inflammatory joint diseases comprise a heterogeneous group of disorders that share in common their propensity to produce destruction of the extracellular matrices of joint cartilage and bone. In addition, the underlying disturbance in immune regulation that is responsible for the localized joint pathology may target extra-articular organs and tissues leading to lung, central nervous system, kidney, cardiovascular, and gastrointestinal system manifestations. Under these circumstances, the generalized systemic inflammatory process may produce generalized effects on bone and connective tissue remodeling that may affect the entire skeleton. Among the inflammatory joint diseases, rheumatoid arthritis, the seronegative spondyloarthropathies, and juvenile rheumatoid arthritis represent excellent models for gaining insights into the effects of local as well as systemic consequences of inflammatory processes on skeletal tissue and cartilage remodeling. Histomorphometric analyses of bone, determination of remodeling indices, assessment of the breakdown products of the matrix components of joint cartilage and bone, and quantitative imaging techniques for assessing bone mass are among the approaches that have been used to assess the effects of the inflammatory joint diseases on local joint structures and generalized skeletal tissue remodeling. This chapter will review the results of these various analytical tools and assays that have been developed to assess the effects of these inflammatory conditions on cartilage and bone remodeling. It also will attempt to correlate the findings from these studies with standard indices used to monitor systemic inflammatory activity and immune system activation.

II. INTRODUCTION

Rheumatoid arthritis (RA) and related inflammatory joint diseases are a clinically diverse group of disorders that share in common their propensity to affect the anatomic components of articular and juxta-articular tissues; of the structurally distinct types of joints, the amphiarthrodial and diarthrodial joints are the sites most frequently affected. The diarthrodial joints are the most common of the articular design patterns. These joints join two opposing bone surfaces that are covered by a specialized hyaline cartilage that provides a low friction articulating interface. The joint cavity is lined by a highly specialized membrane termed the synovium. This membrane is the sight of production of synovial fluid that provides the nutritional requirements for the articular cartilage and also "lubricates" the cartilage surfaces. In most forms of inflammatory arthritis, this lining membrane is the site of the initial inflammatory process. In contrast to the diartrodial joints, amphiarthroses lack a true joint cavity and synovial lining and are characterized by a fibrocartilaginous union that joins the two opposing bone surfaces. These joints are best represented by the intervertebral discs.

Many of the inflammatory joint diseases are accompanied by generalized systemic symptoms, such as fatigue, weight loss, and fever, that may dominate the clinical picture. In addition, the underlying disturbance in immune regulation that is responsible for the localized joint pathology may target extra-articular organs and tissues leading to lung, central nervous system, kidney, cardiovascular, and gastrointestinal system manifestations. Under these circumstances, the generalized systemic inflammatory process may produce generalized effects on bone and connective tissue remodeling that may affect the entire skeleton.

III. EFFECTS OF JOINT INFLAMMATION ON SKELETAL REMODELING

Among the inflammatory joint diseases, rheumatoid arthritis (RA), the seronegative spondyloarthropathies, and juvenile rheumatoid arthritis represent excellent models for gaining insights into the effects of local inflammatory processes as well as systemic consequences of these processes on skeletal tissue and cartilage remodeling. The effects of RA on skeletal tissues and indices of bone remodeling will be discussed first.

A. Rheumatoid Arthritis

Although RA may manifest as a systemic disorder, the hallmark of this condition is the presence of a symmetrical inflammatory polyarthritis that targets the proximal small joints of the hands, wrists, elbows, shoulders, knees, ankles, and feet. The synovial lining of diarthrodial joints is the initial target of the inflammatory joint pathology. This lesion is characterized by proliferation of the synovial lining cells and infiltration of the tissue by inflammatory cells, including lymphocytes, plasma cells, endothelial cells, and activated macrophages [1–3]. With the growth and expansion of the synovial lining, there is eventual extension of the inflammatory tissue mass to the adjacent articular cartilage with progressive overgrowth of the articular surface and formation of the so-called pannus, which is derived from the Greek word meaning "covering" or "mantle". At the interface between the RA synovium and articular cartilage, tongues of proliferating cells can be seen penetrating the extracellular matrix of the cartilage. The specific cellular and biochemical mechanisms that account for the disruption of the integrity of the cartilage matrix and the release of soluble components that can be used to monitor these events are reviewed in the subsequent sections. Similarly, at the interface between the inflamed synovial tissues and adjacent subchondral bone, there is evidence of local activation of bone resorption with destruction of the mineralized bone matrix. The effects of the RA synovial lesion on bone remodeling will be discussed first.

B. Bone Disease Associated with Rheumatoid Arthritis

Three principal forms of bone disease have been described in patients with RA. The first is characterized by focal bone loss affecting the immediate subchondral bone and bone at the joint margins. This gives rise to the "bone erosions" that are characteristic of RA and related forms of inflammatory arthritis. The second form of bone disease is manifested by the development of periarticular osteopenia adjacent to inflamed joints. The third form of bone disease in patients with RA is the presence of generalized osteoporosis involving the axial and appendicular skeleton [4–6].

1. FOCAL SUBCHONDRAL AND MARGINAL BONE EROSIONS

The earliest skeletal lesions are localized to the sites where the inflamed synovial tissue comes into direct contact with the marginal bone surfaces. Focal resorption of the bone matrix leads to excavation of the bone surface which produces the characteristic cystic bone erosions that can be detected radiographically. In addition, the synovial tissue may penetrate the subchondral bone plate, permitting invasion of the marrow spaces. The inflammatory tissue may then undermine the bone plate and produce additional focal areas of subchondral bone loss.

Important insights into the pathogenesis of the progressive focal bone erosions and subchondral osteolysis that characterizes the synovial lesion of RA have been provided by the studies of Bromley and Woolley [7, 8]. They noted the presence of increased numbers of multinucleated cells with phenotypic features of osteoclasts localized to osteolytic lacunae at the junction of the subchondral bone and the adjacent marrow space. Multinucleated cells expressing abundant tartrate-resistant acid phosphatase activity were also present adjacent to the calcified cartilage matrix and they identified these cells as "chondroclasts" [7]. These so-called chondroclasts were observed in 30% of the specimens from large joints such as the knee where they appeared to make a major contribution to the subchondral bone erosions. Interestingly, the researchers rarely observed these cells in specimens from small joints, and they speculated that the mechanisms associated with small joint pathology in RA might differ from those affecting the large joints. Allard *et al.* [9] have made similar speculations regarding the differential mechanism of focal bone loss in large and small joints.

Characterization of cells isolated from RA synovial tissues has provided further support for the concept that cells with phenotypic features and functional activities of authentic osteoclasts are responsible for at least a component of the focal bone resorption that characterizes the RA synovial lesion [10, 11]. This does not preclude the possibility that macrophages or macrophage polykaryons present in the synovial lesions also have the capacity to resorb bone. Studies by several authors have demonstrated that macrophages and macrophage polykaryons have the ability to resorb bone, although their resorptive capacity is much lower than that of osteoclasts [11, 12].

Studies *in vitro* using explant cultures of synovial tissues from patients with RA also support the concept that mononuclear cells derived from synovial tissues from patients with RA can differentiate into cells expressing an osteoclastic phenotype, including the enhanced capacity to resorb bone. In these studies, synovial fragments from patients with RA were digested and the dispersed cells added to bone slices in the presence or absence of the rat osteoblast-like cell line UMR 106. Addition of $1,25(OH)_2$ vitamin D_3 and human macrophage-colony stimulating factor (M-CSF) resulted in differentiation of CD11b- and CD14-positive mononuclear cells into multinucleated cells expressing tartrate-resistant acid phosphatase activity, calcitonin receptor, and vitronectin receptor that were capable of extensive bone resorption [13]. These results suggest the possibility that the RA synovium represents a site to which osteoclast precursor cells of monocyte-macrophage lineage are recruited in response to the local inflammatory mediators. In the presence of appropriate stimuli, these cells have the capacity to differentiate into authentic osteoclasts that in turn mediate the local bone resorptive process.

Characterization of the phenotype of the cells at the bone-pannus junction has been hampered by the lack of a suitable marker to definitively identify osteoclasts and to distinguish these cells from other cells of macrophage lineage or other bone cell types. Our laboratory has cloned the human calcitonin receptor and utilized reagents developed from this cDNA to characterize the phenotype of the mono- and multinucleated cells in resorptive lacunae at the bone-pannus interface in samples from patients with RA [14–16]. These studies confirm that the multinucleated (and some mononuclear cells) in resorption lacunae express abundant calcitonin receptor mRNA, adding further support to the concept that

they are functionally indistinguishable from authentic osteoclasts. These cells also were examined for the expression of mRNA encoding the parathyroid hormone receptor, and no message was detected. These findings are consistent with the observations of others who speculate that parathyroid hormone does not act directly on osteoclasts but rather mediates its effects on early osteoclast progenitors or acts indirectly via effects on osteoblast lineage and/or marrow stromal cells [17–19]. Figure 1A demonstrates the presence of calcitonin receptor-positive osteoclast-like multinucleated cells at the bone-pannus interface from a patient with RA. Figure 1B is a plain radiograph demonstrating a bone erosion of the proximal interphalageal joint associated with the invading rheumatoid synovial pannus.

2. PERIARTICULAR BONE LOSS

Loss of bone adjacent to inflamed joints is the radiographic hallmark of inflammatory joint disorders such as RA. These radiographic changes are usually associated with sites of active synovitis. The bone loss typically occurs early in the course of RA and usually precedes the appearance of focal bone erosions. Shimizo *et al.* [20] performed histomorphometric analyses of bone samples obtained from patients undergoing joint arthroplasty to gain insights into the cellular mechanisms responsible for the periarticular bone loss in patients with RA. Their analyses revealed evidence of increased bone remodeling with an increase both in bone formation and in resorption indices. Local production of proinflammatory mediators that affect bone remodeling, hypervascularity of the synovium, and joint immobilization have been implicated as possible mechanisms responsible for periarticular abnormalities in RA joints [3, 21–26]. Figure 2 is a plain radiograph of the hand from a patient with early RA revealing periarticular bone loss affecting the metacarphalangeal joints.

3. GENERALIZED BONE LOSS

Numerous studies have established that, in addition to the local effects of the inflammatory process on juxta-articular bone, patients with RA have a lower bone mineral density (BMD) and an increased risk of fracture compared to age-matched controls [27–30]. The decrease in bone mass affects the axial spine and appendicular bone, which are not located near synovial-lined joints, suggesting that the local joint pathology is associated with a generalized systemic effect [26, 31–38]. Further evidence that RA adversely affects skeletal remodeling is provided by the study of bone density in monozygotic twins (one with RA and one without RA). These analyses revealed a significant reduction in BMD in the lumbar spine (4.6%), femoral neck (9.7%), and total body (5.7%) in the twin with RA [39].

Multiple confounding factors have hampered the investigation of the pathogenetic mechanisms responsible for the generalized bone loss observed in patients with RA. These include the influence of patient sex, age, mobility, disease

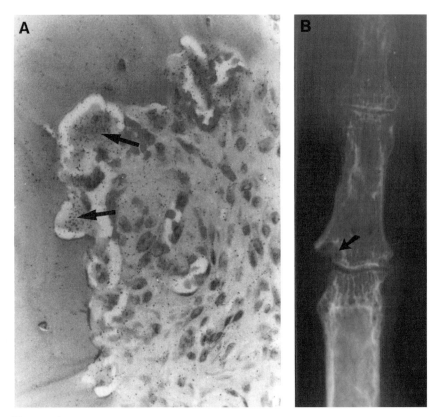

FIGURE 1   (A) This low power photomicrograph demonstrates the interface between the pannus
and the adjacent mineralized bone from a patient with RA. *In situ* hybridization with a radiolabeled
anti-sense cDNA probe from the human calcitonin receptor has been used to demonstrate the presence
of abundant mRNA for the calcitonin receptor in the multinucleated osteoclast-like cells (arrows) on
the bone surface. (B) This plan radiograph demonstrates a bone erosion of the proximal interphalageal
joint (arrow) associated with the invading rheumatoid synovial pannus.

activity and duration, and the concomitant use of immunosuppressive therapies and/or glucocorticoids, all of which
are known to have profound and independent effects on bone
metabolism. Among these factors, disease activity and duration appear to be of particular importance with respect to the
risk for reduced bone mass [40]. In a longitudinal prospective
study, Gough and coworkers [28] concluded that significant
amounts of generalized skeletal bone were lost early in RA
and that this loss was associated with disease activity. These
findings support the previous observations of Als *et al.* [41]
who also noted a significant decrease in bone mass during
the early phases of RA. Further evidence of the impact of
disease activity on bone mass is provided by the studies of
Sambrook *et al.* [32] who showed that two measures of disease activity, joint count and C reactive protein (CRP), correlated with trabecular bone loss in the lumbosacral spine. In
addition, epidemiologic studies have consistently shown the
relationship between physical activity and functional level
and bone density in patients with RA. For example, using the
Framingham activity index (as a measure of functional status), Sambrook *et al.* [34] observed that the level of physical

activity correlated with femoral neck bone mineral density in
a series of patients with RA. These findings were corroborated
by Gough *et al.* [28], who showed an association between disability level (based on the Health Assessment Questionnaire)
and bone loss in the femoral neck and axial spine.

Several different approaches have been used to study the
pathogenesis of the generalized bone loss associated with
RA. Histomorphometric analysis of bone biopsies from patients with RA indicate that the reduced bone mass observed
is related to a decrease in bone formation rather than an increase in bone resorption [38, 42, 43]. However, contradictory findings have been obtained in studies using biochemical markers of bone turnover [44, 45]. For example, Gough
and coworkers [46] evaluated 232 patients who had RA for
less than 2 years. They showed that the urinary markers of
bone resorption, pyridinoline and deoxypyridinoline cross-
links, correlated with the change in BMD at all sites during
the 2 year study and that these markers of resorption were increased in subjects with RA compared to age-matched control
subjects. Similar observations have been made by several
other investigators [27, 45, 47–50]. Excretion of both markers

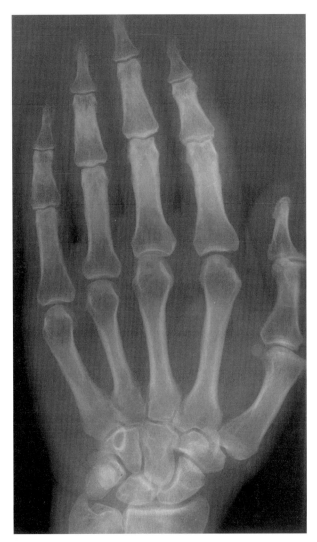

FIGURE 2   This plain radiograph of early RA reveals periarticular bone loss affecting the metacarphalangeal joints.

patients with RA. For example, Hall *et al.* [44] examined the effects of hormone replacement therapy on markers of bone metabolism in 106 postmenopausal women with RA who were treated with or without glucocorticoids. They found that the serum osteocalcin levels tended to be lower in the RA subjects with or without glucocorticoid treatment compared to control subjects. Urinary deoxypyridinoline and CTx (which measures a peptide fragment of type I collagen breakdown) were elevated in glucocoticoid-treated subjects with RA compared to the untreated RA patients and controls. After hormone replacement therapy, urinary CTx excretion decreased significantly both in the steroid-treated and in the nontreated group and these changes correlated with 2-year changes in BMD. Saag *et al.* [51] examined the effects of alendronate therapy on the prevention and treatment of glucocorticoid-induced osteoporosis in a heterogeneous group of 477 patients that included a large number of individuals with RA. The researchers demonstrated that the urinary excretion of N-telopeptides of type I collagen decreased by 60% and serum alkaline phosphatase concentrations decreased by 27% in alendronate-treated subjects. These findings correlated with an increase in bone mass and a decrease in fracture risk.

C. Seronegative Spondyloarthropathies

The seronegative spondyloarthropathies include ankylosing spondylitis, reactive arthritis, Reiter's syndrome, spondylitis and arthritis associated with psoriasis or inflammatory bowel disease, and juvenile-onset spondyloarthropathy. These disorders encompass a broad range of multisystem inflammatory disorders in which the spine, peripheral joints, periarticular structures, or all three sites are involved. The joint inflammation that accompanies these disorders exhibits many of the same histopathological features that characterize the joint pathology in RA, including synovial hyperplasia, lymphoid infiltration, and pannus formation. Joint margin and subchondral erosions and cartilage destruction often are seen, although the inflammation may be restricted to only a few isolated joints. The pattern of distribution is typically asymmetrical, affecting proximal as well as distal joints such as the distal interphalageal joints that are not typically affected in RA. Inflammation of the enthesis (sites of tendinous or ligamentous attachment to bone), especially in the axial spine, is the pathological hallmark of the spondyloarthropathies, and this feature distinguishes this group of disorders from the other inflammatory arthridites.

The earliest focal joint pathology in patients with spondyloartyhropathies most often presents as a localized zone of bone resorption that initially affects the insertion sites of juxta-articular tendon or ligamentous insertions. These enthesopathic erosions are detectable radiographically as localized zones of radiolucency. In contrast to the joint pathology

was increased significantly in the patients with active disease who lost bone quickly. The levels of these urinary markers were highly correlated with CRP but not with serum levels of interleukin-6 (IL-6) or interleukin-1 (IL-1). In the final regression analysis, serial CRP was more closely correlated with BMD change than with any of the other markers. Bone formation indices, as assessed by measurement of serum alkaline phosphatase and procollagen I carboxyterminal propeptide (PICP) levels, were not significantly suppressed, suggesting that suppression of bone formation was marginal and not a dominant factor contributing to the accelerated bone loss in RA subjects. Of interest, on an individual basis, the trend was for patients presenting with active RA to have low bone formation indices and then for the levels to rise rapidly if the disease activity was suppressed.

Indices of bone remodeling also have been used to assess the effects of treatments on generalized bone loss in in RA in which the inflammatory process ultimately leads to progressive bone loss without evidence of bone repair, in patients with spondyloarthropathies, the initial destructive bone lesion may lead to calcification and ossification of the enthesis in the later stages of the disease process.

Braun *et al.* [52] used immunohistological and *in situ* hybridization techniques to study the inflamed sacroiliac joints of patients with spondylitis to gain insights into the biochemical and cellular mechanisms involved in the tendency of the joint inflammation to lead to excessive bone formation. In these studies, computer assisted tomography was used to obtain biopsies of the sacroiliac joints in five patients with ankylosing spondylitis. Analysis of synovial tissue revealed dense infiltrates of T lymphocytes, consisting of both CD4-positive and CD8-positive cells, and CD14-positive macrophages. Localized nodules containing active foci of endochondral ossification were noted within the pannus, a finding not observed in synovial tissues from patients with RA. *In situ* hybridization identified abundant message for TNF-α (but not IL1-β) within the inflammatory cells. Of interest, with respect to the tendency for the development of ossification at the sites of joint inflammation, the message for TGF-β_2 was found in close proximity to the regions of new bone formation. These findings suggest the possibility that local production of growth factors by the inflammatory tissues may induce the new bone formation that gives rise to ossification and eventual bony ankylosis of the sacroiliac joints that occur in some individuals with spondyloarthropathies. A similar process could account for the development of syndesmophytes that characterize the spinal pathology. In the spine, the initial lesion consists of inflammatory granulation tissue at the junction of the annulus fibrosis of the intervertebral disc and the margin of the vertebral bone. Replacement of the outer annular fibers of the intervertebral discs with bone by mechanisms similar to those described by Braun and coworkers [52] could lead eventually to formation of syndesmophytes with resultant ankylosis of the adjoining vertebral bodies.

Although individuals with spondyloarthopathies exhibit a tendency towards the development of localized regions of new bone formation at sites of enthesopathic peripheral joint and spine inflammation, many patients exhibit evidence of marked osteopenia of the spinal column. The bone loss that occurs following bony ankylosis of the spine is a common feature often ascribed to spinal immobility [53]. Will *et al.* [54] evaluated twenty-five patients with early ankylosing spondylitis using dual photon absorptiometry and compared them to age- and sex-matched controls. The researchers observed a significant reduction in bone mineral density in the lumbosacral spine and hip in the spondylitis cohort. Of interest, these changes occurred even in the absence of bony ankylosis. Based on these observations, Will *et al.* concluded that bone loss occurred early in disease before the development of spinal immobility. They speculated that local adverse effects of inflammatory mediators released from the sites of

joint pathology, rather than immobilization, were responsible for the progressive bone loss.

Ralston *et al.* [55] studied the pathogenesis of spontaneous spinal insufficiency fractures in patients with ankylosing spondylitis. Of 111 patients with ankylosing spondylitis evaluated prospectively, fifteen developed radiographic evidence of vertebral compression fractures. Interestingly, bone mineral density of the appendicular skeleton as assessed by single photon absorptiometry was normal. These findings suggest that osteoporosis in these patients is primarily localized to the axial spine. These observations are supported by the findings of Devogelaer *et al.* [56] who used a variety of techniques, including standard radiographs, single and dual energy absorptiometry, and quantitative computer tomography.

D. Juvenile Rheumatoid Arthritis (JRA)

Numerous authors have noted the often dramatic adverse effects of JRA and related forms of inflammatory arthritis on linear growth and acquisition of skeletal mass in children [57, 58]. Hillman *et al.* [59] analyzed biochemical markers of bone remodeling and total body calcium in 44 children with active polyarticular or oligoarticular JRA. Their findings indicated a low bone formation rate with an overall reduction in bone turnover. There was no evidence for an increase in bone resorption rates. Hopp *et al.* [60] studied spinal bone density in 20 children with active JRA using dual photon absorptiometry to assess bone mass. They noted that bone density was reduced in postpubertal girls compared with healthy controls. These observations provide good evidence of the adverse effect of inflammation on skeletal accretion during puberty. Because of their normal rapid increase in skeletal mass, adolescents with active joint disease may be particularly vulnerable to the impact of the inflammatory process on their capacity to achieve expected peak bone mass. Surprisingly, when prepubertal girls with inflammatory joint disease were evaluated, they did not differ from controls at any of the sites measured. This could be related to effects of treatment on the activity of the disease in this group.

Reed and co-workers [61] evaluated radial BMD and serum osteocalcin levels in children with JRA. Over a 3 year period, the researchers noted that improvement in disease activity was associated with an increase of serum osteocalcin to normal levels. In contrast, in children with persistent joint inflammation, serum osteocalcin and BMD remained below normal. These findings provide further evidence of an adverse systemic effect of the underlying inflammatory joint disease on skeletal remodeling. The changes in serum osteocalcin levels are consistent with a suppression of bone formation, and the findings suggest that the effects of the suppression of bone formation in children, especially during the pubertal grow period, may have an adverse effect on the achievement of normal peak bone mass. That this decrease in bone mass predisposes children to an increased risk of fracture in adulthood is supported by several studies [62, 63].

Several proinflammatory cytokines and their receptors have been implicated in the disturbance of local as well as generalized bone remodeling in children with JRA. Serum levels of the soluble receptor for TNF-α, the soluble form of the IL-2 receptor, and IL-6 have been shown to correlate with markers of inflammation (ESR, CRP), indicating an association of these markers with disease activity. The highest levels of these mediators were observed in patients with active systemic disease or with polyarthritis [64]. Similar observations also have been made in adults with RA and related forms of inflammatory arthritis.

IV. EFFECTS OF JOINT INFLAMMATION ON CARTILAGE REMODELING

The subchondral bone is covered by articular cartilage that consists of chondrocytes embedded in a specialized extracellular matrix containing collagens and proteoglycans that are somewhat unique to this tissue. Within the tissue there are no blood vessels, nerves, or lymphatics, and nutrition for the chondrocytes is derived by diffusion both from the blood supply in the subchondral bone and from the synovial fluid. Under normal conditions, chondrocyte proliferation is limited and penetration of other cell types from the joint space or subchondral bone is restricted. The chondrocytes actively maintain a stable equilibrium between synthesis and degradation of matrix components [65]. During aging and in inflammatory and degenerative joint diseases, such as RA and osteoarthritis (OA), this stable equilibrium is disrupted and the rate of loss of collagens and proteoglycans from the matrix exceeds the rate of deposition of newly synthesized molecules [65]. This state of disequilibrium leads to the progressive loss of articular cartilage and disruption of normal joint function.

A. Cartilage Loss in Rheumatoid Arthritis

Cartilage destruction in RA occurs primarily in areas contiguous with the proliferating synovial pannus [66, 67] and to some extent at the cartilage surface exposed to synovial fluid [68, 69] due to the release and activation of proteinases from the synovial cells and polymorphonuclear leukocytes, respectively. In early RA, loss of proteoglycan occurs throughout the cartilage matrix and is not limited to the synovial-pannus junction, and selective damage to type II collagen fibrils can be observed in mid- and deep zones [69, 70]. Thus, proteolytic degradation products of matrix components have been considered both as diagnostic markers of cartilage damage and as potential autoantigens in the induction and mainte-

nance of RA and related inflammatory joint diseases such as ankylosing spondylitis [71–74].

B. Systemic Markers of Cartilage Metabolism in Rheumatoid Arthritis

Molecular markers in body fluids are useful for identifying local and systemic metabolic changes, monitoring the effects of cytokines and therapeutic agents on cartilage metabolism, and predicting the rate of joint destruction in joint disease. Cartilage contains a number of components that undergo change in RA [75]. Molecules originating from the articular cartilage, including aggrecan fragments, which contain chondroitin sulfate and keratan sulfate, type II collagen fragments, collagen pyridinoline cross-links, and cartilage oligomeric protein (COMP), usually are released as degradation products as a result of catabolic processes. Levels of cartilage proteoglycan components, including the keratan-sulfate rich domain and G1 and G2 globular domains of aggrecan and link protein, are higher in synovial fluids than in sera in patients with inflammatory joint diseases such as RA, psoriasis, ankylosing spondylitis, and JRA, and in patients after injury [76–84]. In these disorders, cellular immunity to these matrix components has also been detected [85, 86]. However, because the catabolic cytokines, IL-1 and TNF-α, not only stimulate degradation but also inhibit synthesis of aggrecan and type II collagen, the levels of cartilage matrix fragments in synovial fluid, serum, and urine may represent the net result of these two processes. To overcome potential problems in interpretation of such analyses, specific antibodies that detect either synthetic or cleavage epitopes have been developed in the 1990s to study biological markers of cartilage metabolism in body fluids.

1. TYPE II COLLAGEN

Antibodies that recognize different epitopes on type II collagen have been used to follow both synthesis and degradation of cartilage collagen. The carboxyterminal collagen II-propeptide (CPII) is released by the activity of C-propeptidase during extracellular fibril formation, and after a short half-life in cartilage ($\sim$12 h), it is released into the circulation. CPII concentrations in body fluids thus reflect the rate of synthesis of cartilage collagen. RA patients have abnormally elevated serum levels of CPII and synovial fluid levels are greater than those in serum [84]. In established RA, CPII levels are inversely related to keratan sulfate levels; keratan sulfate is a marker of degradation. The first evidence of increased degradation of type II collagen in RA articular cartilage *in situ* was provided by Dodge and Poole [69]. Specific antibodies that detect increased denaturation of the triple helix have been developed and used to detect type II collagen cleavage in OA articular cartilage [87, 88].

Collagen degradation also has been studied by monitoring the urinary excretion of pyridinoline cross-links. The hydroxylysyl pyridinoline, referred to as pyridinoline, is the most common cross-link of cartilage, but it is also present in bone, which also contains lysyl pyridinoline (deoxypyridinoline) cross-links. There are reports that the levels of pyridinoline, but not of the deoxypyridinoline cross-link, are elevated in RA urine and serum, and that they are greatest in severe or late RA than in inactive disease or OA [45, 47, 48, 89–91]. In one study examining cross-links in synovial fluid, high levels of pyridinoline were found in synovial fluid from RA patients, but deoxypyridinoline was not detected [50]. Although it is unclear whether the pyridinoline:deoxypyridinoline ratio can be used as a marker for which tissue is under attack [92], it is of potential use in identifying the severity of destruction of cartilage and/or adjacent bone and the response to therapy [93]. A report that tranexamic acid, an inhibitor of plasminogen activation, reduces collagen cross-link formation in RA indicates that collagen cross-link formation is a clinically relevant measure of joint tissue destruction [94].

2. AGGRECAN

Fragments of the large aggregating proteoglycan aggrecan and several of its epitopes now can be measured in synovial fluid and serum. The highest levels of the chondroitin sulfate region of the core protein are observed in the synovial fluid of patients with reactive arthritis [95]. Another aggrecan epitope, the hyaluronic acid binding region (HABr) or G1 domain, is released in small amounts in patients with this condition. In RA, an inverse relationship exists between these two epitopes, with dominance of aggrecan release in early and HABr in late destructive disease [96]. Chondroitin sulfate epitopes in the G3 domain of aggrecan, such as those recognized by monoclonal antibody 846 [97], are useful serum markers because they are released under pathologic conditions. Fragments of aggrecan bearing the 846 epitope reflect the degradation of newly synthesized aggrecan molecules and serum levels are frequently elevated in patients with chronic RA [83]. However, very low levels are found in RA patients with rapid erosive disease; in this condition the 846 epitope appears to represent increased aggrecan synthesis, thereby reflecting an attempt at repair and a possibly favorable prognosis [84]. An inverse correlation between the 846 epitope and indices of inflammation, CRP and ESR, suggests an indirect relationship between cartilage repair and inflammation [84]. Similarly, the monoclonal antibody 3B3 detects a neoepitope on chondroitin-6-sulfate chains in synovial fluid which correlates inversely with the extent of articular cartilage damage in RA, OA, and acute knee injury [98–100].

In RA, circulating levels of keratan sulfate generally are decreased, possibly reflecting changes in systemic aggrecan synthesis [81, 83]. Although serum keratan sulfate levels have been found to correlate with the severity of articular damage in RA measured radiographically [76, 101], synovial fluid levels have been found to correlate inversely and may reflect a decrease in cartilage mass in chronic RA [99]. Keratan sulfate, measured by monoclonal antibody 5D4 and ratios of chondroitin-6- to chondroitin-4-sulfate (due to higher levels of the latter [102], were found to be lower in synovial fluids from RA patients than in those from healthy subjects or OA patients [99, 103]. It was proposed that these components may be markers of susceptibility of articular cartilage to early damage in arthritis [99]. Although extensive degradation in RA cartilage can be demonstrated by direct analysis of proteoglycans using these and other specific antibodies [104], assay of a single marker in body fluids may not be sufficient to predict the severity of cartilage proteoglycan damage.

The involvement of metalloproteinases (MMPs) in the degradation of cartilage collagens and proteoglycans in RA is well established. The MMPs of the collagenase and stromelysin families have been given greatest attention because they specifically degrade native collagens and proteoglycans, respectively, and active stromelysin also serves as an activator of latent collagenases. Degradation products of type II collagen [105, 106], as well as aggrecan [77, 78], can be detected in the synovial fluid of RA patients. MMPs have been localized in regions of cartilage degradation [107] and have been shown to be elevated in synovial fluids [108–110] and sera [111, 112] of RA patients. The levels of TIMP-1 are also increased in RA synovial fluids and sera [109, 110, 112], possibly reflecting an endogenous corrective response to the increased levels of active MMPs. Synovial fluid levels of collagenase correlate with the degree of synovial inflammation, but not with CRP [113]. Serum stromelysin (MMP-3) levels correlate with CRP and ESR [111] and thus may reflect inflammatory episodes. However, it is unclear whether serum MMP levels also reflect tissue destruction within synovial joints. Most of the MMP activity in the synovial fluid originates from the synovium in RA, although there is evidence of intrinsic chondrolytic activity by chondrocytes at the cartilage-pannus junction as well as in deeper zones of cartilage matrix in a minority of RA specimens [114]. Serum levels of both MMP-1 and MMP-3 are decreased by therapy with the anti-TNF-α antibody cA2, and MMP-3 levels correlate with CRP levels in RA patients [115]. Although MMPs in synovial fluid or serum may not be specific markers for cartilage degradation per se, antibodies that recognize type II collagen cleavage epitopes are currently under development.

Attention has been focused on the enzymes responsible for aggrecan degradation [116]. Patients with early stage RA who exhibit high concentrations of aggrecan fragments in synovial fluid progress more rapidly towards joint destruction than patients with low concentrations of aggrecan [71]. At least seven specific cleavage sites have been defined in the protein core of aggrecan. Highly specific antipeptide antibodies that recognize catabolic sites within the interglobular G1 domain of aggrecan have been developed as sensitive markers for following disease course and activity and response to therapy. Efforts have been focused on developing antibodies that recognize the aggrecan G1 fragments resulting from cleavage between amino acid residues Asn341 and Phe342, the MMP cleavage site [117, 118], and between Glu373, and Ala 374, the "aggrecanase" cleavage site [119, 120]. Both MMP-8 [121] and membrane type I-MMP (MT1-MMP) [122] have been reported to cleave aggrecan at both cleavage sites. Antibodies that detect N- or C-terminal epitopes on either MMP- or aggrecanase-generated G1 fragments have been used to show elevated levels of fragments resulting from both activities in RA cartilage [123] and in synovial fluids [124]. These studies confirm earlier work showing elevated levels of aggrecanase-generated fragmentsin RA synovial fluids [125]. The combined evidence indicates that both MMPs and aggrecanase activities may be important in aggrecan degradation, because fragments generated by both types of activities are found in RA synovial fluids, and that fragments produced by one type of activity are resistant to further cleavage by the other activity [124].

The presence in the RA joint of other proteinases that can degrade cartilage proteoglycans adds further complexity to the clinical picture. Serine proteinase activities due to urokinase-type plasminogen activator and elastase, which also interact with the MMP proteolytic cascade, have been found to be elevated in RA synovial fluids [126, 127]. The cysteine proteinases, cathepsins L and D, are expressed at high levels in rheumatoid synovium [128].

3. OTHER CARTILAGE MATRIX PROTEINS

Several novel cartilage matrix proteins are not unique to cartilage but have been investigated as markers of tissue damage in RA. Cartilage oligomeric matrix protein (COMP) is a pentameric extracellular matrix protein with subunit size of 100–110 kDa. It is primarily localized in the chondrocyte territorial matrix but is also found in synovium, tendon, and ligament. Like aggrecan, COMP is released into the synovial fluid in reactive arthritis and RA but it is more concentrated in the serum, thus giving a synovial fluid:serum ratio of 10. High serum levels in early RA may reflect an aggressive destructive form of the disease [84, 129]. Studies in vitro showed that TGF-β1 increased COMP mRNA synthesis, and IL-1β counteracted this increase [130]. The human cartilage glycoprotein-39 (HC-gp39) [131], also termed YKL-40 [132], is a major secretory product of articular chondrocytes as well as synovial cells. Similar to COMP, the synovial fluid:serum ratio of HC-gp39 is 15, and elevated levels are observed in inflammatory joint disease. Because synovial cells can contribute to the pools of COMP and HC-gp39 released into the circulation, the increased levels of these markers in synovial fluid and serum are likely markers of inflammatory synovitis, as well as of cartilage destruction.

C. Local Markers of Cartilage Metabolism in Rheumatoid Arthritis

Our understanding of basic cellular mechanisms regulating chondrocyte responses to inflammatory mediators has been inferred from numerous studies in vitro using cultures of cartilage fragments or isolated chondrocytes. Much of this information is also relevant to OA and is supported by studies in animal models [133, 134]. Less information has been derived from direct analysis of cartilage or chondrocytes obtained from RA patients in which cartilage damage is extensive.

1. CYTOKINES AND CYTOKINE-INDUCED MARKERS

The prominent role of proinflammatory cytokines in destruction of cartilage matrix in RA is well supported by current evidence. Of the cytokines released in RA synovial joint, IL-1 and TNF-α are considered to be of major importance in inflammatory tissue destruction. They induce the synthesis of MMPs and other proteinases, prostaglandin E_2 (PGE$_2$) due to increased cyclooxygenase (COX)-2 activity, nitric oxide, and other proinflammatory cytokines such as IL-6, leukemia inhibitory factor (LIF), and IL-8 [135–141]. IL-17, a T-lymphocyte product, also stimulates production of proinflammatory cytokines and has effects on chondrocytes that are similar to the effects of IL-1 [142, 143]. These local markers can be measured in synovial fluids and are regarded as potential targets for therapeutic agents such as proteinase inhibitors, cytokine antagonists, cytokine receptor blocking antibodies, and nonsteroidal inflammatory drugs, including selective cyclooxygenase (COX) inhibitors [144–147]. Thus many new therapeutic agents, which are considered immunomodulators and affect synovial cell function, may also affect chondrocyte function. Chondrocytes are capable of expressing several inflammatory markers, including inducible nitric oxide synthetase (iNOS), cyclooxygenase-2 (COX-2), soluble phospholipase A2 (sPLA2), and collagenase-3 (MMP-13), when stimulated by IL-1 alone or in combination with TNF-α [148–153]. In chondrocyte cultures, the responses to IL-1 appear to depend on the differentiated phenotype, but they may also be observed in synovial cell cultures. Thus, their use as cartilage-specific diagnostic tools or therapeutic indicators would require analysis in situ using cartilage biopsies.

Other cytokine-induced cellular markers are the early response genes and other nuclear factors, which function as transcription factors, including NF-κB, Egr-1, and AP-1. Nuclear factors have been localized in the rheumatoid synovial membrane [154–157] and are likely important in IL-1-regulated processes in cartilage, such as induction of MMP expression and downregulation of cartilage–specific matrix genes [158, 159]. Transcription factors that might serve as more specific markers of chondrocyte phenotype include scleraxis, SOX9 and HoxC-8, which are important regulators of chondrogenesis during development [160–164]; however, they have not been studied in the context of the rheumatoid joint.

2. ADHESION MOLECULES

Adhesion molecules play a prominent role in inflammatory diseases. These molecules are involved in the recruitment of leukocytes from the circulation and their interaction with other cell types, including macrophages, dendritic cells, and fibroblasts, within the inflamed tissue [165]. Principal families of adhesion molecules involved are the selectins, the integrins, the immunoglobulin supergene family, and variants of the CD44 family. Although many of these molecules are common to different inflammatory sites, as is their expression on circulating cells in different rheumatic conditions, tissue-specific differences in expression of certain molecules have been found. Many of the prominent adhesion proteins expressed in the inflamed rheumatoid synovium are also expressed in cartilage. For example, VCAM-1 and ICAM-1, members of the immunoglobulin family, are expressed by human articular chondrocytes and their expression is upregulated by cytokines. Specific roles for CD44 [166] and anchorin CII (annexin V) [167] in cell-matrix interactions in cartilage also have been determined. Several members of the integrin family are expressed by chondrocytes. For example, the $\alpha 1 \beta 1$ integrin functions as a receptor for types II and VI collagen, and the $\alpha 5 \beta 1$ integrin serves as a chondrocyte fibronectin receptor [168]. However, these integrins and the other adhesion molecules described above are not unique to chondrocytes, and therefore, their use as specific markers of cartilage metabolism is limited. Whether the cloned $\alpha 10$ integrin subunit [169], which is expressed in cartilage and mediates binding to type II collagen, will provide a more specific and clinically useful cartilage marker awaits further study.

References

1. Fassbender, H. G. (1983). Histomorphological basis of articular cartilage destruction in rheumatoid arthritis. *Collagen Relat. Dis.* **3**, 141–155.
2. Krane, S. M., Conca, W., Stephenson, M. L., Amento, E. P., and Goldring, M. B. (1990). Mechanisms of matrix degradation in rheumatoid arthritis. *Ann. N.Y. Acad. Sci.* **580**, 340–354.
3. Harris, E. D. J. (1990). Rheumatoid arthritis. Pathophysiology and implications for therapy. *N. Engl. J. Med.* **322**, 1277–1289.
4. Deodhar, A. A., and Woolf, A. D. (1996). Bone mass measurement and bone metabolism in rheumatoid arthritis: A review. *Br. J. Rheumatol.* **35**, 309–322.
5. Goldring, S. R. (1996). Osteoporosis and rheumatic diseases. *In* "Primer on the Metabolic Bone Diseases and Disorders and Mineral Metabolism" (M. J. Favus, ed.), 3rd ed., pp. 299–301. Lippincott-Raven, Philadelphia.
6. Goldring, S. R., and Polisson, R. P. (1998). Bone disease in rheumatological disorders. *In* "Metabolic Bone Disease" (L. Avioli and S. M. Krane, eds.), 2nd ed., pp., 621–635. Academic Press, San Diego, CA.
7. Bromley, M., and Woolley, D. E. (1984). Chondroclasts and osteoclasts at subchondral sites of erosions in the rheumatoid joint *Arthritis Rheum.* **27**, 968–975.
8. Bromley, M., and Woolley, D. E. (1984). Histopathology of the rheumatoid lesion. Identification of cell types at sites of cartilage erosion. *Arthritis Rheum.* **27**, 857–863.
9. Allard, S. A., Muirden, K. D., and Maini, R. N. (1991). Correlation of histopathological features of pannus with patterns of damage in different joints in rheumatoid arthritis. *Ann. Rheum. Dis.* **50**, 278–283.
10. Ashton, B. A., Ashton, I. K., Marshall, M. J., and Butler, R. C. (1993). Localization of vitronectin receptor immunoreactivity and tartrate resistant acid phosphatase activity in synovium from patients with inflammatory with degenrative arthritis. *Ann. Rheum. Dis.* **52**, 133–137.
11. Chang, J. S., Quinn, J. M., Demaziere, A., Bulstrode, C. J., Francis, M. J., Duthie, R. B., and Athanasou, N. A. (1992). Bone resorption by cells isolated from rheumatoid synovium. *Ann. Rheum. Dis.* **51**, 1223–1229.
12. Chambers, T. J., Thomson, B. M., and Fuller, K. (1984). Resorption of bone by isolated rabbit osteoclasts. *J. Cell Sci.* **66**, 383–399.
13. Fujikawa, Y., Sabokbar, A., Neale, S., and Athanasou, N. A. (1993). Human osteoclast formation and bone resorption by monocytes and synovial macrophages in rheumatoid arthritis. *Ann. Rheum. Dis.* **55**, 816–822.
14. Gravallese, E. M., Harada, Y., Wang, J.-T., Gorn, A., Thornhill, T., and Goldring, S. R. (1998). Identification of cell types responsible for bone resorption in rheumatoid arthritis and juvenile rheumatoid arthritis. *Am. J. Pathol.* **152**, 943–951.
15. Gorn, A. H., Lin, H. Y., Yamin, M., Auron, P. E., Flannery, M. R., Tapp, D. R., Manning, C. A., Lodish, H. F., Krane, S. M., and Goldring, S. R. (1992). The cloning, characterization and expression of a human calcitonin receptor from an ovarian carcinoma cell line. *J. Clin. Invest.* **90**, 1726–1735.
16. Gorn, A. H., Rudolph, S. M., Flannery, M. R., Morton, C., Weremowicz, S., Wang, J.-T., Krane, S. M., and Goldring, S. R. (1995). Expression of two human skeletal calcitonin receptor isoforms cloned from a giant cell tumor of bone. *J. Clin. Invest.* **95**, 2680–2691.
17. Rodan, G. A., and Martin, T. J. (1981). Role of osteoblasts in hormonal control of bone resorption—a hypothesis. *Calcif. Tissue Int.* **33**, 349–351.
18. Raisz, L. G. (1988). Local and systemic factors in the pathogenesis of osteoporosis. *N. Engl. J. Med.* **318**, 818–828.
19. Suda, T., Takahashi, N., and Martin, T. J. (1992). Modulation of osteoclast differentiation. *Endocr. Rev.* **13**, 66–80.
20. Shimizo, S., Shiozawa, S., Shiozawa, K., Imura, S., and Fugita, T. (1985). Quantitative histological studies on the pathogenesis of periarticular osteoporosis in rheumatoid arthritis. *Arthritis Rheum.* **28**, 25–31.
21. Deleuran, B. W., Chu, C. Q., Field, M., Brennan, F. M., Katsikis, P., Feldmann, M., and Maini, R. N. (1992). Localization of interleukin-1a, type 1 interleukin-1 receptor and interleukin-1 receptor antagonis in the synovial membrane and cartilage/pannus junction in rhumatoid arthritis. *Br. J. Rheumatol.* **31**, 801–809.
22. Firestein, G. S., Alcaro-Garcia, J. M., and Maki, R. (1990). Quantitative analysis of cytokine gene expression in rheumatoid arthritis. *J. Immunol.* **144**, 3347–3353.
23. Chu, C. Q., Field, M., Feldmann, M., and Maini, R. N. (1991). Localization of tumour necrosis factor-a in synovial tissue and at the cartilage-pannus junction in patients with rheumatoid arthritis. *Arthritis Rheum.* **34**, 1125–1132.
24. Chu, C. Q., Feldmann, M., Allard, S., Abney, E., and Maini, R. N. (1992). Detection of cytokines at the cartilage/pannus junction in patients with rheumatoid arthritis: implications for the role of cytokines in cartilage destruction and repair. *Br. J. Rheumatol.* **32**, 653–661.
25. Mazess, R. B., and Whedon, G. D. (1983). Immobilization and bone. *Calcif. Tissue Int.* **32**, 265–267.

26. Joffe, I., and Epstein, S. (1991). Osteoporosis associated with rheumatoid arthritis: Pathogenesis and management. *Semin. Arthritis Rheum.* **20**, 256–272.

27. Spector, T. D., Hall, G. M., McCloskey, E. V., and Kanis, J. A. (1993). Risk of vertebral fracture in women with rheumatoid arthritis. *Br. Med. J.* **306**, 558.

28. Gough, A. K., Lilley, J., Eyre, S., Holdin, R., and Emery, P. (1994). Generalized bone loss in patients with rheumatoid arthritis. *Lancet* **344**, 23–27.

29. Hooyman, J. R., Melton, L. J., Nelson, A. M., O'Fallon, W. M., and Riggs, B. L. (1984). Fractures after rheumatoid arthritis. A population-based study. *Arthritis Rheum.* **27**, 1353–1361.

30. Beat, A. M., Bloch, D. A., and Fries, J. F. (1991). Predictors of fractures in early rheumatoid arthritis. *J. Rheumatol.* **18**, 804–808.

31. Lane, N. E., and Goldring, S. R. (1998). Bone loss in rheumatoid arthritis: What role does inflammation play. *J. Rheumatol.* **7**, 1251–1253.

32. Sambrook, P. N., Ansell, B. M., Foster, S., Gumpel, J. M., Hesp, R., and Reeve, J. (1985). Bone turnover in early rheumatoid arthritis. 2. Longitudinal bone density studies. *Ann. Rheum. Dis.* **44**, 580–584.

33. Sambrook, P. N., Eisman, J. A., Yeates, M. G., Pocock, N. A., Eberl, S., and Champion, G. D. (1986). Osteoporosis in rheumatoid arthritis: Safety of low-dose corticosteroids. *Ann. Rheum. Dis.* **45**, 950–953.

34. Sambrook, P. N., Eisman, A., Champion, G., Yeates, M. G., Pocock, N. A., and Eberl, S. (1987). Determinants of axial bone loss in rheumatoid arthritis. *Arthritis Rheum.* **30**, 721–728.

35. Sambrook, P., Birmingham, J., Kelly, P., Kempler, S., Freund, J., and Eisman, J. (1992). Postmenopausal bone loss in rheumatoid arthritis: Effects of estrogens and androgens. *J. Rheum.* **19**, 357–361.

36. Peel, N. F., Eastell, R., and Russell, R. G. G. (1991). Osteoporosis in rheumatoid arthritis—the laboratory perspective. *Br. J. Rheum.* **30**, 84–85.

37. Woolf, A. D. (1991). Osteoporosis in rheumatoid arthritis—the clinical viewpoint. *Br. J. Rheum.* **30**, 82–84.

38. Compston, J. E., Vedi, S., Croucher, P. I., Garrahan, N. J., and O'Sullivan, M. M. (1994). Bone turnover in non-steroid treated rheumatoid arthritis. *Ann. Rheum. Dis.* **53**, 163–166.

39. Sambrook, P. N., Spector, T. D., Seeman, E., Bellamy, N., Buchanan, R. R. C., Duffy, D. L., Martin, N. G., Prince, R., Owen, E., Silman, A. J., and Eisman, J. A. (1995). Osteoporosis in rheumatoid arthritis: A monozygotic co-twin control study. *Arthritis Rheum.* **38**, 806–809.

40. Laan, R. F., van Riel, P. L., and van de Putte, L. B. (1992). Bone mass in patients with rheumatoid arthritis. *Ann. Rheum. Dis.* **51**, 826–832.

41. Als, O. S., Gotfredsen, A., Riis, B. J., and Christisnsen, C. (1985). Are disease duration and degree of functional impairment determinants of bone loss in rheumatoid arthritis? *Ann. Rheum. Dis.* **44**, 406–411.

42. Kroger, H., Arnala, I., and Alhava, E. M. (1991). Bone remodeling in osteoporosis associated with rheumatoid arthritis. *Calcif. Tissue Int.* **49**, S90.

43. Mellish, R. W. E., O'Sullivan, M. M., Garrahan, N. J., and Compston, J. E. (1987). Iliac crest trabecular bone mass and structure in patients with non-steroid treated rheumatoid arthritis. *Ann. Rheum. Dis.* **46**, 830–836.

44. Hall, G. M., Spector, T. D., and Delmas, P. D. (1995). Markers of bone metabolism in postmenopausal women with rheumatoid arthritis. Effects of corticosteroids and hormone replacement therapy. *Arthritis Rheum.* **38**, 902–906.

45. Gough, A. K., Peel, N. F., Eastell, R., Holder, R. L., Lilley, J., and Emery, P. (1994). Excretion of pyridinium crosslinks correlates with disease activity and appendicular bone loss in early rheumatoid arthritis. *Ann. Rheum. Dis.* **53**, 14–17.

46. Gough, A., Sambrook, P., Devlin, J., Huissoon, A., Njeh, C., Robbins, S., Nguyen, T., and Emery, P. (1998). Osteoclastic activation is the principal mechanism leading to secondary osteoporosis in rheumatoid arthritis. *J. Rheumatol.* **7**, 1282–1289.

47. Black, D., Marabani, M., Sturrock, R. D., and Robins, S. P. (1989). Urinary excretion of the hydroxypyridinium cross links of collagen in patients with rheumatoid arthritis. *Ann. Rheum. Dis.* **48**, 641–644.

48. Robins, S. P., Stewart, P., Astbury, C., and Bird, H. A. (1986). Measurement of the cross linking compound, pyridinoline, in urine as an index of collagen degradation in joint disease. *Ann. Rheum. Dis.* **45**, 969–973.

49. Siebel, M. J., Duncan, A., and Robins, S. P. (1989). Urinary hydroxypyridinium crosslinks provide indices of cartilage and bone involvement in arthritis disease. *J. Rheumatol.* **16**, 964–970.

50. Sinigaglia, L., Varenna, M., Binelli, L., Bartucci, F., Arrigoni, M., Ferrara, R., and Abbiati, G. (1995). Urinary and synovial pyridinium crosslink concentrations in patients with rheumatoid arthritis and osteoarthritis. *Ann. Rheum. Dis.* **54**, 144–147.

51. Saag, K. G., Emkey, R., Schnitzer, T. J., Brown, J. P., Hawkins, F., Goemaere, S., Thamsborg, G., Liberman, U. A., Delmas, P. D., Malice, M.-P., Czachur, M., and Daifotis, A. G. (1998). Alendronate for the prevention and treatment of glucocorticoid-induced osteoporosis. *N. Engl. J. Med.* **339**, 292–299.

52. Braun, J., Bollow, M., Neure, L., Seipelt, E., Seyrekbasan, F., Herbst, H., Eggens, U., Distler, A., and Sieper, J. (1995). Use of immunohistologic and in situ hybridization techniques in the examination of sacroiliac joint biopsy specimens from patients with ankylosing spondylitis. *Arthritis Rheum.* **4**, 499–505.

53. Spencer, D. G., Park, W. M., Dick, H. M., Papazoglou, S. N., and Buchanan, W. W. (1979). Radiological manifestations in 200 patients with ankylosing spondylitis: correlation with clinical features and HLA-B27. *J. Rheumatol.* **6**, 305–315.

54. Will, R., Bhalla, A., Palmer, R., Ring, F., and Calin, A. (1989). Osteoporosis in early ankylosing spondylitis: a primary pathological event? *Lancet* **23**, 1483–1485.

55. Ralston, S. H., Urquhart, G. D., Brzeski, M., and Sturrock, R. D. (1990). Prevalence of vertebral compression fractures due to osteoporosis in ankylosing spondylitis. *Br. Med. J.* **300**, 563–565.

56. Devogelaer, J.-P., Maldague, B., Malghem, J., and de Deuxchaisnes, C. N. (1992). Appendicular and vertebral bone mass in ankylosing spondylitis. A comparison of plain radiographs with single- and dual-photon absorptiometry and with quantitative computed tomography. *Arthritis Rheum.* **35**, 1062–1067.

57. Ansell, B. M., and Bywaters, E. G. L. (1956). Growth in Still's disease. *Ann. Rheum. Dis.* **15**, 295–318.

58. Bernstein, B. H., Stobie, D., Singsen, B. H., Koster-King, K., Kornreich, H. K., and Hanson, V. (1977). Growth retardation in juvenile rheumatoid arthritis (JRA). *Arthritis Rheum.* **20**, 212–216.

59. Hillman, L., Cassidy, J. T., Johnson, L., Lee, D., and Allen, S. (1994). Vitamin D metabolism and bone mineralization in children with juvenile rheumatoid arthritis *J. Pediatr.* **124**, 910–916.

60. Hopp, R., Degan, J. A., Gallagher, J. C., and Cassidy, J. T. (1991). Estimation of bone mineral density in children with juvenile rheumatoid arthritis. *J. Rheumatol.* **18**, 1235–1239.

61. Reed, A., Haugen, M., Pachman, L., and Langman, C. (1993). Repair of osteopenia in children with juvenile rheumatoid arthritis. *J. Pediatr.* **122**, 693–696.

62. Badley, B. W. D., and Ansell, B. M. (1960). Fractures in Still's disease. *Ann. Rheum. Dis.* **19**, 135–138.

63. Varonos, S., Ansell, B. M., and Reeve, J. (1987). Vertebral collapse in juvenile chronic arthritis: its relationship with glucocorticoid therapy. *Calcif. Tissue Int.* **41**, 75–78.

64. Reeve, J., Loftus, J., Hesp, R., Ansell, B. M., Wright, D. J., and Woo, P. M. (1993). Biochemical prediction of changes in spinal bone mass in juvenile chronic (or rheumatoid) arthritis treated with glucocorticoids. *J. Rheum.* **20**, 1189–1195.

65. Poole, A. R. (1993). Cartilage in health and disease. *In* "Arthritis and Allied Conditions: A Textbook of Rheumatology" (D. J. McCarty and W. P. Koopman, eds.), pp. 279–333. Lea & Febiger, Philadelphia.

66. Kobayashi, I., and Ziff, M. (1975). Electron microscopic studies of the cartilage-pannus junction in rheumatoid arthritis. *Arthritis Rheum.* **18**, 475–483.

67. Woolley, D. E., Crossley, M. J., and Evanson, J. M. (1977). Collagenase at sites of cartilage erosion in the rheumatoid joint. *Arthritis Rheum.* **20**, 1231–1239.

68. Kimura, H., Tateishi, H. J., and Ziff, M. (1977). Surface ultrastructure of rheumatoid articular cartilage. *Arthritis Rheum.* **20**, 1085–1098.

69. Dodge, G. R., and Poole, A. R. (1989). Immunohistochemical detection and immunochemical analysis of type II collagen degradation in human normal, rheumatoid, and osteoarthritic articular cartilages and in explants of bovine articular cartilage cultured with interleukin 1. *J. Clin. Invest.* **83**, 647–661.

70. Mitchell, N. S., and Shepard, N. (1978). Changes in proteoglycan and collagen in cartilage in rheumatoid arthritis. *J. Bone J. Surg., Am. Vol.,* **60A**, 349–354.

71. Saxne, T., and Heinegard, D. (1995). Matrix proteins: Potentials as body fluid markers of changes in the metabolism of cartilage and bone in arthritis. *J. Rheumatol.* **43**, (Suppl.), 71–74.

72. Leroux, J. Y., Guerassimov, A., Cartman, A., Delaunay, N., Webber, C., Rosenberg, L. C., Banerjee, S., and Poole, A. R. (1996). Immunity to the G1 globular domain of the cartilage proteoglycan aggrecan can induce inflammatory erosive polyarthritis and spondylitis in BALB/c mice but immunity to G1 is inhibited by covalently bound keratan sulfate in vitro and in vivo. *J. Clin. Invest.* **97**, 621–632.

73. Kingsley, G., and Panayi, G. S. (1997). Joint destruction in rheumatoid arthritis: Biological bases. *Clin. Exp. Rheumatol.* **15**, S3–S14.

74. Cremer, M. A., Rosloniec, E. F., and Kang, A. H. (1998). The cartilage collagens: A review of their structure, organization, and role in the pathogenesis of experimental arthritis in animals and in human rheumatic disease. *J. Mol. Med.* **76**, 275–288.

75. Poole, A. R., and Dieppe, P. (1994). Biological markers in rheumatoid arthritis. *Semin. Arthritis Rheum.* **23**, 17–31.

76. Thonar, E. J., Lenz, M. E., Klintworth, G. K., Caterson, B., Pachman, L. M., Glickman, P., Katz, R., Huff, J., and Kuettner, K. E. (1985). Quantification of keratan sulfate in blood as a marker of cartilage catabolism. *Arthritis Rheum.* **28**, 1367–1376.

77. Saxne, T., Heinegard, D., and Wollheim, F. A. (1987). Cartilage proteoglycans in synovial fluid and serum in patients with inflammatory joint disease. Relation to systemic treatment. *Arthritis Rheum.* **30**, 972–979.

78. Witter, J., Roughley, P. J., Webber, C., Roberts, N., Keystone, E., and Poole, A. R. (1987). The immunologic detection and characterization of cartilage proteoglycan degradation products in synovial fluids of patients with arthritis. *Arthritis Rheum.* **30**, 519–529.

79. Ratcliffe, A., Doherty, M., Maini, R. N., and Hardingham, T. E. (1988). Increased concentrations of proteoglycan components in the synovial fluids of patients with acute but not chronic joint disease. *Ann. Rheum. Dis.* **47**, 826–832.

80. Lohmander, L. S., Dahlberg, L., Ryd, L., and Heinegard, D. (1989). Increased levels of proteoglycan fragments in knee joint fluid after injury. *Arthritis. Rheum.* **32**, 1434–1442.

81. Poole, A. R., Witter, J., Roberts, N., Piccolo, F., Brandt, R., Paquin, J., and Baron, M. (1990). Inflammation and cartilage metabolism in rheumatoid arthritis. Studies of the blood markers hyaluronic acid, orosomucoid, and keratan sulfate. *Arthritis Rheum.* **33**, 790–799.

82. Silverman, B., Cawston, T. E., Page-Thomas, D. P., Dingle, J. T., and Hazleman, B. L. (1990). The sulphated glycosaminoglycan levels in synovial fluid aspirates in patients with acute and chronic joint disease. *Br. J. Rheumatol.* **29**, 340–344.

83. Poole, A. R., Ionescu, M., Swan, A., and Dieppe, P. A. (1994). Changes in cartilage metabolism in arthritis are reflected by altered serum and synovial fluid levels of the cartilage proteoglycan aggrecan. Implications for pathogenesis. *J. Clin. Invest.* **94**, 25–33.

84. Mansson, B., Carey, D., Alini, M., Ionescu, M., Rosenberg, L. C., Poole, A. R., Heinegard, D., and Saxne, T. (1995). Cartilage and bone metabolism in rheumatoid arthritis. Differences between rapid and slow progression of disease identified by serum markers of cartilage metabolism *J. Clin. Invest.* **95**, 1071–1077.

85. Guerassimov, A., Duffy, C., Zhang, Y., Banerjee, S., Leroux, J. Y., Reimann, A., Webber, C., Delaunay, N., Vipparti, V., Ronbeck, L., Cartman, A., Arsenault, L., Rosenberg, L. C., and Poole, A. R. (1997). Immunity to cartilage link protein in patients with juvenile rheumatoid arthritis. *J. Rheumatol.* **24**, 959–964.

86. Guerassimov, A., Zhang, Y., Banerjee, S., Cartman, A., Leroux, J. Y., Rosenberg, L. C., Esdaile, J., Fitzcharles, M. A., and Poole, A. R. (1998). Cellular immunity to the G1 domain of cartilage proteoglycan aggrecan is enhanced in patients with rheumatoid arthritis but only after removal of keratan sulfate. *Arthritis Rheum.* **41**, 1019–1025.

87. Billinghurst, R. C., Dahlberg, L., Ionescu, M., Reiner, A., Bourne, R., Rorabeck, C., Mitchell, P., Hambor, J., Diekmann, O., Tschesche, H., Chen, J., Van Wart, H., and Poole, A. R. (1997). Enhanced cleavage of type II collagen by collagenases in osteoarthritic articular cartilage. *J. Clin. Invest.* **99**, 1534–1545.

88. Hollander, A. P., Heathfield, T. F., Webber, C., Iwata, Y., Bourne, R., Rorabeck, C., and Poole, A. R. (1994). Increased damage to type II collagen in osteoarthritic articular cartilage detected by a new immunoassay. *J. Clin. Invest.* **93**, 1722–1732.

89. Seibel, M. J., Duncan, A., and Robins, S. P. (1989). Urinary hydroxypyridinium crosslinks provide indices of cartilage and bone involvement in arthritic diseases. *J. Rheumatol.* **16**, 964–970.

90. Astbury, C., Bird, H. A., McLaren, A. M., and Robins, S. P. (1994). Urinary excretion of pyridium crosslinks of collagen correlated with joint damage in arthritis. *Br. J. Rheumatol.* **33**, 11–15.

91. Hein, G., Franke, S., Muller, A., Braunig, E., Eidner, T., and Stein, G. (1997). The determination of pyridinium crosslinks in urine and serum as a possible marker of cartilage degradation in rheumatoid arthritis. *Clin. Rheumatol.* **16**, 167–172.

92. Takahashi, M., Kushida, K., Hoshino, H., Suzuki, M., Sano, M., Miyamoto, S., and Inoue, T. (1996). Concentrations of pyridinoline and deoxypyridinoline in joint tissues from patients with osteoarthritis or rheumatoid arthritis. *Ann. Rheum. Dis.* **55**, 324–327.

93. Greenwald, R. A. (1996). Monitoring collagen degradation in patients with arthritis. The search for suitable surrogates. *Arthritis Rheum.* **39**, 1455–1465.

94. Ronday, H. K., Te Koppele, J. M., Greenwald, R. A., Moak, S. A., De Roos, J. A., Dijkmans, B. A., Breedveld, F. C., and Verheijen, J. H. (1998). Tranexamic acid, an inhibitor of plasminogen activation, reduces urinary collagen cross-link excretion in both experimental and rheumatoid arthritis. *Br. J. Rheumatol.* **37**, 34–38.

95. Saxne, T., Glennas, A., Kvien, T. K., Melby, K., and Heinegard, D. (1993). Release of cartilage macromolecules into the synovial fluid in patients with acute and prolonged phases of reactive arthritis. *Arthritis Rheum.* **36**, 20–25.

96. Saxne, T., and Heinegard, D. (1992). Synovial fluid analysis of two groups of proteoglycan epitopes distinguishes early and late cartilage lesions. *Arthritis Rheum.* **35**, 385–390.

97. Rizkalla, G., Reiner, A., Bogoch, E., and Poole, A. R. (1992). Studies of the articular cartilage proteoglycan aggrecan in health and osteoarthritis. Evidence for molecular heterogeneity and extensive molecular changes in disease. *J. Clin. Invest.* **90**, 2268–2277.

98. Slater, R. R., Jr., Bayliss, M. T., Lachiewicz, P. F., Visco, D. M., and Caterson, B. (1995). Monoclonal antibodies that detect biochemical markers of arthritis in humans. *Arthritis Rheum.* **38**, 655–659.

99. Sharif, M., Osborne, D. J., Meadows, K., Woodhouse, S. M., Colvin, E. M., Shepstone, L., and Dieppe, P. A. (1996). The relevance of chondroitin and keratan sulphate markers in normal and arthritic synovial fluid. *Br. J. Rheumatol.* **35**, 951–957.

100. Bello, A. E., Garrett, W. E., Jr., Wang, H., Lohnes, J., DeLong, E., Caterson, B., and Kraus, V. B. (1997). Comparison of synovial

fluid cartilage marker concentrations and chondral damage assessed arthroscopically in acute knee injury. *Osteoarthritis Cartilage* **5**, 419–426.

101. Haraoui, B., Thonar, E. J., Martel-Pelletier, J., Goulet, J. R., Raynauld, J. P., Ouellet, M., and Pelletier, J. P. (1994). Serum keratan sulfate levels in rheumatoid arthritis: Inverse correlation with radiographic staging. *J. Rheumatol.* **21**, 813–817.

102. Shinmei, M., Miyauchi, S., Machida, A., and Miyazaki, K. (1992). Quantitation of chondroitin-4-sulfate and chondroitin-6-sulfate in pathological joint fluid. *Arthritis Rheum.* **35**, 1304–1308.

103. Belcher, C., Yaqub, R., Fawthrop, F., Bayliss, M., and Doherty, M. (1997). Synovial fluid chondroitin and keratan sulphate epitopes, glycosaminoglycans, and hyaluronan in arthritic and normal knees. *Ann. Rheum. Dis.* **56**, 299–307.

104. Cs-Szabo, G., Roughley, P. J., Plaas, A. H., and Glant, T. T. (1995). Large and small proteoglycans of osteoarthritic and rheumatoid articular cartilage. *Arthritis Rheum.* **38**, 660–668.

105. Cheung, H. S., Ryan, L. M., Kozin, F., and McCarty, D. J. (1980). Identification of collagen subtypes in synovial fluid sediments from arthritic patients. *Am. J. Med.* **68**, 73–79.

106. Moreland, L. W., Stewart, T., Gay, R. E., Huang, G. Q., McGee, N., and Gay, S. (1989). Immunohistologic demonstration of type II collagen in synovial fluid phagocytes of osteoarthritis and rheumatoid arthritis patients. *Arthritis Rheum.* **32**, 1458–1464.

107. Hembry, R. M., Bagga, M. R., Reynolds, J. J., and Hamblen, D. L. (1995). Immunolocalisation studies on six matrix metalloproteinases and their inhibitors, TIMP-1 and TIMP-2, in synovia from patients with osteo- and rheumatoid arthritis. *Ann. Rheum. Dis.* **54**, 25–32.

108. Walakovits, L. A., Moore, V. L., Bhardwaj, N., Gallick, G. S., and Lark, M. W. (1992). Detection of stromelysin and collagenase in synovial fluid from patients with rheumatoid arthritis and posttraumatic knee injury. *Arthritis Rheum.* **35**, 35–42.

109. Clark, I. M., Powell, L. K., Ramsey, S., Hazleman, B. L., and Cawston, T. E. (1993). The measurement of collagenase, tissue inhibitor of metalloproteinases (TIMP), and collagenase-TIMP complex in synovial fluids from patients with osteoarthritis and rheumatoid arthritis. *Arthritis Rheum.* **36**, 372–379.

110. Ahrens, D., Koch, A. E., Pope, R. M., Stein-Picarella, M., and Niedbala, M. J. (1996). Expression of matrix metalloproteinase 9 (96-kd gelatinase B) in human rheumatoid arthritis. *Arthritis Rheum.* **39**, 1576–1587.

111. Manicourt, D. H., Fujimoto, N., Obata, K., and Thonar, E. J. (1995). Levels of circulating collagenase, stromelysin-1, and tissue inhibitor of matrix metalloproteinases 1 in patients with rheumatoid arthritis. Relationship to serum levels of antigenic keratan sulfate and systemic parameters of inflammation. *Arthritis Rheum.* **38**, 1031–1039.

112. Yoshihara, Y., Obata, K., Fujimoto, N., Yamashita, K., Hayakawa, T., and Shinmei, M. (1995). Increased levels of stromelysin-1 and tissue inhibitor of metalloproteinases-1 in sera from patients with rheumatoid arthritis. *Arthritis Rheum.* **38**, 969–975.

113. Maeda, S., Sawai, T., Uzuki, M., Takahashi, Y., Omoto, H., Seki, M., and Sakurai, M. (1995). Determination of interstitial collagenase (MMP-1) in patients with rheumatoid arthritis. *Ann. Rheum. Dis.* **54**, 970–975.

114. Woolley, D. E., and Tetlow, L. C. (1997). Observations on the microenvironmental nature of cartilage degradation in rheumatoid arthritis. *Ann. Rheum. Dis.* **56**, 151–161.

115. Brennan, F. M., Browne, K. A., Green, P. A., Jaspar, J. M., Maini, R. N., and Feldmann, M. (1997). Reduction of serum matrix metalloproteinase 1 and matrix metalloproteinase 3 in rheumatoid arthritis patients following anti-tumour necrosis factor-α (cA2) therapy. *Br. J. Rheumatol.* **36**, 643–650.

116. Lark, M. W., Bayne, E. K., and Lohmander, L. S. (1995). Aggrecan degradation in osteoarthritis and rheumatoid arthritis. *Acta Orthop. Scand. (Suppl. 266)*, **66**, 92–97.

117. Lark, M. W., Williams, H., Hoernner, L. A., Weidner, J., Ayala, J. M., Harper, C. F., Christen, A., Olszewski, J., Konteatis, Z., Webber, R., and Rumford, R. A. (1995). Quantification of a matrix metalloproteinase-generated aggrecan G1 fragment using monospecific anti-peptide serum. *Biochem. J.* **307**, 245–252.

118. Fosang, A. J., Last, K., Gardiner, P., Jackson, D. C., and Brown, L. (1995). Development of a cleavage-site-specific monoclonal antibody for detecting metalloproteinase-derived aggrecan fragments: Detection of fragments in human synovial fluids. *Biochem. J.* **310**, 337–343.

119. Hughes, C. E., Caterson, B., Fosang, A. J., Roughley, P. J., and Mort, J. S. (1995). Monoclonal antibodies that specifically recognize neoepitope sequences generated by 'aggrecanase' and matrix metalloproteinase cleavage of aggrecan: Application to catabolism in situ and in vitro. *Biochem. J.* **305**, 799–804.

120. Lark, M. W., Gordy, J. T., Weidner, J. R., Ayala, J., Kimura, J. H., Williams, H. R., Mumford, R. A., Flannery, C. R., Carlson, S. S., Iwata, M., and Sandy, J. D. (1995). Cell-mediated catabolism of aggrecan. Evidence that cleavage at the "aggrecanase" site (Glu373-Ala374) is a primary event in proteolysis of the interglobular domain. *J. Biol. Chem.* **270**, 2550–2556.

121. Fosang, A. J., Last, K., Neame, P. J., Murphy, G., Knauper, V., Tschesche, H., Hughes, C. E., Caterson, B., and Hardingham, T. E. (1994). Neutrophil collagenase (MMP-8) cleaves at the aggrecanase site E373-A374 in the interglobular domain of cartilage aggrecan. *Biochem. J.* **304**, 347–351.

122. Buttner, F. H., Hughes, C. E., Margerie, D., Lichte, A., Tschesche, H., Caterson, B., and Bartnik, E. (1998). Membrane type 1 matrix metalloproteinase (MT1-MMP) cleaves the recombinant aggrecan substrate rAgg1mut at the 'aggrecanase' and the MMP sites. Characterization of MT1-MMP catabolic activities on the interglobular domain of aggrecan. *Biochem. J.* **333**, 159–165.

123. Lark, M. W., Bayne, E. K., Flanagan, J., Harper, C. F., Hoerrner, L. A., Hutchinson, N. I. Singer, I. I., Donatelli, S. A., Weidner, J. R., Williams, H. R., Mumford, R. A., and Lohmander, L. S. (1997). Aggrecan degradation in human cartilage. Evidence for both matrix metalloproteinase and aggrecanase activity in normal, osteoarthritic, and rheumatoid joints. *J. Clin. Invest.* **100**, 93–106.

124. Fosang, A. J., Last, K., and Maciewicz, R. A. (1996). Aggrecan is degraded by matrix metalloproteinases in human arthritis. Evidence that matrix metalloproteinase and aggrecanase activities can be independent. *J. Clin. Invest.* **98**, 2292–2292.

125. Lohmander, L. S., Neame, P. J., and Sandy, J. D. (1993). The structure of aggrecan fragments in human synovial fluid. Evidence that aggrecanase mediates cartilage degradation in inflammatory joint disease, joint injury, and osteoarthritis. *Arthritis Rheum.* **36**, 1214–1222.

126. Chevalier, X., Groult, N., Texier, J. M., Larget-Piet, B., and Hornebeck, W. (1996). Elastase activity in cartilage extracts and synovial fluids from subjects with osteoarthritis or rheumatoid arthritis: The prominent role of metalloproteinases. *Clin. Exp. Rheumatol.* **14**, 235–241.

127. Saxne, T., Lecander, I., and Geborek, P. (1993). Plasminogen activators and plasminogen activator inhibitors in synovial fluid. Difference between inflammatory joint disorders and osteoarthritis. *J. Rheumatol.* **20**, 91–96.

128. Keyszer, G. M., Heer, A. H., Kriegsmann, J., Geiler, T., Trabandt, A., Keysser, M., Gay, R. E., and Gay, S. (1995). Comparative analysis of cathepsin L, cathepsin D, and collagenase messenger RNA expression in synovial tissues of patients with rheumatoid arthritis and osteoarthritis, by in situ hybridization. *Arthritis Rheum.* **38**, 976–984.

129. Forslind, K., Eberhardt, K., Jonsson, A., and Saxne, T. (1992). Increased serum concentrations of cartilage oligometric matrix protein. A prognostic marker in early rheumatoid arthritis. *Br. J. Rheumatol.* **31**, 593–598.

130. Recklies, A. D., Baillargeon, L., and White, C. (1998). Regulation of cartilage oligomeric matrix protein synthesis in human synovial cells and articular chondrocytes. *Arthritis Rheum.* **41**, 997–1006.

131. Hakala, B. E., White, C., and Recklies, A. D. (1993). Human cartilage gp-39, a major secretory product of articular chondrocytes and synovial cells, is a mammalian member of a chitinase protein family. *J. Biol. Chem.* **268**, 25803–25810.

132. Johansen, J. S., Jensen, H. S., and Price, P. A. (1993). A new biochemical marker of joint injury. Analysis of YKL-40 in serum and synovial fluid. *Br. J. Rheumatol.* **32**, 949–955.

133. van den Berg, W. B. (1997). Lessons for joint destruction from animal models. *Curr. Opin. Rheumatol.* **9**, 221–228.

134. Goldring, M. B. (1999). The role of cytokines as inflammatory mediators in osteoarthritis: Lessons from animal models. *Connect. Tissue Res.* **40**, 1–11.

135. Goldring, M. B. (1993). Degradation of articular cartilage in culture: Regulatory factors. *In* "Joint Cartilage Degradation: Basic and Clinical Aspects" (J. F. Woessner, Jr. and D. S. Howell, eds.), pp. 281–345. Dekker, New York.

136. Feldmann, M., Brennan, F. M., and Maini, R. N. (1996). Role of cytokines in rheumatoid arthritis. *Annu. Rev. Immunol.* **14**, 397–440.

137. Moulton, P. J. (1996). Inflammatory joint disease: The role of cytokines, cyclooxygenases and reactive oxygen species. *Br. J. Biomed. Sci.* **53**, 317–324.

138. Crofford, L. J. (1997). COX-1 and COX-2 tissue expression: Implications and predictions. *J. Rheumatol.* **24**, 15–19.

139. Hauselmann, H. J. (1997). Mechanisms of cartilage destruction and novel nonsurgical therapeutic strategies to retard cartilage injury in rheumatoid arthritis. *Curr. Opin. Rheumatol.* **9**, 241–250.

140. Stichtenoth, D. O., and Frolich, J. C. (1998). Nitric oxide and inflammatory joint diseases. *Br. J. Rheumatol.* **37**, 246–257.

141. Clancy, R. M., Amin, A. R., and Abramson, S. B. (1998). The role of nitric oxide in inflammation and immunity. *Arthritis Rheum.* **41**, 1141–1151.

142. Jovanovic, D. V., Di Battista, J. A., Martel-Pelletier, J., Jolicoeur, F. C., He, Y., Zhang, M., Mineau, F., and Pelletier, J. P. (1998). IL-17 stimulates the production and expression of proinflammatory cytokines, IL-β and TNF-α, by human macrophages. *J. Immunol.* **160**, 3513–3521.

143. Attur, M. G., Patel, R. N., Abramson, S. B., and Amin, A. R. (1997). Interleukin-17 upregulation of nitric oxide production in human osteoarthritis cartilage. *Arthritis Rheum.* **40**, 1050–1053.

144. Vincenti, M. P., Clark, I. M., and Brinckerhoff, C. E. (1994). Using inhibitors of metalloproteinases to treat arthritis. Easier said than done? *Arthritis Rheum.* **37**, 1115–1126.

145. Arend, W. P., and Dayer, J.-M. (1995). Inhibition of the production and effects of interleukin-1 and tumor necrosis factor α in rheumatoid arthritis. *Arthritis Rheum.* **38**, 151–160.

146. Feldmann, M., Brennan, F., Paleolog, E., Taylor, P., and Maini, R. N. (1997). Anti-tumor necrosis factor α therapy of rheumatoid arthritis. Mechanism of action. *Eur. Cytokine Network* **8**, 297–300.

147. Vane, J. R., and Botting, R. M. (1997). Mechanism of action of aspirin-like drugs. *Semin. Arthritis Rheum.* **26**, 2–10.

148. Blanco, F. J., Geng, Y., and Lotz, M. (1995). Differentiation-dependent effects of IL-1 and TGF-β on human articular chondrocyte proliferation are related to inducible nitric oxide synthase expression. *J. Immunol.* **154**, 4018–4026.

149. Geng, Y., Blanco, F. J., Cornelisson, M., and Lotz, M. (1995). Regulation of cyclooxygenase-2 expression in normal human articular chondrocytes. *J. Immunol.* **155**, 796–801.

150. Berenbaum, F., Jacques, C., Thomas, G., Corvol, M. T., Bereziat, G., and Masliah, J. (1996). Synergistic effect of IL-1β and TNFα on prostaglandin E$_2$ production by articular chondrocytes. Involvement of cyclooxygenase without PLA2 stimulation. *Exp. Cell Res.* **222**, 379–384.

151. Jacques, C., Bereziat, G., Humbert, L., Corvol, M., Olivier, J. L., Masliah, J., and Berenbaum, F. (1997). Post-transcriptional effect of IGF-1 on IL-1 beta-induced type II secreted phospholipase A2 gene expression in rabbit articular chondrocytes. *J. Clin. Invest.* **99**, 1864–1872.

152. Reboul, P., Pelletier, J. P., Tardif, G., Cloutier, J. M., and Martel-Pelletier, J. (1996). The new collagenase, collagenase-3, is expressed and synthesized by human chondrocytes but not by synoviocytes. A role in osteoarthritis. *J. Clin. Invest.* **97**, 2011–2019.

153. Goldring, M. B., and Berenbaum, F. (1999). Human chondrocyte culture models for studying cyclooxygenase expression and prostaglandin regulation of collagen gene expression. *Osteoarthritis Cartilage* **7** (in press).

154. Handel, M. L., McMorrow, L. B., and Gravallese, E. M. (1995). Nuclear factor-kB in rheumatoid synovium. Localization of p50 and p65. *Arthritis Rheum.* **38**, 1762–1770.

155. Muller-Ladner, U., Kriegsmann, J., Gay, R. E., and Gay, S. (1995). Oncogenes in rheumatoid arthritis. *Rheum. Dis. Clin. North Am.* **21**, 675–690.

156. Roivainen, A., Soderstrom, K. -O., Pirila, L., Aro, H., Kortekangas, P., Merilahti-Palo, R., Yli-Jama, T., Toivanen, A., and Toivanen, P. (1996). Oncoprotein expression in human synovial tissue: An immunohistochemical study of different types of arthritis. *Br. J. Rheumatol.* **35**, 933–942.

157. Muller-Ladner, U., Gay, R. E., and Gay, S. (1998). Molecular biology of cartilage and bone destruction. *Curr. Opin. Rheumatol.* **10**, 212–219.

158. Vincenti, M. P., Coon, C. I., and Brinckerhoff, C. E. (1998). Nuclear factor kB/p50 activates an element in the distal matrix metalloproteinase 1 promoter in interleukin-1 β-stimulated synovial fibroblasts. *Arthritis Rheum.* **41**, 1987–1994.

159. Benbow, U., and Brinckerhoff, C. E. (1997). The AP-1 site and MMP gene regulation: What is all the fuss about? *Matrix Biol.* **15**, 519–526.

160. Reddi, A. H. (1995). Cartilage morphogenesis: Role of bone and cartilage morphogenetic proteins, homeobox genes and extracellular matrix. *Matrix Biol.* **14**, 599–606.

161. Cerjesi, P., Brown, D., Ligon, K. L., Lyons, G. E., Copeland, N. G., Gilbert, D. J., Jenkins, N. A., and Olson, E. N. (1995). Scleraxis: A basic helix-loop-helix protein that prefigures skeletal formation during mouse embryogenesis. *Development* **121**, 1099–1110.

162. Mundlos, S., and Olsen, B. R. (1997). Heritable diseases of the skeleton. Part I: Molecular insights into skeletal development-transcription factors and signaling pathways. *FASEB J.* **11**, 125–132.

163. Lefebvre, V., and de Crombrugghe, B. (1998). Toward understanding SOX9 function in chondrocyte differentiation. *Matrix Biol.* **16**, 529–540.

164. Yueh, Y. G., Gardner, D. P., and Kappen, C. (1998). Evidence for regulation of cartilage differentiation by the homeobox gene *Hoxc-8*. *Proc. Natl. Acad. Sci. U.S.A.* **95**, 9956–9961.

165. Mojcik, C. F., and Shevach, E. M. (1997). Adhesion molecules. A rheumatologic perspective. *Arthritis Rheum.* **40**, 991–1004.

166. Knudson, C. B. (1993). Hyaluronan receptor-directed assembly of chondrocyte pericellular matrix. *J. Cell Biol.* **120**, 825–834.

167. Mollenhauer, J., Bee, J. A., Lizarbe, M. A., and von der Mark, K. (1984). Role of anchorin CII, a 31,000-mol-wt membrane protein, in the interaction of chondrocytes with type II collagen. *J. Cell Biol.* **98**, 1572–1579.

168. Loeser, R. F., Carlson, C. S., and McGee, M. P. (1995). Expression of β1 integrins by cultured articular chondrocytes and in osteoarthritic cartilage. *Exp. Cell Res.* **217**, 248–257.

169. Camper, L., Hellman, U., and Lundgren-Akerlund, E. (1998). Isolation, cloning, and sequence analysis of the integrin subunit α10, a β1-associated collagen binding integrin expressed on chondrocytes. *J. Biol. Chem.* **273**, 20383–20389.

CHAPTER 45

Osteoarthritis and Degenerative Spine Pathologies

KRISTINA ÅKESSON   Department of Orthopedics, Malmö University Hospital, S-205 02 Malmö, Sweden

I. INTRODUCTION

Osteoarthritis is one of the most common diseases affecting the musculoskeletal system, causing pain, decreased mobility, and reduced quality of life for the individual patient. It is a heterogeneous and complex joint disease, which, in severe cases, may result in progressive joint destruction and ultimately may lead to joint replacement surgery in major joints. The onset of the disease is usually insidious, occurring long before it can be detected with current clinical and diagnostic methods. Subsequently, permanent and irreversible damage of the joint have often occurred by the time the clinical diagnosis is made. Thus, it is highly desirable to develop sensitive and reliable methods for early diagnosis and prognostication of disease progress and to design appropriate therapies to avoid the need for joint replacement surgery.

Advances in the knowledge of bone and cartilage biochemistry and physiology have provided important insights into bone and cartilage composition and metabolism, and thereby, also into the pathogenesis of osteoarthritis and re-lated degenerative joint diseases. In this regard, it is now apparent that the early biochemical changes in osteoarthritis include increased release of degradation products and increased production of reparative molecules from the bone and cartilage matrix. Consequently, it is conceivable that the release of these products may be indicators of abnormalities in bone and cartilage, and biochemical assays of these compounds may be used to detect and/or monitor development of joint disease, including osteoarthritis.

There are currently a number of biochemical assays that can readily detect bone and cartilage matrix molecules in serum, urine, and synovial fluid. Some of these biochemical markers may have the potential to serve as diagnostic aids to evaluate disease progress and response to treatment in joint diseases. However, despite rapid development in this area, most marker assays are still at the level of research, which again reflects the complexity of the problem and the difficulties in defining osteoarthritis [1].

In this chapter, I will discuss the potential utility of biochemical markers to evaluate osteoarthritis patients; detailed

637

descriptions of each marker are presented in other chapters. To facilitate the understanding of the rationale and the value of biochemical markers in osteoarthritic joint disease, a brief background of the epidemiology, etiology, and currently available diagnositic methods is included.

II. CHARACTERISTICS OF OSTEOARTHRITIS (OA)

Osteoarthritis may affect any of the peripheral joints as well as the joints of the axial skeleton. The small joints of the hands and the knee and hip joints are most frequently involved, while other joints such as the shoulders, elbows, wrists, and ankles are more likely to be spared, even in generalized osteoarthritis [2]. In spinal osteoarthritis, changes occur both in the intervertebral disc space, with disc degeneration, and in the small facet joints. Thus, osteoarthritic changes may be limited to one single major joint or may be described as generalized, commonly including multiple small joints with or without engagement of large joints.

The occurrence of osteoarthritis usually begins in the fifth decade of life, with increasing prevalence and incidence with advancing age. Radiographic changes in the finger joints are evident in 10% of individuals by 40–49 years of age, while as many as 70–90% of women above 70 years of age shows signs of finger joint osteoarthritis. Most surveys of hip osteoarthritis indicate a prevalence of 3–4% in populations over 55 years of age, with a similar distribution between men and women. Bilateral changes occur in about one-third of the cases. Thus, osteoarthritis of the hip is a major contributor to the 250,000 total joint replacements of the hip undertaken in the U.S. each year.

Osteoarthritis of the knee joint is more common, with a reported prevalence of radiographic changes ranging from 4 to 30% in populations over 45 years of age; there is an even further age-related increase above age 75 (40–60%), with a predominance of women suffering [2].

Only limited information is available on the natural course of osteoarthritis. This relates to the inconsistent correlation between radiographic changes and clinical symptoms, causing difficulties in the assesment of disease progression, and to the fact that arthritic pain is accepted as part of aging. However, it is well known that osteoarthritis may either lead to rapidly deteriorating joint integrity or be observed as a fairly stable condition. In osteoarthritis of the hip, radiographic progression was seen in two-thirds of the cases over an 11 year period [3], while radiographic progression in a study of knee osteoarthritis was seen in about 30% of the patients during a similar observation period [4].

III. ETIOLOGY

Ample evidence suggests a multifactorial etiology of osteoarthritis by combinations of biomechanical, biochemical,

and genetic factors. However, the initial event that triggers the pathological process is unclear and it is still being debated whether the initial changes occur in the synovium, the cartilage, the subchondral bone, or concurrently in all of these compartments. Even if it is assumed that the synovial involvement is secondary, one can not rule out the possibility that synovial secretion of substances, including resorptive cytokines, could by themselves influence the disease process [5].

Factors interfering with the biomechanical properties of the joint are risk factors for the development of osteoarthritis in weight-bearing joints, particularly the hip and the knee. Congenital and developmental deformities, although relatively rare, confer a high risk of osteoarthritis at an early age. Obesity, joint trauma, and certain repetitive loading patterns (often occupation-related) have also been shown to be associated with an increase in osteoarthritis [6, 7]. Pertaining to this, the knee joint is, for mechanical reasons, more vulnerable to injury than the hip, and instability or incongruity from ligamentous or meniscus injury is related to an increased incidence of osteoarthritis [8].

Hereditary factors also play a role in the development of osteoarthritis (especially generalized osteoarthritis). Familial forms have been identified, and in some instances, are related to specific mutations in genes that regulate matrix production. Indeed, a mutation in the gene encoding type II procollagen (COL2A1) has been linked to the disease in rare familial types of osteoarthritis [9]. However, considering the heterogeniety of the disease, it seems highly unlikely that alteration in one or even several genes can solely account for the overall genetic influence on the development of osteoarthritis.

From a biochemical view point, it is generally accepted that the osteoarthritic process includes alterations in the normal balance between synthesis and degradation of the articular cartilage and/or the subchondral bone. On the other hand, it is less known whether the primary deficiency is inadequate cellular response to normal tissue demand or insufficient cellular response to supranormal demand from mechanical loading or injury. Nevertheless, the metabolic disturbance of bone and/or cartilage turnover leads to increased release of degradation products primarily into the synovial fluid, but also into serum. The subsequent repair response could induce elevated levels of anabolic molecules, some of which may not be incorporated into the matrix but instead may be released into the joint space (i.e., synovial fluid) or the circulation. Therefore, measurements of the levels of these degradation products and/or repair molecules may yield important information regarding the progression of the disease.

Past clinical observations suggest that impairment of the normal coupling between degradation and repair in bone and cartilage can be either continuously progressive or haltered at any time after process initiation. Accordingly, in some patients, radiographically evident osteoarthritis may stabilize with only marginal changes over observational periods of ten years or more, while in another patient with similar baseline changes, the disease may rapidly progress to end-stage joint destruction with in 6–12 months. This implies that regulatory and disease-limiting mechanisms are as complex as the initiating forces and may involve various inter- and intracellular signal transduction mediators and/or local regulators.

IV. TREATMENT OPTIONS

Currently available treatment options for osteoarthritis focus on symptom relief; whereas truly disease-modifying agents or methods are lacking. Thus, the basic therapy includes common analgesics, nonsteroidal anti-inflammatory drugs, physical therapy, walking aids, and eventually, in severe cases, joint replacement surgery. However, future research perspectives encompass strategies ranging from alteration of disease progression, and thereby limitation of joint damage by pharmacological interventions of local or systemic agents, to cartilage transplants.

V. CURRENT DIAGNOSTIC PROCEDURES

In order to evaluate the degree of joint affection, a number of diagnostic tools are available. However, in most cases these require a rather advanced disease state for reliable diagnosis and identification. Aside from clinical assessments, the most widely used and accepted method relies on standardized radiographic assessment of the joint space and of the secondary periarticular changes in peripheral joints [10, 11]. Lower extremity joints are preferably evaluated on weight-bearing films to enhance correct staging and sequential evaluation. Relative insensitivity during early stages of disease and high inter-observer variation on radiographic film interpretation are, nevertheless, major limitations to using radiography diagnostically. Furthermore, evaluation of degenerative changes of the spine imposes specific considerations because there is no distinct correlation between radiographically observed degenerative changes and clinical symptoms.

To overcome these limitations, scintimetric methods using technetium-99 labeled diphosphonate may be valuable tools, at least for peripheral joints, as was shown by Dieppe *et al.* [12]. In this study, the investigators showed a good correlation between subchondral technetium retention and disease progression over five years in patients with established OA.

Several new technologies for osteoarthritis detection, such as digitalization of X-rays and magnetic resonance imaging, are rapidly evolving. These methodologies are extensively computerized techniques, which allow for postexposure manipulation to enhance the evaluation of pathologies. These methods have the potential of becoming important auxiliary, or even primary, diagnostic methods for identifying early cartilage deficiencies, but they need further validation to confirm the clinical and pathological significance of identified aberrations [13, 14].

Most major peripheral joints also are accessible to arthroscopy, with the knee joint most commonly examined. Despite the fact that arthroscopy is not primarily a diagnostic tool, but rather a treatment procedure, this method provides a direct means to identify both major and minor intra-articular lesions and pathological changes. Even so, the significance of the findings for future development of osteoarthritis is only partially known, and factors such as previous meniscectomy, severe instability, and intra-articular fracture are linked to osteoarthritis [8, 15].

VI. BIOCHEMICAL ASPECTS OF OSTEOARTHRITIS

The biochemical alterations caused by osteoarthritis involve the dynamic processes of two completely different but adjacent and partially interconnected tissues: bone and cartilage. Throughout the body, bone is the predominant tissue, constituting 20–25% of the body weight, while cartilage-covered joint surfaces comprise less than a few percent. The normal skeletal bone turnover rate is relatively slow and is estimated to average about 10% per year, with a higher activity in trabecular bone (15–20%) and a lower activity in cortical bone (3–5%) [16]; no such estimation for cartilage turnover is available. In contrast to cartilage, bone tissue is highly vascularized, which promotes rapid exchange of nutrients, ions, and other substances. This also renders the bone tissue susceptible to systemic regulators, including various hormones and mediators such as PTH, 1,25-dihydroxy vitamin D, growth factors, cytokines, mechanical load, or microinjuries [17, 18]. Cartilage depends on diffusion for nutrition and for release of waste products. Normal exchange requires an intact cartilage surface and pressure variation from joint loading. Thus, in addition to mechanical loading, factors such as local enzyme and cytokine release are probably of greater importance than systemic regulators for cartilage turnover. However, putative locally acting regulators such as insulin-like growth factors and cytokines do not uniquely affect either bone or cartilage turnover but affect both, whereas certain enzymes and their inhibitors are tissue-specific.

Bone consists mainly of collagen type I; cartilage mainly contains collagen type II, but additional collagen types are present in various amounts (type VI, IX, X, and XI). The collagen fibrils are similarly synthesized but the final structural assembly differs, giving each type tissue-specific properties of tensile strength and ability to withstand loading forces. In bone, structural solidity is provided by matrix mineralization from precipitation of hydroxyapatite, whereas in cartilage, the firm elasticity results from large proteoglycans responsive to osmotic and loading pressures. In addition, a number of other collagenous and noncollagenous proteins are incorporated into the bone and cartilage matrix.

Bone resorption relies on osteoclasts creating a suitable environment by locally increasing the acidity and by secreting proteinases. Osteoblasts, on the other hand, are specifically related to bone formation or restoration and produce a number of essential proteins in addition to collagen. In cartilage, the chondrocytes are responsible for both the production of new matrix proteins and enzymes related to cartilage degradation. The particular cellular production and the resulting composition of cartilage (type of collagen and proteoglycan content) appears to vary with the distance from the cartilage surface; the surface layers are also affected by enzymes and cytokines produced by synovial cells [19].

Assuming that bone and cartilage turnover under normal circumstances remains at a fairly steady state, products released during tissue breakdown, bone resorption, and cartilage degradation could be used as markers for the catabolic events. During the anabolic phase, osteoblasts and chondrocytes are actively producing collagens and other proteins to be incorporated in the newly synthesized matrix. Surplus products or fragments released into serum or synovial fluid may then be used as markers of bone and cartilage formation. In states of disease, alteration of marker levels should provide insight into the metabolic disturbances in a particular bone and joint disorder. With regard to osteoarthritis, the ideal biochemical marker or markers should (1) detect joint damage at an earlier stage than conventional methods, (2) provide information on disease activity and progressive joint damage, and (3) predict future illness and course of disease.

None of the available biochemical markers for bone or cartilage are able to supply this information and in view of the complexity of the osteoarthritic disease, clinically useful biochemical markers are not to be expected to be found in the near future. Nevertheless, research on biochemical markers has increased our knowledge of the underlying metabolic changes occurring during joint injury and during joint destruction in both osteoarthritis and rheumatoid arthritis.

In the following section, each one of the potentially useful markers for bone and for cartilage will be reviewed separately (Table I).

VII. MARKERS OF BONE TURNOVER

The rationale for using markers primarily regarded as markers of bone formation and bone resorption is obviously

TABLE I.   Potential Biochemical Markers of Bone and Joint Tissue Turnover in Osteoarthritis

Primary tissue source	Marker	Assayed in
Bone	Osteocalcin	Serum + sf
	Bone specific alkaline phosphatase	Serum
	Type I collagen C-propeptide	Serum
	Pyridinoline cross-links	Urine + sf
	Pyridinoline	
	Deoxypyridinoline	
	Pyridinoline cross-linking telopeptides	Urine + serum
	Bone sialoprotein	Serum
Cartilage	Aggrecan	Serum + sf
	Protein fragments	
	Keratan sulfate	
	Chondroitin sulfate	
	Cartilage oligomeric matrix protein (COMP)	Serum + sf
	Type II collagen C-propeptide	Serum + sf
Cartilage and/or synovium	Matrix metalloproteinases and inhibitors	Serum + sf
	Stromelysin (MMP-3)	
	Interstitial collagenase (MMP-1)	
	Tissue inhibitors of metalloproteinases (TIMP)	
Synovium	Hyaluronic acid	Serum
	Type III collagen N-propeptide	Serum + sf

Note: sf, synovial fluid.

related to the fact that bone and cartilage form an integrated tissue compartment where processes involving the interface affect both tissues. The pronounced juxta-articular skeletal involvement in advanced osteoarthritis also indicates an early affect on bone tissue, while observations of structural differences (i.e., bone mass, geometry, cortical width) may suggest a general skeletal difference in this population. In addition, it is possible that the initial changes in the osteoarthritis process emanate form the subchondral bone.

A. Osteocalcin

Osteocalcin is one of the most abundant noncollagenous proteins of bone matrix and is synthesized by the osteoblasts [18]. Osteocalcin is incorporated in the extracellular matrix and is regarded as bone-specific, as the small amount present in dentin is negligible, but its precise function remains unknown. Serum osteocalcin is most often used to evaluate bone turnover in osteoporosis and is regarded as a valid marker of bone formation [20, 21] (see Chapter 3 in this book).

It has been suggested that there is an inverse relationship between osteoarthritis and osteoporosis, with a higher bone mass in patients with osteoarthritis [22]. Subsequenty, if OA represents the antipode of osteoporosis, a protective effect could possibly be inferred and a shift in bone turnover anticipated. In a study of postmenopausal women with generalized osteoarthritis, osteocalcin was moderately but significantly increased compared with age- and sex-matched controls [23]. Even so, the increase was similar to that of postmenopausal women with osteoporosis, despite the higher bone mineral density in women with osteoarthritis [24]. In order to test bone metabolic differences as a possible underlying cause of the increased bone mass in osteoarthritis, the responsiveness to 1,25-dihydroxyvitamin D_3, a stimulator of osteocalcin synthesis and bone formation, was explored. The stimulatory effect of short-term 1,25-dihydroxyvitamin D_3 administration on osteocalcin production was, however, similar in patients with OA and osteoporosis [24]. Still, quantitative and qualitative differences are observed, and Raymaekers et al. [25] showed increased osteocalcin content in iliac crest bone from patients with osteoarthritis, corresponding to a shift towards higher densities in the mineralization profile.

Few studies have been conducted comparing serum osteocalcin and synovial fluid osteocalcin levels in knee osteoarthritis; the few that have been done report diverging results [26–28]. In a study by Sharif et al. [29] synovial fluid concentrations of osteocalcin correlated with abnormalities on scintigraphic scans and the osteocalcin level was related to scintigraphically assessed severity of joint affection (Fig. 1). This is the only study linking osteocalcin to osteoarthritis disease severity, suggesting that subchondral bone involvement

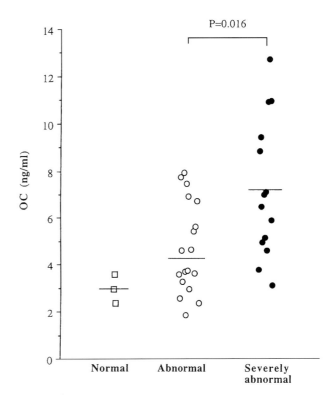

FIGURE 1   Synovial fluid osteocalcin (OC) levels in osteoarthritis patients by category of results on scintigraphy scan. Median concentration indicated by bars. Reprinted from Sharif et al. [29], with permission.

may lead to an increased release of osteocalcin into the synovial fluid. In addition, synovial fluid osteocalcin was almost completely gammacarboxylated in the osteoarthritis patients compared with patients with rheumatoid arthritis [30].

B. Serum Alkaline Phosphatase

The skeletal isoform of alkaline phosphatase is a membrane-bound protein with enzymatic activity (see Chapter 9). Despite this, the release mechanism and the function remain to be elucidated. A study using combinations of monoclonal antibodies shows a 52% increase in serum bone-specific alkaline phosphatase after menopause [31]. Alkaline phosphatase has only briefly been assessed in studies of osteoarthritis. Assessing biochemical markers in patients with spinal osteoarthritis, Peel et al. [32] found a decrease in bone-specific alkaline phosphatase in women with spinal osteoarthritis compared to women without spinal osteoarthritis in a population-based setting. The decrease in bone-specific alkaline phosphatase was 19%. In this study, spinal osteoarthritis was associated with a generalized increase in BMD [32]. In contrast to this, the bone content of alkaline phosphatase was significantly elevated in femoral heads from women with osteoarthritis of the hip compared with controls [33].

C. Type I Collagen Carboxy-Propepetide

During collagen type I synthesis by the osteblasts, the amino- and carboxy-terminal extension peptides are split off. The intact terminal fragments are released into circulation prior to extracellular fibril formation [34] (see Chapters 1 and 2). Studies indicate that PICP may be used as a marker of bone formation, but that is has a questionable sensitivity in identifying subtle alterations of bone turnover [35]. So far, this potential marker has not been evaluated in relation to osteoarthritis.

D. Pyridinoline Cross-Links

Pyridinoline and deoxypyridinoline represent specific degradation products of mature collagen. The pyridinium cross-links interconnect collagen molecules within the extracellular matrix, thus pyridinium cross-links are present in most connective tissues [19]. However, the reported distribution varies depending on tissue type: pyridinoline is primarily present in cartilage, but is also found in bone collagen, whereas deoxypyridinoline is predominant in bone and dentine [36]. Theoretically, deoxypyridinoline should therefore be the more suitable marker of bone resorption; it has indeed been shown to correlate positively with other indicies of bone resorption, and inversely, with bone mass in osteoporosis [31]. The cross-linking telopeptide regions, C-telopeptide to helix and N-telopeptide to helix, have emerged as potential markers of bone resorption and are measurable either in serum or in urine. To date, evaluation of these markers is focused on the assessment of osteoporosis and antiresorptive therapies [19] (see also Chapters 2 and 28 in this book).

In a study assessing the relative amounts of pyridinoline and deoxypyridinoline in subchondral bone, articular cartilage, and synovium, the relative content of PYR:DPD was 3:1 in bone, 25:1 in synovium, and 50:1 in cartilage [37]. These ratios were similar to those found in patients with rheumatoid arthritis [37]. The only significant difference was a higher cartilage content of deoxypyridinoline in osteoarthritis.

Most studies report increased urinary concentrations of pyridinoline and deoxypyridinoline in both single joint and generalized osteoarthritis compared to healthy subjects [38–42]. However, in a report by Hellio le Graverand *et al.* [43] including 114 patients, pyridinoline and deoxypyridinoline excretion did not differ from controls, regardless of whether the patient suffered from hip, knee, or generalized osteoarthritis (Fig. 2). Nevertheless, patients judged to have severe or end-stage osteoarthritis had higher excretion of pyridinolines compared to patients with early osteoarthritis, while the PYD:DPD ratio remained unchanged.

It would be desirable to use biochemical markers as a severity index, and several studies are assessing pyridinoline

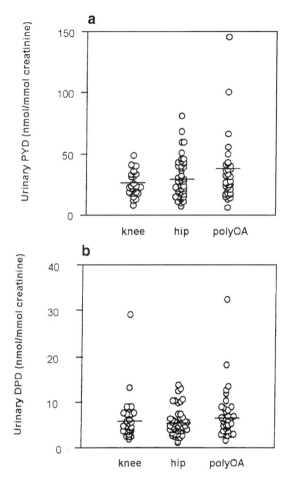

FIGURE 2 Urinary excretion of pyridinoline (PYD) and deoxypyridinoline (DPD) in osteoarthritis subgroups (knee, n = 31; hip, n = 47; generalized, n = 36). Reprinted from Hellio le Graverand *et al.* [43] (1996). *Br. J. Rheum.* **35**, 1091–1095, by permission of Oxford University Press.

excretion in relation to joint destruction. Pyridinoline and deoxypyridinoline were identified as weak markers of disease severity according to X-ray staging of knee osteoarthritis in 60-year old women (r = 0.39 and 0.33 respectively) [41]. Contrary to this, Astbury *et al.* [42] found no difference in pyridinoline and deoxypyridinoline levels relative to the degree of joint involvement in osteoarthritis, but a significant correlation to disease severity in rheumatoid arthritis was found. Furthermore, MacDonald *et al.* [44] found that patients with osteoarthritis of the knee had a higher excretion of deoxypyridinoline compared to patients with generalized osteoarthritis and hip osteoarthritis, but the levels were not correlated to clinical indices of disease in these 39 subjects.

Synovial concentrations of pyridinoline and deoxypyridinoline were measured in 20 patients with osteoarthritis; pyridinoline was about 30% of urinary concentrations and deoxypyridinoline was below the detection limit in all samples. This finding of pyridinoline, but not of deoxypyridinoline, in synovial fluid may suggest that in cases of joint disease, pyridinoline excretion could also derive from breakdown of collagen other than bone collagen (possibly cartilage collagen) [45].

E. Bone Sialoprotein

Bone sialoprotein (BSP) is a phosphorylated glycoprotein containing sialic acid, with suggested cell adhesive properties [46]. BSP is specific for bone and is enriched in the immediate subchondral bone. Serum BSP is increased in states of high turnover and in one study, it was shown to correlate with bone resorption markers [47] (see Chapters 4 and 28). In symptomatic hip osteoarthritis, serum BSP increased significantly during the first year by 63%. This increase was correlated with osteophyte formation, sclerosis, and a radiographic severity index, but not with joint space narrowing assessed by a digitized image analyzer, which was intended as the measure of disease progression [48]. In patients with knee joint abnormalities detectable on bone scan, BSP was elevated compared to scan-negative patients; however, the serum level was not correlated with the extent of abnormalities [49]. BSP also was not a useful tool in predicting disease progress from baseline values, but progressive disease resulted in significantly increased levels in progressors at follow-up three years later [50].

The inconsistency of the findings is not surprising in view of the heterogeniety of the disease and the fact that the study populations include a certain disparity, even if using specific selection criteria defining osteoarthritis. Because the disorder includes both single joint disease and polyarticular involvement, it is more likely that a generalized joint and skeletal affection leads to a larger effect on the biochemical markers measured in serum, and urine as these markers relate to changes in bone turnover of the entire skeleton.

VIII. MARKERS OF CARTILAGE TURNOVER

Acute, and in many circumstances, chronic, joint damage induces an increase in synovial fluid production. Thus, synovial fluid should have high concentrations of degradation products from cartilage breakdown, both after acute trauma to the joint surface and during degenerative processes. Subsequent activation of repair mechanisms may lead to release of unincorporated matrix molecules into the synovial space. Assessment of synovial fluid concentrations of molecular markers of cartilage turnover may provide unique insight into the local joint process. In addition, because of systemic elimination of molecules related to cartilage degeneration and regeneration, these molecules are detectable both in serum

and in urine, but may then signify more general changes in body cartilage turnover.

A. Aggrecan

Aggrecan is the major aggregating proteoglycan present in cartilage tissue. Attached to the core protein are glucosaminoglycan side chains containing keratan sulfate or chondroitin sulfate. Aggrecan is attached to hyaluronic acid through a link protein. Degradation includes cleavage of the chondroitin and keratan sulfate-containing regions, as well as cleavage of the core protein at different sites and release of these fragments into body fluids. Several different epitopes are used to identify core protein fragments as well as the glucosaminoglycan side chains. Some studies also suggest that some of these epitopes, especially those related to chondroitin sulfate, may instead be indicators of aggrecan neosynthesis [51, 52] (see Chapters 5 and 21 in this book).

B. Aggrecan Protein Fragments

Aggrecan protein fragments have been assessed in several studies, most often in those evaluating knee osteoarthritis which present the possibility of studying both synovial fluid and serum levels of aggrecan fragments. Knee trauma usually invokes an acute increase in synovial fluid. Thus, using a trauma model, Lohmander et al. [53] showed a rapid increase in proteoglycan fragment concentration in synovial fluid immediately after trauma. After this initial increase, the levels of proteoclycan fragments fell within a few months; however, a significant elevation persisted in many patients for several years after injury. Additional observartions report increased release of proteoglycan fragments in early stages of osteoarthritis without radiographic changes, and an inverse relationship to osteoarthritis scores have been noted [54, 55] (Fig. 3).

C. Keratan Sulfate

Keratan sulfate epitopes have been proposed as additional markers for cartilage damage (see Chapters 21 and 31). The earliest study by Thonar et al. [56] using a monoclonal antibody specific for keratan sulfate showed increased levels of keratan sulfate in 24 patients with osteoarthritis compared to normal adults. Further studies have confirmd the results, and in a comprehensive study including 125 well-characterized patients with knee osteoarthritis, serum keratan sulfate levels were increased, despite a wide variation in the serum levels in the osteoarthritis population (with men having higher serum levels than women) [57]. Synovial fluid keratan sulfate was measured in knee aspirates and was increased over the serum levels in patients with osteoarthritis; however, there was no

Proteoglycan (ug/ml)

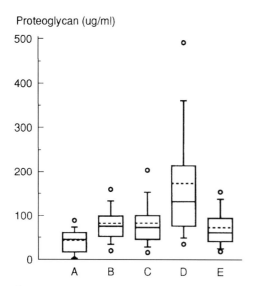

FIGURE 3   The distribution of proteoglycan fragments in joint fluid. (A) 16 healthy knees, (B) 123 cruciate ligament injuries; (C) menicus tears or ruptures; (D) 43 pyrophosphate arthritis; and (E) 135 knees with osteoarthritis. Reprinted from Dahlberg *et al.* [55], with permission.

correlation between serum and synovial fluid concentrations. Serum keratan sulfate levels correlated weakly with the number of joints involved, whereas there was no correlation with clinical disease measure. In an interesting study evaluating a non-weight bearing joint, the gleno-humeral joint, synovial keratan sulfate was elevated in joints with moderate and advanced osteoarthritis as classified during arthroscopy [58]. Further attempts to assess the synovial keratan sulfate level in relation to disease activity or severity have been made, but no association between the two was apparent when using scintigraphic abnormalities as an activity measure in knee osteoarthritis [29].

Polyarticular involvement, as compared to single joint osteoarthritis, may also be a sign of more severe disease and thus a greater release of keratan sulfate could be expected. Nevertheless, in a study involving 137 women, the serum keratan sulfate concentration was unrelated to joint involvement and, in contrast to other studies, the levels were comparable to those in the control group [59]. Thus, the value of keratan sulfate as a diagnostic or severity index remains questionable.

In order to investigate the prognostic value of keratan sulfate, serum keratan sulfate was measured at baseline and after five years in patients with knee osteoarthritis. However, at follow-up no difference was obvious in the baseline levels between those who were to progress radiographically after five years and those who remained stationary [60].

D. Chondroitin Sulfate

Chondroitin sulfate epitopes are present on the largest of intact aggrecan molecules. One of the epitopes, 846, has been

suggested to indicate increased cartilage turnover and cartilage neosynthesis, while epitopes more proximal to the globular domain presumably relate to degradation. The serum levels of chondroitin sulfate epitope 846 were increased by 19% in osteoarthritis patients, whereas the elevation was 56% in patients with rheumatoid arthritis. This finding may indicate a more systemic joint involvement in rheumatoid arthritis. Conversely, the synovial levels were highest in the osteoarthritis patients, particularly in those with the longest disease duration and the most pronounced joint destruction [52].

Chondroitin sulfate epitope 3B3 is not present in normal articular cartilage and synovial fluid but is released early in the osteoarthritic process or in a close temporal relationship to joint injury, as demonstrated in human knee synovial fluid [61, 62]. Chondroitin sulfate epitope 3B3 has also been used to evaluate osteoarthritis of the gleno-humeral joint. Synovial fluid concentrations of epitope 3B3 distinguished normal from diseased joints (osteoarthritis grade II-IV), but did not separeate the different stages [58]. On the other hand, no association with disease activity, as judged by scintimetric abnormalities, was found in knee osteoarthritis using an antibody identifying the same epitope (3B3) in synovial fluid [29].

E. Cartilage Oligomeric Matrix Protein

Cartilage oligomeric matrix protein (COMP) is a noncollagenous protein present in the extracellular matrix, with the highest amounts present in articular cartilage [63]. Despite the unknown function of this protein, it has earned interest as a potential marker of tissue damage because it is highly specific for cartilage (see Chapter 5).

In an initial study by Saxne and Heinegård [64] normal serum concentrations of COMP were found in patients with osteoarthritis. In this study it was also noted that COMP was unrelated to age. The comparison of synovial fluid content did not include controls; instead, it was found that the different types of arthritis had similar joint levels of COMP, with the exception of elevated levels in advanced rheumatoid arthritis. Controlled studies have been undertaken and increased COMP levels have been found in joint fluids of patients with early-stage knee osteoarthritis, as compared to patients with advanced changes and healthy controls [54, 65]. During the three year follow-up period, patients with initial knee pain progressing to radiographically evident osteoarthritis showed increasing concentrations of serum COMP, while nonprogressors did not [50]. In order to further evaluate the usefulness of COMP to monitor disease progression, 57 patients with knee osteoarthritis were followed for five years. The change in serum COMP during the first year follow-up was significantly larger in subsequent progressors compared to nonprogressors [66] (Fig. 4). In addition, in a report on hip osteoarthritis, serum COMP also appeared to be a predictor of progressive joint damage in the hip joint [67].

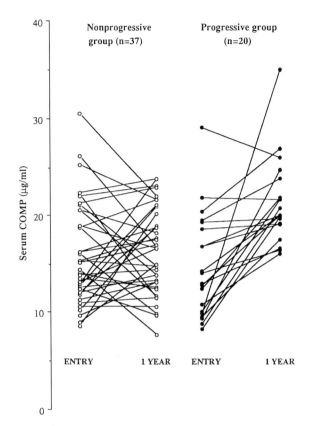

FIGURE 4 Changes in serum cartilage oligomeric matrix protein (COMP) levels over one year in patients with progressive and nonprogressive knee osteoarthritis. Reprinted from Sharif *et al.* [66] (1995). *Br. J. Rheum.* **34**, 306–310, by permission of Oxford University Press.

F. Type II Collagen Carboxy-Propeptide

As previously mentioned, the procollagen extention peptides are split of during collagen type I synthesis and released into body fluids prior to aggregation of the collagen molecules. Measurements of procollagen propeptides should therefore represent newly produced collagen and thereby reflect collagen neosynthesis. Increased collagen type II production may be part of the normal repair process of minor injuries or be an expression of excessive reparative response, as is the possibility in early osteoarthritis. In support of this, several studies have shown increased levels of PIICP in joint fluid of patients with knee osteoarthritis [68–70]. The synovial increase of PIICP was most pronounced in early and midstage osteoarthritis, but decreased in final stage osteoarthritis. In addition, PIIPC correlated positively with BMI, another independent risk factor for osteoarthritis.

G. Matrix Metalloproteinases and Their Inhibitors

The matrix metalloproteinases (MMPs) consisist of a family of 13 enzymes active under both physiological and

pathological conditions of cartilage turnover. The various enzymes, synthesized both by chondrocytes and by synovial cells, are activated during different steps in collagen degradation, with collagenase having the unique ability to cleave the triple helical type II collagen [71]. Other members of the family are gelatinase and stromelysin. The activity of these potent enzymes is regulated by specific tissue inhibitors of metalloproteinases (TIMPs) (see Chapter 10).

Collagenase (MMP-1), stromelysin (MMP-3), and TIMP release have been evaluated in a variety of synovial fluid samples representing normal individuals and patients with different types of knee injury, as well as patients with primary osteoarthritis. The concentrations of metalloproteinases was elevated in all types of knee pathology, with stromelysin showing the differentiating ability. Moreover, a relatively higher increase in the concentration of MMP compared to TIMP is suggested to indicate a potential risk for further cartilage destruction [72]. A persistent elevation of joint fluid levels of stromelysin and TIMP, for many years, is also seen after acute knee injury [73]. Furthermore, subchondral bone tissue from subjects suffering from osteoarthritis of the hip shows increased content of metalloproteinases (gelatinase A/MMP-2) as compared to normal or osteoporotic bone, again indicating the interaction between cellular activity of bone and cartilage [33].

H. Hyaluronic Acid

Hyaluronic acid, a linear polysaccharide, is synthesized by a number of cells, including synovial lining cells. The synthesis is enhanced by most inflammatory mediators, such as cytokines, prostaglandins, cAMP, and growth factors. Situations activating these factors induce increased production of hyaluronic acid. Thus, increased synovial fluid and serum levels can be expected after joint trauma and with degenerative changes. The information on hyaluronic acid in relation to osteoarthritis is limited. One study assessing hyaluronic acid in association with disease progress suggests that hyaluronic acid may predict outcome in knee osteoarthritis [60].

I. Summary

In view of the heterogeniety of OA, the inconsistency of results when evaluating the disease by various biochemical markers is not surprising. First of all, a certain disparity in the study populations is inevitable; despite the use of specific diagnostic or selection criteria, the distinction between single joint or multiple joint involvement may not always be obvious. Even so, osteoarthritis of a major joint may be a sign of a general skeletal engagement and a systemic bone and joint disorder, which could possibly influence the levels of biochemical markers of bone turnover. In this respect, it should be remembered that markers assayed in serum and urine reflect the entire turnover of bone, cartilage, or other connective tissues, whereas synovial fluid measurements provide information on the metabolic activity of the specific joint. It is also important to recognize that either measurement only gives a glimpse of a dynamic process that we inaccurately may interpret as a steady state. Measurements of marker concentrations in joint fluid are attractive, because they provide information about the immediate metabolic activity of the affected joint. Synovial fluid measurements are almost exclusively performed on patients with knee osteoarthritis, because this joint is easily accessible and because knee joint damage often causes a marked fluid effusion. Thus, the knee joint is an excellent model for research, whereas the potential clinical utility of synovial fluid assessment from other joints to evaluate disease activity may be limited.

In this regard, validated and reliable serum or urine markers are desirable. Biochemical markers of bone turnover have, so far, been tested in large population-based settings and normative data are available, but such information to a large extent is lacking for cartilage markers. This may also be one of the limitations in the reported studies; control groups are often relatively small and this especially true for studies reporting on synovial fluid concentrations, thus comparisons are often made with rheumatoid arthritis. Given that one or several of the cartilage markers may emerge as clinically useful tools to monitor joint disease, progression, or therapeutic interventions, it is necessary to include further studies to provide normative information on patient (age, gender, etc.), time (diurnal) and assay-related variability.

IX. CONCLUSIONS

Greater understanding of the underlying processes of bone and cartilage turnover in joint diseases has been gained through the assessment of biochemical marker molecules of bone and cartilage metabolism in synovial fluid, serum, and urine. Tissue-specific molecular markers provide a means to simultaneously study normal degradation and repair processes, as well as pathological states that are inaccessible by other methods. Despite the extensive work and the increased knowledge obtained from biochemical markers of skeletal and connective tissue origin, the search for more refined markers with the propensity of a wider clinical use must be continued.

References

1. Dieppe, P. (1989). Osteoarthritis: Definitions and criteria. *Ann. Rheum. Dis.* **48**, 531–532.
2. Petersson, I. F. (1996). Occurrence of osteoarthritis of the peripheral joints in European populations. *Ann. Rheum. Dis.* **55**, 659–664.
3. Danielsson, L. G. (1964). Incidence and prognosis of coxarthrosis. *Acta Orthop. Scand.* **66**, 9–87.
4. Spector, T. D., Dacre, J. E., Harris, P. A., and Huskisson, E. C. (1992). Radiographical progression of osteoarthritis: An 11 year follow up study of the knee. *Ann. Rheum. Dis.* **51**, 1107–1110.
5. Westcott, D. I., Webb, G. R., Warnock, M. G., Sims, J. V., and Elson, C. J. (1997). Alteration of cartilage metabolism by cells from osteoarthritic bone. *Arthritis Rheum.* **40**, 1282–1291.
6. Cooper, C., Campbell, L., Byng, P., Croft, P., and Coggon, D. (1995). Occupational activity and the risk of hip osteoarthritis. *Ann. Rheum. Dis.* **55**, 680–682.
7. Vingård, E. (1995). Osteoarthrosis of the knee and physical load from occupation. *Ann. Rheum. Dis.* **55**, 677–679.
8. Roos, H., Lindberg, H., Gardsell, P., Lohmander, L. S., and Wingstrand, H. (1994). The prevalence of gonarthrosis and its relation to meniscectomy in former soccer players. *Am. J. Sports Med.* **22**, 219–222.
9. Vikkula, M., Palotie, A., Ritvaniemi, P., Ott, J., Ala-Kokko, L., *et al.* (1993). Early onset osteoarthritis linked to the type II procollagen gene; detailed clinical phenotype and further analysis of the gene. *Arthritis Rheum.* **36**, 401–409.
10. Kjellgren, J. H., Jeffrey, M., and Ball, J. (1963). "Atlas of Standard Radiographs," Vol. 2 Blackwell Scientific, Oxford.
11. Ahlbäck, S. (1968). Osteoarthrosis of the knee: A radiographic investigation. *Acta Radiol.* **277** (Suppl.), 7–72.
12. Dieppe, P., Cushnaghan, J., Young, P., and Kirwan, J. (1993). Prediction of the progression of joint space narrowing in osteoarthritis of the knee by bone scintigraphy. *Ann. Rheum. Dis.* **52**, 557–563.
13. McAlindon, T. E. M., Watt, I, McCrae, F., Goddard, P., and Dieppe, P. A. (1991). Magnetic resonance imaging in osteoarthritis of the knee: Correlation with radiographic and scintigraphic findings. *Ann. Rheum. Dis.* **50**, 514–519.
14. Blackburn, W. D. J., Chivers, S. and Bernreuter, W. (1996). Cartilage imaging in osteoarthritis. *Semin. Arthritis Rheum.* **25**, 273–281.
15. Lane, N. E. (1995). Physical activity at leisure and risk of osteoarthritis. *Ann. Rheum. Dis.* **55**, 682–684.
16. Parfitt, A. M. (1993). The physiological and clinical significance of bone histomorphometric data. In "Bone Histomorphometry. Techniques and Interpretations" (R. Recker, ed.), pp. 143–223. CRC Press, Boca Raton, FL.
17. Rodan, G. A., and Martin, T. J. (1981). Role of osteoclasts in hormonal control of bone resorption—a hypothesis. *Calcif. Tissue Int.* **33**, 349–351.
18. Price, P. A. (1985). Vitamin K-dependent formation of bone Gla protein and its function. *Vitam. Horm.* **42**, 65–107.
19. Eyre, D. R. (1995). The specificity of collagen cross-links as markers of bone and connective tissue degradation. *Acta Orthop. Scand.* **66** (Suppl.), 166–170.
20. Akesson, K. (1995). Biochemical markers of bone turnover. A review. *Acta Orthop. Scand.* **66**, 376–386.
21. Delmas, P. D. (1995). Biochemical markers of bone turnover. *Acta Orthop. Scand.* **66** (Suppl.), 176–182.
22. Dequeker, J. (1985). The relationship between osteoporosis and osteoarthritis. *Clin. Rheum. Dis.* **11**, 271–296.
23. Gevers, G., Dequeker, J., Geusens, P., Verstraeten, A., and Vanderschueren, D. (1988). Serum bone Gla protein (osteocalcin) and other markers of bone mineral metabolism in postmenopausal osteoporosis and osteoarthritis. *J. Orthop. Rheum.* **1**, 22–27.
24. Geusens, P., Vanderschueren, D., Verstraeten, A., Dequeker, J., Devos, P., and Bouillon, R. (1991). Short-term course of 1,25(OH)$_2$D$_3$ stimulates osteoblasts but not osteoclasts in osteoporosis and osteoarthritis. *Calcif. Tissue Int.* **49**, 168–173.
25. Raymaekers, G., Aerssens, J., Van den Eynde, R., Peeters, J., Geusens, P., Devos, P., and Dequeker, J. (1992). Alterations of the mineralization

profile and osteocalcin concentrations in osteoarthritic cortical iliac crest bone. *Calcif. Tissue Int.* **51**, 269–275.

26. Champion, G. V., Delmas, P. D., and Dieppe, P. A. (1989). Serum and synovial fluid osteocalcin (bone Gla protein) levels in joint diseases. *Br. J. Rheum.* **28**, 393–398.

27. Poole, A. R., Ionescu, M. S., Swan, A., Campion, G., Rosenberg, L. C., and Dieppe, P. (1991). Analysis of cartilage and bone molecules and hyaluronic acid in synovial fluid and peripheral blood of patients with arthritis. *Trans. Combined Meet. Orthop. Res. Soci.* Banf, Alberta, Canada.

28. Mattei, J. P., Ferrera, V., Boutsen, T., Franceschi, J. P., Botti, D., De Boissezon, C., Kaphan, G., and Roux, H. (1992). Serum and synovial fluid osteocalcin in rheumatic disease. *Int. J. Clin. Pharmacol. Res.* **12**, 103–107.

29. Sharif, M., George, E., and Dieppe, P. A. (1995). Correlation between synovial fluid markers of cartilage and bone turnover and scintigraphic scan abnormalities in osteoarthritis of the knee. *Arthritis Rheum.* **38**, 78–81.

30. Fairney, A., Patel, K. V., Hollings, N. P., and Seifert, M. H. (1990). Abnormal osteocalcin binding in rheumatoid arthritis. *Ann. Rheum. Dis.* **49**, 229–230.

31. Garnero, P., Sornay-Rendu, E., Chapuy, M-C., and Delmas, P. D. (1996). Increased bone turnover in late postmenopausal women is a major determinant of osteoporosis. *J. Bone Miner. Res.* **11**, 337–349.

32. Peel, N. F. A., Barrington, N. A., Blumsohn, A., Clowell, A., Hannon, R., and Eastell, R. (1995). Bone mineral density and bone turnover in spinal osteoarthrosis. *Ann. Rheum. Dis.* **54**, 867–871.

33. Mansell, J. P., Tarlton, J. F., and Bailey, A. J. (1997). Biochemical evidence for altered subchondral bone collagen metabolism in osteoarthritis of the hip. *Br. J. Rheum.* **36**, 16–19.

34. Risteli, J., Niemi, S., Kauppila, S., Melkko, J., and Risteli, L. (1995). Collagen propeptides as indicators of collagen assembly. *Acta Orthop. Scand.* **66** (Suppl.), 183–188.

35. Charles, P., Mosekilde, L., Risteli, J., Risteli, L., and Eriksen, E. F. (1994). Assessment of bone remodeling using biochemical indicators of type I collagen synthesis and degradation: Relationship to calcium kinetics. *Bone Miner.* **24**, 81–94.

36. Eyre, D. R. (1991). The collagens of articular cartilage. *Semin. Arthritis Rheum.* **21**, 2–11.

37. Takahashi, M., Kushida, K., Hoshino, H., Suzuki, M., Sano, M., Miyamoto, S., and Inoue, T. (1996). Concentrations of pyridinoline and deoxypyridinoline in joint tissue from patients with osteoarthritis and rheumatoid arthritis. *Ann. Rheum. Dis.* **55**, 324–327.

38. Robins, S., Stewart, P., Astbury, C., and Bird, H. A. (1986). Measurement of the cross linking compound, pyridinoline, in urine as an index of collagen degradation in joint disease. *Ann. Rheum. Dis.* **45**, 969–973.

39. Black, D., Duncan, A., and Robins, S. P. (1988). Quantitative analysis of the pyridinium crosslinks of collagen in urine using ion-paired reversed-phase high-performance liquid chromatography. *Anat. Biochem.* **169**, 197–203.

40. Seibel, M. J., Duncan, A., and Robins, S. P. (1989). Urinary hydroxypyridinium crosslinks provide indices of cartilage and bone involvement in arthritic diseases. *J. Rheumatol.* **16**, 964–970.

41. Thompson, P. W., Spector, T. D., James, I. T., Henderson, E., and Hart, D. J. (1992). Urinary collagen crosslinks reflect the radiographic severity of knee osteoarthritis. *Br. J. Rheum.* **31**, 759–761.

42. Astbury, C., Bird, H. A., McLaren, A. M., and Robins, S. P. (1994). Urinary excretion of pyridinium crosslinks of collagen correlated with joint damage in arthritis. *Br. J. Rheum.* **33**, 11–15.

43. Hellio le Graverand, M. P., Tron, A. M., Ichou, M., Dallard, M. C., Richard, M., Uebelhart, D., and Vignon, E. (1996). Assessment of urinary hydroxypyridinium cross-links measurement in osteoarthritis. *Br. J. Rheum.* **35**, 1091–1095.

44. MacDonald, A. G., McHenry, P., Robins, P., and Reid, D. M. (1994). Relationship of urinary pyridinium crosslinks to disease extent and activity in osteoarthritis. *Br. J. Rheum.* **33**, 16–19.

45. Sinigaglia, L., Varenna, M., Binelli, L., Bartucci, F., Arrigoni, M., Ferrara, R., and Abbiati, G. (1995). Urinary and synovial pyridinium crosslink concentrations in patients with rheumatoid arthritis and osteoarthritis. *Ann. Rheum. Dis.* **54**, 144–147.

46. Oldberg, Å., Franzén, A., and Heinegård, D. (1988). The primary structure of a cell-binding bone sialoprotein. *J. Biol. Chem.* **36**, 19430–19432.

47. Seibel, M. J., Woitge, H. W., Pecherstorfer, M., Karmatschek, K., Horn, E., Ludwig, H., Armbruster, F. P., and Ziegler, R. (1996). Serum immunoreactive bone sialoprotein as a new marker of bone turnover in metabolic and malignant bone disease. *J. Clin. Endocrinol. Metab.* **81**, 3289–3294.

48. Conrozier, T., Shan, C., Saxen, T., Mathieu P., Pipemo, M., and Vignon, E. (1997). Serum level of bone sialoprotein correlates with subchondral bone changes in hip osteoarthritis. *Osteoarthritis Cartilage.* **5** (Suppl.), 49.

49. Petersson, I. F., Boegård, T., Heinegård, D., Dahlström, J., Svensson, B., and Saxne, T. (1998). Bone scan and serum markers of bone and cartilage in patients with knee pain and osteoarthritis. *Osteoarthritis Cartilage* **6**, 33–39.

50. Petersson, I. F., Boegård, T., Svensson, B., Heinegård, D., and Saxne, T. (1998). Changes in cartilage and bone metabolism identified by serum markers in early osteoarthritis of the knee joint. *Br. J. Rheumatol.* **37**, 46–50.

51. Poole, A. R., and Dieppe, P. (1994) Biological markers in rheumatoid arthritis. *Semin. Arthritis Rheum.* **23**, 17–31.

52. Poole, A. R., Ionescu, M. S., Swan, A., and Dieppe, P. (1994). Changes in cartilage metabolism in arthritis are reflected by altered serum and synovial fluid levels of the cartilage proteoglycan aggrecan. Implications for pathogenesis. *J. Clin. Invest.* **94**, 25–33.

53. Lohmander, L. S., Dahlberg, L., Ryd, L., and Heinegård, D. (1989). Increased levels of proteoglycan fragments in knee joint fluid after injury. *Arthritis Rheum.* **32**, 1434–1442.

54. Lohmander, L. S., Saxne, T., and Heinegård, D. K. (1994). Release of cartilage oligomeric matrix protein (COMP) into joint fluid after knee injury and in osteoarthritis. *Ann. Rheum. Dis.* **53**, 8–13.

55. Dahlberg, L., Ryd, L., Heinegård, D., and Lohmander, L. S. (1992). Proteoglycan fragments in joint fluid; influence of arthrosis and inflammation. *Acta Orthop. Scand.* **63**, 417–423.

56. Thonar, E. J.-M. A., Lenz, M. E., Klinworth, G. K., Caterson, B., Pachman, L. M., Glickman, P., Katz, R., Huff, J., and Kuettner, K. E. (1985). Quantification of keratan sulfate in blood as a marker of cartilage catabolism. *Arthritis Rheum.* **28**, 1365–1376.

57. Campion, G. V., McCrae, F., Schnitzer, T. J., Lenz, M. E., Dieppe, P. A., and Thonar, E. J.-M. A. (1991). Levels of keratan sulfate in the serum and synovial fluid of patients with osteoarthiritis of the knee. *Arthritis Rheum.* **35**, 1254.

58. Ratcliffe, A., Flatow, E. L., Roth, N., Saed-Nejad, F., and Bigliani, L. U. (1996). Biochemical markers in synovial fluid identify early osteoarthritis of the glenohumeral joint. *Clin. Orthop.* **330**, 45–53.

59. Spector, T. D., Woodward, L., Hall, G. M., Hammond, A., Williams, A., Butler, M. G., James, I. T., Hart, D. J., Thompson, P. W., and Scott, D. L. (1992). Keratan sulphate in rheumatoid arthritis, osteoarthritis, and inflammatory diseases. *Ann. Rheum. Dis.* **51**, 1134–1137.

60. Sharif, M., George, E., Shepstone, L., Knudson, W., Thonar, E. J.-M. A., Cushnaghan, J., and Dieppe, P. (1995). Serum hyaluronic acid level as a predictor of disease progression in osteoarthritis of the knee. *Arthritis Rheum.* **38**, 760–767.

61. Slater, R. R., Bayliss, M. T., Lachiewicz, P. F., Visco, D., and Caterson, B. (1995). Monoclonal antibodies that detect biochemical markers of arthritis in humans. *Arthritis Rheum.* **38**, 655–659.

62. Ratcliffe, A., Grelsamer, R. P., Kiernan, H., Saed-Nejad, F., and Visco, D. (1995). High levels of aggrecan aggregate components are present in synovial fluids from human knee joints with chronic injury or osteoarthrosis. *Acta Orthop. Scand.* **66** (Suppl.), 111–115.

63. Hedbom, E., Antonsson, P., Hjerpe, A., Aeschlimann, D., Paulsson, M., Rosa-Pimentel, E., Sommarin, Y., Wendel, M., Oldberg, Å., and Heinegård, D. (1992). Cartilage matrix proteins. An acidic oligomeric protein (COMP) detected only in cartilage. *J. Biol. Chem.* **267**, 6132–6136.

64. Saxne, T., and Heinegård, D. (1992). Cartilage of oligomeric matrix protein: A novel marker of cartilage turnover detectable in synovial fluid and blood. *Br. J. Rheum.* **31**, 583–591.

65. Petersson, I. F., Sandquist, L., Svensson, B., and Saxne, T. (1997). Cartilage markers in synovial fluid in symptomatic knee osteoarthritis. *Ann. Rheum. Dis.* **56**, 64–67.

66. Sharif, M., Saxne, T., Shepstone, L., Kirwan, J. R., Elson, C. J., Heinegård, D., and Dieppe, P. A. (1995). Relationship between serum cartilage oligomeric matrix protein levels and disease progression in osteoarthritis of the knee joint. *Br. J. Rheum.* **34**, 306–310.

67. Conrozier, T., Shan, C., Saxne, T., Mathieu, P., Pipemo, M., and Vignon, E. (1997). Serum level of cartilage oligomeric matrix protein appears to predict joint space narrowing progression in hip osteoarthritis. *Osteoarthirits Cartilage* **5** (Suppl.), 48.

68. Shinmei, M., Kobayshi, T., Yoshihara, Y., and Samura, A. (1995). Significance of the levels of carboxy terminal type II procollagen peptide, chondroitin sulfate isomers, tissue inhibitors of metalloproteinases, and metalloproteinases in osteoarthritis joint fluid. *J Rheumatol.* **43** (Suppl.), 78–81.

69. Lohmander, L. S., Yoshihara, Y., Roos, H., Kobayashi, T., Yamada, H., and Shinmei, M. (1996). Procollagen II C-propeptide in joint fluid: Changes in concentration with age, time after knee injury and osteoarthritis. *J. Rheumatol.* **23**, 1765–1769.

70. Kobayashi, T., Yoshihara, Y., Samura, A., Yamada, H., Shinmai, M., Roos, H., and Lohmander, L. S. (1997). Synovial fluid concentrations of the C-propetide of type II collagen correlates with body mass index in primary knee osteoarthritis. *Ann. Rheum. Dis.* **56**, 500–503.

71. Murphy, G. (1995). Matrix metalloproteinases and their inhibitors. *Acta Orthop. Scand.* **66** (Suppl.), 55–60.

72. Lohmander, L. S., Hoerrner, L. A., and Lark, M. W. (1993). Metalloproteinases, tissue inhibitor, and proteoglycan fragments in knee synovial fluid in human osteoarthritis. *Arthritis Rheum.* **36**, 181–189.

73. Dahlberg, L., Fridén, T., Roos, H., Lark, M. W., and Lohmander, L. S. (1994). A longitudinal study of cartilage matrix metabolism in patients with cruciate ligament injury: Synovial fluid concentrations of aggrecan fragments, stromelysin-1 and tissue inhibitor of metalloproteinase-1. *Br. J. Rheumatol.* **33**, 1107–1111.

CHAPTER 46

Normal and Abnormal Skeletal Growth

JOSEPH M. GERTNER Serono Laboratories, Norwell, Massachusetts 02061

I. INTRODUCTION

From birth to the end of the pubertal period of growth, the healthy child increases in length by about three fold, undergoes sharp changes in the relative proportions of limb, body, and head size, and accumulates large quantities of calcium and phosphate within the skeleton. In this chapter I will review the normal course of these changes and examine the mechanisms that control them and the methods used to assess their progress. I will discuss some of the major pathological processes that can affect childhood growth, referring to their pathophysiological basis and to associated biochemical and radiological features which can help in diagnosis.

II. THE STRUCTURE OF THE EPIPHYSEAL GROWTH PLATE

Skeletal growth in long bones depends on the proliferation of cartilage cells in the epiphyseal growth plate. As the columns of chondrocytes grow outwards from the growth plate, they mature and eventually die while their surrounding matrix mineralizes. A zone of each growth plate is constantly in the process of maturation, with mineralization occurring in the surrounding matrix. Under the influence of hormones and local factors, the balance of proliferation and maturation eventually shifts in the direction of maturation, resulting in reduction in the width of the zone of proliferating chondrocytes until the epiphysis fuses and the growth plate is eliminated. These events occur in a defined sequence, permitting assessment of skeletal maturity by observation of the sites at which fusion has occurred. The growth hormone/IGF-I axis and androgens appear to promote proliferation, whereas thyroid hormone and estrogens [1] are major factors in the induction of epiphyseal fusion; the latter can be used therapeutically to limit the height of pathologically tall adolescents [2]. Local factors which operate to promote epiphyseal fusion include the basic fibroblast growth factors [3] and retinoic acid receptor agonists. Clinically, the participation of these systems can be appreciated by reference to the epiphyseal distortion that occurs in achondroplasia (due to an activating mutation in the FGF3 receptor) and to the premature epiphyseal fusion described after excessive exposure to retinoids such as etretinate [4].

649

III. HORMONAL CONTROL OF SKELETAL GROWTH

The major hormonal systems directly affecting skeletal growth are the growth hormone (GH)-insulin-like growth factor (IGF) axis, the gonadal axis, and the pituitary-thyroid axis. While glucocorticoid excess (Cushing syndrome) severely limits skeletal growth, there is little evidence that deficiencies in the production of cortisol lead to significant growth failure.

As its name implies, GH, or somatropin, is a major stimulant of postnatal somatic growth. Fetal growth, on the other hand, is much less, if at all, dependent on the GH-IGF-I axis. GH is a pleiotropic 191-amino acid peptide (MW 22 KDa) hormone secreted by the somatotrophes of the anterior pituitary. Secretory bursts are driven by growth hormone-releasing hormone (GHRH) from the medial hypothalamus [5] and are influenced by the inhibitory action of somatostatin and possibly by another stimulatory system acting on the growth hormone releasing secretagogue receptors [6].

Growth hormone interacts with a specific cytokine receptor. A major action of growth hormone at many of the sites at which it operates, including the skeletal growth plate, is to induce the release of insulin-like growth factor I (IGF-I), formerly called somatomedin-C. This substance, which resembles proinsulin structurally and acts through receptors homologous with the insulin receptor, may act both as an endocrine and a paracrine hormone. The products of the GH-IGF-I system induce proliferation without marked maturation of the epiphyseal growth plate and thus induce linear skeletal growth which lasts until sex hormone-mediated epiphyseal closure. The relative extent to which these actions are a function of locally-produced versus circulating IGF-I and the nature of any direct action of GH at that site remain topics for research [7].

As in the case of growth hormone, important evidence for the participation of the thyroid hormones, thyroxine (T4) and triiodothyronine (T3), in skeletal growth comes from observation of states of hormone deficiency. T3, the active metabolite, enters its target cells and signals via a nuclear receptor of the steroid hormone-retinoic acid receptor class. It appears to be necessary both for proliferation and for maturation of the growth plate, so that childhood hypothyroidism results in a profound slowing of linear growth and of epiphyseal maturation.

The third class of hormones influencing skeletal growth is that of the sex hormones, testosterone and estradiol, and their derivatives. Largely absent between infancy and puberty, these hormones are produced in abundance during and after puberty and promote both proliferation and maturation in the epiphyseal growth plate. The "pure" actions of sex hormones on the skeleton are hard to define because of the increased activity of the GH-IGF I axis and of insulin during puberty and because of the convertibility by aromatization of testosterone to estrogens. Traditionally, it was believed that both male and female gonadal hormones promoted epiphyseal proliferation and fusion. However, it has been observed that growth rates can be reduced when boys with high testostrone levels are treated with an aromatase inhibitor [8] which reduces estrogen, but not androgen, levels. In addition, males who lack aromatase or functional estrogen receptors [1] manifest delayed epiphyseal fusion. These observations suggest that even in males it is estrogenic hormones that play a key role in epiphyseal growth and fusion and in the ultimate limitation of the adolescent growth spurt.

IV. FETAL SKELETAL DEVELOPMENT

A. Histogenesis and Organogenesis of the Skeleton

The skeleton and the homeostatic control systems for the skeletal minerals (calcium and phosphate) develop in the protected intrauterine environment. However, most of the functions of the skeleton, such as the protection of vulnerable organs, the anchoring of muscles, the maintenance of the body's shape against gravity, and the provision of a metabolic buffer of calcium and phosphate, are not needed until delivery. The development of the skeleton depends on the integration of events directing cells derived from primitive mesenchyme to produce bone matrix, to mineralize that matrix, and then to remodel the resulting bone. This whole process is under complex genetic control and depends on a tight integration of cellular events within the developing skeleton and with the systems that transport and accumulate mineral for deposition within the skeleton.

The precursors of bone cells begin to form at about five weeks of gestation from membranes or rods of mesenchymal cells. Intramembranous bone forms the sides and vault of the skull and the clavicles while endochondral ossification accounts for most of the remaining bones, particularly those of the developing limbs. In both forms of ossification, osteoprogenitor cells condense, mature into alkaline phosphatase-positive osteoblasts, secrete an extracellular ground substance, and begin to mineralize. A network of collagen fibers forms the framework upon which the first bony trabeculae mineralize to form the so-called primary spongiosa. Secondary foci of ossification that will eventually become epiphyseal centers differentiate from mesenchyme in an analogous manner. Remodelling of the skeleton begins as soon as the primary spongiosa is formed, with osteoclasts resorbing existing bone while osteoblasts form new bone.

B. Ionic and Hormonal Effects on the Fetal Skeleton

The mineralization process itself depends on the controlled delivery of calcium and phosphate to the sites of ossification and on the local effects of the calcitropic hormones, parathyroid hormone (PTH), calcitriol (1,25-dihydroxyvitamin D), and calcitonin. Calcium and phosphorus are transported across the placenta against a concentration gradient which appears as early as 12 weeks. The quantity of mineral transported increases sharply until late in the last trimester, by which time the fetus is accumulating up to 85 mg/kg/d of phosphorus and 150 mg/kg/d of calcium. Placental calcium transport depends on the availability of calcitriol and the parathyroid hormone-related peptide, PTHrP. There are no known intrinsic disorders of the placenta that specifically limit fetal calcium and phosphorus accumulation, but mineral deficiency may accompany the general fetal malnutrition characteristic of placental insufficiency. Pathological consequences can also arise from disordered transplacental calcium transport when calcium concentrations in the maternal serum are too high or too low.

V. POSTNATAL SKELETAL GROWTH

A. Measurement and Reference Sources

As for any physiological variable, accurate measurement is essential for tracking normal processes and for discovering and understanding abnormalities. Skull circumference is measured with a tape at the level of the largest (occipitofrontal) diameter. Because children up to the age of two to three years can not cooperate adequately with a measurement of standing height, stature is measured while they are supine on an adjustable frame which supports the back. The head is placed against a stop at one end while the sliding pointer is brought up to the feet, held plantigrade in gentle traction by an assistant. The generally accepted method of measuring stature in older children is that of Tanner and Whitehouse. To ensure repeatability, the head is placed at a standardized attitude while mild upward traction is applied to the sides of the head. The child stands on the baseboard of the measuring device, which is usually mounted on the wall. A horizontal pointer sliding on vertical tracks is then brought down into firm contact with the vertex. The distance from the ground to the vertex can be read on a fixed ruler or on a rotating indicator which shows the distance travelled by the horizontal pointer from a fixed calibration point.

In this way, many surveys of the height of normal children have been made with the subsequent generation of smooth curves plotting the height distribution for each age against age. Because the genetic and environmental influences on growth across regions change with time, such curves are made in many countries, with regular updates as required by circumstances. In the United States, this work is the responsibility of the National Health, Education, and Nutrition Survey (NHANES). In 1998, NHANES is analyzing results of its fourth survey. Most growth charts used in the U.S.

disseminated by health care organizations and commerical firms are derived from earlier NHANES data [9].

Because the rate, or "velocity," of growth is also often of interest in clinical situations, curves of percentiles for this parameter have been developed. These date are inherently less reliable and less standardized than height information. The period over which the growth rate information is measured (e.g., six months versus one year) significantly affects the values, as does the choice of longitudinal versus cross-sectional input data. In addition, small measurement errors are more likely to increase the variability of height velocity data than are similar errors in the measurement of stature (or height "distance"). These topics are well discussed, along with the presentation of U.S. longitudinal data, by Tanner and Davies [10]. The phases of childhood growth, by distance and velocity, are illustrated in Figure 1.

Knemometry is a research method designed to make very accurate measurements of the length of single bones, which can then be used to observe the short-term effects of local or systemic interventions that might affect growth. The limb containing the bone in question is fixed in a metal frame while the ends of the measuring device are accurately placed

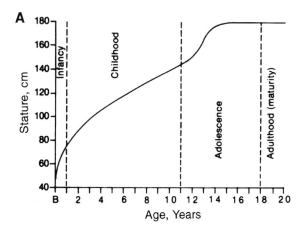

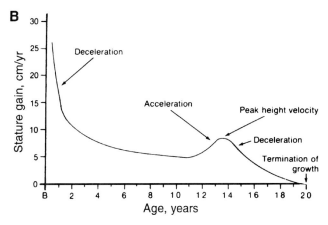

FIGURE 1 The phases of childhood growth, by (A) distance and (B) velocity. From Rallison, 1986. Reprinted by permission of Burgess International Group, Inc., Burgess Publishing, Minneapolis.

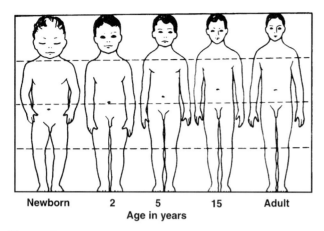

Newborn   2   5   15   Adult
Age in years

FIGURE 2   Changing body proportions during childhood growth. From Rallison, 1986. Reprinted by permission of Burgess International Group, Inc., Burgess Publishing, Minneapolis.

against bony landmarks. The distance between the landmarks is then measured with a micrometer. Although theoretically attractive, this approach has few adherents and is little used.

B. Body Proportion and Its Changes through the Growth Period

The newborn infant has a relatively large head and limbs which are, by adult standards, disproportionally short relative to the rest of the body (Fig. 2). Accurate measurement of the proportions of the skeleton, and the availability of tables of normal values throughout childhood, permit the detection of abnormal patterns of growth and help in the diagnosis of their cause. Conventionally, the upper segment of the skeleton is defined as the region between the vertex of the skull and the upper margin of the symphysis pubis; The lower segment runs from the symphysis to the base of the heel (tarsus). These distances can be measured directly in the recumbant position using a tape. Alternatively, the child's height can be measured when he is sitting, with the back extended against a baseboard. In this case the vertex to rump distance represents the upper segment and the lower segment is calculated as the difference between sitting and standing height. Another method to determine skeletal proportions is to compare arm span to height, as in Leonardo Da Vinci's famous drawing, knowing that in the mature adult, arm span is equal to about 98% of stature. However, because some conditions affect growth in the lower limbs much more severly than those in the upper, direct upper and lower segment measurement is preferable to the use of arm span.

C. Zero to Three Years

Infancy is the period of most rapid skeletal growth, not only in relative terms but also in absolute terms. Table I shows the normal occipito-frontal skull circumference, length, and annualized growth rate from birth to three years at six month intervals.

D. Prepuberty

From about three years of age until the onset of puberty, children of both sexes grow at a slowly decelerating rate with no major systematic fluctuations (see Fig. 2), although there may be a small growth spurt at around age eight and a distinct deceleration immediately before puberty.

E. Puberty and the Sexual Dimorphism in Skeletal Growth

During puberty, both sexes show a sharp increase in growth rate followed by epiphyseal fusion and the complete cessation of growth. The average age for the start and peak of the pubertal growth spurt, as for all manifestations of puberty, is

TABLE I.   Growth in the First Three Years

Age (months)	Occipito-frontal skull circumference (cm)	Length (cm)	Growth velocity (cm/yr) over the preceding three months)
Birth	34.0	50.0	–
6	42.8	66.1	32.2
12	45.8	74.6	17.0
18	47.2	81.0	12.8
24	48.0	86.7	11.4
30	48.5	91.6	9.8
36	49.0	05.9	8.6

Note the rapid fall-off in the growth rates for skull circumference and length. (Data from Hamill *et al.* [9].)

lower in girls than in boys. The peak velocity and duration of the growth spurt are also less in girls than in boys, resulting in the 13 cm mean difference in adult height between men and women. It is the high degree of variability observed in the magnitude and duration of the pubertal growth spurt that renders prediction of adult height so inaccurate.

VI. THE CONTROL OF MINERAL ACCRETION DURING SKELETAL GROWTH

The full grown fetus at term contains about 21 g (range, 13–33 g) of calcium [11]. During growth, this increases steadily to the 1000 g seen in the typical adult. The factors that control the accumulation of calcium into the skeleton during the growth period have been examined by calcium balance techniques, by the use of nonradioactive isotopic calcium tracers [12], and by longitudinal and cross-sectional imaging of bone mineral density [13].

The consensus emerging from these observations is that calcium accumulation is particularly intense during puberty. The precise role of the hormonal changes of puberty in promoting the influx and retention of calcium is unclear, but a pubertal rise in calcitriol levels has been well described and presumably contributes to the process (Fig. 3).

VII. QUANTITATIVE IMAGING DURING SKELETAL GROWTH

Radiology provides powerful tools for tracking skeletal development. These have developed in tandem with progress in technology and the availability of standardized age and sex-related norms.

A. The Assessment of Skeletal Maturity

Skeletal growth depends on the multiplication and maturation of cells within the cartilaginous growth plate and the orderly transition of the surrounding matrix into bone. As the epiphyseal growth plate matures, its shape and width change in a predictable fashion. Eventually fusion of the epiphysis occurs and the radiologically visible "gap" between the epiphysis and its corresponding metaphysis is eliminated.

The peripheral small limb bones mature from cartilage in a similar manner but, lacking a shaft, undergo mineralization and maturation without epiphyseal fusion.

By radiological observation of the bones of the hand and wrist in a large number of normal children, Greulich and Pyle [14] and Tanner *et al.* [15] were able to define many specific developmental stages for each observed bone and to assign a sex-specific mean age at which each stage was reached. By relating the appearance of a child's hand and wrist bones to the corresponding developmental stages shown in these authors' pictorial atlas, the clinician can assign a maturational age to each individual bone. Taking a mean of these maturational ages gives an overall skeletal age, or "bone age," that provides a remarkable degree of insight into the skeletal development of the child examined. While the process of reading bone ages requires skill and patience, it is widely used to assess an individual's prognosis for growth and eventual adult height and as part of the evaluation of hormonal and metabolic disorders which may impact the skeleton.

The use of bone age to assess and predict skeletal development is limited by certain inherent weaknesses of the method. The available data are limited by the genetic and environmental characteristics of the American and British children in the original surveys, published in 1950 and 1975 which can not be repeated because of changed views on the propriety of exposing healthy children to X-rays. Even with a large survey of normal children there will always be

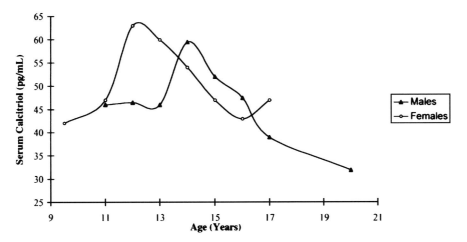

FIGURE 3   Changes in calcitriol levels during growth (after Aksnes and Aarskog). Note the resemblance of this curve to the growth velocity/age curve in Figure 1.

underrepresentation of "outliers" and unusual cases which are, however, precisely the type of child for whom diagnostic evaluation is often required. Finally, the method of reading the shapes of hand bones has a subjective component, leading to disagreement even between experienced observers. Without adequate training, or the provision of adequate time for each examination, the results can be very misleading.

For a child of any given age and height, adult stature depends on a variety of factors of which current height, skeletal age, and sex are the most important. Using the Greulich and Pyle [14] bone age atlas, height prediction algorithms published as a table were produced in 1952 by Bayley and Pinneau [16] and are widely used in the 1990s. Recognizing that other factors, including parental height and relative body weight, also contributed to the prediction, more elaborate predictive equations were developed by Tanner and Whitehouse and by the Fels Institute [17]. Use of these methods involves more computation than the Bayley-Pinneau method but they have been incorporated into popular computer programs used to predict adult height. All these methods for predicting adult stature are considerably limited in accuracy and are more useful for surveys and research than for clinical use in individual children.

B. The Quantification of Bone Mineral Content in Children

The two methods that can provide usable data on bone density in children are dual-energy densitometry (DXA) [18] and quantitative computed tomography (qCT).

1. DUAL ENERGY X-RAY ABSORPTIOMETRY (DXA)

Relatively cheap, delivering a low radiation dose, and with an increasing body of normative data for children, DXA is the most widely used method to measure bone density. The big drawback of DXA bone densitometry in children is that the method actually measures the attenuation of an X-ray beam across a projected cross-section of bone. This attenuation depends not only on the actual density of skeletal mineral but also on the dimensions of the bone along the axis of the X-ray beam and in the plane perpendicular to that beam. These dimensions and their relation to one another change through childhood so that corrections based on the child's height and weight have to be applied to the machine's output [19].

2. QUANTITATIVE COMPUTED TOMOGRAPHY (qCT)

Quantitative computed tomography (qCT) gives a true bone density (mass/unit volume). However, both cost and radiation dose preclude the study of large numbers of children using techniques devised for detailed imaging, so much less normative data are available. Low radiation methods for qCT in children do exist and this method still has potential importance [13].

VIII. BIOCHEMICAL MARKERS OF SKELETAL GROWTH

Histomorphometric studies show that children's bones are active by adult standards not only in the epiphyses but also in the cortical and trabecular regions of the established bone. As a corollary of this activity, all well-established markers of bone formation and resorption are increased in childhood; the graph of activity against age often bears a striking similarity to the growth velocity curve. This phenomenon was first observed in the longer-established markers such as alkaline phosphatase and urinary hydroxyproline exretion and has since been extended to osteocalcin (Fig. 4) and to markers

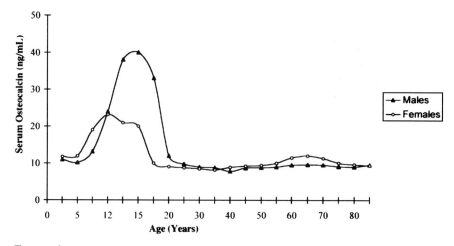

FIGURE 4   Changes in serum osteocalcin levels during growth (after Hauschka). Note the resemblance of this curve to the growth velocity/age curve in Figure 1.

TABLE II. Conditions Classified as Proportionate Growth Failure

Condition	Etiology[a]	Diagnostic test
Growth hormone deficiency	Hypothalamic or pituitary dysfunction	Low serum GH after stimulation
Growth hormone resistance	Mutation of GH receptor	High GH, low IGF-I and GHBP
Hypothyroidism	Congenital or autoimmune	Low thyroxine, high TSH
Turner syndrome (gonadal dysgenesis)	Monosomy X	Karyotype
Cushing syndrome	Endogenous or iatrogenic glucocorticoid excess	High urinary cortisol (endogenous), Medical history (iatrogenic)
Inflammatory bowel disease	?	Intestinal radiology, endoscopy, and biopsy
Hypogonadism	Most often temporary, as in "constitutional delay"	Low gonadal hormone levels; Gonadotropin levels variable according to cause

[a] Only the clinically most common conditions are listed.

of collagen formation and breakdown such as serum PICP and NCPT and urinary pyridinium cross-links and N-terminal type I collagen telopeptide. It is always important to bear in mind when investigating children with suspected bone disease that very high levels of such markers are quite normal in pediatric samples relative to those of adults.

IX. ABNORMAL PATTERNS OF SKELETAL GROWTH

Abnormalities of growth form a major part of the clinical practice of pediatic endocrinology and have given insights into the normal mechanisms whereby skeletal growth is promoted and controlled. Although states of excessive growth may bring considerable distress and can indicate severe pathology [20], only growth failure, which is much more common, will be considered in this section. Before the causes of growth failure were well understood, the various disorders were divided into proportionate and disproportionate growth failure, a classification which remains useful both in the clinic and for an appreciation of the underlying pathophysiology.

A. Proportionate Growth Failure

This term refers to shortness in which the body proportions, specifically the upper:lower segment or the arm span: height ratio, are close to normal. Some deviation may occur because of delayed skeletal maturation which causes the relationship of body proportions to be similar to that seen in a child younger than the patient. The most common causes of this type of shortness are the polygenic influences which lead

to familial shortness and constitutional delay of growth. The latter also appears to be a familial condition in which both skeletal and sexual maturation are significantly delayed. The consequent delayed skeletal maturation can be diagnosed radiologically and provides a good prognosis since a growth spurt which is late but normal in magnitude can lead to adult stature within the normal range. In contrast, familial shortness does not imply a delay in bone age and the affected child can be expected to become a short adult, following the pattern of parents and/or other family members.

Most of the defects of the hormonal axes described in Section III as influencing proliferation and maturation of growth plate cartilage are classified under proportionate short stature, as are some genetic syndromes, most notably Turner syndrome. A listing of some of these conditions is given in Table II.

B. Disproportionate Growth Failure

Disproportionate growth failure occurs when a disorder of bone growth predominantly affects the limbs or the axial skeleton. Although subtle disproportion can occur in systemic hormonal diseases such as hypothyroidism or hypogonadism, the more striking cases occur in intrinsic diseases of bone development. Disorders in which limb shortening predominates include the epiphyseal dysplasias, achondroplasia (in which the epiphyseal proliferation is disrupted by constitutive activation of the fibroblast growth factor 3 receptor [21]), and disorders of mineralization including nutritional and metabolic (hypophosphatemic) rickets. Abnormally long limbs relative to the trunk are seen in Marfan syndrome and in males with Klinefelter syndrome. Maldevelopment of the vertebrae in the various spondylar dysplasias can lead to disproportion through truncal shortening. In clinical practice, however, this form of disproportion is most often due to spinal irradiation used to treat central nervous system or hematologic malignancy during childhood.

C. Disease-Specific Growth Curves

Growth curves for some of the more common conditions affecting linear growth are available. The growth of children with achondroplasia or with Downs, Turner, or Marfan syndrome can be followed using such disease-specific curves. Although it might be somewhat reassuring to see that a child's growth pattern is "expected" for his or her disease, it is often more relevant to use the standard growth curves as a basis for comparison with the healthy population.

References

1. Smith, E. P., Williams, T. C., Lubahn, D., Korach, K. S., Boyd, J., Frank, G. R., Takahashi, H., Cohen, R. M., and Specker, B. (1994), Estrogen resistance caused by a mutation in the estrogen-receptor gene in a man. *N. Engl. J. Med.* **331**, 1056–1061.
2. Binder, G., Grauer, M. L., Wehner, A. V., Wehner, F., and Ranke, M. B. (1997). Outcome in tall stature. Final height and psychological aspects in 220 patients with and without treatment. *Eur. J. Pediatr.* **156**, 905–910.
3. Baron, J., Klein, K. O., Yanovski, J. A., Novosad, J. A., Bacher, J. D., Bolander, M. E., and Cutler, G. B., Jr. (1994). Induction of growth plate cartilage ossification by basic fibroblast growth factor. *Endocrinology* **135**, 2790–2793.
4. Prendiville, J., Bingham, E. A., and Burrows, D. (1986). Premature epiphyseal closure—a complication of etretinate therapy in children. *J. Am. Acad. Dermatol.* **15**, 1259–1262.
5. Hartman, M. L., Veldhuis, J. D., and Thorner, M. O. (1993). Normal control of growth hormone secretion. *Horm. Res.* **40**, 37–47.
6. Howard, A. D., Feighner, S. D., Cully, D. F., Arena, J. P., Liberator, P. A., Rosenblum, C. I., Hamelin, M., Hreniuk, D. L., Palyha, O. C., Anderson, J. *et al.* A receptor in pituitary and hypothalamus that functions in growth hormone release. *Science* **273**, 974–977.
7. Ohlsson, C., Bengtsson, B. A., Isaksson, O. G., Andreassen, T. T., and Slootweg, M. C. (1998). Growth hormone and bone. *Endocr. Rev.* **19**, 55–79.
8. Cutler, G. B. (1997). The role of estrogen in bone growth and maturation during childhood and adolescence. *Steroid Biochem. Mol. Biol.* **61**, 141–144.
9. Hamill, P. V., Drizd, T. A., Johnson, C. L., Reed, R. B., Roche, A. F., and Moore, W. M. (1979). Physical growth: National Center for Health Statistics percentiles. *Am. J. Clin. Nut.* **32**, 607–629.
10. Tanner, J. M., and Davies, P. S. W. (1985). Clinical longitudinal standards for height and height velocity in North American children. *J. Pediatr.* **107**, 317–329.
11. Crowley, S., Trivedi, P., Risteli, L., Risteli, J., Hindmarsh, P. C., and Brook, C. G. (1998). Collagen metabolism and growth in prepubertal children with asthma treated with inhaled steroids. *J. Pediatr.* **132**, 409–413.
12. Abrams, S. A., O'Brien, K. O., and Stuff, J. E. (1996). Changes in calcium kinetics associated with menarche. *J. Clin. Endocrinol. Metab.* **81**, 2017–2020.
13. Gilsanz, V. (1998). Bone density in children: A review of the available techniques and indications. *Eur. J. Radiol.* **26**, 177–182.
14. Greulich, W. W., and Pyle, S. E. (1959). "Radiographic Atlas of Skeletal Development of the Hand and Wrist," 2nd ed. Stanford University Press, Stanford, CA.
15. Tanner, J. M., Whitehouse, R. H., Marshall, W. A. *et al.* (1975). "Assessment of Skeletal Maturity and Prediction of Adult Height." Academic Press, London.
16. Bayley, N., and Pinneau, S. R. (1952). Tables for predicting adult heights from skeletal ages: Revised for use with the Gruelich-Pyle hand system. *J. Pediatr.* **40**, 432–441.
17. Roche, A. F., Wainer, H., and Thissen, D. (1975). The RWT method for the prediction of adult stature. *Pediatrics* **56**, 1028–1033.
18. Glastre, C., Braillon, P., David, L., Cochat, P., Meunier, P. J., and Delmas, P. D. (1990). Measurement of bone mineral content of the lumbar spine by dual energy x-ray absorptiometry in normal children: Correlations with growth parameters. *J. Clin. Endocrinol. Metab.* **70**, 1330–1333.
19. Friedl, K. E., Vogel, J. A., Marchitelli, L. J., and Kubel, S. L. (1993). Assessment of regional body composition changes by dual-energy X-ray absorptiometry. *Basic Life Sci.* **60**, 99–103.
20. Gertner, J. M., Hintz, R. L., and Rosenfeld, R. G., eds. (1987). In "Disorders of Growth," pp. 213–221. Churchill-Livingstone, New York.
21. Naski, M. C., Wang, Q., Xu, J., and Ornitz, D. M., (1996). Graded activation of fibroblast growth factor receptor 3 by mutations causing achondroplasia and thanatophoric dysplasia. *Nat. Genet.* **13**, 233–237.

Index

S

ISBN 0-12-634840-5

90018

9 780126 348408